Pharmacological and Chemical Synonyms

Pharmacological and Chemical Synonyms

A COLLECTION OF NAMES OF DRUGS, PESTICIDES
AND OTHER COMPOUNDS DRAWN FROM
THE MEDICAL LITERATURE OF THE WORLD

Compiled by

E. E. J. MARLER, M.D., M.Sc., Ph.D.

SIXTH EDITION

1976

EXCERPTA MEDICA, AMSTERDAM - OXFORD

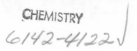

© Excerpta Medica 1976

ISBN Excerpta Medica 90 219 0298 2
ISBN Elsevier North-Holland 0 444 15195 8

Library of Congress Cataloging in Publication Data
Marler, E   E   J
    Pharmacological and chemical synonyms.
     1.   Drugs- -Dictionaries.   I.   Title.   [DNLM:
1.   Dictionaries, chemical.   2.   Dictionaries,
pharmaceutic.   QV13 M347p]
RS51.M3   1976   615'.1'03   76-20594
ISBN 0-444-15195-8 (American Elsevier)

Publisher:

Excerpta Medica
305 Keizersgracht
Amsterdam
P.O. Box 1126

Sole Distributors for the USA and Canada:

Elsevier North-Holland, Inc.
52 Vanderbilt Avenue
New York, N.Y. 10017

Printed in The Netherlands by Casparie b.v., Alkmaar

Foreword

This alphabetical compilation of names used for drugs, pesticides and other substances of pharmacological or biochemical interest (chemical compounds or well-defined biological products) is a 'dictionary' and makes no claim to official status. Its special features are:

Consistent chemical nomenclature: Systematic, unambiguous, fully-numbered names are given wherever possible. The practice of the leading *chemical* abstracting journals has been followed, except that inverted order is not used (this was used in the earliest editions of PCS, but non-chemical readers found it too confusing).

Alternative chemical names: These are included for some more complex compounds, which can be systematically named in a number of ways.

International scope, as far as possible.

Extensive cross-indexing.

Up to date (covering INN list No. 35).

TYPES OF NAMES

(A) *Non-proprietary (common) names*
   (1) *Chemical names*
   (2) *Abbreviated chemical names*
   (3) *Source names*, i.e. names referring to the (biological) origin of compounds such as hormones and plant alkaloids.
   (4) *Pharmacological names* (variously termed "approved", "official" or "generic" names).
   List of such non-proprietary names for *general* use are issued periodically by:
   (a) the WHO, under the designation recINN (= recommended International Non-proprietary Name) or pINN (= proposed International Non-proprietary Name).
   (b) National bodies in various countries, including Great Britain (BAN), the United States (USAN), France (DCF) and the Scandinavian countries (NFN).
   The names in categories (a) and (b) are often identical or differ only slightly in spelling.
   (5) *Pesticide names.* These are common names assigned by international (ISO) and/or national (BSI, ANSI etc.) standardization organizations to compounds used as pesticides. Some of these compounds also have a pharmacological (INN) name, in which case the latter name is used as heading.
   (6) Other non-proprietary names (trivial names) not classifiable in any of the above categories, e.g. those derived from names of places or persons.

(*B*) *Proprietary names*

These are in fact *not* names of chemical compounds as such and their use in this way is improper. They are registered trade-marks. Such a name is the property of the registering manufacturer and *is applicable only to the product* (with or without additives) *produced and/or marketed by him*. Its use as if it were a common name is unjustifiable, being

(*a*) unintentional advertising,
(*b*) infringement of a legal right,
(*c*) confusing (resulting in the indexing of a single substance under separate headings).

Unfortunately this misuse of trade-names is still very common and it is for that reason that a number of trade-names have been included in this list.

(*C*) *Research code numbers*

ARRANGEMENT OF THE ALPHABETICAL LIST

Headings: Each substance has *one single heading* (printed in capital letters). This is always a non-proprietary name. It is followed by a list of all *synonyms* known to us: first the chemical and other non-proprietary names in alphabetical order, then research code number(s), and finally as many trade-names as we have been able to trace. For some well-known drugs, however, which have been known for 20 years or longer (included in the earliest INN lists) the trade-names are no longer collected under the heading, as was done in earlier editions. This, together with the omission of some obsolete material, was necessary to provide space for the large amount of new material, without making the book unmanageably large.

References: Each of the above-mentioned synonyms has its own entry referring to the heading, in the form: X . . . . See Y . . . .

Indication of status of name: (See also above under TYPES OF NAMES)
*** = recINN
** = pINN
* = (*a*) BAN, USAN, DCF or NFN name
      (*b*) pesticide name
(tr) = name transliterated from the Russian (or other Cyrillic) alphabet
no marking = chemical name; common name without official status; research code number
inverted commas = names known or believed to be trade-marks.

CHOICE OF ENTRIES

As a general rule the INN name (if any) is used as heading (for pesticides the ISO name), but sometimes one of the national names or the chemical name has been used. The choice is then *purely arbitrary* and has usually been based on the practical consideration of which name arrived first in our card-index. The alternatives are given as references.

Multiple products: It is obviously impossible to include all the trade-names that refer to products containing more than one active substance. The few which have been included refer to drugs commonly used in the form of mixtures of 2 agents (e.g. the "pill"). Only the active components are mentioned, not the proportions in which they are present.

Vitamins: For the well-known vitamins only the chemical and other non-proprietary names are listed; the trade-names (which are usually self-evident and seldom used in medical literature) are not included. Synthetic derivatives with vitaminic action are given with all their synonyms (including the trade-names).

Biological products: Substances of incompletely defined chemical composition are included only if they have been given a pharmacological (approved, generic, official) name.

SPELLING

The spelling of all names (including official and trade-marks) has been 'translated' into American spelling. We apologise for this liberty but experience has shown that where some names are spelt, for instance, Sulf... and others Sulph..., the result is highly confusing for the reader. Where necessary a note to this effect has been placed at the appropriate point in the alphabetical list.

REMARKS

Proprietary names

Trade-marks have been included in this list for the convenience of readers because they are so often given in the literature without statement of the chemical composition or approved name, or are *misused* as though they were common names. It is obviously impossible to trace all the trade-names in use in different countries. The inclusion of such a name is purely a matter of the chance of its having come to our notice and inclusion or non-inclusion *does not imply any recommendation or the reverse.*

The reference 'X ...'. See Y where 'X' is a trade-name and Y a heading means simply that the drug Y is the *active component* of the proprietary product 'X ...'. This list does not provide any information as to additives or excipients which may be included under the trade-mark, nor does it give any statement about concentration or form (tablet, solution for injection, etc.).

A name which is in some countries a non-proprietary name may be a registered trade-mark in others. This is a difficulty for us in view of our attempt at international scope. We have endeavoured to avoid it as best we can, and where we have failed we must ask for the indulgence of the persons or bodies concerned, pointing out once more that this is a *compilation without official status.*

Soviet names

Some of these are trade-marks elsewhere. Such names have not been used as headings. Soviet names for products described only in literature from the USSR have been regarded as non-proprietary and used as headings. They are marked (tr).

Use of inverted commas

While we have attempted to distinguish proprietary (or possibly proprietary) from non-proprietary names in this way, we cannot guarantee that no mistakes have been made in this respect:

(*a*) The fact that a name is printed *without* inverted commas *does not exclude the possibility that it may have been registered as a trade-mark in some part of the world.* We are confident, however, that such cases are not numerous.

(*b*) The fact that a name is printed in inverted commas does not *necessarily* mean that it is a registered trade-mark. To be on the safe side, however, our rule has been 'when in doubt use inverted commas'.

A

A-1 *see* Ethymidine.
A-2 *see* Pyrophos.
A-15 *see* Schradan.
A-16 *see* Ambucetamide.
A-21 *see* Isoprenaline *and* Ketobemidone.
A-66 *see* Phenmetrazine.
A-101 *see* Demethyldiazepam.
A-102 *see* Temazepam.
A-118 *see* Sultroponium.
A-124 *see* Phenytoin with diazepam.
A-145 *see* Promazine.
A-163 *see* Triaziquone.
A-272 *see* Rutamycin.
A-301 *see* Norgestrienone.
A-350 *see* Aminochlorthenoxazine.
A-377 *see* Chlortetracycline.
A-1981-12 *see* Prodilidine.
A-2205 *see* Profadol.
A-2371 *see* Mithramycin.
A-2655 *see* Dioxamate.
A-7283 *see* Guanoctine.
A-8103 *see* Pipobroman.
A-8999 *see* Aspartocin.
A-12253A *see* Nebramycin.
A-16612 *see* Teroxalene.
A-16900 *see* Teflurane.
A-19120 *see* Pargyline.
A-19757 *see* Encyprate.
A-20968 *see* Piposulfan.
A-22370 *see* Trimetozine.
A-27053 *see* Carbocromen.
A-30400 *see* Pemoline with magnesium hydroxide.
A-31528 *see* Pemoline with magnesium hydroxide.
A-41304 *see* Desoximetasone.
A-732179 *see* Intermedin.
'Aafac' *see* Prothoate.
'Aarane' *see* Disodium cromoglicate.
'Aasevin' *see* Carbaril.
'Aasystem' *see* Thiometon.
'AAT' *see* Parathion.
'Aatrex' *see* Atrazine.
AB-01 *see* Bemegride.
AB-42 *see* Cyacetacide.
AB-100 *see* Uredepa.
AB-103 *see* Benzodepa.
AB-132 *see* Meturedepa.
AB-35616 *see* Dipotassium clorazepate.
'Abacin' *see* Co-trimoxazole.
'Abactrim' *see* Co-trimoxazole.
'Abadole' *see* Aminothiazole.
'Abalgin' *see* Dextropropoxyphene.
'Abar' *see* Leptophos.
'Abate' *see* Temefos.
'Abboticine' *see* Erythromycin ethyl succinate.
Abbott 35616 *see* Dipotassium clorazepate.
Abbott 36581 *see* Butamirate citrate.
Abbott 38414 *see* Ancrod.
Abbott 38579 *see* Protirelin.
Abbott 44090 *see* Sodium valproate.

'Abequito' *see* Nimidane.
ABEQUOSE (3-desoxy-D-fucose).
'Aberel' *see* Tretinoin.
'Abicol' *see* Reserpine with bendroflumethiazide.
'Abirol' *see* Metandienone.
'Abminthic' *see* Dithiazanine.
ABOB *see* Moroxydine.
'Abrastol' *see* Calcinaphthol.
Abrine *see* Methyltryptophan.
ABSINTHOL (3-thujanone; tanaceton; thujone; thuyon).
'Abstem' *see* Calcium carbimide citrate.
'Abstinyl' *see* Disulfiram.
'Abten' *see* Alseroxylon.
'Abuphenine' *see* Butetamate.
AC-17 *see* Carbazochrome sodium sulfonate.
AC-32 *see* Clinolamide.
AC-223 *see* Melinamide.
AC-528 *see* Dioxation.
AC-601 *see* Buramate.
AC-695 *see* Ethotoin.
AC-1075 *see* Cytarabine.
AC-1198 *see* Dimethadione.
AC-1802 *see* Aprindine.
AC-2770 *see* Gitoformate.
AC-3810 *see* Bamifylline.
AC-12402 *see* Chlorbicyclen.
'Acabel' *see* Bevonium metilsulfate.
Acamylophenine *see* Camylofin.
ACAPRAZINE** (*N*-[3-[4-(2,5-dichlorophenyl)piperazin-1-yl]propyl]acetamide; 1-(3-acetamidopropyl)-4-(2,5-dichlorophenyl)piperazine).
'Acaprin' *see* Quinuronium sulfate.
'Acapron' *see* Quinuronium sulfate.
'Acaralate' *see* Chloropropylate.
'Acarol' *see* Bromopropylate.
'Accent' *see* Sodium glutamate.
'Accothion' *see* Fenitrothion.
ACEBROCHOL*** (acetodibromodihydrocholesterol; 5,6β-dibromo-5α-cholestan-3β-ol acetate).
ACEBURIC ACID*** (4-hydroxybutyric acid acetate; 4-acetoxybutyric acid).
ACEBUTOLOL*** ((±)-1-(2-acetyl-4-butyramidophenoxy)-3-isopropylaminopropan-2-ol; (±)-*N*-[3-acetyl-4-(2-hydroxy-3-isopropylaminopropoxy)phenyl]butyramide; (±)-3'-acetyl-4'-(2-hydroxy-3-isopropylaminopropoxy)butyranilide; *N*-[3-acetyl-4-[2-hydroxy-3-(1-methylethylamino)propoxy]phenyl]butanamide; IL-17803A; M&B-17803A; 'sectral').
ACECARBROMAL*** (1-acetyl-3-(2-bromo-2-ethylbutyryl)urea; acetylbromodiethylacetylurea; acetylcarbromal).
ACECARBROMAL WITH PARACETAMOL ('apromal').
ACECLIDINE*** (3-quinuclidinol acetate; 'glaucostat').

1

ACECLIDINE WITH EPINEPHRINE ('glaucadrin').

ACEDAPSONE*** (4′,4‴-sulfonylbis(acetanilide); 4,4′-diacetamidodiphenyl sulfone; *p*,*p*′-sulfonyldiacetanilide; acetyldiphenasone; diacetyldapsone; diacetyldiaphenylsulfone; sulfadiamine; sulfodiamine; BF-103; CI-556; F-1399; DADDS; 'atilon', 'hansolar', 'rodilone').
See also Cycloguanil embonate with acedapsone.

ACEDIASULFONE MORPHOLINE SALT ('bentrofene').

ACEDIASULFONE SODIUM*** (4-amino-4′-carboxymethylaminodiphenyl sulfone Na salt; diaminodiphenylsulfone-*N*-acetic acid Na salt; *N*-(*p*-sulfanilylphenyl)glycine sodium; 'ciloprine').

'Acedicon' *see* Thebacon.

'Acedist' *see* Bromophenophos.

'Acedoxin' *see* Acetyldigitoxin.

ACEFURTIAMINE*** (*S*-ester of thio-2-furoic acid with *N*-(4-amino-2-methylpyrimidin-5-ylmethyl)-*N*-(4-hydroxy-2-mercapto-1-methyl-1-butenyl)formamide *O*-glycolate acetate).

ACEFYLLINE PIPERAZINE*** (piperazine theophyllin-7-ylacetate; theophylline-piperazine acetate; theophylline-piperazine ethanoate; acepifylline; 'etaphylline', 'etophylate').

ACEGLATONE*** (D-glucaric acid 1,4:6,3-dilactone diacetate; saccharic acid 1,4:6,3-dilactone diacetate; 'glucaron').

ACEGLUTAMIDE*** (N^2-acetyl-L-glutamine; L-2-acetamido-4-carbamoylbutyric acid; 'aventol').

ACEGLUTAMIDE ALUMINIUM HYDROXIDE COMPLEX (KW-110).

ACEMETACIN*** (indometacin ester with glycolic acid; glycolic acid indometacin (ester) derivative).

Acemethadone *see* Acetylmethadol.

'Acemydrite' *see* Buzepide.

Acenocoumarin* *see* Acenocoumarol.

ACENOCOUMAROL*** (3-[2-acetyl-1-(*p*-nitrophenyl)ethyl]-4-hydroxycoumarin; 3-(α-acetonyl-*p*-nitrobenzyl)-4-hydroxycoumarin; acenocoumarin; nicoumalone; G-23350, 'sinthrome', 'sintrom').

ACEPERONE*** (4-(4-acetamidomethyl-4-phenylpiperid-1-yl)-4′-fluorobutyrophenone; 4-acetamidomethyl-1-[3-(*p*-fluorobenzoyl)propyl]piperidine; acetobutone; R-3448).

ACEPHATE* (*O*,*S*-dimethyl acetylphosphoramidothioate; 'orthene').

Acephenazine* *see* Acetophenazine.

Acepiphylline* *see* Acefylline piperazine.

'Acepramin' *see* Aminocaproic acid.

ACEPROMAZINE*** (2-acetyl-10-(3-dimethylaminopropyl)phenothiazine; 10-(3-dimethylaminopropyl)phenothiazin-3-yl methyl ketone; acetylpromazine; acetazine; 'soprintin'; 'vetranquil').
See also Etorphine with acepromazine.

ACEPROMAZINE MALEATE (CB-1522; 'anatran', 'anergan', 'atravet', 'lisergan', 'notensil', 'plegicil', 'plegicin', 'plegicyl', 'soprontin').

ACEPROMETAZINE*** (2-acetyl-10-(2-dimethylaminopropyl)phenothiazine; 10-(2-dimethylaminopropyl)phenothiazin-3-yl methyl ketone).

ACEPROMETAZINE WITH MEPROBAMATE ('mepronizine').

ACEQUINOLINE*** (7-methoxy-2,4-dimethyl-3-quinolyl methyl ketone; 3-acetyl-7-methoxy-2,4-dimethylquinoline).

Acesal (tr) *see* Acetylsalicylic acid.

ACESULFAME*** (6-methyl-1,2,3-oxathiazin-4(3H)-one 2,2-dioxide; acetosulfam).

ACETAL (1,1-diethoxyethane; diethylaldehyde; acetaldehyde diethylacetal; acetol; ethylidene diethyl ether).

ACETALDEHYDE (ethanal).

Acetaldehyde diethylacetal *see* Acetal.

Acetaldol *see* Aldol.

5-Acetamido-3-acetamidomethyl-2,4,6-triiodobenzoic acid *see* Iodamide.

Acetamidoacetic acid *see* Aceturic acid.

4-Acetamido-4′-aminodiphenyl sulfone *see* Acetyldapsone.

ACETAMIDOAZOTOLUENE (4-acetamido-2′,3-dimethylazobenzene; *N*-acetyl-4-(*o*-tolylazo)-*o*-toluidine; azodermin).

***p*-Acetamidobenzaldehyde thiosemicarbazone** *see* Thiacetazone.

***p*-Acetamidobenzoic acid inosine dimethylamino-2-propanol complex** *see* Methisoprinol.

Acetamidocaproic acid *see* Acexamic acid.

2-Acetamido-4-carbamoylbutyric acid *see* Aceglutamide.

1-Acetamido-5-cyanopyrimidin-4-one *see* Ciapilome.

7-Acetamido-6,7-dihydro-1,2,3,10-tetramethoxybenzo(a)heptalen-9(5H)-one *see* Colchicine.

4-Acetamido-2-ethoxybenzoic acid methyl ester *see* Ethopabate.

2-Acetamidoethyl 2-(4-chlorophenyl)-2-(3-trifluoromethylphenoxy)acetate *see* Halofenate.

***S*-2-ACETAMIDOETHYL *O*,*O*-DIMETHYL PHOSPHORODITHIOATE** (DAEP; 'amiphos').

2-Acetamidofluorene *see* Fluorenylacetamide.

4-Acetamido-15-glucopyranosyloxy-13,14-dimethoxy-8-methylthio-7-oxotricyclo-(10.4.0.0⁵,¹¹)hexadeca-1(12),5,8,10,13,15-hexaene *see* Thiocolchicoside.

3-Acetamido-5-glycolamido-2,4,6-triiodobenzoic acid *see* Ioxotrizoic acid.

6-Acetamidohexanoic acid *see* Acexamic acid.

5-Acetamido-*N*-(2-hydroxyethyl)-2,4,6-triiodoisophthalamic acid *see* Ioxitalamic acid.

2-Acetamido-4-mercaptobutyric acid *see* Acetylhomocysteine.

2-Acetamido-4-mercaptobutyric acid clofibrate ester *see* Serfibrate.

p-Acetamido-*m*-methoxybenzaldehyde thiosemicarbazone *see* Amithizone.

3-Acetamido-5-(*N*-methylacetamido)-2,4,6-triiodobenzoic acid *see* Metrizoic acid.

4-Acetamidomethyl-1-[3-(*p*-fluorobenzoyl)propyl]piperidine *see* Aceperone.

4-(4-Acetamidomethyl-4-phenylpiperid-1-yl)-4′-fluorobutyrophenone *see* Aceperone.

m-Acetamidophenol *see* Metacetamol.

p-Acetamidophenol *see* Paracetamol.

1-(*p*-Acetamidophenoxy)-3-isopropylamino-2-propanol *see* Practolol.

N-[(*p*-Acetamidophenoxymethyl)-carbonyl]-α-methyl-*m*-(trifluoromethyl)phenethylamine *see* Flucetorex.

1-(*p*-Acetamidophenoxy)-2,2,2-trichloroethanol *see* Cloracetadol.

p-Acetamidophenyl acetate *see* Diacetamate.

p-Acetamidophenyl 2-acetoxybenzoate *see* Benorilate.

p-Acetamidophenyl *O*-acetylsalicylate *see* Benorilate.

1-Acetamidophenyl-4-(3-dimethylaminopropyl)piperazine *see* Piperamide.

4-Acetamidophenyl salicylate *see* Acetaminosalol.

4-Acetamidophenyl salicylate acetate *see* Benorilate.

1-(3-Acetamidopropyl)-4-(2,5-dichlorophenyl)piperazine *see* Acaprazine.

Acetamidosalol *see* Acetaminosalol.

3-Acetamido-2,4,6-triiodobenzoic acid *see* Acetrizoic acid.

2-[3-Acetamido-2,4,6-triiodo-5-(*N*-methylacetamido)benzamido]-2-deoxy-D-glucose *see* Metrizamide.

3-Acetamido-2,4,6-triiodo-5-(*N*-methylacetamido)benzoic acid *see* Metrizoic acid.

5-Acetamido-2,4,6-triiodo-*N*-[(methylcarbamoyl)methyl]isophthalamidic acid *see* Ioglicic acid.

5-Acetamido-2,4,6-triiodo-*N*-methylisophthalamic acid *see* Iotalamic acid.

2-[2-(3-Acetamido-2,4,6-triiodophenoxy)-ethoxymethyl]butyric acid *see* Iopronic acid.

Acetaminophen* *see* Paracetamol.

ACETAMINOSALOL*** (4-acetamidophenyl salicylate; 4′-hydroxyacetanilide salicylate; acetamidosalol; acetaminosal; salophenum; 'cetosalol', 'cetosal', 'phenetsal').

ACETANILIDE (*N*-phenylacetamide; *N*-acetylaniline; antifebrin).

Acetarsenic acid *see* Arsonoacetic acid.

ACETARSOL*** (*N*-acetyl-4-hydroxy-*m*-arsanilic acid; 3-acetamido-4-hydroxybenzenearsonic acid; acetarsone; acetphenarsine; Ehrlich 594; osarsol).

Acetarsone *see* Acetarsol.

Acetarsonic acid *see* Arsonoacetic acid.

'Acetasal' *see* Choline salicylate.

Acetasol *see* Acetopyrine.

Acetate-replacing factor *see* Thioctic acid.

Acetazine *see* Acepromazine.

ACETAZOLAMIDE*** (5-acetamido-2-sulfamoyl-1,3,4-thiadiazole; acetazoleamide; compound 6063; diacarb; 'diamox', 'diluran', 'diomax', 'diuramide', 'diutazol', 'edemox', 'eumicton', 'fonurit', 'glaucomide', 'natrionex', 'nephramid', 'renamid').

ACETERGAMINE*** ((+)-*N*-acetyl-9,10-dihydrolysergamine; *N*-acetyl-8β-aminomethyl-6-methyl-10a-ergoline; (+)-*N*-(6-methylergolin-8β-ylmethyl)acetamide).

ACETERGAMINE TARTRATE (VUFB-6683; 'deprenon').

'Acetexa' *see* Nortriptyline.

ACETIAMINE*** ([*N*-(4-amino-2-methylpyrimidin-5-yl)methyl]-*N*-(4-hydroxy-2-mercapto-1-methyl-1-butenyl)formamide *O*,*S*-diacetate).

ACETIC ACID (ethanoic acid).

Acetic acid 5-nitrofurfurylidenehydrazide *see* Nihydrazone.

Acetic acid phenylhydrazide *see* Acetylphenylhydrazine.

'Acetiodone' *see* Sodium acetrizoate.

ACETIROMATE** (4-(4-hydroxy-3-iodophenoxy)-3,5-diiodobenzoic acid acetate).

Acetoarsinic acid *see* Arsonoacetic acid.

Acetobutone *see* Aceperone.

'Acetochlorone' *see* Chlorbutol.

Acetocinnamone *see* Benzylideneacetone.

ACETOHEXAMIDE*** (1-(*p*-acetylbenzenesulfonyl)-3-cyclohexylurea; 1-[(*p*-acetylphenyl)sulfonyl]-3-cyclohexylurea; 'dimelor', 'dymelor', 'ordimel').

ACETOHYDROXAMIC ACID (*N*-hydroxyacetamide).

ACETOIN (3-hydroxy-2-butanone; acetyl methyl carbinol).

Acetol *see* Acetal; Hydroxyacetone.

Acetol salicylate *see* Salicyl acetol.

Acetomenadione *see* Acetomenaphthone.

ACETOMENAPHTHONE* (2-methyl-1,4-naphthalenediol diacetate; acetomenadione; menadiol diacetate; vitamin K₄).

Acetomenophen *see* Paracetamol.

ACETOMEROCTOL* (2-acetoxymercuri-4-(1,1,3,3-tetramethylbutyl)phenol; 'merbak').

ACETOMESIDIDE (2′,4′,6′-trimethylacetanilide; acetylmesidine).

Acetomorphine *see* Diamorphine.

ACETONE (2-propanone).

Acetone bis(3,5-di-*tert*-butyl-4-hydroxyphenyl)mercaptole *see* Probucol.

Acetone-chloroform *see* Chlorbutol.

ACETONITRILE (ethane nitrile; methyl cyanide).

3-(α-Acetonylbenzyl)-4-hydroxycoumarin *see* Warfarin.

3-(α-Acetonyl-*p*-chlorobenzyl)-4-hydroxycoumarin *see* Coumachlor.

3-(α-Acetonylfurfuryl)-4-hydroxycoumarin *see* Coumafuryl.

3-(α-Acetonyl-*p*-nitrobenzyl)-4-hydroxycoumarin *see* Acenocoumarol.

2-Acetonylpiperidine *see* Isopelletierine.

ACETOPHENAZINE*** (2-acetyl-10-[3-[4-

3

(2-hydroxyethyl)piperazin-1-yl]propyl]-phenothiazine; 10-[3-[4-(2-hydroxyethyl)-piperazin-1-yl]propyl]phenothiazin-2-yl methyl ketone; acephenazine).

ACETOPHENAZINE DIMALEATE (aceto-phenazine maleate; Sch-6673; 'tindal').

p-**Acetophenetidide** *see* Phenacetin.

Acetophenetidin* *see* Phenacetin.

'Acetophenidin' *see* Phenacetin.

Acetophenomethane *see* Bisacodyl.

ACETOPHENONE (methyl phenyl ketone; hypnone).

Acetopherane* *see* Phacetoperan.

ACETOPYRINE (phenazone acetylsalicylate; acetasal).

ACETORPHINE** (5-acetoxy-1,2,3,3a,8,9-hexahydro-2α-(1(R)-hydroxy-1-methyl-butyl)-3-methoxy-12-methyl-3,9a-etheno-9, 9b-iminoethanophenanthro(4,5-bcd)furan; O^3-acetyl-7,8-dihydro-7α-(1(R)-hydroxy-1-methylbutyl)-O^6-methyl-6,14-*endo*-ethenomorphine; 3-*O*-acetyl-7α-(1(R)-hydroxy-1-methylbutyl)tetrahydro-6,14-*endo*-ethenooripavine; 6,7,8,14-tetrahydro-7α-(1-hydroxy-1-methylbutyl)-6,14-*endo*-ethenooripavine 3-acetate; 3-*O*-acetyl-19-propylnorvinol; tetrahydro-7α-(1-hydroxy-1-methylbutyl)-6,14-*endo*-ethenooripavine 3-acetate; etorphine acetate; M-183).

Acetosal *see* Acetylsalicylic acid.

Acetosulfam *see* Acesulfame.

Acetosulfaminum *see* Sulfacetamide.

Acetosulfone* *see* Sulfadiasulfone.

ACETOTOLUIDIDE(S) (*N*-acetyltolu-idine(s); *ar*-methylacetanilide(s)).

Acetovanillone *see* Apocynin.

Acetoxatrine *see* Acoxatrine.

5-Acetoxy-3-(2-aminoethyl)-1-(*p*-methoxy-benzyl)-2-methylindole *see* Hydroxin-dasate.

1-Acetoxy-6-aminooctahydroindolizine *see* Slaframine.

α-Acetoxy-α-benzylhydrocinnamic acid 2-piperid-1-ylethyl ester *see* Fenperate.

4-Acetoxybutyric acid *see* Aceburic acid.

17α-Acetoxy-6-chloro-6-dehydroprogest-erone *see* Chlormadinone.

2-Acetoxy-4'-chloro-3,5-diiodobenzanilide *see* Clioxanide.

21-Acetoxy-3-(2-chloroethoxy)-9α-fluoro-6-formyl-11β-hydroxy-16α,17α-iso-propylidenedioxypregna-3,5-dien-20-one *see* Formocortal.

8-Acetoxy-5-chloroquinoline *see* Cloxiquine acetate.

(11β,16α)-21-Acetoxy-16,17-[cyclopentyl-idenebis(oxy)]-9-fluoro-11-hydr-oxypregna-1,4-diene-3,20-dione *see* Amcinonide.

17α-Acetoxy-6-dehydro-16-methylene-progesterone *see* 17α-Hydroxy-16-methyl-enepregna-4,6-diene-3,20-dione acetate.

4-Acetoxy-2',4'-dibromo-6'-[[(cyclohexyl)-(methyl)amino]methyl]-3-methoxy-benzanilide *see* Brovanexine.

2-Acetoxy-3-diethylcarbamoyl-9,10-dime-thoxy-1,2,3,4,6,7-hexahydro(11bH)-

benzo(a)quinolizine *see* Benzquinamide.

10-Acetoxy-9,10-dihydro-8,8-dimethyl-9-(α-methylbutyryloxy)benzodipyran-2-one *see* Visnadine.

4'-Acetoxy-3',4'-dihydro-3'-(2-methyl-butyryloxy)seselin *see* Visnadine.

3-Acetoxy-6-dimethylamino-4,4-diphenyl-heptane *see* Acetylmethadol.

4-Acetoxy-β-dimethylamino-2-isopropyl-5-methylphenetole *see* Moxisylyte.

5-Acetoxy-*N*,*N*-dimethyl-4,4-diphenyl-2-heptylamine *see* Acetylmethadol.

4-Acetoxy-*N*,1-dimethyl-3,3-diphenyl-hexylamine *see* Noracymethadol.

(2-Acetoxyethyl)(2-chloroethyl)methyl-amine *see* Acetylcholine mustard.

(+)-17-Acetoxy-13-ethyl-18,19-dinor-17α-pregn-4-en-20-yn-3-one oxime *see* Norgestimate.

17-Acetoxy-3,3-ethylenedioxy-6-methyl-pregn-5-en-20-one *see* Edrogestone.

10-[3-[1-(2-Acetoxyethyl)piperazin-4-yl]-propyl]-2-chlorophenothiazine *see* Thiopropazate.

4-Acetoxy-4'-fluorobiphenyl-3-carboxylic acid *see* Flufenisal.

21-Acetoxy-9-fluoro-11β-hydroxy-2'-methyl-5'βH-pregna-1,4-dieno(17,16-d)-oxazole-3,20-dione *see* Fluazacort.

5-Acetoxy-1,2,3,3a,8,9-hexahydro-2α-(1(R)-hydroxy-1-methylbutyl)-3-methoxy-12-methyl-3,9a-etheno-9,9b-iminoethanophenanthro(4,5-bcd)furan *see* Acetorphine.

3-Acetoxy-4-hydroxy-2-(*p*-methoxyben-zyl)pyrrolidine *see* Anisomycin.

21-Acetoxy-3α-hydroxy-5α-pregnane-11,20-dione *see* Alfadolone acetate.

2-(4-Acetoxy-2-isopropyl-5-methylphen-oxy)-*N*,*N*-dimethylethylamine *see* Moxisylyte.

ACETOXYLIDIDE(S) (*N*-acetylxylidine(s); *ar*,*ar*-dimethylacetanilide(s)).

3-Acetoxymethyl-7-(5-amino-5-carboxy-valeramido)-2-cephem-2-carboxylic acid *see* Cephalosporin C.

(±)-α-3-Acetoxy-6-methylamino-4,4-diphenylheptane *see* Noracymethadol.

3-Acetoxymethyl-2-cephem-2-carboxylic acid *see* Cephalosporanic acid.

Acetoxymethyl 4-(2-chloro-*m*-toluidino)-thiophene-3-carboxylate *see* Aclantate.

3-Acetoxymethyl-7-(2-cyanoacetamido)-2-cephem-2-carboxylic acid *see* Cefa-cetrile.

17-Acetoxy-11β-methyl-19-norpregn-4-ene-3,20-dione *see* Norgestomet.

3-Acetoxymethyl-7-(2-phenylacetamido)-2-cephem-2-carboxylic acid *see* Cefa-loram.

Acetoxymethyl 6-phenylacetamidopeni-cillanate *see* Penamecillin.

17α-Acetoxy-6α-methylprogesterone *see* Medroxyprogesterone acetate.

3-Acetoxymethyl-7-[2-(pyrid-4-ylthio)-acetamido]-2-cephem-2-carboxylic acid *see* Cefapirin.

3-Acetoxymethyl-7-(2-thien-2-ylacet-
amido)-2-cephem-2-carboxylic acid *see*
Cefalotin.
3β-Acetoxy-11-oxoolean-12-en-30-oic aci l
cinnamyl ester *see* Cinoxolone.
Acetoxypregnenolone *see* Pregnenolone
acetate.
3-Acetoxyquinuclidine *see* Aceclidine.
4-Acetoxythymol dimethylaminoethyl
ether *see* Moxisylyte.
2-(Acetoxythymoxy)-*N*,*N*-dimethylethyl-
amine *see* Moxisylyte.
4-Acetoxy-*N*,*N*,1-trimethyl-3,3-diphenyl-
hexylamine *see* Acetylmethadol.
1-(4-Acetoxy-2,3,5-trimethylphenoxy)-3-
isopropylamino-2-propanol *see* Trimepranol.
Acetoxytriphenylstannane *see* Fentin
acetate.
Acetparaphenalide *see* Phenacetin.
Acetphenarsine *see* Acetarsol.
ACETPHENOLISATIN * (3,3-bis(*p*-acetoxy-
phenyl)isatin; 3,3-bis(*p*-acetoxyphenyl)-
oxindole; bisatin; diacetoxydiphenylisatin;
diacetyldiphenolisatin; diacetyldihydroxyphenylisatin; diasatin; diphesatine; endophenolphthalein; isaphenin; 'acetalax',
'asitin', 'brocatine', 'cirotyl', 'cirrotyl', 'con-
tax', 'disacetine', 'inlax', 'isacen', 'isaphen',
'isazen', 'isocrin', 'laxo-isatin', 'leacen',
'lisagal', 'nourilax', 'novolax', 'promassolax',
'prulet', 'purgacen').
ACETPYROGALL * (1,2,3-triacetoxyben-
zene; pyrogallol triacetate; 'lenigallol',
'pyracetol').
ACETRIZOIC ACID * (3-acetamido-2,4,6-
triiodobenzoic acid; 'triumbren', 'urokolin').
See also Ethyl acetrizoate; Meglumine
acetrizoate; Sodium acetrizoate.
ACETRYPTINE *** (5-acetyl-3-(2-amino-
ethyl)indole; 5-acetyltryptamine; 3-(2-
aminoethyl)indol-5-yl methyl ketone; 2-(5-
acetylindol-3-yl)ethylamine).
Acetsulfanilamide *see* Sulfacetamide.
Acetsulfonum *see* Sulfadiasulfone.
ACETURIC ACID (acetamidoacetic acid; *N*-
acetylglycine; ethanoylaminoethanoic acid).
See also Closiramine aceturate.
ACETYLACETONE (2,4-pentanedione).
Acetylaminocaproic acid *see* Acexamic
acid.
5-Acetyl-3-(2-aminoethyl)indole *see*
Acetryptine.
2-Acetylaminofluorene *see* Fluorenylacetamide.
(+)-*N*-Acetyl-8β-aminomethyl-6-methyl-
10a-ergoline *see* Acetergamine.
N-Acetyl-*m*-aminophenol *see* Metacetamol.
N-Acetyl-*p*-aminophenol *see* Paracetamol.
Acetyl-*p*-aminosalol *see* Acetaminosalol.
3-(Acetylamino)-2,4,6-triiodo-5-
[[[[(methylamino)carbonyl]methyl]-
amino]carbonyl]benzoic acid *see* Ioglicic
acid.
N-Acetyl-*N*-(3-amino-2,4,6-triiodophenyl)-
2-methyl-β-alanine *see* Iocetamic acid.
17-Acetylandrostane *see* Pregnan-20-one.

1-(*p*-Acetylbenzenesulfonyl)-3-cyclo-
hexylurea *see* Acetohexamide.
N-Acetyl-*S*-(2-benzoylpropyl)cysteine *see*
Bencisteine.
N-Acetyl-3-[(2-benzoylpropyl)thio]alanine
see Bencisteine.
N-Acetyl-*p*-[bis(2-chloroethyl)amino]-
phenylalanine ethyl ester *see* Phenaphan.
N-[*N*-Acetyl-3-[*p*-[bis(2-chloroethyl)-
amino]phenyl]alanyl]-DL-valine ethyl
ester *see* Asaline.
Acetylbromdiethylacetylurea *see* Acecarbromal.
Acetylbromdiethylurea *see* Carbromal.
1-Acetyl-3-(2-bromo-2-ethylbutyryl)urea
see Acecarbromal.
3-[3-Acetyl-4-[3-(*tert*-butylamino)-2-
hydroxypropoxy]phenyl]-1,1-diethyl-
urea *see* Celiprolol.
3-Acetyl-5-*sec*-butyl-4-hydroxy-3-pyrrolin-
2-one *see* Tenuazonic acid.
α-Acetyl-5-*sec*-butyltetramic acid *see*
Tenuazonic acid.
1-(2-Acetyl-4-butyramidophenoxy)-3-
isopropylaminopropan-2-ol *see* Acebutolol.
Acetyl carbinol *see* Hydroxyacetone.
Acetylcarbocholine *see* 3,3-Dimethylbutyl
acetate.
N-Acetyl-*N*-(2-carboxypropyl)-2,4,6-tri-
iodo-*m*-phenylenediamine *see* Iocetamic
acid.
Acetylcarbromal *see* Acecarbromal.
(3-Acetyl-5-chloro-2-hydroxybenzyl)-
diethyl(2-phenoxyethyl)ammonium
3-hydroxy-2-naphthoate *see* Difezil.
3-[2-Acetyl-1-(*p*-chlorophenyl)ethyl]-4-
hydroxycoumarin *see* Coumachlor.
17β-Acetyl-6-chloro-1β,1a,2β,8β,9α,10,11,
12,13,14α,15,16β,16a,17-tetradecahydro-
10β,13β-dimethyl-3H-dicyclopropa(1,2:
16,17)cyclopenta(a)phenanthren-3-one
see Gestaclone.
ACETYLCHOLINE CHLORIDE ***
((2-acetoxyethyl)trimethylammonium
bromide or chloride; choline acetate; ACh).
ACETYLCHOLINE MUSTARD (2-[(2-
chloroethyl)methylamino]ethyl acetate;
(2-acetoxyethyl)(2-chloroethyl)methyl-
amine; methyl-2-acetoxyethyl-2'-chloro-
ethylamine).
'Acetylcodone' *see* Thebacon.
ACETYLCRESOTIC ACID (2-acetoxy-5-
methylbenzoic acid; 'cresopyrine', 'ervasin').
ACETYLCYSTEINE *** (*N*-acetyl-L-cysteine;
NSC-111180; 'airbron', 'broncholysin', 'fluimucil', 'mucomyst', 'mucosolvin', 'NAC').
ACETYLDAPSONE (4-acetamido-4-amino-
diphenyl sulfone; sulfone *N*-acetate; acetyldiaphenylsulfone).
Acetyldiaphenylsulfone *see* Acetyldapsone.
1-[2-Acetyl-4-[(diethylcarbamoyl)amino]-
phenoxy]-3-(*tert*-butylamino)-2-propanol
see Celiprolol.
1-Acetyl-*N*,*N*-diethyllysergamide *see*
Acetyllysergide.
ACETYLDIGITOXIN *** (3β,14β-dihydroxy-

5

5β-card-20(22)-enolide 3-(4'''-acetyltridigitoxoside); 4'''-acetyldigitoxin; α-acetyldigitoxin; 'acedoxin', 'acylanid')

β-**ACETYLDIGOXIN** (3β,12,14-trihydroxy-5β-card-20(22)-enolide 3-(4'''-acetyltridigitoxoside); acetyl-12-hydroxydigitoxin; desglucolanatoside C; 'acygoxin', 'cedigocin', 'cedigoxin', 'dioxanin', 'lanadigin', 'lanatilin', 'novodigal', 'sandolanid').

β-**ACETYLDIGOXIN WITH DILAZEP** ('cormelian digotab').

Acetyldihydrocodeinone see Thebacon.

O^3-**Acetyl-7,8-dihydro-7α-(1(R)-hydroxy-1-methylbutyl)-O^6-methyl-6,14-endo-ethenomorphine** see Acetorphine.

N-**Acetyl-9,10-dihydrolysergamine** see Acetergamine.

Acetyldimepheptanol see Acetylmethadol.

2-Acetyl-10-(2-dimethylaminopropyl)-phenothiazine see Aceprometazine.

2-Acetyl-10-(3-dimethylaminopropyl)-phenothiazine see Acepromazine.

N^1-**Acetyl-N^1-(3,4-dimethylisoxazol-5-yl)sulfanilamide** see Acetylsulfafurazole.

Acetyldiphenasone see Acedapsone.

ACETYLENE (ethine; ethyne; 'narcylene').

Acetylenecarboxylic acid see Propiolic acid.

Acetylene tetrachloride see Tetrachloroethane.

17-Acetylestratriene see 19-Norpregnatrien-20-one.

4-(2-Acetylethyl)-1,2-diphenyl-3,5-pyrazolidinedione see Kebuzone.

Acetylformaldehyde see Methylglyoxal.

Acetylformic acid see Pyruvic acid.

3-(2-Acetyl-1-furan-2-ylethyl)-4-hydroxycoumarin see Coumafuryl.

ACETYLGITALOXIN (16-formylacetylgitoxin).

16-ACETYLGITOXIN ('resorptol').

Acetylglutamine see Aceglutamide.

(1S,3S)-3-Acetyl-1,2,3,4,6,11-hexahydro-3,5,12-trihydroxy-10-methoxy-6,11-dioxo-1-naphthacenyl 3-amino-2,3,6-trideoxy-α-L-lyxo-hexopyranoside see Daunorubicin.

ACETYLHOMOCYSTEINE (2-acetamido-4-mercaptobutyric acid; N-acetylhomocysteine).

N-**Acetylhomocysteine clofibrate** see Serfibrate.

ACETYLHOMOCYSTEINE THIOLACTONE (N-acetyl-DL-homocysteine thiolactone).

ACETYLHOMOCYSTEINE THIOLACTONE WITH CYSTEINE AND FRUCTOSE ('reducdyn').

Acetyl-12-hydroxydigitoxin see Acetyldigoxin.

1-Acetyl-2-(3-hydroxy-3,3-diphenylpropionyl)hydrazine see Diphoxazide.

2-Acetyl-10-[3-[4-(2-hydroxyethyl)piperazin-1-yl]propyl]phenothiazine see Acetophenazine.

2-Acetyl-10-[3-[4-(2-hydroxyethyl)piperid-

1-yl]propyl]phenothiazine see Piperacetazine.

N-[p-**Acetyl-β-hydroxy-α-(hydroxymethyl)phenethyl]-2,2-dichloroacetamide** see Cetofenicol.

3'-Acetyl-4'-(2-hydroxy-3-isopropylaminopropoxy)butyranilide see Acebutolol.

N-[3-**Acetyl-4-(2-hydroxy-3-isopropylaminopropoxy)phenyl]butyramide** see Acebutolol.

3-O-Acetyl-7α-(1(R)-hydroxy-1-methylbutyl)tetrahydro-6,14-endo-ethenooripavine see Acetorphine.

N-[3-**Acetyl-4-[2-hydroxy-3-(1-methylethylamino)propoxy]phenyl]butanamide** see Acebutolol.

2-Acetyl-5-hydroxy-3-oxo-4-hexenoic acid δ-lactone see Dehydroacetic acid.

N-**Acetylhydroxyproline** see Oxaceprol.

1-Acetyl-4-hydroxy-L-proline see Oxaceprol.

2-Acetylimino-3-(2-hydroxy-2-thien-2-ylethyl)thiazoline see Antazonite.

5-Acetylimino-4-methyl-2-sulfamoyl-1,3,4-thiadiazoline see Methazolamide.

2-(5-Acetylindol-3-yl)ethylamine see Acetryptine.

Acetylleucine monoethanolamine salt see Ethanolamine acetylleucinate.

1-Acetyllysergic acid diethylamide see Acetyllysergide.

ACETYLLYSERGIDE (1-acetyllysergic acid diethylamide; 1-acetyl-N,N-diethyllysergamide).

N-**Acetylmerphalan valine peptide ethyl ester** see Asaline.

Acetylmetacresol* see m-Cresyl acetate.

ACETYLMETHADOL*** (3-acetoxy-6-dimethylamino-4,4-diphenylheptane; 5-acetoxy-N,N-dimethyl-4,4-diphenyl-2-heptylamine; 4-acetoxy-N,N,1-trimethyl-3,3-diphenylhexylamine; acetyldimepheptanol; acemethadone; dimepheptanol acetate; methadyl acetate).
See also Alphacetylmethadol; Betacetylmethadol; Levacetylmethadol.

N-**ACETYLMETHIONINE** (methionine acetate; 'methionamine', 'thiomedon').

ACETYLMETHIONINE CHOLINE SALT ('hepsan').

3-Acetyl-7-methoxy-2,4-dimethylquinoline see Acequinoline.

N^1-**Acetyl-N^1-(3-methoxypyrazin-2-yl)-sulfanilamide** see Acetylsulfalene.

N-**Acetyl-5-methoxytryptamine** see Melatonin.

Acetyl methyl carbinol see Acetoin.

Acetyl-β-methylcholine see Methacholine.

N^1-**Acetyl-N^1-(5-methylisoxazol-3-yl)sulfanilamide** see Acetylsulfamethoxazole.

N-**Acetyl-O-methylserotonin** see Melatonin.

N^1-**Acetyl-N^1-(p-nitrophenyl)sulfanilamide** see Sulfanitran.

4-[(p-Acetylphenoxy)acetyl]morpholine p-oxime see Mofoxime.

1-[(p-Acetylphenoxy)acetyl]]piperidine p-oxime see Pifoxime.

1-(p-Acetylphenyl)-2-dichloroacetamido-

1,3-propanediol *see* Cetofenicol.

ACETYLPHENYLHYDRAZINE (acetic acid phenylhydrazide; hydracetin; 'pyrodin').

Acetylphenylsalicylate *see* Acetylsalol.

1-[(*p*-Acetylphenyl)sulfonyl]-3-cyclohexylurea *see* Acetohexamide.

Acetylphosphoramidothioic acid dimethyl ester *see* Acephate.

Acetylpromazine *see* Acepromazine.

3-Acetylpropionic acid *see* Levulinic acid.

3-*O*-Acetyl-19-propylnorvinol *see* Acetorphine.

4-Acetylpyrogallol *see* Gallacetophenone.

N-**Acetylsalicylamide** *see* Salacetamide.

ACETYLSALICYLIC ACID (salicylic acid acetate; acesal; acetosal; acetysal; 'aspirin' (trademark in some countries, nonproprietary name in others)).
See also below and Acetopyrine; Acetylsalol; Aloxiprin; APC; Calcium acetylsalicylate; Carbasalate calcium; Chlormezanone with acetylsalicylic acid; Lysine acetylsalicylate; Magnesium acetylsalicylate; Methyl acetylsalicylate; Phenprobamate with acetylsalicylic acid; Sodium bicarbonate acetylsalicylate.

Acetylsalicylic acid paracetamol ester *see* Benorilate.

ACETYLSALICYLIC ACID WITH ALUMINIUM MAGNESIUM HYDROXIDE ('ascriptin').

ACETYLSALICYLIC ACID WITH ASCORBIC ACID ('boxazin').

ACETYLSALICYLIC ACID WITH PARACETAMOL ('safaprin', 'safpryn').

ACETYLSALICYLSALICYLIC ACID (salsalate acetate; 'diplosal acetate').

ACETYLSALOL (acetylphenylsalicylate; phenyl acetylsalicylate; 'spiroform', 'vesipin', 'vesipyrin').

Acetylsarcolysylvaline ethyl ester *see* Asaline.

N-**Acetylserotonin methyl ether** *see* Melatonin.

Acetylsilicocholine *see* 2-(Trimethylsilylethyl) acetate.

ACETYLSULFAFURAZOLE (*N*¹-acetyl-*N*¹-(3,4-dimethylisoxazol-5-yl)sulfanilamide; acetylsulfisoxazole; 'lipogantrisin').

ACETYLSULFALENE (*N*¹-acetyl-*N*¹-(3-methoxypyrazin-2-yl)sulfanilamide; acetylsulfamethoxypyrazine; RP-11589).

ACETYLSULFAMETHOXAZOLE (*N*¹-acetyl-*N*¹-(5-methylisoxazol-3-yl)sulfanilamide; acetylsulfisomezole; 'sinomin acetyl').

Acetylsulfamethoxypyrazine *see* Acetylsulfalene.

*N*¹-**Acetylsulfanilamide** *see* Sulfacetamide.

(*V*¹-**Acetyl-6-sulfanilylmetanilamido)-sodium** *see* Sulfadiasulfone sodium.

Acetylsulfisomezole *see* Acetylsulfamethoxazole.

Acetylsulfisoxazole *see* Acetylsulfafurazole.

3-*O*-Acetyltetrahydro-7*α*-(1-hydroxy-1-methylbutyl-6,14-*endo*-ethenooripavine *see* Acetorphine.

7*α*-Acetylthioandrost-4-en-3-one-17*β*-ol-17*α*-ylpropionic acid *γ*-lactone *see* Spironolactone.

ACETYLTHIOCHOLINE ((2-mercaptoethyl)trimethylammonium hydroxide acetate; thiocholine acetate; ACS).

α-**Acetylthio-4′,5′-dihydrospiro(androst-4-ene-17,2′(3′H)-furan)-3-one acetate** *see* Spiroxasone.

3-(7*α*-Acetylthio-17*β*-hydroxy-3-oxoandrost-4-en-17*α*-yl)propionic acid lactone *see* Spironolactone.

3-(3-Acetylthio-7-methoxycarbonylheptyldithio)-4-[*N*-(4-amino-2-methylpyrimid-5-ylmethyl)formamido]pent-3-en-1-ol *see* Octotiamine.

5-Acetyltryptamine *see* Acetryptine.

Acetysal (tr) *see* Acetylsalicylic acid.

ACEVALTRATE* (3,4-dihydroxy-3a,4-dihydrospiro(benzofuran-2(3H),2′-oxirane)-6-methanol 6-acetate 3(or 4)-isovalerate 4(or 3)-(3-hydroxy-3-methylbutyrate acetate); 1,7a-dihydro-1,6-dihydroxyspiro-(cyclopenta(c)pyran-7(6H),2′-oxirane)-4-methanol 4-acetate 1(or 6)-isovalerate 6(or 1)-(3-hydroxy-3-methylbutyrate acetate)).
See also Valepotriate.

ACEXAMIC ACID* (6-acetamidohexanoic acid; acetamidocaproic acid; acetylaminocaproic acid; 'plastenan').
See also Prednisolone acexamate; Sodium acexamate.

'**Achromin**' *see* Hydroquinone.

'**Aciban**' *see* Calcium caseinate.

Acid blue CI-92 *see* Anazolene sodium.

Acid fuchsine *see* Fuchsine sulfonates.

'**Acidol**' *see* Betaine hydrochloride.

'**Acimetion**' *see* Methionine.

Acinitrazole* *see* Aminitrozole.

Acinitrozole *see* Aminitrozole.

'**Acinormal**' *see* Aluminium Mg Na silicate.

Aciphenochinolinum *see* Cinchophen.

ACIPIMOX* (5-methylpyrazinecarboxylic acid 4-oxide).

'**Aciquel**' *see* Potassium glucaldrate.

'**Acisorban**' *see* Aluminium Na silicate.

'**Acket**' *see* Salicylamide.

ACL-59 *see* Troclosene potassium.

ACL-60 *see* Troclosene sodium.

ACL-85 *see* Symclosene.

'**Aclan**' *see* Aklomide with sulfanitran.

ACLANTATE* (4-(2-chloro-*m*-toluidino)-thiophene-3-carboxylic acid hydroxymethyl ester acetate ester; *N*-(3-carboxythien-4-yl)-2-chloro-*m*-toluidine acetoxymethyl ester; acetoxymethyl 4-(2-chloro-*m*-toluidino)thiophene-3-carboxylate).

Acoantherin *see* Ouabain.

'**Acodeen**' *see* Butamirate citrate.

'**Acoin**' *see* Guanicaine.

ACONIAZIDE* (isonicotinic acid [*o*-(carboxymethoxy)benzylidene]hydrazide; *N*′-(*o*-carboxymethoxybenzylidene)isoniazid; isonicotinoylhydrazone of *o*-carboxymethoxybenzaldehyde; 'phenoxalid').

Acopyrine *see* Acetopyrine.

ACOXATRINE*** ((±)-N-[1-(1,4-benzo-dioxan-2-ylmethyl)-4-phenylpiperid-4-ylmethyl]acetamide; (±)-4-(N-acetyl-aminomethyl)-1-(1,4-benzodioxan-2-ylmethyl)-4-phenylpiperidine; acetoxa-trine).
'Acramidine' see Aminoacridine.
'Acramine' see Aminoacridine.
'Acrex' see Dinobuton.
Acrichine (tr) see Mepacrine.
'Acricid' see Binapacryl.
ACRIDAN (9,10-dihydroacridine).
ACRIDINE (10-azaanthracene; dibenzo(b,e)-pyridine).
ACRIDINE ORANGE (3,6-bis(dimethyl-amino)acridine).
ACRIDINIC ACID (2,3-quinolinedicarb-oxylic acid).
N-(2-Acridin-9-ylethyl)amphetamine see Acridorex.
N-(2-Acridin-9-ylethyl)-α-methylphen-ethylamine see Acridorex.
ACRIDOREX*** (9-[2-(α-methylphenethyl-amino)ethyl]acridine; N-(2-acridin-9-yl-ethyl)-α-methylphenethylamine; N-(2-acridin-9-ylethyl)amphetamine).
Acriflavine* see Acriflavinium.
ACRIFLAVINIUM CHLORIDE*** (mixture of 3,6-diamino-10-methylacridinium chlor-ide and 3,6-diaminoacridine (proflavine) as hydrochlorides; acriflavine; euflavine; xanthacridine).
'Acriflex' see Aminoacridine.
'Acrinol' see Ethacridine.
'Acrinolin' see Ethacridine.
Acriquine (tr) see Mepacrine.
'Acrisan' see Aminoacridine.
ACRISORCIN*** (9-aminoacridine com-pound with 4-hexylresorcinol; aminacrin 4-hexylresorcinolate; 'akrinol').
'Acrisuxin' see Ethosuximide with mepacrine.
'Acrizane' see Phenacridan.
ACROCINONIDE*** (triamcinolone cyclic 16,17-acetal with acrolein).
'Acrol' see Diaminophenol.
'Acrolactine' see Ethacridine.
ACROLEIN (acrylyl aldehyde; propenal).
ACRONINE*** (3,12-dihydro-6-methoxy-3,3,12-trimethyl-7H-pyrano(2,3-c)acridin-7-one; acronycine; L-42339).
'Acronize' see Chlortetracycline.
Acronycine see Acronine.
'Acrosyl' see Cresol(s).
ACRYLIC ACID (propenoic acid; vinylfor-mic acid).
Acrylic acid polymer cross-linked with allyl sucrose see Carbomer.
ACRYLONITRILE (cyanoethylene; propene nitrile; vinyl cyanide; 'fumigrain', 'ventox').
ACRYLOPHENONE (phenyl vinyl ketone).
Acrylyl aldehyde see Acrolein.
ACS see Acetylthiocholine.
'Actamol' see Mebanazine.
ACTAPLANIN** (glycopeptide antibiotic from *Actinoplanes* str. ATCC 23342).
'Actasal' see Choline salicylate.
'Actase' see Fibrinolysin.

'Actebral' see Cyprodenate.
'Actellic' see Pirimiphos methyl.
'Actemil' see Etofylline nicotinate.
'Acterol' see Nimorazole.
ACTH (adrenocorticotrophin; corticotrophin; corticotropin; 'reachtin', 'solacthyl').
ACTH analogs see Codactide; Norleusactide; Seractide; Tetracosactide; Tosactide.
ACTH human synthetic see Tosactide.
'Actidil' see Triprolidine.
'Actidione' see Cycloheximide.
'Actifed' see Pseudoephedrine with tri-prolidine.
'Actilin' see Framycetin.
ACTINOBOLIN (antibiotic from *Str. griseo-viridus* var. *atrofaciens*; NSC-31083).
Actinochinol* see Actinoquinol.
'Actinochrysin' see Cactinomycin.
Actinomyces flavochromogenes var. heliomycini, antibiotic see Heliomycin.
Actinomyces griseoruber var. beromy-cini, antibiotic see Beromycin.
Actinomyces levoris, antibiotic see Levorin.
Actinomyces olivoreticuli, antibiotic see Olivomycin.
Actinomyces violaceus, antibiotic see Violarin.
Actinomycin C* see Cactinomycin.
Actinomycin D* see Dactinomycin.
ACTINOQUINOL*** (8-ethoxy-5-quinoline-sulfonic acid; actinochinol; aktinokinol). *See also* Sodium actinoquinol.
Actinospectocin see Spectinomycin.
'Actocortin' see Hydrocortisone 21-sodium phosphate.
ACTODIGIN*** (3β-(β-D-glucopyranosyl-oxy)-14,23-dihydroxy-24-nor-5β,14β-chol-20(22)-en-21-oic acid γ-lactone; AY-22241).
'Actomol' see Mebanazine.
'Actosin' see Warfarin.
'Actospar' see Sparteine.
'Actozine' see Phenprobamate.
'Actrapid' see Neutral insulin injection.
'Actril' see Ioxynil.
'Actril D' see Ioxynil plus (2,4-dichlorophen-oxy)acetic acid.
'Actriol' see Epiestriol.
'Acutran' see Amfechloral.
'Acygoxin' see Acetyldigoxin.
'Acylanid' see Acetyldigitoxin.
AD-122 see Atropine octyl bromide.
'Ada' see Aluminium glycinate.
'Adalate' see Nifedipine.
1-Adamantanamine see Amantadine.
ADAMANTANE (diamantane; tricyclo-(3.3.1³,⁷)decane).
N-(1-Adamantanecarbonyl)-3,4-dihydr-oxyphenethylamine see Dopamantine.
Adamantane-1-carboxylic acid estren-olone ester see Bolmantalate.
ADAMANTOYLCYTARABINE (cytarabine 5'-(1-adamantanecarboxylate); AdOCA).
1-Adamantylamine see Amantadine.
1-Adamant-1-ylazetidine-2-carboxylic acid see Carmantadine.
N-Adamant-1-yl-2-(2-dimethylamino-ethoxy)acetamide see Tromantadine.

8

Adamon see Bornyl dibromodihydrocinnamate.

'Adamon' see Ciclonium bromide.

Adamsite see Phenarsazine chloride.

'Adapin' see Doxepin.

'Adaptinol' see Xantofyl palmitate.

'Adazine' see Triflupromazine.

'Adbiol' see Bufetolol.

'Adchnon' see Adrenochrome guanylhydrazone.

'Adcortyl' see Triamcinolone.

'Adebit' see Buformin.

'Ademil' see Flumethiazide.

'Ademol' see Hydroflumethiazide.

ADENINE (6-aminopurine; vitamin B₄).

Adenine arabinoside see Vidarabine.

Adenine 3-deoxyriboside see Cordycepin.

ADENINE HYDROCHLORIDE ('leuco-4').

Adenine psicofuranoside see Angustmycin C.

Adenine riboside see Adenosine.

ADENOSINE (adenine riboside).

ADENOSINE DIPHOSPHATE (ADP).

Adenosine monophosphate see Adenosine phosphate.

ADENOSINE PHOSPHATE*** (adenosine 5-phosphate; adenosine monophosphate; adenylic acid; 5'-adenylic acid; A5MP; AMP; MAP; ergadenylic acid; 'adenovite', 'cardimone', 'cardiomone', 'glutadenyl', 'lycedan', 'mono-phosaden', 'my-B-den', 'myoston', 'phosaden').

ADENOSINE 3',5'-PHOSPHATE (adenyl cyclate; cyclic AMP; CAMP; cyclic adenylate).

ADENOSINE PHOSPHATES ('levadenyl').

Adenosine 5'-pyrophosphate inner salt 5'-ester with 3-carbamoyl-1-β-D-ribofuranosylpyridinium hydroxide see Nadide.

ADENOSINE TRIPHOSPHATE (adenylpyrophosphoric acid; ATP; 'adynol', 'glucobasin', 'striadyne', 'stryadine', 'triadenyl').

Adenosylcobamide see Cobamamide.

'Adenovite' see Adenosine phosphate.

Adenyl cyclate see Adenosine 3',5'-phosphate.

4-Aden-9-yl-2,3-dihydroxybutyric acid see Eritadenine.

5'-Adenylic acid see Adenosine phosphate.

Adenylic acid sparteine salt see Sparteine adenylate.

Adenylpyrophosphoric acid see Adenosine triphosphate.

'Adepril' see Amitriptyline.

'Aderman' see Phenylmercuric borate.

Adermine see Pyridoxine.

'Adermykon' see Chlorphenesin.

ADICILLIN*** (6-(D-5-amino-5-carboxyvaleramido)penicillanic acid; (+)-adicillin; penicillin N; (4-amino-4-carboxybutyl)-penicillin; α-aminoadipic penicillin; cephalosporin N; synnematin B).

(–)-ADICILLIN (6-L-(5-amino-5-carboxyvaleramido)penicillanic acid; isopenicillin N).

'Adigal' see Lanatoside A.

'Adipan' see Amphetamine.

'Adipex' see Methamphetamine.

'Adipex-neu' see Phentermine resin.

ADIPHENINE*** (2-diethylaminoethyl 2,2-diphenylacetate; difacil; spasmolytin; 'patrovina', 'rophene', 'trasentin', 'vagospasmyl').

ADIPIC ACID (1,4-butanedicarboxylic acid; hexanedioic acid).

Adipic acid bis(3-carboxy-2,4,6-triiodoanilide) see Adipiodone.

Adipic acid bis[3-carboxy-2,4,6-triiodo-5-(N-methylcarboxamido)anilide] see Iocarmic acid.

ADIPIODONE*** (N,N'-adipoylbis(3-amino-2,4,6-triiodobenzoic acid); N,N'-adipoyldi-(3-carboxy-2,4,6-triiodoaniline); 3,3'-(adipoyldiimino)bis(2,4,6-triiodobenzoic acid); adipic acid bis(3-carboxy-2,4,6-triiodoanilide); bilignost; iodipamide; 'cavumbren', 'ultrabil').

ADIPIODONE MEGLUMINE (adipiodone methylglucamine; bis(N-methylglucamine) salt of adipiodone; iodipamide methylglucamine; methylglucamine iodipamide; 'cholospect', 'endografin', 'intrabilix', 'radioselectan biliare', 'transbilix').

See also Meglumine diatrizoate with adipiodone meglumine.

Adipiodone methylglucamine see Adipiodone meglumine.

ADIPIODONE SODIUM (adipiodone disodium salt; sodium iodipamide; Be-426; 'biligrafin', 'cholografin').

Adipoylbis(aminotriiodobenzoic acid) see Adipiodone.

3,3'-(Adipoyldiimino)bis(2,4,6-triiodobenzoic acid) see Adipiodone.

5,5'-(Adipoyldiimino)bis(2,4,6-triiodo-N-methylisophthalamic acid) see Iocarmic acid.

'Adiprazine' see Piperazine adipate.

'Adiuretin' see Desmopressin.

ADNAMINE (2,3,7,8-tetrahydroxy-5-(methylaminomethyl)dibenzo(a,e)cycloheptatriene).

'Adobiol' see Bufetolol.

AdOCA see Adamantoylcytarabine.

'Adoisine' see Warfarin-deanol.

'ADONA' see Carbazochrome sodium sulfonate.

'Adopon' see Camylofin.

'Adrenalin' see Epinephrine.

Adrenaline* see Epinephrine.

ADRENALONE** (3',4'-dihydroxy-2-methylaminoacetophenone; adrenone; methylaminoacetopyrocatechol).

ADRENOCHROME (3-hydroxy-1-methyl-5,6-indoledione; AC-17; 'omega').

ADRENOCHROME GUANYLHYDRAZONE (adrenochrome monoguanylhydrazone; 'adchnon').

ADRENOCHROME GUANYLHYDRAZONE MESILATE (adrenochrome guanylhydrazone methanesulfonate; 'S-adchnon').

Adrenochrome semicarbazone see Carbazochrome.

ADRENOLUTIN (3,5,6-trihydroxy-1-

9

methylindole; 5,6-dihydroxy-1-methyl-indoxyl).

'Adrenosem' see Carbazochrome salicylate.
'Adrenoxyl' see Carbazochrome.
'Adrestat' see Carbazochrome salicylate.
Adriamycin see Doxorubicin.
'Adriblastina' see Doxorubicin.
'Adroyd' see Oxymetholone.
ADS-3 see Aminophenazone with bamethan.
'Adsorbon' see Magnesium trisilicate.
'Aducin' see Sodium dibunate.
'Adumbran' see Oxazepam.
'Adurix' see Clopamide.
'Adynol' see Adenosine triphosphate.
AE-705-W see Neutramycin.
Aecachinum see Quinine ethyl carbonate.
'Aerbron' see Proxazole.
'Aerial grammoxone' see Paraquat metil-sulfate.
'Aerogastol' see Diphenylpyraline.
Aeron (tr) see Atropine camphorate with scopolamine camphorate.
'Aeropax' see Dimeticone.
'Aero-ped' see Phenylmercuric nitrate.
'Aerosol OT' see Sodium dioctyl sulfo-succinate.
'Aerosporin' see Polymyxin B.
Aesculetin see Esculetin.
Aesculin see Esculin.
AESCULUS HIPPOCASTANUM EXTRACT (horse chestnut extract; 'venostasin').
AET see (2-Aminoethyl)isothiuronium bromide.
Aetaphen see Oxedrine.
Aeth.... see Eth....
'Aethoxysklerol' see Polidocanol.
Aetian see 5β-Androstane.
Aetio.... see Etio....
AF-2 see Furylfuramide.
AF-634 see Proxazole citrate.
AF-864 see Benzydamine.
AF-983 see Bendazac sodium.
AF-1161 see Trazodone.
'Afadiol' see Aluminium histidinate with magnesium hydroxide.
'Afalon' see Linuron.
'Afenil' see Calcium chloride urea.
'Afodial' see Aluminium histidinate.
'Afos' see Mecarbam.
Afoxanide see Rafoxanide.
'Afragil' see Mobecarb with pibecarb.
'Afrin' see Oxymetazoline.
'Afugan' see Pyrazophos.
AG-3 see Carbocromen.
Agarin see Muscimol.
AGARIC ACID (agaricin; laricic acid; agaricic acid; agaricinic acid; hexadecylcitric acid).
'Agasten' see Clemastine.
'Agedal' see Noxiptiline.
'Agena' see Benzalkonium chloride.
'Agene' see Nitrogen trichloride.
'Agerite alba' see Monobenzone.
Agkistrodon rhodostoma venom see Ancrod.
'Agliral' see Glycyclamide.

'Agluco' see Carbutamide.
'Aglunat' see Lanatoside A.
AGMATINE (1-(4-aminobutyl)guanidine; 4-guanidobutylamine).
AGN-197 see Pifenate.
AGN-616 see Fantridone.
AGN-1414 see Mitotenamine.
'Agofell' see Diisopromine.
'Agofollin' see Estradiol dipropionate.
'Agolene' see Menbutone magnesium.
'Agontan' see Diiodotyrosine.
Agr-1240 see Minaprine.
'Agrisil' see Trichloronat.
AH-2 see Methapyrilene.
AH-3 see 2-(2-Benzylphenoxy)triethylamine.
AH-289 see Chlorcyclizine.
AH-853 see p-Methyldiphenhydramine.
AH-3232 see Dipotassium clorazepate.
AH-3365 see Salbutamol.
AH-3923 see Salmefamol.
AH-5158A see Labetalol.
AH-8165D see Fazadinium bromide.
AHR-85 see Methocarbamol.
AHR-223 see Methoxydone.
AHR-224 see Pyroxamine.
AHR-233 see Mephenoxalone.
AHR-438 see Metaxalone.
AHR-483 see Hexopyrronium bromide.
AHR-504 see Glycopyrronium bromide.
AHR-619 see Doxapram.
AHR-712 see Butaperazine.
AHR-857 see Sulfametoxydiazine.
AHR-965 see Fenfluramine.
AHR-1680 see Fenpipalone.
AHR-2277 see Lenperone.
AHR-3070-C see Metoclopramide.
'Ahypnon' see Bemegride.
AI-306 see Broxyquinoline.
AI-307 see Broxyquinoline with broxaldine.
'Aicamine' see Orazamide.
'Aimax' see Metallibure.
'Airbron' see Acetylcysteine.
'Airol' see Tretinoin.
'Ajatin' see Benzododecinium.
Ajmalicine see Raubasine.
AJMALINE (pseudobrucine; neoajmaline; rauwolfin; 'cardiorhythmine', 'gilurtymal', 'tachmalin').
AJMALINE CHLOROACETATE see Lorajmine.
AK-123 see Flavoxate.
'Akaritox' see Tetradifon.
'Akineton' see Biperiden.
'Akinophyl' see Biperiden.
AKLOMIDE*** (2-chloro-4-nitrobenzamide; 'novastat').
AKLOMIDE WITH SULFANITRAN ('aclan', 'novostat').
Akrichin (tr) see Mepacrine.
'Akrinol' see Acrisorcin.
'Akrinor' see Cafedrine with theodrenaline.
'Aktiferrin' see Iron-serine complex.
Aktinokinol see Actinoquinol.
AL-0361 see Oxyfenamate.
AL-0559 see Fenamole.
AL-842 see Deterenol.
ALACHLOR* (2-chloro-N-(2,6-diethyl-

10

phenyl)-*N*-(methoxyphenyl)acetamide;
N-(2-chloroacetyl)-2,6-diethyl-*N*-(methoxy-methyl)aniline; 'alochlor', 'lasso').
'Alacortril' *see* Fluperolone.
'Aladione' *see* Diftalone.
Ala²⁶-gly²⁷-ser³¹-α¹⁻³⁹-corticotrophin *see* Seractide.
'Alamine' *see* Aluminium glycinate.
'Alanap' *see* Naptalam.
ALANINE (2-aminopropionic acid; α-alanine).
β-ALANINE (3-aminopropionic acid).
ALANOSINE (L(–)-2-amino-3-(*N*-nitroso-hydroxylamino)propionic acid).
Alant camphor *see* Alantolactone.
Alantidanhydride *see* Alantolactone.
Alantin *see* Inulin.
ALANTOLACTONE (alant camphor; alan-tidanhydride; elecamphane; helenin; inula camphor; 'eupatal').
Alant starch *see* Inulin.
Alanylglycylisoleucinylvalylserine *see* Peptide 67-82.
N-(β-Alanyl)-1-methylhistidine *see* Anserine.
N-(β-Alanyl)-2-methylhistidine *see* Ophi-dine.
'Alar' *see* Daminozide.
'Alaxa' *see* Bisacodyl.
ALAZANINE TRICLOFENATE***
(mixture of 1 mol. 3-ethyl-2-[3-(3-ethyl-2-benzothiazolinylidene)propenyl]benzothia-zolium 2,4,5-trichlorophenate and 2 mol. 2,4,5-trichlorophenol).
'Albamycin' *see* Novobiocin.
ALBENDAZOLE** (methyl 5-(propylthio)-benzimidazole-2-carbamate).
'Albicort' *see* Triamcinolone acetonide.
'Albiotic' *see* Lincomycin.
'Albocresil' *see* Methylenedi(*m*-cresol-sulfonic acid) polymer.
ALBOMYCIN (tr) (an antibiotic from *Actino-myces subtropicus*, identical with grisein).
'Albone' *see* Hydrogen peroxide.
'Albothyl' *see* Methylenedi(*m*-cresolsulfonic acid) polymer.
ALBUMIN TANNATE (albutannin; tannal-bumin; 'eldoform', 'entero-norm', 'tannalbin').
Albutannin *see* Albumin tannate.
Albuterol* *see* Salbutamol.
ALBUTOIN*** (3-allyl-5-isobutyl-2-thiohy-dantoin; Bax-422-Z; 'co-ord', 'euprax').
ALCA *see* Alcloxa.
'Alcaine' *see* Proxymetacaine.
Alcanfor *see* Camphor.
Alcapton *see* Homogentisic acid.
Alcaptonic acid *see* Homogentisic acid.
'Alchloquin' *see* Clioquinol.
ALCLOFENAC*** (2-(4-allyloxy-3-chloro-phenyl)acetic acid; 'mervan', 'mirvan', 'neoston', 'prinalgin').
ALCLOXA*** (chlorotetrahydroxy[(2-hydroxy-5-oxo-2-imidazolin-4-yl)ureato]-dialuminium; aluminium chlorohydroxy allantoinate; ALCA; RC-173).
'Alcobon' *see* Fluocytosine.
Alcohol *see* Ethanol.

'Alcopar' *see* Bephenium.
'Alcotine' *see* Aluminium nicotinate.
ALCURONIUM CHLORIDE*** (*N*,*N*′-dial-lylnortoxiferinium dichloride; *N*,*N*′-diallyl-bisnortoxiferine dichloride; alcuronium dichloride; allnortoxiferin; DANT; Ro-4-3816; 'alloferin').
ALD-25 *see* Ethyllysergide.
ALDA *see* Aldioxa.
'Aldactide' *see* Hydroflumethiazide with spironolactone.
'Aldactone' *see* Spironolactone.
Aldadiene *see* Canrenoate potassium.
'Aldarsone' *see* Phenarsone.
'Aldecin' *see* Beclometasone dipropionate.
'Alderlin' *see* Pronetalol.
ALDESULFONE SODIUM*** (4,4′-di-aminodiphenyl sulfone formaldehyde sulf-oxylate sodium salt; sodium sulfonylbis(*p*-phenyleneimino)dimethanesulfinate; sulf-oxone sodium; 'diasone', 'diazon', 'novo-trone').
ALDICARB* (2-methyl-2-(methylthio)-propanal *O*-[(methylamino)carbonyl]-oxime; 2-methyl-2-(methylthio)propion-aldehyde *O*-(methylcarbamoyl)oxime; 'temick', 'temik').
'Aldinamide' *see* Pyrazinamide.
ALDIOXA*** (dihydroxy[(2-hydroxy-5-oxo-2-imidazolin-4-yl)ureato]aluminium; aluminium dihydroxy allantoinate; ALDA; RC-172).
'Aldocorten' *see* Aldosterone.
ALDOL (β-hydroxybutyraldehyde; acetaldol).
'Aldomet' *see* Methyldopa.
'Aldomet ester' *see* Methyldopate.
'Aldometil' *see* Methyldopa.
'Aldoril' *see* Methyldopa with hydrochloro-thiazide.
ALDOSTERONE*** (11β,21-dihydroxy-3,20-dioxo-4-pregnen-18-al; 17α-pregn-4-en-18-al-11β,21-diol-3,20-dione; 18-formyl-4-pregnene-11β,21-diol-3,20-dione; 11β,21-dihydroxypregn-4-ene-3,18,20-trione; elec-trocortin; 18-oxocorticosterone; 'aldocor-ten').
'Aldozone' *see* Butizide with spironolactone.
ALDRIN (1,2,3,4,10,10-hexachloro-1,4,4a,5, 8,8a-hexahydro-1,4:5,8-dimethanonaph-thalene *endo-exo* form; HHDN; 'octalene', 'seedrin').
Aldrin *endo-endo* **isomer** *see* Isodrin.
'Aldrisone' *see* Endrisone.
'Alentin' *see* Carbutamide.
'Alergosan' *see* Chloropyramine.
'Alertol' *see* Pipradrol.
Aletamine* *see* Alfetamine.
ALETHEINE (β-alanylmercaptamine; β-alanylcysteamine; dipeptide of β-alanine and 2-mercaptoethylamine).
'Aleudrine' *see* Isoprenaline.
'Aleukon' *see* Chlornaphazine.
'Alevaire' *see* Tyloxapol.
'Alexan' *see* Cytarabine.
ALEXIDINE*** (1,1′-hexamethylenebis[5-(2-ethylhexyl)biguanide]; WIN-21904).
ALFADOLONE*** (3α,21-dihydroxy-5α-

11

pregnane-11,20-dione; 5α-pregnane-3α-diol-11,20-dione; alphadolone; GR-2/1574).

ALFADOLONE ACETATE (21-acetoxy-3α-hydroxy-5α-pregnane-11,20-dione).

ALFADOLONE ACETATE WITH ALFAXALONE (CT-1341; 'alfatesin', 'althesin').

'Alfadryl' *see* Moxastin.

'Alfasol' *see* Algestone acetonide.

Alfasone *see* Algestone.

Alfasone acetophenide *see* Algestone acetofenide.

'Alfatesin' *see* Alfadolone acetate with alfaxalone.

ALFAXALONE* (3α-hydroxy-5α-pregnane-11,20-dione; 5α-pregnan-3α-ol-11,20-dione; alphaxalone; GR-2/234).
See also Alfadolone acetate with alfaxalone.

'Alfenamin' *see* Aluminium flufenamate.

'Alferin' *see* Warfarin.

Alfetadrin* *see* Alfetamine.

ALFETAMINE (α-allylphenethylamine; aletamine; alfetadrin; NDR-5061A).

'Alflorone' *see* Fludrocortisone acetate.

'Alfuran' *see* Nitrofurantoin.

'Algaphan' *see* Dextropropoxyphene.

ALGELDRATE (hydrated aluminium hydroxide; colloidal aluminium hydroxide; hydracoll; W-4600).
See also Dimeticone with algeldrate; Glycalox; Sucralox.

ALGELDRATE WITH CALCIUM CARBONATE ('solugastril').

'Algeril' *see* Propiram fumarate.

'Algesal suractive' *see* Myrtecaine.

ALGESTONE* (16α,17-dihydroxypregn-4-ene-3,20-dione; 16,17-dihydroxyprogesterone; alfasone; alphasone).

ALGESTONE ACETOFENIDE (algestone cyclic acetal with acetophenone; algestone acetophenide; alfasone acetophenide; DPA; SQ-15010; 'deloxadrate', 'neo-alfasol').

ALGESTONE ACETOFENIDE WITH ESTRADIOL ENANTATE ('deladroxate').

ALGESTONE ACETONIDE* (16α,17α-isopropylidenedioxypregn-4-ene-3,20-dione; algestone cyclic acetal with acetone; alfasone acetonide; W-3395; 'alfasol').

'Algin' *see* Sodium alginate.

Alginates *see* Calcium alginate; Sodium alginate.

ALGINIC ACID (norgine; 'kelacid').

'Alglyn' *see* Aluminium glycinate.

'Alhydex' *see* Glutaral.

ALIBENDOL* (5-allyl-N-(2-hydroxyethyl)-3-methoxysalicylamide).

'Alicap' *see* Chlorbufam plus pyrazon.

'Alidine' *see* Anileridine.

'Alimax' *see* Metallibure.

ALIMEMAZINE* (10-(3-dimethylamino-2-methylpropyl)phenothiazine; methylpromazine; trimeprazine; RP-6549; 'valledrine', 'vanectyl', 'variagil').

ALIMEMAZINE TARTRATE ('nedeltran', 'panectyl', 'repeltin', 'temaril', 'temaryl', 'teralen', 'theralene', 'vallergan').

Alimemazine S,S-dioxide *see* Oxomemazine.

'Alinamin' *see* Prosultiame.

ALIPAMIDE* (4-chloro-3-sulfamoylbenzoic acid 2,2-dimethylhydrazide; CI-546; D-1721).

'Alipur' *see* Chlorbufam plus cycluron.

Alisobumal* *see* Butalbital.

'Alival' *see* Nomifensin.

'Alivin' *see* Penethamate.

ALIZARIN (1,2-dihydroxyanthraquinone).

Alizarin yellow *see* Gallacetophenone.

'Alkacitron' *see* Disodium hydrogen citrate.

'Alkalovert' *see* Phytic acid.

'Alkam' *see* Aluminium glycinate.

ALKAVERVIR* (standardized preparation of *Veratrum viride* alkaloids; 'veriloid').

'Alkeran' *see* Melphalan.

'Alkron' *see* Parathion.

Alkylbenzyldimethylammonium chlorides *see* Benzalkonium.

Alkyldimethyl(3,4-dichlorobenzyl)ammonium chlorides *see* Aralkonium.

Allacyl (tr) *see* Aminometradine.

ALLANTOIN (5-ureidohydantoin; glyoxyldiureide; 'alphosyl', 'cordiamin').

'Allardorm' *see* Butethal.

Allatsil (tr) *see* Aminometradine.

'Allegron' *see* Nortriptyline.

ALLENOIC ACID (6-hydroxy-2-naphthalenepropionic acid).

'Allercur' *see* Clemizole.

Allergan-211 *see* Idoxuridine.

'Allergisan' *see* Chlorpheniramine maleate.

'Allergosil' *see* Ethane-1,2-disulfonic acid.

ALLETHRIN* (3-allyl-2-methyl-4-oxo-2-cyclopenten-1-yl chrysanthemate; 2-methyl-4-oxo-3-(2-propenyl)-2-cyclopenten-1-yl 2,2-dimethyl-3-(2-methyl-1-propenyl)-cyclopropanecarboxylate; allyl cinerin; pallethrine; 'presyn').
See also Bioallethrin.

ALLETORPHINE* (N-allyl-7,8-dihydro-7α-(1(R)-hydroxy-1-methylbutyl-O⁶-methyl-6,14-*endo*-ethenonormorphine; 17-allyl-17-demethyl-7α-((R)-1-hydroxy-1-methylbutyl)-6,14-*endo*-ethenotetrahydro-oripavine; N-allylnoretorphine; R & S 218-M).

ALLIDOCHLOR* (2-chloro-N,N-dipropenyl-acetamide; N,N-diallyl-2-chloroacetamide; N-(2-chloroacetyl)diallylamine; CDAA; 'randox').

ALLICIN (allyl allylthiosulphinate ester).

ALLIN (S-allyl-L-cysteine sulfoxide).

'Allional' *see* Allopyrine.

'Allisan' *see* Dicloran.

Allisat (tr) *see* Allium sativum.

ALLITHIAMINE (N-[2-(allyldithio)-4-hydroxy-1-methyl-1-butenyl]-N-(4-amino-2-methylpyrimidin-5-ylmethyl)formamide thiamine allyl disulfide).

ALLIUM SATIVUM (garlic; allisat).

Allnortoxiferin *see* Alcuronium.

ALLOBARBITAL* (5,5-diallylbarbituric acid; allobarbitone; diallylbarbital; diallymal).
See also Aminophenazone with allobarbital.

Allobarbitone* *see* Allobarbital.

ALLOCLAMIDE*** (2-allyloxy-4-chloro-*N*-(2-diethylaminoethyl)benzamide; CE-264; 'hexacol').

ALLOCUPREIDE SODIUM*** (*m*-[1-(3-allyl-*S*-cupropseudothioureido)]benzoic acid Na salt; *S*-copper deriv. of *m*-[[(allylimino)-mercaptomethyl]amino]benzoic acid Na salt; 3-(allylcuprothioureido)benzoic acid Na salt; cuproallylthiourea-*m*-benzoic acid Na salt; cupradyl; cupralylnatrium; cupralylsodium; cuprothiosinamine *m*-benzoate sodium; 'cupralene', 'cuprelon', 'cuprion', 'ebesal').

'Alloferine' *see* Alcuronium chloride.

ALLOIMPERATORIN (9-hydroxy-4-(3-methyl-2-butenyl)-7H-furo(3,2-g)(1)benzopyran-7-one).

Allomaleic acid *see* Fumaric acid.

ALLOMETHADIONE*** (3-allyl-5-methyl-2,4-oxazolidinedione; aloxidone; 'allydione', 'malazol', 'malidone'.)

'Allonal' *see* Allopyrine.

Allophanamide *see* Biuret.

ALLOPHANIC ACID (carbamoylcarbamic acid).

Allopregnane *see* 5α-Pregnane.

Allopropylbarbital* *see* Aprobarbital.

'Allopur' *see* Allopurinol.

ALLOPURINOL** (1H-pyrazolo(3,4-d)pyrimidin-4-ol; 4-hydroxypyrazolo(3,4-d)pyrimidine; BW-56-185; HPP; NSC-1390; 'allopur', 'allural', 'apurin', 'bleminol', 'cellidrin', 'epidropal', 'foligan', 'gichtex', 'milurit', 'urosin', 'zyloprim', 'zyloric').

ALLOPYRINE (aprobarbital derivative of amidopyrine; 'allional', 'allonal', 'alphadorm', 'barbadon', 'barprine', 'icobudon', 'sedipral').

Allorphine *see* Nalorphine.

ALLOXAN (2,4,5,6(1H,3H)-pyrimidinetetrone; mesoxalylurea; ENT-7169).

ALLOXANTIN (alloxanylalloxan; 5,5'-dihydroxy-5,5'-bibarbituric acid; 5,5'-dihydroxyhydurilic acid; uroxin).

Alloxazine mononucleotide *see* Flavin mononucleotide.

'Alltox' *see* Camphechlor.

'Allydione' *see* Allomethadione.

Allylacetic acid *see* 4-Pentenoic acid.

ALLYL ALCOHOL (2-propen-1-ol).

ALLYLAMINE (2-propenylamine).

1-Allyl-6-amino-3-ethyluracil *see* Aminometradine.

2-(Allylamino)-4-thiazolecarboxylic acid 3-(5-nitro-2-furyl)allylidene)hydrazide *see* Nifuralide.

1-(2-Allylamino-1,3-thiazol-4-yl)-6-(5-nitro-2-furyl)-1-oxo-2,3-diaza-3,5-hexadiene *see* Nifuralide.

m-[1-(3-Allyl-*S*-auropseudothioureido)]-benzoic acid *see* Sodium auroallylthioureidobenzoate.

Allylbarbital* *see* Butalbital.

Allylbarbituric acid* *see* Butalbital.

5-Allyl-5-(2-bromoallyl)barbituric acid *see* Brallobarbital.

5-ALLYL-5-BUTYLBARBITURIC ACID

('idobutal').

Allylcatechol methylene ether *see* Safrole.

N[1]**-Allyl-4-chloro-6-(3-hydroxy-2-butenylideneamino)-1,3-benzenedisulfonamide** *see* Ambuside.

Allyl cinerin *see* Allethrin.

m-[1-(3-Allyl-*S*-cupropseudothioureido)]-benzoic acid *see* Allocupreide sodium.

5-Allyl-5-cyclohexen-1-yl-2-thiobarbituric acid *see* Thialbarbital.

5-Allyl-5-cyclopenten-1-ylbarbituric acid *see* Cyclopentobarbital.

17-Allyl-17-demethyl-7α-((R)-1-hydroxy-1-methylbutyl)-6,14-*endo*-ethenotetrahydrooripavine *see* Alletorphine.

Allyldiethylacetamide *see* 2,2-Diethyl-4-pentenoic amide.

N-**Allyl-7,8-dihydro-7α-(1(R)-hydroxy-1-methylbutyl)-O**[6]**-methyl-6,14-*endo*-ethenonormorphine** *see* Alletorphine.

5-Allyl-5-(2,2-dimethylpropyl)barbituric acid *see* Nealbarbital.

17-Allyl-4,5α-epoxy-3,14-dihydroxymorphinan-6-one *see* Naloxone.

ALLYLESTRENOL*** (17α-allyl-4-estren-17β-ol; 3-desoxy-19-nortestosterone; allyloestrenol; 'gestanin', 'gestanon').

ALLYLESTRENOL TARTRATE ('turinal').

5-Allyl-3-ethylbarbituric acid *see* Ethallymal.

ALLYLGLYCINE (2-amino-4-pentenoic acid).

5-Allyl-*N*-(2-hydroxyethyl)-3-methoxysalicylamide *see* Alibendol.

1-Allyl-2-(2-hydroxy-3-isopropylaminopropoxy)benzene *see* Alprenolol.

N-**Allyl-3-hydroxymorphinan** *see* Levallorphan.

N-**Allyl-14-hydroxynordihydromorphinone** *see* Naloxone.

5-Allyl-5-(2-hydroxypropyl)barbituric acid *see* Proxibarbal.

Allyliminomercaptomethylbenzoic acid *S*-copper derivative *see* Allocupreide.

Allyliminomercaptomethylbenzoic acid *S*-gold derivative *see* Sodium auroallylthioureidobenzoate.

5-Allyl-5-isoamyl-2-thiobarbituric acid *see* Thiamylal.

5-Allyl-5-isobutylbarbituric acid *see* Butalbital.

5-Allyl-5-isobutyl-2-thiobarbituric acid *see* Buthalital.

5-Allyl-5-isobutyl-2-thiohydantoin *see* Albutoin.

5-Allyl-5-isopropylbarbituric acid *see* Aprobarbital.

5-Allyl-5-isopropyl-1-methylbarbituric acid *see* Enallylpropymal.

ALLYL ISOTHIOCYANATE (mustard oil).

Allylmercaptomethylpenicillin *see* Almecillin.

1-Allyl-3-methoxy-4,5-methylenedioxybenzene *see* Myristicin.

2-(4-ALLYL-2-METHOXYPHENOXY)-*N,N*-DIETHYLACETAMIDE (4-allyl-2-methoxyphenoxyacetic acid diethylamide;

13

G-29505; 'detrovel', 'estil', 'eunal').

5-Allyl-5-(1-methylbutyl)barbituric acid
see Secobarbital.

5-Allyl-5-(1-methylbutyl)-2-thiobarbituric acid *see* Thiamylal.

4-Allyl-1,4-methylenedioxybenzene *see*
Safrole.

5-Allyl-1-methyl-5-(1-methyl-2-pentenyl)-barbituric acid *see* Methohexital.

3-Allyl-5-methyl-2,4-oxazolidinedione *see*
Allomethadione.

3-Allyl-2-methyl-4-oxo-2-cyclopenten-1-yl chrysanthemate *see* Allethrin.

3-Allyl-1-methyl-4-phenyl-4-propionoxy-piperidine *see* Allylprodine.

5-Allyl-5-(1-methylpropyl)barbituric acid
see Talbutal.

5-Allyl-5-(2-methylpropyl)barbituric acid
see Butalbital.

5-Allyl-5-(2-methylpropyl)-2-thiobar-bituric acid *see* Buthalital.

α-Allyl-N-methyl-3,4,5-trimethoxyphen-ethylamine *see* Trimoxamine.

5-Allyl-5-neopentylbarbituric acid *see*
Nealbarbital.

N-Allylnoratropine *see* Naltropine.

N-Allylnoretorphine *see* Alletorphine.

N-Allylnormorphine *see* Nalorphine.

N-Allylnoroxymorphone *see* Naloxone.

Allyloestrenol* *see* Allylestrenol.

2-(Allyloxyamino)-7-chloro-5-(o-chloro-phenyl)-3H-1,4-benzodiazepine *see*
Uldazepam.

2-Allyloxy-4-chloro-N-(2-diethylamino-ethyl)benzamide *see* Alloclamide.

2-(4-Allyloxy-3-chlorophenyl)acetic acid
see Alclofenac.

2-Allyloxy-N-(2-diethylaminoethyl)-4-trifluoromethylbenzamide *see*
Flualamide.

2-Allyloxy-N-(2-diethylaminoethyl)-α,α,α-trifluoro-p-toluamide *see* Flualamide.

3-(o-Allyloxyphenoxy)-2-hydroxy-N-iso-propyl-1-propylamine *see* Oxprenolol.

1-(o-Allyloxyphenoxy)-3-isopropylamino-propan-2-ol *see* Oxprenolol.

2-ALLYL-4-PENTENOIC ACID (diallyl-acetic acid).
See also Bismuth 2-allyl-4-pentenoate.

α-Allylphenethylamine *see* Alfetamine.

1-(o-Allylphenoxy)-3-isopropylamino-propan-2-ol *see* Alprenolol.

5-ALLYL-5-PHENYLBARBITURIC ACID
('alphasem', 'alpheba', 'alphenal', 'alphe-nate', 'lubergal', 'phenyral', 'prophenal').

2-ALLYL-2-PHENYL-4-PENTENOIC ACID (2-phenyl-2-prop-2-enyl-4-pentenoic acid; phenyldiallylacetic acid).

2-(4-Allylpiperazin-1-yl)-4-amino-6,7-dimethoxyquinazoline *see* Quinazosin.

ALLYLPRODINE* (3-allyl-1-methyl-4-phenyl-4-propionoxypiperidine; Ro-2-7113).

Allylpyrocatechol methylene ether *see*
Safrole.

2-Allylsulfamoyl-5-chloro-4-sulfamoyl-N-(3-hydroxy-2-butenylidene)aniline
see Ambuside.

12-Allyl-7,7a,8,9-tetrahydro-3,7a-dihydr-oxy(4aH)-8,9c-iminoethanophenanthro-(4,5-bcd)furan-5(6H)-one *see* Naloxone.

6-[2-(Allylthio)acetamido]penicillanic acid *see* Almecillin.

3-Allylthiomethyl-6-chloro-3,4-dihydro-2-methyl-7-sulfamoyl-(2H)1,2,4-benzo-thiadiazine 1,1-dioxide *see* Methalthiazide.

3-Allylthiomethyl-6-chloro-3,4-dihydro-7-sulfamoyl-(2H)1,2,4-benzothiadiazine 1,1-dioxide *see* Altizide.

Allylthiomethylpenicillin *see* Almecillin.

Allylthiosulfinic acid allyl ester *see* Allicin.

1-Allyl-2-thiourea *see* Thiosinamine.

1-Allyl-2,4,5-trimethoxybenzene *see*
Eusarone.

α-Allyl-3,4,5-trimethoxy-N-methylphen-ethylamine *see* Trimoxamine.

Allypropymal* *see* Aprobarbital.

ALMADRATE SULFATE** (aluminium magnesium hydroxide oxide sulfate hydrate; dimagnesium tetraaluminium hydroxide oxide sulfate hydrate; W-4425).

ALMECILLIN** (6-[2-(allylthio)acetamido]-penicillanic acid; allylthiomethylpenicillin; allylmercaptomethylpenicillin; penicillin O).

'Almederm' *see* Hexachlorophene.

ALMESTRONE** (3-hydroxy-7α-methyl-estra-1,3,5(10)-trien-17-one; 7α-methyl-estra-1,3,5(10)-trien-3-ol-17-one).

'Alminate' *see* Aluminium glycinate.

'Almora' *see* Magnesium gluconate.

'Alochlor' *see* Alachlor.

'Alodan' *see* Chlorbicyclen *and* Pethidine.

ALOE-EMODIN (1,8-dihydroxy-3-hydroxy-methylanthraquinone; 3-hydroxymethyl-dianthone; 3-hydroxymethylchrysazin; rhabarberone).

'Alofen' *see* Promazine.

ALOGLUTAMOL (tris(hydroxymethyl)-aminomethane gluconate dihydroxy aluminate; trometamol gluconate alumin-ate; 'tasto').

ALONIMID** (2,3-dihydrospiro(naphthal-ene-1(4H),3'-piperidine)-2',4,6'-trione).

'Alotec' *see* Orciprenaline.

'Aloxidone' *see* Allomethadione.

ALOXIPRIN** (polymeric condensation product of aluminium oxide and acetylsali-cylic acid; 'palaprin', 'paloxin').

'Aloxyn' *see* 8-Quinolinol.

'Alpen' *see* Pheneticillin.

ALPERTINE** (ethyl 5,6-dimethoxy-3-[2-(4-phenylpiperazin-1-yl)ethyl]indole-2-carboxylate; 1-[2-[2-(ethoxycarbonyl)-5,6-dimethoxyindol-3-yl]ethyl]-4-phenyl-piperazine).

Alpha amylase* *see* α-Amylase.

ALPHACETYLMETHADOL** (α-3-acet-oxy-6-dimethylamino-4,4-diphenylhept-ane).
See also Acetylmethadol.

Alphadolone* *see* Alfadolone.

'Alphadorm' *see* Allopyrine.

'Alphadrol' *see* Fluprednisolone.

'Alphadryl' *see* Moxastin.

Alphahypophamine *see* Oxytocin.

14

ALPHAMEPRODINE*** (α-3-ethyl-1-methyl-4-phenyl-4-propionoxypiperidine).

ALPHAMETHADOL*** (α-6-dimethyl-amino-4,4-diphenyl-3-heptanol).
See also Dimepheptanol.

Alpha methyl dopa *see* Methyldopa.

'Alphamucase' *see* Chymotrypsin with chondroitinase.

ALPHAPRODINE*** (α-1,3-dimethyl-4-phenyl-4-propionoxypiperidine; anadol; Nu-1196; 'nisentil', 'prisilidene').

'Alphaquil' *see* 1-Phenylpropyl carbamate.

'Alpharesidol' *see* Hydroxocobalamin.

'Alphasem' *see* 5-Allyl-5-phenylbarbituric acid.

'Alphasol MA' *see* Sodium dihexyl sulfosuccinate.

'Alphasol OT' *see* Sodium dioctyl sulfosuccinate.

Alphasone *see* Algestone.

'Alphatron' *see* Radon.

'Alphazurine 2G' *see* Patent blue.

'Alpheba' *see* 5-Allyl-5-phenylbarbituric acid.

'Alphenal' *see* 5-Allyl-5-phenylbarbituric acid.

'Alphenate' *see* 5-Allyl-5-phenylbarbituric acid.

'Alphintren' *see* Chymotrypsin.

Alphol *see* 1-Naphthyl salicylate.

'Alphosyl' *see* Allantoin.

'Alphozone' *see* Succinyl peroxide.

ALPRAZOLAM** (8-chloro-1-methyl-6-phenyl-4H-s-triazolo(4,3-a)(1,4)benzo-diazepine; U-31889).

ALPRENOLOL*** (1-(o-allylphenoxy)-3-isopropylaminopropan-2-ol; 1-allyl-2-(2-hydroxy-3-isopropylaminopropoxy)-benzene; alprenolol hydrochloride; H-56/28; 'apliobal', 'aptine', 'gubernal').

ALRESTATIN** (sodium 1,3-dioxo-1H-benz-(de)isoquinoline-2(3H)-acetate).

ALSEROXYLON* (fractionally purified extract of *Rauwolfia serpentina*; 'abten', 'koglucoid', 'rautensin', 'rauwiloid').

'Altafur' *see* Furaltadone.

'Altan' *see* Dantron.

'Altest' *see* Sulfosalicylic acid.

'Althesin' *see* Alfadolone acetate with alfaxalone.

Althiazide* *see* Altizide.

ALTIZIDE*** (3-allylthiomethyl-6-chloro-3,4-dihydro(2H)-1,2,4-benzothiadiazine-7-sulfonamide 1,1-dioxide; althiazide; P-1779).

'Altodel' *see* Kinoprene.

'Altodor' *see* Etamsylate.

'Altorick' *see* Triprene.

'Altosid' *see* Methoprene.

'Alubasine' *see* Aluminium glycinate.

Alufibrate *see* Aluminium clofibrate.

'Alugan' *see* Bromociclen.

'Aluglycin' *see* Aluminium glycinate.

ALUMINIUM ACETATE (Al subacetate; basic Al acetate; Essigsaure tonerde; 'essitol', 'eston', 'lenicet', 'subeston').

Aluminium aminoacetate *see* Aluminium glycinate.

Aluminium chlorohydroxy allantoinate *see* Alcloxa.

ALUMINIUM CLOFIBRATE** (bis[2-(p-chlorophenoxy)-2-methylpropionato]-hydroxyaluminium; alufibrate).

Aluminium dextran sulfate complex *see* Detralfate.

Aluminium dihydroxyallantoinate *see* Aldioxa.

ALUMINIUM FLUFENAMATE (aluminium (α,α,α-trifluoro-m-tolyl)anthranilate; 'alfenamin').

ALUMINIUM GLYCINATE (basic Al aminoacetate; dihydroxy aluminium amino-acetate; 'ada', 'alamine', 'alglyn', 'alkam', 'alminate', 'alubasine', 'aluglycine', 'alzi-nox', 'aspogen', 'dimothyn', 'doraxamin', 'elcosal', 'robalate', 'tabnet', 'ulpepsan').

ALUMINIUM HISTIDINATE (aluminium L-histidinate; 'afodial').

ALUMINIUM HISTIDINATE WITH MAGNESIUM HYDROXIDE (K-3717; 'afadiol').

Aluminium hydroxide *see also* Aceglutamide hydroxide complex.

Aluminium hydroxide, colloidal *see* Algeldrate.

Aluminium hydroxide-glycerol complex polymer *see* Glycalox.

Aluminium hydroxide-sucrose complex polymer *see* Sucralox.

ALUMINIUM MAGNESIUM GLYCINATE (hydroxyaluminium magnesium amino-acetate; HAMA; 'glycamine-AM').

ALUMINIUM MAGNESIUM HYDROXIDE (magnesium aluminium hydroxide; 'maalox').
See also Acetylsalicylic acid with aluminium magnesium hydroxide.

Aluminium magnesium hydroxide carbonate hydrate *see* Hydrotalcite.

Aluminium magnesium hydroxide oxide sulfate *see* Almadrate sulfate.

ALUMINIUM MAGNESIUM SODIUM SILICATE ('acinormal', 'veegum').

ALUMINIUM 2-NAPHTHOLDISULFO-NATE (aluminol; 'alumnol').

ALUMINIUM NICOTINATE ('alcotine').

ALUMINIUM OXYCHLORIDE ('hidrofugal').

ALUMINIUM PHOSPHATE ('aluphos', 'phosphalgel').

ALUMINIUM PHOSPHIDE ('delicia').

ALUMINIUM PHOSPHIDE WITH AM-MONIUM CARBAMATE ('phostoxin').

ALUMINIUM PHOSPHOSULFATE ('col-Al').

ALUMINIUM SALICYLATE (Al subsalicyl-ate; basic Al salicylate; 'alunozal', 'basal-Noury', 'salumin').

Aluminium sodium phosphate (basic) *see* Kasal.

ALUMINIUM SODIUM SILICATE ('acisorban', 'alusil', 'enelbin', 'kaylene', 'ludozan', 'neutralon').

Aluminium sucrose hydrogen sulfate basic salt *see* Sucralfate.

ALUMINIUM SULFANILATE ('sulfalumin').

Aluminium (α,α,α-**trifluoro-m-tolyl**)-**anthranilate** see Aluminium flufenamate.

Aluminol see Aluminium naphtholdisulfonate.

'Alumnol' see Aluminium naphtholdisulfonate.

'Alunozal' see Aluminium salicylate.

'Alupent' see Orciprenaline.

'Aluphos' see Aluminium phosphate.

'Alurene' see Chlorothiazide.

'Alusil' see Aluminium sodium silicate.

ALVERINE** (N,N-bis(3-phenylpropyl)-ethylamine; N-ethyl-3,3'-diphenyldipropyl-amine; dipropyline; gamatran; phenprop-amine).

ALVERINE CITRATE* ('fugipaverin', 'phenopropyl', 'profenil', 'sestron', 'spaco-lin', 'spasmacol', 'spasmaverine', 'supavan').

'Alvinine' see Xenysalate.

'Alvit-55' see Dieldrin.

'Alvodine' see Piminodine esilate.

'Alvonal' see Strophanthin.

'Alvothane' see Hexachloroethane.

'Alvyl' see Polyvinyl alcohol.

'Alypin' see Amydricaine.

'Alzinox' see Aluminium glycinate.

AM-109 see Methitural.

AM-684-beta see Relomycin.

'Amabevan' see Carbarsone.

'Amadil' see Paracetamol.

AMADINONE* (6-chloro-17-hydroxy-19-norpregna-4,6-diene-3,20-dione; 6-chloro-19-norpregna-4,6-diene-17-ol-3,20-dione).

'Amandacide' see Calcium mandelate.

AMANOZINE* (2-amino-4-anilino-s-tri-azine; N-phenylformoguanamine; amano-zine hydrochloride; W-1191-2; 'urofort').

AMANTADINE** (1-adamantanamine; 1-adamantylamine; amantadine hydro-chloride; 1-aminoadamantane; EXP-105-1; 'amantan', 'mantadan', 'mantadix', 'matadan', 'symmetrel', 'viregyt', 'virofral').

'Amantan' see Amantadine.

AMANTOCILLIN* (6-(3-amino-1-adamantanecarboxamido)penicillanic acid; 3-aminoadamant-1-yl-penicillin).

AMARANTH* (Bordeaux S; chiefly the tri-Na salt of 2-hydroxy-1-(4-sulphonaphth-1-ylazo)naphthalene-3,6-disulfonic acid).

AMARINE (2,4,5-triphenyl-2-imidazoline).

Ambathizon* see Thiacetazone.

AMBAZONE* (1,4-benzoquinone amidino-hydrazine thiosemicarbazone hydrate; ben-zoquinone guanylhydrazone thiosemicarba-zone; 'iversal').

Ambegon* see Ambenonium chloride.

'Amben' see p-Aminobenzoic acid.

AMBENONIUM CHLORIDE* (bis(2-chlorobenzylchloride) of N,N'-bis(2-di-ethylaminoethyl)oxamide; [oxalylbis(imino-ethylene)]bis[(o-chlorobenzyl)diethylam-monium chloride]; ambestigmin; ambegon; WIN-8077; 'mysuran', 'mytelase').

AMBENOXAN* (2-[[2-(2-methoxy-ethoxy)ethyl]aminomethyl]-1,4-benzo-dioxan; N-[2-(2-methoxyethoxy)ethyl]-1,4-benzodioxan-2-methylamine).

Ambestigmin* see Ambenonium chloride.

'Ambilhar' see Niridazole.

'Amblosin' see Ampicillin.

'Amboclorin' see Chlorambucil.

'Ambodryl' see Bromazine.

AMBOMYCIN** (antibiotic from Str. ambo-faciens; diazomycin C; duazomycin C; NSC-10270).

'Ambravein' see Pipacycline.

AMBROXOL* (trans-4-[(2-amino-3,5-dibromobenzyl)amino]cyclohexanol; 2-amino-3,5-dibromo-N-(trans-4-hydroxy-cyclohexyl)benzylamine; 3,5-dibromo-Nα-(trans-4-hydroxycyclohexyl)toluene-α,2-diamine; trans-N-(2-amino-3,5-dibromo-benzyl)-4-hydroxycyclohexylamine; NA-872).

AMBUCAINE* (2-diethylaminoethyl ester of 4-amino-2-butoxybenzoic acid; benoxin-ate; WIN-3706; 'dorsacaine', 'sympocaine').

AMBUCETAMIDE* (2-dibutylamino-2-(p-methoxyphenyl)acetamide; 2-dibutyl-amino-4'-methoxyacetanilide; dibutamide; A-16; 'meritin').

Ambuphylline* see Bufylline.

AMBUSIDE* (N¹-allyl-4-chloro-6-(3-hydr-oxy-2-butenylideneamino)-1,3-benzene-disulfonamide; 5-allylsulfamoyl-2-chloro-4-(3-hydroxybut-2-enylideneamino)-benzenesulfonamide; 2-allylsulfamoyl-5-chloro-4-sulfamoyl-N-(3-hydroxy-2-butenylidene)aniline; EX-4810; 'hydrion', 'novohydrin').

AMBUTONIUM BROMIDE* ((3-carba-moyl-3,3-diphenylpropyl)ethyldimethyl-ammonium bromide; R-100).

'Ambylan' see Apramycin.

AMCA see Tranexamic acid.

AMCHA see Tranexamic acid.

'Amchafibrin' see Tranexamic acid.

AMCINAFAL* (triamcinolone cyclic 6,17-acetal with 3-pentanone).

AMCINAFIDE* (triamcinolone cyclic 6,17-acetal with acetophenone).

AMCINONIDE* (9-fluoro-11β,16α,17,21-tetrahydroxypregna-1,4-diene-3,20-dione 16,17-cyclic cyclopentanone acetal 21-acetate; (11β,16α)-21-acetoxy-16,17-[cyclopentylidenebis(oxy)]-9-fluoro-11-hydroxypregna-1,4-diene-3,20-dione; triamcinolone cyclic 16,17-acetal with cyclopentanone, 21-acetate).

'Amdelate' see Ammonium mandelate.

'Amebacilin' see Fumagillin.

'Amebacillin' see Fumagillin.

'Amebarsin' see Difetarsone.

'Amebil' see Clioquinol.

'Amecytine' see Mitomycin.

AMEDALIN* (3-methyl-3-(3-methylamino-propyl)-1-phenyl-2-indolinone; UK-3540).

'Amenyl' see Chlormadinone acetate with ethinylestradiol.

'Americaine' see Benzocaine.

'Amertan' see Thiomersal tannate.

Ametazole* see Betazole.

AMETHOBENZEPINE (11-(2-dimethyl-

16

aminoethoxy)-6,11-dihydrodibenz(b,e)-
thiepine fumarate).
Amethocaine* *see* Tetracaine.
'Amethone' *see* Amolanone.
'Amethopterin' *see* Methotrexate.
'Ametox' *see* Sodium thiosulfate.
AMETRYN* (2-ethylamino-4-isopropyl-
amino-6-(methylthio)-*s*-triazine; *N*-ethyl-
N'-(1-methylethyl)-6-(methylthio)-1,3,5-
triazine-2,4-diamine; 'gesapax').
'Ametycin' *see* Mitomycin.
AMFEBUTAMONE** ((±)-2-*tert*-butyl-
amino-3'-chloropropiophenone).
AMFECLORAL*** (α-methyl-*N*-(2,2,2-
trichloroethylidene)phenethylamine;
1-phenyl-2-(2,2,2-trichloroethylidene-
amino)propane; amphechloral; 'acutran').
AMFEPENTOREX*** (*N*,α-dimethyl-*p*-
pentylphenethylamine; *N*-methyl-*p*-pentyl-
amphetamine; CB-2201; 'proligne').
AMFEPRAMONE** (2-diethylaminopropio-
phenone; α-diethylaminopropiophenone;
1-benzoyltriethylamine; diethylpropion;
diethylpropion hydrochloride; T-712;
'apisate', 'derfon', 'diepropon', 'dobesin',
'effilon', 'frekentine', 'natorexic', 'obesitex',
'regenon', 'tenuate', 'tepanil', 'tylinal').
Amfetyline *see* Fenetylline.
'Amfipen' *see* Ampicillin.
'Amfodyne' *see* Imidecyl iodine.
AMFOMYCIN** (antibiotic from *Str. canus*;
amphomycin; 'ecomytrin').
AMFONELIC ACID*** (7-benzyl-1-ethyl-
1,4-dihydro-4-oxo-1,8-naphthyridine-3-
carboxylic acid; WIN-25978).
'Amiben' *see* Chloramben.
'Amicar' *see* Aminocaproic acid.
AMICARBALIDE*** (3,3'-diamidino-
carbanilide; 1,3-bis(*m*-amidinophenyl)urea).
AMICARBALIDE ISETIONATE (amicarbalide di(ethanol-2-sulfonate); amicarbalide diisethionate; 'diampron').
AMICIBONE*** (benzyl 1-(2-hexahydro-
1H-azepin-1-ylethyl)-2-oxocyclohexanecarb-
oxylate).
AMICLORAL* (6-*O*-(2,2,2-trichloro-1-
hydroxyethyl)-α-D-glucopyranose 1→4
polymer with α-D-glucopyranose;
SK&F-39186).
AMICYCLINE*** (9-amino-4-dimethyl-
amino-1,4,4a,5,5a,6,11,12a-octahydro-
3,10,12,12a-tetrahydroxy-1,11-dioxonaph-
thacene-2-carboxamide).
AMIDAPSONE*** ((*p*-sulfanilylphenyl)-
urea; *p*-amino-*p*-ureidodiphenyl sulfone;
N-carbamoyldapsone).
'Amidazophen' *see* Aminophenazone.
Amidazotoluene *see* Aminoazotoluene.
Amide PP *see* Nicotinamide.
AMIDEFRINE MESILATE*** (3'-(1-hydr-
oxy-2-methylaminoethyl)methanesul-
fonanilide methanesulfonate; amidephrine
mesylate; MJ-5190; 'fentrinol').
Amidephrine mesylate *see* Amidefrine
mesilate.
N-(**4-(Amidinoamidino)piperazin-1-yl-
methyl)tetracycline** *see* Guamecycline.

9-(*p*-Amidinobenzylidene)fluorene *see*
Renytoline.
**1-Amidino-3-(3-chloro-4-cyanophenyl)-
urea** *see* Cloguanamile.
***N*-Amidino-3,5-diamino-6-chloropyrazin-
amide** *see* Amiloride.
***N*-Amidino-3,5-diamino-6-chloropyraz-
inecarboxamide** *see* Amiloride.
***N''*-(2-Amidinoethyl)-4-formamido-
1,1',1''-trimethyl-*N*,4':*N'*,4''-ter(pyrrole-
2-carboxamide)** *see* Stallimycin.
***N*-Amidinoglycine** *see* Glycocyamine.
1-Amidino-3-(*p*-nitrophenyl)urea *see*
Nitroguanil.
*N*⁵**-Amidinoornithine** *see* Arginine.
Amidinopenicillin HX *see* Mecillinam.
**8-[3-(*m*-Amidinophenyl)-2-triazeno]-3-
amino-5-ethyl-6-phenylphenanthridin-
ium chloride** *see* Isometamidium chloride.
***N*-Amidinoputrescine** *see* Agmatine.
*N*¹**-Amidinosulfanilamide** *see* Sulfaguanid-
ine.
2-Amidino-1,2,3,4-tetrahydroisoquinoline
see Debrisoquine.
AMIDITHION* (*s*-[2-[(2-methoxyethyl)-
amino]-1-oxoethyl]*O*,*O*-dimethyl phos-
phorodithioate; 'thiocron').
Amidofebrin *see* Aminophenazone.
Amidofen (tr) *see* Aminophenazone.
'Amidofos' *see* Dimethoate.
'Amidol' *see* Diaminophenol.
Amidoline *see* Etomidoline.
Amidone* *see* Methadone.
Amidophen (tr) *see* Aminophenazone.
Amidopyrazoline *see* Aminophenazone.
Amidopyrine *see* Aminophenazone.
Amidotrizoate *see* Sodium diatrizoate.
Amidotrizoic acid *see* Diatrizoic acid.
'Amidozol' *see* Sulfasomizole.
Amidozone *see* Aminophenazone.
AMIFLOVERINE*** (2-(3,5-diethoxyphen-
oxy)triethylamine; 5-(2-diethylamino-
ethoxy)-1,3-diethoxybenzene).
AMIKACIN** (*O*-3-amino-3-deoxy-α-D-
glucopyranosyl(1→4)-*O*-[6-amino-6-
deoxy-α-D-glucopyranosyl(1→6)]-*N*³-
(4-amino-L-2-hydroxybutyryl)-2-deoxy-L-
streptamine; (2*S*)-4-amino-*N*-[(1*R*,2*S*,3*S*,
4*R*,5*S*)-5-amino-2-(3-amino-3-deoxy-α-D-
glucopyranosyloxy)-4-(6-amino-6-deoxy-
α-D-glucopyranosyloxy)-3-hydroxycyclo-
hexyl]-2-hydroxybutyramide; amikacin
sulfate; BBK-8; 'amikin', 'biklin').
'Amikapron' *see* Tranexamic acid.
AMIKHELLIN (9-diethylaminoethoxy-4-
hydroxy-7-methyl-5H-furo(3,2-g)(1)benzo-
pyran-5-one; 8-diethylaminoethoxy-5-
hydroxy-2-methylfurano-6,7-chromone;
F-19; 'nokhel').
'Amikin' *see* Amikacin.
AMILOMER** (product of reaction of
starch with epichlorohydrin).
AMILORIDE*** (*N*-amidino-3,5-diamino-6-
chloropyrazinecarboxamide; 2,6-diamino-
3-carboguanidino-5-chloropyrazine;
amipramizide; desmethylpipazuroylguanidine; amipramidine; guanamprazine;

DCP; MK-870; 'colectril', 'midamor', 'modamide').
AMILORIDE WITH HYDROCHLORO-THIAZIDE ('moduretic').
'Amilyt' *see* Benzoquinonium.
'Amimethyline' *see* Protriptyline.
'Amimycin' *see* Oleandomycin.
Aminacrin* *see* Aminoacridine.
'Aminacyl-B-PAS' *see* Calcium benzamido-salicylate.
Aminarsone *see* Carbarsone.
Aminarsonic acid *see* Arsanilic acid.
Aminazin (tr) *see* Chlorpromazine.
'Amindan' *see* Sulfanilamide sulfosalicylate.
AMINDOCATE** (2-dimethylaminoethyl 1-(2-dimethylaminoethyl)-2,3-dimethyl-indole-5-carboxylate; deanol ester with 1-(2-dimethylaminoethyl)-2,3-dimethyl-indole-5-carboxylic acid).
Amine oxidase *see* Monoamine oxidase.
Aminic acid *see* Formic acid.
AMINITROZOLE*** (2-acetamido-5-nitro-thiazole; acinitrazole; acinitrozole; 'enhep-tin-A', 'pleocide', 'trichocid', 'trichorad', 'trichoral', 'tritheon').
Aminoacetic acid*** *see* Glycine.
N-(2-Aminoacetyl)-β-hydroxy-2,5-dimethoxyphenethylamine *see* Mido-drine.
N-(Aminoacetyl)-p-phenetidine *see* Phenocoll.
Aminoacrichine *see* Aminoacriquine.
AMINOACRIDINE*** (9-aminoacridine; 5-aminoacridine; aminacrin; monacrine; 'acramidine', 'acramine', 'acriflex', 'acrisan', 'cimlac', 'minocrin', 'trichojel').
Aminoacridine 4-hexylresorcinolate *see* Acrisorcin.
AMINOACRIQUINE (tr) (2-amino-3-chloro-9-(4-diethylamino-1-methylbutylamino)-7-methoxyacridine; aminoacrichine).
1-Aminoadamantane *see* Amantadine.
6-(3-Amino-1-adamantanecarboxamido)-penicillanic acid *see* Amantocillin.
3-Aminoadamantyl-1-penicillin *see* Amantocillin.
α-Aminoadipic penicillin *see* Adicillin.
α-Aminoadipic cephalosporin *see* Cephalosporin C.
2-Amino-4-(2-amino-2-carboxyethylthio)-butyric acid *see* Cystathionine.
4-O-[3α-Amino-6α-[(4-amino-4-deoxy-α-D-glucopyranosyl)oxy]-2,3,4,4aβ,6,7,8,8aα-octahydro-8β-hydroxy-7β-(methylamino)pyrano(3,2-b)pyran-2α-yl]-2-deoxy-D-streptamine *see* Apramycin.
5-Amino-6-(7-amino-5,8-dihydro-6-meth-oxy-5,8-dioxoquinolin-2-yl)-4-(2-hydr-oxy-3,4-dimethoxyphenyl)-3-methyl-picolinic acid *see* Streptonigrin.
5-Amino-6-(7-amino-5,8-dihydro-6-methoxy-5,8-dioxo-2-quinolyl)-4-(2-hydroxy-3,4-dimethoxyphenyl)-3-methylpicolinic acid *see* Rufocromo-mycin.
3-Amino-8-[(2-amino-6-methylpyrimidin-4-yl)amino]-6-(p-aminophenyl)-5-

methylphenanthridinium bromide 1′-methobromide *see* Pyritidium bromide.
8-Amino-6-(p-aminophenyl)-5-methyl-phenanthridinium chloride *see* Phenidium chloride.
AMINOANFOL (4-amino-4-desoxypteroyl-aspartic acid).
Aminoanthracene *see* Anthramine.
4-AMINOANTIPYRINE (4-amino-2,3-dimethyl-1-phenyl-3-pyrazolin-5-one; 4-aminophenazone; 'ampyrone').
4-Amino-1-arabinofuranosyl-1,2-dihydro-2-pyrimidinone *see* Cytarabine.
2-Amino-4-arsenosophenol *see* Oxophenar-sine.
p-AMINOAZOBENZENE (p-phenylazo-aniline).
AMINOAZOTOLUENE (4-amino-2′,3-dimethylazobenzene; 4-(o-tolylazo)-o-toluidine; 2-amino-5-azotoluene; amid-azotoluene; non-staining scarlet).
5-Aminobarbituric acid *see* Uramil.
'Aminobenz' *see* Orthocaine.
p-Aminobenzenearsonic acid *see* Arsanilic acid.
p-Aminobenzenephosphonic acid *see* Phosphanilic acid.
p-AMINOBENZENESTIBONIC ACID ('pentastib').
p-Aminobenzenestibonic acid salts *see* Ethylstibamine; Stibamine.
p-Aminobenzenesulfocyanamide *see* Sulcymide.
m-Aminobenzenesulfonamide *see* Metanil-amide.
o-Aminobenzenesulfonamide *see* Orthanil-amide.
p-Aminobenzenesulfonamide *see* Sulfanil-amide.
p-Aminobenzenesulfonoxymethylamide-N-D-glucoside sodium sulfite *see* Glucosulfamide.
o-Aminobenzoic acid *see* Anthranilic acid.
p-AMINOBENZOIC ACID (PAB; PABA; pabacidum; vitamin B_x; vitamin H).
p-Aminobenzoic acid esters *see* Amoxecaine; Benzocaine; Butamin; Butethamine; Buto-caine; Butylcaine; Dimethocaine; Isobutyl-caine; Leucinocaine; Naepaine; Procaine; Propylcaine; Risocaine.
m-Aminobenzoic acid ethyl ester *see* Ethyl m-aminobenzoate.
p-Aminobenzoic acid salts *see* Potassium p-aminobenzoate; Sodium p-aminobenzoate.
2-Amino-6-benzyl-3-ethoxycarbonyl-4,5,6,7-tetrahydrothieno(2,3-c)pyridine *see* Tinoridine.
α-Aminobenzylpenicillin *see* Ampicillin.
p-Aminobenzylpenicillin *see* Penicillin T.
4-Amino-N-(1-benzylpiperid-4-yl)-5-chloro-o-anisamide *see* Clebopride.
2-Amino-6-benzyl-4,5,6,7-tetrahydro-thieno(2,3-c)pyridine-3-carboxylic acid ethyl ester *see* Tinoridine.
Aminobiphenyl *see* Biphenylamine.
5-Amino-1-(bisdimethylaminophosphor-yl)-3-phenyl-1,2,4-triazole *see* Triamiphos.

5-Amino-1,3-bis(2-ethylhexyl)-5-methyl-hexahydropyrimidine see Hexetidine.

4-Amino-5-bromo-*N*-(2-diethylamino-ethyl)-*o*-anisamide see Bromopride.

4-Amino-5-bromo-*N*-(2-diethylamino-ethyl)-2-methoxybenzamide see Bromopride.

5-Amino-4-bromo-2-phenylpyridazin-3(2H)-one see Brompyrazon.

3-Amino-4-butoxybenzoic acid 2-(2-di-ethylaminoethoxy)ethyl ester see Betoxycaine.

3-Amino-2-butoxybenzoic acid diethyl-aminoethyl ester see Metabutoxycaine.

4-Amino-2-butoxybenzoic acid diethyl-aminoethyl ester see Ambucaine.

4-Amino-3-butoxybenzoic acid diethyl-aminoethyl ester see Oxybuprocaine.

***p*-Amino-α-(*sec*-butylaminomethyl)benzyl alcohol** see Amiterol.

4-Amino-α-(*tert*-butylaminomethyl)-3,5-dichlorobenzyl alcohol see Clenbuterol.

4-Amino-6-*tert*-butyl-3-(methylthio)-*as*-triazin-5(4H)-one see Metribuzin.

3-(2-Aminobutyl)indole see Etryptamine.

5-Amino-*N*-butyl-2-prop-2-ynyloxy-benzamide see Parsalamide.

4-AMINO-*N*-BUTYL-1,2,5-SELENADI-AZOLE-3-CARBOXAMIDE (NSC-86047).

4-AMINOBUTYRIC ACID (γ-aminobutyric acid; GABA).

4-Aminobutyric acid lactam see 2-Pyrroli-dinone.

***N*-(4-Aminobutyryl)histidine** see Homo-carnosine.

***N*-(4-Aminobutyryl)-1-methylhistidine** see Homoanserine.

AMINOCAPROIC ACID* (6-amino-hexanoic acid; ε-aminocaproic acid; epsilon-aminocaproic acid; EACA; CL-10304; CY-116; JD-177; 'acepramin', 'amicar', 'capramol', 'caproamin', 'caprocid', 'capro-lest', 'eaca', 'ekaprol', 'epsicapron', 'hemo-caprol', 'ipsilon', 'kaprolsin').

α-Aminocaproic acid see Norleucine.

Aminocaproic lactam see Caprolactam.

AMINOCARB* (4-dimethylamino-*m*-tolyl methylcarbamate; 4-dimethylamino-3-methylphenyl methylcarbamate; arprocarb; 'matacil').

6-Amino-8-carbamoyloxymethyl-1,1a,2,8,8a,8b-hexahydro-8a-methoxy-1,5-dimethylazirino(2',3':3,4)pyrrolo(1,2-a)indole-4,7-dione see Porfiromycin.

4-Amino-4-carboxybutylpenicillin see Adicillin.

2-(2-Amino-2-carboxyethyl)-*N*,*N*-bis(2-chloroethyl)-4-nitrophenethylamine see Nitrocaphane.

2-(2-Amino-2-carboxyethyl)-*N*,*N*-bis(2-chloroethyl)phenethylamine see Ocaphane.

2[2-(2-Amino-4-carboxyethyl)-2'-nitro-phenyl]-2',2''-dichlorotriethylamine see Nitrocaphane.

2-[2-(2-Amino-2-carboxyethyl)phenyl]-2',2''-dichlorotriethylamine see Ocaphane.

N²-((+)-5-Amino-5-carboxypentylamino-methyl)tetracycline see Lymecycline.

3-Amino-*N*-(α-carboxyphenethyl)succin-amic acid *N*-methyl ester see Aspartame.

7-(5-Amino-5-carboxyvaleramido)-cephalosporanic acid see Cephalosporin C.

6-D-(5-Amino-5-carboxyvaleramido)-penicillanic acid see Adicillin.

6-L-(5-Amino-5-carboxyvaleramido)-penicillanic acid see (−)-Adicillin.

Aminochinuride see Aminoquinuride.

3-Amino-4-chlorobenzoic acid 2-dimethyl-aminoethyl ester see Clormecaine.

2-Amino-5-chlorobenzoxazole see Zoxazol-amine.

4-Amino-5-chloro-*N*-(2-diethylamino-ethyl)-*o*-anisamide see Metoclopramide.

4-Amino-5-chloro-*N*-(2-diethylamino-ethyl)-2-methoxybenzamide see Metoclopramide.

2-Amino-3-chloro-9-(4-diethylamino-1-methylbutylamino)-7-methoxyacrid-ine see Aminoacriquine.

6-Amino-2-(2-chloroethyl)-2,3-dihydro-1,3-benzoxazin-4-one see Aminochlorthen-oxazine.

4-(4-Amino-5-chloro-2-methoxy-benzamido)-1-benzylpiperidine see Clebopride.

4-Amino-3-(*p*-chlorophenyl)butyric acid see Baclofen.

2-Amino-5-(*p*-chlorophenyl)-2-oxazoline see Clominorex.

5-Amino-4-chloro-2-phenylpyridazin-3(2H)-one see Pyrazon.

AMINOCHLORTHENOXAZINE (6-amino-2-(2-chloroethyl)-2,3-dihydro-1,3-benzox-azin-4-one; A-350; ICI-350).
See also Aminophenazone with amino-chlorthenoxazine.

7-[2-Amino-2-(1,4-cyclohexadien-1-yl)-acetamido]-3-methyl-2-cephem-2-carboxylic acid see Cefradine.

6-(2-Amino-2-(1,4-cyclohexadien-1-yl)-acetamido)penicillanic acid see Epicillin.

6-(1-Aminocyclohexanecarboxamido)-penicillanic acid see Ciclacillin.

2-Amino-*N*-cyclohexyl-3,5-dibromo-*N*-methylbenzylamine see Bromhexine.

(1-Aminocyclohexyl)penicillin see Ciclacillin.

1-Aminocyclopentanecarboxylic acid see Cycloleucine.

'Aminodal' see Sodium theophyllin-7-yl-acetate.

1-Amino-1-deoxy-D-glucitol see Glucamine.

2-Amino-2-deoxy-β-D-glucopyranose see Glucosamine.

O-3-Amino-3-deoxy-α-D-glucopyranosyl-(1→4)-O-[6-amino-6-deoxy-α-D-gluco-pyranosyl-(1→6)] N³-(4-amino-L-2-hydroxybutyryl)-2-deoxy-L-streptamine see Amikacin.

O-6-Amino-6-deoxy-α-D-glucopyranosyl-(1→4)-O-[3-deoxy-4-C-methyl-3-(methylamino)-β-L-arabinopyranosyl-

(1→6)]-2-deoxy-D-**streptamine** *see* Betamicin.

L-*O*-(3-**Amino-3-deoxy-α-D-glucopyranosyl**)-(1→4)-*O*-[2,6-diamino-2,6-dideoxy-α-D-glucopyranosyl-(1→6)]-2-deoxy-streptamine *see* Bekanamycin.

O-3-**Amino-3-deoxy-α-D-glucopyranosyl**-(1→4)-*O*-[2,6-diamino-2,3,4,6-tetra-deoxy-α-D-*erythro*-**hexopyranosyl**-(1→6)]-2-deoxy-L-**streptamine** *see* Dibekacin.

O-3-**Amino-3-deoxy-α-D-glucopyranosyl**-(1→4)-*O*-[2,6-diamino-2,3,6-trideoxy-α-D-*ribo*-**hexopyranosyl**-(1→6)]-2-deoxy-streptamine *see* Tobramycin.

2-**Amino-2-deoxy-D-glucose** *see* Glucosamine.

2′-**Amino-2′-deoxykanamycin** *see* Kanendomycin.

9-(3-**Amino-3-deoxy-β-D-ribofuranosyl**)-6-**dimethylaminopurine** *see* Puromycin mononucleoside.

trans-[(2-**Amino-3,5-dibromobenzyl**)-**amino**]**cyclohexanol** *see* Ambroxol.

N-(2-**Amino-3,5-dibromobenzyl**)-*N*-**cyclohexylmethylamine** *see* Bromhexine.

trans-*N*-(2-**Amino-3,5-dibromobenzyl**)-4-**hydroxycyclohexylamine** *see* Ambroxol.

N-(2-**Amino-3,5-dibromobenzyl**)-*N*-**methylcyclohexylamine** *see* Bromhexine.

2-**Amino-3,5-dibromo-*N*-cyclohexyl-*N*-methylbenzylamine** *see* Bromhexine.

2-**Amino-3,5-dibromo-*N*-(*trans*-4-hydroxycyclohexyl)benzylamine** *see* Ambroxol.

3-**Amino-2,5-dichlorobenzoic acid** *see* Chloramben.

1-(4-**Amino-3,5-dichlorophenyl**)-2-*tert*-**butylaminoethanol** *see* Clenbuterol.

O-2-**Amino-2,3-dideoxy-α-D-ribohexopyranosyl**-(1→4)-*O*-[*O*-α-D-**mannopyranosyl**-(1→4)-*O*-2,6-diamino-2,6-dideoxy-β-L-**idopyranosyl**-(1→3)-β-D-**ribofuranosyl**-(1→5)]-2-deoxy-D-**streptamine** *see* Lividomycin.

o-**Amino-*N*-(2-diethylaminoethyl)benzamide** *see* Orthoprocainamide.

2-**Amino-4′-diethylaminoethyl-*o*-benzotoluidide** *see* Atolide.

6-**Amino-1,2-dihydro-1-hydroxy-2-imino-4-piperid-1-ylpyrimidine** *see* Minoxidil.

α-**Amino-2,5-dihydro-5-methyl-2-furanacetic acid** *see* Furanomycin.

2-**Amino-3′,4′-dihydroxyacetophenone** *see* Noradrenalone.

2-**Amino-3-(3,4-dihydroxyphenyl)-2-methylpropionic acid** *see* Methyldopa.

2-**Amino-6-(dihydroxypropyl)-4-hydroxypteridine** *see* Biopteridin.

2-**Amino-3-(3,5-diiodo-4-hydroxyphenyl)-propionic acid** *see* Diiodotyrosine.

3-(3-**Amino-4,6-diiodophenyl)-β-alanine** *see* Betazine.

4-**Amino-6,7-dimethoxy-2-[4-(2-furoyl)-piperazin-1-yl]quinazoline** *see* Prazosin.

2-**Amino-*N*-(2,5-dimethoxy-β-hydroxyphenethyl)acetamide** *see* Midodrine.

2-**Amino-1-(2,5-dimethoxy-4-methyl-phenyl)propane** *see* 2,5-Dimethoxy-4-methylamphetamine.

1-(4-**Amino-6,7-dimethoxyquinazolin-2-yl**)-4-(2-furoyl)**piperazine** *see* Prazosin.

4-**Amino-6,7-dimethoxyquinoline** *see* Amiquinsin.

4-**Amino-6-(1,1-dimethylethyl)-3-(methylthio)-1,2,4-triazin-5(4H)-one** *see* Metribuzin.

2-**Amino-7,7-dimethyl-6-hydroxypurine** *see* Herbipolin.

4-**Amino-2,3-dimethyl-1-phenyl-3-pyrazolin-5-one** *see* 4-Aminoantipyrine.

Aminodiphenyl *see* Biphenylamine.

α-**Aminodiphenylethane** *see* Stilbylamine.

3-**Amino-1,1-dithien-2-ylbut-1-ene** *see* Thiambutene.

4-**Amino-1-dodecylquinaldinium acetate** *see* Laurolinium.

2-**Aminoethaneselenol** *see* Selenomercaptamine.

2-**Aminoethanesulfinic acid** *see* Hypotaurine.

2-**Aminoethanesulfonic acid** *see* Taurine.

Aminoethanol nitrate *see* Itramin.

α-(1-**Aminoethyl**)-*m*-**hydroxybenzyl alcohol** *see* Metaraminol.

3-(2-**Aminoethyl**)-5-**hydroxy-1-(*p*-methoxybenzyl)-2-methylindole** *see* Hydroxindasol.

2-(2-**Aminoethyl**)**imidazole** *see* 2-Imidazoleethylamine.

4-(2-**Aminoethyl**)**imidazole** *see* Histamine.

3-(2-**Aminoethyl**)**indole** *see* Tryptamine.

3-(2-**Aminoethyl**)**indol-5-yl methyl ketone** *see* Acetryptine.

S-(2-**AMINOETHYL)ISOTHIURONIUM BROMIDE HYDROBROMIDE** (2-(2-aminoethyl)-2-thiopseudourea-HBr; AET; ethylisothiuronium bromide; ethiron; ethyrone; etiron; NSC-22877; 'antiradon', 'surrectan').

3-(2-**Aminoethyl**)-1-(*p*-methoxybenzyl)-2-**methylindol-5-ol** *see* Hydroxindasol.

2-**Aminoethyl nitrate** *see* Itramin.

p-(2-**Aminoethyl**)**phenol** *see* Tyramine.

α-(1-**Aminoethyl**)**protocatechuyl alcohol** *see* Corbadrine.

3-(2-**Aminoethyl**)**pyrazole** *see* Betazole.

4-(2-**Aminoethyl**)**pyrocatechol** *see* Dopamine.

2-**Aminoethyl sodium thiophosphate** *see* Cystafos.

2-(2-**Aminoethyl**)-4-(**ethylthio**)**butyric acid** *see* Ethionine.

2-(2-**Aminoethyl**)-2-**thiopseudourea hydrobromide** *see* *S*-(2-Aminoethyl)isothiuronium bromide.

2-**Amino-6-[(*p*-fluorobenzyl)amino]-3-pyridinecarbamic acid ethyl ester** *see* Flupirtine.

4-**Amino-5-fluoro-1,2-dihydropyrimidin-2-one** *see* Flucytosine.

Aminoform *see* Methenamine.

Aminoformaldehyde *see* Methenamine.

Aminoformamidine *see* Guanidine.

6-**Amino-9-(L-1,2-furopyranosenyl)purine**

see Angustmycin A.

Aminoglutaramic acids *see* Glutamine; Isoglutamine.

2-Aminoglutaric acid *see* Glutamic acid.

AMINOGLUTETHIMIDE*** (2-(*p*-aminophenyl)-2-ethylglutarimide; 'elipten', 'eliptin').

Aminoglyoxylic acid *see* Oxamic acid.

AMINOGUANIDINE (guanylhydrazine).

2-Amino-5-guanidovaleric acid *see* Arginine.

2-Aminoheptane *see* Tuaminoheptane.

6-Amino-1,1a,2,8,8a,8b-hexahydro-8-hydroxymethyl-8a-methoxy-1,5-dimethylazirino(2′,3′:3,4)pyrrolo(1,2-a)-indole-4,7-dione *see* Porfiromycin.

6-Amino-1,1a,2,8,8a,8b-hexahydro-8-hydroxymethyl-8a-methoxy-5-methylazirino(2′,3′:3,4)pyrrolo(1,2-a)indole-4,7-dione carbamate *see* Mitomycin.

2-Aminohexanoic acid *see* Norleucine.

6-Aminohexanoic acid *see* Aminocaproic acid.

α-(1-Aminohexyl)benzhydrol *see* Hexapradol.

***p*-Aminohippurate** *see* Sodium *p*-aminohippurate.

2-Aminohydracrylic acid *see* Serine.

α-Aminohydrocinnamic acid *see* Phenylalanine.

3-Amino-4-hydroxybenzenearsonic acid *N*-methanal sulfoxylate *see* Phenarsone sulfoxylate.

4-Amino-3-hydroxybenzoic acid methyl ester *see* Orthocaine.

α-Amino-*p*-hydroxybenzyl penicillin *see* Amoxicillin.

2-Amino-3-hydroxybutyric acid *see* Threonine.

2-Amino-4-hydroxybutyric acid *see* Homoserine.

3-AMINO-4-HYDROXYBUTYRIC ACID (β-amino-γ-hydroxybutyric acid; GOBAB).

4-AMINO-3-HYDROXYBUTYRIC ACID (γ-amino-β-hydroxybutyric acid; 3-hydroxyGABA; GABOB; 'gamibetol', 'ganibetal').

Aminohydroxycaproic acid *see* Hexahomoserine.

5-Amino-4-(2-hydroxy-3,4-dimethoxyphenyl)-6-(5-hydroxy-4-methoxy-2,2-dimethyl-2H-imidazo(4,5-h)quinolin-8-yl)-3-methylpicolinic acid *see* Isopropylideneazastreptonigrin.

2-Amino-4-hydroxy-3,3-dimethylbutyric acid *see* Pantonine.

α-Amino-*p*-hydroxyhydrocinnamic acid *see* Tyrosine.

1-[4-Amino-2-hydroxy-4-(hydroxyimino)-butoxy]naphthalene *see* Nadoxolol.

α-Amino-3-hydroxy-5-isoxazoleacetic acid *see* Ibotenic acid.

4-Amino-5-hydroxymethyl-2-methylpyrimidine *see* Toxopyrimidine.

2-Amino-2-hydroxymethyl-1,3-propanediol *see* Trometamol.

6-Amino-1-hydroxyoctahydroindolizine

acetate *see* Slaframine.

2-Amino-3-(3-hydroxy-4-oxopyrid-1-yl)-propionic acid *see* Leucenol.

(6*R*,7*R*)-7-(*R*)-2-Amino-2-[*p*-hydroxyphenyl)acetamido]-3-methyl-2-cephem-2-carboxylic acid *see* Cefadroxil.

7-[2-Amino-2-(*p*-hydroxyphenyl)-acetamido]-3-[[(5-methyl-1,3,4-thiadiazol-2-yl)thio]methyl]-2-cephem-2-carboxylic acid *see* Cefaparole.

6-[D(−)-2-Amino-2-(*p*-hydroxyphenyl)-acetamido]penicillanic acid *see* Amoxicillin.

7-(2-Amino-2-(*p*-hydroxyphenylacetamido)-3-[*v*-triazol-4-ylthio)methyl]-2-cephem-2-carboxylic acid *see* Cefatrizine.

[6*R*-[6α,7β(*R*)]]-7-[[Amino-(4-hydroxyphenyl)acetyl]amino]-3-methyl-2-cephem-2-carboxylic acid *see* Cefadroxil.

***m*-Amino-*p*-hydroxyphenylarsenoxide** *see* Oxophenarsine.

1-Amino-1-(3-hydroxyphenyl)ethanol *see* Norfenefrine.

2-Amino-3-hydroxypropionic acid *see* Serine.

3-Amino-2-hydroxypropionic acid *see* Isoserine.

3-AMINO-2-HYDROXYPROPYL *p*-BUTYLAMINOBENZOATE ('tussicain').

***p*-[(2-Amino-4-hydroxy-6-pteridylmethyl)-amino]benzoic acid** *see* Pteroic acid.

2-Amino-6-hydroxypurine *see* Guanine.

6-Amino-2-hydroxypurine *see* Isoguanine.

α-Amino-(3-hydroxy-4-pyridinone)-propionic acid *see* Leucenol.

2-Amino-3-hydroxy-2′-(2,3,4-trihydroxybenzyl)propionohydrazide *see* Benserazide.

2-Amino-4-hydroxy-6-trihydroxypropylpteridine *see* Neopterin.

2-Aminohypoxanthine *see* Guanine.

5-AMINO-4-IMIDAZOLECARBOXAMIDE *N*-CARBAMOYL ASPARTATE (5-amino-4-imidazolecarboxamide ureidosuccinate; 'carbaica').

5-Aminoimidazole-4-carboxamide orotate *see* Orazamide.

2-Amino-3-imidazolylpropionic acid *see* Histidine.

7-Amino-3-imino(3H)phenothiazine *see* Thionine.

2-Amino-3-indolepropionic acid *see* Tryptophan.

α-Aminoisocaproic acid *see* Leucine.

Aminoisometradine *see* Amisometradine.

β-Aminoisopropylbenzene *see* Phentermine.

4-Amino-3-isoxazolidinedione *see* Cycloserine.

3-Aminolactic acid *see* Isoserine.

2-Amino-4-mercaptobutyric acid *see* Homocysteine.

2-Amino-3-mercaptopropionic acid *see* Cysteine.

2-Amino-6-mercaptopurine *see* Tioguanine.

2-Amino-4-methoxybutyric acid *see* Methoxinine.

3-Amino-*N*-(α-methoxycarbonyl-

phenethyl)succinamic acid *see* Aspartame.

3'-(L-α-Amino-*p*-methoxyhydrocinnama-mido)-3'-deoxy-*N*,*N*-dimethyladenosine *see* Puromycin.

4-Amino-2-methoxy-5-pyrimidine-methanol *see* Bacimethrin.

9-Amino-4-methylacridine *see* Methyl-aminacrin.

***p*-Aminomethylbenzenesulfonamide** *see* Mafenide.

1-(3-Amino-4-methylbenzenesulfonyl)-3-cyclohexylurea *see* Metahexamide.

***p*-AMINOMETHYLBENZOIC ACID** (α-amino-*p*-toluic acid; PAMBA; 'gumbix', 'styptopur').

α-Aminomethylbenzyl alcohol *see* Phenyl-ethanolamine.

3'-Amino-4'-methylcaprophenone *O*-(2-aminoethyl)oxime *see* Caproxamine.

β-Aminomethyl-*p*-chlorohydrocinnamic acid *see* Baclofen.

4-Aminomethylcyclohexanecarboxylic acid *see* Tranexamic acid.

α-Amino-β-(2-methylenecyclopropane)-propionic acid *see* Hypoglycin A.

3-Aminomethyl-7-fluoro-1-phenyl-isochroman *see* Fenisorex.

2-Amino-6-methylheptane *see* Octodrine.

6-Amino-2-methyl-2-heptanol *see* Hept-aminol.

3'-Amino-4'-methylhexanophenone *O*-(2-aminoethyl)oxime *see* Caproxamine.

α-Aminomethyl-*m*-hydroxybenzyl alcohol *see* Norfenefrine.

α-Aminomethyl-*p*-hydroxybenzyl alcohol *see* Octopamine.

α-Aminomethyl-4-hydroxy-3-methoxy-benzyl alcohol *see* Normetanephrine.

4-Aminomethyl-5-hydroxy-6-methyl-3-pyridinemethanol *see* Pyridoxamine.

5-Aminomethyl-3-isoxazolol *see* Muscimol.

6-Amino-3-methyl-1-(2-methylallyl)-uracil *see* Amisometradine.

8β-Aminomethyl-6-methyl-10a-ergoline *see* Dihydrolysergamine.

2-Amino-6-(1-methyl-4-nitroimidazol-5-ylthio)purine *see* Tiamiprine.

2-Amino-4-methyl-1-pentanol *see* Leucinol.

***p*-Amino-*N*-(1-methyl-2-phenylethyl)-phenylacetamide** *see* Fepracet.

3-Amino-4-methylphenyl pentyl ketone *O*-(2-aminoethyl)oxime *see* Caproxamine.

4-Aminomethyl-6-methyl-2-phenyl-3-pyridazin-one *see* Metamfazone.

***p*-Amino-α-[(1-methylpropyl)amino-methyl]benzyl alcohol** *see* Amiterol.

(2-Amino-2-methylpropyl)benzene *see* Phentermine.

3-(Aminomethyl)pyridine *see* Picolamine.

***N*-(2-Amino-6-methylpyrid-3-ylmethyl)-3,4,5-trimethoxybenzamide** *see* Trimetamide.

4-Amino-2-methyl-5-pyrimidineme-thanol *see* Toxopyrimidine.

***N*-(4-Amino-2-methylpyrimidin-5-ylmethyl)-*N*-[(2-(allyldithio)-4-**

hydroxy-1-methyl-1-butenyl]-formamide *see* Allithiamine.

3-(4-Amino-2-methylpyrimidin-5-yl-methyl)-5-(2-chloroethyl)-4-methyl-thiazolium chloride *see* Beclotiamine.

4-*N*-(4-Amino-2-methylpyrimidin-5-yl-methyl)formamido-3-(benzoylthio)-pent-3-enyl benzoate *see* Bentiamine.

4-*N*-(4-Amino-2-methylpyrimidin-5-yl-methyl)formamido-3-(benzoylthio)-pent-3-enyl phosphate *see* Benfotiamine.

8-[[2-[*N*-(4-Amino-2-methylpyrimidin-5-ylmethyl)formamido]-1-(2-hydroxy-ethyl)propenyl]dithio]-6-mercapto-octanoic acid methyl ester acetate *see* Octotiamine.

1-(4-Amino-2-methylpyrimidin-5-yl-methyl)-3-(2-hydroxyethyl)-2-methyl-pyridinium bromide *see* Pyrithiamine.

***N*-(4-Amino-2-methylpyrimidin-5-yl-methyl)-*N*-(4-hydroxy-2-mercapto-1-methyl-1-butenyl)formamide *S*-ben-zoate *O*-phosphate** *see* Benfotiamine.

***N*-(4-Amino-2-methylpyrimidin-5-yl-methyl)-*N*-(4-hydroxy-2-mercapto-1-methyl-1-butenyl)formamide *O*,*S*-di-benzoate** *see* Bentiamine.

***N*-(4-Amino-2-methylpyrimidin-5-yl-methyl)-*N*-(4-hydroxy-2-mercapto-1-methyl-1-butenyl)formamide ethyl carbonate *S*-ester with ethyl thiocar-bonate** *see* Cetotiamine.

***N*-(4-Amino-2-methylpyrimidin-5-yl-methyl)-*N*-(4-hydroxy-2-mercapto-1-methyl-1-butenyl)formamide *O*-gly-colate acetate *S*-ester with thio-2-furoic acid** *see* Acefurtiamine.

***N*-(4-Amino-2-methylpyrimidin-5-yl-methyl)-*N*-[4-hydroxy-1-methyl-2-(propyldithio)-1-butenyl]formamide** *see* Prosultiamine.

***N*-(4-Amino-2-methylpyrimidin-5-yl-methyl)-*N*-[4-hydroxy-1-methyl-2-(tetrahydrofurfuryldithio)-1-butenyl]-formamide** *see* Fursultiamine.

***N*-(4-Amino-2-methylpyrimidin-5-yl-methyl)-*N*-[1-(2-oxo-1,3-oxathian-4-ylidene)ethyl]formamide** *see* Cycoti-amine.

2-Amino-4-(methylselenyl)butyric acid *see* Selenomethionine.

2-Amino-4-(methylsulfinyl)butyric acid *see* Methionine sulfoxide.

5-Aminomethyl-2,3,7,8-tetrahydroxy-dibenzo(a,e)cycloheptatriene *see* Noradnamine.

2-Amino-4-(methylthio)butyric acid *see* Methionine.

2-Amino-2-(methylthio)-5-pyrimidine-methanol *see* Methioprim.

2-Amino-3-methylvaleric acid *see* Isoleucine.

2-Amino-4-methylvaleric acid *see* Leucine.

AMINOMETRADINE*** (1-allyl-6-amino-3-ethyl-1,2,3,4-tetrahydro-2,4-pyrimidine-dione; 1-allyl-6-amino-3-ethyluracil; al-lacyl; allatsil; aminometramide; 'catapyrin', 'katapirin', 'mictine', 'mincard').

Aminometramide* *see* Aminometradine.

4-Amino-1-naphthalenesulfonic acid *see* Naphthionic acid.

4-Amino-1-naphthoic acid diethylamino-ethyl ester *see* Naphthocaine.

6-AMINONICOTINAMIDE (6-AN; NSC-21206).

3-Amino-6-(5-nitrofurfurylidenemethyl)-1,2,4-triazine *see* Furalazine.

3-Amino-6-[2-(5-nitrofuryl)vinyl]-pyridazine *see* Nifurprazine.

3-Amino-6-[2-(5-nitro-2-furyl)vinyl]-*as*-triazine *see* Furalazine.

L(−)-**2-Amino-3-(*N*-nitrosohydroxyl-amino)propionic acid** *see* Alanosine.

2-Amino-1-octadecanol *see* Sphingine.

2-Amino-4-octadecene-1,3-diol *see* Sphingosine.

(−)-**13β-Amino-5,6,7,8,9,10,11α,12-octa-hydro-5α-methyl-5,11-methanobenzo-cyclodecen-3-ol** *see* Dezocine.

Amino oxidase *see* Monoamine oxidase.

Aminooxoacetic acid *see* Oxamic acid.

α-**Aminooxy-6-bromo-*m*-cresol** *see* Brocresine.

5-(Aminooxymethyl)-2-bromophenol *see* Brocresine.

AMINOPENTAMIDE* (4-dimethylamino-2,2-diphenylvaleramide; BL-139; 'centrine').

2-Aminopentanedioic acid *see* Glutamic acid.

2-Amino-4-pentenoic acid *see* Allylglycine.

N-**[5-[3-[(5-Aminopentyl)hydroxycarba-moyl]propionamido]pentyl]-3-[[5-(*N*-hydroxyacetamido)pentyl]carbamoyl]-propionylhydroxamic acid** *see* Deferoxamine.

Aminophan *see* Cinchophen.

4-Aminophenazone *see* 4-Aminoantipyrine.

AMINOPHENAZONE**** (4-(dimethyl-amino)-2,3-dimethyl-1-phenyl-3-pyrazolin-5-one; 4-dimethylaminophenazone; 4-di-methylaminoantipyrine; amidofebrin; amidofen; amidophen; amidopyrine; amidopyrazoline; amidozone; aminopyrine; aminopyrazolin; 'amidazophen', 'anafe-brina', 'aneuxol', 'brufacon', 'brufalgin', 'brufaneuxol', 'dimapyrin', 'dipyrin', 'febri-nina', 'novamidon', 'piridol', 'pyradone', 'pyramidon', 'pyramon', 'pyrodin').

AMINOPHENAZONE ASCORBATE ('vaditon').

AMINOPHENAZONE CYCLAMATE****** (aminophenazone cyclohexylsulfamate).

Aminophenazone cyclohexylsulfamate *see* Aminophenazone cyclamate.

AMINOPHENAZONE ETHYL SALICYLATE ('latepyrine').

AMINOPHENAZONE-FORMALDEHYDE SODIUM SULFOXYLATE ('dimenaz-one').

AMINOPHENAZONE GENTISATE ('gentamidon', 'pirissal').

AMINOPHENAZONE WITH ALLO-BARBITAL ('cibalgin', 'pabialgin').

AMINOPHENAZONE WITH AMINO-

CHLORTHENOXAZINE ('dereuma').

AMINOPHENAZONE WITH BAMETHAN (ADS-3; 'prontylin').

AMINOPHENAZONE WITH 1,2-DIPHENYL-3,5-PYRAZOLIDINE-DIONE ('osadrin').

AMINOPHENAZONE WITH PHENYL-BUTAZONE ('butapyrine', 'irgapyrin', 'pyra-elmedal').

1-(*p*-Aminophenethyl)-4-phenylisoni-pecotic acid ethyl ester *see* Anileridine.

(−)-**3-(*p*-Aminophenethyl)-2,3,4,5-tetra-hydro-8-methoxy-2-methyl-1*H*-3-benzazepine** *see* Anilopam.

N-**(5-*p*-Aminophenoxypentyl)phthalimide** *see* Amphotalide.

Aminophenurobutane* *see* Carbutamide.

7-(α-Aminophenylacetamido)cephalo-sporanic acid *see* Cefaloglycin.

7-((+)-2-Amino-2-phenylacetamido)-3-methyl-2-cephem-2-carboxylic acid *see* Cefalexin.

6-(α-Aminophenylacetamido)penicillanic acid *see* Ampicillin.

p-**Aminophenylacetic acid phenyliso-propylamide** *see* Fepracet.

2-Amino-2-phenylacetophenone *see* Desylamine.

N-(*p*-**Aminophenylacetyl)amphetamine** *see* Fepracet.

p-**Aminophenyl 2-aminothiazol-5-yl sulfone** *see* Thiazolsulfone.

1-(*p*-Aminophenyl)-2-*sec*-butylamino)-benzyl alcohol *see* Amiterol.

α-*p*-**Aminophenyl-α-ethylglutarimide** *see* Aminoglutethimide.

2-Amino-5-phenyl-2-oxazolinone *see* Aminorex.

α-**Aminophenylpenicillin** *see* Ampicillin.

2-Amino-3-phenylpropionic acid *see* Phenylalanine.

1-(*m*-Aminophenyl)-2(1*H*)-pyridinone *see* Amphenidone.

N-[*p*-(*p*-**Aminophenylsulfonyl)phenyl]-glycine** *see* Acediasulfone.

5-Amino-1-phenyl-1*H*-tetrazole *see* Fenamole.

P-**(5-Amino-3-phenyl-1,2,4-triazol-1-yl)-*N,N,N',N'*-phosphonic diamide** *see* Triamiphos.

Aminophosphine oxide *see* Phosphinic amide.

AMINOPHYLLINE**** (theophylline-ethylene-diamine; theophyllamine).

3α-Amino-5α-pregnan-2-ol *see* Funtumidine.

AMINOPROMAZINE**** (10-(2,3-bisdime-thylaminopropyl)phenothiazine; imino-promazine; proquamezine; tetrame-prozine).

AMINOPROMAZINE FUMARATE (A-124; RP-3828; 'jenotone', 'lispamol', 'lispasmol', 'lorusil').

3-AMINOPROPIONITRILE (β-amino-propionitrile; BAPN; lathyrus factor).

3-Amino-4-propoxybenzoic acid diethyl-aminoethyl ester *see* Proxymetacaine.

4-Amino-2-propoxybenzoic acid diethyl-

aminoethyl ester *see* Propoxycaine.
1-(2-Aminopropoxy)-2,6-xylene *see* Mexiletine.
2-(2-Aminopropoxy)-*m*-xylene *see* Mexiletine.
1-(3-Aminopropyl)-1,3-dihydro-*N*,3,3-tri-methyl-1-phenylbenzo(c)thiophene *see* Talsupram.
2-(1-Aminopropyl)-2-indanol *see* Indanorex.
***m*-(1-Aminopropyl)phenol** *see* α-Methyl-*m*-tyramine.
***N*-(3-Aminopropyl)putrescine** *see* Spermidine.
1-(4-Amino-2-propylpyrimidin-5-ylme-thyl)-2-picolinium chloride-HCl *see* Amprolinium.
6-Amino-9-(β-D-psicofuranosyl)purine *see* Angustmycin C.
AMINOPTERIN SODIUM*** (*N*-[*p*-[(2,4-diaminopterid-6-ylmethyl)amino]benzoyl]-glutamic acid sodium salt; 4-amino-4-desoxyfolic acid sodium salt; antifolic acid; APGA; NSC-739).
2-Aminopurine-6-thiol *see* Tioguanine.
4-(6-Aminopurin-9-yl)-4-deoxy-D-erythronic acid *see* Eritadenine.
4-(6-Aminopurin-9-yl)-2,3-dihydroxy-butyric acid *see* Eritadenine.
'Aminopyrazolin' *see* Aminophenazone.
Aminopyrine* *see* Aminophenazone.
4-Amino-7H-pyrrolo(2,3-d)pyrimidine riboside *see* 7-Deazaadenosine.
Aminoquin *see* Pamaquin.
AMINOQUINOL*** (7-chloro-2-(o-chloro-styryl)-4-[(4-diethylamino-1-methylbutyl)-amino]quinoline).
AMINOQUINURIDE (1,3-bis(4-amino-2-methylquinolin-6-yl)urea; 6,6′-carbonylbis-(2-methyl-4-aminoquinoline); amino-chinuride; 'revasa', 'surfen').
AMINOREX*** (2-amino-5-phenyl-2-oxazo-line; McN-742).
AMINOREX FUMARATE ('apiquel', 'meno-cil').
7-Amino-3-(β-D-ribofuranosyl)pyrazolo-(4,3-d)pyrimidine *see* Formycin A.
AMINOSALICYLIC ACID* (4-aminosali-cylic acid; *p*-aminosalicylic acid; amino-salylum; PAS; PASA; PASK).
See also Calcium aminosalicylate; Fenamisal; Hydroxyprocaine; Pasiniazid; Pheniramine aminosalicylate; Potassium aminosalicylate.
AMINOSALICYLIC ACID HYDRAZIDE (4-aminosalicylic acid hydrazide; 'pasdra-zide').
AMINOSALICYLIC ACID WITH ASCORBIC ACID ('pascorbic').
***p*-Aminosalol** *see* Fenamisal.
Aminosalylum *see* Aminosalicylic acid.
4-AMINO-1,2,5-SELENADIAZOLE-3-CARBOXYLIC ACID (NSC-84531).
Aminosidin *see* Paromomycin.
'Aminosin' *see* Thiosinamine.
Aminosine *see* Chlorpromazine.
2-Aminosuccinamic acid *see* Asparagine.
2-Aminosuccinamide *see* Aspartamide.
2-Aminosuccinic acid *see* Aspartic acid.

4-Amino-4′-succinylaminodiphenyl sulfone *see* Succinyldapsone.
8-Amino-1,2,3,4-tetrahydro-2-methyl-4-phenylisoquinoline *see* Nomifensine.
4-Amino-2,2,5,5-tetrakis(trifluoro-methyl)-3-imidazoline *see* Midaflur.
2-Aminotetralin *see* Tetrahydro-2-naphthyl-amine.
AMINOTHIAZOLE*** (2-aminothiazole; 2-thiazylamine).
AMINOTHIAZOLE HYDROGEN SUCCINATE ('morbasin', 'thyrosan').
AMINOTHIAZOLE MALEATE (RP-2921; 'abadole', 'basedol').
2-Amino-2-thiazoline phenylbutazone salt *see* Thiazolinobutazone.
***p*-Aminothiolobenzoic acid diethylamino-ethyl ester** *see* Thiocaine.
α-Amino-*p*-toluic acid *see* *p*-Aminomethyl-benzoic acid.
3-Amino-*p*-tolyl pentyl ketone *O*-(2-aminoethyl)oxime *see* Caproxamine.
Aminotrate phosphate* *see* Trolnitrate.
3-Amino-1H-1,2,4-triazole *see* Amitrole.
4-Amino-3,5,6-trichloropicolinic acid *see* Picloram.
4-Amino-3,5,6-trichloropyridine-2-carboxylic acid *see* Picloram.
(8*S*,10*S*)-10[(3-Amino-2,3,6-trideoxy-α-L-*lyxo*-hexopyranosyl)oxy]-8-glycolyl-7,8,9,10-tetrahydro-6,8,11-trihydroxy-1-methoxy-5,12-naphthacenedione *see* Doxorubicin.
1-(3-Amino-4,5,6-triethoxyphthalid-3-yl)-1,2,3,4-tetrahydro-8-methoxy-2-methyl-6,7-methylenedioxyisoquinoline *see* Tritoqualine.
7-Amino-4,5,6-triethoxy-(5,6,7,8-tetra-hydro-4-methoxy-6-methyl-1,3-dioxolo-(4,5-g)isoquinolin-5-yl)phthalidol *see* Tritoqualine.
2-Amino-5-(α,α,α-trifluoro-*p*-tolyl)-2-oxazoline *see* Fluminorex.
30-Amino-3,14,25-trihydroxy-3,9,14,20,25-pentaazatriacontane-2,10,13,21,24-pentaone *see* Deferoxamine.
***N*-(3-Amino-2,4,6-triiodobenzoyl)-*N*-phenyl-β-alanine** *see* Iobenzamic acid.
3-[(3-Amino-2,4,6-triiodobenzoyl)phenyl-amino]propionic acid *see* Iobenzamic acid.
2-(3-Amino-2,4,6-triiodobenzyl)butyric acid *see* Iopanoic acid.
3′-Amino-2,4,6-triiodo-*N*-methylglutar-anilic acid *see* Iomeglamic acid.
3-[*N*-(3-Amino-2,4,6-triiodophenyl)acet-amido]-2-methylpropionic acid *see* Iocetamic acid.
3-(3-Amino-2,4,6-triiodophenyl)-2-ethyl-propionic acid *see* Iopanoic acid.
4-[*N*-(3-Amino-2,4,6-triiodophenyl)-*N*-methylcarbamoyl)butyric acid *see* Iomeglamic acid.
***N*-(3-Amino-2,4,6-triiodophenyl)-*N*-methylglutaramic acid** *see* Iomeglamic acid.
4-(4-Amino-6,7,8-trimethoxyquinazolin-2-

yl)piperazine-1-carboxylic acid 2-hydroxy-2-methylpropyl ester *see* Trimazosin.

Aminourea *see* Semicarbazide.

***p*-Amino-*p*′-ureidodiphenylsulfone** *see* Amidapsone.

2-Aminovaleric acid *see* Norvaline.

'Aminoweidnerit' *see* Methenamine thiocyanate.

'Aminoxidin' *see* Paromomycin.

AMINOXYTRIPHENE*** (3-dimethylamino-1,1,2-tris(*p*-methoxyphenyl)-1-propene; 2,3,3-tris(*p*-methoxyphenyl)-*N*,*N*-dimethylallylamine; amotriphene; WIN-5494; 'myordil').

Aminoxytropine tropate *see* Atropine oxide.

AMIODARONE*** (2-butyl-3-[4-(2-diethylaminoethoxy)-3,5-diiodobenzoyl)benzofuran; 2-butyl-3-benzofuranyl 4-(2-diethylaminoethoxy)-3,5-diiodophenyl ketone; L-3428; SK & F-33134A; 'cordarone').

AMIODOXYL BENZOATE* (ammonium *o*-iodoxybenzoate; 'arthrytin', 'oxo-ate').

AMIPERONE** (4-(*p*-chlorophenyl)-1-[3-(*p*-fluorobenzoyl)propyl]-*N*,*N*-dimethylisonipecotamide; 4-[4-(*p*-chlorophenyl)-4-di-methylcarbamoylpiperid-1-yl]-4′-fluoro-butyrophenone; R-2962).

AMIPHENAZOLE*** (2,4-diamino-5-phenyl-thiazole; DAPT; daftazol; fenamizol; phenamizole; DHA-245; 'daptazole').

'Amiphos' *see* 2-Acetamidoethyl dimethyl phosphorodithioate.

Amipramidine *see* Amiloride.

Amipramizide *see* Amiloride.

AMIQUINSIN*** (4-amino-6,7-dimethoxy-quinoline; amiquinsin hydrochloride; U-935).

AMISOMETRADINE*** (6-amino-1,2,3,4-tetrahydro-3-methyl-1-(2-methylallyl)-2,4-pyrimidinedione; 6-amino-3-methyl-1-(2-methylallyl)uracil; aminoisometradine; 'rolicton').

AMITEROL*** ((±)-*p*-amino-α-*sec*-butyl-aminomethyl)benzyl alcohol; (±)-*p*-amino-α-[(1-methylpropyl)aminomethyl]benzyl alcohol; (±)-1-(*p*-aminophenyl)-2-*sec*-butylaminoethanol).

Amithiozone* *see* Thiacetazone.

AMITHIZONE (tr) (*p*-acetamido-*m*-methoxy-benzaldehyde thiosemicarbazone; amitizon; SHCH-85).

Amitizon (tr) *see* Amithizone.

AMITON* (*S*-(2-diethylaminoethyl)-*O*,*O*-diethyl phosphorothioate; DSDP; 'inferno', 'metramas', 'tetram').

'Amitrene' *see* Dexamphetamine.

AMITRIPTYLINE*** (5-(3-dimethylamino-propylidene)-10,11-dihydro-5H-dibenzo-(a,d)cycloheptene; 3-(3-dimethylamino-propylidene)-5H-dibenzo(a,d)1,4-cyclo-heptadiene; 10,11-dihydro-*N*,*N*-dimethyl-5H-dibenzo(a,d)cycloheptene-Δ⁵,γ-propyl-amine; proheptadiene; N-750 SA; Ro-4-1575; 'adepril', 'elavil', 'horizon', 'laroxyl', 'lentizol', 'redomex', 'redormex', 'saroten', 'sarotex', 'tepercin', 'tryptanol', 'tryptizol').

AMITRIPTYLINE *N*-OXIDE ('dano').

AMITRIPTYLINE WITH CHLORDIA-ZEPOXIDE ('limbitrol').

AMITRIPTYLINE WITH PERPHEN-AZINE ('etrafon', 'limbatril', 'mutabon', 'mutanxion', 'mutaspline', 'triavil').

Amitrol *see* Amitrole.

AMITROLE* (3-amino-1H-1,2,4-triazole; 1H-1,2,4-triazol-3-amine; amitrol; 3A-T; ATA; 'amizol', 'cytrol', 'ustinex PA', 'weedazol').

AMIXETRINE*** (1-(β-isopentyloxy-phenethyl)pyrrolidine; 1-[2-(3-methyl-butoxy)-2-phenylethyl]pyrrolidine; 1-(2-isoamyloxy-2-phenylethyl)pyrrolidine; CERM-898; 'somagest').

'Amizepin' *see* Carbamazepine.

Amizil *see* Benactyzine.

'Amizine' *see* Simazine.

'Amizol' *see* Amitrole.

Amizole *see* Sulfamidopyrine.

Ammicardin *see* Khellin.

'Ammidin' *see* Pentosalen.

Amminosidine *see* Paromomycin.

Ammoidin *see* Methoxsalen.

'Ammoket' *see* Ammonium mandelate.

Ammonium bithiolicum *see* Ammonium sulfobituminate.

Ammonium camphocarbonate *see* Camphoramine.

Ammonium camphocarboxylate *see* Camphoramine.

Ammonium 3-camphocarboxylate *see* Camphoramine.

Ammonium ichthosulfonate *see* Ammonium sulfobituminate.

Ammonium *o*-iodoxybenzoate *see* Amiodoxyl benzoate.

AMMONIUM MANDELATE ('amdelate', 'ammoket', 'mandicid', 'manduryl')

Ammonium 2-oxobornane-3-carboxylate *see* Camphoramine.

AMMONIUM PHTHALAMATE (ammonium *o*-carbamoylbenzoate; 'spirogen').

AMMONIUM SULFOBITUMINATE (ammonium sulfobituminosum; ammonium sulfoichthyolate; ammonium bithiolicum; ammonium ichthosulfonate; bithyolum; bituminolum; ichthammonium; ichthosulfol).

Ammonium sulfobituminosum *see* Ammonium sulfobituminate.

Ammonium sulfoichthyolate *see* Ammonium sulfobituminate.

'Ammophylline' *see* Aminophylline.

'Ammorid' *see* Methylbenzethonium.

'A.M.N.' *see* Flavin mononucleotide.

AMOBARBITAL** (5-ethyl-5-isoamylbar-bituric acid; 5-ethyl-5-(3-methylbutyl)bar-bituric acid; 5-ethyl-5-isopentylbarbituric acid; amylobarbitone; barbamyl; pentymal; amobarbital sodium; 'amytal', 'beotol', 'dorlotin', 'dorminal', 'dormytal', 'eunoctal', 'hypnamil', 'isomyl', 'isomytal', 'mudeka', 'somnal', 'stadadorm').

AMOBARBITAL WITH SCOPOLAMINE METHYL NITRATE ('veryl').

AMODIAQUINE*** (4-(7-chloro-4-quinolyl-amino)-α-diethylamino-o-cresol; 7-chloro-4-(3-diethylaminomethyl-4-hydroxyanilino)-quinoline; SN-10751; 'amodiaquin', 'CAM-AQI', 'camoquin', 'camoquinal', 'flavoquine', 'miaquine').

AMODIAQUINE WITH PRIMAQUINE ('camoprim').

'Amoebal' see Arsthinol.

'Amoebin' see Ethacridine.

'Amoenol' see Clioquinol.

AMOGASTRIN** (N-carboxy-L-tryptophyl-L-methioninyl-L-α-aspartyl-3-phenyl-L-alaninamide N-tert-pentyl ester).

AMOLANONE** (3-(2-diethylaminoethyl)-3-phenyl-2-benzofuranone; 4-diethylamino-2-(o-hydroxyphenyl)-2-phenylbutyric acid lactone; AP-43; 'amethone').

AMOPROXAN*** (α-isopentyloxymethyl-4-morpholineëthanol 3,4,5-trimethoxybenzoate; 4-(2-hydroxy-3-isopentyloxypropyl)-morpholine 3,4,5-trimethoxybenzoate ester; N-[3-isoamyloxy-2-(3,4,5-trimethoxybenzoyloxy)propyl]morpholine; CERM-730).

AMOPYROQUINE*** (7-chloro-4-(4-hydroxy-3-pyrrolidin-1-ylmethylanilino)-quinoline; 4-(7-chloroquinolin-4-ylamino)-α-pyrrolidin-1-yl-o-cresol; PAM-780; 'propoquin').

Amotriphene see Aminoxytriphene.

AMOXAPINE*** (2-chloro-11-piperazin-1-yldibenz(b,f)(1,4)oxazepine; CL-67772).

AMOXECAINE** (N,N',N'-triethyl-N-(2-hydroxyethyl)ethylenediamine p-aminobenzoate ester; 2-[(2-diethylaminoethyl)-ethylamino]ethyl p-aminobenzoate; RP-2856; 'locastine').

AMOXICILLIN*** (6-[D(−)-2-amino-2-(p-hydroxyphenyl) acetamido] penicillanic acid; 6-((−)-α-amino-4-hydroxyphenyl-acetamido) penicillanic acid; α-amino-p-hydroxybenzyl penicillin; amoxycillin; BRL-2333; 'amoxid', 'amoxil', 'clamoxyl', 'hiconcil', 'larocin', 'larotid').

'Amoxid' see Amoxicillin.

'Amoxil' see Amoxicillin.

Amoxycillin* see Amoxicillin.

AMOXYDRAMINE CAMSILATE*** (N,N-dimethyl-2-(diphenylmethoxy)ethylamine N-oxide 2-oxo-10-bornanesulfonate; amy-oxydramine camphorsulfonate; diphenhydramine N-oxide camsylate; diphenhydramine aminoxide camsylate).

AMOXYDRAMINE UNDECENATE ('mykestron').

AMP see Rifampicin.

5-AMP see Adenosine phosphate.

A5MP see Adenosine phosphate.

'Ampazine' see Promazine.

Amphaethamine see Amphetamine.

Amphechloral* see Amfechloral.

AMPHENIDONE*** (1-(m-aminophenyl)-2-(1H)-pyridinone; 'dornwal').

AMPHETAMINE*** ((±)-amphetamine; (±)-α-methylphenethylamine; 2-amino-1-phenylpropane; β-phenylisopropylamine; amphaethamine; phenamine; amphetamine

base, phosphate or sulphate).

(+)-Amphetamine see Dexamphetamine.

(−)-Amphetamine see Levamfetamine.

Amphetamine p-aminophenylacetate see Fepracet.

(±)-AMPHETAMINE p-CHLORO-PHENOXYACETATE ('satietyl').

Amphetamine-pyridoxine condensation product see Pyridoxiphen.

AMPHETAMINIL (2-[(1-methyl-2-phenyl-ethyl)amino]-2-phenylacetonitrile; 2-(α-methylphenethylamino)-2-phenylaceto-nitrile; 2-phenyl-2-(phenylisopropylamino)-acetonitrile; N-(α-cyanobenzyl)amphet-amine; AN-1; 'aponeuron').

Amphetyline see Fenetylline.

'Amphocortrin' see Amfomycin.

'Amphocycline' see Hexacycline with amphotericin B.

'Amphodyne' see Imidecyl iodine.

Amphomycin* see Amfomycin.

AMPHOTALIDE*** (N-(5-p-aminophenoxy-pentyl)phthalimide; M & B-1948-A).

AMPHOTERICIN B*** (antibiotic from Str. nodosus; 'amphozone', 'fungitin', 'fungizone'). See also Hexacycline with amphotericin B; Tetracycline with amphotericin B.

'Amphotropine' see Hexacamphamine.

'Amphozone' see Amphotericin B.

'Ampibel' see Ampicillin.

AMPICILLIN*** (D(−)-6-(α-aminophenyl-acetamido)penicillanic acid; 6-(2-amino-2-phenylacetamido)penicillanic acid; α-aminobenzylpenicillin; ampicillin trihy-drate; AY-6108; BRL-1341; P-50; Wy-5103; 'amblosin', 'amfipen', 'ampibel', 'amplital', 'binotal', 'britacil', 'cymbi', 'deripen', 'doktacillin', 'fortapen', 'omnipen', 'penbritin', 'penbristol', 'penbrock', 'penicline', 'penorsin', 'pensyn', 'pentrexyl', 'plitrexyl', 'polycillin', 'qidamp', 'semicillin', 'suractin' 'totacillin', 'totapen', 'vericyline', 'viccillin').

Ampicillin ester with ethyl 2-hydroxy-ethyl carbonate see Bacampicillin.

AMPICILLIN GUAIACYLDIETHYL-AMINOACETATE ('diampicicol').

Ampicillin hydroxymethyl ester pivalate see Pivampicillin.

Ampicillin phthalidyl ester see Talampicillin.

AMPICILLIN SODIUM (sodium ampicillin; 'penbritin-S', 'polycillin N').

AMPICILLIN TRIHYDRATE (AY-6108; 'principen').

AMPICILLIN WITH CLOXACILLIN ('ampiclox', 'ampiox', 'cloxamp', 'tupen').

AMPICILLIN WITH DICLOXACILLIN (HI-56; 'ampiplus', 'cervantal', 'diamplicil', 'duplexcillin', 'totocillin').

AMPICILLIN WITH FLUCLOXACILLIN ('magnapen').

AMPICILLIN WITH OXACILLIN ('cervantal parenteral').

AMPICILLIN WITH OXYPHENBUTAZ-ONE ('ampifenil').

'Ampiclox' see Ampicillin with cloxacillin.

'**Ampifenil**' *see* Ampicillin with oxyphenbutazone.

'**Ampiox**' *see* Ampicillin with cloxacillin.

'**Ampiplus**' *see* Ampicillin with dicloxacillin.

'**Amplicaine**' *see* Octacaine.

'**Amplidione**' *see* Oxazidione.

'**Amplital**' *see* Ampicillin.

'**Ampliuril**' *see* Benziodarone.

'**Amplivix**' *see* Benziodarone.

AMPROLIUM*** (1-(4-amino-2-propylpyrimidin-5-ylmethyl)-2-picolinium chloride-HCl; 'amprolmix', 'anticoccid').

'**Amprolmix**' *see* Amprolium.

AMPROTROPINE* (3-diethylamino-2,2-dimethylpropyl tropate; AP-4-7; 'syntropan').

AMPYRIMINE*** (5-phenylpyrimido(4,5-d)pyrimidine-2,4,7-triamine; 2,4,7-triamino-5-phenylpyrimido(4,5-d)pyrimidine).

'**Ampyrone**' *see* 4-Aminoantipyrine.

AMPYZINE** (2-dimethylaminopyrazine; ampyzine sulfate; W-3580-B).

AMQUINATE*** (methyl 7-diethylamino-4-hydroxy-6-propyl-3-quinolinecarboxylate).

AMSONIC ACID* (3,3'-diaminostilbene-2,2'-disulfonic acid).
See also Chlorphenoctium amsonate.

'**Amuno**' *see* Indometacin.

'**Amycycline**' *see* Chlortetracycline with α-amylase.

AMYDRICAINE (benzoate of 1-dimethylamino-2-(dimethylaminomethyl)-2-butanol; benzoate of tetramethyldiaminodimethyl ethyl carbinol; 'alypin', 'benzopropyl').

Amygdalic acid *see* Mandelic acid.

AMYGDALIN (mandelonitrile gentiobioside).

AMYGDALOPHENIN (*N*-mandelyl-*p*-phenetidine).

tert-**Amyl alcohol** *see* 2-Methyl-2-butanol.

2-Amylaminoethyl *p*-aminobenzoate *see* Naepaine.

α-AMYLASE (alpha amylase; 'buclamase', 'fortizyme', 'maxilase', 'oramyl').
See also Chlortetracycline with α-amylase.

'**Amylcaine**' *see* Naepaine.

5-*sec*-Amyl-5-(bromoallyl)barbituric acid *see* 5-(2-Bromoallyl)-5-(1-methylbutyl)-barbituric acid.

Amyleine *see* Amylocaine.

Amylene *see* Pentene.

AMYLENE CHLORAL (condensation product of chloral and 2-methyl-2-butanol; 'dormiol').

Amylene hydrate *see* 2-Methyl-2-butanol.

Amyl mercaptan *see* 1-Pentanethiol.

AMYLMETACRESOL* (amyl-*m*-cresol; 5-methyl-2-pentylphenol; 6-pentyl-*m*-cresol; *in* 'strepsils').

AMYL NITRITE (isoamyl nitrite; 'aspiral', 'frenodosa', 'isomyl nitrite', 'nitramyl', 'vaporole').

Amylobarbitone* *see* Amobarbital.

AMYLOCAINE (benzoate of 1-dimethylamino-2-methyl-2-butanol; benzoate of dimethylaminomethyl ethyl methyl carbinol; amyleine; 'stovaine').

Amylopectin sodium sulfate *see* Sodium amylosulfate.

Amylosulfate *see* Sodium amylosulfate.

Amylpenicillin *see* Penicillin F.

'**Amylsine**' *see* Naepaine.

'**Amytal**' *see* Amobarbital.

AN-1 *see* Amphetaminil.

AN-148 *see* Methadone.

AN-448 *see* Mazindol.

AN-1317 *see* Perimetazine.

AN-1320 *see* Fumaria officinalis.

AN-1324 *see* Glybuzole.

'**Anabactyl**' *see* Carbenicillin.

ANABASEINE (3,4,5,6-tetrahydro-2-pyrid-3-ylpyridine; 3,4,5,6-tetrahydro-2,3'-bipyridine).

ANABASINE (2-pyrid-3-ylpiperidine; 1,2,3,4,5,6-hexahydro-2,3'-bipyridine; neonicotine).

'**Anabile**' *see* Ox bile.

'**Anabolex**' *see* Androstanolone.

Anadol(tr) *see* Alphaprodine.

'**Anadrol**' *see* Oxymetholone.

'**Anadur**' *see* Nandrolone (*p*-hexyloxy)hydrocinnamate.

'**Anaestheform**' *see* Benzocaine.

'**Anaesthesin**' *see* Benzocaine.

'**Anafebrina**' *see* Aminophenazone.

'**Anaflex**' *see* Polynoxylin.

'**Anafranil**' *see* Clomipramine.

ANAGESTONE*** (17-hydroxy-6α-methylpregn-4-en-20-one).

ANAGESTONE ACETATE (3-deoxy-17α-hydroxy-6α-methylprogesterone acetate).

ANAGESTONE ACETATE WITH MESTRANOL (MI-860; 'preventa').

'**Analeptin**' *see* Oxedrine.

'**Analexin**' *see* Fenyramidol.

Analgésine *see* Phenazone.

Analgin (tr) *see* Novaminsulfon.

'**Analjol**' *see* Methyl acetylsalicylate.

'**Analutos**' *see* Calcium acetylsalicylate.

'**Ananase**' *see* Bromelains.

'**Anapolon**' *see* Oxymetholone.

'**Anaprel**' *see* Rescinnamine.

Anaprilin (tr) *see* Propranolol.

'**Anarcon**' *see* Nalorphine.

'**Anastil**' *see* Guaiacol.

'**Anasyth**' *see* Stanozolol.

'**Anatensol**' *see* Fluphenazine.

'**Anathrombase**' *see* Dicoumarol.

'**Anatran**' *see* Acepromazine.

Anautine* *see* Diphenhydramine.

'**Anavar**' *see* Oxandrolone.

ANAZOCINE** (9-*syn*-methoxy-3-methyl-9-phenyl-3-azabicyclo(3.3.1)nonane; 9-*syn*-methoxy-3-methyl-9-phenylisogranatanine; 4β-methoxy-1-methyl-4α-phenyl-3α,5α-propanopiperidine; azabicyclane).

ANAZOLENE SODIUM** (4-(4-anilino-5-sulfonaphth-1-ylazo)-5-hydroxy-2,7-naphthalenedisulfonic acid trisodium salt; trisodium 4'-anilino-8-hydroxy-1,1'-azonaphthalene-3,5',6-trisulfonate; sodium anazolene; sodium anoxynaphthonate; CI-92; 'coomassie blue', 'wofazurin').

'**Ancaris**' *see* Thenium closilate.

'**Ancef**' *see* Cefazolin.

Anchoic acid *see* Azelaic acid.
ANCITABINE** ((2R,3R,3aS,9aR)-2,3,3a,9a-tetrahydro-3-hydroxy-6-imino-6H-furo-(2′,3′:4,5)oxazolo(3,2-a)pyrimidine-2-methanol; 2,2′-anhydro-1β-D-arabino-furanosylcytosine; anhydro-ara C; 2,2′-anhydrocytarabine; 2,2′-cyclo-1β-D-arabinofuranosylcytosine; cyclocytidine; 2,2′-O-cyclocytidine; 2,2′-c-ara C; 2,2′-cyclocytarabine).
ANCITABINE ACETATE (NSC-129220).
'Ancobon' *see* Flucytosine.
'Ancolan' *see* Meclozine.
'Anconcen' *see* Chlormadinone acetate with mestranol.
'Ancotil' *see* Flucytosine.
ANCROD** (anticoagulant (defibrinating) fraction from *Agkistrodon rhodostoma* venom; Abbott-38414; 'arvin', 'venacil').
'Ancylol' *see* Disophenol.
ANCYMIDOL* (α-(p-anisyl)-α-cyclopropyl-5-pyrimidinemethanol; α-cyclopropyl-α-(p-methoxyphenyl)-5-pyrimidinemethanol; EL-531).
'Ancyte' *see* Piposulfan.
'Andantol' *see* Isothipendyl.
'Andradurin' *see* Testosterone 3-(p-hexyloxy)-hydrocinnamate.
'Andramine' *see* Hexobendine.
'Androcur' *see* Cyproterone acetate.
'Androdurin' *see* Testosterone ketolaurate.
Androfurazanol *see* Furazabol.
Androisoxazole *see* 17β-Hydroxy-17α-methyl-5α-androstano(3,2-c)isoxazole.
'Androlone' *see* Androstanolone.
Androsta-1,4-dien-17β-ol-3-one *see* Boldenone.
Androsta-4,6-dien-17β-ol-3-one-17α-yl-propionic acid *see* Canrenoic acid.
'Androstalone' *see* Mestanolone.
Androstanazole *see* Stanozolol.
5α-ANDROSTANE (androstane; etioallocholane; NSC-49000).
5β-ANDROSTANE (etiocholane; aetian; etian).
ANDROSTANOLONE* (5α-androstan-17β-ol-3-one; stanolone; dihydrotestosterone; 17β-hydroxy-5α-androstan-3-one; 5α-dihydrotestosterone; 'anabolex', 'androlone', 'cristerona', 'neodrol', 'proteina', 'stanaprol', 'stanoprol').
5α-Androstan-3α-ol-17-one *see* Androsterone.
5α-ANDROSTAN-3β-OL-17-ONE (isoandrosterone; epiandrosterone; 3-hydroxy-etioallocholan-17-one).
5β-ANDROSTAN-3α-OL-17-ONE (3α-hydroxy-5β-androstan-17-one; etiocholanone; 5-isoandrosterone).
5α-Androstan-17β-ol-3-one *see* Androstanolone.
Androst-4-en-17α-ol-3-one *see* Epitestosterone.
4-Androsten-17β-ol-3-one *see* Testosterone.
Androst-5-en-3β-ol-17-one *see* Prasterone.
ANDROSTERONE (5α-androstan-3α-ol-17-one; 3α-hydroxy-5α-androstan-17-one).
'Anelmid' *see* Dithiazanine.

ANEMONIN (1,2-dihydroxy-1,2-cyclobutane-diacrylic acid dilactone).
'Anergan' *see* Acepromazine.
'Anergex' *see* Poisonoak extract.
'Anesthesin' *see* Benzocaine.
'Anesthone' *see* Benzocaine.
ANETHOLE (1-methoxy-4-propenylbenzene; p-propenylanisole; anise camphor).
ANETHOLE TRITHIONE (5-(p-methoxy-phenyl)-1,2-dithiole-3-thione; 3-(p-anisyl)-trithione; trithio-p-methoxyphenylpropene; 1-(p-methoxyphenyl)-4,5-dithia-1-cyclopent-ene-3-thione; SK&F-1717; 'felviten', 'hepasulfo', 'heporal', 'sulfralem', 'sulfarlem', 'tiotrifar', 'trithio').
Aneurine *see* Thiamine.
'Aneuxol' *see* Aminophenazone.
'Anexate' *see* Mefenorex.
'Anfix' *see* Formothion.
ANG-66 *see* Diacetoxyscirpenol.
ANGELIC ACID (cis-α,β-dimethylacrylic acid).
α-ANGELICA LACTONE (4-hydroxy-3-pentenoic acid γ-lactone; β,γ-angelica lactone; △²-angelica lactone).
β-ANGELICA LACTONE (4-hydroxy-2-pentenoic acid γ-lactone; α,β-angelica lactone; △¹-angelica lactone).
ANGELICIN (2H-furo(2,3-h)-1-benzopyran-2-one; 7,8-furocoumarin; 4-hydroxy-5-benzofuranacrylic acid γ-lactone).
'Anghirol' *see* Cynarin.
'Angicid' *see* Sulfanilamide.
'Angicone' *see* Bismuth valproate.
'Anginin' *see* 2,6-Pyridinedimethanol bis-(methylcarbamate).
'Angio-conray' *see* Sodium iotalamate.
'Angiografin' *see* Meglumine diatrizoate.
'Angiombrine' *see* Meglumine acetrizoate.
ANGIOTENSIN(S) (angiotonin(s); hyper-tensin(s).
β-ANGIOTENSIN-II (Ba-33902).
ANGIOTENSINAMIDE* (N-[1-[N-[N-(N-(N-(N²-asparaginylarginyl)valyl)tyro-syl)valyl]histidyl]propyl]-3-phenylalanine; val₅-hypertensin II-asp-β-amide; angioten-sin amide; 'hypertensin-Ciba').
Angiotonin *see* Angiotensin.
'Angioxin' *see* 2,6-Pyridinedimethanol bis-(methylcarbamate).
'Angioxyl' *see* Kallidinogenase.
'Angitrit' *see* Trolnitrate.
'Angolon' *see* Imolamine.
Anguidin *see* Diacetoxyscirpenol.
ANGUSTMYCIN A (6-amino-9-(L-1,2-furo-pyranosenyl)purine).
ANGUSTMYCIN C (6-amino-9-(β-D-psico-furanosyl)purine; 9-D-psicofuranosyl ade-nine; 'psicofuranine').
'Anhaline' *see* Hordenine.
2,2′-Anhydro-1-β-D-arabinofuranosyl-cytosine *see* Ancitabine.
Anhydro-ara-C *see* Ancitabine.
Anhydro-4,4′-bis(diethylamino)-5″-hydr-oxytriphenylmethanol-2″,4″-disulfonic acid sodium salt *see* Patent blue.
Anhydro-4,4′-bis(diethylamino)triphenyl-

28

methanol-2″,4″-disulfonic acid sodium salt *see* Sulfan blue.

N^1,N^1-**Anhydrobis(2-hydroxyethyl)-biguanide** *see* Moroxydine.

2,2′-Anhydrocytarabine *see* Ancitabine.

3,6-Anhydro-4-O-β-D-galactopyranosyl-α-D-galactopyranose 2,4′-bis(potassium/sodium sulfate)(1→3′)polysaccharide *see* Poligeenan.

Anhydrogitalin *see* Gitoxin.

Anhydroglucochloral *see* Chloralose.

Anhydrohydroxynorprogesterone *see* Norethisterone.

ANHYDROMETHYLENECITRIC ACID ((β-hydroxymethyl)tricarballylic acid γ-lactone).
See also Sodium anhydromethylenecitrate; Salicylic acid anhydromethylenecitrate.

'Anhydron' *see* Cyclothiazide.

ANICAINE (tr) (2-piperid-1-ylethyl diphenylacetate; anikain).

ANIDOXIME** (3-diethylamino-1-phenyl-1-propanone O-([(4-methoxyphenyl)amino]carbonyl]oxime; 3-diethylaminopropiophenone O-[[(p-methoxyphenyl)amino]carbonyl]oxime; bamoxine; BRL-11870; E-142).

ANILAMATE*** (salicylanilide methylcarbamate).

ANILAZINE* (4,6-dichloro-2-(o-chloroanilino)-s-triazine; 4,6-dichloro-N-(2-chlorophenyl)-1,3,5-triazin-2-amine; 'dyrene', 'kemate').

ANILERIDINE*** (ethyl 1-(p-aminophenethyl)-4-phenylisonipecotate; 1-[2-(p-aminophenyl)ethyl]-4-carbethoxy-4-phenylpiperidine; MK-89; 'alidine', 'leritin').

ANILINE (aminobenzene; benzenamine; phenylamine).

Aniline violet *see* Crystal violet.

2-[(Anilinocarbonyl)oxy]-N-ethyl-propionamide *see* Carbetamide.

1-(2-Anilinoethyl)-4-[4,4-bis(p-fluorophenyl)butyl]piperazine *see* Difluanazine.

1-(2-Anilinoethyl)-4-(2-diethylaminoethoxy)-4-phenylpiperidine *see* Diamocaine.

4-Anilino-8-hydroxy-1,1′-azonaphthalene-3,5′,6-trisulfonic acid trisodium salt *see* Anazolene sodium.

2-Anilinomethyl-2-imidazoline *see* Phenamazoline.

1-(3-Anilinopropyl)-4-phenylisonipecotic acid *see* Piminodine.

4-(4-Anilino-5-sulfonaphth-1-ylazo)-5-hydroxy-2,7-naphthalenedisulfonic acid trisodium salt *see* Anazolene sodium.

ANILOPAM** ((−)-3-(p-aminophenethyl)-2,3,4,5-tetrahydro-8-methoxy-2-methyl-1H-3-benzazepine).

ANILPYRINE (acetanilide-phenazone condensation product).

Animal galactose factor *see* Orotic acid.

'Animert' *see* Tetrasul.

ANISACRIL*** (2-(o-methoxyphenyl)-3,3-diphenylacrylic acid).

ANISALDEHYDE (p-methoxybenzaldehyde).

ANISAMIDE(S) (methoxybenzamide(s)).

1-[p-[2-(o-Anisamido)ethyl]benzenesulfonyl]-3-cyclopentylurea *see* Glipentide.

Anise camphor *see* Anethole.

ANISIC ACID (p-methoxybenzoic acid).

m-**Anisic acid 3-piperid-1-ylpropyl ester** *see* Pribecaine.

ANISIDINE(S) (ar-methoxyaniline(s)).

ANISINDIONE*** (2-(p-anisyl)-1,3-indandione; 2-(p-methoxyphenyl)-1,3-indandione; 'miradon', 'unidone').

ANISOLE (methoxybenzene; methyl phenyl ether).

ANISOMYCIN* (3-acetoxy-4-hydroxy-2-(p-methoxybenzyl)pyrrolidine; PA-106; 'flagicidin').

ANISOPERIDONE* (4′-methoxy-4-(4-phenylpiperid-1-yl)butyrophenone; 1-[3-(p-methoxybenzoyl)propyl]-4-phenylpiperidine; R-1647).

ANISOPIROL*** (±)-α-(p-fluorophenyl-4-(o-methoxyphenyl)-1-piperazinebutanol).

Anisotropine methylbromide* *see* Octatropine methyl bromide.

3-(p-Anisoyl)-3-bromoacrylic acid *see* Bromebric acid.

1-(p-Anisoyl)-1-(3,4-dichlorophenyl)-3,3-dimethylurea *see* Anisuron.

3-(p-Anisoyl)-6-methoxy-2-methylindole-1-acetic acid *see* Duometacin.

ANISURON* (1-(p-anisoyl)-1-(3,4-dichlorophenyl)-3,3-dimethylurea; N-(3,4-dichlorophenyl)-N-(dimethylaminocarbamoyl)-p-anisamide; N-(3,4-dichlorophenyl)-N-[(dimethylamino)carbonyl]-4-methoxybenzamide; 1-(3,4-dichlorophenyl)-1-(p-methoxybenzoyl)-3,3-dimethylurea; methoxymarc; metoxymarc).

α-(p-**Anisyl)-α-cyclopropyl-5-pyrimidinemethanol** *see* Ancymidol.

2-(p-Anisyl)-1-[p-(2-diethylaminoethoxy)phenyl]-1-phenylethanol *see* Ethamoxytriphetol.

3-(p-Anisyl)trithione *see* Anethole trithione.

'Aniten' *see* Flurenol-butyl.

'Ankilostin' *see* Tetrachloroethylene.

'Anobesina' *see* Dinex sodium.

'Anodynon' *see* Chloroethane.

ANOL (p-(1-propenyl)phenol).

'Anovan' *see* Phendimetrazine.

'Anovlar' *see* Norethisterone acetate with ethinylestradiol.

ANP-235 *see* Meclofenoxate.

ANP-297 *see* Mefexamide.

ANP-3401 *see* Cinametic acid.

'Anquil' *see* Benperidol *and* Reserpine.

'Ansadol' *see* Salicylamide.

ANSERINE (N-(β-alanyl)-1-methylhistidine).

'Ansolysen' *see* Pentolonium.

'Ansopal' *see* Chloral hydrate acetylglycinamide.

'Anspor' *see* Cefradine.

'Antabus' *see* Disulfiram.

'Antabuse' *see* Disulfiram.

'Antacid' *see* Citric acid.

'Antacidin' *see* Calcium saccharate.

ANTAFENITE*** ((±)-5,6-dihydro-6-phenylimidazo(2,1-b)thiazole).
'Antagosan' see Aprotinin.
'Antagothyroil' see Thiouracil.
'Antallin' see Sodium calcium edetate.
'Antalvic' see Dextropropoxyphene.
'Antamin' see Diphenhydramine ascorbate.
'Antapentan' see Phendimetrazine.
'Antasol' see Fluphenazine.
ANTAZOLINE*** (2-(N-benzylanilinomethyl)-2-imidazoline; imidamine; phenazoline; M-5512; PM-265).
ANTAZONITE** ((±)-N-[3-(2-hydroxy-2-thien-2-ylethyl)-4-thiazolin-2-ylidene]-acetamide; 2-acetylimino-2-(2-hydroxy-2-thien-2-ylethyl)thiazoline; R-6438).
ANTELMYCIN*** (antibiotic from *Str. longissimus*; anthelmycin; L-33876).
'Antemovis' see Serotonin creatinine sulfate.
'Antepar' see Piperazine citrate.
'Antergan' see Phenbenzamine.
'Anthalazine' see Piperazine.
Anthelmycin* see Antelmycin.
'Anthelvet' see Tetramisole.
'Anthio' see Formothion.
'Anthiphen' see Dichlorophen.
Anthralin* see Dithranol.
2-ANTHRAMINE (2-aminoanthracene).
Anthramycin* see Antramycin.
ANTHRANILIC ACID (o-aminobenzoic acid).
Anthranol see 9-Anthrol.
β-Anthranoylalanine see Kynurenine.
Anthrapurol see Dantron.
ANTHRAROBIN (1,2,9-anthratriol; 1,2-dihydroxy-9-anthrol; 1,2-dihydroxyanthranol; desoxyalizarin; leucoalizarin).
1,2,9-Anthratriol see Anthrarobin.
1,8,9-Anthratriol see Dithranol.
Anthridonium chloride* see Isometamidium chloride.
9-ANTHROL (9-hydroxyanthracene; anthranol).
ANTHRONE (9,10-dihydro-9-oxoanthracene; carbothrone).
Anthropodeoxycholic acid see Chenodeoxycholic acid.
Antialopecia factor see Inositol.
Antibiotic 452-7 see Violarin.
Antibiotic 899 see Staphylomycin.
Antibiotic 1719 see Azotomycin.
Antibiotic PAA 155 see Indolmycin.
ANTIBIOTIN (avidin).
'Anticarie' see Hexachlorobenzene.
'Antichlor' see Sodium thiosulfate.
'Anticoccid' see Amprolium.
'Antideprin' see Imipramine.
Antidiuretic hormone see Vasopressin.
'Antidrase' see Diclofenamide.
ANTIENITE*** ((±)-5,6-dihydro-6-thien-2-ylimidazo(2,1-b)thiazole; R-814).
Antierythrite see Erythritol.
Antifebrin see Acetanilide.
'Antifoam A' see Dimeticone.
'Antiformin' see Sodium hypochlorite.
Antigastrin see 2-Phenyl-2-pyrid-2-ylthioacetamide.

'Antigest' see 17α-Hydroxy-16-methylene-pregna-4,6-diene-3,20-dione acetate with mestranol.
Antihemorrhagic vitamin see Phytomenadione.
'Antihydral' see Methenamine.
Antiinflammatory hormone see Hydrocortisone.
'Antilon' see Eterobarb.
'Antilysin' see Aprotinin.
'Antimalarine' see Plasmocide.
'Antiminth' see Pyrantel embonate.
Antimony compounds see following entries, Methylglucamine antimonate and under Stib . . . .
Antimony sodium bis(pyrocatechol-2,4-disulfonate) see Stibophen.
Antimony sodium dimercaptosuccinate see Sodium stibocaptate.
Antimony sodium gluconate see Sodium antimonyl gluconate; Sodium stibogluconate.
ANTIMONYL POTASSIUM TARTRATE (potassium antimony tartrate; tartar emetic; APT; PAT).
'Antimosan' see Stibophen.
'Antin' see Phenyltoloxamine.
'Antinonin' see Dinitro-o-cresol.
'Antio' see Formothion.
Antipernicious anemia factor see Cyanocobalamin.
'Antiphen' see Dichlorophen.
'Anti-pica' see Fluanisone.
Antipyrine see Phenazone.
(Antipyrinylisobutylamino)methane sulfonate see Dibupyrone.
N-[(Antipyrinylisopropylamino)methyl]-nicotinamide see Niprofazone.
N-Antipyrinylnicotinamide see Nifenazon.
'Antiradon' see (Aminoethyl)isothiuronium.
Antispectacled eye factor see Inositol.
Anti-sprout see Propham.
Antisterility vitamin see Tocopherol.
Antistiffness factor see Stigmasterol.
'Antisukrin' see Carbutamide.
'Antitanil' see Dihydrotachysterol.
ANTITHEINE (tr) (N^1-methylimidazole-4,5-dicarboxylic acid diethyldiamide).
'Antithermin' see Levulinic acid phenylhydrazone.
Antiulcer vitamin see Vitamin U.
Antivitamin K$_3$ see 2-Chloro-1,4-naphthoquinone.
Antorfin (tr) see Nalorphine.
Antorphine (tr) see Nalorphine.
'Antracol' see Propineb.
ANTRAFENINE** (2-[4-(α,α,α-trifluoro-m-tolyl)piperazin-1-yl]ethyl N-[7-(trifluoromethyl)-4-quinolyl]anthranilate.
ANTRAMYCIN** (5,10,11,11a-tetrahydro-9,11-dihydroxy-8-methyl-5-oxo-1H-pyrrolo-(2,1-c)(1,4)benzodiazepine-trans-2-acrylamide; anthramycin).
Antrapurol see Dantron.
'Antrenyl' see Oxyphenonium bromide.
Antridonium see Isometamidium.
'Antroidin' see Chorionic gonadotrophin.

'**Antrycide**' *see* Quinapyramine.
'**Antrypol**' *see* Suramin.
ANTU* (1-naphth-1-yl-2-thiourea;
α-naphthylthiourea; 'anturat', 'bantu',
'krysid', 'milogard', 'rattrack').
'**Antupex**' *see* Tipepidine.
'**Anturan**' *see* Sulfinpyrazone.
'**Anturat**' *see* Antu.
'**Anucaine**' *see* Procaine.
'**Anugesic**' *see* Pramocaine.
'**Anvene**' *see* Mytatrienediol.
'**Anvitoff**' *see* Tranexamic acid.
'**Anxitol**' *see* Medazepam.
'**Anzol**' *see* Benzethonium.
'**Aolept**' *see* Periciazine.
'**Aolet**' *see* Periciazine.
'**Aovin**' *see* Troleandomycin.
AP-14 *see* Difamizole.
AP-43 *see* Amolanone.
AP-67 *see* Chlorthenoxazin.
AP-350 *see* Aminochlorthenoxazin.
AP-407 *see* Amprotropine.
'**Apacarb**' *see* Propoxur.
'**Apamide**' *see* Paracetamol.
'**APAP**' *see* Paracetamol.
'**Apaurin**' *see* Diazepam.
Apazone *see* Azapropazone.
APC (acetylsalicylic acid, caffeine & phenace-
tin; ascophen; citramon; novocephalgin).
APD *see* Detralfate.
'**Apesan**' *see* Carisoprodol.
APGA *see* Aminopterin.
'**Aphamite**' *see* Parathion.
'**Aphlozyme**' *see* Chymotrypsin.
APHOLATE (2,2,4,4,6,6-hexakis(1-aziri-
dinyl)-2,2,4,4,6,6-hexahydro-1,3,5,2,4,6-
triazatriphosphorine; hexakis(1-aziridinyl)
phosphonitrilate; ENT-26316; NSC-26812).
'**Aphoxide**' *see* Tepa.
Aphrodine *see* Yohimbine.
'**Aphthiria**' *see* Lindane.
'**Apicosan**' *see* Bee venom.
APICYCLINE** (4-(2-hydroxyethyl)-α-tetra-
cyclinyl-1-piperazineacetic acid; *N*-[[4-(2-
hydroxyethyl)piperazin-1-yl]carboxy-
methyl]tetracycline; RIT-1140; 'traserit').
APIGENIN (4′,5,7-trihydroxyflavone; 5,7-di-
hydroxy-2-(*p*-hydroxyphenyl)chromone;
'versulin').
Apilit (tr) *see* Bee venom.
APIOLE (2,5-dimethoxysafrole; 4-allyl-3,6-
dimethoxy-1,2-methylenedioxybenzene;
parsley camphor).
'**Apiquel**' *see* Aminorex.
'**Apisate**' *see* Amfepramone.
'**Apliobal**' *see* Alprenolol.
'**Aplodan**' *see* Creatinolphosphate.
APOATROPINE (atropamine; atropyl-
tropeine).
Apocupreine *see* Apoquinine.
APOCYNIN (acetovanillone; 4′-hydroxy-3′-
methoxyacetophenone).
'**Apodrine**' *see* Norephedrine.
Apoephedrine *see* Norephedrine.
Apolate *see* Sodium apolate.
APOMORPHINE (10,11-dihydroxy-6-
methyl-4H-dibenzo(de,g)quinoline; 10,11-

dihydroxyaporphine).
APOMORPHINE METHYL BROMIDE
('bromophin', 'euporphin').
Apomorphine 10-methyl ether *see* Mor-
phothebaine.
'**Aponal**' *see* Doxepin.
'**Aponeuron**' *see* Amphetaminil.
'**Apophedrine**' *see* Norephedrine.
APOPINENE (6,6-dimethyl-2-norpinene;
6,6-dimethylbicyclo(3,1,1)hept-2-ene).
APOQUININE (apocupreine; demethylated
quinine).
APORPHINE (6-methyl-4H-dibenzo(de,g)-
quinoline).
'**Apothesine**' *see* Cinnacaine.
'**Apothyrin**' *see* Diiodotyrosine.
'**Apralan**' *see* Apramycin.
APRAMYCIN** (4-*O*-[3α-amino-6α-[(4-
amino-4-deoxy-α-D-glucopyranosyl)oxy]-
2,3,4,4aβ,6,7,8,8aα-octahydro-8β-
hydroxy-7β-(methylamino)pyrano(3,2-b)-
pyran-2α-yl]-2-deoxy-D-streptamine;
EL-857; 'ambylan', 'apralan').
APRENAL (tr) (*N*-(3-diethylaminopropyl)-
2,2-diphenylacetamide; diphenylacetic acid
diethylaminopropylamide).
'**Apresoline**' *see* Hydralazine.
Apressin (tr) *see* Hydralazine.
APRINDINE*** (*N*-(3-diethylaminopropyl)-
N-phenyl-2-indanamine; *N*-(2,3-dihydro-
1H-inden-2-yl)-*N*′,*N*′-diethyl-1,3-
propanediamine; AC-1802; 'fibocil',
'fiboran').
'**Aprinox**' *see* Bendroflumethiazide.
'**Apritox**' *see* Trichloronat.
APROBARBITAL*** (5-allyl-5-isopropylbar-
bituric acid; allypropymal; allopropylbar-
bital; aprobarbital sodium).
'**Aprobit**' *see* Promethazine hydroxyethyl
chloride.
APROFENE*** (2-diethylaminoethyl 2,2-di-
phenylpropionate; aprophen; 'spasmadryl').
'**Apromal**' *see* Acetylcarbromal with
paracetamol.
APRONAL (1-(2-isopropyl-3-pentenoyl)urea;
allylisopropylacetylurea; apronalid;
'sedormid').
Apronalid *see* Apronal.
Aprophen (tr) *see* Aprofene.
'**Aprosone**' *see* 4-Chloro-2-methylphenoxy)-
acetic acid.
APROTININ** (kallikrein-trypsin inhibitor;
Frey inhibitor; RP-9921; 'antagosan',
'antilysin', 'contrical', 'contrykal',
'trascolan', 'trasylol', 'zymofren').
APT *see* Antimonyl potassium tartrate.
'**Aptine**' *see* Alprenolol.
APTOCAINE*** (*N*-(2-pyrrolidin-1-yl-
propionyl)-*o*-toluidine; 2′-methyl-2-pyr-
rolidin-1-ylpropionanilide; 2-methyl-2-
pyrrolidin-1-yl-*o*-acetotoluidide; aptocaine
hydrochloride; 'pirothesin').
'**Aptrol**' *see* *p*-Methylamphetamine.
'**Apurin**' *see* Allopurinol.
APY-606 *see* Spiclomazine.
'**Apyron**' *see* Calcium acetylsalicylate; Mag-
nesium acetylsalicylate.

AQ-110 *see* Tretoquinol.
AQL-208 *see* Tretoquinol.
'Aquachloral' *see* Chloral hydrate.
'Aquacide' *see* Diquat.
'Aqualose' *see* Polyoxyl lanolin.
'Aquamollin' *see* Tetrasodium edetate.
'Aquamox' *see* Quinethazone.
'Aquaphor' *see* Xipamide.
'Aquatensen' *see* Methyclothiazide.
'Aquedux' *see* Clofenamide.
'Aquex' *see* Clopamide.
AQUOCOBALAMIN (vitamin B₁₂ᵦ).
  See also Hydroxocobalamin.
Aquocobinamide cyanide *see* Cyanocobalamin.
Ara-A *see* Vidarabine.
9β-ᴅ-Arabinofuranosyladenine *see*
  Vidarabine.
Arabinofuranosylcytosine *see* Cytarabine.
Arabinofuranosyl-5-fluorocytosine *see*
  Flucytosine arabinoside.
Arabinofuranosylguanine *see* Guanine
  arabinoside.
Arabinofuranosylpurine-6-thiol *see*
  Mercaptopurine arabinoside.
Araboascorbic acid *see* Isoascorbic acid.
Ara-C *see* Cytarabine.
Arachic acid *see* Arachidic acid.
ARACHIDIC ACID (eicosanoic acid; arachic
  acid).
ARACHIDONIC ACID (5,8,11,14-eicosatetraenoic acid).
ARACHIS OIL* (ground-nut oil; nut oil;
  peanut oil).
ARACHIS OIL EMULSION ('prosparol').
Ara-CMP *see* Cytarabine 5'-phosphate.
Ara-cytidine *see* Cytarabine.
'Aracytine' *see* Cytarabine.
Ara-FC *see* Flucytosine arabinoside.
Ara-G *see* Guanine arabinoside.
'Aralen' *see* Chloroquine.
ARALKONIUM CHLORIDE* (alkyldimethyl(3,4-dichlorobenzyl)ammonium
  chloride(s); 'dynaltone', 'dynium chloride').
'Aramercur' *see* Chlormerodrin.
'Aramine' *see* Metaraminol.
'Aramite' *see* tert-Butylphenoxyisopropyl
  chloroethyl sulfite.
ARANOTIN* (5,5a,13,13a-tetrahydro-5,13-
  dihydroxy-8H,16H-7a,15a-epidithio-7H,
  15H-bisoxepino(3',4':4,5)pyrrolo(1,2-a:
  1',2'-d)pyrazine-7,15-dione 5-acetate;
  L-53183).
'Aranthol' *see* N-Methylheptaminol.
'Arasan' *see* Thiram.
'Arathane' *see* Dinocap.
ARBAPROSTIL* ((E,Z)-(1R,2R,3R)-7-[3-
  hydroxy-2-[(3R)-(3-hydroxy-3-methyl-1-
  octenyl)]-5-oxocyclopentyl]hepten-5-oic
  acid).
Arbutin *see* Hydroquinone glucopyranoside.
'Arcanax' *see* Hydroxyzine.
ARC-I-K-1 *see* Metofoline.
'Arcobutine' *see* Mofebutazone.
'Arcolax' *see* Ispagula.
'Arcomonol' *see* Mofebutazone.
'Arcosal' *see* Tolbutamide.

'Arcton 6' *see* Dichlorodifluoromethane.
'Arcton 33' *see* Cryofluorane.
'Arcton 63' *see* Trichlorotrifluoroethane.
'Arcylate' *see* Sodium sulfosalicylate.
ARDF-26 *see* Gliquidone.
ARDMA *see* Puromycin aminonucleoside.
ARECAIDINE (1-methyl-1,2,5,6-tetrahydronicotinic acid; arecaine).
Arecaidine methyl ester *see* Arecoline.
Arecaine *see* Arecaidine.
Arecaline *see* Arecoline.
ARECOLINE (methyl 1,2,5,6-tetrahydro-1-
  methylnicotinate; arecaidine methyl ester;
  arecaline).
ARECOLINE-ACETARSOL (molecular
  compound of arecoline with acetarsol:
  'cestarsol', 'drocarbil', 'neumural',
  'tenoban').
'Arentyl' *see* Nortriptyline.
'Aresin' *see* Monolinuron.
'Aretit' *see* Dinoseb acetate.
'Arezine' *see* Monolinuron.
'Arfonad' *see* Trimetaphan camsilate.
'Argicillin' *see* Methocidin.
ARGININE*** (ʟ(+)-arginine; 2-amino-5-
  guanidovaleric acid; N⁵-amidinoornithine).
  See also Indometacin arginine salt.
ARGININE ASPARTATE ('sargenor').
ARGININE GLUTAMATE* (ʟ(+)-glutamic
  acid compound with ʟ(+)-arginine (1:1);
  'modumate').
ARGININE MALATE ('rocmaline').
ARGININE OXOGLURATE (arginine
  2-oxoglutarate; 'eucol').
8-Arginineoxytocin *see* Argiprestocin.
8-Argininevasopressin *see* Argipressin.
Arginine vasotocin *see* Argiprestocin.
ARGIPRESSIN* (8-argininevasopressin;
  AVP).
ARGIPRESTOCIN*** (8-arginineoxytocin;
  arginine vasotocin; vasotocin).
'Arichin' *see* Mepacrine.
'Aristocort' *see* Triamcinolone diacetate.
'Aristodan' *see* Triamcinolone.
'Aristoderm' *see* Triamcinolone acetonide.
ARISTOLOCHIC ACID (8-methoxy-3,4-
  methylenedioxy-10-nitrophenanthrene-1-
  carboxylic acid; 'descresept', 'tardolyt').
'Aristosol' *see* Triamcinolone acetonide
  sodium phosphate.
'Aristospan' *see* Triamcinolone hexacetonide.
'Arkitropin' *see* Homatropine methyl
  bromide.
'Arlacel(s)' *see under* Sorbitan(s).
'Arlef' *see* Flufenamic acid.
'Arlidin' *see* Buphenine.
'Arlytene' *see* Moxisylyte.
'Armazal' *see* Cyacetacide.
ARMIN (tr) (ethyl p-nitrophenyl ethylphosphonate; ethylethoxyphosphoryl p-nitrophenolate).
'Arocan' *see* Hexacamphamine.
'Aroclor' *see* Polychlorinated biphenyl
  mixture; Polychlorinated terphenyl mixture.
'Aroxine' *see* Forminitrazole.
'Arpezine' *see* Piperazine.
Arprocarb *see* Aminocarb *and* Propoxur.

'Arrhenal' see Disodium methanearsonate.
ARSACETIN (*N*-acetylarsanilic acid).
ARSACETIN SODIUM (sodium *N*-acetyl-arsanilate; 'arsanthran').
ARSANILIC ACID** (4-aminobenzene-arsonic acid).
m-**ARSANILIC ACID** (3-aminobenzene-arsonic acid).
o-**ARSANILIC ACID** (2-aminobenzene-arsonic acid).
'Arsanthran' see Arsacetin sodium.
'Arsemetine' see Emetine-acetarsol.
'Arsenamide' see Thiacetarsamide.
ARSENIC TRIOXIDE (arsenious acid; arsenious anhydride; arsenious oxide; white arsenic).
Arsenious acid see Arsenic trioxide.
Arsenious anhydride see Arsenic trioxide.
Arsenious oxide see Arsenic trioxide.
ARSENOBENZENE (arsenodibenzene; 'arzene').
Arsenophenolamine see Arsphenamine.
'Arsenyl' see Disodium methanearsonate.
'Arsinyl' see Disodium methanearsonate.
'Arsobal' see Melarsoprol.
ARSONOACETIC ACID (acetarsenic acid; acetarsonic acid; acetoarsinic acid).
ARSPHENAMINE* (3,3'-diamino-4,4'-dihydroxyarsenobenzene-diHCl; arsenophenolamine; arsphenolamine; Ehrlich 606; Ehrlich-Hatta preparation; NSC-3097; 'salvarsan').
Arsphendichloride see Dichlorophenarsine.
Arsphenolamine see Arsphenamine.
Arsphenoxide see Oxophenarsine.
ARSTHINOL** (cyclic 3-hydroxypropylene ester of 3-acetamido-4-hydroxydithiobenzenearsonous acid; 2-(3-acetamido-4-hydroxyphenyl)-1,3-dithia-2-arsacyclopentane-4-methanol; mercaptoarsenol; 'amoebal', 'balarsan', 'balarsen').
'Arsynal' see Disodium methanearsonate.
'Artalan' see Thiopropazate.
'Artamin' see Penicillamine.
'Artane' see Trihexyphenidyl.
Arterenol see Noradrenaline.
'Arthriticin' see Piperazine.
'Arthropan' see Choline salicylate.
'Arthrytin' see Amiodoxyl benzoate.
'Artosin' see Tolbutamide.
'Artricid' see Niflumic acid.
'Artrochin' see Chloroquine.
'Arvin' see Ancrod.
'Arvynol' see Ethchlorvynol.
'Arylid' see 4',5-Dichlorosalicylanilide.
'Arzene' see Arsenobenzene.
AS XVII see Trospium chloride.
AS-716 see Thenalidine.
AS-17665 see Nifurthiazole.
ASA-226 see Chlorazanil.
Asahina see Naringenin.
'Asahydrin' see Chlormerodrin.
ASALINE (tr) (*N*-[*N*-acetyl-3-[*p*-(bis(2-chloroethyl)amino)phenyl]alanyl]-DL-valine ethyl ester; *N*-acetylmerphalan valine peptide ethyl ester; *N*-(*N*-acetyl-DL-sarcolysyl)-DL-valine ethyl ester).

'Asaprol' see Calcinaphthol.
Asarabacca camphor see Asarone.
'Asarinin' see Sesamin.
ASARONE (*trans*-1-propenyl-2,4,5-trimethoxybenzene; asarabacca camphor; asarum).
β-**ASARONE** (*cis*-1-propenyl-2,4,5-trimethoxybenzene).
Asarum see Asarone.
'ASC-4' see Dibromsalan with tribromsalan.
'Ascabin' see Benzyl benzoate.
'Ascabiol' see Benzyl benzoate.
'Ascal' see Calcium acetylsalicylate.
'Ascarex' see Piperazine citrate.
'Ascaricum' see Ascaridole.
ASCARIDOLE (1,4-peroxido-2*p*-menthene; askaridol; 'ascaricum', 'ascarisin', 'vermidrageletten').
'Ascarisin' see Ascaridole.
ASCARYLOSE (3,6-bisdeoxy-L-mannose).
'Asciatine' see Butylchloralamidopyrine.
Ascophen (tr) see APC.
ASCORBIC ACID*** (enolic form of 3-oxo-L-gulofuranolactone; vitamin C; cevitamic acid; hexuronic acid; avitamic acid; xyloascorbic acid).
See also Acetylsalicylic acid with ascorbic acid; Dehydroascorbic acid; Galascorbin; Isoascorbic acid; Paracetamol with ascorbic acid; Potassium ascorbate-tannin complex; Sodium ascorbate; Tetracycline with ascorbic acid.
ASCORBIC ACID HYDROGEN PEROXIDE CUPRIC COMPLEX ('ascoxal').
ASCORBIC ACID-NICOTINAMIDE COMPLEX ('nicastubin', 'nicoscorbine').
ASCORBIC ACID-PYRIDOXINE COMPLEX ('pyridoscorbin').
ASCORBIC ACID WITH DISODIUM FRUCTOSE 1,6-DIPHOSPHATE ('fructergyl').
Ascorbo-2-phenylcinchoninic acid see Strontium ascorbophenylcinchoninate.
'Ascorphylline' see Choline theophyllinate *and* Etofylline.
'Ascoxal' see Ascorbic acid hydrogen peroxide cupric complex.
'Ascriptin' see Acetylsalicylic acid with aluminium magnesium hydroxide.
Asebogenol see Phloretin.
Asebotin see Phlorizin.
'Aseptanide' see Triclocarban.
'Aseptol' see 2-Phenolsulfanic acid.
'Aseptorid' see Sulfatolamide.
'Asevin' see Carbaril.
'Asferryl' see Iron arsenotartrate.
ASIATIC ACID (2,3,23-trihydroxyurs-12-en-28-oic acid).
ASIATICOSIDE (asiatic acid glycoside; 'madecassol').
'Asilone' see Dimeticone.
'Asipol' see Diphenylpiperidinopropane.
Askaridol see Ascaridole.
ASL-279 see Dopamine.
'Aslavital' see Procaine with vitamins.
'Asmapax' see Ephedrine resinate.

33

Asnase *see* L-Asparaginase.

'Aspaminol' *see* 1,1-Diphenyl-3-piperid-1-yl-1-butanol.

L-**ASPARAGINASE** (L-asparagine aminohydrolase from *Esch. coli* cultures; asnase; colaspase; ATCC-9367; Fb-6366; NSC-109229; 'crasnitin', 'kidrolase', 'krasnitin').

ASPARAGINE (2-aminosuccinamic acid; aspartamic acid).

L-**Asparagine aminohydrolase** *see* L-Asparaginase.

Asparaginic acid *see* Aspartic acid.

'Aspardoxine' *see* Pyridoxine aspartate.

ASPARTAME*** (3-amino-*N*-(α-carboxyphenethyl)succinamic acid *N*-methyl ester; 3-amino-*N*-(α-methoxycarbonylphenethyl)-succinamic acid; L-aspartyl-L-phenylalanine methyl ester; 'equa', 'trisweet').

Aspartamic acid *see* Asparagine.

ASPARTAMIDE (2-aminosuccinamide).

ASPARTIC ACID** (aminosuccinic acid).
See also Arginine aspartate; Ferrous aspartate; Magnesium aspartate; Ornithine aspartate; Potassium aspartate; Pyridoxine aspartate.

25-L-Aspartic acid-26-L-alanine-27-glycine-30-L-glutamine-30-L-serine α$^{1-39}$-**corticotrophin**(pig) *see* Seractide.

ASPARTOCIN** (antibiotic from *Str. griseus* var. *spiralis*; (A-8999).

L-**Aspartyl-L-phenylalanine methyl ester** *see* Aspartame.

L-**Aspartyl-L-tyrosyl-L-methionylglycyl-L-tryptophyl-L-methionyl-L-aspartyl-phenyl-L-alaninamide hydrogen sulfate (ester)** *see* Sincalide.

'Aspegic' *see* Lysine acetylsalicylate.

Aspergillin O *see* Brinase.

Aspergillus fumigatus, antibiotic, *see* Fumagillin.

Aspergillus giganteus, antibiotic, *see* Nifungin.

Aspergillus glaucus, antibiotic, *see* Mitosper.

Aspergillus ochraceus, fibrinolytic enzyme, *see* Ocrase.

Aspergillus oryzae, fibrinolytic enzyme, *see* Brinase.

Aspergillus restrictus, antibiotic, *see* Mitogillin.

ASPERLIN*** (6,7-epoxy-4,5-dihydroxy-2-octenoic acid δ-lactone acetate; 6-(1,2-epoxypropyl)-5,6-dihydro-5-hydroxy-2H-pyran-2-one acetate; U-13933).

ASPIDINOL (2′,6′-dihydroxy-4′-methoxy-3′-methylbutyrophenone; 4-butyryl-2-methyl-phloroglucinol-1-methyl ether).

'Aspiral' *see* Amyl nitrite.

'Aspirin' *see* Acetylsalicylic acid.

'Aspogen' *see* Aluminium glycinate.

'Aspriodine' *see* Iodoacetylsalicylic acid.

Asta-4828 *see* Trofosfamide.

Asta-4942 *see* Ifosfamide.

Asta C-4898 *see* Dilazep.

'Asterit' *see* Chloroxylenol.

'Asterol' *see* Dimazole.

'Asthmalitan' *see* Isoetarine.

'Asthmolysin' *see* Diprophylline.

'Astiban' *see* Sodium stibocaptate.

'Astiban acid' *see* Stibocaptic acid.

'Astinon' *see* Fludrocortisone acetate.

'Astomol' *see* Mebanazine.

'Astonin' *see* Fludrocortisone.

Astra-1512 *see* Prilocaine.

Astra-1572 *see* Iron sorbitex.

Astra-3476 *see* Ciclonium bromide.

Astra-4241 *see* Imiclopazine.

'Astrafer' *see* Dextriferron.

'Astrobain' *see* Ouabain.

'Astrumal' *see* Potassium perchlorate.

'Asturidon' *see* Secbutabarbital.

'Astyryl' *see* Glycarsamide.

'Asuccin' *see* Succinic acid.

ASULAM*** (methyl [(*p*-aminophenyl)-sulfonyl]carbamate; methyl sulfanilyl-carbamate; 'asulox').

'Asulox' *see* Asulam.

'Asuntol' *see* Coumafos.

'Asverin' *see* Tipepidine.

3A-T *see* Amitrole.

AT-7 *see* Hexachlorophene.

'AT-10' *see* Dihydrotachysterol.

AT-17 *see* Dimemorfan.

AT-101 *see* Isosorbide.

AT-581 *see* Ocaphane.

AT-1258 *see* Nitrocaphane.

ATA *see* Amitrole.

'Atamine' *see* Mepyramine.

'Ataractan' *see* Azacyclonol.

'Atarax' *see* Hydroxyzine.

ATCC-9376 *see* L-Asparaginase.

'Atelor' *see* Dimazole.

'Atelora' *see* Dimazole.

ATENOLOL** (*p*-(2-hydroxy-3-isopropyl-aminopropoxy)phenylacetamide; 1-(*p*-carbamoylmethylphenoxy)-3-isopropyl-amino-2-propanol; ICI-66082; 'tenormine').

'Atensine' *see* Diazepam.

'Aterosol' *see* Clofibrate.

'Atgard' *see* Dichlorvos.

'Atherolip' *see* Clofibrate.

'Atheropront' *see* Clofibrate.

'Athyromazole' *see* Carbimazole.

'Atilon' *see* Acedapsone.

'Ativan' *see* Lorazepam.

'Atlasetox' *see* Demephion-O plus Demephion-S.

ATOLIDE*** (2-amino-4′-diethylamino-*o*-benzotoluidide).

'Atonyl' *see* Carbachol.

'Atorel' *see* Inosine.

'Atoxatrin' *see* Homatropine methyl nitrate.

ATP *see* Adenosine triphosphate.

'Atractyl' *see* Isoamyl mandelate.

'Atratan' *see* Atropine tannate.

'Atratol' *see* Atrazine.

ATRATON*** (*N*-ethyl-6-methoxy-*N*′-(1-methylethyl)-1,3,5-triazine-2,4-diamine; 2-ethylamino-4-isopropylamino-6-methoxy-*s*-triazine; atratone; 'gestamin').

Atratone *see* Atraton.

'Atravet' *see* Acepromazine.

'Atraxin' *see* Meprobamate.

ATRAZINE*** (2-chloro-4-ethylamino-6-isopropylamino-s-triazine; 6-chloro-N-ethyl-N'-(1-methylethyl)-1,3,5-triazine-2,4-diamine; G-30027; W-6693; 'aatrex', 'atratol', 'gesaprim', 'hungazin').

Atremon (tr) see Chromocarb.

'Atrilon 5' see Propatyl nitrate.

'Atrinal' see Atropine sulfuric ester.

'Atriphos' see Adenosine triphosphate.

Atrochin see Scopolamine.

'Atrol' see Deanol.

ATROLACTAMIDE (α-methylmandel-amide; 2-hydroxy-2-phenylpropionamide; M-144; 'themisone').

ATROLACTIC ACID (α-methylmandelic acid; α-phenyllactic acid; 2-hydroxy-2-phenylpropionic acid).

Atrolactic acid tropine ester see Pseudo-atropine.

ATROMENTIN (3,6-bis(p-hydroxyphenyl)-2,5-dihydroxy-p-benzoquinone).

ATROMEPINE*** (tropine (−)-α-methyl-tropate; tropine 2-methyl-2-phenylhydr-acrylate; (−)-3α-tropanyl 2-methyl-2-phenylhydracrylate; levomepate; 'normo-spas').

(+)-ATROMEPINE (TMT).

(−)-Atromepine see Atromepine.

'Atromid' see Clofibrate with androsterone.

'Atromidin' see Clofibrate.

'Atromid-S' see Clofibrate.

Atropamine see Apoatropine.

ATROPINE (tropine DL-tropate; atropine sulfate).
See also below and Diphenoxylate with atropine.

Atropine p-biphenylylmethyl bromide see Xenytropium.

ATROPINE CAMPHORATE WITH SCOPOLAMINE CAMPHORATE ('aeron').

Atropine L-isomer see Hyoscyamine.

ATROPINE METHOBROMIDE (8-methyl-atropinium bromide; atropine methyl bromide; tropin; 'mintussin').

ATROPINE METHONITRATE*** (8-methylatropinium nitrate; atropine methyl nitrate; 'ekomine', 'eumydrin', 'harvatrate', 'metanite', 'metropine', 'pylostrophin').

Atropine methyl bromide see Atropine methobromide.

Atropine methyl nitrate see Atropine metho-nitrate.

ATROPINE OCTYL BROMIDE (octyl-atropinium bromide; AD-122).

ATROPINE OXIDE*** (atropine N-oxide; atropine aminoxide; atropine oxide hydro-chloride; aminoxytropine tropate: genatro-pine; 'tropino', 'xtro').

Atropine propionate ester see Prampine.

ATROPINE SULFATE ESTER ('atrinal').

ATROPINE TANNATE ('atratan').

Atropyltropeine see Apoatropine.

Atroquin see Scopolamine.

DL-Atroscine see Hyoscine.

L-Atroscine see Scopolamine.

'Atrovent' see Ipratropium bromide.

'Atumin' see Dicycloverine.

'Aturbal' see Phenglutarimide.

'Aturbane' see Phenglutarimide.

'Augmentin' see Tiformin.

'Auraloin' see Barbaloin.

'Auramine' see Aurothioglucose.

AURANOFIN** ((1-thio-β-D-glucopyrano-sato)(triethylphosphine)gold 2,3,4,6-tetra-acetate.

AURANTIIN (naringenin 7-rutoside; narin-genin 7-rhamnoglucoside; isohesperidin; naringin; naringoside).

'Aurcoloid-198' see Gold([198]Au) colloidal.

'Aureocina' see Chlortetracycline.

'Aureomycin' see Chlortetracycline.

'Aureoquin' see Quinetalate.

'Aureotan' see Aurothioglucose.

'Auricidin' see Sodium aurotiosulfate.

Auroallylthioureidobenzoate see Sodium auroallylthioureidobenzoate.

'Aurolin' see Sodium aurotiosulfate.

α-Auromercaptoacetanilide see Aurothio-glycanide.

'Auromyose' see Aurothioglucose.

'Auropex' see Sodium aurotiosulfate.

'Auropin' see Sodium aurotiosulfate.

'Aurosan' see Sodium aurotiosulfate.

AUROTHIOGLUCOSE* (S-gold deriv. of thioglucose; 'aureotan', 'auromyose', 'aurumine', 'oronol', 'romosol', 'solganal-B').

AUROTHIOGLYCANIDE*** (α-auromer-captoacetanilide; S-gold derivative of 2-mercaptoacetanilide; 'lauron').

Aurothiomalate see Sodium aurothiomalate.

'Aurothion' see Sodium aurotiosulfate.

Aurothiosinamine-m-benzoic acid see Sodium auroallylthioureidobenzoate.

Aurothiosulfate see Sodium aurotiosulfate.

'Aurumine' see Aurothioglucose.

'Autan' see Diethyltoluamide.

'Auxiloson' see Dexamethasone isonicotinate.

'Auxisone' see Dexamethasone isonicotinate.

'Avacan' see Camylofin.

'Avadex' see Diallate.

'Avadex BW' see Triallate.

'Avafortan' see Camylofin with novamin-sulfon.

'Avantin' see 2-Propanol.

'Avatec' see Lasalocid.

'Avazyme' see Chymotrypsin.

'Aventol' see Aceglutamide.

'Aventyl' see Nortriptyline.

'Aversan' see Disulfiram.

'Aviamide-6' see Policapram.

'Avicol' see Chlorphentermine.

'Avicol SL' see Cloforex.

'Avidin' see Antibiotin.

'Aviester' see Pegoterate.

'Avil' see Pheniramine p-aminosalicylate.

'Avinar' see Uredepa.

'Avipron' see Chlorphentermine.

Avitamic acid see Ascorbic acid.

'Avlocardyl' see Propranolol.

'Avloclor' see Chloroquine.

'Avlosulfon' see Dapsone.

'Avlosulfone-EOS' see Dapsonedisulfonic acid disodium salt.

'Avolin' see Dimethyl phthalate.

'**Avomine**' *see* Promethazine teoclate.
AVOPARCIN*** (glycopeptide antibiotic from *Str. candidus*).
Avorin *see* Frangulin.
AVP *see* Argipressin.
AW-142333 *see* Perlapine.
AW-142446 *see* Clodazone.
'**Axeen**' *see* Proxibarbal.
Axerophthal *see* Retinal.
Axerophthol *see* Retinol.
'**Axiquel**' *see* Valnoctamide.
AY-5312 *see* Chlorhexidine.
AY-5406-1 *see* Benactyzine.
AY-5710 *see* Magaldrate.
AY-5810 *see* Pentapiperium metilsulfate.
AY-6108 *see* Ampicillin.
AY-8682 *see* Cyheptamide.
AY-11440 *see* Clogestone acetate.
AY-17611 *see* Digitoxigenin hemisuccinate.
AY-20385 *see* Nequinate.
AY-20694 *see* Dexpropranolol.
AY-21011 *see* Practolol.
AY-21367 *see* Furobufen.
AY-21554 *see* Talopram.
AY-22214 *see* Taclamine.
AY-22241 *see* Actodigin.
AY-22469 *see* Deprostil.
AY-23028 *see* Butaclamol.
AY-23289 *see* Prodolic acid.
AY-23713 *see* Pirandamine.
AY-23946 *see* Tandamine.
AY-56031 *see* Prothipendyl.
AY-61122 *see* Metallibure.
AY-61123 *see* Clofibrate.
AY-62013 *see* Etoglucid.
AY-62014 *see* Butriptyline.
AY-62021 *see* Clopenthixol.
AY-62022 *see* Medrogestone.
AY-64043 *see* Propranolol.
'**Ayphylline**' *see* Diprophylline.
AZ-8 *see* Guaiazulene.
10-Azaanthracene *see* Acridine.
5-Aza-10-arsenaanthracene *see* Phenarsazine.
Azabicyclane *see* Anazocine.
3-AZABICYCLO(3.3.1)NONANE (3,5-propanopiperidine; isogranatanine).
9-Azabicyclo(3.3.1)nonane *see* Granatanine.
9-Azabicyclo(3.3.1)nonan-3-ol *see* Granatoline.
1-Azabicyclo(2.2.2)octane *see* Quinuclidine.
8-Azabicyclo(3.2.1)octane *see* Nortropane.
1-(3-Azabicyclo(3.3.0)oct-3-yl)-3-(*p*-toluenesulfonyl)urea *see* Gliclazide.
AZABON** (3-sulfanilyl-3-azabicyclo(3.2.2)-nonane).
AZABUPERONE** (4'-fluoro-4-(hexahydropyrrolo(1,2-a)pyrazin-2(1H)-yl)butyrophenone; 2-[3-(*p*-fluorobenzoyl)propyl]-hexahydropyrrolo(1,2-a)pyrazine).
AZACLORINE** (2-chloro-10-[3-(hexahydropyrrolo(1,2-a)pyrazin-2(1H)-yl)-propionyl]phenothiazine; 2(1H)-[2-[(2-chlorophenothiazin-10-yl)carbonyl]ethyl]-hexahydropyrrolo(1,2-a)pyrazine; 2-chloro-phenothiazin-10-yl 2-(hexahydropyrrolo-(1,2-a)pyrazin-2(1H)-yl)ethyl ketone.)

'**Azacon**' *see* Prothipendyl.
'**Azacortid**' *see* Fluazacort.
AZACOSTEROL*** (17β-[(3-dimethylamino-propyl)methylamino]androst-5-en-3β-ol; azacosterol dihydrochloride; azacosterol hydrochloride; 20,25-diazacholesterol dihydrochloride; SC-12937; 'ornitrol').
Azacycloheptane *see* Hexamethylenimine.
Azacycloheptatriene *see* Azepine.
2-(Azacycloheptyl)ethyl *m*-nitrophenyl ketone *see* Fenitron.
AZACYCLONOL*** (α,α-diphenyl-α-piperid-4-ylmethanol; α-(4-piperidyl)benzhydrol; α,α-diphenyl-4-piperidinemethanol; 'ataractan', 'calmeran', 'frenquel', 'Mer-17', 'psychosan').
Azacyclooctane *see* Heptamethylenimine.
1-[2-(1-Azacyclooctyl)ethyl]guanidine *see* Guanethidine.
Azacyclopropane *see* Aziridine.
5-AZACYTIDINE (4-amino-*s*-triazin-2-one riboside; NSC-102816).
AZAFEN (tr) (10-methyl-2-(4-methylpiper-azin-1-yl)-3,4-diazaphenoxazine; azaphen).
AZAFTOCINE** (10-(3-(hexahydropyrrolo-(1,2-a)pyrazin-2(1H)-yl)propionyl)-2-trifluoromethylphenothiazine; hexahydro-2(1H)-(2-((2-trifluoromethylphenothiazin-10-yl)carbonyl)ethyl)pyrrolo(1,2-a)-pyrazine; 2-(hexahydropyrrolo(1,2-a)-pyrazin-2(1H)-yl)ethyl 2-trifluoromethyl-phenothiazin-10-yl ketone).
8-AZAGUANINE (5-amino-7-hydroxy-1H-*v*-triazolo(4,5-d)pyrimidine; NSC-749; 'azan', 'guanazolo').
'**Azak**' *see* Terbucarb.
AZALOMYCIN*** (azalomycin F; antibiotic from *Str. hygroscopicus* var. *azalomyceticus*).
Azalomycin F* *see* Azalomycin.
Azamethone *see* Azamethonium.
AZAMETHONIUM BROMIDE*** (or **CHLORIDE**) (3-methyl-3-azapentane-1,5-bis(dimethylethylammonium bromide); [(methylimino)diethylene]bis(ethyldi-methylammonium bromide); *N,N,N',N'',N''*-pentamethyldiethylenetriamine dietho-bromide; azamethone; azapenthyleneam-monium; pentamethazene; pentamine; C-9295; P-9295; 'ganlion', 'pendiomid').
Azamin *see* Melamine.
'**Azan**' *see* Azaguanine.
AZANATOR*** (5-(1-methyl-4-piperidylid-ene)-5H-(1)benzopyrano(2,3-b)pyridine).
AZANATOR MALEATE* (azanator (Z)-2-butanedioate (1:1); azanator maleate (1:1); Sch-15280).
5-AZAOROTIC ACID (*s*-triazine-2,4-dione-6-carboxylic acid).
3-Azapentane-1,5-diamine *see* Diethyl-enetriamine.
Azapenthyleneammonium *see* Azame-thonium.
AZAPERONE*** (4'-fluoro-4-(4-pyrid-2-yl)-piperazin-1-yl)butyrophenone; 1-[3-(*p*-fluorobenzoyl)propyl]-4-pyrid-2-ylpiper-azine; R-1929; 'stresnil', 'suicalm').
AZAPETINE* (6-allyl-6,7-dihydro(5H)di-

benz(c,e)azepine; azapetine phosphate; Ro-2-3248; 'azephine', 'ilidar').

Azaphen *see* Azafen.

1-Azaphenothiazine *see* Pyrido(3,2-b)(1,4)-benzothiazine.

AZAPROCIN*** (3-cinnamyl-8-propionyl-3,8-diazabicyclo(3.2.1)octane).

AZAPROPAZONE*** (5-dimethylamino-9-methyl-2-propyl-1H-pyrazolo(1,2-a)(1,2,4)-benzotriazine-1,3(2H)-dione; cinnopropazone; 3-(dimethylamino)-1,2-dihydro-7-methyl-1,2-(propylmalonyl)-1,2,4-benzotriazine; apazone; Mi-85; 'prolixan 300', 'rheumox', 'sinnamin').

8-AZAPURINE (*v*-triazolo(3,4-d)pyrimidine).

AZAPYRROLIDINIUM (3-methyl-3-azapentamethylene-1,5-bis(1-methylpyrrolidinium salt(s)); bis[2-(1-methylpyrrolidinium)ethyl]methylamine).

AZAQUINZOLE*** (1,3,4,6,7,11b-hexahydro-2H-pyrazino(2,1-a)isoquinoline).

AZARIBINE*** (2-(β-D-ribofuranosyl-*as*-triazine-3,5(2H,4H)-dione 2′,3′,5′-triacetate; 2′,3′,5′,tri-*O*-acetyl-6-azauridine; riboazauracil; azauracil riboside triacetate; azauridine triacetate; CB-304; 'triazure').

AZASERINE*** (L-serine diazoacetate ester; diazoacetylserine; *O*-diazoacetyl-L-serine; AZS; NSC-742).

AZASPIRIUM CHLORIDE** (8,9-dihydro-4,11-dimethoxy-9-methylene-5-oxospiro-[5H-furo(3′,2′:6,7)(1)benzopyrano(3,2-c)-pyridine-7(6H),1′-piperidinium] chloride).

[2-(6-Azaspiro(2.5)oct-6-yl)ethyl]guanidine *see* Spirgetine.

AZATADINE*** (6,11-dihydro-11-(1-methylpiperid-4-ylidene)-5H-benzo(5,6)cyclohepta(1,2-b)pyridine).

AZATADINE MALEATE ('idulian').

AZATEPA*** (*P,P*-bis(1-aziridinyl)-*N*-ethyl-*N*-(1,3,4-thiadiazol-2-yl)phosphinic amide; azetepa; CL-25477).

3-Aza-1-thiaazulen-2-one *see* Cycloheptathiazol-2-one.

1-Aza-4-thia-2,3,5,6-dibenzocycloheptadiene *see* 10,11-Dihydrodibenzo(b,f)(1,4)-thiazepine.

AZATHIOPRINE*** (6-(1-methyl-4-nitroimidazol-5-ylthio)purine; NSC-39084; BW-57-322; 'imuran', 'imurel').

AZATHYMIDINE (6-azathymine desoxyriboside).

AZATHYMINE (6-methyl-1,4,6-triazine-3,5(2H,4H)dione; NSC-3426).

AZAURACIL (2,3,4,5-tetrahydro-1,2,4-triazine-3,5-dione; *as*-triazine-3,5(2H,4H)-dione; 6-AZ; AzU; NSC-3425).

AZAURIDINE (2-β-D-ribofuranosyl-*as*-triazine-3,5(2H,4H)-dione; 6-azauracil riboside; AzUR; NSC-32074).

Azauridine triacetate *see* Azaribine.

AZELAIC ACID (1,7-heptanedicarboxylic acid; anchoic acid; lepargylic acid; nonanedioic acid).

'Azephine' *see* Azapetine.

Azepinamide *see* Glypinamide.

AZEPINE (azacycloheptatriene).

Azetepa* *see* Azatepa.

AZIDAMFENICOL*** (D(−)-*threo*-2-azido-*N*-[β-hydroxy-α-(hydroxymethyl)-*p*-nitrophenethyl]acetamide; D(−)-*threo*-2-azido-acetamido-1-(*p*-nitrophenyl)-1,3-propanediol; azido-amphenicol; 'leukomycin-*N*′).

Azidithion *see* Menazon.

2-Azidoacetamido-1-(*p*-nitrophenyl)-1,3-propanediol *see* Azidamfenicol.

Azido-amphenicol *see* Azidamfenicol.

D-(−)-(α-Azidobenzyl)penicillin *see* Azidocillin.

AZIDOCILLIN*** (6-D(−)-2-azido-2-phenylacetamido)penicillanic acid; D-(−)-(α-azidobenzyl)penicillin; BRL-2534; SPC-297-D; 'globacillin', 'nalpen', 'purapen').

2-Azido-4-isopropylamino-6-(methylthio)-*s*-triazine *see* Aziprotryne.

4-Azido-*N*-(1-methylethyl)-6-(methylthio)-1,3,5-triazin-2-amine *see* Aziprotryne.

6-(2-Azido-2-phenylacetamido)penicillanic acid *see* Azidocillin.

Azidophosphonic bisdimethylamide *see* Mazidox.

Azindole *see* Benzimidazole.

Azinepurine *see* Pteridine.

AZINPHOS-ETHYL* (*O,O*-diethyl *S*-(4-oxobenzotriazin-3-ylmethyl) phosphorodithioate; *O,O*-diethyl phosphorodithioate *S*-ester with 3-(mercaptomethyl)-1,2,3-benzotriazin-4(3H)-one; benzotriazinylmethyldithiophosphoric acid diethyl ester; triazotion; 'ethyl-gusathion', 'ethyl guthion', 'gusathion A').

AZINPHOS-METHYL* (*O,O*-dimethyl *S*-(4-oxobenzotriazin-3-ylmethyl) phosphorodithioate; *O,O*-dimethyl phosphorodithioate *S*-ester with 3-(mercaptomethyl)-1,2,3-benzotriazin-4(3H)-one; benzotriazinylmethyldithiophosphoric acid dimethyl ester; Bayer-17147; methylthiazothion; methyltriazotion; 'gusathion', 'gusathion M', 'guthion', 'methyl guthion').

AZINPHOS-METHYL PLUS DEMETON-S-METHYLSULFON ('gusathion-MS').

AZINTAMIDE*** (2-(6-chloropyridazin-3-ylthio)-*N,N*-diethylacetamide; ST-9067).

AZIPROTRYNE* (2-azido-4-isopropylamino-6-(methylthio)-*s*-triazine; 4-azido-*N*-(1-methylethyl)-6-(methylthio)-1,3,5-triazin-2-amine; C-7019; 'brassoran', 'mesoranil').

AZIRIDINE (ethylenimine; azacyclopropane; dimethylenimine).

1-AZIRIDINECARBOXYLIC ACID (*N,N*-ethylenecarbamic acid).

1-AZIRIDINEETHANOL (1-(2-hydroxyethyl)aziridine; 2-aziridin-1-ylethanol; hydroxyimine).

Aziridine polymer with diepoxybutane *see* Polyetadene.

2-Aziridin-1-ylethanol *see* 1-Aziridineethanol.

AZLOCILLIN* (6-[D-2-(2-oxoimidazoline-1-carboxamido)-2-phenylacetamido]penicillanic acid; BAY e 6905).

'Azoangin' *see* Chrysoidine citrate.

AZOBENZENE (azodibenzene; phenylazobenzene).

1,1'-Azobis(chloroformamidine) *see* Chlorazodin.

1,1'-Azobis (*N,N*-**dimethylformamide**) *see* Diamide.

1,1'-Azobisformamide *see* Azoformamide.

1,1'-Azobis(3-methyl-2-phenyl-1H-imidazo(1,2-a)pyridinium bromide) *see* Fazadinium bromide.

'Azochloramide' *see* Chlorazodin.

'Azodermin' *see* Acetamidoazotoluene.

p,p'-**Azodibenzoic acid bis(diethylamino-ethyl) ester** *see* Azoprocaine.

Azodicarbonamide *see* Azoformamide.

'Azodrin' *see* Monocrotophos.

'Azodyne' *see* Phenazopyridine.

Azoester *see* Methyl phenyldiazenecarboxylate.

AZOFORMAMIDE (1,1'-azobisformamide; azodicarbonamide; dicarbamoyldiimide).

'Azohel' *see* Chrysoidine citrate.

'Azoiodine' *see* Chrysoidine dihydriodide.

'Azojod' *see* Chrysoidine dihydriodide.

AZOLIMINE*** (2-imino-3-methyl-1-phenyl-4-imidazolidinone).

AZOLINIC ACID *see* Cinoxacin.

Azoniaspiro(3α-benzilyloxynortropane-8,1'-pyrrolidine) chloride *see* Trospium chloride.

Azophen *see* Phenazone.

Azophenylene *see* Phenazine.

AZOPROCAINE (4,4'-bis(2-diethylamino-carbethoxy)azobenzene; bis(2-diethyl-aminoethyl ester) of *p,p'*-azodibenzoic acid).

AZOPYRIDINE (azodipyridine; pyridylazo-pyridine).

'Azopyrine' *see* Salazosulfapyridine.

'Azorhodan' *see* Chrysoidine thiocyanate.

Azo rubine *see* Carmoisine.

Azorubrum *see* Bordeaux B.

AZOSEMIDE** (2-chloro-5-(1H-tetrazol-5-yl)-*N*⁴-2-thenylsulfanilamide; 2-[[3-chloro-4-sulfamoyl-6-(1H-tetrazol-5-yl)anilino]methyl]thiophene; 5-[4-chloro-5-sulfamoyl-2-(2-thenylamino)phenyl]-1H-tetrazole).

AZOSULFAMIDE (*N*⁴-(7-acetamido-3,6-disulfo-1-hydroxy-2-naphthaleneazo)sulfanilamide; 'drometil', 'neoprontosil', 'prontosil S', 'prontosil soluble').

AZOTHOATE* (*O*-[4-[(4-chlorophenyl)-azo]phenyl] *O,O*-dimethyl phosphorothioate; 4-chloro-4'-[(dimethoxyphosphinothioyl)oxy]azobenzene; 'slam').

AZOTOMYCIN*** (antibiotic from *Str. ambofaciens*; duazomycin B; antibiotic 1719; NSC-56654).

Azotoyperite *see* Chlormethine.

Azovan blue* *see* Evans blue.

Azoxodone (tr) *see* Pemoline.

AZS *see* Azaserine.

'Azudimidine' *see* Salazosulfadimidine.

AZULENE (cyclopentacycloheptene).

'Azulfidine' *see* Salazosulfapyridine.

'Azulon' *see* Guaiazulene.

AZURE A (3-amino-7-dimethylaminophen-azathionium chloride; *asym*. dimethylthionine chloride).

AZURE B (3-methylamino-7-dimethylamino-phenazathionium chloride; trimethylthionine chloride).

AZURE C (3-amino-7-methylaminophenaza-thionium chloride; methylthionine chloride).

AZURESIN* (complex of azure A with a carbacrylamine cation-exchange resin; 'diagnex-blue').

B

B-22 *see* Propham.
B-23 *see* Tifenamil.
B-44-P *see* Streptovaricin.
B-80 *see* Ibuprofen.
B-100 *see* Methaqualone.
B-346 *see* Prenylamine.
B-360 *see* Paroxypropione.
B-518 *see* Cyclophosphamide.
B-663 *see* Clofazimine.
B-907 *see* Pyrithione sodium.
B-1420 *see* Propanidid.
B-1500 *see* Mefruside.
B-5833 *see* Camazepam.
B-10610 *see* Meglumine iodoxamate.
B-35251 *see* Mitocromin.
B-64114 *see* Bumadizone.
BA-4164-8 *see* Diflumidone.

BA-4223 *see* Triflumidate.
Ba-5473 *see* Oxyphenonium.
Ba-5968 *see* Hydralazine.
Ba-10370 *see* Sulfachloropyridazine.
Ba-11391 *see* Xylometazoline.
Ba-18605 *see* Sulfapyrazole.
Ba-21401 *see* Tribenoside.
Ba-29038 *see* Boldenone undecenoate.
Ba-29837 *see* Deferoxamine.
Ba-30803 *see* Benzoctamine.
Ba-30920 *see* Tetracosactide.
Ba-31458 *see* Gestadienol acetate.
Ba-32644 *see* Niridazole.
Ba-33112 *see* Deferoxamine mesilate.
Ba-33902 *see* β-Angiotensin II.
Ba-34276 *see* Maprotiline.
Ba-34647 *see* Baclofen.

Ba-36278A *see* Cefacetrile.
Ba-39089 *see* Oxprenolol.
Ba-41795 *see* Codactide.
Ba-42915 *see* Tetracosactide zinc phosphate complex.
'Babesan' *see* Quinuronium sulfate.
'Baburon' *see* Quinuronium sulfate.
BACAMPICILLIN*** (ampicillin ester with ethyl 2-hydroxyethyl carbonate; 'penglobe').
'Bacarate' *see* Phendimetrazine.
'Bacdip' *see* Quintiofos.
Bacillosporin *see* Polymyxin.
Bacillus brevis, antibiotics *see* Gramicidin; Tyrothricin.
Bacillus cereus, enzyme *see* Penicillinase.
Bacillus colistinus var. polymyxa, antibiotic *see* Colistin.
Bacillus polymyxa, antibiotics *see* Colistin; Polymyxin B.
Bacillus subtilis, antibiotics *see* Bacitracin; Fluvomycin.
Bacillus subtilis, enzymes *see* Sutilains.
BACIMETHRIN (4-amino-5-hydroxymethyl-2-methoxypyrimidine; 4-amino-2-methoxy-5-pyrimidinemethanol).
BACITRACIN*** (basic polypeptide from *B. subtilis*).
See also Neomycin with bacitracin.
BACLOFEN*** (4-amino-3-(*p*-chlorophenyl)butyric acid; β-aminomethyl-*p*-chlorohydrocinnamic acid; β-(4-chlorophenyl)-GABA; Ba-34647; C-34647-Ba; 'lioresal').
'Bactocill' *see* Oxacillin.
'Bactol' *see* Clioquinol.
'Bactrim' *see* Co-trimoxazole.
'Bactrimel' *see* Co-trimoxazole.
'Badional' *see* Sulfathiourea.
'Baktolan' *see* Chlorocresol.
BAL *see* Dimercaprol.
'Balan' *see* Benfluralin.
'Balarsen' *see* Arsthinol.
'Baldon' *see* Dimethylthiambutene.
'Baltix' *see* Clofedanol.
'Balusil' *see* Proguanil.
BAMBERMYCIN** (antibiotic from *Str. bambergiensis*; bambermycins; moenomycin; 'flavomycin').
Bambermycins* *see* Bambermycin.
BAMETHAN*** (α-butylaminomethyl-*p*-hydroxybenzylalcohol; 2-butylamino-1-(*p*-hydroxyphenylethanol); bamethan sulfate; BOL; 'bupatol', 'butylsympathol', 'vasculat', 'vasculit').
See also Aminophenazone with bamethan.
BAMETHAN WITH INOSITOL NICOTINATE ('vasculnicol').
BAMIFYLLINE*** (8-benzyl-7-[2-[ethyl(2-hydroxyethyl)amino]ethyl]theophylline; bamifylline hydrochloride; benzetamofylline; AC-3810; BAX-2739z; CB-8102; 'trentadil').
BAMIPINE*** (4-(*N*-benzylanilino)-1-methylpiperidine; *N*-(1-methylpiperid-4-yl)-*N*-phenylbenzylamine; 'soventol').
Bamoxine* *see* Anidoxime.
'Bancaris' *see* Thenium closilate.
'Bandol' *see* Carbifene.

Banisterine *see* Harmine.
'Banistyl' *see* Dimetotiazine.
'Banminth' *see* Pyrantel tartrate.
'Banminth II' *see* Morantel tartrate.
'Banocide' *see* Diethylcarbamazine.
'Banol' *see* Carbanolate.
'Banthine' *see* Methantheline.
'Bantu' *see* Antu.
'Banvel' *see* Dicamba.
'Banvel D' *see* Dicamba dimethylamine.
'Banvel T' *see* Tricamba.
BAPN *see* Aminopropionitrile.
Baptitoxine *see* Cytisine.
BAQD-10 *see* Dequalinium.
'Barbadon' *see* Allopyrine.
BARBALOIN (*Aloe vera* glycoside; auraloin; curaçaolin).
Barbamate *see* Barban.
'Barbamon' *see* Barbipyrine.
Barbamyl (tr) *see* Amobarbital.
BARBAN* (4-chlorobut-2-yn-1-yl *m*-chlorocarbanilate; 4-chlorobut-2-yn-1-yl *N*-(*m*-chlorophenyl)carbamate; barbamate; chlorinat; klorinat; 'carbyne').
BARBEXACLONE** (1-cyclohexyl-2-methylaminopropyl 5-ethyl-5-phenylbarbiturate; compound of phenobarbital with *N*,α-dimethylcyclohexaneëthylamine; propylhexedrine phenobarbital compound; phenomitur; P-841; 'maliasin'). †
BARBIPYRINE (barbital deriv. of aminophenazone; pyrabarbital; verodon; 'barbamon', 'deltyl', 'peralga', 'veramon', 'veropyrin', 'verum').
BARBITAL*** (5,5-diethylbarbituric acid; barbitone; diemal; barbital sodium).
Barbitone* *see* Barbital.
BARBITURIC ACID (malonylurea; hexahydro-2,4,6-pyrimidinetrione).
'Barbonin' *see* Ethaverine.
'Barbosec' *see* Secobarbital.
'Baron' *see* Erbon.
'Barosil' *see* Dimeticone.
BAROTAL (5-(2-butenyl)-5-ethylbarbituric acid; 5-crotyl-5-ethylbarbituric acid; 'kalypnon').
'Barprine' *see* Allopyrine.
'Barquinol' *see* Clioquinol.
'BAS' *see* Benanserin.
BAS-3179F *see* Diethyltoluamide.
BAS-3510H *see* Bentazon.
'Basal-Noury' *see* Aluminium salicylate.
'Basamid' *see* Dazomet.
'Basanor' *see* Brompyrazon plus isonoruron.
'Basedol' *see* Aminothiazole.
'Basergin' *see* Ergometrine.
'Basfitox' *see* Buturon plus isonoruron.
'Basofortina' *see* Methylergometrine.
'Basolest' *see* Carbimazole.
'Basudin' *see* Dimpylate.
BATHOCUPROINE (2,9-dimethyl-4,7-diphenyl-1,10-phenanthroline sodium disulfonate; BSC).
BATHOPHENANTHROLINE (4,7-diphenyl-1,10-phenanthroline).
BATILOL** (3-octadecyloxy-1,2-propanediol; batyl alcohol).

'Batrafen' *see* Ciclopirox.
BATROXOBIN*** (thrombin-like enzyme from venom of *Bothrops atrox*; ST-25; 'defibrase').
BATROXOBIN WITH HEPARIN ('darkinal', 'diabtyl').
Batyl alcohol *see* Batilol.
Bax-422-Z *see* Albutoin.
Bax-1400-Z *see* Dimethadione.
BAX-1515 *see* Sutilains.
BAX-1526 *see* Chymopapain.
BAX-2739-Z *see* Bamifylline.
'Baxacor' *see* Etafenone.
'Baxarytmon' *see* Propafenone.
BAY.... *see also* Bayer....
BAY-1470 *see* Xylazine.
BAY-1521 *see* Noxiptyline.
BAY-4503 *see* Propiram fumarate.
BAY-41831 *see* Fenitrothion.
Bay-9002 *see* Naftalofos.
Bay-9015 *see* Niclofolan.
Bay-79770 *see* Chloraniformethan.
Bay-94337 *see* Metribuzin.
BAY a-1040 *see* Nifedipine.
BAY b-5097 *see* Clotrimazole.
BAY b-5369 *see* Carbenicillin.
BAY e-6905 *see* Azlocillin.
BAY f-1353 *see* Mezlocillin.
BAY-Va-1470 *see* Xylazine.
'Baycaine' *see* Tolycaine.
'Baycaron' *see* Mefruside.
'Baycid' *see* Fenthion.
'Baycillin' *see* Propicillin.
Bayer.... *see also* BAY....
Bayer-21/199 *see* Coumafos.
Bayer-73 *see* Clonitralide.
Bayer-186 *see* Clofedanol.
Bayer-205 *see* Suramin.
Bayer-693 *see* Ethylstibamine.
Bayer-1213 *see* Levomepromazine.
Bayer-1355 *see* Fencarbamide.
Bayer-1362 *see* Butaperazine.
Bayer-1420 *see* Propanidid.
Bayer-1470 *see* Xylazine.
Bayer-2349 *see* Metrifonate.
Bayer-2353 *see* Niclosamide.
Bayer-3231 *see* Triaziquone.
Bayer-3504 *see* Polyvinylpyridine *N*-oxide.
Bayer-5360 *see* Metronidazole.
Bayer-5400 *see* Sulfametoxydiazine.
Bayer-8169 *see* Demeton-O plus demeton-S.
Bayer-9002 *see* Naftalofos.
Bayer-9015 *see* Nicofolan.
Bayer-17147 *see* Azinphosmethyl.
Bayer-25141 *see* Fensulfothion.
Bayer-29493 *see* Fenthion.
Bayer-37344 *see* Methiocarb.
Bayer-38819 *see* Bis(*p*-chlorophenyl) acet-imidoylphosphoramidothioate.
Bayer-39007 *see* Propoxur.
Bayer-41831 *see* Fenitrothion.
Bayer-45515 *see* Parathion methyl.
Bayer-A-124 *see* Aminopromazine.
Bayer-L-13/59 *see* Metrifonate.
Bayer-S-1752 *see* Fenthion.
'Bayercillin' *see* Propicillin.
'Baygon' *see* Propoxur.

'Bayluscide' *see* Clonitralide.
'Bayrena' *see* Sulfametoxydiazine.
'Bayrusil' *see* Quinalphos.
'Bayten' *see* Fenthion.
'Baytex' *see* Fenthion.
'Baythion' *see* Phoxim.
'Baytinal' *see* Buthalital.
BBA *see* Benzylidenebutyric acid.
BBK-8 *see* Amikacin.
'B-B-S' *see* Benzyl benzoate.
BC-17 *see* Iodoxamic acid.
BC-40 *see* Hexadistigmine.
BC-48 *see* Demecarium.
BC-51 *see* Distigmine.
BC-105 *see* Pizotifen.
(−)-BC-2627 *see* Butorphanol.
BCNU *see* Carmustine.
BCP *see* Bucolome.
BCS *see* Bathocuproine.
BDH-312 *see* Mephenesin.
BDH-1298 *see* Megestrol.
BDH-1921 *see* Melengestrol.
BE-419 *see* Ioglycamic acid.
BE-426 *see* Adipiodone.
Be-724-A *see* Bendroflumethiazide.
'Beaprine' *see* Carsalam.
'Beatiline' *see* Benactyzine.
'Beatol' *see* Amobarbital.
BEBEERINE (D-bebeerine; chondodendrine; chondrodendrine; pelosine).
'Becantal' *see* Sodium dibunate.
'Becantex' *see* Sodium dibunate.
Becanthone* *see* Becantone.
BECANTONE** (1-[[2-ethyl-(2-hydroxy-2-methylpropyl)amino]ethylamino]-4-methylthioxanthen-9-one; becanthone; WIN-13820).
'Becantyl' *see* Sodium dibunate.
'Becilan' *see* Pyridoxine.
BECLAMIDE** (*N*-benzyl-3-chloropropion-amide; benzchlorpropamide; chloracon; chloroethylphenamide; 'hibicon', 'nydrane', 'posedrine').
BECLOBRATE** (ethyl (±)-2-[[α-(*p*-chlorophenyl)-*p*-tolyl]oxy]-2-methyl-butyrate).
BECLOMETASONE*** (9α-chloro-16β-methylprednisolone; 9-chloro-11β,17,21-trihydroxy-16β-methylpregna-1,4-diene-3,20-dione; 9-chloro-16β-methylpregna-1,4-diene-11β,17,21-triol-3,20-dione; beclomethasone).
BECLOMETASONE DIPROPIONATE* (beclometasone 17,21-dipropionate; 9-chloro-11β-hydroxy-16β-methyl-17,21-bis(1-oxopropoxy)pregna-1,4-diene-3,20-dione; Sch-18020W; 'aldecin', 'beconase', 'becotide', 'clenil', 'propaderm', 'sanasth-myl').
Beclomethasone* *see* Beclometasone.
'Beclomycin' *see* Colistin.
BECLOTIAMINE*** (3-(4-amino-2-methyl-pyrimidin-5-ylmethyl)-5-(2-chloroethyl)-4-methylthiazolium chloride; chloroethyl-thiamine; 'cocciden').
'Beconase' *see* Beclometasone dipropionate.
'Becotide' *see* Beclometasone dipropionate.

BEE VENOM ('apicosan', 'apilit', 'forapin', 'melittin').

BEFURALINE** (1-(2-benzofuranylcarbonyl)-4-benzylpiperazine; 2-[(4-benzylpiperazin-1-yl)carbonyl]benzofuran).

BEHENIC ACID (docosanoic acid).

Bei-1293 *see* Xipamide.

BEIH *see* Nialamide.

'Bekadid' *see* Hydrocodone.

BEKANAMYCIN** (L-*O*-3-amino-α-D-glucopyranosyl-(1→4)-*O*-[2,6-diamino-2,6-dideoxy-α-D-glucopyranosyl-(1→6)]-2-deoxystreptamine; kanamycin B).

'Belcomycin' *see* Colistin.

'Belfacillin' *see* Meticillin.

'Belfene' *see* Diphenylpyraline.

'Belganyl' *see* Suramin.

'Bellacristin' *see* Belladonnin.

BELLADONNIN (isatropic acid ditropine ester; isatropyldidtropeine; C-45; 'bellacristin').

'Belosin' *see* Camylofin.

BELOXAMIDE** (*N*-benzyloxy-*N*-(3-phenylpropyl)acetamide; W-1372).

'Bemaphate' *see* Chloroquine.

'Bemarsal' *see* Difetarsone.

BEMEGRIDE** (3-ethyl-3-methylglutarimide; β-ethyl-β-methylglutarimide; 4-ethyl-4-methyl-2,6-piperidinedione; AB-01; NP-13; 'ahypnon', 'eukraton', 'malysol', 'megimide', 'methetharimide', 'mikedimide').

BEMETIZIDE** (6-chloro-3,4-dihydro-3-(α-methylbenzyl)-2H-1,2,4-benzothiadiazine 7-sulfonamide 1,1-dioxide; 6-chloro-3,4-dihydro-3-(1-phenylethyl)-7-sulfamoyl-2H-1,2,4-benzothiadiazine 1,1-dioxide; Diu-60).

Bemidone *see* Hydroxypethidine.

BENACTYZINE** (2-diethylaminoethyl benzilate; benactyzine hydrochloride; amizil; diazil; WIN-5606; 'beatiline', 'cafron', 'cevanol', 'finalin', 'fobex', 'lucidil', 'neuroleptone', 'nutinal', 'parasan', 'parpon', 'phoebex', 'phobex', 'procalm', 'suavitil', 'valladan').

See also Meprobamate with benactyzine.

Benactyzine methobromide *see* Methylbenactyzium bromide.

'Benadryl' *see* Diphenhydramine.

BENANSERIN* (1-benzyl-5-methoxy-2-methyltryptamine-HCl; benzyldimethylserotonin; benzyl antiserotonin; serotonin benzyl analogue; Woolley's antiserotonin; 'BAS').

BENAPRIZINE** (2-(ethylpropylamino)-ethyl benzilate; benaprizine; BRL-1288; 'brizin').

Benapryzine* *see* Benaprizine.

BENAZOLIN* (4-chloro-2-oxo-3(2H)-benzothiazoleacetic acid; 3-(carboxymethyl)-4-chlorobenzothiazol-2(3H)-one; 'cornox CWK', 'ley cornox', 'legumex extra', 'tricornox').

Benazoline* *see* Metizoline.

Bencaine (tr) *see* Diethylaminoethyl benzoate.

Benchinox *see* Benquinox.

BENCISTEINE** (*N*-acetyl-3-[(2-benzoylpropyl)thio]alanine; *N*-acetyl-*S*-(2-benzoylpropyl)cysteine).

Bencurine *see* Gallamine.

BENCYCLANE** (1-benzyl-1-(3-dimethylaminopropoxy)cycloheptane; 3-(1-benzylcycloheptyloxy)-*N,N*-dimethylpropylamine; benzcyclan; 'dilangio', 'ludilat').

BENCYCLANE FUROATE (Egyt-201; 'fludilat', 'galidor', 'halidor').

BENDAZAC** (2-(1-benzyl-1H-indazol-3-yloxy)acetic acid; 'bendazolic acid').

BENDAZAC SODIUM (AF-983; 'versus').

BENDAZOL** (2-benzylbenzimidazole; dibazole; 'tromasedan').

'Bendazolic acid' *see* Bendazac.

BENDIOCARB* (2,2-dimethyl-1,3-benzodioxol-4-yl methylcarbamate; NC-6897; OMS-1394; 'ficam').

'Bendralan' *see* Pheneticillin.

Bendrofluazide* *see* Bendroflumethiazide.

BENDROFLUMETHIAZIDE** (3-benzyl-3,4-dihydro-6-trifluoromethyl-2H-1,2,4-benzothiadiazine-7-sulfonamide 1,1-dioxide; 3-benzyl-3,4-dihydro-7-sulfamoyl-6-trifluoromethyl-1,2,4-benzothiadiazine 1,1-dioxide; benzylhydroflumethiazide; benzydroflumethiazide; bendrofluazide; Be-724-A; FT-81; 'aprinox', 'berkozide', 'centonuron', 'centyl', 'leocentyl', 'naturetin', 'naturine', 'neo-naclex', 'neorontyl', 'poliuron', 'pluryl', 'salures').

See also Reserpine with bendroflumethiazide.

'Benedorm' *see* Pyrithyldione.

Benefin *see* Benfluralin.

'Benemid' *see* Probenecid.

'Benetazone' *see* Tribuzone.

BENETHAMINE PENICILLIN** (*N*-benzyl-2-phenylethylamine salt of penicillin G; benzylpenicillin salt of *N*-benzylphenethylamine; *N*-benzylphenethylamine-6-(phenylacetamido)penicillanate).

BENFLUOREX* (2-[(α-methyl-*m*-trifluoromethylphenethyl)amino]ethanol benzoate (ester); *N*-(2-benzoyloxyethyl)-*m*-trifluoromethylamphetamine; benzoyloxyfenfluramine; S-992).

BENFLURALIN* (*N*-butyl-*N*-ethyl-2,6-dinitro-4-(trifluoromethyl)aniline; *N*-butyl-*N*-ethyl-α,α,α-trifluoro-2,6-dinitro-*p*-toluidine; benefin; bethrodine; 'balan', 'binnell', 'quilan').

BENFOSFORMIN** (disodium [(benzylamidino)amidino]phosphoramidate monohydrate; 5-benzyl-1-phosphorylbiguanide monosodium salt; JAV-852).

BENFOTIAMINE** (4-*N*-(4-amino-2-methylpyrimid-5-ylmethyl)formamido-3-(benzoylthio)pent-3-enyl phosphate; *N*-(4-amino-2-methylpyrimidin-5-ylmethyl)-*N*-(4-hydroxy-2-mercapto-1-methyl-1-butenyl)formamide *S*-benzoate *O*-phosphate; *S*-benzoylthiamine *O*-phosphate; 'bietamine').

BENFURODIL HEMISUCCINATE** (2-(1-hydroxyethyl)-β-hydroxymethyl-3-methyl-5-benzofuranacrylic acid γ-lactone hydrogen succinate; 'eucilat').

BENHEPAZONE*** (1-benzyl-2(1H)-cyclo-heptimidazolone).

'Ben-hex' see Lindane.

Benhexol see Orphenadrine.

'Benisol' see Benzalkonium.

'Benisone' see Betamethasone benzoate.

'Benlate' see Benomyl.

'Benlate T' see Benomyl plus thiram.

'Benlo' see Benzyl benzoate.

'Benlotex' see Benzyl benzoate.

BENMOXIN*** (benzoic acid 2-(α-methyl-benzyl)hydrazide; 1-benzoyl-2-(α-methyl-benzyl)hydrazine).

BENOMYL* (methyl 1-(butylcarbamoyl)-benzimidazole-2-carbamate; [1-[(butyl-amino)carbonyl]-1H-benzimidazol-2-yl]-carbamic acid methyl ester; 'benlate').

BENOMYL PLUS THIRAM ('benlate T').

'Benoquin' see Monobenzone.

'Benoril' see Benorilate.

BENORILATE*** (p-acetamidophenyl 2-acetoxybenzoate; 4-acetamidophenyl salicylate acetate; paracetamol acetyl-salicylate; benorylate; p-acetamidophenyl O-acetylsalicylate; fenasprate; WIN-11450; 'benoril', 'benortan').

See also Acetylsalicylic acid with par-acetamol.

'Benortan' see Benorilate.

BENORTERONE*** (17β-hydroxy-17-methyl-B-norandrost-4-en-3-one; 17-meth-yl-B-norandrost-4-en-17β-ol-3-one; 17α-methyl-B-nortestosterone; SK&F-7692).

Benorylate* see Benorilate.

BENOXAFOS*** (S-(5,7-dichlorobenz-oxazol-2-ylmethyl) O,O-diethyl phos-phorodithioate).

BENOXAPROFEN** (2-[2-(p-chlorophen-yl)benzoxazol-5-yl]propionic acid; 5-(1-carboxyethyl)-2-(p-chlorophenyl)benzox-azole; 2-(p-chlorophenyl)-α-methyl-5-benzoxazoleacetic acid; LRCL-3794).

Benoxinate see Ambucaine.

Benoxiquine see Benzoxiquine.

BENPERIDOL** (4'-fluoro-4-[4-(2-oxobenz-imidazolin-1-yl)piperid-1-yl]butyrophen-one; 1-[1-[4-(p-fluorophenyl)-4-oxobutyl]-piperidin-4-yl]-2-benzimidazolinone; 1-[1-[3-(p-fluorobenzoyl)propyl]piperid-4-yl]-2-benzimidazolinone; benzoperidol; benz-peridol; CB-8089; McN-JR-4584; R-4584; 'anquil', 'frenactyl', 'glianimon').

BENPROPERINE*** (1-[2-(2-benzyl-phenoxy)-1-methylethyl]piperidine; 1-(2-benzylphenoxy)-2-piperid-1-ylpropane; benproperine phosphate; 'pirexyl').

BENQUINOX* (benzoic acid [(4-hydroxy-imino)-2,5-cyclohexadien-1-ylidene]-hydrazide; COBH; QBH; benchinox; cerenox; 'ceredon').

BENQUINOX PLUS METHYL-THIOXOARSINE ('rhizoctol').

BENRIXATE*** (4-benzyl-1-piperidine-carboxylic acid 2-diethylaminoethyl ester; 2-diethylaminoethyl 4-benzyl-1-piperidine-carboxylate; 2-diethylaminoethyl 4-benzyl-pipecolinate).

BENSALAN*** (N-(p-bromobenzyl)-3,5-dibromosalicylamide; 3,5-dibromo-N-(p-bromobenzyl)salicylamide).

BENSERAZIDE*** (DL-serine 2-(2,3,4-tri-hydroxybenzyl)hydrazide; DL-2-amino-3-hydroxy-2'-(2,3,4-trihydroxybenzyl)-propionohydrazide; serazide; Ro 04-4602; Ro 4-4602).

See also Levodopa with benserazide.

BENSULDAZIC ACID*** (5-benzyldihydro-6-thioxo-2H-1,3,5-thiadiazine-3(4H)-acetic acid).

Bensulfamide see Mafenide.

BENSULFENE (dibenzoyl disulfide; benzoyl disulfide; 'septiolan').

BENSULIDE* (S-[2-(benzenesulfonamido)-ethyl] O,O-diisopropyl phosphorodithioate; O,O-bis(1-methylethyl) S-[2-[(phenyl-sulfonyl)amino]ethyl] phosphorodithioate; N-[2-[(diisopropoxyphosphinothioyl)thio]-ethyl]benzenesulfonamide; 'betasan', 'prefar').

Bensylyt* see Phenoxybenzamine.

BENTAZEPAM*** (1,3,6,7,8,9-hexahydro-5-phenyl-2H-(1)benzothieno(2,3-e)1,4-diazepin-2-one; 1,2-dihydro-5-phenyl-6,7-tetramethylene-3H-thieno(2,3-e)(1,4)diaz-epin-2-one; CI-718; QM-6008; 'thiadipon').

BENTAZON* (3-isopropyl-1H-2,1,3-benzo-thiadiazin-4(3H)-one 2,2-dioxide; 3-(1-methylethyl)-1H-2,1,3-benzothiadiazin-4(3H)-one 2,2-dioxide; BAS-3510H).

BENTHIOCARB (S-(p-chlorophenyl) diethylcarbamothioate; 'saturn').

BENTIAMINE*** (4-(N-4-amino-2-methyl-pyrimid-5-ylmethyl)formamido-3-(benzo-ylthio)pent-3-enyl benzoate; N-(4-amino-2-methylpyrimidin-5-ylmethyl)-N-(4-hy-droxy-2-mercapto-1-methyl-1-butenyl)-formamide O,S-dibenzoate; 'nevriton').

BENTIPIMINE*** (1-[2-(o-chloro-α-phenyl-benzylthio)ethyl]-4-(o-methylbenzyl)-piperazine; 1-[2-(o-chlorobenzhydrylthio)-ethyl]-4-(o-methylbenzyl)piperazine).

'Bentonyl' see Trolnitrate.

'Bentrofene' see Acediasulfone morpholine salt.

'Bentyl' see Dicycloverine.

'Bentylol' see Dicycloverine.

BENURESTAT** (2-(p-chlorobenzamido)-acetohydroxamic acid; 4-chloro-N-[2-(hydroxyamino)-2-oxoethyl]benzamide; EU-2826).

'Benuride' see Ethylphenacemide.

'Ben-U-ron 500' see Paracetamol.

'Benvil' see Tybamate.

'Benylate' see Benzyl benzoate.

'Benzabor' see Dimethylamine trichloro-benzoate.

'Benzac' see Dimethylamine trichloro-benzoate.

Benzacine (tr) see Deanol benzilate.

'Benzacyl' see Calcium benzamidosalicylate; Sodium benzamidosalicylate.

Benzalacetone see Benzylideneacetone.

Benzalbutyramide see Benzylidenebutyramide.

β-**Benzalbutyric acid** see 3-Benzylidene-
butyric acid.

BENZALDEHYDE-4-CARBOXYLIC ACID
(*p*-formylbenzoic acid).

BENZALDEHYDE-3-SULFONIC ACID
(*m*-sulfobenzaldehyde).

'Benzalin' see Nitrazepam.

BENZALKONIUM CHLORIDE*
(mixture of alkylbenzyldimethylammonium
chlorides; C-4; 'agena', 'benasept',
'benisol', 'BTC', 'cequartyl', 'desivon',
'drapolene', 'germinol', 'germitol',
'killavon', 'laudammonium', 'lorakon',
'merphene', 'natusan', 'onix-BTC', 'osvan',
'PQR', 'quatommon', 'roccal', 'rodalon',
'sanisol', 'steramine', 'throsil', 'urgo',
'zephiran', 'zephirol', 'zinol').

'Benzamelid' see Isobutylcaine.

BENZAMIDE (benzoic acid amide).

N-[2-[6-**Benzamido-2-chlorobenzyl)meth-
ylamino]acetyl]morpholine** see
Fominoben.

α-**Benzamido-***p*-[2-(diethylamino)ethoxy]-
N,*N*-dipropylhydrocinnamamide** see
Tiropramide.

4-**Benzamido-***N*,*N*-dipropylglutaramic
acid** see Proglumide.

4-**Benzamido-1-(2-indol-3-ylethyl)-
piperidine** see Indoramin.

3-[2-(4-**Benzamidopiperid-1-yl)ethyl]-
indole** see Indoramin.

4-**BENZAMIDOSALICYLIC ACID**
(4-benzoylaminosalicylic acid).
See also Calcium benzamidosalicylate;
Sodium benzamidosalicylate.

Benzamine see Eucaine.

Benzamine blue see Trypan blue.

Benzamon (tr) see Furfuryltrimethylammonium benzenesulfonate.

BENZAMYL (tr) (1-benzoyl-5-ethyl-5-iso-
amylbarbituric acid; *N*-benzoylamobar-
bital; *N*-benzoylbarbamyl).

Benzanidine (tr) see Betanidine.

BENZANILIDE (benzoic acid anilide; *N*-
benzoylaniline; *N*-phenylbenzamide).

'Benzapas' see Calcium benzamidosalicylate.

BENZARONE* (2-ethyl-3-(4-hydroxy-
benzoyl)benzofuran; 2-ethylbenzofuran-3-
yl 4-hydroxyphenyl ketone; L-2197;
'fragivix').

Benzarone diethylaminoethyl ether see
Etabenzarone.

BENZATHINE (*N*,*N*'-dibenzylethylenedi-
amine; DBED).

Benzathine benzylpenicillin* see Benzathine penicillin.

BENZATHINE PENICILLIN* (*N*,*N*-dibenz-
ylethylenediamine-dipenicillin G; benzethacil; benzathine benzylpenicillin;
penicillinbenzatin; pendepon; 'bica-penicillin', 'bicillin', 'cepacilina', 'cillenta',
'debecylina', 'dibencil', 'dibencillin', 'dura-
penita', 'duropenin', 'extencilline', 'longacilina', 'longicid', 'neolin', 'penadure', 'pen-
di-ben', 'penditan', 'penduran', 'penidural',
'penidure', 'permapen', 'tardocillin',
'tardomyocel').

BENZATHINE PENICILLIN V (*N*,*N*-di-
benzylethylenediamine-dipenicillin V;
'biphecillin', 'ostrocilline').

BENZATHINE TENUAZONATE (*N*,*N*'-di-
benzylethylenediamine derivative of 3-
acetyl-5-*sec*-butyl-4-hydroxy-3-pyrrolin-2-
one; NSC-82260).

BENZATROPINE* (tropine benzhydryl
ether; 3-(diphenylmethoxy)tropane; benzotropine; benztropine).

BENZATROPINE MESILATE (benzatropine methanesulfonate; MK-02;
'cobrentin', 'cogentin').

1-**Benzazole** see Indole.

Benzazolin see Tolazoline.

Benzazone-VII (tr) see 5-Nitro-2-furaldehyde
thiosemicarbazone.

BENZBROMARONE* (3-(3,5-dibromo-4-
hydroxybenzoyl)-2-ethylbenzofuran; 3,5-
dibromo-4-hydroxyphenyl 2-ethylbenzo-
furan-3-yl ketone; L-2214; 'desuric',
'minuric', 'uricovac').

Benzcarbimine see Benzodepa.

Benzchinamide* see Benzquinamide.

Benzchlorpropamide see Beclamide.

Benzcurine see Gallamine.

Benzcyclan see Bencyclane.

'Benzedrex' see Propylhexedrine.

'Benzedrine' see Amphetamine.

'Benzelia' see Benzyl benzoate.

Benzenamine see Aniline.

Benzene carbonitrile see Benzonitrile.

o-**Benzenedicarboxylic acid** see Phthalic
acid.

m-**Benzenedicarboxylic acid** see Isophthalic
acid.

p-**Benzenedicarboxylic acid** see Terephthalic acid.

Benzenehexachlor see Lindane.

Benzene hexachloride see Lindane.

Benzenemethanol see Benzyl alcohol.

BENZENESTIBONIC ACID (phenylstibinic
acid).

S-[2-(**Benzenesulfonamido)ethyl**] *O*,*O*-
diisopropyl phosphorodithioate see
Bensulide.

2-**Benzenesulfonamido-1,3,4-thiadiazole-
5-sulfonamide** see Benzolamide.

Benzenesulfonic acid esters and salts see
Besilate(s).

2-**Benzenesulfonyl-5-***tert*-butyl-1,3,4-thia-
diazole** see Glybuzole.

BENZESTROL* (2,4-bis(*p*-hydroxyphen-
yl)-3-ethylhexane; 4,4'-(1,2-diethyl-3-
methyltrimethylene)diphenol; 1,3-bis(*p*-
hydroxyphenyl)-1,2-diethyl-3-methyl-
propane; benzoestrol; octestrol; 'ocestrol',
'octofollin').

Benzetamophylline see Bamifylline.

Benzethacil* see Benzathine penicillin.

BENZETHIDINE* (ethyl ester of 1-(2-
benzyloxyethyl)-4-phenylisonipecotic acid;
ethyl 1-(2-benzyloxyethyl)-4-phenylpiper-
idine-4-carboxylate).

BENZETHONIUM CHLORIDE* (benzyl-
dimethyl-[2-[2-(*p*-1,1,3,3-tetramethylbutyl-

phenoxy)ethoxy]ethyl]ammonium chloride; 'ammorid', 'anzol', 'hyamine 1622', 'phemeride', 'phemerol', 'quatrachlor', 'septin', 'solamine', 'teramine').

BENZETIMIDE** (($\pm$)-2-(1-benzylpiperid-4-yl)-2-phenylglutarimide; 1-benzyl-4-(2,6-dioxo-3-phenylpiperid-3-yl)piperidine; benzetimide hydrochloride; McN-JR-4919-11; R-4929; 'dioxatrine', 'spasmentral').
See also Dexetimide.

'Benzevan' *see* Benzyl benzoate.

Benzhexachlor *see* Lindane.

Benzhexol* *see* Trihexyphenidyl.

Benzhydramine *see* Diphenhydramine.

Benzhydrazide *see* Benzohydrazide.

BENZHYDROL (diphenylmethanol; diphenyl carbinol).

BENZHYDRYLAMINE (α-phenylbenzylamine).

BENZHYDRYLAMINE PENICILLINATE ('orencil', 'penidryl').

Benzhydrylcinnamylpiperazine *see* Cinnarizine.

N-**(2-Benzhydrylethyl)-1-phenylethylamine** *see* Fendiline.

1-Benzhydryl-4-[2-(2-hydroxyethoxy)-ethyl]piperazine *see* Decloxizine.

2-Benzhydrylidenebutylamine *see* Etifelmine.

4-Benzhydrylidene-2,5-cyclohexadien-1-one *see* Fuchsone.

3-Benzhydrylidene-1,1-diethyl-2-methylpyrrolidinium bromide *see* Prifinium bromide.

4-Benzhydrylidene-1,1-dimethylpiperidinium methylsulfate *see* Diphemanil.

1-Benzhydrylimidazole-5-carboxylic acid ethyl ester *see* Etomidate.

(2-Benzhydrylisopropyl)ethyldimethylammonium bromide *see* Emepronium bromide.

1-Benzhydryl-4-methylpiperazine *see* Cyclizine.

2-Benzhydryloxy-*N*,*N*-dimethylethylamine *see* Diphenhydramine.

2-Benzhydryloxy-*N*,*N*-dimethylethylamine *N*-oxide *see* Amyoxydramine.

N-**(2-Benzhydryloxyethyl)-*N*-methylcinnamylamine** *see* Cinfenine.

3-Benzhydryloxy-8-ethylnortropane *see* Etybenzatropine.

1-(2-Benzhydryloxyethyl)piperidine *see* Perastin.

4-Benzhydryloxy-1-methylpiperidine *see* Diphenylpyraline.

4-Benzhydryloxy-1-methylpiperidine chlorotheophyllinate *see* Piprinhydrinate.

2-Benzhydryl-1′-phenyldiethylamine *see* Fendiline.

1-Benzhydryl-4-piperonylpiperazine *see* Medibazine.

BENZIDINE (4,4′-diaminobiphenyl).

BENZIL (bibenzoyl; dibenzoyl; diphenylglyoxal; diphenyl diketone).

BENZILAMIDE (benzilic acid amide).

BENZILIC ACID (diphenylglycolic acid;

α-phenylmandelic acid; diphenylhydroxyacetic acid).

Benzilic acid esters *see* Benactyzine; Benaprizine; Difemerine; Metamizil; Methylbenactyzium bromide; Metindizate; Pipethanate; Triclazate.

BENZILONIUM BROMIDE*** (1,1-diethyl-3-hydroxypyrrolidinium benzilate; 1-ethyl-3-pyrrolidinol benzilate ethobromide; CI-379; PU-239; 'minelcin', 'portyn', 'pyrbenine', 'ulcoban').

8α-Benziloyloxy-6,10-ethano-5-azoniaspiro(4,5)decane chloride *see* Trospium chloride.

(2-Benziloyloxyethyl)dimethylethylammonium bromide *see* Lachesine.

BENZIMIDAZOLE (1,3-benzodiazole; azindole; benziminazole; benzoglyoxaline; *N*,*N*′-methenyl-*o*-phenylenediamine).

Benzimidazole-2-carbamic acid ethyl ester *see* Lobendazole.

Benzimidazole-1,3-dimethanol-2-thione *see* Thibenzazoline.

Benziminazole *see* Benzimidazole.

Benzindamine* *see* Benzydamine.

BENZINDOPYRINE*** (1-benzyl-3-(2-pyrid-4-ylethyl)indole; benzindopyrine hydrochloride; pyrbenzindole; IN-461).

'Benzinoform' *see* Carbon tetrachloride.

BENZIODARONE*** (2-ethylbenzofuran-3-yl 4-hydroxy-3,5-diiodophenyl ketone; 2-ethyl-3-(4-hydroxy-3,5-diiodobenzoyl)-benzofuran; 2-ethyl-3-(4-hydroxy-3,5-diiodobenzoyl)coumarone; L-2329; 'ampliuril', 'amplivix', 'cardivix', 'retrangor').

Benzmalacene *see* Benzmalecene.

BENZMALECENE*** (*N*-[2,3-bis(*p*-chlorophenyl)-1-methylpropyl]maleamic acid α-form; MK-135; benzmalacene).

BENZNIDAZOLE** (*N*-benzyl-2-nitroimidazole-1-acetamide; 1-[(*N*-benzylcarbamoyl)methyl]-2-nitroimidazole; *N*-[[(2-nitroimidazol-1-yl)methyl]carbonyl]benzylamine; Ro 7-1051).

Benzoaric acid *see* Ellagic acid.

BENZOBARBITAL*** (1-benzoyl-5-ethyl-5-phenylbarbituric acid; *N*-benzoylphenobarbital; benzonal).

'Benzo blue' *see* Trypan blue.

BENZOCAINE* (ethyl *p*-aminobenzoate; ethoform; norcaine; 'americaine', 'anaesthesin', 'anaesthoform', 'anaesthone', 'euphagin', 'orthesin', 'parathesin', 'rhaetocaine', 'subcutin').

'Benzochloryl' *see* DDT.

BENZO(b)CHRYSENE (3,4-benzotetraphene; 3,4-benzotetraphine).

BENZOCLIDINE** (3-quinuclidinyl benzoate (ester); 3-benzoyloxyquinuclidine; oxylidine).

Benzoctametamina *see* Benzoctamine.

BENZOCTAMINE*** (*N*-methyl-9,10-ethanoanthracene-9(10H)-methylamine; 1-methylaminomethyldibenzo(b,e)bicyclo-(2.2.2)octadiene; benzoctametamina; benzoctamine hydrochloride; Ba-30803;

44

C-30803-Ba; 'tacitin').

Benzoctarpomine *see* Maprotiline.

3α-[(5H-Benzo(4,5)cyclohepta(1,2-b)-pyridyl)-5-oxy]tropane *see* Tropirine.

BENZODEPA*** (benzyl bis(1-aziridinyl)-phosphinylcarbamate; bis(1-aziridinyl)-benzyloxycarbonylaminophosphine oxide; benzcarbimine; AB-103; NSC-37096; 'dualar').

1,2-Benzodiazine *see* Cinnoline.

1,4-Benzodiazine *see* Quinoxaline.

1,3-Benzodiazole *see* Benzimidazole.

1,4-BENZODIOXAN (1,4-benzodioxane; 1,2-ethylenedioxybenzene).

Benzodioxane *see* Benzodioxan; Piperoxan.

1-(1,4-Benzodioxan-2-ylmethyl)-1-benzyl-hydrazine *see* Domoxin.

(1,4-Benzodioxan-2-ylmethyl)guanidine *see* Guanoxan.

(1,4-Benzodioxan-6-ylmethyl)guanidine *see* Guabenxan.

8-(1,4-Benzodioxan-2-ylmethyl)-1-phenyl-1,3,8-triazaspiro(4,5)decan-4-one *see* Spiroxatrine.

1,3-BENZODIOXOLE (1,2-methylene-dioxybenzene).

1-(1,3-Benzodioxol-5-yl)-4,4-dimethyl-1-penten-3-ol *see* Stiripentol.

BENZODODECINIUM CHLORIDE*** (benzyldodecyldimethylammonium chloride; benzyllauryldimethylammonium chloride; 'ajatin', 'otocone', 'sterinol').

'Benzoechtrosa' *see* Chlorazole fast pink.

Benzoestrol *see* Benzestrol.

BENZOFURAN (coumarone).

1-(2-Benzofurancarbonyl)-4-benzyl-piperazine *see* Benfuraline.

2-Benzofurancarboxylic acid *see* Coumarilic acid.

α-Benzofuran-2-yl p-chlorobenzyl alcohol *see* Cloridarol.

N-Benzofuran-2-ylmethyl-N',N'-dimethyl-N-pyrid-2-ylethylenediamine *see* Etofuradine.

BENZOFURAZAN (2,1,3-benzoxadiazole).

BENZOFURAZAN N-OXIDE (benzofuroxan).

Benzofuroxan *see* Benzofurazan N-oxide.

2-Benzofuryl p-chlorophenyl carbinol *see* Cloridarol.

Benzoglyoxaline *see* Benzimidazole.

BENZOHYDRAZIDE (benzoic acid hydrazide; benzhydrazide; benzoylhydrazine).

BENZOHYDROXAMIC ACID (N-benzoyl-hydroxylamine).

BENZOIC ACID (carboxybenzene; dracylic acid; phenylformic acid).

Benzoic acid anhydride with 3-chloro-N-ethoxy-2,6-dimethoxybenzene-carboximidic acid *see* Benzoximate.

Benzoic acid hydrazide *see* Benzohydrazide.

Benzoic acid [(4-hydroxyimino)-2,5-cyclohexadien-1-ylidene]hydrazide *see* Benquinox.

Benzoic acid 2-(α-methylbenzyl)hydrazide *see* Benmoxin.

Benzoic acid salts *see* Lithium benzoate;

Sodium benzoate.

o-Benzoic sulfimide *see* Saccharin.

BENZOIN (α-hydroxy-α-phenylaceto-phenone; benzoyl phenyl carbinol; 2-hydroxy-1,2-diphenylethanone).

Benzol *see* Benzene.

BENZOLAMIDE (2-benzenesulfonamido-1,3,4-thiadiazole-5-sulfonamide; CL-11366; W-1803).

Benzolin (tr) *see* Tolazoline.

Benzomate *see* Benzoximate.

6,7-BENZOMORPHAN (2,6-methano-1,2,3,4,5,6-hexahydro-3-benzazocine).

Benzonal (tr) *see* Benzobarbital.

Benzonaphthol *see* 2-Naphthyl benzoate.

BENZONATATE*** (2-(ω-methoxyocta-ethyleneoxy)ethyl p-butylaminobenzoate; nonaethyleneglycolmethyl ester of p-butyl-aminobenzoic acid; 2,5,8,11,14,17,20,23,26-nonoxaoctacosan-28-ol p-butylaminoben-zoate; benzonatinum; benzononatine; Egyt-13; KM-65; 'exangit', 'tessalon').

Benzonatinum *see* Benzonatate.

BENZONITRILE (cyanobenzene; benzene carbonitrile; phenyl cyanide).

Benzononatine *see* Benzonatate.

Benzoparadiazine *see* Quinoxaline.

Benzoperidol *see* Benperidol.

BENZOPHENONE (diphenyl ketone).

'Benzopropyl' *see* Amydricaine.

Benzopteridinedione *see* Isoalloxazine.

Benzo(a)pyrazine *see* Quinoxaline.

BENZOPYRAZONE (4-(3-oxo-3-phenyl-propyl)-1,2-diphenyl-3,5-pyrazolidine-dione; 4-(2-benzoylethyl)-1,2-diphenyl-3,5-pyrazolidinedione).

BENZO(a)PYRENE (3,4-benzpyrene).

BENZO(e)PYRENE (1,2-benzpyrene).

Benzo(d)pyridazine *see* Phthalazine.

Benzo(b)pyridine *see* Quinoline.

Benzo(a)pyrimidine *see* Quinazoline.

BENZOPYRINE (phenazone benzoate; anti-pyrine benzoate).

Benzopyrinium *see* Benzpyrinium.

2,3-Benzopyrrole *see* Indole.

BENZOPYRRONIUM BROMIDE*** (1,1-dimethyl-3-hydroxypyrrolidinium bromide benzilate).

Benzoquinamide *see* Benzquinamide.

o-BENZOQUINONE (1,2-benzoquinone).

p-BENZOQUINONE (1,4-benzoquinone; quinone; 1,4-cyclohexadienedione).

p-Benzoquinone guanylhydrazone thiosemicarbazone *see* Ambazone.

BENZOQUINONIUM CHLORIDE* (bis-(benzylchloride) of 2,5-bis(3-diethylamino-propylamino)-p-benzoquinone; WIN-2747; 'amilyt', 'mytolon').

'Benzoral' *see* Polybenzarsol.

Benzosalicin *see* Salicin benzoate.

Benzostigmin *see* Benzpyrinium.

o-Benzosulfimide *see* Saccharin.

Benzotetraphene *see* Benzochrysene.

Benzotetraphine *see* Benzochrysene.

Benzotetrazine *see* Pteridine.

1-Benzothiazol-2-yl-1,3-dimethylurea *see* Methabenzthiazuron.

45

1-Benzothiazol-2-yl-3-methylurea *see* Benzthiazuron.

BENZO(b)THIEN-4-YL METHYLCARBAMATE (Mc-A-600; OMS-708; 'mobam').

Benzotriazinylmethyldithiophosphoric acid diethyl ester *see* Azinphos-ethyl.

Benzotriazinylmethyldithiophosphoric acid dimethyl ester *see* Azinphos-methyl.

BENZOTRIPT** (N-(p-chlorobenzoyl)-L-tryptophan; 2-(p-chlorobenzamido)-3-indolepropionic acid; N-(1-carboxy-2-indol-3-ylethyl)-p-chlorobenzamide).

Benzotropine *see* Benzatropine.

2,1,3-Benzoxadiazole *see* Benzofurazan.

N-Benzoxazol-2-yl-N-benzyl-N',N'-dimethylethylenediamine *see* Oxadimedine.

2-Benzoxazolyl N-methyldithio-1-naphthalenecarbamate *see* Naftoxate.

Benzoxazone *see* Caroxazone.

BENZOXIMATE* (anhydride of benzoic acid with 3-chloro-N-ethoxy-2,6-dimethoxybenzenecarboximidic acid; benzomate; 'citrazon').

BENZOXIQUINE*** (8-quinolinol benzoate ester; 8-benzoyloxyquinoline; benoxiquine; 'dioxyline').

Benzoylaminosalicylic acid *see* Benzamidosalicylic acid.

N-Benzoylamobarbital *see* Benzamyl.

N-Benzoylaniline *see* Benzanilide.

N-Benzoylbarbamyl *see* Benzamyl.

5-Benzoyl-2-benzimidazolecarbamic acid methyl ester *see* Mebendazole.

Benzoyl carbinol *see* 2-Hydroxyacetophenone.

5-Benzoyl-2-(1-carboxyethyl)thiophene *see* Tiaprofenic acid.

1-Benzoyl-1-(3,4-dichlorophenyl)-3,3-dimethylurea *see* Phenobenzuron.

3'-Benzoyl-1,1-difluoromethanesulfonanilide *see* Diflumidone.

Benzoyl disulfide *see* Bensulfene.

1-[[1-(2-Benzoylethyl)benzimidazol-2-yl]-methyl]-4-cinnamylpiperazine *see* Cinprazole.

1-(2-Benzoylethyl)-2-[(4-cinnamyl-piperazin-1-yl)methyl]benzimidazole *see* Cinprazole.

4-(2-Benzoylethyl)-1,2-diphenyl-3,5-pyrazolidinedione *see* Benzopyrazone.

1-Benzoyl-5-ethyl-5-isoamylbarbituric acid *see* Benzamyl.

1-Benzoyl-5-ethyl-5-phenylbarbituric acid *see* Benzobarbital.

'Benzoyl-flagyl' *see* Metronidazole benzoate.

5-Benzoylhexahydro-1H-furo(3,4-c)-pyrrole *see* Octazamide.

m-Benzoylhydratropic acid *see* Ketoprofen.

N-Benzoylhydroxylamine *see* Benzohydroxamic acid.

5-Benzoyl-4-hydroxy-2-methoxybenzenesulfonic acid *see* Sulisobenzone.

1-Benzoyl-2-(α-methylbenzyl)hydrazine *see* Benmoxin.

1-Benzoylmethyl-3-(m-hydroxyphenyl)-

1,3-dimethylpiperidine *see* Myfadol.

5-Benzoyl-α-methyl-2-thiopheneacetic acid *see* Tiaprofenic acid.

N-(2-Benzoyloxyethyl)-m-trifluoro methylamphetamine *see* Benfluorex.

Benzoyloxyfenfluramine *see* Benfluorex.

8-Benzoyloxyquinoline *see* Benzoxiquine.

3-Benzoyloxyquinuclidine *see* Benzoclidine.

Benzoylpas calcium* *see* Calcium benzamidosalicylate.

BENZOYL PEROXIDE* (dibenzoyl peroxide).

N-Benzoylphenobarbital *see* Benzobarbital.

2-(3-Benzoylphenyl)propionic acid *see* Ketoprofen.

BENZOYLPROP-ETHYL* (ethyl N-benzoyl-N-(3,4-dichlorophenyl)-L-alanine; N-(3,4-dichlorophenyl)-N-[1-(ethoxycarbonyl)ethyl]benzamide; WL-17731; 'shellsol A').

N¹-Benzoylsulfanilamide *see* Sulfabenzamide.

Benzoylthiamine disulfide *see* Bisbentiamine.

S-Benzoylthiamine O-phosphate *see* Benfotiamine.

2-(5-Benzoylthien-2-yl)propionic acid *see* Tiaprofenic acid.

1-Benzoyltriethylamine *see* Amfepramone.

m-Benzoyl-N-trifluoromethylsulfonylcarbanilic acid ethyl ester *see* Triflumidate.

'Benzperidine' *see* Perastine.

Benzperidol *see* Benperidol.

BENZPHETAMINE*** (N-benzyl-N,α-dimethylphenethylamine; N-benzyl-N-methylamphetamine; N-benzylmethamphetamine; 'didrex', 'inappetyl').

Benzphetamine oxide *see* Oxifentorex.

BENZPIPERYLONE*** (4-benzyl-1-(1-methylpiperid-4-yl)-3-phenyl-3-pyrazolin-5-one; KB-95; 'reublonil').

1,2-Benzpyrene *see* Benzo(e)pyrene.

3,4-Benzpyrene *see* Benzo(a)pyrene.

BENZPYRINIUM BROMIDE*** (1-benzyl-3-hydroxypyridinium bromide dimethylcarbamate; benzopyrinium; benzostigmine; benzstigmine; 'stigmenine', 'stigmonine').

BENZQUINAMIDE*** (N,N-diethyl-1,3,4,6, 7,11b-hexahydro-2-hydroxy-9,10-dimethoxy(2H)benzo(a)quinolizine-3-carboxamide acetate; 2-acetoxy-3-diethylcarbamoyl-9,10-dimethoxyhexahydrobenzo(a)quinolizine; benzochinamide; benzoquinamide; P-2647; 'emete-con', 'quantril').

Benzstigmine *see* Benzpyrinium.

BENZTHIAZIDE*** (3-benzylthiomethyl-6-chloro-7-sulfamoyl-1,2,4-(4H)benzothiadiazine 1,1-dioxide; benzylthiomethylchlorothiazide; P-1393; 'exna', 'fovane', 'naclex', 'urese').

See also Methoserpidine with benzthiazide.

BENZTHIAZIDE WITH TRIAMTERENE ('dytide').

BENZTHIAZURON* (1-benzothiazol-2-yl-3-methylurea; 2-(methylcarbamido)benzothiazole; 'gatnon').

'Benzthiozone' *see* Thiacetazone.

Benztropine* *see* Benzatropine.

BENZYDAMINE*** (1-benzyl-3-(3-dimethylaminopropoxy)(1H)indazole; benzindamine; benzydamine hydrochloride; AF-864; C-1523; 'imotryl', 'tantum').

BENZYDAMINE PHENYLBUTAZONE-5-ENOLATE (LS-701; 'butazidamina').

BENZYDAMINE WITH ERYTHROMYCIN (ER-72; 'eriflogin').

BENZYDAMINE WITH HEXAMIDINE ISETIONATE (C-1605; 'hexo-imotryl').

BENZYDAMINE WITH TETRACYCLINE ('tantum biotic').

Benzydroflumethiazide *see* Bendroflumethiazide.

2-Benzylacetic acid *see* Hydrocinnamic acid.

BENZYL ALCOHOL*** (benzenemethanol; phenyl carbinol; phenmethylol).

[(Benzylamidino)amidino]phosphoramidic acid disodium salt *see* Benfosformin.

4-Benzylamino-2-methyl(7H)pyrrolo-(2,3-d)pyrimidine *see* Rolodine.

2-(N-Benzylanilino)acetamidoxime *see* Cetoxime.

1-[2-(N-Benzylanilino)-3-isobutoxypropyl]pyrrolidine *see* Bepridil.

4-(N-Benzylanilino)-1-methylpiperidine *see* Bamipine.

Benzyl antiserotonin *see* Benanserin.

2-Benzylbenzimidazole *see* Bendazol.

BENZYL BENZOATE (peruscabin; 'ascabin', 'ascabiol', 'B-B-S', 'benlo', 'benlotex', 'benylate', 'benzelia', 'benzevan', 'benzylets', 'cabiol', 'colebenz', 'mykomed', 'novoscabian', 'novoscabin', 'peruol', 'proscabin', 'scabinol', 'scobenol', 'spasmodin', 'spastussin', 'vanzoate', 'venzonate', 'zonol').

Benzyl bis(1-aziridinyl)phosphinylcarbamate *see* Benzodepa.

2-Benzyl-3-butylamino-5-carboxybenzenesulfonamide *see* Besunide.

4-Benzyl-3-butylamino-5-sulfamoylbenzoic acid *see* Besunide.

Benzylcarbamoylethanol *see* Buramate.

Benzylcarbamoylethylisoniazid *see* Nialamide.

1-[(N-Benzylcarbamoyl)methyl]-2-nitroimidazole *see* Benznidazole.

2-Benzyl-4-chlorophenol *see* Clorofene.

N-Benzyl-3-chloropropionamide *see* Beclamide.

Benzyl cinnamate *see* Cinnamein.

1-Benzyl-2(1H)-cycloheptimidazolinone *see* Benhepazone.

3-(1-Benzylcycloheptyloxy)-N,N-dimethylpropylamine *see* Bencyclane.

N-Benzylcyclopropanecarbamic acid ethyl ester *see* Encymate.

Benzyl(2-diethylaminoethyl)malonic acid diethyl ester *see* Diethyl benzyl(2-diethylaminoethyl)malonate.

Benzyldiethyl(tetramethylbutylphenoxyethyl)ammonium chloride *see* Octafonium.

Benzyldiethyl(2,6-xylylcarbamoylmethyl)ammonium benzoate *see* Denatonium.

Benzyl 9,10-dihydro-1-methyl-(+)-lysergamine-N-carboxylate *see* Metergoline.

5-Benzyl-4,5-dihydro-4-oxo-1H-1,2,5-benzotriazepine-3-carboxamidoxime *see* Trizoxime.

5-Benzyldihydro-6-thioxo-2H-1,3,5-thiadiazine-3(4H)-acetic acid *see* Bensuldazic acid.

3-Benzyl-3,4-dihydro-6-trifluoromethyl-2H-1,2,4-benzothiadiazine-7-sulfonamide 1,1-dioxide *see* Bendroflumethiazide.

S-BENZYL O,O-DIISOPROPYL PHOSPHOROTHIOATE ('kitazin P').

2-[Benzyl(2-dimethylaminoethyl)amino]-benzoxazole *see* Oxadimedine.

4-Benzyl-2-(2-dimethylaminoethyl)-1(2H)-phthalazinone *see* Talastine.

4-Benzyl-1-(2-dimethylaminoethyl)-piperidine *see* Pimetine.

1-Benzyl-1-(3-dimethylaminopropoxy)-cycloheptane *see* Bencyclane.

1-Benzyl-3-(3-dimethylaminopropoxy)-indazole *see* Benzydamine.

1-Benzyl-2,3-dimethylguanidine *see* Betanidine.

1-Benzyl-2,3-dimethylindole-5-carboxylic acid dimethylaminoethyl ester *see* Indocate.

Benzyldimethyl(octylcresoxyethoxyethyl)ammonium chloride *see* Methylbenzethonium chloride.

N-Benzyl-N,α-dimethylphenethylamine *see* Benzphetamine.

N-Benzyl-N,α-dimethylphenethylamine N-oxide *see* Oxifentorex.

Benzyldimethyl(phenoxyethyl)ammonium ion *see* Bephenium.

N-Benzyl-N',N'-dimethyl-N-phenylethylenediamine *see* Phenbenzamine.

N-Benzyl-N',N'-dimethyl-N-pyrid-2-ylethylenediamine *see* Tripelennamine.

Benzyldimethylserotonin *see* Benanserin.

Benzyldimethyl(tetramethylbutylphenoxyethoxyethyl)ammonium chloride *see* Benzethonium chloride.

Benzyldimethyl(tetramethylbutyltoloxyethoxyethyl)ammonium chloride *see* Methylbenzethonium chloride.

1-Benzyl-4-(2,6-dioxo-3-phenylpiperid-3-yl)piperidine *see* Benzetimide.

Benzyldodecyldimethylammonium chloride *see* Benzododecinium chloride.

Benzyl[2-(p-dodecoylphenoxy)ethyl]-dimethylammonium chloride *see* Lauralkonium chloride.

7-Benzyl-1-ethyl-1,4-dihydro-4-oxo-1,8-naphthyridine-3-carboxylic acid *see* Amfonelic acid.

1-Benzyl-3-ethyl-6,7-dimethoxyisoquinoline *see* Moxaverine.

8-Benzyl-7-[2-[ethyl(2-hydroxyethyl)-amino]ethyl]theophylline *see* Bamifylline.

S-BENZYL O-ETHYL PHENYLPHOSPHONOTHIOATE ('inezin').

α-Benzyl-N-ethyltetrahydrofurylamine

see Zylofuramine.

5-Benzylfuran-3-ylmethyl 2,2-dimethyl-3-(2-methyl-1-propenyl)cyclopropane-carboxylate
cis-(+)-, *see* Cismethrin.
cis, trans-(±)-, *see* Resmethrin.
trans-(+)-, *see* Bioresmethrin.

trans-(±)-5-Benzylfuran-3-ylmethyl 3-(3-methoxy-2-methyl-3-oxo-1-propenyl)-2,2-dimethylcyclopropane-carboxylate *see* Pyresmethrin.

Benzylfuroline *see* Resmethrin.

5-Benzyl-3-furylmethyl chrysanthemate
cis-(+)-, *see* Cismethrin.
cis, trans-(±)-, *see* Resmethrin.
trans-(+)-, *see* Bioresmethrin.

Benzylglucofuranoside *see* Tribenoside.

Benzylhexadecyldimethylammonium chloride *see* Cetalkonium chloride.

Benzylhydroflumethiazide *see* Bendro-flumethiazide.

Benzyl *p*-hydroxybenzoate *see* Benzyl paraben.

4-Benzyl-1-[3-hydroxy-3-(*p*-hydroxy-phenyl)prop-2-yl]piperidine *see* Ifenprodil.

O-Benzylhydroxylamine *see* Benzyloxy-amine.

BENZYL(HYDROXYMETHYL)-DIMETHYLAMMONIUM CHLORIDE DODECYLCARBAMATE ('urolocide').

4-Benzyl-α-(*p*-hydroxyphenyl)-β-methyl-1-piperidineethanol *see* Ifenprodil.

1-Benzyl-3-hydroxypyridinium bromide dimethylcarbamate *see* Benzpyrinium.

BENZYLIDENEACETONE (4-phenyl-3-buten-2-one; acetocinnamone; benzal acetone; cinnamyl methyl ketone; methyl styryl ketone).

3-BENZYLIDENEBUTYRAMIDE (β-benzalbutyramide).

3-BENZYLIDENEBUTYRIC ACID (β-benzalbutyric acid; 3-methyl-4-phenyl-3-butenoic acid; BBA).

N¹-BENZYLIDENEISONIAZID (benzaldehydeisonicotinoylhydrazone; 'isoteben').

4-Benzylidene-5,6,7,8-tetrahydro-1,3(2H, 4H)-isoquinolinedione *see* Tesimide.

2-Benzyl-2-imidazoline *see* Tolazoline.

2-(1-Benzyl-1H-indazol-3-yloxy)acetic acid *see* Bendazac.

Benzyllauryldimethylammonium chloride *see* Benzododecinium chloride.

N-Benzylmethamphetamine *see* Benz-phetamine.

N-Benzylmethamphetamine N-oxide *see* Oxifentorex.

N-Benzyl-N-methylamphetamine *see* Benzphetamine.

1-Benzyl-2-(5-methylisoxazol-3-ylcarbon-yl)hydrazine *see* Isocarboxazid.

α-Benzyl-β-methyl-α-phenyl-1-pyrrol-idinepropanol acetate *see* Pyrrolifene.

4-Benzyl-1-(1-methylpiperid-4-yl)-3-phenyl-3-pyrazolin-5-one *see* Benzpiperylone.

N-Benzyl-N-methyl-2-propynylamine *see*

Pargyline.

BENZYLMORPHINE (morphine benzyl ether; 'peronine').

Benzylmorphine myristyl ester *see* Myrophine.

BENZYL NICOTINATE ('pycaril').
See also Dexamethasone with benzyl nicotinate.

N-Benzyl-2-nitroimidazole-1-acetamide *see* Benznidazole.

1-Benzyl-2-oxocyclohexanepropionic acid *see* Hexacyprone.

BENZYLOXYAMINE (O-benzylhydroxyl-amine).

7-Benzyloxy-6-butyl-1,4-dihydro-4-oxo-quinoline-3-carboxylic acid methyl ester *see* Nequinate.

7-Benzyloxy-6-butyl-4-hydroxy-3-quinol-inecarboxylic acid methyl ester *see* Nequinate.

3-Benzyloxy-6-hydroxy-N-methyl-4,5-epoxymorphin-7-ene tetradecanoate ester *see* Myrophine.

3-Benzyloxy-N-methyl-6-myristyloxy-4,5-epoxymorphin-7-ene *see* Myrophine.

p-Benzyloxyphenol *see* Monobenzone.

N-Benzyloxy-N-(3-phenylpropyl)acet-amide *see* Beloxamide.

BENZYL PARABEN (benzyl *p*-hydroxyben-zoate; 'nipabenzyl').

Benzylpenicillin *see* Penicillin G.

N-Benzylphenethylamine 6-(phenylacet-amido)penicillanate *see* Benethamine penicillin.

O-BENZYLPHENOL (α-phenol-o-cresol; 'delegol').

1-[2-(2-Benzylphenoxy)-1-methylethyl]-piperidine *see* Benproperine.

1-(2-Benzylphenoxy)-2-piperid-1-yl-propane *see* Benproperine.

2-(2-Benzylphenoxy)TRIETHYL-AMINE (2-benzylphenyl 2-diethylamino-ethyl ether; AH₃; CI-072).

(Benzylphenylaminoethyl)ethyldimethyl-ammonium bromide *see* Phenbenzamine ethobromide.

Benzylphenyl carbamate *see* Diphenan.

2-Benzylphenyl 2-diethylaminoethyl ether *see* Benzylphenoxytriethylamine.

Benzylphenylurethan *see* Diphenan.

5-Benzyl-1-phosphorylbiguanide mono-sodium salt *see* Benfosformin.

4-Benzylpipecolinic acid 2-diethylamino-ethyl ester *see* Benrixate.

2-[(4-Benzylpiperazin-1-yl)carbonyl]-benzofuran *see* Befuraline.

4-Benzyl-1-piperidinecarboxylic acid 2-diethylaminoethyl ester *see* Benrixate.

α-[1-(4-Benzylpiperid-1-yl)ethyl]-*p*-hydroxybenzyl alcohol *see* Ifenprodil.

2-(4-Benzylpiperid-1-yl)-1-(*p*-hydroxy-phenyl)-1-propanol *see* Ifenprodil.

2-(1-Benzylpiperid-4-yl)-2-phenylglutar-imide *see* Benzetimide.

Benzylpivaloylhydrazine *see* Pivhydrazine.

2-Benzyl-2-propylamine *see* Phentermine.

1-Benzyl-3-(2-pyrid-4-ylethyl)indole *see*

Benzindopyrine.
BENZYL SUCCINATE (succinic acid mono-benzyl ester).
See also Calcium benzyl succinate; Dibenzyl succinate; Sodium benzyl succinate.
BENZYLSULFAMIDE*** (4-benzylamino-benzenesulfonamide; N^4-benzylsulfanil-amide; M&B-125; RP-46).
Benzylsulfanilamide *see* Benzylsulfamide.
p-**Benzylsulfonamidobenzoic acid** *see* Carinamide.
5-Benzyl-1,3,4,5-tetrahydro-2-methyl-2H-pyrido(4,3-b)indole *see* Mebhydrolin.
1-Benzyl-2,3,4,9-tetrahydro(1H)pyrido-(3,4-b)indole *see* Fenharmane.
S-**Benzyl thiobenzoate** *see* Tibenzate.
BENZYL THIOCYANATE (benzylrhoda-nide; 'solvat').
3-Benzylthiomethyl-6-chloro-3,4-dihydro-7-sulfamoylbenzothiadiazine dioxide *see* Hydrobentizide.
3-Benzylthiomethyl-6-chloro-7-sulfa-moylbenzothiadiazine dioxide *see* Benzthiazide.
Benzylthiomethylchlorothiazide *see* Benzthiazide.
Benzyl(trimethylacetyl)hydrazine *see* Pivhydrazine.
'**Beosit**' *see* Endosulfan.
'**Bepanthen**' *see* Dexpanthenol.
'**Bepaprone**' *see* β-Propiolactone.
'**Beparin**' *see* β-Heparin.
Beperiden *see* Biperiden.
BEPHENIUM HYDROXYNAPHTHO-ATE*** (benzyldimethyl(2-phenoxyethyl)-ammonium 3-hydroxy-2-naphthoate; bephenium embonate; naftamon; 'alcopar').
BEPIASTINE*** (6-(2-dimethylaminoethyl)-pyrido(2,3-b)(1,5)benzothiazepin-5(6H)-one).
BEPRIDIL** (1-[2-(*N*-benzylanilino)-3-isobutoxypropyl]pyrrolidine).
'**Beprochin**' *see* Pamaquin.
'**Beracillin**' *see* Penicillamine.
'**Berberal N**' *see* Berberin with neomycin.
BERBERIN WITH NEOMYCIN ('berberal-N').
BERBINE (5,6,13,13a-tetrahydro(8H)-dibenzo(a,g)quinolizine; tetrahydroproto-berberine).
'**Berenil**' *see* Diminazene.
'**Berkdopa**' *see* Levodopa.
'**Berkfurin**' *see* Nitrofurantoin.
'**Berkmycen**' *see* Oxytetracycline.
'**Berkomin**' *see* Imipramine.
'**Berkozide**' *see* Bendroflumethiazide.
'**Berlicetin**' *see* Chloramphenicol.
'**Berocillin**' *see* Pivampicillin.
BEROMYCIN (tr) (antibiotic (anthracycline derivative) from *Actinomyces griseoruber* var. *beromycini*).
'**Berotec**' *see* Fenoterol.
BERYTHROMYCIN** (12-deoxyerythro-mycin; erythromycin B).
'**Beserol**' *see* Chlormezanone with par-acetamol.
'**Beserol 500**' *see* Chlormezanone with

novaminsulfon.
BESILATE(S)** (benzenesulfonate(s); besylate(s)).
See also Dichlorophenyl besilate; Hexa-methonium besilate.
'**Beston**' *see* Bisbentiamine.
BESUNIDE** (3-butylamino-α-phenyl-5-sulfamoyl-*p*-toluic acid; 4-benzyl-3-butyl-amino-5-sulfamoylbenzoic acid; 3-benzyl-3-butylamino-5-carboxybenzenesulfonamide).
Besylate(s)* *see* Besilate(s).
'**Betacaine**' *see* Eucaine.
'**Beta-cardone**' *see* Sotalol.
BETACETYLMETHADOL*** (β-3-acetoxy-6-dimethylamino-4,4-diphenylheptane).
See also Acetylmethadol.
'**Beta-chlor**' *see* Chloral betaine.
'**Beta-corlan**' *see* Betamethasone sodium phosphate.
'**Betadine**' *see* Povidone-iodine.
'**Betadorm**' *see* Carbromal with diphen-hydramine.
'**Betadran**' *see* Bupranolol.
'**Betadrenol**' *see* Bupranolol.
'**Betafluorene**' *see* Dexamethasone succinate.
BETAHISTINE*** (2-(2-methylaminoethyl)-pyridine; PT-9; 'betaserc', 'serc'). †
Beta-hypophamine *see* Vasopressin.
Betainchloralum* *see* Chloral betaine.
BETAINE HYDROCHLORIDE (lycine; oxyneurine; trimethylglycine-HCl; 'acidol').
'**Betajel**' *see* Ispagula.
'**Betaloc**' *see* Metoprolol.
'**Betalone**' *see* Meprednisone.
BETAMEPRODINE*** (β-3-ethyl-1-methyl-4-phenyl-4-propionoxypiperidine).
BETAMETHADOL*** (β-6-dimethylamino-4,4-diphenyl-3-heptanol).
See also Dimepheptanol.
BETAMETHASONE*** (9α-fluoro-16β-methyl-1,4-pregnadiene-11β,17α,21-triol-3,20-dione; 9α-fluoro-11β,17,21-trihydr-oxy-16β-methylpregna-1,4-diene-3,20-dione; 9α-fluoro-16β-methylprednisolone; betamethasone phosphate; flubenisolone; 'betnelan', 'betnesol', 'celestene', 'celestone', 'rinderon').
BETAMETHASONE ACETATE WITH BETAMETHASONE SODIUM PHOS-PHATE ('celestene-chronodose', 'celestone-soluspan').
Betamethasone 21-acetate 17-isobutyrate *see* Betamethasone acibutate.
Betamethasone 21-acetate 17-(2-methyl-propionate) *see* Betamethasone acibutate.
BETAMETHASONE ACIBUTATE*** (betamethasone 21-acetate 17-isobutyrate; betamethasone 21-acetate 17-(2-methyl-propionate); GR2/541).
BETAMETHASONE ADAMANTOATE ('betsovet').
BETAMETHASONE BENZOATE* (beta-methasone 17-benzoate; 'benisone', 'fluobate').
BETAMETHASONE DIPROPIONATE (S-8440; Sch-11460; 'diproderm', 'dipro-sone').

Betamethasone disodium phosphate *see* Betamethasone sodium phosphate.

BETAMETHASONE SODIUM PHOSPHATE (betamethasone disodium phosphate; 'beta-corlan', 'celestan-soluble').

BETAMETHASONE VALERATE (betamethasone 17-valerate ester; 'betneval', 'betnovate', 'bextasol', 'ecoval 70', 'retenema', 'valisone').

Betamezid (tr) *see* Pivhydrazine.

BETAMICIN* (*O*-6-amino-6-deoxy-α-D-glucopyranosyl-(1→4)-*O*-[3-deoxy-4-*C*-methyl-3-(methylamino)-β-L-arabino-pyranosyl-(1→6)]-2-deoxy-D-streptamine; betamicin sulfate; Sch-14342).

BETAMINE (tr) (3-(3-amino-4,6-diiodophenyl)-β-alanine).

'Betanal' *see* Phenmedipham.

'Beta-neg' *see* Propranolol.

BETANIDINE** (1-benzyl-2,3-dimethyl-guanidine; bethanidine sulfate; benzanidine; BW-467C60; 'esbatal').

'Betapar' *see* Meprednisone.

BETAPRODINE*** (β-1,3-dimethyl-4-phenyl-4-propionoxypiperidine). *See also* Alphaprodine.

'Betaprone' *see* Propiolactone.

Betapyrimidum *see* Nikethamide.

'Betaquil' *see* 2-Phenylpropyl carbamate.

'Betares' *see* Propranolol.

Betasan *see* Bensulide.

'Betaserc' *see* Betahistine.

Betasin (tr) *see* Betazine.

BETAZINE (tr) (3-(4-hydroxy-3,5-diiodophenyl)-β-alanine; diiodo-β-tyrosine; betasin).

BETAZOLE** (3-(2-aminoethyl)pyrazole; ametazole; 'gastramine', 'histalog').

BETHANECHOL* (carbamyl-β-methylcholine; (2-hydroxypropyl)trimethylammonium chloride carbamate; (2-carbamoyloxypropyl)trimethylammonium chloride; 'mecothane', 'muscaran', 'myocholine', 'myotonine', 'urecholine').

Bethanidine* *see* Betanidine.

Bethrodine *see* Benfluralin.

Betitol *see* Inositol.

'Betnelan' *see* Betamethasone.

'Betnesol' *see* Betamethasone.

'Betneval' *see* Betamethasone valerate.

'Betnovate' *see* Betamethasone valerate.

Betol *see* 2-Naphthyl salicylate.

'Betoral' *see* Phenformin.

Betoxicaine* *see* Betoxycaine.

BETOXYCAINE*** (2-(2-diethylaminoethoxy)ethyl 3-amino-4-butoxybenzoate; betoxicaine; 'millicaine').

'Betsovet' *see* Betamethasone adamantoate.

Betula oil *see* Methyl salicylate.

'Beveno' *see* Cyclovalone.

'Bevidine' *see* Povidone-iodine.

Bevonium methylsulfate* *see* Bevonium metilsulfate.

BEVONIUM METILSULFATE*** (2-hydroxymethyl-1,1-dimethylpiperidinium methyl sulfate benzilate; bevonium methylsulfate; piribenzil; CG-201; 'acabel').

'Bextasol' *see* Betamethasone valerate.

BEZAFIBRATE** (2-[*p*-[2-(*p*-chlorobenzamido)ethyl]phenoxy]-2-methylpropionic acid; BM-15075).

BEZITRAMIDE*** (1-[1-(2-cyano-3,3-diphenylpropyl)piperid-4-yl]-3-propionyl-2-benzimidazolinone; 1-(2-cyano-3,3-diphenylpropyl)-4-(2-oxo-3-propionylbenzimidazolin-1-yl)piperidine; R-4845; 'burgodin').

BF-103 *see* Acedapsone.

BFP *see* Dimefox.

BFPO *see* Dimefox.

BH-135 *see* Tolpentamide.

BHA *see* Butylated hydroxyanisole.

γ-BHC *see* Lindane.

BHC with DDT *see* Lindane with DDT.

BHT *see* Butylated hydroxytoluene.

4′,‴4-Biacetophenone-2,2″-bis[dimethyl-(2-hydroxyethyl)ammonium bromide] *see* Hemicholinium.

Biacetyl *see* 2,3-Butanedione.

BIALAMICOL*** (3,3′-diallyl-5,5′-bis(diethylaminomethyl)-4,4′-dihydroxybiphenyl; 6,6′-diallyl-2,2′-bis(diethylaminomethyl)-4,4′-biphenol; (5,5′-diallyl-α,α′-bis(diethylamino)-*m*,*m*′-bitolyl-4,4′-diol; 6,6′-diallyl-α,α′-bis(diethylamino)-4,4′-bi-*o*-cresol; bialamicol dihydrochloride; biallylamicol; biethylamicol; CI-301; CT-871; PAA-701; SN-6771; 'camoform').

Biallylamicol *see* Bialamicol.

'Biamine' *see* Thiamine.

5,5′-Bibarbituric acid *see* Hydurilic acid.

Bibenzone* *see* Bibenzonium bromide.

BIBENZONIUM BROMIDE*** ([2-(1,2-diphenylethoxy)ethyl]trimethylammonium bromide; bibenzone; diphenetholine; 'lysobex', 'medipectol', 'sedobex', 'thoragol').

BIBENZYL (1,2-diphenylethane).

BIBROCATHOL*** (bismuth tetrabromopyrocatechate; 'noviform', 'novoform').

Bibrophen *see* Bismuth tribromphenate.

'Bica-penicillin' *see* Benzathine penicillin.

'Bicarnesine' *see* Bicarnitine.

BICARNITINE (carnitine carnitinate; dicarnitine; 'bicarnesine').

'Bicillin' *see* Benzathine penicillin.

'Bicine' *see* *N*,*N*-Bis(2-hydroxyethyl)glycine.

'Biciron' *see* Tramazoline.

BICLOFIBRATE*** (2,2-bis(*p*-chlorophenoxy)acetic acid 1-methylpyrrolidin-2-ylmethyl ester; 1-methylpyrrolidin-2-ylmethyl bis(*p*-chlorophenoxy)acetate).

BICLOTYMOL*** (2,2′-methylenebis(6-chlorothymol); 'hexpneumine').

'Bicolon' *see* Dimeticone.

'Bicor' *see* Terodiline.

'Bicortone' *see* Prednisone.

BICP *see* Chlorbufam.

Bicyclo(2.2.1)heptane *see* Norbornane.

Bicyclo(2.2.1)hept-2-ene *see* Norbornene.

[2-[1-((2.2.1)Bicyclohept-2-en-5-yl)-1-phenylethoxy]ethyl]diethylmethylammonium bromide *see* Ciclonium bromide.

1-(Bicyclo(2.2.1)hept-5-en-2-yl)-1-phenyl-

3-piperid-1-yl-1-propanol *see* Biperiden.
(BICYCLOHEXYL)-1-CARBOXYLIC ACID (1-cyclohexylcyclohexanecarboxylic acid).
(Bicyclohexyl)-1-carboxylic acid 2-diethylaminoethyl ester *see* Dicycloverine.
(Bicyclohexyl)-1-carboxylic acid 2-piperid-1-ylethyl ester *see* Dihexyverine.
'Bidex' *see* Chlorhexidine.
BIDIMAZIUM IODIDE*** (4-biphenyl-4-yl-2-(4-dimethylaminostyryl)-3-methyl-thiazolium iodide).
'Bidisin' *see* Chlorfenprop-methyl.
'Bidizole' *see* Sulfasomizole.
'Bidrin' *see* Dicrotophos.
'Biebrich scarlet medicinal R' *see* Scarlet red.
'Bietamine' *see* Benfotiamine.
BIETAMIVERINE*** (2-diethylaminoethyl α-phenyl-1-piperidineacetate; 'novosparol', 'spasmoparid').
BIETASERPINE** (1-(2-diethylaminoethyl)-reserpine; DL-152).
BIETASERPINE WITH HYDRO-CHLOROTHIAZIDE ('pleiatensin').
Biethylamicol *see* Bialamicol.
'Bi-euglucon' *see* Glibenclamide with phenformin.
BIFLURANOL*** (*erythro*-4,4′-(1-ethyl-2-methylethylene)bis(2-fluorophenol); *erythro*-2,3-bis-(3-fluoro-4-hydroxyphenyl)-pentane; BX-341).
'Bifteral' *see* Lactulose.
Bigitalin *see* Gitoxin.
Biguamor (tr) *see* Moroxydine.
BIGUANIDE (amidinoguanidine; diguanide; formamidinylimiourea; guanylguanidine).
Bigumal *see* Proguanil.
'Bihypnal' *see* Dichloralphenazone.
Biioquinol *see* Quinine iodobismuthate.
'Bilagol' *see* Diisopromine.
'Bilarcil' *see* Metrifonate.
'Bilevon' *see* Niclofolan.
'Bilharcid' *see* Piperazine diantimonyl tartrate.
Bilignost (tr) *see* Adipiodone.
'Biligrafin' *see* Adipiodone.
'Biligram' *see* Ioglycamide.
'Bilijodon' *see* Iopanoic acid.
Bilineurine *see* Choline.
'Biliodyl' *see* Phenobutiodil.
'Bilipolin' *see* Ioglycamide.
'Biliton' *see* Dehydrocholic acid.
'Bilitox' *see* Cupric chloride.
Bilitrast (tr) *see* Pheniodol.
'Bilivistan' *see* Ioglycamide with sodium ioglycamate.
'Bilobran' *see* Dodine.
'Bilopaque' *see* Sodium tyropanoate.
'Biloptin' *see* Sodium ipodate.
BIMETOPYROL (4,5-bis(*p*-methoxyphenyl)-2-methylpyrrole).
2,2′-Bimorphine *see* Pseudomorphine.
BIN-7 *see* Usnic acid sodium salt.
Binan (tr) *see* Usnic acid sodium salt.
BINAPACRYL*** (2-*sec*-butyl-4,6-dinitrophenyl senecioate; 2-*sec*-butyl-4,6-dinitro-phenyl 3-methylcrotonate; 2-*sec*-butyl-4,6-dinitrophenyl 3,3-dimethylacrylate; 2-(1-methylpropyl)-4,6-dinitrophenyl-3-methyl-2-butenoate; dinoseb senecioate; 'acricid', 'endosan', 'morocide').
'Binartrina' *see* Oxyphenbutazone with propetamide.
'Binasol' *see* Bismuth sodium tartrate.
'Binazin' *see* Todralazine.
BINIRAMYCIN*** (antibiotic from *Str. bikiniensis*).
'Binnell' *see* Benfluralin.
'Binotal' *see* Ampicillin.
BIOALLETHRIN* (*trans*-(+)-2-methyl-4-oxo-3-(2-propenyl)-2-cyclopenten-1-yl 2,2-dimethyl-3-(2-methyl-1-propenyl)-cyclopentanecarboxylate; *trans*-(+)-allethrin; EA-3054; ENT-16275).
See also Allethrin.
'Biobasal AG' *see* Histaglobin.
'Biobase' *see* Carbenoxolone sodium.
'Biocetab' *see* Cetrimonium.
BIOCHANIN A (5,7-dihydroxy-4′-methoxy-isoflavone).
'Biocholine' *see* Choline.
'Biocidan' *see* Cethexonium.
'Biocodone' *see* Hydrocodone.
'Biocolina' *see* Choline.
Biocolorin *see* Esculin.
'Biocytin' *see* Biotinyllysine.
'Biodramine' *see* Dimenhydrinate.
'Bioepiderm' *see* Biotin.
'Biogastrone' *see* Carbenoxolone.
'Biogest' *see* 6-Chloro-17α-hydroxy-16-methylenepregna-4,6-diene-3,20-dione with mestranol.
'Bio-met' *see* Bis(tributyltin) oxide.
Biomitsin (tr) *see* Chlortetracycline.
'Biomorphyl' *see* Hydromorphone.
Biomycin *see* Chlortetracycline.
'Bional' *see* Carbenoxolone.
BIOPROPAZEPAN (tetrahydro-1H-1,4-diazepine-1,4(5H)-dipropanol; homo-piperazine-1,4-dipropanol).
Biopropazepan bis(3,4,5-trimethoxy-benzoate) *see* Dilazep.
BIOPTERIDIN (2-amino-6-(dihydroxy-propyl)-4-hydroxypteridine).
'Bioquin' *see* 8-Quinolinol.
'Bioral' *see* Carbenoxolone sodium.
BIORESMETHRIN* (*trans*-(+)-5-benzyl-furan-3-ylmethyl 2,2-dimethyl-3-(2-methyl-1-propenyl)cyclopropanecarboxylate; NRDC-107).
See also Cismethrin; Resmethrin.
Bios-I *see* Biotin.
Bios-II *see* Inositol.
'Biosept' *see* Cetylpyridinium bromide.
'Biosone' *see* Enoxolone.
'Biostat' *see* Oxytetracycline.
Biosterol *see* Retinol.
'Biotexin' *see* Novobiocin.
BIOTIN** (*cis*-tetrahydro-2-oxothieno(3,4)-imidazoline-4-valeric acid; hexahydro-2-oxo(1H)thieno(3,4)imidazole-4-valeric acid; coenzyme R; vitamin B_w; vitamin H; bios-I; 'bioepiderm').

BIOTINYLLYSINE (*N*-biotinyl-L-lysine; 'biocytin').

Biovetin (tr) *see* Chlortetracycline.

Biovit-40 (tr) *see* Chlortetracycline.

Bioxone *see* Chlormethazole.

BiPC *see* Chlorbufam.

BIPERIDEN*** (α-(bicyclo(2.2.1)hept-5-en-2-yl)-α-phenyl-1-piperidinepropanol; 1-(bicyclo(2.2.1)hept-5-en-2-yl)-1-phenyl-3-piperid-1-yl-1-propanol; α-5-norbornen-2-yl-α-phenyl-1-piperidinepropanol; beperiden; LM-203A; 'akineton'; 'akinophyl').

BIPHASIC INSULIN INJECTION* (suspended insulin crystals in solution of insulin buffered at pH 7; 'insulin novo rapitard').

'Biphecillin' *see* Benzathine penicillin V.

'Biphenabid' *see* Probucol.

'Biphenal' *see* Hydroxypethidine.

Biphenamine* *see* Xenysalate.

BIPHENYL (diphenyl; phenylbenzene; 'dinyl').

[1,1'-Biphenyl]-4-acetic acid *see* Biphenylylacetic acid.

BIPHENYLAMINE (aminobiphenyl; aminodiphenyl).

2,2'-Biphenyldicarboxylic acid *see* Diphenic acid.

Biphenylenebis(diphenyltetrazolium chloride) *see* Neotetrazolium.

p,p'-**Biphenylenebisglyoxal** *see* Xenygloxal.

Biphenylene oxide *see* Dibenzofuran.

Biphenylethylacetic acid *see* Biphenylylbutyric acid.

BIPHENYLYLACETIC ACID (2-(*p*-biphenylyl)acetic acid; [1,1'-biphenyl]-4-acetic acid; xenylacetic acid).

Biphenylylacetic acid 2-fluoroethyl ester *see* Fluenetil.

4,4'-Biphenylylbisazo(1-naphthylamine-4-sulfonic acid) *see* Congo red.

2-(*p*-Biphenylyl)butyric acid *see* Xenbucin.

2-(*p*-Biphenylyl)butyric acid salt with *trans*-**4-phenylcyclohexylamine** *see* Butixirate.

3-(4-Biphenylylcarbonyl)propionic acid *see* Fenbufen.

4,4'-Biphenylyldiglyoxyl aldehyde *see* Xenygloxal.

4-Biphenyl-4-yl-2-(4-dimethylaminostyryl)-3-methylthiazolium iodide *see* Bidimazium iodide.

4-Biphenylylethylacetic acid *see* Xenbucin.

4-(4-Biphenylyl)-3-ethyl-2-(*p*-pyrrolidin-1-ylstyryl)thiazolium iodide *see* Pretamazium iodide.

2-(*p*-Biphenylyl)-4-hexenoic acid *see* Xenhexenic acid.

8-(*p*-Biphenylylmethyl)atropinium bromide *see* Xenytropium.

4-Biphenylyl methylcarbamate *see* Paxamate.

2-(*p*-Biphenylyl)thiolobutyric acid diethylaminoethyl ester *see* Xenthiorate.

BIPIPERIDINE (dipiperidyl).

2,2'-Bipseudoindoxyl *see* Indigotin.

BIPYRIDINE (dipyridyl; pyridylpyridine).

BIQ-16 *see* Hedaquinium.

'Birlane' *see* Clofenvinfos.

(−)-α-**Bisabolol** *see* Levomenol.

2,2'-Bis(4-acetamidophenoxy)ethyl ether *see* Diamfenetide.

2,2-Bis(4-acetoxyphenyl)-2H-1,4-benzoxazin-3(4H)-one *see* Bisoxatin diacetate.

Bis(*p*-acetoxyphenyl)cyclohexylidenemethane *see* Cyclofenil.

2-[Bis(*p*-acetoxyphenyl)methyl]pyridine *see* Bisacodyl.

1α,7α-Bis(acetylthio)-17α-methylandrost-4-en-17β-ol-3-one *see* Tiomesterone.

BISACODYL** (2-[bis(*p*-acetoxyphenyl)methyl]pyridine; 4,4'-pyrid-2-ylmethylenediphenol diacetate; 4,4'-diacetoxy-α-(2-pyridyl)diphenylmethane; diacetate of 2-(*p,p'*-dihydroxybenzhydryl)pyridine; acetophenomethane; 'alaxa', 'ducolax', 'dulcolan', 'dulcolax', 'godalax', 'nourilax N', 'perilax', 'toilax').

BISACODYL WITH DIMETICONE ('laxbene').

BISACODYL TANNEX* (complex of bisacodyl with tannins; 'clysodrast').

Bis[2-(*N*-adamant-1-yl-*N*-methylamino)ethyl] succinate dimethiodide *see* Diadonium iodide.

1,5-Bis(*p*-allylmethylaminophenyl)-3-pentanone dimethobromide *see* 1,5-Diphenyl-3-oxopentamethylene-*p,p'*-bis-(allyldimethylammonium bromide).

1,3-Bis(4-amidino-2-bromophenoxy)propane *see* Dibrompropamidine.

Bis(*p*-amidinophenyl)ether *see* Phenamidine.

1,3-Bis(*p*-amidinophenyl)triazene *see* Diminazene.

1,3-Bis(*m*-amidinophenyl)urea *see* Amicarbalide.

1,3-Bis(4-amino-2-methylquinolin-6-yl)urea *see* Aminoquinuride.

Bis(*p*-aminophenyl) sulfone *see* Dapsone.

N,N'-Bis(3-aminopropyl)putrescine *see* Spermine.

4,4'-Bis(1-amino-4-sulfonaphth-2-ylazo)biphenyl *see* Congo red.

1,2-Bis(*p*-arsonophenylamino)ethane *see* Difetarsone.

N,N'-Bis(*p*-arsonophenyl)ethylenediamine *see* Difetarsone.

Bisatin *see* Acetphenolisatin.

Bis(1-aziridinyl)benzyloxycarbonylaminophosphine oxide *see* Benzodepa.

2,4-Bis(1-aziridinyl)-6-chloropyrimidine *see* Ethymidine.

Bis(1-aziridinyl)(cyclohexylamino)phosphine sulfide *see* Hexaphosphamide.

2,5-Bis(1-aziridinyl)-3,6-dipropoxy-*p*-benzoquinone *see* Inproquone.

Bis(1-aziridinyl)ethoxycarbonylaminophosphine oxide *see* Uredepa.

Bis(1-aziridinyl)-*N*-ethyl-*N*-(1,3,4-thiadiazol-2-yl)phosphinic amide *see* Azetepa.

2,5-Bis(1-aziridinyl)-3-(2-hydroxy-1-

methoxyethyl)-6-methyl-*p*-benzoquinone carbamate *see* Carboquone.

Bis(1-aziridinyl)phosphinylcarbamic acid esters *see* Benzodepa; Meturedepa; Uredepa.

BISBENDAZOLE*** (bis[1-(1-methyl-benzimidazol-2-yl)ethyl] tetrathio-*p*-benzenedicarbamate).

BISBENTIAMINE*** (*N,N'*-[dithiobis[2-(2-hydroxyethyl)-1-methylvinylene]]bis[*N*-[(4-amino-2-methylpyrimidin-5-yl)methyl]-formamide]benzoate; *N,N'*-[dithiobis[2-(2-benzoyloxyethyl)-1-methylvinylene]]bis-[*N*-(4-amino-2-methylpyrimidin-5-yl-methyl)formamide]; benzoylthiamine disulfide; 'beston').

1,4-Bis[(*N,N'*-bisethylene)diamidothio-phosphoryl]piperazine *see* Thiodipin.

2,6-Bis[bis(2-hydroxyethyl)amino]-4,8-bis(1-piperidyl)pyrimido(5,4-d)pyrimidine *see* Dipyridamole.

2,2-Bis(*p*-bromophenyl)glycolic acid isopropyl ester *see* Bromopropylate.

1,4-Bis(3-bromopropionyl)piperazine *see* Pipobroman.

5-[Bis[2-(2-butoxyethoxy)ethoxy]meth-yl]-1,3-benzodioxole *see* Piperonal bis[2-(2-butoxyethoxy)ethyl]acetal.

1,3-Bis(3-butoxy-2-hydroxypropyl)pheno-barbital dicarbamate *see* Difebarbamate.

2,2-Bis(carbamoyloxymethyl)-3-methyl-pentane *see* Mebutamate.

1,3-Bis(carbamoylthio)-*N,N*-dimethyl-2-propylamine *see* Cartap.

1,2-Bis(3-carbethoxy-2-thioureido)-benzene *see* Thiophanate.

1,2-Bis(3-carbomethoxy-2-thioureido)-benzene *see* Thiophanate methyl.

5,7-Bis(carboxymethoxy)flavone *see* Flavodic acid.

1,3-Bis(2-carboxy-4-oxobenzopyran-5-yloxy)-2-propanol *see* Cromoglicic acid.

1,3-Bis(2-carboxy-4-oxochromen-5-yloxy)-propan-2-ol *see* Cromoglicic acid.

Bis(*o*-carboxyphenyl) salicylate *see* Succinylsalicylic acid.

1,3-Bis(*p*-chlorobenzylideneamino)-guanidine *see* Robenidine.

2-[Bis(2-chloroethyl)amino-3-(2-chloro-ethyl)tetrahydro-2H-1,3,2-oxaphosphor-ine 2-oxide *see* Trofosfamide.

3-[2-[2-[Bis(2-chloroethyl)amino]ethyl]-4-nitrophenyl]alanine *see* Nitrocaphane.

3-[*o*-[2-[Bis(2-chloroethyl)amino]ethyl]-phenyl]alanine *see* Ocaphane.

5-[Bis(2-chloroethyl)amino]-6-methyl-uracil *see* Dopan.

p-[Bis(2-chloroethyl)amino]-*N*-nicotinoyl-phenylalanine ethyl ester *see* Nicosin.

2-[Bis(2-chloroethyl)amino]-(2H)1,3,2-oxaphosphorinane 2-oxide *see* Cyclo-phosphamide.

p-[Bis(2-chloroethyl)amino]phenylacet-amidobenzoic acid ethyl ester *see* Phenastezin.

2-[*p*-[Bis(2-chloroethyl)amino]phenyl-acetamido]-3-imidazol-4-ylpropionic

acid methyl ester *see* Hisphen.

2-[*p*-[Bis(2-chloroethyl)amino]phenyl-acetamido]-4-(methylthio)butyric acid ethyl ester *see* Phenamet.

2-[*p*-[Bis(2-chloroethyl)amino]phenyl-acetamido]-3-phenylpropionic acid *see* Lofenal.

p-[Bis(2-chloroethyl)amino]phenylacetic acid *see* Chlorphenacyl.

p-[Bis(2-chloroethyl)amino]phenylacetic acid cholesteryl ester *see* Phenesterin.

N-[*p*-[Bis(2-chloroethyl)amino]phenyl-acetyl]-L-histidine methyl ester *see* Hisphen.

N-[*p*-[Bis(2-chloroethyl)amino]phenyl-acetyl]methionine ethyl ester *see* Phenamet.

N-[*p*-[Bis(2-chloroethyl)amino]phenyl-acetyl]-DL-phenylalanine *see* Lofenal.

DL-3-[*o*-[Bis(2-chloroethyl)amino]phenyl]-alanine *see* *o*-Sarcolysin.

DL-3-[*m*-[Bis(2-chloroethyl)amino]phenyl]-alanine *see* *m*-Sarcolysin.

DL-3-[*p*-[Bis(2-chloroethyl)amino]phenyl]-alanine *see* Sarcolysin.

D-3-[*p*-[Bis(2-chloroethyl)amino]phenyl]-alanine *see* Medphalan.

L-3-[*p*-[Bis(2-chloroethyl)amino]phenyl]-alanine *see* Melphalan.

L-3-[*m*-[Bis(2-chloroethyl)amino]phenyl]-alanine peptide complex *see* Pepti-chemio.

4-[*p*-[Bis(2-chloroethyl)amino]phenyl]-butyric acid *see* Chlorambucil.

4-[*p*-[Bis(2-chloroethyl)amino]phenyl]-butyric acid prednisolone 21-ester *see* Prednimustine.

2-[*p*-(Bis(2-chloroethyl)amino]phenyl)-ethyl acetate *see* Phenester.

DL-3-[*p*-[Bis(2-chloroethyl)amino]phenyl]-*N*-formylalanine *see* Formylsarcolysin.

5-[Bis(2-chloroethyl)amino]uracil *see* Uramustine.

Bis(2-chloroethyl)carbamic acid 3-ester with estradiol *see* Estramustine.

Bis(2-chloroethyl) (3-chloro-4-methyl-coumarin-7-yl) phosphate *see* Haloxon.

N,N-Bis(2-chloroethyl)-2-chloro-1-propyl-amine *see* Novembichin.

N,N-Bis(2-chloroethyl)-4-methoxy-3-methyl-1-naphthylamine *see* Mito-clomine.

N,N-Bis(2-chloroethyl)methylamine *see* Chlormethine.

Bis(2-chloroethyl)-2-naphthylamine *see* Chlornaphazine.

1,3-Bis(2-chloroethyl)-1-nitrosourea *see* Carmustine.

N,N-Bis(2-chloroethyl)phosphorodiam-idic acid esters *see* Cyclophosphamide; Defosfamide.

N,N-Bis(2-chloroethyl)-*N,O'*-propylene-phosphoric diamide *see* Cyclophospham-ide.

Bis(2-chloroethyl) sulfide *see* Mustard gas.

3,12-Bis(2-chloroethyl)-3,6,9,12-tetraza-dispiro(5.5.5)hexadecane *see*

53

Spirazidine.

2,6-Bis(5-chloro-2-hydroxybenzyl)-4-chlorophenol see Trichlorophen.

Bis(5-chloro-2-hydroxyphenyl) sulfide see Fenticlor.

3,12-Bis(3-chloro-2-hydroxypropyl)-3,12-diaza-6,9-diazoniadispiro(5.2.5.2)hexadecane dichloride see Prospidium chloride.

N,N³-**Bis(3-chloro-2-hydroxypropyl)-*N,N²*-dispirotripiperazine dichloride** see Prospidium chloride.

2,2-Bis(*p*-chlorophenoxy)acetic acid 1-methylpiperid-4-yl ester see Lifibrate.

2,2-Bis(*p*-chlorophenoxy)acetic acid 1-methylpyrrolidin-2-ylmethyl ester see Biclofibrate.

BIS(*p*-CHLOROPHENOXY)METHANE (DCPM; K-1875; 'neotran').

Bis[2-(*p*-chlorophenoxy)-2-methylpropionato]hydroxyaluminium see Aluminium clofibrate.

Bis[2-(*p*-chlorophenoxy)-2-methylpropionato]magnesium see Magnesium clofibrate.

O,O-**BIS(*p*-CHLOROPHENYL) *N*-ACETIMIDOYLPHOSPHORAMIDOTHIOATE** (Bayer-38819; 'gophicide').

1,4-Bis[*N*¹-[*N*¹-(*p*-chlorophenyl)amidino]-amidino]piperazine see Picloxydine.

α,α-**Bis(*p*-chlorophenyl)cyclopropanemethanol** see Proclonol.

2,2-Bis(*p*-chlorophenyl)glycolic acid ethyl ester see Chlorobenzilate.

2,2-Bis(*p*-chlorophenyl)glycolic acid isopropyl ester see Chloropropylate.

O,O-**Bis(*p*-chlorophenyl)(1-iminoethyl)phosphoramidothioate** see Phosacetim.

Bis(*p*-chlorophenyl) methyl carbinol see Chlorfenethol.

N-[2,3-**Bis(*p*-chlorophenyl)-1-methylpropyl]maleamic acid** see Benzmalecene.

α,α-**Bis(*p*-chlorophenyl)-3-pyridinemethanol** see Parinol.

Biscumarol see Dicoumarol.

4,4'-Bis[*p*-(13-cyclopentyltridecanamido)-phenyl] sulfone see Chaulmosulfone.

6,7-Bis(cyclopropylmethoxy)-4-hydroxyquinoline-3-carboxylic acid ethyl ester see Ciproquinate.

BisDEAEfluorenone see Tilorone.

3,6-Bisdeoxy-L-mannose see Ascarylose.

1,4-Bis(diaziridinylphosphinylidyne)-piperazine see Dipin.

2,2-Bis(3,5-di-*tert*-butyl-4-hydroxyphenyl)-acetic acid see Terbuficin.

Bisdichlorohydroxyphenyl sulfide see Bithionol.

Bis(2,4-dichlorophenyl)iodonium chloride see Feniodium chloride.

2,6-Bis(diethanolamino)-4,8-dipiperidino-pyrimido(5,4-d)pyrimidine see Dipyridamole.

Bis[*S*-(diethoxyphosphinothioyl)mercapto]methane see Ethion.

2,7-Bis(2-diethylaminoethoxy)fluoren-9-one see Tilorone.

6,7-Bis(2-diethylaminoethoxy)-4-methyl-coumarin see Oxamarin.

2,2-Bis(2-diethylaminoethyl)-1-cyclohexyl-1-phenylethane see Phenetamine.

2,4-Bis(diethylamino)-6-hydrazino-*s*-triazine see Meladrazine.

Bis(diethylaminomethyl)diallylbiphenol see Bialamicol.

4-[3,5-Bis(diethylaminomethyl)-4-hydroxyanilino]-7-chloroquinoline see Cycloquine.

Bis(diethylthiocarbamyl) disulfide see Disulfiram.

Bis(diethylthiocarbamyl) sulfide see Monosulfiram.

2,3-Bis(3,4-dihydroxybenzyl)butane see Nordihydroguaiaretic acid.

1,4-Bis(3,4-dihydroxyphenyl)butane see Nordihydroguaiaretic acid.

N,N'-**Bis[2-(3,4-dihydroxyphenyl)-2-hydroxyethyl]hexamethylenediamine** see Hexoprenaline.

Bis(dimethylamido)fluorophosphate see Dimefox.

3,6-Bis(dimethylamino)acridine see Acridine orange.

Bis(2-dimethylaminoethyl) succinate bisethochloride see Suxethonium.

Bis(2-dimethylaminoethyl) succinate bismethochloride see Suxamethonium.

Bis(dimethylamido)fluorophosphine oxide see Dimefox.

1,3-Bis(dimethylamino)-2-propanol dimethiodide see Prolonium.

10-[2,3-Bis(dimethylamino)propyl]-phenothiazine see Aminopromazine.

Bis(2,2-dimethyl-1-aziridinyl)phosphinylcarbamic acid ethyl ester see Meturedepa.

S,S'-**Bis(dimethylcarbamodithioato)zinc** see Ziram.

Bis(dimethylcarbamoyl)diimide see Diamide.

2,6-Bis(1,1-dimethylethyl)-4-methylphenyl methylcarbamate see Terbucarb.

1,1'-Bis(3,5-dimethylmorpholinocarbonylmethyl)-4,4'-bipyridinium dichloride see Morfamquat.

1,1'-Bis[2-(3,5-dimethylmorpholino)-2-oxoethyl]-4,4'-bipyridinium dichloride see Morfamquat.

N,N-**Bis[2-[*N*-(α,α-dimethylphenethyl)-*N*-methylacetamido]methyl]-2-hydroxyethylamine** see Oxetacaine.

Bis[3-(2,5-dimethylpyrrolidin-1-yl)propyl]hexadecylmethylammonium bromide see Pirralkonium bromide.

Bis(dimethylthiocarbamyl) disulfide see Thiram.

1,3-Bis(3,5-dioxopiperazin-1-yl)propane see Razoxane.

1,1'-Bis(2,3-epoxypropyl)-4,4'-bipiperidine see Epipropidine.

1,4-Bis(2,3-epoxypropyl)piperazine see Epoxypropylpiperazine.

'Biseptol' see Cotrimoxazole.

1,2-Bis(3-ethoxycarbonyl-2-thioureido)-

benzene *see* Thiophanate.

Bis(2-ethoxyethyl) ether *see* Trioxaun-
decane.

N,N′-**Bis**(*p*-**ethoxyphenyl)acetamidine**
see Phenacaine.

4,6-Bis(ethylamino)-2-chloro-*s*-triazine
see Simazine.

Bis(ethyleniminosulfonyl)propane *see*
1,1′-(Trimethylenedisulfonyl)bisaziridine.

**2,6-Bis(2-ethylhexyl)hexahydro-7α-
methyl(1H)imidazo(1,5-c)imidazole**
see Hexedine.

N[1],*N*[3]-**Bis(2-ethylhexyl)-2-methyl-1,2,3-
propanetriamine** *see* Propoctamine.

**Bis(*N*-ethylidenethreoninato) hydrogen
diaquoferrate (II)** *see* Ferrotrenine.

Bis(ethylxanthogen) *see* Dixanthogen.

BISFENAZONE[***] (3-[[(2,3-dimethyl-5-oxo-
1-phenyl-3-pyrazolin-4-yl)amino]methyl]-
4-isopropyl-2-methyl-1-phenyl-3-pyrazolin-
5-one).

erythro-**2,3-Bis(3-fluoro-4-hydroxyphenyl)-
pentane** *see* Bifluranol.

**1-[4,4-Bis(*p*-fluorophenyl)butyl]-4-(5-
chloro-2-oxobenzimidazolin-1-yl)-
piperidine** *see* Clopimozide.

**1-[4,4-Bis(*p*-fluorophenyl)butyl]-4-(4-
chloro-α,α,α-trifluoro-*m*-tolyl)-4-piper-
idinol** *see* Penfluridol.

**1-[4,4-Bis(*p*-fluorophenyl)butyl]-4-(2-
oxobenzimidazolin-1-yl)piperidine** *see*
Pimozide.

**8-[4,4-Bis(*p*-fluorophenyl)butyl]-1-phenyl-
1,3,8-triazaspiro(4,5)-decan-4-one** *see*
Fluspirilene.

**[4-[4,4-Bis(*p*-fluorophenyl)butyl]piper-
azin-1-yl]-2′,6′-acetoxylidide** *see*
Lidoflazine.

**1-[1-[4,4-Bis(*p*-fluorophenyl)butyl]-
piperid-4-yl]-2-benzimidazolinone** *see*
Pimozide.

**1-[1-[4,4-Bis(*p*-fluorophenyl)butyl]-
piperid-4-yl]-5-chlorobenzimidazolin-
2-one** *see* Clopimozide.

**2-[Bis(*p*-fluorophenyl)methoxy]ethyl-
amine** *see* Flunamine.

**1-[Bis(*p*-fluorophenyl)methyl]-4-
cinnamylpiperazine** *see* Flunarizine.

**1,3-Bis(4-formylpyridinium)propane
dibromide dioxime** *see* Trimedoxime.

'Bisguadine' *see* Alexidine.

Bishydroxycoumarin[*] *see* Dicoumarol.

**2-[Bis(2-hydroxyethyl)amino]-4,5-di-
phenyloxazole** *see* Ditazole.

**8-[Bis(2-hydroxyethyl)aminomethyl]-
6,7-dihydroxy-4-methylcoumarin** *see*
Esculamine.

**4-[Bis(2-hydroxyethyl)amino]-2-(5-nitro-
fur-2-yl)quinazoline** *see* Nifurquinazol.

N,N-**BIS(2-HYDROXYETHYL)GLYCINE**
(diethylolglycine; 'Fe-3-specific', 'bicine').

**1,4-Bis(2-hydroxyethyl)piperazine
bis(2-phenylbutyrate)** *see* Febuverine.

Bis(2-hydroxyethyl) sulfide *see* Thiodiglycol.

**2,4-Bis(1-hydroxyethyl)-1,3,5,8-tetra-
methylporphine-6,7-dipropionic acid**

see Hematoporphyrin.

1,10-Bis(2-hydroxyethylthio)decane *see*
Tiadenol.

**Bis(3-hydroxy-4-hydroxymethyl-2-meth-
ylpyrid-5-ylmethyl) disulfide** *see*
Pyritinol.

**Bis(4-hydroxyimino-1-methylpyridinium
methyl ether) dichloride** *see* Obidoxime.

**1,3-Bis(4-hydroxyiminomethylpyridi-
nium)propane dibromide** *see* Trimedoxime.

**3-[Bis(hydroxymethyl)amino]-6-[2-(5-
nitro-2-furyl)ethenyl]-1,2,4-triazine** *see*
Di(hydroxymethyl)furalazine.

**3-[Bis(hydroxymethyl)amino]-6-[2-(5-
nitro-2-furyl)vinyl]-1,2,4-triazine** *see*
Di(hydroxymethyl)furalazine.

**1,3-Bis(hydroxymethyl)benzimidazole-2-
thione** *see* Thibenzazoline.

**1,1-Bis(hydroxymethyl)cyclopentane
carbanilate** *see* Cyclarbamate.

**2,2-Bis(hydroxymethyl)-1,3-dihydroxy-
propane** *see* Pentaerythritol.

**5,6-Bis(hydroxymethyl)-1,2,3,4,7,7-hexa-
chloronorbornene sulfite** *see* Endosulfan.

**4,5-Bis(hydroxymethyl)-3-hydroxy-α-
picoline** *see* Pyridoxine.

**[4,5-Bis(hydroxymethyl)-2-methylpyrid-
3-yloxy]glycolic acid compound with
2-[(5-hydroxy-4-hydroxymethylpyrid-
3-yl)methoxy]glycolic acid** *see*
Piridoxilate.

**3,4-Bis(*p*-hydroxy-*m*-methylphenyl)-
hexane** *see* Methestrol.

N,N′-**Bis(1-hydroxymethylpropyl)ethyl-
enediamine** *see* Ethambutol.

**2,6-Bis(hydroxymethyl)pyridyl bis-
(methylcarbamate)** *see* 2,6-Pyridinedi-
methanol bis(methylcarbamate).

**5,5-Bis(hydroxymethyl)-2-trichlorometh-
yl-1,3-dioxane** *see* Pentrichloral.

1,3-BIS(HYDROXYMETHYL)UREA
(dimethylolurea; 'methural').

**3,3-Bis(*p*-hydroxyphenyl)-2,1-benzoxa-
thiole 1,1-dioxide** *see* Phenolsulfonphthalein.

**2,2-Bis(*p*-hydroxyphenyl)-1,4-benzoxazin-
3-one** *see* Bisoxatin.

**Bis(*p*-hydroxyphenyl)cyclohexylidene-
methane diacetate** *see* Cyclofenil.

**1,3-Bis(*p*-hydroxyphenyl)-1,2-diethyl-3-
methylpropane** *see* Benzestrol.

**3,6-Bis(*p*-hydroxyphenyl)-2,5-dihydroxy-
p-benzoquinone** *see* Atromentin.

**1,4-Bis(*p*-hydroxyphenyl)-2,3-diisocyana-
to-1,3-butadiene** *see* Xanthocillin X.

1,3-Bis(*p*-hydroxyphenyl)-3-ethylhexane
see Benzestrol.

trans-**3,4-Bis(*p*-hydroxyphenyl)-3-hexene**
see Diethylstilbestrol.

**3,4-BIS(*p*-HYDROXYPHENYL)-2-
HEXENE** (pseudostilbestrol).

3,3-Bis(*p*-hydroxyphenyl)-2-indolinone
see Oxyphenisatine.

o-**[Bis(*p*-hydroxyphenyl)methyl]benzyl
alcohol** *see* Phenolphthalol.

4-(Bis(*p*-hydroxyphenyl)methylene)-2,5-

55

cyclohexadien-1-one *see* Roseolic acid.
3,3-Bis(*p*-hydroxyphenyl)-7-methyl-2-indolinone bis(hydrogen sulfate) *see* Sulisatin.
2,3-Bis(*p*-hydroxyphenyl)oxindole *see* Oxyphenisatine.
3,3-Bis(*p*-hydroxyphenyl)phthalide *see* Phenolphthalein.
1,4-Bis(3-hydroxypropionyl)piperazine dimesylate *see* Piposulfan.
Bis(1-hydroxy-2(1H)-pyridinethionato)zinc *see* Pyrithione zinc.
1,3-Bis(1-hydroxy-2,2,2-trichloroethoxy)-3-*o*-toloxypropane *see* Toloxychlorinol.
3,3′-Bis(2-imidazolin-2-yl)carbanilide *see* Imidocarb.
4,4′-Bis(isopentyloxy)thiocarbanilide *see* Tiocarlide.
Bis(isopropylamino)fluorophosphine oxide *see* Mipafox.
4,6-Bis(isopropylamino)-2-methoxy-*s*-triazine *see* Prometon.
4,6-Bis(isopropylamino)-2-(methylthio)-*s*-triazine *see* Prometryn.
1,6-Bis(methanesulfonyl)mannitol *see* Mannityl dimesilate.
1,4-Bis(methanesulfonyloxy)butane *see* Busulfan.
2,4-Bis(methanesulfonyloxy)pentane *see* Dimethyltrimethylene mesilate.
1,2-Bis(3-methoxycarbonyl-2-thioureido)-benzene *see* Thiophanate methyl.
Bis(6-methoxy-1-phenazinol-5,10-dioxidato-*O*¹,*O*¹⁰)copper *see* Cuprimyxin.
1,1-Bis(*p*-methoxyphenyl)-2,2-dimethyl-propane *see* Dianisylneopentane.
1,3-Bis(*p*-methoxyphenyl)-2-(*p*-ethoxy-phenyl)guanidine *see* Guanicaine.
2,3-Bis(*p*-methoxyphenyl)indole *see* Indoxole.
4,5-Bis(*p*-methoxyphenyl)-2-methyl-pyrrole *see* Bimetopyrol.
4,5-Bis(*p*-methoxyphenyl)-2-trifluoro-methylimidazole *see* Flumizole.
1,4-Bis(2-methoxy-4-propylphenoxy-acetyl)piperazine *see* Simetride.
Bis(1-methylamyl) sodium sulfosuccin-ate *see* Sodium dihexyl sulfosuccinate.
Bis[1-(1-methylbenzimidazol-2-yl)ethyl] tetrathio-*p*-benzenedicarbamate *see* Bisbendazole.
2,6-Bis(3,4-methylenedioxyphenyl)-3,7-dioxabicyclo(3.3.0)octane *see* Sesamin.
N,*N*′-Bis(1-methylethyl)-6-(methylthio)-1,3,5-triazine-2,4-diamine *see* Prometryn.
O,*O*-Bis(1-methylethyl) *S*-[2-[(phenyl-sulfonyl)amino]ethyl] phosphorodi-thioate *see* Bensulide.
N,*N*′-Bis(1-methylethyl)phosphorodi-amidic fluoride *see* Mipafox.
1,4-Bis(α-methylphenethyl)piperazine *see* Diphenazine.
N,*N*-Bis[*N*-methyl-*N*-(phenyl-*tert*-butyl)-acetamido]-2-hydroxyethylamine *see* Oxetacaine.
2-[Bis(*N*-methyl-*N*-phenyl-*tert*-butyl-carbamoylmethyl)amino]ethanol *see*

Oxetacaine.
3,4-Bis(*m*-methyl-*p*-propionoxyphenyl)-hexane *see* Methestrol dipropionate.
2-[2-[Bis(1-methylpropyl)amino]-1-hydroxyethyl]-1-(*o*-chlorobenzyl-pyrrole) *see* Viminol.
Bis(2-methylpropyl)carbamothioic acid *S*-ethyl ester *see* Butylate.
1,6-Bis(methylsulfonyl)mannitol *see* Mannityl dimesilate.
N,*N*′-Bis(morpholinocarbonyl)-*N*,*N*′-dibutylethylenediamine *see* Dimorpholamine.
5,7-Bis(2-morpholinoethoxy)-4-methyl-coumarin *see* Moxicoumone.
BISMUTH 2-ALLYL-4-PENTENOATE (bismuth diallylacetate; 'medobis').
BISMUTH CARBONATE (basic bismuth carbonate; Bi oxycarbonate; Bi subcarbon-ate; $2Bi_2O_3 \cdot 2CO_2 \cdot H_2O$).
BISMUTH CHLORIDE (basic bismuth chloride; bismuth oxychloride; bismuth subchloride; bismuthyl chloride).
BISMUTH CHRYSOPHANATE (basic bismuth chrysophanate; 4,5-dihydroxy-2-methylanthraquinone Bi salt; 'dermol').
Bismuth diallylacetate *see* Bismuth 2-allyl-4-pentenoate.
Bismuth dipropylacetate *see* Bismuth valproate.
BISMUTH GALLATE* (basic bismuth gallate; Bi oxygallate; Bi subgallate; gallabis; 'dermatol', 'helcosol').
Bismuth glycolylarsanilate *see* Glycobiarsol.
BISMUTH HYDROXIDE (hydrated Bi oxide; 'bismon').
Bismuth hydroxide 6-methyl-8-quinolinol compound *see* Mebiquine.
Bismuth iodide *see* Bismuth sodium iodide.
BISMUTH NITRATE (basic bismuth nitrate; bismuth oxynitrate; bismuth sub-nitrate; magisterium bismuthi).
See also Camylofin with bismuth nitrate.
Bismuth oxide *see* Bismuth hydroxide.
Bismuth oxycarbonate *see* Bismuth carbon-ate.
Bismuth oxychloride *see* Bismuth chloride.
Bismuth oxygallate *see* Bismuth gallate.
Bismuth oxynitrate *see* Bismuth nitrate.
Bismuth oxysalicylate *see* Bismuth salicylate.
Bismuth 2-propylvalerate *see* Bismuth valproate.
BISMUTH SALICYLATE (basic bismuth salicylate; bismuth oxysalicylate; bismuth subsalicylate).
BISMUTH SODIUM ACID TARTRATE (soluble bismuth tartrate).
BISMUTH SODIUM IODIDE (sodium iodobismuthate; 'aniobi', 'bismjol', 'iodo-bismutol').
BISMUTH SODIUM NEUTRAL TARTRATE (bismuthyl tartrate; Na tartrobismuthate; 'binasol', 'sigmuth', 'sobita').
Bismuth subcarbonate *see* Bismuth carbon-ate.
Bismuth subchloride *see* Bismuth chloride.

Bismuth subgallate see Bismuth gallate.
Bismuth subnitrate see Bismuth nitrate.
Bismuth subsalicylate see Bismuth salicylate.
BISMUTH TARTRATE(S) see Bismuth potassium sodium tartrate; Bismuth sodium acid tartrate; Bismuth sodium neutral tartrate.
Bismuth tetrabromopyrocatechuate see Bibrocathol.
BISMUTH TRIBROMOPHENATE (bromphenol bismuth; bromphenobis; bibrophenum; 'sigmaform', 'xeroform').
Bismuth tryparsamide see Tryparsamide bismuth salt.
BISMUTH VALPROATE (bismuth 2-propylvalerate; bismuth dipropylacetate; 'angicone', 'suppangin').
'Bismuthol' see Bismuth salicylate.
Bismuthoxy *p-N*-**glycolylarsanilate** see Glycobiarsol.
Bismuthyl tartrate see Bismuth sodium neutral tartrate.
1,4-Bis[2-(2-naphth-1-ylpropionyloxy)-ethyl]piperazine see Nafiverine.
1,5-Bis(5-nitro-2-furyl)-1,4-pentadien-3-one amidinohydrazone see Nitrovin.
BISOBRIN*** (1,1'-tetramethylenebis-(1,2,3,4-tetrahydro-6,7-dimethoxyiso-quinoline)).
BISOBRIN LACTATE* (meso-1,1'-tetra-methylenebis(1,2,3,4-tetrahydro-6,7-dimethoxyisoquinoline) dilactate; EN-1661L).
'Bisolvomycin' see Bromhexine with oxytetracycline.
'Bisolvon' see Bromhexine.
'Bisolvonamide' see Bromhexine with sulfadiazine.
BISORCIC** (N^2,N^5-diacetyl-L-ornithine; L-2,5-diacetamidovaleric acid).
BISOXATIN*** (2,2-bis(*p*-hydroxyphenyl)-2H-1,4-benzoxazin-3(4H)-one; 2,2-bis(*p*-hydroxyphenyl)-2,3-dihydro-1,4-benzoxazin-3-one; La-271; 'wylaxin').
Bisoxatin acetate* see Bisoxatin diacetate.
BISOXATIN DIACETATE* (2,2-bis(*p*-acetoxyphenyl)-2H-1,4-benzoxazin-3(4H)-one; bisoxatin acetate; La-271a; Wy-8138; 'maratan', 'talsis').
Bis(1,2,2,6,6-pentamethylpiperid-4-yl)succinate see Suxemerid.
1,4-Bis(2-phenylbutyryloxyethyl)piperazine see Febuverine.
1,1-Bis(phenylcarbamoyloxymethyl)-cyclopentane see Cyclarbamate.
1,4-Bis(phenylisopropyl)piperazine see Diphenazine.
N,N-**Bis(3-phenylpropyl)ethylamine** see Alverine.
1,4-Bis(3-phenylprop-2-yl)piperazine see Diphenazine.
2,6-Bis(*p*-pyrrolidin-1-ylstyryl)-1-ethylpyridinium iodide see Stilbazium iodide.
Bis(8-quinolinato-N^2,O^8)copper see Oxine-copper.

'Bisteril' see Phenazopyridine.
Bis(*N,N,N',N'*-tetramethylphosphoro-diamidic) anhydride see Schradan.
2,6-Bis(2-thenylidene)cyclohexanone see Tenylidone.
1,1-Bis(2-thienyl)-3-diethylamino-1-butene see Diethylthiambutene.
Bis(thymol iodide) see Dithymol diodide.
'Bistreptase' see Streptodornase with streptokinase.
BIS(TRIBUTYLTIN) OXIDE ('bio-met', 'fungi-ban', 'hollicide', 'lastanox', 'sun-nitt', 'T.B.T.O.', 'tin anti-slime').
Bis(2,2,2-trichloroethyl) carbamate see Cloretate.
1,3-Bis(2,2,2-trichloro-1-hydroxyethyl)-urea see Dicloralurea.
1,4-BIS(TRICHLOROMETHYL)BENZ-ENE (hexachloro-*p*-xylene; 'chloxyl', 'hetol').
Bis(2,2,2-trifluoroethyl)ether see Flurotyl.
N,N'-**Bis[3-(3,4,5-trimethoxybenzoyloxy)-propyl]-*N,N'*-dimethylethylenediamine** see Hexobendine.
'Bistrimin' see Phenyltoloxamine.
Bis[tris(*p*-aminophenyl)methylium] 4,4'-methylenebis(3-hydroxy-2-naphthoate) see Pararosaniline embonate.
Bistropamide see Tropicamide.
'Bithion' see Temefos.
BITHIONOL** (2,2'-thiobis(4,6-dichloro-phenol); 2,2'-thiobis(4,6-dichlorophenox-ide); bis(3,5-dichloro-2-hydroxyphenyl) sulfide; tetrachlorodihydroxydiphenyl sulfide; D-26; TBP; XL-7).
Bithionolate sodium* see Sodium bitionolate.
BITHIONOL SULFOXIDE ('bitin S', 'disto-5', 'neo-distol').
Bithymoldiiodide see Dithymol diiodide.
Bithyolum see Ammonium sulfobituminate.
'Bitin S' see Bithionol sulfoxide.
BITIPAZONE*** (2,3-butanedione bis[4-(2-piperid-1-ylethyl)thiosemicarbazone]).
BITOLTEROL** (4-[2-(*tert*-butylamino)-1-hydroxyethyl]-*o*-phenylene di-*p*-toluate).
3,3'-BITOLYL (3,3'-dimethylbiphenyl).
BITOSCANATE*** (*p*-phenylene bis(isothio-cyanate); phenylene diisothiocyanate; HOE-16842; Hö-16842; L-6842; 'jonit', 'yonit').
'Bitrex' see Denatonium.
BIURET (allophanamide; allophanic acid amide; carbamylurea; ureidoformamide).
'Bivelin' see Dihydroergotoxine with leucinocaine mesilate.
BL-5 see Cyclocumarol.
BL-139 see Aminopentamide.
BL-191 see Pentoxifylline.
'Bladafum' see Sulfotep.
'Bladan' see Parathion.
'Bladan 393' see Sulfotep.
'Bladex' see Cyanazine.
'Blattanex' see Propoxur.
'Bledocaine' see Prilocaine.
'Bleminol' see Allopurinol.
'Blenoxane' see Bleomycin.
BLEOMYCIN** (antibiotic from *Str. verti-*

cillus; bleomycin A; bleomycin sulfate; NSC-125066; 'blenoxane').

Bleomycin A* *see* Bleomycin.

'Bloat guard' *see* Poloxalene.

'Blocadren' *see* Timolol maleate.

'Blockaine' *see* Propoxycaine.

BL-P-152 *see* Pheneticillin.

BL-P-804 *see* Hetacillin.

BL-P 1322 *see* Cefapirin.

BL-P-1462 *see* Suncillin sodium.

BL-R743 *see* Intrazole.

BL-S578 *see* Cefadroxil.

BLUENSOMYCIN*** (antibiotic from *Str. bluensis*).

Blue tetrazolium *see* Tetrazolium blue.

'Blue VRS' *see* Sulphan blue.

'Blutene' *see* Tolonium.

BM-15075 *see* Bezafibrate.

BMIH *see* Isocarboxazid.

'B-nine' *see* Daminozide.

'Bocasan' *see* Sodium perborate.

BOEA *see* Ethyl biscoumacetate.

'Bogadin-TM' *see* Ibogaine.

'Bogalite' *see* Formaldehyde sodium sulfoxylate.

BOL *see* Bamethan.

Bol-148 *see* Bromolysergide.

BOLANDIOL*** (estr-4-ene-3β,17β-diol).

BOLANDIOL DIPROPIONATE** (SC-7525).

BOLASTERONE*** (7α,17-dimethylandrost-4-en-17β-ol-3-one; 17β-hydroxy-7α,17-dimethylandrosten-4-en-3-one; 7α,17-dimethyltestosterone; U-19763; 'myagen').

BOLAZINE** (17β-hydroxy-2α-methyl-5α-androstan-3-one azine).

BOLDENONE*** (17β-hydroxyandrosta-1,4-dien-3-one; androsta-1,4-dien-17β-ol-3-one).

BOLDENONE UNDECENOATE (boldenone undec-10-enoate; Ba-29038; C-29038).

BOLDINE (2,9-dihydroxy-1,10-dimethoxy-6-methyl-4H-dibenzo(de,g)quinoline; 2,9-dihydroxy-1,10-dimethoxyaporphine).

BOLENOL** (17α-ethyl-5-estren-17-ol; 19-nor-17α-pregn-5-en-17-ol).

Boletic acid *see* Fumaric acid.

'Bolfo' *see* Propoxur.

'Bolfortan' *see* Testosterone nicotinate.

BOLMANTALATE*** (estr-4-en-17β-ol-3-one adamantane-1-carboxylate; 17β-hydroxyestr-4-en-3-one 1-adamantanecarboxylate; 19-nortestosterone adamantane-1-carboxylate; nandrolone adamantane-1-carboxylate).

'Bona' *see* 3-Hydroxy-2-naphthoic acid.

'Bonadoxin' *see* Meclozine.

Bonafton (tr) *see* Bonaphthone.

'Bonaid' *see* Buquinolate.

'Bonamine' *see* Meclozine.

'Bonapar' *see* Fenyramidol.

BONAPHTHONE (tr) (6-bromo-1,2-naphthoquinone; bonafton).

'Bonifen' *see* Pyritinol.

'Bonine' *see* Meclozine.

'Bonjela' *see* Cetalkonium.

'Bonoform' *see* Tetrachloroethane.

'Bonomycin' *see* Sancycline.

'Bontourist' *see* Dimenhydrinate.

BOP *see* Bromopregnenetrione.

Boracic acid *see* Boric acid.

BORAX (Na tetraborate; Na biborate; Na borate; Na pyroborate; $Na_2B_4O_7 \cdot 10H_2O$).

BORDEAUX B (azorubrum; chiefly the di-Na salt of 2-hydroxy-1-(naphth-1-ylazo)-3,6-naphthalenedisulphonic acid).

Bordeaux S *see* Amaranth.

'Borgal' *see* Sulfadoxine with trimethoprim.

BORIC ACID (orthoboric acid; boracic acid; H_3BO_3).
See also Borax; Boroglyceride; Ethyl borate; Methenamine borate; Magnesium borate; Procaine borate; Sodium perborate.

2-BORNANAMINE (isobornylamine).

BORNANE (camphane; 1,7,7-trimethyl-bicyclo(2.2.1)heptane; 1,7,7-trimethyl-norbornane).

2-Bornanol *see* Borneol.

2-Bornanone *see* Camphor.

BORNAPRINE** (3-diethylaminopropyl 2-phenylbicyclo(2.2.1)heptane-2-carboxylate; 2-phenylnorbornane-2-carboxylic acid 3-diethylaminopropyl ester; 'sormodren').

Bornene chlorination product *see* Campheclor.

BORNEOL (2-bornanol; 2-hydroxybornane; 2-hydroxycamphane; 2-camphanol; bornyl alcohol; camphol; Malayan camphor).

Bornyl alcohol *see* Borneol.

BORNYL DIBROMODIHYDROCIN-NAMATE (adamon).

'Borocarpine' *see* Pilocarpine.

BOROGLYCERIDE (boric acid-glycerol paste; boroglycerin; boroglycerol; 'glacialin', 'glyboral').
See also Glyceryl triborate.

Borohexamine *see* Methenamine borate.

Borosalicylic acid copper salt *see* Copper borosalicylate.

'Borovertine' *see* Methenamine borate.

Bothrops atrox venom, enzyme *see* Batroxobin.

BOTIACRINE*** (S-(2-dimethylaminoethyl) 9,9-dimethyl-10-acridancarbothioate; 9,9-dimethylacridan-10-carbothioic acid 2-dimethylaminoethyl thioester; deanol ester of 9,9-dimethyl-10-acridancarbothioic acid).

'Botran' *see* Dicloran.

'Bourbonal' *see* Homovanillin.

'Bourbonal-INH' *see* Homovanillidene-isoniazid.

'Bovisynchron' *see* Chlormadinone.

'Boxazin' *see* Acetylsalicylic acid with ascorbic acid.

BOXIDINE** (1-[2-(4'-trifluoromethyl-biphenyl-4-yloxy)ethyl]pyrrolidine; 3-pyrrolidin-1-yl-4'-(α,α,α-trifluoro-p-tolyl)propiophenone; 4-trifluoromethyl-4'-(2-pyrrolidin-1-ylethoxy)biphenyl; CL-65205).

BP-400 *see* Pimethixene.

BP-1184 *see* Guanoctine.

'B-paracipan' *see* Calcium benzamidosalicylate.

'**B-PAS**' *see* Calcium benzamidosalicylate; Sodium benzamidosalicylate.
'**B.P.L.**' *see* β-Propiolactone.
BR-18 *see* Pipoxolan.
BR-700 *see* Fentiazac.
BR-750 *see* Guanabenz.
'**Bradilan**' *see* Nicofuranose.
'**Bradosol**' *see* Domiphen bromide.
BRADYKININ (kallidin II).
Bradykinyl-isoleucyl-tyrosine *O*-sulfate *see* Phyllokinin.
'**Bradyl 250**' *see* Nadoxolol.
BRALLOBARBITAL (5-allyl-5-(2-bromoallyl)barbituric acid; UCB-5033; 'vesperone').
'**Brassicol**' *see* Quintozene.
BRASSIDIC ACID (*trans*-13-docosenoic acid).
'**Brassoran**' *see* Aziprotryne.
'**Bravo**' *see* Chlorothalonil.
'**Braxoron**' *see* Bromopregnenetrione.
'**Bredon**' *see* Oxolamine.
Brenzschleimsäure *see* Furoic acid.
Brenztraubensäure *see* Pyruvic acid.
'**Brestan**' *see* Fentin acetate.
'**Brethine**' *see* Terbutaline.
BRETYLIUM TOSILATE*** ((*o*-bromobenzyl)ethyldimethylammonium *p*-toluenesulfonate; bretylium tosylate; ornid; BW-373C57; 'darenthin').
Bretylium tosylate* *see* Bretylium tosilate.
'**Brevatonal**' *see* Oxydipentonium chloride.
'**Brevicurarium**' *see* Piprocurarium.
'**Brevidil E**' *see* Suxethonium.
'**Brevidil M**' *see* Suxamethonium.
'**Brevital**' *see* Methohexital.
'**Bricanyl**' *see* Terbutaline.
'**Bridal**' *see* Phenbenzamine.
'**Brietal**' *see* Methohexital.
'**Brij**' *see* Lauromacrogol.
BRILLIANT GREEN* (anhydro-4,4'-bis-(diethylamino)triphenylmethane oxalate; anhydrobis(*p*-diethylaminophenyl)phenylmethanol oxalate; diamond green G; emerald green; ethyl green; fast green J; malachite green G; solid green; viride nitens; CI-662).
'**Brinaldix**' *see* Clopamide.
BRINASE*** (fibrinolytic enzyme from *Asp. oryzae*; mould fibrinolysin; aspergillin O).
'**Brinastase**' *see* Chymotrypsin with trypsin.
BRINDOXIME*** (2-[[(6,8-dibromo-9H-indeno(2,1-d)pyrimidin-9-ylidene)amino]oxy]-*N*-(2-dimethylaminoethyl)propionamide; *N*-[2-[[(6,8-dibromo-9H-indeno-(2,1-d)pyrimidin-9-ylidene)amino]oxy]propionyl]-*N'*,*N'*-dimethylethylenediamine; 6,8-dibromo-9-oxo-9H-indeno(2,1-d)-pyrimidine *O*-[1-[[(2-dimethylaminoethyl)amino]carbonyl]ethyl]oxime).
'**Brinerdine**' *see* Reserpine with clopamide & dihydroergocristine.
'**Bripadon**' *see* Fluoresone.
'**Briserin**' *see* Reserpine with clopamide & dihydroergocristine.
'**Bristab**' *see* Hydroflumethiazide.
'**Bristaciclina A**' *see* Hexacycline.
'**Bristacin**' *see* Rolitetracycline.

'**Bristain**' *see* Phenyltoloxamine.
'**Bristamine**' *see* Phenyltoloxamine.
'**Bristamycin**' *see* Erythromycin stearate.
'**Bristocef**' *see* Cefapirin.
'**Bristopen**' *see* Oxacillin.
'**Britacil**' *see* Ampicillin.
British antilewisite *see* Dimercaprol.
'**Brizin**' *see* Benaprizine.
BRL-152 *see* Pheneticillin.
BRL-284 *see* Levopropicillin.
BRL-556 *see* Oxypyrronium bromide.
BRL-804 *see* Hetacillin.
BRL-1241 *see* Meticillin.
BRL-1288 *see* Benaprizine.
BRL-1341 *see* Ampicillin.
BRL-1621 *see* Cloxacillin.
BRL-1702 *see* Dicloxacillin.
BRL-2039 *see* Flucloxacillin.
BRL-2064 *see* Carbenicillin.
BRL-2288 *see* Ticarcillin.
BRL-2333 *see* Amoxicillin.
BRL-2534 *see* Azidocillin.
BRL-3000 *see* Penicillin G, purified.
BRL-3475 *see* Carfecillin.
BRL-8988 *see* Talampicillin.
BRL-11870 *see* Anidoxime.
BRL-13856 *see* Clopirac.
BRL-50216 *see* Clociguanil.
Brobenzoxaldine* *see* Broxaldine.
'**Brocadisipal**' *see* Orphenadrine.
'**Brocadopa**' *see* Levodopa.
'**Brocalcin**' *see* Calcium bromide-lactobionate.
'**Brocasipal**' *see* Orphenadrine.
'**Brocide**' *see* Dichloroethylene.
'**Brocillin**' *see* Propicillin.
BROCRESINE*** (α-(aminooxy)-6-bromo-*m*-cresol; 5-(aminooxymethyl)-2-bromophenol; 4-bromo-3-hydroxybenzyloxyamine; *O*-(*p*-bromo-*m*-hydroxybenzyl)hydroxylamine; CL-54998; NSD-1055; brocresine phosphate; 'contramine').
'**Brofene**' *see* Bromofos.
BROFEZIL** (2-[4-(*p*-bromophenyl)thiazol-2-yl]propionic acid; 4-(*p*-bromophenyl)-α-methyl-2-thiazoleacetic acid; brofezil sodium; ICI-54594).
BROFOXINE** (6-bromo-1,4-dihydro-4,4-dimethyl-2H-3,1-benzoxazin-2-one).
'**Brolene**' *see* Dibrompropamidine isetionate.
'**Brolitene**' *see* Idrocilamide.
'**Brolon**' *see* Bromopregnenetrione.
BROMACIL* (5-bromo-3-*sec*-butyl-6-methyluracil; 5-bromo-6-methyl-3-(1-methylpropyl)-2,4-(1H,3H)pyrimidinedione; 'hyvar X').
BROMACRYLIDE*** (*N*-(3-bromopropionamidomethyl)acrylamide).
Bromadal *see* Carbromal.
'**Bromadryl**' *see* Embramine.
BROMAL (tribromoacetaldehyde).
'**Bromalin**' *see* Methenamine ethobromide.
BROMAMIDE*** (3-(*p*-bromoanilino)-*N*,*N*-dimethylpropionamide).
Bromanautine *see* Diphenhydramine bromotheophyllinate.
BROMANIL (2,3,5,6-tetrabromo-*p*-benzo-

quinone).

'Bromat' *see* Cetrimonium.

BROMAZEPAM*** (7-bromo-1,3-dihydro-5-pyrid-2-yl-2H-1,4-benzodiazepin-2-one; Ro 5-3350; 'lexatin', 'lexotan').

BROMAZEPAM WITH CLIDINIUM BROMIDE (Ro 10-7453).

BROMAZINE*** (2-(*p*-bromo-α-phenylbenzyloxy)-*N*,*N*-dimethylethylamine; 2-(*p*-bromobenzhydryloxy)-*N*,*N*-dimethylethylamine; bromodiphenhydramine; 'ambodryl', 'bromo-benadryl', 'deserol', 'histabromazine').

'Bromchlophos' *see* Naled.

BROMCHLORENONE*** (6-bromo-5-chloro-2-benzoxazolinone; 'vinyzene').

Bromdiethylacetylurea *see* Carbromal.

Bromdylamine *see* Brompheniramine.

BROMEBRIC ACID*** (*cis*-3-bromo-3-(*p*-methoxybenzoyl)acrylic acid; (E)-3-*p*-anisoyl-3-bromoacrylic acid; MBBA; 'cytembena', 'cytoval').

BROMELAINS*** (mixture of proteolytic enzymes from *Ananas comosus*; bromelin(s); 'ananase', 'deazin', 'extranase', 'traumanase').
See also Tetracycline with bromelains.

Bromelin *see* Bromelains.

BROMETENAMINE*** (equimolecular complex of bromoform and hexamethylenetetramine; methenamine bromoform complex).

BROMETHOL* (2,2,2-tribromoethanol; ethabrome; ethobrome; narkolan).

Bromethylformin *see* Methenamine ethobromide.

'Bromeval' *see* Bromisoval.

'Bromex' *see* Naled.

Bromfenoxim *see* Bromofenoxim.

BROMHEXINE*** (3,5-dibromo-*N*α-cyclohexyl-*N*α-methyltoluene-α,2-diamine; 2-amino-3,5-dibromo-*N*-cyclohexyl-*N*-methylbenzylamine; *N*-(2-amino-3,5-dibromobenzyl)-*N*-methylcyclohexylamine; (2-amino-3,5-dibromobenzyl)-*N*-cyclohexyl-*N*-methylamine; bromobenzonium; bromhexine hydrochloride; Na-274; 'bisolvon', 'quat').

BROMHEXINE WITH FOMINOBEN ('P9-tus').

BROMHEXINE WITH OXYTETRACYCLINE ('bisolvomycin').

BROMHEXINE WITH SULFADIAZINE ('bisolvonamide').

'Brominal' *see* Bromoxynil.

BROMINDIONE*** (2-(*p*-bromophenyl)-1,3-indandione; bromophenindione; brophenadion; 'circladin', 'fluidemin', 'halinone').

'Brominil' *see* Bromoxynil.

BROMISOVAL** (1-(2-bromo-3-methylbutyryl)urea; α-bromoisovalerylurea; bromoisopropylacetylurea; bromeval; bromurea; bromvaletone; bromvalerylurea; bromvalurea; BVU).
See also Carbromal with bromisoval.

5-(2-Bromoallyl)-5-*sec*-butylbarbituric acid *see* Butallylonal.

5-(2-Bromoallyl)-5-isopropylbarbituric acid *see* Propallylonal.

5-(2-Bromoallyl)-5-isopropyl-1-methylbarbituric acid *see* Enibomal.

5-(2-BROMOALLYL)-5-(1-METHYLBUTYL)BARBITURIC ACID (5-*sec*-amyl-5-(2-bromoallyl)barbituric acid; R-239; 'rectidon', 'recton', 'sigmodal').

5-(2-Bromoallyl)-5-(1-methylpropyl)-barbituric acid *see* Butallylonal.

3-(*p*-Bromoanilino)-*N*,*N*-dimethylpropionamide *see* Bromamide.

Bromoaprobarbital *see* Propallylonal.

'Bromo-benadryl' *see* Bromazine.

2-(*p*-Bromobenzhydryloxy)-*N*,*N*-dimethylethylamine *see* Bromazine.

Bromobenzonium *see* Bromhexine.

***p*-Bromobenzothiohydroxamic acid S-(2-diethylaminoethyl)ester** *see* Dietixim.

(Bromobenzyl) (chloroisopropylmethylphenoxypropyl)dimethylammonium chloride *see* Halopenium chloride.

N-(*p*-Bromobenzyl)-3,5-dibromosalicylamide *see* Bensalan.

(*o*-Bromobenzyl)ethyldimethylammonium *p*-toluenesulfonate *see* Bretylium tosilate.

4-Bromo-α-(4-bromophenyl)-α-hydroxybenzeneacetic acid 1-methylethyl ester *see* Bromopropylate.

4'-Bromo-3-*tert*-butyl-2-hydroxy-6-methyl-5-nitro-2'-(trifluoromethyl)benzanilide *see* Bromoxanide.

5-Bromo-3-*sec*-butyl-6-methyluracil *see* Bromacil.

4'-Bromo-3-*tert*-butyl-α',α',α'-trifluoro-5-nitro-2-cresoto-*o*-toluidide *see* Bromoxanide.

6-Bromo-5-chloro-2-benzoxazolinone *see* Bromchlorenone.

5-Bromo-3-[(2-chloroethyl)ethylaminomethyl]benzo(b)thiophene *see* Mitotenamine.

5-Bromo-*N*-(2-chloroethyl)-*N*-ethylbenzo(b)thiophene-3-methylamine *see* Mitotenamine.

7-Bromo-6-chlorofebrifugine *see* Halofuginone.

7-Bromo-6-chloro[3-(3-hydroxypiperid-2-yl)acetonyl]-4(3H)-quinazolinone *see* Halofuginone.

1-(4-Bromo-3-chlorophenyl)-3-methoxy-3-methylurea *see* Chlorbromuron.

5-BROMO-4'-CHLOROSALICYLAMIDE (5-bromosalicyl-4-chloroanilide; 'salifungin').

2-Bromo-2-chloro-1,1,1-trifluoroethane *see* Halothane.

Bromochromium *see* Merbromin.

BROMOCICLEN*** (5-bromomethyl-1,2,3,4,7,7-hexachloro-2-norbornene; bromocyclen; 'alugan', 'bromodan').

'Bromocoll' *see* Gelatin bromotannate.

5-Bromo-2,3-cresotamide *see* Brosotamide.

BROMOCRIPTINE*** (2-bromoergocryptine; (5'α)-2-bromo-12'-hydroxy-2'-(1-methylethyl)-5'-(2-methylpropyl)-

ergotaman-3′,6′,18-trione; CB-154; NSC-169774).

BROMOCRIPTINE MESILATE (bromocriptine methanesulfonate; 'parlodel').

Bromocyclen* *see* Bromociclen.

'Bromodan' *see* Bromociclen.

5-Bromo-2′-deoxyuridine *see* Broxuridine.

***O*-(4-Bromo-2,4-dichlorophenyl) *O,O*-diethyl phosphorothioate** *see* Bromofosethyl.

4-Bromo-2,5-dichlorophenyl dimethyl phosphorothioate *see* Bromofos.

***O*-(4-Bromo-2,5-dichlorophenyl) *O*-methyl phenylphosphonothioate** *see* Leptophos.

Bromodiethylacetylurea *see* Carbromal.

6-Bromo-1,4-dihydro-4,4-dimethyl-2H-3,1-benzoxazin-2-one *see* Brofoxine.

7-Bromo-3,4-dihydro-2(1H)-isoquinolinecarboxamidine sulfate *see* Guanisoquin.

7-Bromo-1,3-dihydro-5-pyrid-2-yl-2H-1,4-benzodiazepin-2-one *see* Bromazepam.

4′-Bromo-2,6-dihydroxybenzanilide *see* Resorantel.

4-(2-Bromo-4,5-dimethoxybenzyl)-4-[2-[2-(6,6-dimethylbicyclo(3.1.1)hept-2-yl)ethoxy]ethyl]morpholinium bromide *see* Pinaverium bromide.

2-[*p*-Bromo-α-(2-dimethylaminoethyl)-benzyl]pyridine *see* Brompheniramine.

2-Bromo-10-(3-dimethylaminopropyl)-phenothiazine *see* Bromopromazine.

Bromodiphenhydramine* *see* Bromazine.

2-Bromoergocryptine *see* Bromocriptine.

2-Bromo-2-ethylbutyramide *see* Carbromide.

***N*-(2-BROMOETHYL)-*N*-ETHYL-1-NAPHTHALENEMETHYLAMINE** (SY-28).

2-Bromo-*N*-ethyl-*N*-isopropylacetamide *see* Ibrotamide.

1-Bromo-2-(*p*-ethylphenyl)-1,2-diphenylethylene *see* Broparestrol.

BROMOFENOXIM* (3,5-dibromo-4-hydroxybenzaldehyde *O*-(2,4-dinitrophenyl)-oxime; bromfenoxim; 'faneron').

17α-Bromo-6α-fluoro-4-pregnene-3,20-dione *see* Haloprogesterone.

17α-Bromo-6α-fluoroprogesterone *see* Haloprogesterone.

BROMOFORM (tribromomethane).

Bromoform-hexamine complex *see* Brometenamine.

'Bromoformin' *see* Methenamine ethobromide.

Bromoform-methenamine complex *see* Brometenamine.

BROMOFOS*** (*O*-(4-bromo-2,5-dichlorophenyl) *O,O*-dimethyl phosphorothioate; bromophos; bromphos; CELA S-1942; 'brofene', 'brophene', 'nexion').

BROMOFOS-ETHYL (*O*-(4-bromo-4,6-dichlorophenyl) *O,O*-diethyl phosphorothioate; bromophos ethyl; 'nexagan').

[3-(5-Bromo-2-furoyloxy)butyl]diethylmethylammonium iodide *see* Fubrogonium iodide.

BROMOHYDRIN (3-bromo-1,2-propanediol; 3-bromopropylene glycol; α-bromohydrin; glycerol α-monobromohydrin).

3-Bromo-6-hydroxybenz-*p*-bromanilide *see* Dibromsalan.

5-Bromo-2-hydroxybenzyl alcohol *see* Bromosaligenin.

***O*-(*p*-Bromo-*m*-hydroxybenzyl)hydroxylamine** *see* Brocresine.

4-Bromo-3-hydroxybenzyloxyamine *see* Brocresine.

5-Bromo-2-hydroxy-3-methylbenzamide *see* Brosotamide.

(5′α)-2-Bromo-12′-hydroxy-2′-(1-methylethyl)-5′-(2-methylpropyl)ergotaman-3′,6′,18-trione *see* Bromocriptine.

Bromoisopropylacetylurea *see* Bromisoval.

5-Bromo-3-isopropyl-6-methyluracil *see* Isocil.

Bromoisovalerylurea *see* Bromisoval.

BROMOLYSERGIDE (D-2-bromo-*N*,*N*-diethyllysergamide bitartrate; Bol-148).

3-Bromo-3-(*p*-methoxybenzoyl)acrylic acid *see* Bromebric acid.

5-Bromomethyl-1,2,3,4,7,7-hexachloro-2-norbornene *see* Bromociclen.

5-Bromo-6-methyl-3-(1-methylethyl)-2,4-(1H,3H)-pyrimidinedione *see* Isocil.

5-Bromo-6-methyl-3-(1-methylpropyl)-2,4-(1H,3H)-pyrimidinedione *see* Bromacil.

5-Bromo-2-methyl-5-nitro-*m*-dioxane *see* Nibroxane.

2-(*p*-Bromo-α-methyl-α-phenylbenzyloxy)-*N*,*N*-dimethylethylamine *see* Embramine.

'Bromomycetin' *see* 1-(*p*-Bromophenyl)-2-dichloroacetamido-1,3-propanediol.

1-BROMO-2-NAPHTHOL ('wormin').

6-Bromo-1,2-naphthoquinone *see* Bonaphthone.

5-Bromonicotinic acid ester with 10-methoxy-1,6-dimethylergoline-8β-methanol *see* Nicergoline.

8β-(5-Bromonicotinoyloxymethyl)-10-methoxy-1,6-dimethylergoline *see* Nicergoline.

Bromonitropropanediol *see* Bronopol.

Bromoperidol *see* Bromperidol.

BROMOPHENAZONE (bromoantipyrine; bromopyrine).

Bromophenindione *see* Bromindione.

BROMOPHENOPHOS (4,4′,6,6′-tetrabromo-3,3′-biphenyldiol 2-dihydrogen phosphate; 'acedist').

2-(*p*-Bromo-α-phenylbenzyloxy)-*N*,*N*-dimethylethylamine *see* Bromazine.

***threo*-1-(*p*-BROMOPHENYL)-2-DICHLOROACETAMIDO-1,3-PROPANEDIOL** ('bromomycetin').

3-(*p*-Bromophenyl)-*N*,*N*-dimethyl-3-pyrid-2-ylpropylamine *see* Brompheniramine.

4-(*p*-Bromophenyl)-1-[3-(*p*-fluorobenzoyl)-propyl]-4-piperidinol *see* Bromperidol.

4-[4-(*p*-Bromophenyl)-4-hydroxypiperid-1-yl]-4′-fluorobutyrophenone *see* Bromperidol.

2-(*p*-**Bromophenyl**)-**1,3-indandione** *see* Bromindione.

5-BROMO-2-PHENYL-1,3-INDANDIONE ('uridione').

1-(*p*-Bromophenyl)-3-methoxy-3-methyl-urea *see* Metobromuron.

4-(*p*-Bromophenyl)-α-methyl-2-thiazole-acetic acid *see* Brofezil.

2-[1-(*p*-Bromophenyl)-1-phenylethoxy]-*N,N*-dimethylethylamine *see* Embramine.

2-[4-(*p*-Bromophenyl)thiazol-2-yl]-propionic acid *see* Brofezil.

'**Bromophin**' *see* Apomorphine methyl bromide.

Bromophos* *see* Bromofos.

9α-BROMO-4-PREGNENE-3,11,20-TRIONE (9α-bromo-11-oxoprogesterone; BOP; 'braxoron', 'brolon', 'broxoron').

BROMOPRIDE*** (4-amino-5-bromo-*N*-(2-diethylaminoethyl)-*o*-anisamide; 4-amino-5-bromo-*N*-(2-diethylaminoethyl)-2-methoxybenzamide).

BROMOPROMAZINE (2-bromo-10-(3-dimethylaminopropyl)phenothiazine).

3-Bromo-1,2-propanediol *see* Bromohydrin.

Bromoprophenpyridamine *see* Bromphen-iramine.

Bromopropionamidomethylacrylamide *see* Bromacrylide.

BROMOPROPYLATE* (isopropyl 2,2-bis(*p*-bromophenyl)glycolate; isopropyl 4,4'-dibromobenzilate; 1-methylethyl 4-bromo-α-(4-bromophenyl)-α-hydroxy-benzeneacetate; phenisobromolate; 'acarol', 'neoron').

Bromopyrine *see* Bromophenazone.

4'-Bromo-γ-resorcylanilide *see* Resorantel.

5-Bromosalicyl-4-chloroanilide *see* 5-Bromo-4'-chlorosalicylanilide.

Bromosulfonphthalein *see* Sulfobrom-phthalein.

2-Bromo-1,1,1,2-tetrafluoroethane *see* Teflurane.

3-Bromo-1,1,2,2-tetrafluoropropane *see* Halopropane.

Bromotrifluoroethyl methyl ether *see* Roflurane.

Bromotriphenylethylene *see* Broparoestrol.

4-(6-Bromoveratryl)-4-[2-[2-(6,6-dimeth-yl-2-norpinyl)ethoxy]ethyl]morpholi-nium bromide *see* Pinaverium bromide.

BROMOXANIDE** (4'-bromo-3-*tert*-butyl-α',α',α'-trifluoro-5-nitro-2-cresoto-*o*-toluid-ide; 4'-bromo-3-*tert*-butyl-2-hydroxy-6-methyl-5-nitro-2'-(trifluoromethyl)-benzanilide).

Bromoxine *see* Broxyquinoline.

BROMOXYNIL* (3,5-dibromo-4-hydroxy-benzonitrile; 'brominal', 'brominil', 'buctril').

BROMPERIDOL*** (4-[4-(*p*-bromophenyl)-4-hydroxypiperid-1-yl]-4'-fluorobutyro-phenone; 4-(*p*-bromophenyl)-1-[3-(*p*-fluorobenzoyl)propyl]-4-piperidinol; bromperidol; R-11333).

BROMPHENIRAMINE*** (3-(*p*-bromo-phenyl)-*N,N*-dimethyl-3-pyrid-2- ylpropyl-amine; 2-[*p*-bromo-α-(2-dimethylamino-ethyl)benzyl]pyridine; bromdylamine; bromoprophenpyridamine; bromprophen pyridamine; parabromdylamine; 'ilvin'). *See also* Dexbrompheniramine.

BROMPHENIRAMINE MALEATE ('dimetane', 'dimotane').

'**Bromphenobis**' *see* Bismuth tribromo-phenate.

Bromphenol bismuth *see* Bismuth tribromo-phenate.

Bromphos *see* Bromofos.

Bromphthalein *see* Sulfobromphthalein.

Bromprophenpyridamine *see* Bromphenir-amine.

BROMPYRAZON* (5-amino-4-bromo-2-phenyl-3(2H)-pyridazinone; brompyra-zone).

BROMPYRAZON PLUS ISONORURON ('basanor').

Brompyrazone *see* Brompyrazon.

BROMSALIGENIN (monobromosalicyl alcohol; 5-bromo-2-hydroxybenzyl alcohol; 'bromsalizol').

'**Bromsalizol**' *see* Bromsaligenin.

'**Bromsulfalein**' *see* Sulfobromphthalein.

Bromsulfophthalein *see* Sulfobrom-phthalein.

'**Bromsulfphthalein**' *see* Sulfobrom-phthalein.

Bromtannigel *see* Gelatin bromotannate.

'**Brom-tetragnost**' *see* Sulfobromphthalein.

'**Bromthalein**' *see* Sulfobromphthalein.

'**Bromural**' *see* Bromisoval.

Bromurea *see* Bromisoval.

Bromvalerylurea *see* Bromisoval.

Bromvaletone *see* Bromisoval.

Bromvalurea *see* Bromisoval.

'**Bronchiol**' *see* Ethyl acetrizoate.

'**Bronchocaine**' *see* Dimethylaminoethyl butylaminosalicylate.

'**Bronchocillin**' *see* Penethamate hydriodide.

'**Bronchodilator-1313**' *see* Phenisonone.

'**Bronchodine**' *see* Codeine.

'**Broncholysin**' *see* Acetylcysteine.

'**Bronchopen**' *see* Penethamate hydriodide.

'**Bronchoselectan**' *see* Sodium acetrizoate.

'**Broncovaleas**' *see* Salbutamol.

BRONOPOL*** (2-bromo-2-nitro-1,3-propanediol).

'**Brontina**' *see* Deptropine.

'**Brontine**' *see* Deptropine.

'**Brontyl**' *see* Proxyphylline.

BROPARESTROL*** (α-bromo-α'-(*p*-ethyl-phenyl)stilbene; 1-bromo-2-(*p*-ethylphenyl)-1,2-diphenylethylene; bromotriphenyl-ethylene; broparoestrol; 'longestrol').

Brophenadion *see* Bromindione.

'**Brophene**' *see* Bromofos.

BROQUINALDOL*** (5,7-dibromo-2-methyl-8-quinolinol; 5,7-dibromo-8-hydr-oxyquinaldine).

BROSOTAMIDE*** (5-bromo-2,3-cresot-amide; 5-bromo-2-hydroxy-3-methyl-benzamide).

BROTIANIDE** (3,4'-dibromo-5-chlorothio-salicylanilide acetate (ester)).

BROVANEXINE** (2',4'-dibromo-α-(cyclohexylmethylamino)-o-vanillotoluidide acetate (ester); 4-acetoxy-2',4'-dibromo-6'-[[(cyclohexyl)(methyl)amino]methyl]-3-methoxybenzanilide).

'Brovon' see Atropine methyl nitrate.

BROXALDINE** (5,7-dibromo-2-methyl-8-quinolinol benzoate; brobenzoxaldine; 5,7-dibromo-8-hydroxyquinaldine).
See also Broxyquinoline with broxaldine.

'Broxil' see Pheneticillin.

'Broxoron' see Bromopregnenetrione.

BROXURIDINE** (5-bromo-2'-deoxy-uridine; BUDR; NSC-38297).

BROXYQUINOLINE*** (5,7-dibromo-8-quinolinol; bromoxine; AI-306; 'dibromo-quin', 'fenilor').

BROXYQUINOLINE WITH BROXAL-DINE (AI-307; 'intestopan', 'phenipan').

BROXYQUINOLINE WITH BROXAL-DINE & CHLOROQUINE DIPHOSPH-ATE ('intestopan-Q').

BROXYQUINOLINE WITH BROXAL-DINE & TETRACYCLINE ('sando-cycline').

'Brucker lens' see Hefilcon A.

'Brufaneuxol' see Aminophenazone.

'Brufen' see Ibuprofen.

'Brulidine' see Dibrompropamidine isetion-ate.

Bruneomycin (tr) see Streptonigrin.

Bryamycin see Thiostrepton.

BS-272 see Proscillaridin with theophylline.

BS-479 see Metacetamol.

BS-556 see Medrylamine.

BS-572 see Cyclandelate.

BS-4231 see Glisoxepide.

BS-5892 see Buformin.

BS-5930 see Orphenadrine.

BS-6748 see Xyloxemine.

BS-6987 see Deptropine.

BS-7020a see Deptropine methobromide.

BS-7029 see Cyheptamide.

BS-7051 see Hepzidine.

BS-7161-D see Pytamine.

BSA see Sulisobenzone.

BSP see Sulfobromphthalein.

BT see Tetrazolium blue.

BT-325 see Sulfaperin.

BT-436 see Dehydroemetine.

BTC see Benzalkonium.

BTS-13622 see Hexaprofen.

BTS-18322 see Flurbiprofen.

'Bubulin' see Metrifonate with atropine and pralidoxime.

BUCAINIDE** (1-hexyl-4-(N-isobutylbenz-imidoyl)piperazine; 1-hexyl-4-[N-(2-methyl-propyl)benzimidoyl]piperazine).

'Bucarban' see Carbutamide.

BUCARPOLATE (2-(2-butoxyethoxy)ethyl piperonylate; 2-(2-butoxyethoxy)ethyl 3,4-methylenedioxybenzoate).

'Buccalsone' see Hydrocortisone sodium succinate.

BUCETIN*** (3-hydroxy-p-butyrophenetid-ide; 4'-ethoxy-3'-hydroxybutyranilide).

'Buclamase' see Amylase.

BUCLIZINE*** (1-(p-tert-butylbenzyl)-4-(p-chlorobenzhydryl)piperazine; 1-(p-tert-butylbenzyl)-4-(p-chloro-α-phenylbenzyl)-piperazine; buclizine hydrochloride; UCB-4445; 'histabutazine', 'longifene', 'retamin', 'softran', 'vibazine').

BUCLOSAMIDE*** (N-butyl-4-chlorosalicyl-amide; 'demycin').

BUCLOSAMIDE WITH SALICYLIC ACID ('jadit').

BUCLOXIC ACID*** (3-(3-chloro-4-cyclohexylbenzoyl)propionic acid; 4-(3-chloro-4-cyclohexylphenyl)-4-oxobutyric acid; 'esfar').
See also Calcium bucloxate.

BUCOLOME*** (5-butyl-1-cyclohexylbar-bituric acid; BCP; 'paramidine').

BUCRILATE*** (isobutyl 2-cyanoacrylate; bucrylate).

'Bucrol' see Carbutamide.

Bucrylate see Bucrilate.

'Buctril' see Bromoxynil.

BUCUMOLOL** (8-[3-(tert-butylamino)-2-hydroxypropoxy]-5-methylcoumarin; 1-(tert-butylamino)-3-(5-methylcoumarin-8-yloxy)-2-propanol; bucumolol hydrochloride; C-3 Sankyo; CS-359).

BUDR see Broxuridine.

BUDRALAZINE*** (4-methyl-3-penten-2-one (1-phthalazinyl)hydrazone; 1-(1,3-dimethylbut-2-enylidene)-2-phthalazin-1-yl-hydrazine; 1-[2-(1,3-dimethylbut-2-enylidene)hydrazino]phthalazine).

'Bufedon' see Buphenine.

Bufenadine* see Bufenadrine.

BUFENADRINE*** (2-(o-tert-butylbenzhydr-yloxy)-N,N-dimethylethylamine; 2-(o-tert-butyl-α-phenylbenzyloxy)-N,N-dimethyl-ethamine; o-tert-butyldiphenhydramine; bufenadine).

BUFENIODE*** (4-hydroxy-3,5-diiodo-α-[1-(1-methyl-3-phenylpropylamino)ethyl]-benzyl alcohol; 'proclival').

BUFETOLOL** (1-tert-butylamino-3-[o-(tetrahydrofurfuryloxy)phenoxy]-2-propanol; 2-[[o-(3-tert-butylamino-2-hydr-oxypropoxy)phenoxy]methyl]tetrahydro-furan; bufetolol hydrochloride; bufuronol; Y-6124; 'adbiol', 'adobiol').

BUFEXAMAC*** (2-(p-butoxyphenyl)aceto-hydroxamic acid; CP-1044-J3; 'droxaryl', 'feximac', 'parfenac').

BUFLOMEDIL*** (2',4',6'-trimethoxy-4-pyrrolidin-1-ylbutyrophenone; 1-[3-(2,4,6-trimethoxybenzoyl)propyl]pyrrolidine; 3-pyrrolidin-1-ylpropyl 2,4,6-trimethoxy-phenyl ketone; LL-1656).

BUFOGENIN*** (14,15β-epoxy-3β-hydroxy-5β-bufa-20,22-dienolide; 'respigon').

BUFORMIN** (1-butylbiguanide; N¹-butyl-biguanide; DBV; BS-5892; H-224; W-37; 'adebit', 'silubin', 'sindiatil', 'tidemol').

'Buformin' see Chlormebuform.

BUFOTENINE (5-hydroxy-N,N-dimethyltryptamine; *N*,*N*-dimethylserotonin; mappine).

BUFROLIN** (6-butyl-1,4,7,10-tetrahydro-4,10-dioxo-1,7-phenanthroline-2,8-dicarboxylic acid).

BUFROLIN SODIUM (bufrolin disodium salt; ICI-74917).

BUFURALOL** (α-(*tert*-butylaminomethyl)-7-ethyl-2-benzofuranmethanol; 2-(2-*tert*-butylamino-1-hydroxyethyl)-7-ethyl-benzofuran; 2-*tert*-butylamino-1-(7-ethyl-benzofuran-2-yl)ethanol; Ro 03-4787).

Bufuronol *see* Bufetolol.

BUFYLLINE* (theophylline-2-amino-2-methylpropan-1-ol; theophylline-amino-isobutanol; theophylline-isobutanolamine; ambuphylline; 'butaphyllamine', 'buthoid').

BULBOCAPNINE (11-hydroxy-10-methoxy-6-methyl-1,2-methylenedioxy-4H-dibenzo-(de,g)quinoline; 11-hydroxy-10-methoxy-1,2-methylenedioxyaporphine).

BUMADIZONE*** (butylmalonic acid mono-(1,2-diphenylhydrazide); B-64114).

BUMADIZONE CALCIUM ('eumotol').

BUMECAINE** (1-butyl-2',4',6'-trimethyl-2-pyrrolidinecarboxanilide; 1-butyl-*N*-(2,4,6-trimethylphenyl)-2-pyrrolidinecarboxamide).

BUMETANIDE*** (3-butylamino-4-phenoxy-5-sulfamoylbenzoic acid; 'burinex').

Bunaftide *see* Bunaftine.

BUNAFTINE*** (*N*-butyl-*N*-(2-diethylaminoethyl)-1-naphthamide; *N*-butyl-*N'*,*N'*-diethyl-*N*-naphth-1-oylethylenediamine; bunaftide).

BUNAMIDINE*** (*N*,*N*-dibutyl-4-hexyloxy-1-naphthamidine; bunamidine hydrochloride; BW-62-415; 'scolaban').

BUNAMIODYL*** (sodium 3-(3-butyramido-2,4,6-triiodophenyl)-2-ethylacrylate; *N*-[5-(2-carboxybut-1-enyl)-2,4,6-triiodophenyl]butyramide; 2-(3-butyramido-3,4,6-triiodophenylmethylene)butyric acid; bunamiodyl sodium; buniodyl; 'orabilex', 'orabilix').

BUNAPSILATE(S)** (3,7-di-*tert*-butyl-naphthalene-1,5-disulfonate(s)).

Buniodyl* *see* Bunamiodyl.

BUNITROLOL*** (*o*-(3-*tert*-butylamino-2-hydroxypropoxy)benzonitrile; 1-*tert*-butylamino-3-(*o*-cyanophenoxy)-2-propanol; 2-nitrilo-*N*-*tert*-butylphenoxypropanolamine; Kö-1366).

BUNOLOL*** ((±)-5-(3-*tert*-butylamino-2-hydroxypropoxy)-3,4-dihydro-1(2H)-naphthalenone).

'Bunt-cure' *see* Hexachlorobenzene.

'Bunt-no-more' *see* Hexachlorobenzene.

'Bupatol' *see* Bamethan.

BUPHENINE*** (*p*-hydroxy-α-[1-(1-methyl-3-phenylpropyl)amino]ethylbenzyl alcohol; 1-(*p*-hydroxyphenyl)-2-(1-methyl-3-phenyl-propylamino)-1-propanol; *p*-hydroxy-*N*-(3-phenylisobutyl)norephedrine; nylidrin; phenyl-*sec*-butylnorsuprifen; SK&F-1700A; 'arlidin', 'bufedon', 'dilatal', 'dilatol', 'dilatropon', 'dilydrin', 'opino', 'perdilatal',

'suprifen-Psb', 'verina').

BUPICOMIDE** (5-butyl-2-pyridine carboxamide; 5-butylpicolinamide; fusaric acid amide; Sch-10595).

BUPIVACAINE*** (*N*-butylpipecolic acid 1,6-xylidide; *N*-butylpipecolic acid 2,6-dimethylanilide; 1-butyl-2',6'-pipecoloxylidide; 1-butyl-2-(2,6-xylylcarbamoyl)piperidine; 1-butyl-2-piperidinecarboxylic acid 2,6-xylidide; bupivacaine hydrochloride; AH-2250; LAC-43; WIN-11318; 'carbostesin', 'marcain').

BUPRANOLOL*** (3-*tert*-butylamino-1-(2-chloro-5-methylphenoxy)-2-propanol; 1-*tert*-butylamino-3-(6-chloro-*m*-toloxy)-2-propanol; KL-255; 'betadran', 'betadrenol').

BUPRENORPHINE*** (21-cyclopropyl-7α-(*S*)-1-hydroxy-1,2,2-trimethylpropyl-6,14-*endo*-ethano-6,7,8,14-tetrahydrooripavine).

BUPROPION* ((±)-1-(3-chlorophenyl)-2-[(1,1-dimethylethyl)amino]-1-propanone; (±)-2-*tert*-butylamino-3'-chloropropiophenone; bupropion hydrochloride; 'wellbatrin').

BUQUINOLATE*** (ethyl 4-hydroxy-6,7-diisobutoxyquinoline-3-carboxylate; U-1093; 'bonaid').

BURAMATE** (2-hydroxyethyl benzylcarbamate; benzylcarbamoylethanol; AC-601; 'hyamate', 'hybamate').

'Burgodin' *see* Bezitramide.

BURIMAMIDE (1-[4-(imidazol-4(5)-yl)-butyl]-3-methylthiourea; 4(5)-[4-(3-methylthioureido)butyl]imidazole).

'Burinex' *see* Bumetanide.

BURODILINE** (1-pyrrolidineethanol 4-butoxy-3,5-dimethoxybenzoate ester; 2-pyrrolidin-1-ylethyl 4-butoxy-3,5-dimethoxybenzoate; 'vasopentol').

'Buronil' *see* Melperone.

'Bursoline' *see* Diglycocoll hydriodide iodine.

'Buscalide' *see* Proglumide with scopolamine butyl bromide.

'Buscapine' *see* Scopolamine butyl bromide.

'Buscolysin' *see* Scopolamine butyl bromide.

'Buscopan' *see* Scopolamine butyl bromide.

'Buscopax' *see* Scopolamine butyl bromide with oxazepam.

BUSPIRONE** (8-[4-[4-(pyrimidin-2-yl)-piperazin-1-yl]butyl]-8-azaspiro(4.5)-decane-7,9-dione; 2-[4-[4-(7,9-dioxo-8-azaspiro(4.5)dec-8-yl)butyl]piperazin-1-yl]pyrimidine; 4-[4-(7,9-dioxo-8-azaspiro-(4.5)dec-8-yl)butyl]-1-pyrimidin-2-ylpiperazine).

BUSULFAN*** (1,4-bis(methanesulfonyloxy)-butane; 1,4-dimethanesulfonyloxybutane; 1,4-butanediol dimethanesulfonate; tetramethylene ester of methanesulfonic acid; tetramethylene dimesilate; busulphan; myelosan; sulfabutin; CB-2041; GT-41; NSC-750; 'citosulfan', 'cytoleukon', 'mablin', 'mielucin', 'misulban', 'mitostan', 'myeloleukon', 'myelucin', 'mylecytan', 'myleran').

Busulphan* *see* Busulfan.

Butabarbital* see Secbutabarbital.
'Butabarpal' see Secbutabarbital.
BUTACAINE** (3-dibutylaminopropyl ester of *p*-aminobenzoic acid; butaprobenz; butacaine sulfate; butocaine; 'butellin', 'butyn', 'elycaine').
BUTACETIN* (4'-*tert*-butoxyacetanilide; BW-63-90; 'tromal').
Butachlor* see Butoclor.
BUTACID (*p*-dibutylsulfamoylbenzoic acid; 'longacid').
'Butacide' see Piperonyl butoxide.
BUTACLAMOL** (3α-*tert*-butyl-2,3,4,4aβ, 8,9,13bα,14-octahydro-1H-benzo(6,7)-cyclohepta(1,2,3-de)pyrido(2,1-a)iso-quinolin-3-ol; butaclamol hydrochloride; AY-23028).
BUTADIAZAMIDE*** (*N*-(5-butyl-1,3,4-thiadiazol-2-yl)-*p*-chlorobenzenesulfon-amide; 5-butyl-2-(*p*-chlorobenzenesulfon-amido)-1,3,4-thiadiazole).
'Butadion' see Phenylbutazone.
BUTALAMINE** (5-(2-dibutylaminoethyl-amino)-3-phenyl-1,2,4-oxadiazole; butal-amine hydrochloride; La-1221; 'adrevil', 'surem', 'surheme').
BUTALBITAL*** (5-allyl-5-(2-methyl-propyl)barbituric acid; 5-allyl-5-isobutyl-barbituric acid; allylbarbital; allyl-barbituric acid; alisobumal; itobarbital; tetrallobarbital; 'sandoptal').
'Butalidon' see Phenylbutazone.
BUTALLYLONAL* (5-(2-bromoallyl)-5-*sec*-butylbarbituric acid (or its sodium deriv-ative); 5-(2-bromoallyl)-5-(1-methylprop-yl)barbituric acid; 'pernocton', 'pernoston', 'sonbutal').
Butamben see Butylcaine.
Butameverine* see Butaverine.
Butamid (tr) see Tolbutamide.
BUTAMIN (3-dimethylamino-1,2-dimethyl-propyl *p*-aminobenzoate hydrochloride; 'totocaine', 'tutokaine').
BUTAMIRATE** (2-(2-diethylaminoethoxy)-ethyl 2-phenylbutyrate; diethylamino-ethoxyethyl phenylethylacetate; butamyr-ate; HH-197).
BUTAMIRATE CITRATE (Abbott-36581; 'acodeen', 'sinecod').
BUTAMISOLE** ((−)-2-methyl-3'-(2,3,5,6-tetrahydroimidazo(2,1-b)thiazol-6-yl)-propionanilide; (−)-2,3,5,6-tetrahydro-6-[3-[(2-methylpropionyl)amino]phenyl]-imidazo(2,1-b)thiazole).
BUTAMOXANE*** (2-butylaminomethyl-1,4-benzodioxan; F-1052).
Butamyrate* see Butamirate.
Butanal see Butyraldehyde.
Butanamide see Butyramide.
1-Butanecarboxylic acid see Valeric acid.
1,4-Butanediamine see Putrescine.
2,3-BUTANEDIONE (biacetyl; diacetyl).
2,3-Butanedione bis(4-(2-piperid-1-yl-ethyl)thiosemicarbazone) see Bitipazone.
2,3-Butanedione oxime see Diacetylmonox-ime.
erythro-**1,2,3,4-Butanetetrol** see Erythritol.

threo-**1,2,3,4-Butanetetrol** see Threitol.
BUTANILICAINE*** (2-butylamino-6'-chloro-*o*-acetotoluidide; *N*-butylamino-acetyl-6-chloro-*o*-toluidine; 'hostacaine').
Butanimide see Succinimide.
BUTANIXIN** (2-(*p*-butylanilino)nicotinic acid).
Butanoic acid see Butyric acid.
1-BUTANOL (butyl alcohol).
2-BUTANOL (*sec*-butyl alcohol).
BUTAPERAZINE** (2-butyryl-10-[3-(4-methylpiperazin-1-yl)propyl]phenothiazine dimaleate; 1-[10-[3-(4-methylpiperazin-1-yl)propyl]phenothiazin-2-yl]-1-butanone; butyrylperazine; AHR-712; Bayer-1362; Riker-595; 'randolectil', 'repoise').
'Butaphyllamine' see Bufylline.
Butaprobenz see Butacaine.
'Butapyrine' see Aminophenazone with phenylbutazone.
BUTAVERINE*** (butyl-3-phenyl-3-piperid-1-ylpropionate; butameverine; 'cemora').
BUTAXAMINE*** (α-(1-*tert*-butylamino-ethyl)-2,5-dimethoxybenzyl alcohol; (±)-*erythro*-2-*tert*-butylamino-1-(2,5-dimethoxy-phenyl)-1-propanol; *N*-*tert*-butylmethox-amine; butoxamine; butoxamine hydro-chloride; BW-64-9).
'Butazidamina' see Benzydamine phenyl-butazone-5-enolate.
'Butazolidine' see Phenylbutazone.
'Butellin' see Butacaine.
2-Butenamide see Crotonamide.
Butenedioic acids see Fumaric acid; Maleic acid.
Butenemal* see Vinbarbital.
'Butenil' see Butethal.
cis-**2-Butenoic acid** see Isocrotonic acid.
trans-**2-Butenoic acid** see Crotonic acid.
5-(2-Butenyl)-5-ethylbarbituric acid see Barotal.
2-(2-Butenyl)-4-hydroxy-3-methyl-2-cyclopenten-1-one esters see Cinerin I; Cinerin II.
Butenylideneisoniazid see Crotoniazide.
1-(2-Butenylidene)-2-isonicotinoylhydr-azine see Crotoniazide.
3-(2-Butenyl)-2-methyl-4-oxo-2-cyclopent-en-1-yl chrysanthemate see Cinerin I.
3-[3-(2-Butenyl)-2-methyl-4-oxo-2-cyclo-penten-1-yl] 1-methyl chrysanthemum-dicarboxylate see Cinerin II.
p-**(2-Buten-2-yl)phenyl acetate** see Fenabutene.
'Butesamid' see Ethyl butylethylmalonate.
'Butesin' see Butylcaine.
BUTETAMATE*** (2-diethylaminoethyl 2-phenylbutyrate; diethylaminoethyl phenyl-ethylacetate; butethamate).
BUTETAMATE CITRATE (butethamate citrate; 'abuphenine', 'convenil', 'fenesina').
BUTETHAL* (5-butyl-5-ethylbarbituric acid; butobarbital; butobarbitone; 'allardorm', 'butenil', 'dormirette', 'etoval', 'longanoct', 'monodorm', 'neonal', 'soneryl', 'supponeryl').
Butethamate* see Butetamate.

65

BUTETHAMINE* (isobutylaminoethyl *p*-aminobenzoate; 'monocaine').

'Butex' *see* Parabens.

BUTHALITAL SODIUM*** (5-allyl-5-(2-methylpropyl)-2-thiobarbituric acid sodium derivative; 5-allyl-5-isobutyl-2-thiobarbituric acid sodium derivative; buthalitone; thialbutone; thialisobumal; thiobutone; 'baytinal', 'narcogen', 'transithal', 'ulbreval').

Buthalitone* *see* Buthalital.

Buthiazide* *see* Butizide.

BUTHIOPURINE (6-(4-carboxybutylthio)-purine; 5-(purin-6-ylthio)valeric acid; NSC-130678; 'cytogran').

'Buthoid' *see* Bufylline.

BUTIBUFEN*** (2-(*p*-isobutylphenyl)butyric acid).

'Butidrate' *see* Butidrine with pentaerythrityl tetranitrate.

BUTIDRINE*** (5,6,7,8-tetrahydro-α-(1-methylpropylaminomethyl)-2-naphthalenemethanol; α-(*sec*-butylaminomethyl)-5,6,7,8-tetrahydro-2-naphthalenemethanol; 2-*sec*-butylamino-1-(5,6,7,8-tetrahydro-2-naphthyl)ethanol; 2-(1-methylpropyl)-1-(5,6,7,8-tetrahydronaphth-2-yl)ethanol; butydrine; hydrobutamine; idrobutamina; 'recetan').

BUTIDRINE WITH PENTAERYTHRITYL TETRANITRATE ('butidrate').

Butilchlorofos (tr) *see* Butonate.

Butilklorophos (tr) *see* Butonate.

BUTIN (3′,4′,7-trihydroxyflavanone).

BUTINOLINE*** (1,1-diphenyl-4-pyrrolidin-1-ylbut-2-yn-1-ol).

'Butipyrine' *see* Butylchloralamidopyrine.

Butirao *see* Buturon.

BUTIROSIN*** (mixture of A and B forms of *O*-[2,6-diamino-2,6-dideoxy-α-D-glucopyranosyl-(1→4)]-*O*-[β-D-xylofuranosyl-(1→5)]-*N*¹-(4-amino-2-hydroxybutyryl)-2-deoxystreptamine).

'Butisol' *see* Secbutabarbital.

'Butisulfina' *see* Carbutamide.

BUTIXIRATE*** (α-ethyl-4-biphenylacetic acid compound with *trans*-4-phenylcyclohexylamine (1:1); xenbucin salt with *trans*-4-phenylcyclohexylamine; *trans*-4-phenylcyclohexylamine 2-(*p*-biphenylyl)butyrate; Mg-5771; 'flectar').

BUTIZIDE** (6-chloro-3,4-dihydro-3-isobutyl-2H-1,2,4-benzothiadiazine-7-sulfonamide 1,1-dioxide; buthiazide; isobutylhydrochlorothiazide; thiabutizide; thiobutazine; 'eunephran', 'saltucin').

BUTIZIDE WITH SPIRONOLACTONE ('aldozone').

Butobarbital *see* Butethal.

Butobarbitone* *see* Butethal.

'Butoben' *see* Butyl paraben.

Butocaine *see* Butacaine.

BUTOCIN (ethyl *N*-[5-(purin-6-ylthio)-valeryl]glycinate; *N*-[1-oxo-5(1H)-(purin-6-ylthio)pentyl]glycine ethyl ester; NSC-172755).

BUTOCLOR* (*N*-butoxymethyl)-2-chloro-2′,6′-diethylacetanilide; *N*-(butoxymethyl)-2-chloro-*N*-(2,6-diethylphenyl)acetamide; *N*-(butoxymethyl)-*N*-(2-chloroacetyl)-2,6-diethylaniline; butachlor; 'machete').

BUTOCTAMIDE** (*N*-(2-ethylhexyl)-3-hydroxybutyramide).

BUTOCTAMIDE HEMISUCCINATE (L-2; M-2H).

Butoforme* *see* Butylcaine.

BUTOMELIDE (tr) (4-butoxy-4′-(4-methylpiperazin-1-yl)thiocarbanilide; 1-[*p*-[3-(*p*-butoxyphenyl)thioureido]phenyl]-4-methylpiperazine).

BUTONATE** (butyric acid ester with dimethyl(2,2,2-trichloro-1-hydroxyethyl)-phosphonate; butilchlorofos; butilklorophos; butylchlorophos; metrifonate butyrate).

BUTOPIPRINE*** (2-butoxyethyl α-phenyl-1-piperidineacetate).

BUTOPYRAMMONIUM IODIDE*** (butyldimethyl(2,3-dimethyl-5-oxo-1-phenyl-3-pyrazolin-4-yl)ammonium iodide; quaternary butyl iodide of aminopyrine).

BUTOPYRONOXYL* (butyl 4,5-dihydro-6,6-dimethyl-4-oxopyran-2-carboxylate; butyl mesityl oxide; indalone).

BUTORPHANOL** ((−)-17-(cyclobutylmethyl)morphinan-3,14-diol; (−)-17-(cyclobutylmethyl)-3,14-dihydroxymorphinan; levo-BC-2627).

Butoxamine* *see* Butaxamine.

4′-*tert*-Butoxyacetanilide *see* Butacetin.

p-**Butoxybenzoic acid 3-diethylamino-1,2-dimethylpropyl ester ethiodide** *see* Quateron.

[3-[(*p*-Butoxybenzoyl)oxy]-2,3-dimethylpropyl]triethylammonium iodide *see* Quateron.

8-(*p*-Butoxybenzyl)-3α-hydroxy-1αH,5αH-tropanium bromide (−)-tropate *see* Butropium bromide.

BUTOXYCARBOXIM* (3-methylsulfonyl-2-butanone *O*-(methylaminocarbonyl)-oxime).

6-Butoxy-3-(2,6-diaminopyrid-3-yl)-azopyridine *see* Neotropin.

2-Butoxy-*N*-(2-diethylaminoethyl)-cinchoninamide *see* Cinchocaine.

4-Butoxy-3,5-dimethoxybenzoic acid 2-pyrrolidin-1-ylethyl ester *see* Burodiline.

4-Butoxy-4′-dimethylamino-2-thiocarbanilide *see* Thiambutosine.

α-[2-(2-Butoxyethoxy)ethoxy]-4,5-methylenedioxy-2-propyltoluene *see* Piperonyl butoxide.

5-[[2-(2-Butoxyethoxy)ethoxy]methyl]-6-propyl-1,3-benzodioxole *see* Piperonyl butoxide.

2-(2-Butoxyethoxy)ethyl 3,4-methylenedioxybenzoate *see* Bucarpolate.

2-(2-Butoxyethoxy)ethyl piperonylate *see* Bucarpolate.

2-Butoxyethyl α-phenyl-1-piperidineacetate *see* Butopiprine.

1-(2-Butoxy-2-hydroxypropyl)-5-ethyl-

5-phenylbarbituric acid carbamate ester *see* Febarbamate.

BUTOXYLATE*** (butyl 1-(3-cyano-3,3-diphenylpropyl)-4-phenylpiperidine-4-carboxylate; butyl 1-(3-cyano-3,3-diphenylpropyl)-4-phenylisonipecotate; butyl-difenoxilate).

1-*tert*-Butoxy-3-methoxy-2-propanol *see* Terbuprol.

N-(Butoxymethyl)-N-(2-chloroacetyl)-2,6-diethylaniline *see* Butoclor.

N-(Butoxymethyl)-2-chloro-2',6'-diethyl-acetanilide *see* Butoclor.

N-(Butoxymethyl)-2-chloro-N-(2,6-diethylphenyl)acetamide *see* Butoclor.

4-Butoxy-4'-(4-methylpiperazin-1-yl)-thiocarbanilide *see* Butomelide.

N-[2-(p-Butoxyphenoxy)acetyl]-N-(2,5-diethoxyphenyl)-N',N'-diethylethyl-enediamine *see* Fenoxedil.

1-[2-[[2-(p-Butoxyphenoxy)acetyl]-(o-methoxyphenyl)amino]ethyl]pyrrolidine *see* Fexicaine.

N-(2-(p-Butoxyphenoxy)acetyl)-N-(2-pyrrolidin-1-ylethyl)-o-anisidine *see* Fexicaine.

2-(p-Butoxyphenoxy)-N-(2,5-diethoxyphenyl)-N-(2-diethylaminoethyl)-acetamide *see* Fenoxedil.

2-(p-Butoxyphenoxy)-N-(o-methoxyphenyl)-N-(2-pyrrolidin-1-ylethyl)acetamide *see* Fexicaine.

1-Butoxy-3-phenoxy-2-propanol *see* Febuprol.

2-(p-Butoxyphenyl)acetohydroxamic acid *see* Bufexamac.

1-(p-Butoxyphenyl)-3-(p-dimethylaminophenyl)-2-thiourea *see* Thiambutosine.

p-Butoxyphenyl 3-morpholinopropyl ether *see* Pramocaine.

1-[p-[3-(p-Butoxyphenyl)thioureido]-phenyl]-4-methylpiperazine *see* Butomelide.

4'-Butoxy-3-piperid-1-ylpropiophenone *see* Dyclonine.

BUTRIPTYLINE*** (5-(3-dimethylamino-2-methylpropyl)-10,11-dihydro-5H-dibenzo-(a,d)cycloheptene; 5-(dimethylaminoiso-butyl)-10,11-dihydro-5H-dibenzo(a,d)-cycloheptene; 10,11-dihydro-N,N,β-tri-methyl-5H-dibenzo(a,d)cycloheptene-5-propylamine; DL-3-(10,11-dihydro-5H-dibenzo(a,d)cyclohepten-5-yl)-2-methyl-propyldimethylamine; DL-butriptyline; butriptyline hydrochloride; AY-62014; 'evadyne').

BUTROPIUM BROMIDE** (8-(p-butoxy-benzyl)-3α-hydroxy-1αH,5αH-tropanium bromide (−)-tropate; 'choliopan').

Butter yellow *see* Dimethylaminoazobenzene.

BUTURON* (1-(p-chlorophenyl)-3-methyl-3-(1-methyl-2-propynyl)urea; butirao; 'butyron', 'eptapur').

BUTURON PLUS ISONORURON ('basfitox').

Butydrine *see* Butidrine.

Butylacetic acid *see* Hexanoic acid.

tert-Butylacetic acid esters and salts *see* Tebutate(s).

Butyl alcohols *see* 1-Butanol; 2-Butanol; 2-Methyl-2-propanol.

N-Butylaminoacetyl-6-chloro-o-toluidine *see* Butanilicaine.

Butyl p-aminobenzoate *see* Butylcaine.

p-Butylaminobenzoic acid 3-amino-2-hydroxypropyl ester *see* 3-Amino-2-hydroxypropyl p-butylaminobenzoate.

p-Butylaminobenzoic acid 2-diethyl-aminoethyl ester *see* 2-Diethylaminoethyl p-butylaminobenzoate.

p-Butylaminobenzoic acid 2-dimethyl-aminoethyl ester *see* Tetracaine.

p-Butylaminobenzoic acid 1-methyl-piperid-4-yl ester *see* Paridocaine.

p-Butylaminobenzoic acid nonoxaocta-cosanol ester *see* Benzonatate.

[1-[(Butylamino)carbonyl]-1H-benzimid-azol-2-yl]carbamic acid methyl ester *see* Benomyl.

2-Butylamino-6'-chloro-o-acetotoluidide *see* Butanilicaine.

3-tert-Butylamino-1-(2-chloro-5-methyl-phenoxy)-2-propanol *see* Bupranolol.

(±)-2-tert-Butylamino-3'-chloropropio-phenone *see* Bupropion.

1-tert-Butylamino-3-(6-chloro-m-toloxy)-2-propanol *see* Bupranolol.

1-tert-Butylamino-3-(o-cyanophenoxy)-2-propanol *see* Bunitrolol.

1-tert-Butylamino-3-[p-(3-cyclohexyl-ureido)phenoxy]-2-propanol *see* Talinolol.

1-tert-Butylamino-3-(o-cyclopentyl-phenoxy)-2-propanol *see* Penbutolol.

1-(tert-Butylamino)-3-(3,4-dihydro-2(1H)-oxoquinolin-5-yl)-2-propanol *see* Carteolol.

2-tert-Butylamino-1-(3,5-dihydroxyphen-yl)ethanol *see* Terbutaline.

2-tert-Butylamino-1-(2,5-dimethoxyphen-yl)-1-propanol *see* Butaxamine.

2-sec-Butylamino-4-ethylamino-6-meth-oxy-s-triazine *see* Secbumeton.

2-tert-Butylamino-4-ethylamino-6-meth-oxy-s-triazine *see* Terbumeton.

2-tert-Butylamino-4-ethylamino-6-(meth-ylthio)-s-triazine *see* Terbutryn.

2-tert-Butylamino-1-(7-ethylbenzofuran-2-yl)ethanol *see* Bufuralol.

α-(1-tert-Butylaminoethyl)-2,5-dimethoxy-benzyl alcohol *see* Butaxamine.

4-Butylamino-1-ethyl-1H-pyrazolo(3,4-b)-pyridine-5-carboxylic acid ethyl ester *see* Cartazolate.

α-Butylamino-p-hydroxybenzyl alcohol *see* Bamethan.

5-(2-tert-Butylamino-1-hydroxyethyl)-N-carbamoyl-2-hydroxyaniline *see* Carbuterol.

2-(2-tert-Butylamino-1-hydroxyethyl)-7-ethylbenzofuran *see* Bufuralol.

6-(2-tert-Butylamino-1-hydroxyethyl)-3-hydroxy-2-(hydroxymethyl)pyridine *see* Pirbuterol.

1-[5-(2-*tert*-Butylamino-1-hydroxyethyl)-2-hydroxyphenyl]urea *see* Carbuterol.

5-(2-*tert*-Butylamino-1-hydroxyethyl-*m*-phenylene diisobutyrate *see* Ibuterol.

4-(2-(*tert*-Butylamino)-1-hydroxyethyl)-*o*-phenylene di-*p*-toluate *see* Bitolterol.

5-(2-*tert*-Butylamino-1-hydroxyethyl)-resorcinol diisobutyrate *see* Ibuterol.

2-*tert*-Butylamino-1-(4-hydroxy-3-hydroxymethylphenyl)ethanol *see* Salbutamol.

2-*tert*-Butylamino-1-(5-hydroxy-6-hydroxymethylpyrid-2-yl)ethanol *see* Pirbuterol.

2-Butylamino-1-(*p*-hydroxyphenyl)-ethanol *see* Bamethan.

o-(3-*tert*-Butylamino-2-hydroxypropoxy)-benzonitrile *see* Bunitrolol.

5-[3-(*tert*-Butylamino)-2-hydroxypropoxy]-3,4-dihydrocarbostyril *see* Carteolol.

5-(3-*tert*-Butylamino-2-hydroxypropoxy)-3,4-dihydro-1(2H)-naphthalenone *see* Bunolol.

8-[3-(*tert*-Butylamino)-2-hydroxypropoxy]-5-methylcoumarin *see* Bucumolol.

3-(3-*tert*-Butylamino-2-hydroxypropoxy)-4-morpholino-1,2,5-thiadiazole *see* Timolol.

2-[[*o*-(3-*tert*-Butylamino-2-hydroxypropoxy)phenoxy]methyl]tetrahydrofuran *see* Bufetolol.

1-[*p*-(3-*tert*-Butylamino-2-hydroxypropoxy)phenyl]-3-cyclohexylurea *see* Talinolol.

1-[3-(*tert*-Butylamino)-2-hydroxypropoxy]-5,6,7,8-tetrahydro-*cis*-6,7-naphthalenediol *see* Nadolol.

Butylaminomethylbenzodioxan *see* Butamoxane.

2-Butylaminomethyl-8-(2-chloroethoxy)-1,4-benzodioxan *see* Chlorethoxybutamoxane.

1-*tert*-Butylamino-3-(5-methylcoumarin-8-yloxy)-2-propanol *see* Bucumolol.

α-(*tert*-Butylaminomethyl)-3,5-dihydroxybenzyl alcohol *see* Terbutaline.

2-Butylaminomethyl-8-ethoxy-1,4-benzodioxan *see* Ethomoxane.

α-(*tert*-Butylaminomethyl)-7-ethyl-2-benzofuranmethanol *see* Bufuralol.

α-Butylaminomethyl-*p*-hydroxybenzyl alcohol *see* Bamethan.

α-(*tert*-Butylaminomethyl)-4-hydroxy-3-hydroxymethylbenzyl alcohol *see* Salbutamol.

α-(*tert*-Butylaminomethyl)-4-hydroxy-3-(methylsulfonylmethyl)benzyl alcohol *see* Sulfonterol.

α⁶-(*tert*-Butylaminomethyl)-3-hydroxy-2,6-pyridinedimethanol *see* Pirbuterol.

α-(*tert*-Butylaminomethyl)-4-hydroxy-3-ureidobenzyl alcohol *see* Carbuterol.

α¹-(*tert*-Butylaminomethyl)-4-hydroxy-*m*-xylene-α,α'-diol *see* Salbutamol.

α-(*sec*-Butylaminomethyl)-5,6,7,8-tetrahydro-2-naphthalenemethanol *see* Butidrine.

1-*tert*-Butylamino-3-(4-morpholino-1,2,5-thiadiazol-3-yloxy)-2-propanol *see* Timolol.

3-Butylamino-4-phenoxy-5-sulfamoylbenzoic acid *see* Bumetanide.

3-Butylamino-α-phenyl-5-sulfamoyl-*p*-toluic acid *see* Besunide.

4-Butylaminosalicylic acid dimethylaminoethyl ester *see* Hydroxytetracaine.

1-(*tert*-Butylamino)-3-[(5,6,7,8-tetrahydro-*cis*-6,7-dihydroxynaphth-1-yl)oxy]-2-propanol *see* Nadolol.

1-*tert*-Butylamino-3-(*o*-(tetrahydrofurfuryloxy)phenoxy)-2-propanol *see* Bufetolol.

2-*sec*-Butylamino-1-(5,6,7,8-tetrahydro-2-naphthyl)ethanol *see* Butidrine.

2-(*p*-Butylanilino)nicotinic acid *see* Butanixin.

BUTYLATE (*S*-ethyl bis(2-methylpropyl)-carbamothioate; 'sutan').

BUTYLATED HYDROXYANISOLE* (mixture of 2-*tert*-butyl-4-methoxyphenol and 3-*tert*-butyl-4-methoxyphenol; 'embanox', 'nipantiox 1-F', 'tenox-BHA').

BUTYLATED HYDROXYTOLUENE (2,6-di*tert*-butyl-*p*-cresol; 2,6-di*tert*-butyl-4-methylphenol; 3,5-di*tert*-butyl-4-hydroxytoluene; BHT; DBPC; 'impruvol', 'ionol', 'vianol').

2-(*o*-*tert*-Butylbenzhydryloxy)-*N*,*N*-dimethylethylamine *see* Bufenadrine.

5-Butyl-2-benzimidazolecarbamic acid methyl ester *see* Parbendazole.

2-Butyl-3-benzofuranyl 4-(2-diethylaminoethoxy)-3,5-diiodophenyl ketone *see* Amiodarone.

α-Butylbenzyl alcohol *see* Fenipentol.

1-(*p*-*tert*-Butylbenzyl)-4-(*p*-chlorobenzhydryl)piperazine *see* Buclizine.

1-Butylbiguanide *see* Buformin.

N-*tert*-Butyl-1,4-butanediamine *see* Dibutadiamin.

'Butyl butex' *see* Butyl paraben.

BUTYLCAINE* (butyl *p*-aminobenzoate; butamben; butoforme; 'butesin', 'planiform', 'scuroform').

tert-Butylcarbamic acid *m*-(dimethylcarbamoylamino)phenyl ester *see* Karbutilate.

1-(Butylcarbamoyl)benzimidazole-2-carbamic acid methyl ester *see* Benomyl.

5-Butyl-5-(2-carbamoyloxyethyl)-barbituric acid carbamate ester *see* Carbubarb.

1-[*m*-(*tert*-Butylcarbamoyloxy)phenyl]-3,3-dimethylurea *see* Karbutilate.

α-Butyl-5-carboxy-2-hydroxybenzyl alcohol *see* Fepentolic acid.

BUTYLCHLORALAMIDOPYRINE (compound of butylchloral hydrate with aminophenazone; butylchloralaminoanalgesine; 'asciatin', 'butipyrine', 'trigemine', 'trigeminin').

Butylchloralaminoanalgesine *see* Butylchloralamidopyrine.

BUTYLCHLORAL HYDRATE* (2,2,3-trichloro-1,1-butanediol; croton-chloral

68

hydrate; trichlorobutylideneglycol).

5-Butyl-2-(*p*-chlorobenzenesulfonamido)-1,3,4-thiadiazole *see* Butadiazamide.

N-Butyl-*N'*-(4-chloro-2-methylphenyl)-*N*-methylformamidine *see* Chlormebuform.

3-*tert*-Butyl-5-chloro-6-methyluracil *see* Terbacil.

4-*tert*-Butyl-2-chlorophenyl methyl *N*-methylphosphoramidate *see* Crufomate.

Butylchlorophos *see* Butonate.

N-Butyl-4-chlorosalicylamide *see* Buclosamide.

Butyl 2-cyanoacrylate *see* Enbucrilate.

5-Butyl-1-cyclohexylbarbituric acid *see* Bucolome.

BUTYL 2,4-DICHLOROPHENOXY-ACETATE ('lironox').

1-Butyl-2-(3,4-dichlorophenylimino)-pyrrolidine *see* Clenpirin.

1-Butyl-3-(3,4-dichlorophenyl)-1-methyl-urea *see* Neburon.

2-Butyl-3-[4-(2-diethylaminoethoxy)-3,3-diiodobenzoyl]benzofuran *see* Amiodarone.

N-Butyl-*N*-(2-diethylaminoethyl)-1-naphthamide *see* Bunaftine.

N-Butyl-*N'*,*N'*-diethyl-*N*-naphth-1-oyl-ethylenediamine *see* Bunaftine.

Butyl difenoxilate *see* Butoxylate.

Butyl 4,5-dihydro-6,6-dimethyl-4-oxo-pyran-2-carboxylate *see* Butopyronoxyl.

4-Butyl-1,2-dihydro-5-hydroxy-1,2-diphenyl-3,6-pyridazinedione *see* Denpidazone.

2-Butyl-1-(2-dimethylaminoethoxy)iso-quinoline *see* Quinisocaine.

5-Butyl-2-(dimethylamino)-4-hydroxy-6-methylpyrimidine *see* Dimethirimol.

5-Butyl-2-dimethylamino-6-methyl-4-pyrimidinol *see* Dimethirimol.

Butyldimethyl(dimethylphenyloxopyr-azolinyl)ammonium iodide *see* Butopyr-ammonium.

2-(4-*tert*-Butyl-2,6-dimethyl-3-hydroxy-benzyl)-2-imidazoline *see* Oxymetazoline.

6-*sec*-Butyl-2,4-dinitrophenol *see* Dinoseb.

2-*sec*-Butyl-4,6-dinitrophenyl 3,3-dimethyl-acrylate *see* Binapacryl.

2-*sec*-Butyl-4,6-dinitrophenyl isopropyl carbonate *see* Dinobuton.

2-*sec*-Butyl-4,6-dinitrophenyl 3-methyl-crotonate *see* Binapacryl.

2-*sec*-Butyl-4,6-dinitrophenyl senecioate *see* Binapacryl.

o-*tert*-Butyldiphenhydramine *see* Bufen-adrine.

N-*tert*-Butyl-3,3-diphenyl-1-methylpropyl-amine *see* Terodiline.

4-Butyl-1,2-diphenyl-3,5-pyrazolidine-dione *see* Phenylbutazone.

5-Butyl-2-ethylamino-4-hydroxy-6-methylpyrimidine *see* Ethirimol.

5-Butyl-2-(ethylamino)-6-methyl-4-pyrimidinol *see* Ethirimol.

5-Butyl-2-ethylbarbituric acid *see* Butethal.

5-*sec*-Butyl-5-ethylbarbituric acid *see* Secbutabarbital.

1-Butyl-2-ethylbiguanide *see* Etoformin.

Butylethylcarbamothioic acid *S*-propyl ester *see* Pebulate.

N-Butyl-*N*-ethyl-2,6-dinitro-4-(trifluoro-methyl)aniline *see* Benfluralin.

2-But-2-yl-2-ethylmalonamic acid ethyl ester *see* Ethyl butylethylmalonamate.

5-*sec*-Butyl-5-ethyl-2-thiobarbituric acid *see* Thiobutabarbital.

N-Butyl-*N*-ethyl-α,α,α-trifluoro-2,6-dinitro-*p*-toluidine *see* Benfluralin.

Butyl 6α-fluoro-11β-hydroxy-16α-methyl-3,20-dioxopregna-1,4-dien-21-oate *see* Fluocortin butyl.

Butyl *p*-hydroxybenzoate *see* Butyl paraben.

α-Butyl-α-hydroxy-4,3-cresotic acid *see* Fepentolic acid.

p-*tert*-Butyl-α-[3-[4-(hydroxydiphenyl-methyl)piperid-1-yl]propyl]benzyl alcohol *see* Terfenadine.

Butyl 9-hydroxy-9H-fluorene-9-carboxyl-ate *see* Flurenol-butyl.

4-Butyl-4-hydroxymethyl-1,2-diphenyl-3,5-pyrazolidinedione *p*-chlorobenzoate ester *see* Feclobuzone.

4-Butyl-4-hydroxymethyl-1,2-diphenyl-3,5-pyrazolidinedione hydrogen succinate *see* Suxibuzone.

4-Butyl-1-(*p*-hydroxyphenyl)-2-phenyl-3,5-pyrazolidinedione *see* Oxyphenbuta-zone.

6-*tert*-Butyl-3-(2-imidazolin-2-ylmethyl)-2,4-dimethylphenol *see* Oxymetazoline.

Butylmalonic acid mono(1,2-diphenyl-hydrazide) *see* Bumadizone.

2-(*p*-Butylmercaptobenzhydrylmercapto)-*N*,*N*-dimethylethylamine *see* Captodiame.

Butyl mesityl oxide *see* Butopyronoxyl.

N-*tert*-Butylmethoxamine *see* Butaxamine.

tert-Butyl-4-methoxyphenols *see* Butylated hydroxyanisole.

3-(*N*-*tert*-Butylmethylamino)-3-methyl-1-butyne *see* Butynamine.

2-*sec*-Butyl-2-methyl-1,3-propanediol carbamate isopropylcarbamate *see* Nisobamate.

2-*sec*-Butyl-2-methyl-1,3-propanediol dicarbamate *see* Mebutamate.

'Butylnorsimpatol' *see* Bamethan.

3α-*tert*-Butyl-2,3,4,4aβ,8,9,13bα,14-octahydro-1H-benzo(6,7)cyclohepta-(1,2,3-de)pyrido(2,1-a)isoquinolin-3-ol *see* Butaclamol.

N-*tert*-Butyloxycarbonyl-β-alanyl-L-tryptophyl-L-methionyl-L-aspartyl-L-phenylalanine amide *see* Pentagastrin.

BUTYL PARABEN (butyl *p*-hydroxybenzo-ate; 'butoben', 'butyl butex', 'nipasol').

BUTYLPHENAMIDE* (*N*-butyl-3-phenyl-salicylamide; 'bynamid').

1-(*p*-*tert*-Butylphenoxy)-3-(*p*-carboxy-phenoxy)-2-propanol *see* Terbufibrol.

2-(*p*-*tert*-Butylphenoxy)cyclohexyl 2-propynyl sulfite *see* Propargite.

p-[3-(*p*-*tert*-Butylphenoxy)-2-hydroxy-

propoxy]benzoic acid *see* Terbufibrol.
2-(*p-tert*-**BUTYLPHENOXY**)**ISOPROPYL**
2-CHLOROETHYL SULFITE (2-(*p-tert*-
butylphenoxy)-1-methylethyl 2-chloro-
ethylsulfite; 2-chloroethyl 2-[4-(1,1-dimeth-
ylethyl)phenoxy]-1-methylethyl sulfite
ester; R-88; 'aramite', 'niagaramite',
'ortho-mite').
2-(*o-tert*-**Butyl-α-phenylbenzyloxy**)-*N*,*N*-
dimethylethylamine *see* Bufenadrine.
α-[**1-[4-**(*p-tert*-**Butylphenyl**)-**4-hydroxy-**
butyl]piperid-4-yl]benzhydrol *see*
Terfenadine.
α-(*p-tert*-**Butylphenyl**)-**4-(hydroxydiphen-**
ylmethyl)-**1-piperidinebutanol** *see*
Terfenadine.
Butyl 3-phenyl-3-piperid-1-ylpropionate
see Butaverine.
4-Butyl-1-phenyl-3,5-pyrazolidinedione
see Mofebutazone.
N-**Butyl-3-phenylsalicylamide** *see* Butylphenamide.
Butyl phthalate *see* Dibutyl phthalate.
5-Butylpicolinamide *see* Bupicomide.
5-Butylpicolinic acid *see* Fusaric acid.
N-**Butylpipecolic acid 2,6-dimethylanilide**
see Bupivacaine.
1-Butyl-2′,6′-pipecoloxylidide *see*
Bupivacaine.
5-Butyl-2-pyridinecarboxamide *see*
Bupicomide.
5-Butylpyridine-2-carboxylic acid *see*
Fusaric acid.
Butylscopolamine *see* Scopolamine butyl
bromide.
'**Butylsympathol**' *see* Bamethan.
6-Butyl-1,4,7,10-tetrahydro-4,10-dioxo-
1,7-phenanthroline-2,8-dicarboxylic
acid *see* Bufrolin.
N-(**5-Butyl-1,3,4-thiadiazol-2-yl**)-*p*-**chloro-**
benzenesulfonamide *see* Butadiazamide.
*N*¹-(**5-*tert*-Butyl-1,3,4-thiadiazol-2-yl**)-
sulfanilamide *see* Glybuzole.
2-[*p*-(Butylthio)-α-phenylbenzylthio]-*N*,*N*-
dimethylethylamine *see* Captodiame.
Butylthiopurine isomer *see* Butyl-
purinethiol.
1-Butyl-3-*p*-toluenesulfonylurea *see* Tolbutamide.
1-Butyl-3-tosylurea *see* Tolbutamide.
N-*tert*-**Butyl-*N*,1,1-trimethyl-2-propynyl-**
amine *see* Butynamine.
1-Butyl-*N*-(2,4,6-trimethylphenyl)-2-
pyrrolidinecarboxamide *see* Bumecaine.
1-Butyl-2′,4′,6′-trimethyl-2-pyrrolidine-
carboxanilide *see* Bumecaine.
Butyl vinyl ether polymer *see* Polyvinox.
1-Butyl-2-(2,6-xylylcarbamoyl)piperidine
see Bupivacaine.
'**Butyn**' *see* Butacaine.
BUTYNAMINE*** (*N*-*tert*-butyl-*N*,1,1-
trimethyl-2-propynylamine; 3-(*N*-*tert*-butyl-
methylamino)-3-methyl-1-butyne).
2-Butynoic acid *see* Tetrolic acid.
BUTYRAMIDE (butyric acid amide;
butanamide).
1-[[*p*-(2-Butyramidoethyl)phenyl]sulfon-

yl]-3-(3-cyclohexen-1-yl)-2-imino-
imidazolidine *see* Glibutimine.
3-(3-Butyramido-2,4,6-triiodophenyl)-2-
ethylacrylic acid *see* Bunamiodyl.
2-(3-Butyramido-3,4,6-triiodophenyl-
methylene)butyric acid *see* Bunamiodyl.
BUTYRIC ACID (butanoic acid).
1-Butyric acid-6-(L-2-aminobutyric acid)-
7-glycineoxytocin *see* Cargutocin.
Butyric acid ester with dimethyl (2,2,2-
trichloro-1-hydroxyethyl)phosphonate
see Butonate.
BUTYRIN (glycerol monobutyrate).
'**Butyron**' *see* Buturon.
Butyrone *see* 4-Heptanone.
p-**BUTYROPHENETIDIDE** (*N*-(*p*-ethoxy-
phenyl)butyramide; *p*-ethoxybutyranilide).
BUTYROPHENONE (phenyl propyl ketone).
BUTYROPIPAZONE (4′-fluoro-4-(4-phenyl-
piperazin-1-yl)butyrophenone; R-1892).
Butyrylacetic acid *see* Oxohexanoic acid.
N-**Butyryl-*p*-[[(3-cyclohexen-1-yl)-2-**
iminoimidazolidin-1-yl]sulfonyl]-
phenethylamine *see* Glibutimine.
3′-(5-Butyryl-2,4-dihydroxy-3,3-dimethyl-
6-oxo-1,4-cyclohexadien-1-ylmethyl)-
2′,6′-dihydroxy-4′-methoxybutyro-
phenone *see* Desaspidin.
4-Butyryl-2-methylphloroglucinol-1-
methyl ether *see* Aspidinol.
2-Butyryl-10-[3-(4-methylpiperazin-1-yl)-
propyl]phenothiazine *see* Butaperazine.
Butyrylperazine *see* Butaperazine.
'**Butysedal**' *see* Tetrabarbital.
Butyvinal *see* Vinylbital.
BUZEPIDE (2,2-diphenyl-4-hexamethyl-
eniminobutyramide; 1-(3-carbamoyl-3,3-
diphenylpropyl)hexamethylenimine;
1-(3-carbamoyl-3,3-diphenylpropyl)-
hexahydroazepine; 1-(3-carbamoyl-3,3-
diphenylpropyl)perhydroazepine; R-658;
'acemydrite').
BUZEPIDE METIODIDE*** (1-(3-
carbamoyl-3,3-diphenylpropyl)hexahydro-
1-methylazepinium iodide; buzepide
methiodide; 4-hexahydroazepin-1-yl-2,2-
diphenylbutyramide methiodide; 4-(*N*-
hexamethylenimino)-2,2-diphenylbutyr-
amide; metazepium iodide; R-661).
BUZEPIDE METIODIDE WITH
HALOPERIDOL ('vesadol').
BVU *see* Bromisoval.
BW-29C48 *see* Pipanone.
BW-33T57 *see* Metisazone.
BW-47-83 *see* Cyclizine.
BW-48/80 *see* Compound 48/80.
BW-49-210 *see* Diaveridine.
BW-50-63 *see* Pyrimethamine.
BW-50-71 *see* Tioguanine.
BW-55-5 *see* Oxipurinol.
BW-56-72 *see* Trimethoprim.
BW-56-158 *see* Allopurinol.
BW-57-223 *see* Lucanthone.
BW-57-322 *see* Azathioprine.
BW-57-323 *see* Tiamiprine.
BW-57C65 *see* Cloguanamile.
BW-58-271 *see* Rolodine.

BW-61-32 *see* Stilbazium iodide.
BW-61-43 *see* Isopropylmethoxamine.
BW-62-415 *see* Bunamidine.
BW-63-90 *see* Butacetin.
BW-64-9 *see* Butaxamine.
BW-79T61 *see* Lucanthone.
BW-139C55 *see* Pentacynium.
BW-233 *see* Lucanthone.
BW-349C59 *see* Moxipraquine.
BW-356C61 *see* Gloxazone.
BW-373C57 *see* Bretylium tosilate.
BW-378C48 *see* Dipipanone.
BW-467C60 *see* Betanidine.
BW-545C64 *see* Xylamidine tosilate.

BW-611C65 *see* Thenium closilate.
BW-50197 *see* Metodiclorofen.
Bwy20 *see* Scopolamine butyl bromide with oxazepam.
BX-311 *see* Cinoxolone.
BX-341 *see* Bifluranol.
BX-363A *see* Cicloxolone disodium.
BY-123 *see* Neomycin with sulfamethizole.
'Byk-M 1' *see* Mephenesin.
Bykomycin (tr) *see* Neomycin with bacitracin.
'Bykonox' *see* Vinylbital.
'Bynamid' *see* Butylphenamide.
BZ 55 *see* Carbutamide.

C

C-3 *see* Capobenic acid.
C-3 Sankyo *see* Bucumolol.
C 4 *see* Benzalkonium.
C 5 *see* Pentamethonium.
C 6 *see* Hexamethonium.
C 10 *see* Decamethonium.
C-16 *see* Poligeenan.
C-45 *see* Belladonnin.
C-197 *see* Strophanthin.
C-209 *see* Dexamethasone with indometacin.
C-283 *see* Nitracrine.
C-1488 *see* Paromomycin.
C-1523 *see* Benzydamine.
C-1605 *see* Benzydamine with hexamidine isetionate.
C-2924 *see* Sodium auroallylthioureidobenzoate.
C-4311/b *see* Methylphenidate.
C-4675 *see* Pentapiperide.
C-5473 *see* Oxyphenonium.
C-5511 *see* Ketobemidone.
C-5581 *see* Phenyltoloxamine.
C-5864-Su *see* Guanethidine.
C-5968 *see* Hydralazine.
C-6866 *see* Chlormethine.
C-7019 *see* Aziprotryne.
C-7115 *see* Ketobemidone.
C-7337 *see* Phentolamine mesilate.
C-7441 *see* Dihydralazine.
C-8514 *see* Chlorphenamidine.
C-9295 *see* Azamethonium.
C-11925 *see* Phanquinone.
C-12669/A *see* Demecolcine.
C-13155 *see* Meladrazine.
C-13437-Su *see* Nafenopin.
C-15095 E *see* Thiambutosine.
C-17309 *see* Metandienone.
C-193901 *see* Clonitazene.
C-22598 *see* Chlormebuform.
C-29038 *see* Boldenone undecenoate.
C-30803-Ba *see* Benzoctamine.
C-30920-Ba *see* Tetracosactide.

C-32644 *see* Niridazole.
C-34276-Ba *see* Maprotiline.
C-34647-Ba *see* Baclofen.
C-36278A-Ba *see* Cefacetrile.
C-39089-Ba *see* Oxprenolol.
C-41795-Ba *see* Codactide.
C-42915-Ba *see* Tetracosactide zinc phosphate complex.
Caa-40 *see* Isoxsuprine.
Cabbagin *see* Vitamin U.
'Cabiol' *see* Benzyl benzoate.
'Ca Chel 330' *see* Calcium trisodium pentetate.
CACODYLIC ACID (dimethylarsinic acid).
'Cacodyl new' *see* Disodium methanearsonate.
CACTINOMYCIN*** (antibiotic from *Str. chrysomallus*; actinomycin C; HBF-386; 'sanamycin').
CADAVERINE (pentamethylenediamine; 1,5-pentanediamine).
'Cadminate' *see* Cadmium succinate.
CADMIUM SUCCINATE ('cadminate').
CADMIUM SULFIDE ('capsebon').
'Caducid' *see* Fluoresone.
CAFAMINOL** (8-[(2-hydroxyethyl)-methylamino]caffeine; 'rhinoptil').
CAFEDRINE** (7-[2-(2-hydroxy-1-methyl-phenethylamino)ethyl]theophylline; norephedrine-theophylline).
CAFEDRINE WITH THEODRENALINE ('H-835'; 'akrinor', 'praxinor', 'voveran').
'Cafergot' *see* Ergotamine tartrate with caffeine.
Caffearin *see* Trigonelline.
CAFFEIC ACID (3,4-dihydroxycinnamic acid).
See also Piperidine caffeate.
CAFFEINE (1,3,7-trimethylxanthine; coffein; guarin; guaranine; methyltheobromine; thein).
Caffeoylquinic acid *see* Chlorogenic acid.
Caffeoylshikimic acid *see* Dactyliferic acid.
'Cafilon' *see* Phenmetrazine teoclate with

N-(2-hydroxyethyl)phenmetrazine-2-phenylbutyrate.

'Cafron' see Benactyzine.

'Caid' see Chlorophacinone.

'Calbroben' see Calcium dibromobehenate.

Calcacetosal see Calcium acetylsalicylate.

'Calcamine' see Dihydrotachysterol.

'Calcibromin' see Calcium bromide-lactobionate.

'Calcibronat' see Calcium bromide-lactobionate.

'Calcicol' see Calcium guaiacolsulfonate.

CALCIFEDIOL*** (9,10-secocholesta-5,7,10(19)-triene-3β,25-diol).

Calciferol* see Ergocalciferol.

'Calcigenol' see Calcium phosphate.

CALCINAPHTHOL (calcium 2-naphthol-1-sulfonate; 'abrastol', 'asaprol').

'Calciobrom' see Calcium bromide-lactobionate.

CALCIODOXYL BENZOATE* (calcium o-iodoxybenzoate; 'calsiod', 'oxo-ate-B').

'Calciofon' see Calcium gluconate.

'Calciostab' see Calcium thiosulfate.

'Calciparin' see Heparin calcium.

'Calcitare' see Calcitonin (pig).

Calcitetramate disodium see Sodium calcium edetate.

CALCITONIN*** (thyrocalcitonin; pig calcitonin; 'calcitare', 'staporos').
See also Salcatonin.

CALCIUM ACETYLSALICYLATE
(calcacetosal; 'analutos', 'apyron', 'ascal', 'calspirin', 'calsprate', 'dispril', 'disprin', 'kalmopyrin', 'kalsetal', 'rasprin', 'regasprin', 'renolon', 'rumarid', 'sinaspril', 'solprin', 'tylcalsin', 'uniprin').

Calcium acetylsalicylate carbamide see Carbasalate calcium.

Calcium acetylsalicylate urea see Carbasalate calcium.

CALCIUM ALGINATE ('calgitex', 'coalgan', 'goalgan', 'kalipin').
See also Sodium alginate.

CALCIUM AMINOSALICYLATE (calcium 4-aminosalicylate; 'PAC', 'pasara calcium', 'pasido-kalcium').

Calcium-4-benzamido-2-hydroxybenzoate see Calcium benzamidosalicylate.

CALCIUM BENZAMIDOSALICYLATE***
(calcium 4-benzoylaminosalicylate; calcium benzoylpas; calcium 4-benzamido-2-hydroxybenzoate; benzoylpascalcium; 'aminacyl B-PAS'; 'benzacyl Ca', 'benzapas', 'B-paracipan', 'B-PAS', 'HP-170', 'pasoyl', 'therapas').
See also Sodium benzamidosalicylate.

CALCIUM BENZOYLPAS* see Calcium benzamidosalicylate.

CALCIUM BENZYL SUCCINATE (succinic acid monobenzyl ester calcium salt).

CALCIUM BENZYL SUCCINATE-p-AMINOBENZOATE DOUBLE SALT ('paramon').

CALCIUM BENZYL SUCCINATE-BENZOATE DOUBLE SALT ('subenon').

CALCIUM BENZYL SUCCINATE-

SALICYLATE DOUBLE SALT ('salisuccyl').

CALCIUM BROMIDE-LACTOBIONATE
(Ca(C$_{12}$H$_{21}$O$_{12}$)$_2$·CaBr$_2$·6H$_2$O; calcium galactoglyconate bromide; 'brocalcin', 'calcibromin', 'calcibronat', 'calciobrom').

CALCIUM BUCLOXATE (CB-804)
See also Bucloxic acid.

CALCIUM CARBAMOYLASPARTATE
(calcium ureidosuccinate; 'pacilan').

Calcium carbaspirin* see Carbasalate calcium.

CALCIUM CARBIMIDE*** (Ca carbylamine; Ca cyanamide; Ca isocyanide; carbodimide calcium; nitrolin).

CALCIUM CARBIMIDE CITRATE
(citrated calcium carbimide; 'abstem', 'dipsan', 'temposil').

Calcium carbylamine see Calcium carbimide.

CALCIUM CASEINATE* ('aciban').

'Calcium-Chefaro' see Calcium glucoheptonate.

CALCIUM CHLORIDE-UREA COMPLEX
('afenil').

CALCIUM CLOFIBRATE** (Ru-19583; 'dabical').
See also Clofibric acid.

'Calcium-Corbière' see Calcium glucoheptonate.

CALCIUM CRESOLSULFONATE(S)
('cresival', 'kresival', 'sirtal').

Calcium cyanamide see Calcium carbimide.

CALCIUM CYCLAMATE (calcium N-cyclohexylsulfamate; 'cyclan', 'sucaryl-calcium').

Calcium N-cyclohexylsulfamate see Calcium cyclamate.

'Calcium-Diasporal' see Calcium levulinate.

CALCIUM DIBROMOBEHENATE
(calcium dibromodocosenate; 'calbroben', 'sabromine').

CALCIUM 2,2-DICHLOROVINYL METHYL PHOSPHATE (dichlorvos demethyl calcium salt).
See also Dichlorvos with calcium 2,2-dichlorovinyl methyl phosphate.

Calcium 2,5-dihydroxybenzenesulfonate see Calcium dobesilate.

CALCIUM DIOCTYL SULFOSUCCINATE
(dioctyl calcium sulfosuccinate; 'surfak').
See also Dantron with calcium dioctyl sulfosuccinate.

Calcium disodium edetate see Sodium calcium edetate.

CALCIUM DOBESILATE*** (calcium 2,5-dihydroxybenzenesulfonate; dobesilate calcium; E-205; MD-205; 'dexium', 'doxium').

'Calcium-Drobena' see Calcium glucoheptonate.

CALCIUM 2-ETHYLBUTYRATE (calcium ethylbutanoate; 'ethanion').
See also Hydroxyzine embonate with calcium 2-ethylbutyrate.

'Calcium-Eupharma' see Ergocalciferol.

CALCIUM FOLINATE*** (calcium N^5-formyltetrahydrofolate; citrovorum factor;

NSC-3590; 'folvite', 'leucovorin').
CALCIUM FRUCTOSE 1,6-DIPHOS-PHATE ('candiolin', 'glucofos').
Calcium galactogluconate bromide see Calcium bromide-lactobionate.
CALCIUM GLUBIONATE* ((D-gluconato)(lactobionato)calcium monohydrate; $(C_{12}H_{21}O_{12} \cdot C_6H_{11}O_7)Ca \cdot H_2O$; calcium gluconogalactobionate; calcium gluconolactobionate).
Calcium D-glucarate see Calcium saccharate.
Calcium glucoheptogluconate see Calcium glucoheptonate.
CALCIUM GLUCOHEPTONATE (calcium hexahydroxyheptonate; calcium glucoheptogluconate; 'calcium-Chefaro', 'calcium-Corbière', 'calcium-Drobena', 'calcium-Sandoz', 'hi-glucon').
CALCIUM GLUCONATE* (solid calcium gluconate; Ca glyconate; Ca gluconicum; $C_{12}H_{22}O_{14}Ca \cdot H_2O$; 'calciofon', 'calcium-Sandoz', 'calglucon', 'glucal', 'glucobiogen', 'kalzan').
Calcium gluconate solutions see Calcium glucoheptonate.
Calcium gluconogalactobionate see Calcium glubionate.
Calcium gluconogalactogluconate see Calcium gluconate.
Calcium gluconolactobionate see Calcium glubionate.
CALCIUM GLUTAMATE ('vivacalcium').
Calcium glyconate see Calcium gluconate.
CALCIUM GUAIACOLSULFONATE ('calcicol', 'gaiacyl').
Calcium hexahydroxyheptonate see Calcium glucoheptonate.
Calcium o-iodoxybenzoate see Calciodoxyl benzoate.
Calcium isocyanide see Calcium carbimide.
CALCIUM LEVULINATE ('calcium-Diasporal', 'calcium-Pharmacon', 'flanthin', 'laevucalcin', 'mil-U-cal', 'neocalcin').
CALCIUM MAGNESIUM PHYTATE (calcium magnesium inositolhexaphosphate; inositocalcium; phytocalcine; 'inosine', 'phytine', 'phytobiase').
CALCIUM MANDELATE ('amandacide', 'camdelate', 'eggopurin', 'mandecal').
CALCIUM METHYL POLYGALACT-URONATE SULFONATE COMPLEX-(ES) (G-31150; R-2055; 'hemeran', 'sistilin', 'sistyline').
Calcium 2-naphthol-1-sulfonate see Calcinaphthol.
'Calcium-Noury' see Sodium calcium edetate.
Calcium octanoate with calcium propionate and sodium and zinc octanoates and propionates see Propionate caprylate mixture.
CALCIUM OLEATE ('collosol calcium').
CALCIUM PANTOTHENATE (calcium salt of N-(2,4-dihydroxy-3,3-dimethyl-butyryl)-β-alanine; 'pancal', 'pantholin', 'pantothaxin').
Calcium pentacemin trisodium see Calcium trisodium pentetate.

'Calcium-Pharmacon' see Calcium levulinate.
CALCIUM PHOSPHATE(S)
acid (Ca hydrogen phosphate).
basic (basic tricalcium phosphate; $3(PO_4)_2 \cdot Ca_3 \cdot CaO$; hydroxyapatite).
neutral (tricalcium phosphate; Ca ortho-phosphate; 'calcigenol').
Calcium polycarbophil see Polycarbophil calcium.
CALCIUM POLYGALACTURONATE(S) ('frenemo').
CALCIUM PROPIONATE ('mycoban').
Calcium propionate with calcium octanoate and sodium and zinc octanoates and propionates see Propionate caprylate mixture.
Calcium propionate with sodium propionate see Propionate compound.
CALCIUM SACCHARATE* (calcium D-glucarate; 'antacidin').
'Calcium-Sandoz' see Calcium gluco-heptonate; Calcium gluconate.
CALCIUM SODIUM FERRICLATE* (monocalcium tetrasodium bis[pentaaqua-[D-gluconato(4-)]tetra-μ-hydroxy-dioxotriferrate(3-)]; ferriclate calcium sodium).
Calcium tetrasodium bis[pentaaqua-[D-gluconato(4-)]tetra-μ-hydroxy-dioxotriferrate(3-)] see Calcium sodium ferriclate.
Calcium theobromsal see Theobromine Ca salicylate.
CALCIUM THIOSULPHATE ('calciostab', 'tecesal').
Calcium trisodium (carboxymethyl-imino)bis(ethylenenitrilo)tetraacetic acid see Calcium trisodium pentetate.
CALCIUM TRISODIUM PENTETATE* (calcium trisodium salt of diethylenetri-aminepentaacetic acid; calcium trisodium (carboxymethylimino)bis(ethylenenitrilo)-tetraacetic acid; trisodium salt of 2,2'-carb-oxymethyliminobis(ethyleniminodiacetic acid) calcium chelate; calcium pentacemin trisodium; pentacine; 'Ca Chel 330', 'ditripentat', 'penthamil').
Calcium ureidosuccinate see Calcium carbamoylaspartate.
'Calgam' see Pangamic acid.
'Calgitex' see Calcium alginate.
'Calgluchin' see Calcium gluconate.
'Calglucon' see Calcium gluconate.
'Calibene' see Suxibuzone.
'Calixin' see Tridemorph.
Callicrein see Kallidinogenase.
'Calmeran' see Azacyclonol.
'Calmonal' see Meclozine.
'Calmpose' see Diazepam.
Calomel see Mercurous chloride.
'Calped' see Phenylmercuric nitrate.
'Calpol' see Paracetamol.
'Calsiod' see Calciodoxyl benzoate.
'Calsol' see Tetrasodium edetate.
'Calspirin' see Calcium acetylsalicylate.
'Calsprate' see Calcium acetylsalicylate.

CALSULFHYDRYL* (aqueous dispersion of Ca complex salts with labile SH group; 'hydrosulphosol').

'Calsynar' *see* Salcatonin.

'Calurin' *see* Carbasalate calcium.

CALUSTERONE*** (17β-hydroxy-7β,17-dimethylandrost-4-en-3-one; 7β,17-dimethylandrost-4-en-17β-ol-3-one; 'methosarb'). †

CALYCOPTERIN (4′,5′-dihydroxy-3,6,7,8-tetramethoxyflavone; thapsin).

'Camalon' *see* Cyclarbamate.

'Camandeline' *see* Calcium mandelate.

'Camatropin' *see* Homatropine methyl bromide.

CAMAZEPAM** (7-chloro-1,3-dihydro-3-hydroxy-1-methyl-5-phenyl-2H-1,4-benzodiazepin-2-one dimethylcarbamate ester; temazepam dimethylcarbamate; B-5833; SB-5833).

CAMBENDAZOLE*** (isopropyl 2-thiazol-4-yl-5-benzimidazolecarbamate; MK-905).

'Cambimycin' *see* Hachimycin.

'Camdelate' *see* Calcium mandelate.

'Camesol 90' *see* Dimethyl sulfoxide.

CAMIVERINE*** (2-phenyl-N-(2-pyrrolidin-1-ylethyl)glycine isopentyl ester; isopentyl 2-phenyl-2-[(2-pyrrolidin-1-ylethyl)amino]acetate).

'Camoform' *see* Bialamicol.

'Camolar' *see* Cycloguanil embonate.

CAMP *see* Adenosine 3′,5′-phosphate.

Camphane *see* Bornane.

2-Camphanol *see* Borneol.

Camphechlor *see* Campheclor.

CAMPHECLOR* (mixture of chlorinated derivatives of bornene; camphechlor; chlorcamphene; chlorinated camphene; chlorphen; kamfochlor; polychlorcamphene; poliklorkamfen; 'alltox', 'chlorten', 'estonox', 'geniphene', 'phenacide', 'phenatox', 'phenphene', 'toxakil', 'toxaphene').

Camphetamide *see* Camphotamide.

Camphidonium *see* Trimethidinium.

Camphocarbonic acid *see* 2-Oxobornane-3-carboxylic acid.

Camphocarboxylic acid *see* 2-Oxobornane-3-carboxylic acid.

Camphol *see* Borneol.

CAMPHONANIC ACID (1,2,2-trimethyl-cyclopentanecarboxylic acid).

CAMPHOR (2-camphanone; 2-oxo-1,7,7-trimethylbicyclo(2.2.1)heptane; alcanfor; 2-oxobornane).

α-CAMPHORAMIC ACID (3-carbamyl-1,2,2-trimethylcyclopentanecarboxylic acid).

CAMPHORAMINE (ammonium 2-oxobornane-3carboxylate; ammonium camphocarbonate; ammonium camphocarboxylate; ammonium 3-camphorcarboxylate).

3-Camphorcarboxylic acid *see* 2-Oxobornane-3-carboxylic acid.

CAMPHORIC ACID (1,2,2-trimethyl-1,3-cyclopentanedicarboxylic acid).

CAMPHORSULFONIC ACID (2-oxobornane-10-sulfonic acid), esters and salts *see* Camsilate(s).

CAMPHOTAMIDE*** (camphosulfonyl-N-methylpyridine-β-diethylcarboxamide; 3-(diethylcarbamoyl)-1-methylpyridinium camphorsulfonate; N′-methylnikethamide camphorsulfonate; camphetamide; camphetamine).

Camphramine *see* Camphotamide.

CAMPTOTHECIN (2-ethyl-9,11-dihydro-8-(hydroxymethyl)-9-oxoindolizino(1,2-b)-quinoline-7-glycolic acid sodium salt; NSC-100880).

CAMSILATE(S)** (camphorsulfonate(s); camsylate(s)).

See also Amoxydramine camsilate; Emetine camsilate; Etamiphyllin camsilate; (Hydroxyanilino)ethanol camsilate; Leptacine camsilate; Trimetaphan camsilate.

Camsylate(s)* *see* Camsilate(s).

CAMYLOFIN*** (isopentyl ester of 2-(2-diethylaminoethylamino)-2-phenylacetic acid; isoamyl ester of 2-(2-diethylaminoethylamino)-2-phenylacetic acid; isopentyl ester of N-(2-diethylaminoethyl)-2-phenylglycine; acamylophenine; 'adopon', 'avacan', 'belosin', 'licosin', 'novospasmin', 'sintespasmil').

CAMYLOFIN WITH BISMUTH NITRATE ('sedomuth').

CAMYLOFIN WITH NOVAMINSULFON ('avafortan').

'Camyna' *see* Tioxolone.

Canadine *see* Tetrahydroberberine.

'Candamide' *see* Lithium carbonate.

'Candaseptic' *see* Chlorocresol.

'Candeptin' *see* Candicidin.

CANDICIDIN** (antibiotic from *Str. griseus*; 'candeptin').

'Candiolin' *see* Calcium fructose 1,6-diphosphate.

Canescine *see* Deserpidine.

'Canesten' *see* Clotrimazole.

Canforemetina *see* Emetine camsilate.

CANNABINOL*** (6,6,9-trimethyl-3-pentylbenzo(c)chromen-1-ol; 6,6,9-trimethyl-3-pentyl-6H-dibenzo(b,d)pyran-1-ol).

CANNABIS (*C. indica*; Indian hemp; marihuana).

Cannabiscetin *see* Myricetin.

Cannogenic acid L-thevetoside *see* Perusitin.

Cannogenin L-thevetoside *see* Peruvoside.

'Canocyl' *see* Magnesium acetylsalicylate.

'Canogard' *see* Dichlorvos.

'Canopar' *see* Thenium closilate.

CANRENOATE POTASSIUM*** (androsta-4,6-dien-17β-ol-3-on-17α-ylpropionic acid potassium salt; 3-(17β-hydroxy-3-oxoandrosta-4,6-dien-17-yl)propionic acid potassium salt; potassium canrenoate; potassium 17-hydroxy-3-oxo-17α-pregna-4,6-diene-21-carboxylate; aldadiene; CB-8109; SC-14266; 'soludactone').

CANRENOIC ACID*** (androsta-4,6-dien-17β-ol-3-on-17α-ylpropionic acid; 3-(17β-hydroxy-3-oxoandrosta-4,6-dien-17-yl)-propionic acid; 17β-hydroxy-3-oxo-17α-pregna-4,6-diene-21-carboxylic acid; 17α-(2-carboxyethyl)-17β-hydroxyandrosta-4,6-

dien-3-one).

Canrenoic acid lactone *see* Canrenone.

Canrenoic acid potassium salt *see* Canrenoate potassium.

CANRENONE** (canrenoic acid γ-lactone; RP-11614; SC-9376).

'Cantabilin' *see* Hymecromone.

CANTHARIDIN (hexahydro-3α,7α-dimethyl-4,7-epoxyisobenzofuran-1,3-dione; exo-1,2-*cis*-dimethyl-3,6-epoxyhexahydrophthalic anhydride; cantharides camphor).

'Cantil' *see* Mepenzolate.

'Cantrex' *see* Kanamycin.

'Cantrol' *see* 4-(4-Chloro-2-methylphenoxy)-butyric acid.

'Caparol' *see* Prometryn.

'Capastat' *see* Capreomycin.

'Capazine' *see* Prochlorperazine.

'Capellin' *see* Phenazone salicylate.

'Capla' *see* Mebutamate.

CAPOBENIC ACID*** (6-(3,4,5-trimethoxybenzamido)hexanoic acid; 6-(3,4,5-trimethoxybenzamido)caproic acid; trimethoxybenzoyl-6-aminocaproic acid; C-3; 'C-tre').
See also Sodium capobenate.

'Capramol' *see* Aminocaproic acid.

CAPREOMYCIN*** (antibiotic from *Str. capreolus*; L-29275; 'capastat', 'caprocin', 'ogostal').

Capric acid *see* Decanoic acid.

Caprine *see* Norleucine.

'Caproamin' *see* Aminocaproic acid.

CAPROCHLORONE (L-4-(o-chlorobenzyl)-5-oxo-4-phenylhexanoic acid; 4-(o-chlorobenzyl)-5-oxo-4-phenylcaproic acid; caproclorone).

'Caprocid' *see* Aminocaproic acid.

'Caprocin' *see* Capreomycin.

Caproclorone *see* Caprochlorone.

'Caprodat' *see* Carisoprodol.

Caproic acid *see* Hexanoic acid.

'Caprokol' *see* Hexylresorcinol.

CAPROLACTAM (hexahydro-2H-azepin-2-one; 2-oxohexamethylenimine; aminocaproic lactam; ε-caprolactam).

Caprolactam polymer *see* Policapram.

'Caprolest' *see* Aminocaproic acid.

Caprophenone *see* Hexanophenone.

'Caprosem' *see* Cloxotestosterone acetate.

CAPROXAMINE*** (E)-3'-amino-4'-methylhexanophenone O-(2-aminoethyl)oxime; 3'-methyl-4'-methylcaprophenone O-(2-aminoethyl)oxime; 3-amino-4-methylphenyl pentyl ketone (2-aminoethyl)oxime; 3-amino-p-tolyl pentyl ketone (2-aminoethyl)oxime; caproxamine sulfate; DU-22550).

Caprylic acid *see* Octanoic acid.

Caprylic alcohol *see* 1-Octanol.

CAPRYLIC COMPOUND* (sodium and zinc octanoates).

CAPSAICIN (decenoic acid vanillylamide; vanillylamide of 9-methylnon-6-enoic acid).

'Capsebon' *see* Cadmium sulfide.

CAPTAFOL* (3a,4,7,7a-tetrahydro-2-[(1,1,2,2-tetrachloroethyl)thio]-1H-isoindole-1,3(2H)-dione; N-[(1,1,2,2-tetrahydroethyl)thio]-4-cyclohexenedicarboximide; N-(tetrachloroethylthio)-△⁴-tetrahydrophthalimide; 'difolatan', 'folcid').

CAPTAFOL PLUS PYRIDINITRIL ('ciluan').

'Captagon' *see* Fenetylline.

CAPTAMINE** (2-dimethylaminoethanethiol; N-(2-mercaptoethyl)dimethylamine; N,N-dimethylmercaptamine; captamine hydrochloride).

CAPTAN* (3a,4,7,7a-tetrahydro-2-[(trichloromethyl)thio]-1H-isoindole-1,3(2H)-dione; cis-N-(trichloromethylthio)-4-cyclohexene-1,2-dicarboximide; N-(trichloromethylthio)-△⁴-tetrahydrophthalimide; SR-406; 'orthocide-406', 'vancide-89').

'Captax' *see* 2-Mercaptobenzothiazole.

CAPTODIAME** (2-(p-butylmercaptobenzhydrylmercapto)-N,N-dimethylethylamine; p-butylthiodiphenylmethyl-2-dimethylaminoethyl sulfide; 2-[p-(butylthio)-α-phenylbenzylthio]-N,N-dimethylethylamine; captodramine hydrochloride; captodramine; 'covatin', 'covatix', 'N 68', 'suvren').

Captodramine* *see* Captodiame.

CAPURIDE*** (N-(2-ethyl-3-methylvaleryl)-urea; McN-X-94; 'pacinox').

CAQ *see* Cloxiquine acetate.

2,2'-c-ara C *see* Ancitabine.

'Caradrin' *see* Proscillaridin.

'Caragard' *see* Terbumeton.

CARAMIPHEN*** (2-diethylaminoethyl ester of 1-phenylcyclopentanecarboxylic acid; caramiphen hydrochloride; merpanit; pentaphene; G-2747; 'panparnit', 'parpanit', 'pentafin').

CARAMIPHEN EDISILATE (caramiphen ethandisulfonate; caramiphen edisylate; 'taoryl', 'toryn').

CARBACHOL** (choline chloride carbamate; carbaminoylcholine; carbamylcholine; carbocholine; 'atonyl', 'carbamed', 'carbolin', 'carcholin', 'cholinergol', 'choryl', 'doryl', 'enterotonin', 'glaumarin', 'iricoline', 'jestryl', 'lentin', 'miostat', 'moryl').

'Carbadal' *see* Carbromal.

Carbadipimidine *see* Carpipramine.

CARBADOX** (methyl 3-(2-quinoxalinylmethylene)carbazate N¹,N⁴-dioxide; GS-6244; 'mecadox').

'Carbaica' *see* 5-Amino-4-imidazolecarboxamide N-carbamoylaspartate.

'Carbamat' *see* Isoprocarb.

CARBAMAZEPINE*** (5H-dibenz(b,f)-azepine-5-carboxamide; G-32883; 'amizepin', 'tegretol').

'Carbamed' *see* Carbachol.

CARBAMIC ACID (aminoformic acid).

Carbamic acid hydrazide *see* Semicarbazide.

Carbamide *see* Urea.

Carbamidine *see* Guanidine.

Carbamimidic acid *see* Pseudourea.
N-**CARBAMOYLASPARTIC ACID**
(ureidosuccinic acid).
See also Calcium carbamoylaspartate.
m-**Carbamoylbenzoic acid** *see* Isophthalamic
acid.
o-**Carbamoylbenzoic acid** *see* Phthalamic
acid.
p-**Carbamoylbenzoic acid** *see* Tere-
phthalamic acid.
4-Carbamoylbutyric acid *see* Glutaramic
acid.
Carbamoylcarbamic acid *see* Allophanic
acid.
Carbamoylcefaloridine *see* Cefalonium.
Carbamoylcholine *see* Carbachol.
CARBAMOYLCYSTEINE (*S*-carbamoyl-L-
cysteine; carbamylcysteine; NSC-102498;
SCC).
Carbamoyldapsone *see* Amidapsone.
**3-Carbamoyl-4-deacetyl-3-de(methoxy-
carbonyl)vincaleukoblastine** *see*
Vindesine.
(**Carbamoyldiphenylpropyl)diisopropyl-
methylammonium iodide** *see* Isopropamide.
(**Carbamoyldiphenylpropyl)ethyl-
dimethylammonium bromide** *see*
Ambutonium.
**1-(3-Carbamoyl-3,3-diphenylpropyl)-
hexahydro-1-methylazepinium iodide**
see Buzepide metiodide.
**1-(3-Carbamoyl-3,3-diphenylpropyl)-
1-methylpiperidinium bromide** *see*
Fenpiverinium bromide.
**4'-Carbamoyl-1-[3-(*p*-fluorobenzoyl)-
propyl]-1,4'-bipiperidine** *see*
Pipamperone.
N-**Carbamoylmaleamic acid** *see* Maleuric
acid.
N-**Carbamoylmalonamic acid** *see*
Malonuric acid.
**3(4H)-Carbamoylmethyl-2H-1,3-
benzoxazin-2-one** *see* Caroxazone.
Carbamoyl-β-methylcholine *see*
Bethanechol.
**1-(*p*-Carbamoylmethylphenoxy)-3-
isopropylamino-2-propanol** *see* Atenolol.
**3-Carbamoyl-1-methylpyridinium
hydroxide** *see* *N*[1]-Methylnicotinamide.
1-Carbamoylmethyl-2-pyrrolidinone *see*
Piracetam.
**4-Carbamoyloxy-1-[3-(*p*-fluorobenzoyl)-
propyl]octahydroquinoline** *see*
Cicarperone.
**4-Carbamoyloxy-1-[4-(*p*-fluorophenyl)-4-
oxobutyl]decahydroquinoline** *see*
Cicarperone.
**3-(Carbamoyloxymethyl)-7-[2-(2-furyl)-2-
(methoxyimino)acetamido]-2-cephem-
2-carboxylic acid** *see* Cefuroxime.
(**2-Carbamoyloxypropyl)trimethyl-
ammonium chloride** *see* Bethanechol.
**2-Carbamoylphenoxyacetic acid tetra-
hydrofuryl ester** *see* Fenamifuril.
**1-[2-(4-Carbamoylphenoxy)ethylamino]-
3-(2-methylphenoxy)-2-propanol** *see*

Tolamolol.
**4-(4-Carbamoyl-4-piperid-1-ylpiperid-1-
yl)-2,2-diphenylbutyronitrile** *see*
Piritramide.
**4-(4-Carbamoyl-4-piperid-1-ylpiperid-1-
yl)-4'-fluorobutyrophenone** *see*
Pipamperone.
**5-[3-[(4-Carbamoyl-4-piperid-1-yl)-
piperid-1-yl]propyl]-10,11-dihydro-5H-
dibenz(b,f)azepine** *see* Carpipramine.
**10[3-(4-Carbamoylpiperid-1-yl)propyl]-
2-chlorophenothiazine** *see* Metopimazine.
**3-(4-Carbamoylpyrid-1-ylmethyl)-7-thien-
2-ylacetamido-8-oxo-5-thia-1-azabi-
cyclo(4.2.0)oct-2-ene-2-carboxylic acid**
see Cefalonium.
**3-Carbamoyl-1-β-D-ribofuranosylpyridi-
nium hydroxide 5'-ester with adenosine 5'-pyrophosphate inner salt** *see*
Nadide.
O-**Carbamoylsalicylic acid lactam** *see*
Carsalam.
'**Carbamult**' *see* Promecarb.
Carbamylcysteine *see* Carbamoylcysteine.
Carbamylurea *see* Biuret.
CARBANILAMIDE (phenylcarbamide;
phenylurea; ureidobenzene).
CARBANILIC ACID (phenylcarbamic acid).
**Carbanilic acid 1-(ethylcarbamoyl)ethyl
ester** *see* Carbetamide.
Carbanilic acid isopropyl ester *see*
Propham.
CARBANILIDE (1,3-diphenylurea).
CARBANOLATE* (2-chloro-4,5-dimethyl-
phenyl methylcarbamate; 6-chloro-3,4-
xylyl methylcarbamate; chlorxylam;
'banol').
CARBANTEL** (1-*p*-chlorophenyl)-3-valer-
imidoylurea).
CARBARIL** (1-naphthyl methylcarbamate; carbaryl; 'asevin', 'karbosep',
'sevin').
CARBARSONE** (*N*-carbamylarsanilic acid;
p-ureidobenzenearsonic acid; aminarsone).
Carbaryl* *see* Carbaril.
CARBASALATE CALCIUM*** (salicylic
acid acetate calcium salt compound (1:1)
with urea; calcium acetylsalicylate-urea;
calcium carbaspirin; carbaspirin calcium;
calcium acetylsalicylate carbamide;
'calurin', 'iromin').
Carbaspirin calcium* *see* Carbasalate
calcium.
'**Carbathion**' *see* Metam-sodium.
CARBAZIC ACID (hydrazinecarboxylic
acid).
See also Carbenzide.
Carbazilquinone *see* Carboquone.
CARBAZOCHROME*** (adrenochrome
semicarbazone; 3-hydroxy-1-methyl-5,6-
indolinedione semicarbazone; 'adrenosem',
'adrenoxyl').
CARBAZOCHROME SALICYLATE***
(mixture of carbazochrome with sodium
salicylate; 'adrenosem', 'adrestat').
**CARBAZOCHROME SODIUM SULFON-
ATE***** (5,6-dihydro-1-methyl-5,6-dioxo-3-

indolinesulfonic acid 5-semicarbazone sodium salt; AC-17; 'ADONA').

CARBAZOCHROME SODIUM SULFONATE WITH CHLORPHENIRAMINE MALEATE ('emex antistaminico').

CARBAZOCHROME WITH TROXERUTIN ('fleboside').

CARBAZOCINE*** (14-cyclopropylmethyl-1,2,3,4,4a,5,6,11-octahydro(5,11b)iminoethano(11bH)benzo(a)carbazole).

CARBAZOLE (dibenzopyrrole; diphenylenimine).

Carbazotic acid see Picric acid.

Carbazylquinone see Carboquone.

CARBENICILLIN*** (α-carboxybenzylpenicillin; N-(2-carboxy-3,3-dimethyl-7-oxo-4-thia-1-azabicyclo(3.2.0)hept-6-yl)-2-phenylmalonamic acid; 6-(phenylmalonamido)penicillanic acid; 6-(2-carboxy-2-phenylacetamido)penicillanic acid; carbenicillin disodium; sodium carbenicillin; Bay b-5369; BRL-2064; CP-15639-2; 'anabactyl', 'fugacillin', 'microcillin', 'pyopen').

Carbenicillin indanyl* see Carindacillin.

CARBENOXOLONE*** (3β-(3-carboxypropionyloxy)-11-oxoolean-12-en-30-oic acid; 3-O-(3-carboxypropionate) ester of 3β-hydroxy-11-oxo-18β-olean-12-en-30-oic acid; 3β-hydroxy-11-oxo-18β-olean-12-en-30-oic acid hydrogen succinate; (3β,20β)-3-(3-carboxy-1-oxopropoxy)-11-oxoolean-12-en-29-oic acid; enoxolone hydrogen succinate).

Carbenoxolone disodium salt see Carbenoxolone sodium.

CARBENOXOLONE SODIUM* (carbenoxolone disodium salt; 'biobase', 'biogastrone', 'bioral', 'duogastrone', 'neogel', 'terulcon').
See also Enoxolone.

CARBENZIDE*** (ethyl 2-(α-methylbenzyl)-1-hydrazinecarboxylate; ethyl 3-(α-methylbenzyl)carbazate; ethyl benzhydrylcarbazate).

CARBESILATE(S)** (p-carboxybenzenesulfonate(s)).

CARBESTROL (3-ethyl-4-(p-methoxyphenyl)-2-methyl-3-cyclohexene-1-carboxylic acid; NSC-19962)

CARBETAMIDE* 2-[(anilinocarbonyl)oxy]-N-ethylpropionamide; N-ethyl-2-[[(phenylamino)carbonyl]oxy]propanamide; 1-(ethylcarbamoylethyl) carbanilate; carbethamide; 'legurame').

Carbetapentane see Pentoxyverine.

Carbethamide see Carbetamide.

2-(α-Carbethoxybenzyl)thiazolidine-4-carboxylic acid see Leucogen.

4-Carbethoxy-1,3-dimethyl-4-phenylhexamethylenimine see Metethoheptazine.

7-(Carbethoxymethoxy)-3-(2-diethylaminoethyl)-4-methylcoumarin see Carbocromen.

7-Carbethoxymethoxyflavone see Efloxate.

2-Carbethoxymethylene-3-methyl-5-piperid-1-yl-4-thiazolidinone see Etozolin.

1-Carbethoxy-3-methyl-2-thioimidazole see Carbimazole.

1-Carbethoxy-2-phthalazinohydrazine see Todralazine.

Carbethoxysyringoyl methyl reserpate see Syrosingopine.

3-Carbethoxy-6,7,8,9-tetrahydro-1,6-dimethyl-4-oxohomopyrimidazole methyl sulfate see Rimazolium metilsulfate.

4-Carbethoxy-α,α,4-triphenyl-1-piperidinebutyronitrile see Diphenoxylate.

CARBETHYL SALICYLATE* (ethyl salicylate carbonate; 'sal-ethyl carbonate').

Carbetidine see Etoxeridine.

'Carbicron' see Dicrotophos.

Carbidine (tr) see Dicarbine.

CARBIDOPA*** ((−)-L-α-hydrazino-3,4-dihydroxy-α-methylhydrocinnamic acid; (−)-L-α-hydrazino-3,4-dihydroxy-α-methylhydrocinnamic acid monohydrate; (S)-α-hydrazino-3,4-dihydroxy-α-methylbenzenepropanoic acid monohydrate; 2-hydrazino-3-(3,4-dihydroxyphenyl)-2-methylpropionic acid; 2-(3,4-dihydroxybenzyl-2-hydrazinopropionic acid; α-hydrazino-α-methyldopa; hydrazinomethyldopa; α-methyldopa hydrazine; MK-486).
See also Levodopa with carbidopa.

CARBIFENE*** (2-ethoxy-N-methyl-N-[2-(methylphenethylamino)ethyl]-2,2-diphenylacetamide; etomide; etymide; carbiphene hydrochloride; SQ-10269; 'bandol', 'jubalon').

CARBIMAZOLE*** (ethyl 3-methyl-2-thioimidazoline-1-carboxylate; 1-carbethoxy-3-methyl-2-thioimidazole; 1-methyl-2-imidazolethiol ethyl carbonate; ethyl methimazolate; 'athyromazole', 'basolest', 'neomercazole', 'neo-thyreostat').

Carbimide calcium see Calcium carbimide.

Carbinamine see Methylamine.

Carbinol see Methanol.

CARBINOXAMINE*** (2-[(p-chlorophenyl)-(2-pyridyl)methoxy]-N,N-dimethylethylamine; 2-dimethylaminoethoxy-2-pyridyl-4-chlorophenylmethane; 2-[(p-chlorophenyl)-2-(dimethylaminoethoxy)methyl]pyridine; 2-[p-chloro-α-(2-dimethylaminoethoxy)benzyl]pyridine; p-chloro-α-pyrid-2-ylbenzyl 2-dimethylaminoethyl ether; paracarbinoxamine).

CARBINOXAMINE MALEATE ('clistin', 'polistine').
See also Rotoxamine.

Carbiphene* see Carbifene.

'Carbitol' see 2-(2-Ethoxyethoxy)ethanol.

8β-Carbobenzyloxyaminomethyl-1-methyl-10α-ergoline see Metergoline.

N-Carbobenzyloxy-9,10-dihydro-1-methyllysergamine see Metergoline.

'Carbocaine' see Mepivacaine.

Carbocholine see Carbachol.

CARBOCISTEINE** (3-[(carboxymethyl)thio]alanine; S-carboxymethylcysteine; 'mucodyne', 'transbronchin').

77

CARBOCISTEINE WITH THEOPHYL-LINE (MJ-12; 'thio-theo').

CARBOCLORAL*** (ethyl (2,2,2-trichloro-1-hydroxyethyl)carbamate; ethyl trichloramate; chloral urethan; CI-336; HY-185; 'somnal', 'ural', 'uraline', 'uralium').

CARBOCROMEN*** (ethyl 3-(2-diethylaminoethyl)-4-methyl-2-oxo(2H)-1-benzopyran-7-yloxyacetate; 7-(carbethoxymethoxy)-3-(2-diethylaminoethyl)-4-methylcoumarin; 3-(2-diethylaminoethyl)-7-(ethoxycarbonylmethoxy)-4-methylcoumarin; chromonar hydrochloride; A-27053; AG-3; Cassella-4489; 'cardiocap', 'intenkordin', 'intensain', 'intercordin').

Carbodimide calcium see Calcium carbimide.

CARBOFENOTION*** (S-[(p-chlorophenylthio)methyl] O,O-diethyl phosphorodithioate; carbophenothion; carbothion; nephocarp; 'garrathion', 'lirotrithion', 'trithion').

CARBOFENOTION METHYL (S-[(p-chlorophenylthio)methyl] O,O-dimethyl phosphorodithioate; carbophenthion methyl; 'methyltrithion').

CARBOFURAN* (2,3-dihydro-2,2-dimethylbenzofuran-7-yl methylcarbamate; NIA-10242; 'furadan').

N⁴-(**Carbo-2-hydroxyethoxy)sulfanilamide** see Sulocarbilate.

Carbolane see Phosfolan.

Carbolic acid see Phenol.

'**Carbolin**' see Carbachol.

β-**Carboline** see 9H-Pyrido(3,4-b)indole.

γ-**Carboline** see 5H-Pyrido(4,3-b)indole.

'**Carbolith**' see Lithium carbonate.

Carbolonium* see Hexcarbacholine.

CARBOMER*** (polymer of acrylic acid cross-linked with allyl sucrose; 'carbopol').

Carbomethene see Ketene.

2-Carbomethoxy-3-benzyloxytropane see Cocaine; Pseudococaine.

6-Carbomethoxy-N-(2-diethylaminoacetyl)-o-toluidine see Tolycaine.

18-Carbomethoxy-12,13-dimethoxyibogamine see Conopharyngine.

4-Carbomethoxy-1,2-dimethyl-4-phenylhexamethylenimine see Metheptazine.

2-Carbomethoxy-4-methyl-3-(α-propylaminopropionylamino)thiophene see Carticaine.

(**Carbomethoxy-1-methylvinyl) dimethyl phosphate** see Mevinphos.

(**1-Carbomethoxy-1-propen-2-yl) dimethyl phosphate** see Mevinphos.

(**3-Carbomethoxypropyl)trimethylammonium chloride** see Carpronium chloride.

CARBOMYCIN** (antibiotic from *Str. halstedii*; 'magnamycin').

'**Carbona**' see Carbon tetrachloride.

Carbon dichloride see Tetrachloroethylene.

Carbon hexachloride see Hexachloroethane.

CARBON TETRACHLORIDE (chlorocarbon; tetrachloromethane; 'carbona', 'benzinoform', 'necatorina', 'phenixin', 'phenoxin', 'phoenixin', 'pyrene', 'seretin', 'thawpit').

Carbonylbis(1-methylquinolinium methosulfate) see Quinuronium.

Carbonyl chloride see Phosgene.

Carbonyldiamide see Urea.

Carbophenothion* see Carbofenotion.

Carbophos (tr) see Malathion.

'**Carbopol**' see Carbomer.

2-(4-Carbopropoxymethyl-2-methoxyphenoxy)-N,N-diethylacetamide see Propanidid.

CARBOQUONE*** (2,5-bis(1-aziridinyl)-3-(2-hydroxy-1-methoxyethyl)-6-methyl-p-benzoquinone carbamate ester; carbazilquinone; carbazylquinone; CS-310; NSC-134679).

'**Carbostesin**' see Bupivacaine.

Carbostibamide see Urea stibamine.

CARBOSTYRIL (2-quinolinol).

'**Carbothiazol**' see Maleylsulfathiazole.

Carbothion see Carbofenotion.

Carbothrone see Anthrone.

'**Carbowaxes**' see Macrogols.

3-Carboxamido-2-chlorobenzenesulfonamide see Sulclamide.

3-Carboxamido-4-hydroxy-α-[(1-methyl-3-phenylpropylamino)methyl]benzyl alcohol see Labetalol.

1-(4-Carboxamidoimidazol-5-yl)-3,3-dimethyltriazene see Dacarbazine.

4-(4-Carboxamido-4-piperid-1-ylpiperid-1-yl)-4'-fluorobutyrophenone see Pipamperone.

10-[3-(4-Carboxamidopiperid-4-yl)propyl]-2-methylsulfonylphenothiazine see Metopimazine.

5-Carboxanilido-2,3-dihydro-6-methyl-1,4-oxathiin see Carboxin.

CARBOXIN* (5-carboxanilido-2,3-dihydro-6-methyl-1,4-oxathiin; 5,6-dihydro-2-methyl-N-phenyl-1,4-oxathiin-3-carboxamide; D-735; DCMO; 'vitavax').

CARBOXIN DIOXIDE (5-carboxanilido-2,3-dihydro-6-methyl-1,4-oxathiin 4,4-dioxide; oxycarboxin; DCMOD; F-461; 'plantavax').

Carboxin monoxide see Carboxin oxide.

CARBOXIN OXIDE (5-carboxanilido-2,3-dihydro-6-methyl-1,4-oxathiin 4-oxide; carboxin monoxide; F-831).

1-(2-Carboxybenzamido)naphthalene see Naptalam.

p-**Carboxybenzenesulfondiethylamide** see Etebenecid.

p-**Carboxybenzenesulfonic acid, esters and salts** see Carbesilate(s).

1-(α-Carboxybenzyl)-1-methylpiperidinium iodide ester with diethyl(hydroxyethoxyethyl)methylammonium iodide see Piprocurarium.

α-**Carboxybenzylpenicillin disodium salt** see Carbenicillin.

6-(4-Carboxybutylthio)purine see Buthiopurine.

1-[3-(2-Carboxybutyl)-2,4,6-triiodophenyl]pyrrolidin-2-one see Iolidonic acid.

(**3-Carboxy-7-chloro-2,3-dihydro-2-hydr-**

oxy-5-phenyl-1H-1,4-benzodiazepin-2-yloxy)potassium *see* Dipotassium clorazepate.

1-[(3-Carboxy-4-chlorophenyl)sulfonyl]-3,5-dimethylpiperidine *see* Tibric acid.

3β-(*cis*-2-Carboxycyclohexylcarbonyloxy)-11-oxoolean-12-en-30-oic acid *see* Cicloxolone.

2-Carboxy-2′,6′-dichloro-3′-methyldiphenylamine *see* Meclofenamic acid.

N-Carboxydihydro-1-methyl-9,10-lysergamine benzyl ester *see* Metergoline.

9-(3-Carboxy-2,3-dihydroxypropyl)-adenine *see* Eritadenine.

2-Carboxy-3,4-dimethoxybenzaldehyde isonicotinoylhydrazone *see* Opiniazide.

N-(2-Carboxy-3,3-dimethyl-7-oxo-4-thia-1-azabicyclo(3.2.0)hept-6-yl)-2-phenylmalonamic acid *see* Carbenicillin.

N-(2-Carboxy-3,3-dimethyl-7-oxo-4-thia-1-azabicyclo(3.2.0)hept-6-yl)-2-phenylmalonamic acid 1-indan-5-yl ester *see* Carindacillin.

N-(2-Carboxy-3,3-dimethyl-7-oxo-4-thia-1-azabicyclo(3.2.0)hept-6-yl)-2-phenylmalonamic acid 1-phenyl ester *see* Carfecillin.

N-(2-Carboxy-3,3-dimethyl-7-oxo-4-thia-1-azabicyclo(3.2.0)hept-6-yl)-3-thiophenemalonamic acid *see* Ticarcillin.

2-Carboxy-1,1-dimethylpyrrolidinium iodide ester with choline iodide *see* Trepirium iodide.

3-[2-(1-Carboxyethoxy)ethoxy]-N-ethyl-2,4,6,-triiodoacetanilide *see* Iolixanic acid.

3-(1-Carboxyethyl)benzophenone *see* Ketoprofen.

2-[*p*-(1-Carboxyethyl)benzoyl]thiophene *see* Suprofen.

2-[(2-Carboxyethyl)carbonyl]dibenzofuran *see* Furobufen.

2-[4-(1-Carboxyethyl)-2-chlorobenzoyl]-thiophene *see* Cliprofen.

5-(1-Carboxyethyl)-2-(*p*-chlorophenyl)-benzoxazole *see* Benoxaprofen.

1-[4-(1-Carboxyethyl)-2-chlorophenyl]-3-pyrroline *see* Pirprofen.

4-(1-Carboxyethyl)-2-chlorophenyl 2-thienyl ketone *see* Cliprofen.

2-Carboxyethyl dibenzofuran-2-yl ketone *see* Furobufen.

17α-(2-Carboxyethyl)-17β-hydroxyandrosta-4,6-dien-3-one *see* Canrenoic acid.

17α-(2-Carboxyethyl)-17β-hydroxyandrosta-4,6-dien-3-one lactone *see* Canrenone.

2-(1-Carboxyethyl)-7-methoxy-10-methylphenothiazine *see* Protizinic acid.

1-[*p*-(1-Carboxyethyl)phenyl]cyclohexene *see* Tetriprofen.

2-[*p*-(1-Carboxyethyl)phenyl]isoindolin-1-one *see* Indoprofen.

2-[*p*-(1-Carboxyethyl)phenyl]phthalimidine *see* Indoprofen.

2-[[(5-Carboxy-5-formamidopentyl)-carbamoyl](2-phenylacetamido)-

methyl]-5,5-dimethyl-4-thiazolidine-carboxylic acid *see* Libecillide.

β-Carboxyglutaric acid *see* Tricarballylic acid.

3-(3-Carboxy-4-hydroxyphenyl)-4,5-dihydro-2-phenyl-3H-benz(e)indole *see* Fendosal.

N-(1-Carboxy-2-indol-3-ylethyl)-*p*-chlorobenzamide *see* Benzotript.

2-Carboxy-4-isopropenyl-3-pyrrolidineacetic acid *see* Kainic acid.

o-Carboxymethoxybenzaldehyde isonicotinoylhydrazone *see* Aconiazide.

Carboxymethylcellulose *see* Sodium carboxymethylcellulose.

3-(Carboxymethyl)-4-chlorobenzothiazol-3(2H)-one *see* Benazolin.

Carboxymethylcysteine *see* Carbocisteine.

(Carboxymethyl)dimethyl(2-hydroxyethyl)ammonium hydroxide inner salt *see* Oxibetaine.

(Carboxymethyl)dimethyl(3-palmitamidopropyl)ammonium hydroxide inner salt *see* Pendecamaine.

(Carboxymethyl)(2-hydroxyethyl)-dimethylammonium hydroxide inner salt *see* Oxibetaine.

Carboxymethyliminobis(ethylenenitrilodiacetic acid) *see* Pentetic acid.

2-Carboxymethyl-10-methylphenothiazine *see* Metiazinic acid.

6-(5-Carboxy-3-methylpent-2-enyl)-7-hydroxy-5-methoxy-4-methylphthalide *see* Mycophenolic acid.

S-(1-Carboxymethylpropyl)cysteine *see* Isovalthine.

1-Carboxymethyltheobromine *see* Theobromin-1-ylacetic acid.

7-Carboxymethyltheophylline sodium salt *see* Sodium 1-theophyllin-7-ylacetate.

3-[(Carboxymethyl)thio]alanine *see* Carbocisteine.

N-Carboxy-3-morpholinosydnone imine ethyl ester *see* Molsidomine.

(3β,20β)-3-(3-Carboxy-1-oxopropoxy)-11-oxoolean-12-en-29-oic acid *see* Carbenoxolone.

1-[[2-Carboxy-8-oxo-7-[(2-thien-2-yl)-acetamido]-5-thia-1-azabicyclo(4.2.0)-oct-2-en-3-yl]methyl]pyridinium hydroxide inner salt *see* Cefaloridine.

N-(*p*-Carboxyphenethyl)-5-chloro-2-methylbenzamide *see* Meglitinide.

o-Carboxyphenoxyacetic acid hydroxymercuripropanolamide *see* Mercuderamide.

1-(2-Carboxyphenoxy)-3-hexyloxy-2-propanol *see* Exiproben.

6-(2-Carboxyphenylacetamido)penicillanic acid *see* Carbenicillin.

4-Carboxy-α-phenyl-2-thiazolidineacetic acid ethyl ester *see* Leucogen.

3-(2-Carboxypropenyl)-2,2-dimethyl-cyclopropanecarboxylic acid *see* Chrysanthemumdicarboxylic acid.

(3-Carboxypropyl)trimethylammonium chloride methyl ester *see* Carpronium chloride.

N-(**3-Carboxypyridin-2-yl**)-α,α,α-**trifluoro-***m*-**toluidine** *see* Niflumic acid.

N-(**3-Carboxypyridin-4-yl**)-α,α,α-**trifluoro-***m*-**toluidine** *see* Triflocin.

6-(3-Carboxy-2-quinoxalinecarbox-amido)penicillanic acid *see* Quinacillin.

3-Carboxyquinoxalin-2-yl-penicillin *see* Quinacillin.

2-(4-Carboxystyryl)-5-nitro-1-vinyl-imidazole *see* Stirimazole.

Carboxysulfamidochrysoidine *see* Sulfachrysoidine.

3-Carboxy-6,7,8,9-tetrahydro-1,6-dimethyl-4-oxo-4H-pyrido(1,2-a)-pyrimidinium methyl sulfate ethyl ester *see* Rimazolium metilsulfate.

4-(4-Carboxytetrahydro-2H-1,3-thiazin-2-yl)-2-hydroxy-5-hydroxymethyl-2-methylpyridine *see* Tiapirinol.

N[1]-(**Carboxythiazolyl**)**sulfanilamide** *see* Sulfacarizole.

6-(α-Carboxy-α-thien-3-ylacetamido)-penicillanic acid *see* Ticarcillin.

N-(**3-Carboxythien-4-yl**)-**2-chloro-***m*-**toluidine acetoxymethyl ester** *see* Aclantate.

3-[Carboxy(trifluoromethylsulfonyl)-amino]benzophenone ethyl ester *see* Triflumidate.

3-Carboxy-α,2,2-trimethylcyclopropane-acrylic acid *see* Chrysanthemumdicarb-oxylic acid.

2-Carboxy-1,1,6-trimethylpiperidinium iodide choline ester iodide *see* Dimecolonium iodide.

2-Carboxy-1,1,6-trimethylpiperidinium iodide ester with diethyl(2-hydroxy-ethyl)methyl)ammonium iodide *see* Dicolinium iodide.

N-**Carboxy**-L-**tryptophyl**-L-**methionyl**-L-α-**aspartyl-3-phenyl**-L-**alaninamide** *N-tert-***pentyl ester** *see* Amogastrin.

Carboxyveratrylideneisoniazid *see* Opiniazide.

Carboxyverazid *see* Opiniazide.

CARBROMAL* (1-(2-bromo-2-ethyl-butyryl)urea; acetylbromodiethylurea; bromdiethylacetylurea; bromodiethyl-acetylurea; bromadal; uradal).

CABROMAL WITH APC (carbromal with acetylsalicylic acid, phenacetin and caffeine; 'contradol').

CARBROMAL WITH BROMISOVAL ('sekundal').

CARBROMAL WITH DIPHENHYDR-AMINE ('betadorm').

CARBROMAL WITH PARACETAMOL ('paidipyrin').

CARBROMIDE (2-bromo-2,2-diethylacet-amide; diethylbromoacetamide; 2-bromo-2-ethylbutyramide).

CARBUBARB* (5-butyl-5-(2-carbamoyl-oxyethyl)barbituric acid carbamate ester).

CARBUTAMIDE* (*N*[1]-(butylcarbamoyl)-sulfanilamide; 1-butyl-3-sulfanilylurea; aminophenurobutane; 'alentin', 'anti-sukrin', 'bucrol', 'butisulfina', 'BZ 55', 'diabesulf', 'diabetal', 'emedan', 'glucidoral', 'invenol', 'midosal', 'nadisan', 'norboral', 'orabetic', 'oranil', 'orasulin', 'talanton', 'U 6987').

CARBUTAMIDE WITH PHENFORMIN ('glucifrene').

CARBUTEROL* (1-[5-(2-*tert*-butyl-amino-1-hydroxyethyl)-2-hydroxyphenyl]-urea; 5-(2-*tert*-butylamino-1-hydroxy-ethyl)-*N*-carbamoyl-2-hydroxyaniline; α-(*tert*-butylaminomethyl)-4-hydroxy-3-ureidobenzyl alcohol; carbuterol hydro-chloride; SK&F-40383).

'Carbyne' *see* Barban.

'Carcholin' *see* Carbachol.

'Cardan' *see* Oxyphencyclimine.

'Cardelmycin' *see* Novobiocin.

'Cardigin' *see* Digitoxin.

'Cardilan' *see* Nicofuranose *and* Magnesium aspartate with potassium aspartate.

'Cardilate' *see* Erythrityl tetranitrate.

'Cardimone' *see* Adenosine phosphate.

'Cardine' *see* Visnadine.

'Cardiocap' *see* Carbocromen.

'Cardiodynamin' *see* Oxedrine.

'Cardiografin' *see* Meglumine diatrizoate.

'Cardio-green' *see* Indocyanine green.

'Cardiolanata' *see* Lanatoside(s).

'Cardiolipol' *see* Niceritrol.

'Cardiomone' *see* Adenosine phosphate.

'Cardiophylin' *see* Aminophylline.

'Cardioquin' *see* Quinidine polygalacturon-ate.

'Cardiorhythmine' *see* Ajmaline.

'Cardiorytmin' *see* Procainamide.

'Cardioverina' *see* Papaverine.

'Cardivix' *see* Benziodarone.

'Cardiwell' *see* Erythrityl tetranitrate.

'Cardrase' *see* Ethoxolamide.

'Cardrax' *see* Ethoxolamide.

'Carduben' *see* Visnadine.

CARFECILLIN* (6-(4-phenoxycarbonyl-phenylacetamido)penicillanic acid; *N*-(2-carboxy-3,3-dimethyl-7-oxo-4-thia-1-azabicyclo(3.2.0)hept-6-yl)-2-phenyl-malonamic acid 1-phenyl ester; carfecillin sodium; carfenicillin; BRL-3475; 'uticillin').

CARFENAZINE* (1-[10-[3-(4-(2-hydroxy-ethyl)-1-piperazinyl)propyl]phenothiazin-2-yl]-1-propanone; 10-[3-[4-(2-hydroxy-ethyl)piperazin-1-yl]propyl]-2-propionyl-phenothiazine; carphenazine).

CARFENAZINE MALEATE* (Wy-2445; 'proketazine').

Carfenicillin *see* Carfecillin.

CARFIMATE* (1-phenyl-2-propynyl carb-amate; α-ethynylbenzyl alcohol carbamate; ethynyl phenyl carbinol carbamate; 'CFC', 'nirvegil', 'nirvotin', 'nirvotinal').

CARGUTOCIN (1-butyric acid-6-(L-2-aminobutyric acid)-7-glycineoxytocin).

'Cariamyl' *see* Heptaminol theophylline-acetate.

'Caridan' *see* Oxyphencyclimine.

CARINAMIDE* (*p*-(benzylsulfonamido)-benzoic acid; *p*-(α-toluenesulfonamido)-

benzoic acid; p'-carboxy-p-toluenesulfon-
anilide; caronamide; 'coronamide', 'retentin', 'staticin').

CARINDACILLIN** (1-indan-5-yl ester of
N-(2-carboxy-3,3-dimethyl-7-oxo-4-thia-1-
azabicyclo(3.2.0)hept-6-yl)-2-phenyl-
malonamic acid; 6-(2-(indan-5-ylcarbonyl)-
2-phenylacetamido)penicillanic acid;
carbenicillin indanyl; carbenicillin indanyl
sodium; indanyl carbenicillin; CP-15464;
'carindapen').

'Carindapen' see Carindacillin.
'Caripeptic' see Papain.
'Carisoma' see Carisoprodol.
CARISOPRODOL*** (2-carbamyloxymeth-
yl-2-isopropylcarbamyloxymethylpentane;
carbamate isopropylcarbamate of 2-methyl-
2-propyl-1,3-propanediol; isopropylmeprobamate; isoprotan; isoprothane;
'apesan', 'caprodat', 'carisoma', 'flexartal',
'rela', 'sanoma', 'soma', 'tonolyt').

'Carlytene' see Moxisylyte.
CARMANTADINE** (1-adamant-1-yl-2-
azetidinecarboxylic acid; Sch-15427).
CARMETIZIDE** (methyl 6-chloro-3,4-
dihydro-2-methyl-7-sulfamoyl-2H-1,2,4-
benzothiadiazine-3-carboxylate 1,1-
dioxide).
CARMOISINE (chiefly the disodium salt of
4-hydroxy-3-(4-sulfonaphth-1-ylazo)-
naphthalene-1-sulfonic acid; azo rubine;
D&C red 10; CI-14720).
'Carmurit' see Etoxazene.
CARMUSTINE*** (1,3-bis(2-chloroethyl)-1-
nitrosourea; BCNU; NSC-409962).
CARNIDAZOLE** (O-methyl [2-(2-methyl-
5-nitroimidazol-1-yl)ethyl]thiocarbamate;
2-(2-methyl-5-nitroimidazol-1-yl)ethyl-
thiocarbamic acid methyl ester). †
CARNITINE (γ-butyro-β-hydroxybetaine;
vitamin B₁; 'novain').
Carnitine carnitinate see Bicarnitine.
CARNOSINE (N-(β-alanyl)histidine).
'Carofur' see Nifurprazine.
'Caroid' see Papain.
Caronamide see Carinamide.
β-Carotene-4,4'-diol dipalmitate see
Xantofyl palmitate.
CAROVERINE** (1-(2-diethylaminoethyl)-
3-(p-methoxybenzyl)-2(1H)-quinoxalinone;
P-201-1).
CAROXAZONE*** (2-oxo-2H-1,3-
benzoxazine-3(4H)-acetamide; 3(4H)-
carbamoylmethyl-2H-1,3-benzoxazin-2-
one; benzoxazone; Fi-6654).
CARPERIDINE*** (ethyl ester of 1-(2-
carbamoylethyl)-4-phenylisonipecotic acid;
ethyl 1-(2-carbamoylethyl)-4-phenylpiper-
idine-4-carboxylate).
CARPERONE*** (isopropylcarbamate ester
of 4'-fluoro-4-(4-hydroxypiperid-1-yl)-
butyrophenone).
Carphenazine* see Carfenazine.
Carphenol see Diphenan.
CARPIPRAMINE*** (1'-[3-(10,11-dihydro-
(5H)dibenz(b,f)azepin-5-yl)propyl]-1,4'-
bipiperidine-4'-carboxamide; 5-[3-[(4-

carbamoyl-4-piperid-1-yl)piperid-1-yl]-
propyl]-10,11-dihydro-5H-dibenz(b,f)-
azepine; carbadipimidine; PZ-1511;
RP-21679; 'defekton').
CARPROFEN** (($\pm$)-6-chloro-α-methyl-
carbazole-2-acetic acid).
CARPRONIUM CHLORIDE*** ((3-carb-
oxypropyl)trimethylammonium chloride
methyl ester; (3-carbomethoxypropyl)-
trimethylammonium chloride).
Carragenan degradation product see
Poligeenan.
CARSALAM*** (2H-1,3-benzoxazine-2,4-
(3H)dione; 3,4-dihydro(2H)-1,3-benzox-
azine-2,4-dione; O-carbamoylsalicylic acid
lactam; 'beaprine', 'veradyne').
CARTAP* (1,3-bis(carbamoylthio)-N,N-
dimethyl-2-propylamine; S,S'-[2-(dimethylamino)-1,3-propanediyl] carbamothioate;
cartap hydrochloride; NTD-2; 'padan').
CARTAZOLATE*** (ethyl 4-butylamino-1-
ethyl-1H-pyrazolo(3,4-b)pyridine-5-
carboxylate).
CARTEOLOL** (5-[3-($tert$-butylamino)-2-
hydroxypropoxy]-3,4-dihydrocarbostyril;
1-($tert$-butylamino)-3-(3,4-dihydro-2(1H)-
oxoquinolin-5-yl)-2-propanol.
CARTICAINE** (4-methyl-3-(2-propyl-
aminopropionamido)-2-thiophenecarb-
oxylic acid methyl ester; methyl 4-methyl-
3-(2-propylaminopropionamido)-2-thio-
phenecarboxylate; 2-carbomethoxy-4-
methyl-3-(α-propionylamino)thiophene;
carticaine hydrochloride; HOE-045;
HOE-40045; 'ultracain').
CARTOX (tr) (carbon dioxide with 10%
ethylene oxide).
'Carudol' see Pyrazinobutazone.
CARVACROL (2-p-cymenol; 2-methyl-5-
isopropylphenol).
'Carvasept' see Chlorocarvacrol.
'Carvasin' see Isosorbide dinitrate.
'Caryolysin' see Chlormethine.
CARZENIDE** (p-carboxybenzenesulfon-
amide; p-sulfamoylbenzoic acid; 'dirnate').
'Carzol' see Formetanate.
CASANTHROL* (purified mixture of
anthranol glycosides from $Cascara$ $sagrada$
'peristim').
'Casantin' see Diethazine.
'Casmalon' see Cyclarbamate.
'Casoron' see Dichlobenil.
Cassella-4489 see Carbocromen.
Cassic acid see Rhein.
'Castrix' see Crimidine.
'Castron' see Pheniprazine.
'Catabex' see Dropropizine.
'Catalin' see 1-Hydroxypyrido(3,2-a)-
phenoxazin-5-one-3-carboxylic acid.
'Catanil' see Chlorpropamide.
'Catapres' see Clonidine.
'Catapresan' see Clonidine.
'Catapyrin' see Aminometradine.
'Catarase' see Chymotrypsin.
Catechin see Catechol.
Catechinic acid see Catechol.
CATECHOL (3,3',4',5,7-pentahydroxy-

flavan; 3,3',4',5,7-flavanpentol; catechin; catechinic acid; catechuic acid).
See also Pyrocatechol.
Catechuic acid *see* Catechol.
Catenulin *see* Paromomycin.
'Cateudyl' *see* Methaqualone.
Cathine *see* Norpseudoephedrine.
'Cathocin' *see* Novobiocin.
'Cathomycin' *see* Novobiocin.
'Catovit' *see* Prolintane.
'Catran' *see* Pheniprazine.
'Catron' *see* Pheniprazine.
'Catroniazid' *see* Pheniprazine.
'Caved S' *see* Deglycyrrhizinized liquorice.
'Caviject' *see* Fusidic acid.
'Cavodil' *see* Pheniprazine.
'Cavoform' *see* Paraformaldehyde.
'Cavolax' *see* Dantron.
'Cavumbren' *see* Adipiodone.
'Caytine' *see* Protokylol.
CB-11 *see* Phenadoxone.
CB-154 *see* Brocriptine.
CB-304 *see* Azaribine.
CB-309 *see* Fenabutene.
CB-804 *see* Calcium bucloxate.
CB-1048 *see* Chlornaphazin.
CB-1181 *see* Butadiene diepoxide.
CB-1314 *see* Metochalcone.
CB-1348 *see* Chlorambucil.
CB-1506 *see* Chloroethyl mesilate.
CB-1522 *see* 2-Fluoroethyl dimesilate.
CB-1528 *see* Ethyl mesilate.
CB-1540 *see* Methyl mesilate.
CB-1592 *see* Chloroethylcysteine.
CB-1639 *see* Cycloleucine.
CB-1678 *see* Propiomazine.
CB-1729 *see* o-Sarcolysin.
CB-2041 *see* Busulfan.
CB-2067 *see* Nonamethylene dimesilate.
CB-2201 *see* Amfepentorex.
CB-2387 *see* Dimethyltrimethylene mesilate.
CB-2511 *see* Mannityl dimesilate.
CB-2562 *see* Erythrityl dimesilate.
CB-3007 *see* Sarcolysin.
CB-3025 *see* Melphalan.
CB-3026 *see* Medphalan.
CB-3208 *see* Formylmelphalan.
CB-3697 *see* Dextrofemine.
CB-4261 *see* Tetrazepam.
CB-4306 *see* Dipotassium clorazepate.
CB-8049 *see* Diphenoxylate.
CB-8053 *see* Thiamphenicol.
CB-8073 *see* Diloxanide furoate.
CB-8080 *see* Etynodiol diacetate.
CB-8089 *see* Benperidol.
CB-8092 *see* Oxazepam.
CB-8102 *see* Bamifylline.
CB-8109 *see* Canrenoate potassium.
CB-8129 *see* Uric acid oxidase.
CB-12025 *see* Nifuralide.
CCC *see* Chlormequat.
CCK-179 *see* Dihydroergotoxine.
CCNU *see* Lomustine.
CD-68 *see* Chlordane.
CDAA *see* Allidochlor.
CDIB *see* Methyl clofenapate.
CDP-choline *see* Citicoline.

CDT *see* Simazine.
CE-264 *see* Alloclamide.
CE-305 *see* Flualamide.
CE-746 *see* Eprazinone.
'Cealysin' *see* Hexamethylolmelamine.
'Cecekin' *see* Cholecystokinin-pancreozymin.
'Cedigocin' *see* Acetyldigoxin.
'Cedigoxin' *see* Acetyldigoxin.
'Cedilanid' *see* Lanatoside C.
'Cedilanid D' *see* Deslanoside.
'Cedi-sanol' *see* Lanatoside C.
'Cedocard' *see* Isosorbide dinitrate.
'Cedona' *see* Deglycyrrhizinized liquorice.
'Cedopurin' *see* Methenamine mandelate.
Cedrarin *see* Orexin.
'Cedulamin' *see* Methenamine mandelate.
'Ceduran' *see* Nitrofurantoin with liquorice.
'Ceepryn' *see* Cetylpyridinium.
CEFACETRILE** (7-(2-cyanoacetamido)-3-(hydroxymethyl)-2-cephem-2-carboxylic acid acetate (ester); 3-(acetoxymethyl)-7-(2-cyanoacetamido)-2-cephem-2-carboxylic acid; 7-(2-cyanoacetamido)cephalosporanic acid; Ba-36278A; C-36278A-Ba; 'celospor').
CEFADROXIL** ([6R-[6α,7β(R)]]-7-[[amino-(4-hydroxyphenyl)acetyl]amino]-3-methyl-2-cephem-2-carboxylic acid; (6R,7R)-7-[(R)-2-amino-2-(p-hydroxyphenyl)acetamido]-3-methyl-2-cephem-2-carboxylic acid; BL-S578).
'Cefadyl' *see* Cefapirin.
CEFALEXIN** (7-(D-2-amino-2-phenylacetamido)-3-methyl-2-cephem-2-carboxylic acid; 7-(D-2-amino-2-phenylacetamido)-3-methyl-8-oxo-5-thia-1-azabicyclo(4.2.0)-oct-2-ene-2-carboxylic acid; cephalexin; L-66873, 'cepexin', 'cepol', 'ceporexin', 'keflex', 'keforal', 'oracef', 'palitex', 'syncl').
CEFALOGLYCIN** (7-(2-amino-2-phenyl-acetamido)-3-hydroxymethyl-8-oxo-5-thia-1-azabicyclo(4.2.0)oct-2-ene-2-carboxylic acid acetate inner salt; 7-(D-α-aminophenyl-acetamido)cephalosporanic acid; cephaloglycin; 'kafacin', 'kefglycin').
'Cefaloject' *see* Cefapirin.
CEFALONIUM** (3-(4-carbamoylpyridyl-methyl)-8-oxo-7-[α-(thien-2-yl)acetamido]-5-thia-1-azabicyclo(4.2.0)oct-2-ene-2-carboxylic acid; cephalonium; carbamoyl-cefalonium).
CEFALORAM** (3-(acetoxymethyl)-8-oxo-7-(phenylacetamido)-5-thia-1-azabicyclo-(4.2.0)oct-2-ene-2-carboxylic acid; 7-phenylacetamidocephalosporanic acid; cephaloram).
CEFALORIDINE** (3-(1-pyridylmethyl)-7-[(2-thienyl)acetamido]-3-cephem-4-carboxylic acid betaine; 3-pyrid-1-ylmethyl-7-thien-2-ylacetamido-8-oxo-5-thia-1-azabicyclo(4.2.0)oct-2-ene-2-carboxylic acid; 1-[[2-carboxy-8-oxo-7-[(2-thien-2-yl)acetamido]-5-thia-1-azabicyclo(4.2.0)oct-2-en-3-yl]methyl]pyridinium hydroxide inner salt; cephaloridine; L-40602; Sch-11527; 'ceporan', 'ceporin', 'ceropan', 'glaxoridin', 'keflodin', 'keflordin', 'kefspor', 'loridine',

CEFALOTIN** (3-(acetoxymethyl)-8-oxo-7-[2-(2-thienyl)acetamido]-5-thia-1-azabicyclo(4.2.0)oct-2-ene-2-carboxylic acid; 7-(2-thienylacetamido)cephalosporanic acid; cephalosporin 871; cephalothin; cefalotin sodium; 'ceporacin', 'cepovenin', 'keflin'). †

CEFAMANDOLE** (7-D-mandelamido-3-[[(1-methyl-1H-tetrazol-5-yl)thio]methyl]-2-cephem-2-carboxylic acid; cephamandole).

'Cefamezin' see Cefazolin.

CEFAPAROLE** ((6R,7R)-7-[(R)-2-amino-2-(p-hydroxyphenyl)acetamido]-3-[[(5-methyl-1,3,4-thiadiazol-2-yl)thio]methyl]-2-cephem-2-carboxylic acid).

CEFAPIRIN** (3-hydroxymethyl-7-[2-(4-pyridylthio)acetamido]-2-cephem-2-carboxylic acid acetate (ester); 3-acetoxymethyl-7-[2-(pyrid-4-ylthio)acetamido]-2-cephem-2-carboxylic acid; 7-[2-(pyrid-4-ylthio)-acetamido]cephalosporanic acid; cefapirin sodium; cephapirin; cephapirin sodium; BL-P 1322; 'bristocef', 'cefadyl', 'cefaloject', 'cefatrex', 'cefatrexyl').

'Cefatrex' see Cefapirin.

'Cefatrexyl' see Cefapirin.

CEFATRIZINE** ((6R,7R)-7-[(R)-2-amino-2-(p-hydroxyphenyl)acetamido]-3-[(v-triazol-4-ylthio)methyl]-2-cephem-2-carboxylic acid).

CEFAZOLIN** (3-[[(5-methyl-1,3,4-thiadiazol-2-yl)thio]methyl]-7-[2-(1H-tetrazol-1-yl)acetamido]-2-cephem-2-carboxylic acid; cefazolin sodium; cephazolin; L-46083; SK&F-41558; 'ancef', 'cefacidal', 'cefamezin', 'celmetin', 'elzogram', 'gramaxin', 'kefzol', 'totacef', 'zolicef').

CEFOXAZOLE** (7-[3-(o-chlorophenyl)-5-methylisoxazole-4-carboxamido]cephalosporanic acid; (6R,7R)-7-[3-(o-chlorophenyl)-5-methylisoxazole-4-carboxamido]-3-(hydroxymethyl)-2-cephem-2-carboxylic acid acetate ester; cephoxazole).

CEFOXITIN*** (3-hydroxymethyl-7-methoxy-7-(2-thien-2-ylacetamido)-2-cephem-2-carboxylic acid carbamate ester; cefoxitin sodium).

CEFRADINE*** (7-[D-2-amino-2-(1,4-cyclohexadien-1-yl)acetamido]-3-methyl-2-cephem-2-carboxylic acid; SQ-11436; 'anspor', 'eskacef', 'maxisporin', 'sefril', 'velosef').

CEFROTIL** ((6R,7R)-3-methyl-7-[2-[p-(1,4,5,6-tetrahydropyrimidin-2-yl)phenyl]acetamido]-2-cephem-2-carboxylic acid).

CEFTEZOLE** ((6R,7R)-7-[2-(1H-tetrazol-1-yl)acetamido]-3-[(1,3,4-thiadiazol-2-ylthio)methyl]-2-cephem-2-carboxylic acid).

CEFUROXIME** ((6R,7R)-3-(carbamoyloxymethyl)-7-[(2Z)-2-(2-furyl)-2-(methoxyimino)acetamido]-2-cephem-2-carboxylic acid; (6R,7R)-7-[2-(2-furyl)glyoxylamido]-3-(hydroxymethyl)-2-cephem-2-carboxylic acid (Z)-mono(O-methyloxime) carbamate ester).

'Ceglunat' see Lanatoside C.

'Celadigal' see Lanatoside C.

CELA S-1942 see Bromofos.

CELA S-2957 see Chlorthiophos.

'Celbenin' see Meticillin.

'Celestan soluble' see Betamethasone sodium phosphate.

'Celestene' see Betamethasone.

'Celestene-chronodose' see Betamethasone acetate with betamethasone sodium phosphate.

'Celestone' see Betamethasone.

'Celiomycin' see Viomycin.

'Celiopaste' see Thallium sulfate.

CELIPROLOL** (3-[3-acetyl-4-[3-(tert-butylamino)-2-hydroxypropoxy]phenyl]-1,1-diethylurea; 1-[2-acetyl-4-[(diethylcarbamoyl)amino]phenoxy]-3-(tert-butylamino)-2-propanol).

CELLABURATE*** (cellulose acetate butyrate).

CELLACEFATE** (a partial mixed acetate and hydrogen phthalate ester of cellulose; cellacephate; cellulose acetophthalate).

Cellacephate* see Cellacefate.

'Cellase-1000' see Cellulase.

'Cellon' see Tetrachloroethane.

'Cellosolve' see 2-Ethoxyethanol.

'Celluflex' see Tricresyl phosphate.

CELLULASE** (concentrate of cellulose-splitting enzymes from Aspergillus niger; 'cellase-1000').

Cellulose see Cellacefate; Hypromellose; Methylcellulose; Oxidized cellulose; Oxidized regenerated cellulose; Sodium carboxymethylcellulose.

Cellulose acetate butyrate see Cellaburate.

Cellulose acetophthalate see Cellacefate.

Cellulose nitrate see Pyroxylin.

Cellulosic acid see Oxidized cellulose.

'Celontin' see Mesuximide.

'Celospor' see Cefacetrile.

'Celtacillin' see Propicillin.

'Celuton' see Sodium acexamate.

'Cemora' see Butaverine.

'Censedal' see Nealbarbital.

'Centalun' see 3,4-Dihydroxy-3-methyl-4-phenyl-1-butyne.

'Centonuron' see Bendroflumethiazide.

'Centracid' see Triclocarban.

'Contractyl' see Promazine.

'Centrine' see Aminopentamide.

Centrophenoxine* see Meclofenoxate.

'Centroton' see Pyrovalerone.

'Centyl' see Bendroflumethiazide.

'Ceolat' see Dimeticone.

'Cepacilina' see Benzathine penicillin.

'Cepacol' see Cetylpyridinium.

'Cepentyl' see N-Cyclopentyllysergamide.

'Cepexin' see Cefalexin.

CEPH see Todralazine.

CEPHAELINE (desmethylemetine; 'sedatussin').

Cephalexin* see Cefalexin.

'Cephalmin' see Thioproperazine mesilate.

Cephaloglycin* see Cefaloglycin.

Cephalonium* see Cefalonium.

Cephaloridine* see Cefaloridine.

CEPHALOSPORANIC ACID (3-acetoxy-methyl-8-oxo-5-thia-1-azabicyclo(4.2.0)oct-2-ene-2-carboxylic acid; 3-acetoxymethyl-cephem-(2)-carboxylic acid; 3-hydroxy-methyl-2-cephem-2-carboxylic acid acetate (ester)).

CEPHALOSPORIN C* (3-acetoxymethyl-7-(5-amino-5-carboxyvaleramido)-8-oxo-5-thia-1-azabicyclo(4.2.0)oct-2-ene-2-carb-oxylic acid; aminoadipyl cephalosporin).

Cephalosporin N *see* Adicillin.

Cephalosporin 871 *see* Cefalotin.

Cephalothin* *see* Cefalotin.

Cephamandole* *see* Cefamandole.

Cephapirin* *see* Cefapirin.

Cephazolin* *see* Cefazolin.

2-CEPHEM-2-CARBOXYLIC ACID (8-oxo-5-thia-1-azabicyclo(4.2.0)oct-2-ene-2-carboxylic acid; 3-cephem-4-carboxylic acid).

3-Cephem-4-carboxylic acid *see* 2-Cephem-2-carboxylic acid.

Cephoxazole* *see* Cefoxazole.

'Cepillina' *see* Meticillin.

'Cepol' *see* Cefalexin.

'Ceporacin' *see* Cefalotin.

'Ceporan' *see* Cefaloridine.

'Ceporexin' *see* Cefalexin.

'Ceporin' *see* Cefaloridine.

'Cepovenin' *see* Cefalotin.

'Cequartyl' *see* Benzalkonium.

Cerasine red *see* Oil scarlet.

'Cercine' *see* Diazepam.

'Cercobin' *see* Thiophanate.

Cerebronic acid *see* 2-Hydroxytetracosanoic acid.

Cerebrostenediol *see* Cholest-5-ene-3,24-diol.

Cerebrostenolone *see* Cholest-5-en-24-ol-3-one.

Cerebrosterol *see* Cholest-5-ene-3,24-diol.

'Ceredon' *see* Benquinox.

'Cerenox' *see* Benquinox.

'Ceresan' *see* Ethylmercuric chloride.

'Ceresan-M' *see* Ethylmercuri-*p*-toluenesul-fonanilide.

CERM-370 *see* Amoproxan.

CERM-898 *see* Amixetrine.

CERM-1290 *see* Scopolamine methyl methosulfate.

CERM-3209 *see* Papaverine adenylate.

'Ceropan' *see* Cefaloridine.

'Certonal' *see* Methaqualone.

'Certonin' *see* Dehydrocholic acid.

'Certrol' *see* Ioxynil.

'Cerubidin' *see* Daunorubicin.

CERULETIDE** (5-oxo-L-prolyl-L-glutamin-yl-L-aspartyl-L-tyrosyl-L-threonylglycyl-L-tryptophyl-L-methionyl-L-aspartyl-L-phenylalaninamide 4-(hydrogen sulfate) ester).

'Cerutil' *see* Meclofenoxate.

'Cervantal oral' *see* Ampicillin with dicloxacillin.

'Cervantal parenteral' *see* Ampicillin with oxacillin.

'Cervilaxin' *see* Relaxin.

'Cervoxan' *see* Deanol acetamidobenzoate.

'Cescan-131' *see* Cesium(^{131}Cs) chloride.

CESIUM(^{131}Cs) CHLORIDE*** ('cescan-131').

'Cestarsol' *see* Arecoline-acetarsol.

'Cetab' *see* Cetrimonium.

CETACEUM (cetyl palmitate; parmaceti; spermaceti; 'hemotabs', 'parmacetyl').

'Cetacillin' *see* Propicillin.

Cetalkon* *see* Cetalkonium.

CETALKONIUM CHLORIDE*** (benzyl-hexadecyldimethylammonium chloride; cetylbenzyldimethylammonium chloride; cetalkon; 'bonjela', 'zettyn').

CETAMIFEN (tr) (ethanolamine salt of 2-phenylbutyric acid; aminoethanol salt of phenylethylacetic acid; cetamiphen).

Cetamiphen (tr) *see* Cetamifen.

'Cetamium' *see* Cetylpyridinium.

Cetanol *see* 1-Hexadecanol.

'Cetarin' *see* Racemorphan.

'Cetavlex' *see* Cetrimonium.

'Cetavlon' *see* Cetrimonium.

CETHEXONIUM BROMIDE (dimethyl-hexadecyl(2-hydroxycyclohexyl)ammo-nium bromide; 'biocidan').

CETIEDIL*** (α-cyclohexyl-3-thiophene-acetic acid 2-(hexahydro-1H-azepin-1-yl)-ethyl ester; 2-(hexahydro-1H-azepin-1-yl)-ethyl α-cyclohexyl-3-thiopheneacetate; α-thien-3-ylcyclohexaneacetic acid 2-hexamethyleniminoethyl ester; 2-hexa-methyleniminoethyl α-thien-2-ylcyclo-hexaneacetate; 2-hexamethyleniminoethyl α-cyclohexyl-3-thiopheneacetate; INO-502; 'stratene').

'Cetiprin' *see* Emepronium.

Cetobemidone *see* Ketobemidone.

CETOFENICOL*** (D-threo-*N*-[*p*-acetyl-β-hydroxy-α-(hydroxymethyl)phenethyl]-2,2-dichloroacetamide; 1-(*p*-acetylphenyl)-2-(dichloroacetamido)-1,3-propanediol; cetophenicol; W-3746).

CETOHEXAZINE*** (4,6-dimethyl-2,3-dihydropyridazin-3(2H)-one; 4,6-dimethyl-3(2H)-pyridazinone).

CETOMACROGOL(S)* (cetyl ethers of macrogols).

CETOMACROGOL 1000*** (polyethylene glycol 1000 monohexadecyl ether; poly-ethylene glycol 1000 monocetyl ether; 'texofors A1P').

Cetophenicol* *see* Cetofenicol.

'Cetosal' *see* Acetaminosalol.

'Cétosalol' *see* Acetaminosalol.

'Ceto-sanol' *see* Lanatoside C.

CETOSTEARYLIC ALCOHOL (mixture of 1-octadecanol and 1-hexadecanol).

CETOTIAMINE*** (*S*-ester of *O*-ethyl thio-carbonate with *N*-(4-amino-2-methyl-pyrimidin-5-ylmethyl)-*N*-(4-hydroxy-2-mercapto-1-methyl-1-butenyl)formamide ethyl carbonate; *O*,*S*-dicarbethoxythiamine; *S*-ethoxycarbonylthiamine; DCET; SECT).

CETOXIME*** (2-(*N*-benzylanilino)acet-amidoxime; cetoxime hydrochloride; 'febramine').

Cetrimide* *see* Cetrimonium.

84

CETRIMONIUM BROMIDE* (or CHLORIDE)** (hexadecyltrimethylammonium bromide; cetyltrimethylammonium bromide; cetrimide; CTAB; 'biocetab', 'bromat', 'cetab', 'cetavlex', 'cetavlon', 'cetylamine', 'cirrasol OD', 'gomaxine', 'lissolamine', 'micol', 'quamonium', 'savlon', 'seboderm', 'vantoc').

CETRIMONIUM PENTACHLORO-PHENATE (hexadecyltrimethylammonium pentachlorophenate; cetryltrimethyl-ammonium pentachlorophenate; TCAP).

Cetyl alcohol see 1-Hexadecanol.

Cetylamine see Hexadecylamine.

'Cetylamine' see Cetrimonium.

'Cetylcide' see Cetrimonium.

Cetylic acid see Palmitic acid.

Cetyl palmitate see Cetaceum.

CETYLPYRIDINIUM BROMIDE* (or CHLORIDE)** (hexadecylpyridinium bromide or chloride; 'biosept', 'ceepryn', 'cepacol', 'cetamium', 'dobendan', 'fixanol C', 'germidine', 'pyrisept', 'sterogenol').

CETYLPYRIDINIUM CHLORIDE WITH HEXETIDINE ('doreperol').

CETYLPYRIDINIUM o-THYMOTINATE (hexadecylpyridinium 3-hydroxy-p-cymene-carboxylate; hexadecylpyridinium-3-iso-propyl-6-methylsalicylate; 'pedyol').

Cetyltrimethylammonium bromide see Cetrimonium.

'Cevanol' see Benactyzine.

CF-318C see Octafluorocyclobutane.

'CFC' see Carfimate.

CFC-12 see Dichlorodifluoromethane.

'CFT' see Diallate.

CG-21 see Fenyramidol oxyphenbutazone salt.

CG-201 see Bevonium metilsulfate.

CG-315 see Tramadol.

CG-635 see Etiroxate.

CG-3117 see Naproxen.

CGP-2175 see Metoprolol tartrate.

CH-3565 see Triclosan.

CH-13437 see Nafenopin.

CHALCONE (chalkone; benzylideneaceto-phenone; 3-phenylacrylophenone; 1,3-diphenyl-2-propen-1-one; phenyl styryl ketone).

CHAULMESTROL (ethyl chaulmoograte).

CHAULMOOGRIC ACID (13-(2-cyclo-penten-1-yl)-tridecanoic acid).

CHAULMOSULFONE* (4,4′-bis(dihydro-chaulmoogrylamino)diphenyl sulfone; 4,4′-bis[p-(13-cyclopentyltridecanamido)-phenyl]sulfone; 4′,4″-sulfonylbis(cyclo-pentanetridecananilide)).

'Chelaton' see Trisodium edetate.

'Chel DTPA' see Pentetic acid.

'Chelen' see Chloroethane.

CHELIDAMIC ACID (1,4-dihydro-4-oxo-2,6-pyridinedicarboxylic acid).

'Chelintox' see Sodium calcium edetate.

'Chemical mace' see 2-Chloroacetophenone.

'Chemiofuran' see Nitrofurantoin.

'Chemipen' see Pheneticillin.

CHENODEOXYCHOLIC ACID

(3α,7α-dihydroxycholanic acid; anthro-podeoxycholic acid; gallodeoxycholic acid; 'chenofalk').

Chenta see 1,2-Diaminocyclohexanetetra-acetic acid.

'Chetovis' see Prasterone.

CHIA see Clorindanic acid.

Chick antidermatitis factor see Pantothenic acid.

Chillifolin* see Quillifolin.

Chin.... See also Quin....

China green see Malachite green.

'Chinaphthol' see Quinaphthol.

Chindecamine* see Quindecamine.

CHINIOFON* (mixture of 8-hydroxy-7-iodo-5-quinolinesulfonic acid with 20% of Na bicarb.; iodoquinoline; meditrene; quiniofon).

Chinocide see Quinocide.

Chinoform see Clioquinol.

CHINOMETHIONAT* (6-methyl-1,3-dithiolo(4,5-b)quinoxalin-2-one; 6-methyl-2,3-quinoxalinedithiol cyclic S,S-dithio-carbonate; quinomethionate; 'forstan', 'morestan').

Chinon see Quinone.

CHINOPYRINE (compound of quinine-HCl with phenazone; quinopyrine).

'Chinoral' see Quinochloral.

'Chinosol' see 8-Quinolinol potassium sulfate.

Chinothionat see Thioquinox.

'Chinoxone' see Oxycinchophen.

'Chinurea' see Quinurea.

Chitosamine see Glucosamine.

Chloditan (tr) see Mitotane.

Chlodofen (tr) see Feniodium chloride.

Chlophedianol* see Clofedanol.

Chlophenadion see Clorindione.

Chlopoxide see Chlordiazepoxide.

Chlopropham see Chlorpropham.

Chlor.... See also Clor....

Chloracetophenone see Chloroacetophenone.

Chloracetoxyquinoline see Cloxiquine acetate.

Chloracizin (tr) see Cloracizin.

Chloracon (tr) see Beclamide.

CHLORACYZINE* (2-chloro-10-(3-diethylaminopropionyl)phenothiazine; 2-chlorophenothiazin-10-yl 2-diethyl-aminoethyl ketone).

'Chloradione' see Chlorophacinone.

CHLORAL (trichloroacetaldehyde).

CHLORAL-AMINOPYRINE (cpd. of aminopyrine and chloral; 'chloralpyrine').

CHLORAL BETAINE* (chloral hydrate-betaine adduct; betain chloralum; cloral betaine; 'betachlor', 'β-chlor', 'somilar').

'Chloraldurat' see Chloral hydrate.

CHLORAL HYDRATE (trichloroacetal-dehyde monohydrate; trichloroethylidene glycol; 2,2,2-trichloro-1,1-ethanediol; 'aquachloral', 'chloraldurat', 'hydral', 'lorinal', 'notec', 'phaldrone', 'rectules', 'somnos', 'sorosil').

See also Butylchloral hydrate; Chloral betaine; Dichloralphenazone.

CHLORAL HYDRATE ACETYLGLYCIN-

AMIDE ('ansopal', 'duphanox').

Chloral hydrocyanide see Chlorocyano-hydrin.

CHLORALODOL*** (2-methyl-4-(2,2,2-trichloro-1-hydroxyethoxy)-2-pentanol; chlorhexadol; 'lora', 'mechloral', 'mecoral').

Chloralosane see α-Chloralose.

CHLORALOSE (1,2-anhydro-1,2-(2,2,2-trichloroethylidenealdehydo)-D-glucose; (*R*)-1,2-*O*-(2,2,2-trichloroethylidene)-α-D-glucofuranose; anhydroglucochloral; glucochloral; glucochloralose).

α-CHLORALOSE (chloralosane; 'dorcalm', 'kalmettum-somniferum', 'somnio').

β-CHLORALOSE (parachloralose).

CHLORALPHENAZONE (compound of 1 mol. phenazone with 1 mol. chloral hydrate; chloralantipyrine; 'hypnal').

'Chloralpyrine' see Chloral-aminopyrine.

Chloral urethan see Carbocloral.

CHLORAMBEN* (3-amino-2,5-dichloro-benzoic acid; 'amiben', 'vegaben').

CHLORAMBUCIL*** (4-[*p*-bis-(2-chloro-ethyl)aminophenyl]butyric acid; chloraminophene; CB-1348; NSC-3088; 'amboclorin', 'ecloril', 'leukeran', 'lin-folysin', 'lympholysin').

Chlorambucil prednisolone 21-ester see Prednimustine.

Chloramide see Tosylchloramide.

'Chloramin' see Chlormethine.

Chloramine-T see Tosylchloramide.

Chloraminophene see Chlorambucil.

Chloramiphene see Clomifene.

CHLORAMPHENICOL*** (D(−)-*threo*-2-(dichloroacetamido)-1-(*p*-nitrophenyl)-1,3-propanediol; D-*threo*-2,2-dichloro-*N*-(β-hydroxy-α-hydroxymethyl-*p*-nitrophen-ethyl)acetamide; laevomycetin; levo-chloramphenicol; levomycetin).

(+)-CHLORAMPHENICOL (dextramycin; dextromycetin).

DL-CHLORAMPHENICOL (synthomycin).

(−)-Chloramphenicol see Chloramphenicol.

CHLORAMPHENICOL HEMISUCCIN-ATE ('solnicol').

CHLORAMPHENICOL HEMISUCCIN-ATE SODIUM SALT ('chlorocid S').

CHLORAMPHENICOL PANTOTHEN-ATE COMPLEX* (cloramfenicol pantotenate complex; PP-036; 'pantofenicol', 'pantovernil').

CHLORAMPHENICOL STEARATE (eusynthomycin; eusintomicine; 'mado-micetina').

CHLORAMPHENICOL WITH OLEAN-DOMYCIN ('chlotaon').

CHLORAMPHENICOL WITH PRED-NISONE ('cortiphenicol').

Chloranautine see Dimenhydrinate.

CHLORANIFORMETHAN (*N*-[1-(3,4-dichloroanilino)2,2,2-trichloroethyl]-formamide; *N*-(2,2,2-trichloro-1-form-amidoethyl)aniline; Bay-79770; XXI/07; 'imugan').

CHLORANIL (2,3,5,6-tetrachloro-*p*-benzo-quinone; 'spergon', 'vulklor').

CHLORANILIC ACID (2,5-dichloro-3,6-dihydroxy-*p*-benzoquinone).

CHLORANOCRYL* (*N*-(3,4-dichloro-phenyl)-2-methyl-2-propenamide; *N*-(3,4-dichlorophenyl)-2-methylacrylamide; 'dicryl').

CHLORASQUIN (*N*-[*p*-[(2,4-diamino-5-chloroquinazolin-6-ylmethyl)amino]-benzoyl]aspartic acid dihydrate; NSC-529861).

CHLORAZANIL*** (2-amino-4-(*p*-chloro-anilino)-*s*-triazine; chlorazinil; ASA-226; 'daquin', 'doclizid-T', 'neo-urofort', 'orpidan', 'orpizin', 'triazurol').

Chlorazin see Chlorazine and Cyclo-guanil.

CHLORAZINE* (6-chloro-2,4-bis(diethyl-amino)-*s*-triazine; 6-chloro-*N*,*N*,*N*′,*N*′-tetraethyl-1,3,5-triazine-2,4-diamine; chlorazin; G-25804).

Chlorazinil see Chlorazanil.

CHLORAZODIN*** (α,α′-azobis(chloro-formamidine); 1,1′-azobis(chloroform-amidine); *N*,*N*-dichloroazodicarbamidine; chloroazodin; 'azochloramid').

CHLORAZOLE FAST PINK ('benzoech-trosa').

CHLORBENOXAMINE*** (1-[2-(*o*-chloro-benzhydryloxy)ethyl]-4-(*o*-methylbenzyl)-piperazine; 1-[2-(*o*-chloro-α-phenylbenzyl-oxy)ethyl]-4-(*o*-methylbenzyl)piperazine; chlorbenzoxyethamine; UCB-1474; 'libratar').

CHLORBENSIDE* (1-chloro-4-[[(4-chloro-phenyl)methyl]thio]benzene; *p*-chloro-benzyl *p*-chlorophenyl sulfide; 1-chloro-4-[(*p*-chlorobenzyl)thio]benzene; 4-chloro-α-[(*p*-chlorophenyl)thio]toluene; 'chlor-paracide', 'chlorsulphacide', 'mitox').

Chlorbenzilate see Chlorobenzilate.

CHLORBETAMIDE*** (*N*-(2,4-dichloro-benzyl)-*N*-(dichloroacetyl)ethanolamine; *N*-(dichloroacetyl)-*N*-(2,4-dichlorobenzyl)-2-hydroxyethylamine; 1,1-dichloro-*N*-(2,4-dichlorobenzyl)-*N*-(2-hydroxyethyl)-acetamide; WIN 5047; 'diantil', 'man-tomide', 'pontalin').

CHLORBICYCLEN* (1,2,3,4,7,7-hexa-chloro-5,6-bis(chloromethyl)bicyclo(2.2.1)-hept-2-ene; 1,4,5,6,7,7-hexachloro-5,6-bis-(chloromethyl)norbornene; AC-12402; 'alodan').

CHLORBROMURON* (1-(4-bromo-3-chlorophenyl)-3-methoxy-3-methylurea; 'maloran').

CHLORBUFAM* (1-methylprop-2-ynyl *m*-chlorocarbanilate; 1-methylprop-2-ynyl *N*-(*m*-chlorophenyl)carbamate; 1-methyl-2-propynyl 3-chlorophenylcarbamate; BICP; BiPC).

CHLORBUFAM PLUS CYCLURON ('alipur').

CHLORBUFAM PLUS PYRAZON ('alicap').

Chlorbutanol see Chlorbutol.

CHLORBUTOL* (acetone-chloroform; trichloroisobutyl alcohol; trichloro-*tert*-

butyl alcohol; 1,1,1-trichloro-2-methyl-2-propanol; chlorbutanol; chlorobutanol; 'acetochlorone', 'chloretone', 'chlortran', 'dentalone', 'methaform', 'mycozol', 'nautisan', 'sedaform').

Chlorcamphene *see* Campheclor.
Chlorcholine *see* Chlormequat.
Chlorcyclamide (tr) *see* Chlorhexamide.
CHLORCYCLIZINE* (1-(*p*-chlorobenzhydryl)-4-methylpiperazine; 1-[α-(*p*-chlorophenyl)benzyl]-4-methylpiperazine; AH 289).
'Chlordan' *see* Chlordane.
CHLORDANE* (1,2,4,5,6,7,8,8-octachloro-2,3,3a,4,7,7a-hexahydro-4,7-methanoindene; compound 1068; CD-68; HCS-3260; M-40; M-410; octachlor; 'chlordan', 'chlorkill', 'octa-klor', 'ortho-klor', 'toxichlor', 'velsicol-1068', 'wydane').
CHLORDANE-KEROSENE MIXTURE ('flit').
Chlordantoin* *see* Clodantoin.
CHLORDECONE* (decachlorooctahydro-1,3,4-metheno-2H-cyclobuta(cd)pentalen-2-one; decachloropentacyclo(3.3.2.0^{2,6}.0^{3,9}.0^{7,10})decan-4-one; 'kepone').
CHLORDIAZEPOXIDE* (7-chloro-2-methylamino-5-phenyl-3H-1,4-benzodiazepine 4-oxide; chlopoxide; methaminodiazepoxide; chlordiazepoxide hydrochloride; Ro-5-0690; 'elenium', 'librium', 'napoton', 'radepur', 'risolid'). *See also* Amitriptyline with chlordiazepoxide.
CHLORDIAZEPOXIDE WITH CLIDINIUM BROMIDE ('librax').
Chlordimeform *see* Chlorphenamidine.
CHLORDIMORINE* (3-chloro-4-[3-(4-morpholino)propoxy]biphenyl; 4-[3-(3-chloro-4-biphenylyloxy)propyl]morpholine).
Chlorepin *see* Clobazam.
'Chloresene' *see* Lindane.
Chlorethamine *see* Chlormethine.
Chlorethazine *see* Chlormethine.
Chlorethiazole *see* Clomethiazole.
CHLORETHOXYBUTAMOXANE (2-butylaminomethyl-8-(2-chloroethoxy)-1,4-benzodioxan).
Chloretin *see* Prynachlor.
'Chloretone' *see* Chlorbutol.
'Chlorextol' *see* Polychlorinated biphenyl mixture.
CHLORFENETHOL* (*p*-chloro-α-(*p*-chlorophenyl)-α-methylbenzyl alcohol; 4-chloro-α-(4-chlorophenyl)-α-methylbenzenemethanol; 4 4'-dichloro-α-methylbenzhydrol; bis(*p*-chlorophenyl) methyl carbinol; *p p'*-dichlorodiphenyl methyl carbinol; CPAS; DCPC; DCPE; DMC; 'dimite', 'micasin').
CHLORFENETHOL PLUS CHLORFENSULFIDE ('milbex').
Chlorfenidim *see* Monuron.
CHLORFENPROP-METHYL* (methyl 3-chloro-3-(*p*-chlorophenyl)propionate; methyl α,4-dichlorobenzenepropanoate; 'bidisin').
CHLORFENSON* (*p*-chlorophenyl *p*-chloro-benzenesulfonate; *p*-chlorophenyl closilate; CPCBS; PCPCBS; chlorofenizon; difenson; metakson; ovex; ovochlor; 'estonmite', 'ovatran', 'ovotran').

Chlorfenvinphos *see* Clofenvinfos.
Chlorfluoran *see* Cryofluorane.
CHLORFLURAZOLE* (4,5-dichloro-2-(trifluoromethyl)-1H-benzimidazole; chlorofluorazole; NC-2983).
Chlorftalidon *see* Chlortalidone.
Chlorguanide *see* Proguanil.
Chlorguanide triazine pamoate *see* Cycloguanil embonate.
Chlorhexadol* *see* Chloralodol.
CHLORHEXAMIDE (1-(*p*-chlorobenzenesulfonyl)-3-cyclohexylurea; chlorcyclamide; 'oradian').
CHLORHEXIDINE* (1,6-bis(*p*-chlorophenyldiguanido)hexane; hexamethylene-1,6-bis[1-(5-*p*-chlorophenyl)biguanide]; 1,1'-hexamethylenebis[5-(*p*-chlorophenyl)-biguanide]; chlorhexidine dihydrochloride; AY-5312; 'bidex', 'chlorohex', 'hibiscrub', 'hibitane', 'nolvascin', 'rotersept', 'sterilon').
CHLORHEXIDINE DIGLUCONATE ('corsodyl', 'hibiscrub').
Chlorhistapyridamine *see* Chlorpheniramine.
Chlorhydroxyquinoline *see* Cloxiquine.
Chloridine (tr) *see* Pyrimethamine.
Chloriguane *see* Proguanil.
Chlorimipramine *see* Clomipramine.
Chlorimpiphenine *see* Imiclopazine.
Chlorinat *see* Barban.
Chlorinated biphenyl mixture *see* Polychlorinated biphenyl mixture.
Chlorinated camphene *see* Campheclor.
CHLORINATED PHENOXYACETIC ACID MIXTURE (chiefly 2,4-dichlorophenoxyacetic acid and 2,4,5-trichlorophenoxyacetic acid; 'hormoslyr').
Chlorindanol* *see* Clorindanol.
'Chlorisept' *see* Cloxiquine.
CHLORISONDAMINE CHLORIDE* (4,5,6,7-tetrachloro-2-(2-dimethylaminoethyl)-2-methylisoindolinium chloride methochloride; 4,5,6,7-tetrachloro-2-(2-dimethylaminoethyl)isoindoline dimethochloride; hisindamone; Su-3088; 'ecolid').
'Chlor-kill' *see* Chlordane.
CHLORMADINONE* (6α-chloropregna-4,6-diene-17α-ol-3,20-dione; 6-chloro-17α-hydroxy-6-dehydroprogesterone; 6-chloro-17α-hydroxypregna-4,6-diene-3,20-dione; 'bovisynchron').
△¹-**Chlormadinone** *see* Delmadione.
CHLORMADINONE ACETATE* (17α-acetoxy-6-chloro-6-dehydroprogesterone; 'clordion', 'gestafortin', 'gestogan', 'lormin', 'luteran', 'menstridyl', 'nacenyl', 'normenon').
CHLORMADINONE ACETATE WITH ETHINYLESTRADIOL ('amenyl').
CHLORMADINONE ACETATE WITH MESTRANOL (S-3850; 'anconcen', 'C-quens', 'eunomin', 'femigen', 'gesta-

mestrol', 'gestranol', 'ovosiston', 'sequens', 'volenyl').

CHLORMEBUFORM * (N-butyl-N'-(4-chloro-2-methylphenyl)-N-methylformamidine; C-22598; 'buformin', 'ektomin').

Chlormeprazine see Prochlorperazine.

CHLORMEQUAT * ((2-chloroethyl)trimethylammonium chloride; 2-chloro-N,N,N-trimethylethanamium chloride; CCC; chlorcholine; chlorocholine chloride; 'cycocel').

CHLORMERODRIN *** ((3-chloromercuri-2-methoxypropyl)urea; chlormeroprin; mercurylurée; promeran; 'aramercur', 'asahydrin', 'diurone', 'katonil', 'mercardox', 'mercloran', 'mercoral', 'merculest', 'neohydrin', 'oramercur', 'oricur').

CHLORMERODRIN-THEOPHYLLINE (theophylline-merodrin; theomedrine; 'mercuron').

Chlormeroprin see Chlormerodrin.

Chlormethazanone see Chlormezanone.

CHLORMETHAZOLE * (2-(3,4-dichlorophenyl)-4-methyl-1,2,4-oxazolidine-3,5-dione; bioxone; methazole; 'probe', 'tunic').

Chlormethazone see Chlormezanone.

Chlormethiazole * see Clomethiazole.

CHLORMETHINE *** (2,2'-dichloro-N-methyldiethylamine, bis(2-chloroethyl)-methylamine; azotoyperite; chlorethamine; chlorethazine; embichin; mechlorethamine; mustine; nitrogen mustard; NM; HN2; stickstofflost; MBA; C-6866; NSC-762; SK-101; TS-160; 'caryolysin', 'chloramin', 'cloramin', 'dema', 'dichloren', 'erasol', 'mebichloramine', 'mitoxine', 'mustargen', 'nitol', 'nitrogranulogen', 'sinalost').

CHLORMETHINE OXIDE (chlormethine aminoxide; chlormethine-N-oxide; HN2O; HN2-oxide; MBAO; NSC-10107; N-oxydlost; XA-2; 'mitomen', 'mustron', 'nitromin', 'ossiamina', 'ossiclorin', 'oxyamine').

Chlormethylenecycline * see Meclocycline.

CHLORMEZANONE *** (2-(p-chlorophenyl)tetrahydro-3-methyl-4H-1,3-thiazine-4-one 1,1-dioxide; 2-(p-chlorophenyl)-3-methyl-4-metathiazanone 1,1-dioxide; chlormethazanone; chlormethazone; 'supotran', 'trancopal').

CHLORMEZANONE WITH ACETYLSALICYLIC ACID ('tranco-gesic').

CHLORMEZANONE WITH NOVAMINSULFON ('beserol 500').

CHLORMIDAZOLE *** (1-(p-chlorobenzyl)-2-methylbenzimidazole; H-115; 'mucopolycid', 'myco-polycid').

CHLORNAPHAZINE *** (N,N-bis(2-chloroethyl)-2-naphthylamine; 2,2'-dichloro-N-(2-naphthyl)diethylamine; chloronaphthine; CB-1048; R-48; 'alukon', 'chlornaftina', 'cloronaftine', 'erysan').

Chlornidine see Clonidine.

2-CHLOROACETOPHENONE (chloracetophenone; α-chloroacetophenone; phenacyl chloride; tear gas; C.N.; 'chemical mace', 'mace').

17-Chloroacetylajmaline see Lorajmine.

N-(2-Chloroacetyl)diallylamine see Allidochlor.

N-(2-Chloroacetyl)-2,6-diethyl-N-(methoxymethyl)aniline see Alachlor.

Chloroamitriptyline see Chlorproheptadiene.

3-(p-Chloroanilino)-10-(p-chlorophenyl)-2,10-dihydro-2-isopropyliminophenazine see Clofazimine.

p-[2-(5-Chloro-o-anisamido)ethyl]benzoic acid see Meglitinide.

1-[p-[2-(5-Chloro-o-anisamido)ethyl]-phenylsulfonyl]-3-cyclohexylurea see Glibenclamide.

Chloroazodin see Chlorazodin.

o-Chlorobenzalmalononitrile see o-Chlorobenzylidenemalononitrile.

2-(p-Chlorobenzamido)acetohydroxamic acid see Benurestat.

2-[p-[2-(p-Chlorobenzamido)ethyl]-phenoxy]-2-methylpropionic acid see Bezafibrate.

2-(p-Chlorobenzamido)-3-indolepropionic acid see Benzotript.

4-Chloro-1,3-benzenedisulfonamide see Clofenamide.

p-Chlorobenzenesulfonic acid, esters and salts see Closilate(s).

1-(p-Chlorobenzenesulfonyl)-3-cyclohexylurea see Chlorhexamide.

1-(p-Chlorobenzenesulfonyl)-3-(p-dimethylaminophenyl)urea see Glyparamide.

1-(p-Chlorobenzenesulfonyl)-3-(hexahydro(1H)azepin-1-yl)urea see Glypinamide.

4-(p-Chlorobenzenesulfonyl)-1,1-pentamethylenesemicarbazone see Chlorpentazide.

1-(p-Chlorobenzenesulfonyl)-3-piperid-1-ylurea see Chlorpentazide.

1-(p-Chlorobenzenesulfonyl)-3-propylurea see Chlorpropamide.

1-(p-Chlorobenzenesulfonyl)-3-pyrrolidin-1-ylurea see Glyclopyramide.

1-(p-Chlorobenzhydryl)-4-cinnamyl-piperazine see Clocinizine.

1-(p-Chlorobenzhydryl)-4-[2-[2-(2-hydroxyethoxy)ethoxy]ethyl]piperazine see Etodroxizine.

1-(p-Chlorobenzhydryl)-4-[2-(2-hydroxyethoxy)ethyl]piperazine see Hydroxyzine.

1-(p-Chlorobenzhydryl)-4-(m-methylbenzyl)piperazine see Meclozine.

1-(p-Chlorobenzhydryl)-4-methyl-1,4-diazacycloheptane see Homochlorcyclizine.

1-(p-Chlorobenzhydryl)-4-methylhomo-piperazine see Homochlorcyclizine.

1-(p-Chlorobenzhydryl)-4-methyl-piperazine see Chlorcyclizine.

1-[2-(o-Chlorobenzhydryloxy)ethyl]-4-(o-methylbenzyl)piperazine see Chlorbenoxamine.

4-[2-(p-Chlorobenzhydryloxy)ethyl]-morpholine see Difencloxamine.

1-[2-(*p*-Chlorobenzhydryloxy)ethyl]-**
piperidine *see* Cloperastine.
3-(*p*-Chlorobenzhydryloxy)-1-methyl-**
pyrrolidine *see* Pyroxamine.
3-(*p*-Chlorobenzhydryloxy)tropane** *see*
Clobenztropine.
1-[2-(*o*-Chlorobenzhydrylthio)ethyl]-4-**
(*o*-methylbenzyl)piperazine *see* Bentipimine.
CHLOROBENZILATE[*] (ethyl 2,2-bis(*p*-
chlorophenyl)glycolate; ethyl 4-chloro-α-
(4-chlorophenyl)-α-hydroxybenzeneacetate;
ethyl 4,4′-dichlorobenzilate; chlorbenzilate;
G-23922; 'folbex').
(Chlorobenzimidazolylmethyl)-
dimethylphenylethylenediamine *see*
Midamaline.
6-Chloro-1,2-benzisothiazolin-3-one *see*
Ticlatone.
***p*-Chlorobenzoic acid ester of 4-butyl-4-**
hydroxymethyl-1,2-diphenyl-3,5-
pyrazolidinedione *see* Feclobuzone.
6-Chloro-2H-1,2,4-benzothiadiazine-7-
sulfonamide 1,1-dioxide *see* Chlorothiazide.
5-Chloro-2-benzoxalinone *see* Chlorzoxazone.
Chlorobenzoxamine *see* Chlorbenzoxamine.
N-(*p*-Chlorobenzoyl)-*N*-(2-hydroxyethyl)-**
3-methyl-2-norbornanemethylamine
see Clocanfamide.
1-(*p*-Chlorobenzoyl)-5-methoxy-2-methyl-
3-indoleacetic acid *see* Indometacin.
3-(*p*-Chlorobenzoyl)-6-methoxy-2-
methyl-1-indoleacetic acid *see*
Clometacin.
2-[2-[1-(*p*-Chlorobenzoyl)-5-methoxy-2-
methylindol-3-yl]acetamido]-2-deoxy-
D-glucose *see* Glucametacin.
5-[3-[(*p*-Chlorobenzoylmethyl)amino]-
propyl]-10,11-dihydro-5H-dibenz(b,f)-
azepine *see* Lofepramine.
N-(*p*-Chlorobenzoylmethyl)-3-(10,11-**
dihydro-5H-dibenz(b,f)azepin-5-yl)-*N*-
methylpropylamine *see* Lofepramine.
2-(*p*-(*p*-Chlorobenzoyl)phenoxy)-2-
methylpropionic acid isopropyl ester
see Fenofibrate.
1-(*p*-Chlorobenzoyl)-3-(1H-tetrazol-3-yl-
methyl)indole *see* Intrazole.
N-(*p*-Chlorobenzoyl)-L-tryptophan** *see*
Benzotript.
Chlorobenztropine *see* Clobenztropine.
((+)-*N*-(*o*-Chlorobenzyl)amphetamine
see Clobenzorex.
1-(*o*-Chlorobenzyl)-2-[2-[bis(1-methyl-
propyl)amino]-1-hydroxyethyl]pyrrole
see Viminol.
***p*-Chlorobenzyl *p*-chlorophenyl sulfide**
see Chlorbenside.
N-(*o*-Chlorobenzyl)dexamphetamine** *see*
Clobenzorex.
1-(*o*-Chlorobenzyl)-α-[(di-*sec*-butylamino)-
methyl]pyrrole-2-methanol *see* Viminol.
α-(*p*-Chlorobenzyl)-*p*-(2-diethylamino-
ethoxy)-*p*′-methylbenzhydrol *see*
Triparanol.

2-(*p*-Chlorobenzyl)-1-(2-diethylamino-
ethyl)-5-nitrobenzimidazole *see*
Clonitazene.
2-[(*p*-Chlorobenzyl)(2-dimethylamino-
ethyl)amino]pyridine *see* Chloropyramine.
N-(*p*-Chlorobenzyl-*N*′,*N*′-dimethyl-*N*-**
pyrid-2-ylethylenediamine *see* Chloropyramine.
o-**CHLOROBENZYLIDENEMALONO-**
NITRILE (*o*-chlorobenzalmalononitrile;
C.S.).
N-(*o*-Chlorobenzyl)-α-methylphenethyl-**
amine *see* Clobenzorex.
3-(*p*-Chlorobenzyl)octahydroquinolizine
see Cloquinozine.
4-(*o*-Chlorobenzyl)-5-oxo-4-phenylhexa-
noic acid *see* Caprochlorone.
N-[2-(*p*-Chlorobenzyl)prop-2-yl]carbamic**
acid ethyl ester *see* Cloforex.
1-(*p*-Chlorobenzyl)-2-pyrrolid-1-ylmethyl-
benzimidazole *see* Clemizole.
1-[α-[*N*-(*o*-Chlorobenzyl)pyrryl]]-2-di-
***sec*-butylamine ethanol** *see* Viminol.
3-(*p*-Chlorobenzyl)quinolizidine *see*
Cloquinozine.
5-(*o*-Chlorobenzyl)-4,5,6,7-tetrahydro-
thieno(3,2-c)pyridine *see* Ticlopidine.
1-[(*p*-Chlorobenzyl)thio]-4-fluorobenzene
see Fluorbenside.
2-[[4′-Chlorobiphenyl-1-yl)acetyl]-1H-
indene-1,3(2H)-dione *see* Chlorophacinone.
2-(4′-Chlorobiphenyl-1-yloxy)-2-methyl-
propionic acid methyl ester *see* Methyl
clofenapate.
4-[3-(3-Chloro-4-biphenylyloxy)propyl]-
morpholine *see* Chlordimorine.
2-Chloro-*N*,*N*-bis(2-chloroethyl)-1-propyl-
amine *see* Novembichin.
2-Chloro-4,6-bis(diethylamino)-*s*-triazine
see Chlorazine.
2-Chloro-4,6-bis(ethylamino)-*s*-triazine
see Simazine.
2-Chloro-4,6-bis(isopropylamino)-*s*-
triazine *see* Propazine.
6-Chloro-*N*,*N*′-bis(1-methylethyl)-1,3,5-
triazine *see* Propazine.
Chlorobutanol[***] *see* Chlorbutol.
4-Chlorobut-2-yn-1-yl *m*-chlorocarbanilate
see Barban.
4-Chlorobut-2-yn-1-yl (*m*-chlorophenyl)-
carbamate *see* Barban.
Chlorocamphamide *see* Clocanfamide.
Chlorocanfamide *see* Clocanfamide.
3-Chloro-5-[3-(4-carbamoyl-4-piperid-1-
ylpiperid-1-yl)propyl]-10,11-dihydro-
5H-dibenz(b,f)azepine *see* Clocapramine.
m-**Chlorocarbanilic acid esters** *see*
Barban; Chlorbufam; Chlorpropham.
m-**Chlorocarbanilic acid 2-chlorobutynyl**
ester *see* Barban.
'Chlorocarbon' *see* Carbon tetrachloride.
CHLOROCARVACROL ('carvasept',
'hadensa', 'tricranolin', 'trikranolin').
Chlorochin *see* Chloroquine.
3′-Chloro-4′-(*p*-chlorobenzoyl)-3,5-

diiodosalicylanilide *see* Salantel.
1-Chloro-4[(*p*-chlorobenzyl)thio]benzene *see* Chlorbenside.
Chloro-(3-chloro-4-cyclohexylphenyl)-acetic acid *see* Fenclorac.
3-[5-Chloro-α-(*p*-chloro-β-hydroxyphenethyl)-2-thenyl]-4-hydroxycoumarin *see* Ticlomarol.
6-Chloro-3-chloromethyl-3,4-dihydro-2-methyl-7-sulfamoylbenzothiadiazine dioxide *see* Methyclothiazide.
N-(*p*-Chloro-α-chloromethylphenacyl)-2,2-dichloroacetamide *see* Cloponone.
3-Chloro-3-(3-chloro-2-nitrophenyl)pyrrole *see* Pyrrolnitrin.
5-Chloro-N-(2-chloro-4-nitrophenyl)-salicylamide *see* Niclosamide.
3'-Chloro-4'-(*p*-chlorophenoxy)-3,5-diiodosalicylanilide *see* Rafoxanide.
7-Chloro-5-(*o*-chlorophenyl)-1,3-dihydro-3-hydroxy-2H-1,4-benzodiazepin-2-one *see* Lorazepam.
4-Chloro-α-(4-chlorophenyl)-α-hydroxybenzeneacetic acid ethyl ester *see* Chlorobenzilate.
4-Chloro-α-(4-chlorophenyl)-α-hydroxybenzeneacetic acid 1-methylethyl ester *see* Chloropropylate.
***p*-Chloro-α-(*p*-chlorophenyl)-α-methylbenzyl alcohol** *see* Chlorfenethol.
1-Chloro-4-[[(4-chlorophenyl)methyl]-thio]benzene *see* Chlorbenside.
8-Chloro-6-(*o*-chlorophenyl)-1-methyl-4H-s-triazolo(4,3-a)(1,4)benzodiazepine *see* Triazolam.
3-Chloro-3-(*p*-chlorophenyl)propionic acid methyl ester *see* Chlorfenpropmethyl.
***p*-Chloro-α-(*p*-chlorophenyl)-α-pyrid-3-ylbenzyl alcohol** *see* Parinol.
10-Chloro-11b-(*o*-chlorophenyl)-2,3,7,11b-tetrahydrooxazolo(3,2-d)(1,4)benzodiazepin-6(5H)-one *see* Cloxazolam.
4-Chloro-α-[(*p*-chlorophenyl)thio]toluene *see* Chlorbenside.
4-Chloro-α-(4-chlorophenyl)-α-trichloromethylbenzenemethanol *see* Dicofol.
***p*-Chloro-α-(*p*-chlorophenyl)-α-trichloromethylbenzyl alcohol** *see* Dicofol.
7-Chloro-2-(*o*-chlorostyryl)-4-[(4-diethylamino-1-methylbutyl)amino]quinoline *see* Aminoquinol.
Chlorocholine chloride *see* Chlormequat.
'Chlorocid S' *see* Chloramphenicol hemisuccinate sodium salt.
CHLOROCRESOL*** (4-chloro-3-methylphenol; *p*-chloro-*m*-cresol; 6-chloro-3-hydroxytoluene; 'baktolan', 'candaseptic', 'parmetol', 'peritonan').
Chlorocrotylmercaptomethylpenicillin *see* Penicillin S.
CHLOROCYANOHYDRIN (chloral hydrocyanide; trichloroacetonitrile).
2-Chloro-6-(1-cyano-1-methylethylamino)-4-ethylamino-s-triazine *see* Cyanazine.
**2-Chloro-8β-(cyanomethyl)-6-methyl-

ergoline *see* Lergotrile.
***exo*-3-Chloro-*endo*-6-cyano-2-norbornanone** *see* 5-Chloro-6-oxo-2-norbornanecarbonitrile.
1-(N-(3-Chloro-4-cyanophenyl)carbamoyl]guanidine *see* Cloguanamile.
Chlorocyclizine *see* Chlorcyclizine.
7-Chloro-5-cyclohexen-1-yl-1,3-dihydro-2H-1,4-benzodiazepin-2-one *see* Nortetrazepam.
7-Chloro-5-cyclohexen-1-yl-1,3-dihydro-1-methyl-2H-1,4-benzodiazepin-2-one *see* Tetrazepam.
3-(3-Chloro-4-cyclohexylbenzoyl)-propionic acid *see* Bucloxic acid.
6-Chloro-2-cyclohexyl-3-oxo-5-isoindolinesulfonamide *see* Clorexolone.
4-(3-Chloro-4-cyclohexylphenyl)-4-oxobutyric acid *see* Bucloxic acid.
5-Chloro-2-cyclohexyl-6-sulfamoylphthalimidine *see* Clorexolone.
6-Chloro-3-cyclopentylmethyl-3,4-dihydro-7-sulfamoylbenzothiadiazine dioxide *see* Cyclopenthiazide.
7-Chloro-2-[(cyclopropylmethyl)amino]-5-phenyl(3H)-1,4-benzodiazepine-4-oxide *see* Cyprazepam.
7-Chloro-1-cyclopropylmethyl-1,3-dihydro-5-phenyl-2H-1,4-benzodiazepin-2-one *see* Prazepam.
6-Chloro-6-dehydro-17α-hydroxyprogesterone *see* Chlormadinone.
7-Chloro-6-demethyl-6-methylenetetracycline *see* Meclocycline.
7-Chloro-6-demethyltetracycline *see* Demeclocycline.
7(S)Chloro-7-deoxylincomycin *see* Clindamycin.
10-Chlorodeserpidine *see* Chloroserpidine.
10-Chloro-11-desmethoxyreserpine *see* Chloroserpidine.
***cis*-4-[3-(2-Chlorodibenz(b,e)oxepin-11(6H)-ylidene)propyl]-1-piperazineethanol** *see* Pinoxepin.
6-Chloro-3-dichloromethyl-3,4-dihydro-7-sulfamoylbenzothiadiazine dioxide *see* Trichlormethiazide.
5-Chloro-2-(2,4-dichlorophenoxy)phenol *see* Triclosan.
2-Chloro-1-(2,4-dichlorophenyl)vinyl diethyl phosphate *see* Clofenvinfos.
6-Chloro-1,6-didehydroretroprogesterone *see* Trengestone.
N-[2-Chloro-1-[(diethoxyphosphinothioyl)thio]ethyl]phthalimide *see* Dialifos.
6-Chloro-3(2H)-[[(diethoxyphosphinothioyl)thio]methyl]benzoxazol-2-one *see* Phosalone.
5-Chloro-2-[*p*-(2-diethylaminoethoxy)-phenyl]benzothiazole *see* Haletazole.
α-Chloro-α'-[*p*-(2-diethylaminoethoxy)phenyl]stilbene *see* Clomifene.
2-Chloro-4-diethylamino-6-ethylamino-s-triazine *see* Trietazine.
2'-Chloro-2-[(2-diethylaminoethyl)ethylamino]acetanilide *see* Clodacaine.
**7-Chloro-1-(2-diethylaminoethyl)-5-(*o*-

fluorophenyl)-1,3-dihydro-2H-1,4-
benzodiazepin-2-one *see* Flurazepam.
6-Chloro-2-diethylamino-4-isopropyl-
amino-*s*-triazine *see* Ipazine.
7-Chloro-4-(4-diethylamino-1-methyl-
butylamino)-3-methylquinoline *see*
Sontoquine.
(2-Chloro-3-diethylamino-1-methyl-3-oxo-
1-propenyl) dimethyl phosphate *see*
Phosphamidon.
2-Chloro-10-(3-diethylaminopropionyl)-
phenothiazine *see* Chloracyzine.
5-Chloro-7-(3-diethylaminopropylamino-
methyl)-8-quinolinol *see* Clamoxyquin.
2-Chloro-10-(3-diethylaminopropyl)-
phenothiazine *see* Chlorproethazine.
[2-Chloro-2-(diethylcarbamoyl)-1-
methylvinyl] dimethyl phosphate *see*
Phosphamidon.
2-Chloro-*N,N*-diethyl-3-hydroxycroton-
amide dimethyl phosphate *see*
Phosphamidon.
6-Chloro-*N,N*-diethyl-*N'*-(1-methylethyl)-
1,3,5-triazine-2,4-diamine *see* Ipazine.
2-Chloro-*N*-(2,6-diethylphenyl)-*N*-
(methoxymethyl)acetamide *see* Alachlor.
6-Chloro-*N,N'*-diethyl-1,3,5-triazine-2,4-
diamine *see* Simazine.
9-Chloro-6α,11β-difluoro-21-hydroxy-16α-
methylpregna-1,4-diene-3,20-dione
see Halocortolone.
9-Chloro-6α,11β-difluoro-16α-methyl-
pregna-1,4-dien-21-ol-3,20-dione *see*
Halocortolone.
Chlorodifon *see* Tetradifon.
3-(2-Chloro-9,10-dihydroacridin-9-yl)-
N,N-dimethylpropylamine *see*
Clomacran.
10-Chloro-5,10-dihydroarsacridine *see*
Phenarsazine chloride.
1'-[3-(3-Chloro-10,11-dihydro-5H-dibenz-
(b,f)azepin-5-yl)propyl][1,4'-bipiper-
idine]-4'-carboxamide *see* Clocapramine.
4'-Chloro-2-[[3-(10,11-dihydro-5H-dibenz-
(b,f)azepin-5-yl)propyl]methylamino]-
acetophenone *see* Lofepramine.
1-(8-Chloro-10,11-dihydrodibenzo(b,f)-
thiepin-10-yl)-4-methylpiperazine *see*
Clorotepine.
S-[2-Chloro-1-(1,3-dihydro-1,3-dioxo-2H-
isoindol-2-yl)ethyl] *O,O*-diethyl
phosphorodithioate *see* Dialifos.
7-Chloro-2,3-dihydro-2,2-dihydroxy-5-
phenyl-1H-1,4-benzodiazepine-3-
carboxylic acid *see* Clorazepic acid.
3-Chloro-10,11-dihydro-5-(3-dimethyl-
aminopropyl)-5H-dibenzo(b,f)azepine
see Clomipramine.
11-Chloro-8,12b-dihydro-2,8-dimethyl-
12b-phenyl-4H(1,3)-oxazino(3,2-d)(1,4)-
benzodiazepine-4,7(6H)-dione *see*
Ketazolam.
7-Chloro-1,3-dihydro-3-hydroxy-1-methyl-
5-phenyl-2H-1,4-benzodiazepin-2-one
see Temazepam.
7-Chloro-1,3-dihydro-3-hydroxy-1-
methyl-5-phenyl-2H-1,4-benzodiazepin-

2-one dimethylcarbamate *see*
Camazepam.
7-Chloro-1,3-dihydro-3-hydroxy-5-phenyl-
2H-1,4-benzodiazepin-2-one *see* Oxazepam.
7-Chloro-3,4-dihydro-10-hydroxy-3-
(α,α,α-trifluoro-*p*-tolyl)-1,9(2H)-
acridandione *see* Floxacrine.
6-Chloro-3,4-dihydro-3-isobutyl-2H-
1,2,4-benzothiadiazine-7-sulfonamide
1,1-dioxide *see* Butizide.
7-Chloro-3,3a-dihydro-2H,9H-isoxazolo-
(3,2-b)(1,3)benzoxazin-9-one *see*
Seclazone.
6-Chloro-3,4-dihydro-3-(α-methylbenzyl)-
2H-1,2,4-benzothiadiazine-7-sulfon-
amide 1,1-dioxide *see* Bemetizide.
7-Chloro-2,3-dihydro-1-methyl-5-phenyl-
1H-1,4-benzodiazepine *see* Medazepam.
7-Chloro-1,3-dihydro-1-methyl-5-phenyl-
2H-1,4-benzodiazepin-2-one *see* Diazepam.
7-Chloro-1,3-dihydro-1-methyl-5-phenyl-
2H-1,4-benzodiazepine-2-thione *see*
Sulazepam.
8-Chloro-10,11-dihydro-10-(4-methyl-
piperazin-1-yl)dibenzo(b,f)thiepine
see Clorotepine.
6-Chloro-3,4-dihydro-2-methyl-7-sulfa-
moyl-2H-1,2,4-benzothiadiazine-3-
carboxylic acid 1,1-dioxide methyl
ester *see* Carmetizide.
6-Chloro-3,4-dihydro-3-(5-norbornen-2-
yl)-7-sulfamoyl-2H-1,2,4-benzothia-
diazine 1,1-dioxide *see* Cyclothiazide.
2-Chloro-10-[3-[4-(dihydro-2(3H)-
oxofuran-3-yl)-4-hydroxypiperid-1-yl]-
propyl]phenothiazine *see* Furomazine.
(7-Chloro-1,3-dihydro-2-oxo-5-phenyl-2H-
1,4-benzodiazepin-1-ylmethyl)dimeth-
ylphosphine oxide *see* Fosazepam.
7-Chloro-1,3-dihydro-5-phenyl-1,4-
benzodiazepin-2-one *see* Demethyldiazepam.
8-Chloro-4,5-dihydro-1-phenyl-3H-1,5-
benzodiazepin-2-one *see* Lofendazam.
7-Chloro-1,3-dihydro-5-phenyl-2H-1,4-
benzodiazepin-2-one 4-oxide *see*
Demoxazepam.
6-Chloro-3,4-dihydro-3-(1-phenylethyl)-
7-sulfamoyl-2H-1,2,4-benzothiadiazine
1,1-dioxide *see* Bemetizide.
7-Chloro-1,3-dihydro-5-phenyl-1-prop-2-
ynyl-2H-1,4-benzodiazepin-2-one *see*
Pinazepam.
7-Chloro-1,3-dihydro-5-phenyl-1-(2,2,2-
trifluoroethyl)-2H-1,4-benzodiazepin-
2-one *see* Halazepam.
6-Chloro-3,4-dihydro-3-succinimidometh-
yl-2H-1,2,4-benzothiadiazine-7-sulfon-
amide 1,1-dioxide *see* Sumetizide.
6-Chloro-3,4-dihydro-7-sulfamoylbenzo-
thiadiazine dioxide *see* Hydrochlorothiazide.
6-Chloro-3,4-dihydro-3-[(2,2,2-trifluoro-
ethyl)thiomethyl]-2H-1,2,4-benzo-
thiadiazine-7-sulfonamide 1,1-dioxide
see Epitizide.

91

6-Chloro-3β,17-dihydroxypregna-4,6-dien-20-one *see* Clogestone.

6α-Chloro-17,21-dihydroxypregna-1,4-diene-3,11,20-trione *see* Chloroprednisone.

7-Chloro-1-(2,3-dihydroxypropyl)-5-(*o*-fluorophenyl)-1,3-dihydro-2H-1,4-benzodiazepin-2-one *see* Proflazepam.

6-Chloro-4-(2,3-dihydroxypropyl)-2-methyl-2H-1,4-benzoxazin-3(4H)-one *see* Diproxadol.

4'-Chloro-3,5-diiodosalicylanilide acetate *see* Clioxanide.

Chlorodimeform *see* Chlorphenamidine.

Chlorodimenol *see* Clobutinol.

4'-Chloro-3,5-dimethoxy-4-(2-morpholino-ethoxy)benzophenone *see* Morclofone.

4-Chloro-4'-[(dimethoxyphosphinothio-yl)oxy]azobenzene *see* Azothoate.

2-[*p*-Chloro-α-(2-dimethylaminoethoxy)-benzyl]pyridine *see* Carbinoxamine; Rotoxamine.

2-Chloro-α-(2-dimethylaminoethyl)-benzhydrol *see* Clofedanol.

2-[*p*-Chloro-α-(2-dimethylaminoethyl)-benzyl]pyridine *see* Chlorpheniramine.

8-Chloro-11-(2-dimethylaminoethyl)-6,11-dihydro-5H-benzo(5,6)cyclohepta-(1,2-b)pyridine *see* Closiramine.

7-Chloro-10-(2-dimethylaminoethyl)-5,10-dihydro-11H-dibenzo(b,e)(1,4)-diazepin-11-one *see* Clobenzepam.

-Chloro-α-(2-dimethylamino-1-methyl-ethyl)-α-methylphenethyl alcohol *see* Clobutinol.

2-Chloro-4-dimethylamino-6-methyl-pyrimidine *see* Crimidine.

7-Chloro-4-dimethylamino-1,4,4a,5,5a,6,11,12a-octahydro-3,6,10,12,12a-penta-hydroxy-N-(hydroxymethyl)-6-methyl-1,11-dioxo-2-naphthacenecarboxamide *see* Clomocycline.

7-Chloro-4-dimethylamino-1,4,4a,5,5a,6,11,12a-octahydro-3,6,10,12,12a-penta-hydroxy-1,11-dioxo-2-naphthacene-carboxamide *see* Demeclocycline.

2-Chloro-10-(3-dimethylaminopropionyl)-phenothiazine *see* Cloracizin.

2-Chloro-9-(3-dimethylaminopropyl)-acridan *see* Clomacran.

3-Chloro-5-(3-dimethylaminopropyl)-10,11-dihydro(5H)dibenzo(b,f)azepine *see* Clomipramine.

3-Chloro-5-(3-dimethylaminopropyl-idene)(5H)dibenzo(a,d)cycloheptene *see* Chlorproheptatriene.

3-Chloro-5-(3-dimethylaminopropyl-idene)-10,11-dihydro(5H)dibenzo(a,d)-cycloheptene *see* Chlorproheptadiene.

3-Chloro-11-[3-(dimethylamino)propyl-idene]-5,6-dihydromorphanthridine *see* Elanzepine.

2-Chloro-10-(3-dimethylaminopropyl-idene)thioxanthene *see* Chlorprothixene.

2-Chloro-10-(3-dimethylaminopropyl)-phenothiazine *see* Chlorpromazine.

5-Chloro-1-(3-dimethylaminopropyl)-3-phenyl-2-benzimidazolinone *see* Clodazon.

6-Chloro-3-(1,2-dimethylbutyl)-3,4-dihydro-7-sulfamoyl-2H-1,2,4-benzo-thiadiazine 1,1-dioxide *see* Melbutizide.

5-Chloro-3-(1,1-dimethylethyl)-6-methyl-2,4(1H,3H)-pyrimidinedione *see* Terbacil.

2-Chloro-4-(1,1-dimethylethyl)phenyl methyl methylphosphoramidate *see* Crufomate.

p-Chloro-α,α-dimethyl-N-(2-hydroxy-ethyl)phenethylamine *see* Etolorex.

o-Chloro-α,α-dimethylphenethylamine *see* Clortermine.

p-Chloro-α,α-dimethylphenethylamine *see* Chlorphentermine.

2-(*p*-Chloro-α,α-dimethylphenethyl-amino)ethanol *see* Etolorex.

2-Chloro-4,5-dimethylphenyl methyl-carbamate *see* Carbanolate.

7-Chloro-1-(dimethylphosphinylmethyl)-1,3-dihydro-5-phenyl-2H-1,4-benzo-diazepin-2-one *see* Fosazepam.

4-Chloro-N-(*cis*-2,6-dimethylpiperid-1-yl)-3-sulfamoylbenzamide *see* Clopamide.

2-Chloro-5-[(3,5-dimethylpiperidino)-sulfonyl]benzoic acid *see* Tibric acid.

2-Chloro-N,N-dimethyl-△9,γ-propylamine *see* Chlorprothixene.

N1-(5-Chloro-2,6-dimethylpyrimidin-4-yl)sulfanilamide *see* Sulfaclomide.

4-Chloro-2',6'-dimethyl-5-sulfamoyl-salicylanilide *see* Xipamide.

3'-Chloro-2,4'-dimethylvaleranilide *see* Pentanochlor.

1-CHLORO-2,4-DINITROBENZENE (dinitrochlorobenzene; DNCB).

4'-Chloro-2,6-dioxocyclohexanecarbo-thioanilide *see* Ontianil.

1-(*o*-Chloro-α,α-diphenylbenzyl)imidazole *see* Clotrimazole.

2-Chloro-1,2-diphenyl-1-[*p*-(2-diethyl-aminoethoxy)phenyl]ethylene *see* Clomifene; Enclomifene; Zuclomifene).

2-[*p*-(2-Chloro-1,2-diphenylvinyl)phen-oxy]triethylamine *see* Clomifene; Enclomifene; Zuclomifene.

2-Chloro-N-N-dipropenylacetamide *see* Allidochlor.

5-Chloro-2,4-disulfamoyltoluene *see* Disulfamide.

4-Chloro-N-1,3-dithietan-2-ylidene-2-methylaniline *see* Nimidane.

1-Chloro-2,3-epoxypropane *see* Epichloro-hydrin.

4-Chloroestr-4-en-17β-ol-3-one *see* Norclostebol.

CHLOROETHANE (ethyl chloride; ether hydrochloric; muriatic ether; 'anodynon', 'chelen', 'chloryl', 'kelene', 'kelin', 'narcotile').

2-CHLOROETHANOL (ethylene chloro-hydrin; glycol chlorohydrin; 'cinecol'). *See also* Chloroethyl mesilate; Chloroethyl salicylate.

3-(2-Chloroethoxy)-6-cyano-9-fluoro-

pregna-3,5-diene-11β,16α,17,21-tetrol-20-one 16,17-acetonide 21-acetate *see* Cicortonide.

3-Chloro-N-ethoxy-2,6-dimethoxybenzenecarboximidic acid anhydride with benzoic acid *see* Benzoximate.

3-(2-Chloroethoxy)-9α-fluoro-6-formyl-3,5-pregnadiene-11β,16α,17α,21-tetrol-20-one 16α,17α-acetonide *see* Formocortal.

3-(2-Chloroethoxy)-9-fluoro-11β,16α,17,21-tetrahydroxy-20-oxopregna-3,5-diene 6-carbonitrile cyclic 16,17-acetal with acetone 21-acetate *see* Cicortonide.

10-Chloro-3-ethoxymethyl-2,3,6,9-tetrahydro-9-oxo-p-dioxino(2,3-g)quinoline-8-carboxylic acid ethyl ester *see* Quincarbate.

2-Chloro-4-ethylamino-6-isopropylamino-s-triazine *see* Atrazine.

6-Chloro-2-ethylamino-4-methyl-4-phenyl-4H-3,1-benzoxazine *see* Etifoxine.

6-Chloro-2-ethylamino-4-phenyl-4H-3,1-benzothiazine *see* Etasuline.

2-[[4-Chloro-6-(ethylamino)-1,3,5-triazin-2-yl]amino]-2-methylpropionitrile *see* Cyanazine.

p-Chloro-α-ethylbenzyl alcohol *see* 1-(p-Chlorophenyl)-1-propanol.

3-(2-Chloroethyl)-2-[bis(2-chloroethyl)-amino]tetrahydro-2H-1,3,2-oxaphosphorine 2-oxide *see* Trofosfamide.

2-Chloroethyl N,N-bis(2-chloroethyl)-N'-(3-hydroxypropyl)phosphorodiamidate *see* Defosfamide.

3-(2-Chloroethyl)-2-(2-chloroethylamino)-2H-1,3,2-oxazaphosphorinane 2-oxide *see* Ifosfamide.

3-(2-Chloroethyl)-2-(2-chloroethylamino)-tetrahydro-2H-1,3,2-oxaphosphorine 2-oxide *see* Ifosfamide.

1-(2-Chloroethyl)-3-cyclohexyl-1-nitrosourea *see* Lomustine.

S-(2-CHLOROETHYL)CYSTEINE (3-(2-chloroethylthio)alanine; CB-1592).

N-(2-Chloroethyl)dibenzylamine *see* Dibenamine.

2-(2-Chloroethyl)-2,3-dihydro-4H-1,3-benzoxazin-4-one *see* Chlorthenoxazine.

6-Chloro-3-ethyl-3,4-dihydro-7-sulfamoylbenzothiadiazine dioxide *see* Ethiazide.

2-Chloroethyl 2-[4-(1,1-dimethylethyl)-phenoxy]-1-methylethyl sulfite ester *see* 2-(p-tert-Butylphenoxy)isopropyl 2-chloroethyl sulfite.

2-CHLOROETHYL ESILATE (2-chloroethyl ethanesulfonate; 2-chloroethyl esylate; NSC-50257).

5-[(2-Chloroethyl)(2-fluoroethyl)amino]-6-methyluracil *see* Ftordopan.

7-Chloro-4-[4-[ethyl(2-hydroxyethyl)-amino]-1-methylbutylamino]quinoline *see* Hydroxychloroquine.

2-CHLOROETHYL MESILATE (2-chloroethyl methanesulfonate; 2-chloroethyl mesylate; CB-1506; NSC-18061).

2-[(2-Chloroethyl)methylamino]ethyl acetate *see* Acetylcholine mustard.

1-(2-Chloroethyl)-3-(4-methylcyclohexyl)-1-nitrosourea *see* Semustine.

6-Chloro-N-ethyl-N'-(1-methylethyl)-1,3,5-triazine-2,4-diamine *see* Atrazine.

N-(2-Chloroethyl)-N-(1-methyl-2-phenoxyethyl)benzylamine *see* Phenoxybenzamine.

5-(2-Chloroethyl)-4-methylthiazole *see* Clomethiazole.

1-(2-CHLOROETHYL)-1-NITROSOUREA (NSC-47547).

5-Chloro-3-ethylpent-4-en-1-yn-3-ol *see* Ethchlorvynol.

1-Chloro-3-ethylpent-1-en-4-yn-3-ol *see* Ethchlorvynol.

Chloroethylphenamide *see* Beclamide.

3-[1-[p-(2-Chloroethyl)phenyl]butyl]-4-hydroxycoumarin *see* Clocoumarol.

3-[p-(2-Chloroethyl)-α-propylbenzyl]-4-hydroxycoumarin *see* Clocoumarol.

2-CHLOROETHYL SALICYLATE (ethylenechlorohydrin salicylate).

7-Chloro-2-ethyl-1,2,3,4-tetrahydro-4-oxo-6-quinazolinesulfonamide *see* Quinethazone.

7-Chloro-2-ethyl-1,2,3,4-tetrahydro-6-sulfamoylquinazolin-4(3H)-one *see* Quinethazone.

Chloroethylthiamine *see* Beclotiamine.

Chloroethylthioalanine *see* Chloroethylcysteine.

(2-Chloroethyl)trimethylammonium chloride *see* Chlormequat.

17α-Chloroethynyl-19-nor-4,9(10)-androstadien-3-one *see* Ethynerone.

Chlorofenizon *see* Chlorfenson.

2-(4-Chloro-4'-fluorobenzhydryloxy)-ethylamine *see* Halonamine.

6-Chloro-3-(p-fluorobenzyl)-3,4-dihydro-(2H)-1,2,4-benzothiadiazine-7-sulfonamide-1,1-dioxide *see* Paraflutizide.

9-Chloro-6α-fluoro-11β,21-dihydroxy-16α-methylpregna-1,4-diene-3,20-dione *see* Clocortolone.

21-Chloro-9α-fluoro-11β,17α-dihydroxy-16α-methylpregna-1,4-diene-3,20-dione *see* Clobetasol.

21-Chloro-9α-fluoro-11β-hydroxy-16α,17α-isopropylidenedioxypregn-4-ene-3,20-dione *see* Halcinonide.

21-Chloro-9α-fluoro-11α-hydroxy-16β-methylpregna-1,4-diene-3,11,20-trione *see* Clobetasone.

9-Chloro-6α-fluoro-16α-methylpregna-1,4-diene-11β,21-diol-3,20-dione *see* Clocortolone.

2-[[p-Chloro-α-(p-fluorophenyl)benzyl]-oxy]ethylamine *see* Halonamine.

7-Chloro-5-(o-fluorophenyl)-2,3-dihydro-1-(2,2,2-trifluoroethyl)-1H-1,4-benzodiazepine *see* Fletazepam.

6-[3-(2-Chloro-6-fluorophenyl)-5-methyl-4-isoxazolecarboxamido]penicillanic acid *see* Flucloxacillin.

3-(2-Chloro-6-fluorophenyl)-5-methylisoxazol-4-ylpenicillin *see* Flucloxacillin.

10-Chloro-11b-(o-fluorophenyl)-2,3,7,11b-tetrahydro-7-(2-hydroxyethyl)oxazolo-(3,2-d)(1,4)benzodiazepin-6(5H)-one *see* Flutazolam.

1-Chloro-4-[[(4-fluorophenyl)thio]-methyl]benzene *see* Fluorbenside.

4-Chloro-α-[(p-fluorophenyl)thio]toluene *see* Fluorbenside.

21-Chloro-9-fluoropregn-4-ene-11β,16α,17-triol,3,20-dione cyclic acetal with acetone *see* Halcinonide.

21-Chloro-9-fluoro-11β,16α,17-trihydroxy-pregn-4-ene-3,20-dione cyclic acetal with acetone *see* Halcinonide.

Chloroflurazole *see* Chlorflurazole.

CHLOROFORM (trichloromethane; formyl terchloride).

Chloroformyl chloride *see* Phosgene.

Chlorofos (tr) *see* Metrifonate.

4-Chloro-N-(2-furfuryl)-5-sulfamoyl-anthranilic acid *see* Furosemide.

CHLOROGENIC ACID (3-caffeoylquinic acid; 3-(3,4-dihydroxycinnamoyl)quinic acid).

Chloroguanide* *see* Proguanil.

Chloroguanil *see* Proguanil.

2-Chloro-10-[3-(hexahydropyrrolo(1,2-a)-pyrazin-2(1H)-yl)propionyl]pheno-thiazine *see* Azaclorine.

'Chlorohex' *see* Chlorhexidine.

Chlorohexidine *see* Chlorhexidine.

CHLOROHYDRIN (3-chloro-1,2-propanediol; 3-chloropropylene glycol; α-chlorohydrin; glycerol α-monochlorohydrin; U-5897).

Chlorohydrin dinitrate *see* Clonitrate.

4-Chloro-N-[2-(hydroxyamino)-2-oxoethyl]benzamide *see* Benurestat.

4-Chloro-17β-hydroxyandrost-4-en-3-one *see* Clostebol.

5-Chloro-2-hydroxydiphenylmethane *see* Clorofene.

4-Chloro-17β-hydroxyestr-4-en-3-one *see* Norclostebol.

7-Chloro-4-[4-(2-hydroxyethylamino)-1-methylbutylamino]quinoline *see* Cletoquine.

2-[[[p-Chloro-N-(2-hydroxyethyl)benz-amido]methyl]-3-methylnorbornane *see* Clocanfamide.

p-Chloro-N-(2-hydroxyethyl)-α,α-dimethylphenethylamine *see* Etolorex.

p-Chloro-N-(2-hydroxyethyl)-N-(3-methylnorborn-2-ylmethyl)benzamide *see* Clocanfamide.

5-Chloro-3-[[[4-(2-hydroxyethyl)-piperazin-1-yl]carbonyl]methyl]-benzothiazolin-2-one *see* Tiaramide.

2-Chloro-9-[3-[4-(2-hydroxyethyl)piperazin-1-yl]propylidene]thioxanthene *see* Clopenthixol.

2-Chloro-10-[3-[4-(2-hydroxyethyl)piperazin-1-yl]propyl]phenothiazine *see* Perphenazine.

7-Chloro-4-hydroxy-5-indancarboxylic acid *see* Clorindanic acid.

2-CHLORO-4-(HYDROXYMERCURI)-PHENOL (hydroxymercurichlorophenol; 'semesan', 'uspulun').

2-Chloro-6-hydroxymercuriphenoxy-acetic acid barbital salt *see* Merbaphen.

4-CHLORO-17β-HYDROXY-17-METHYL-1,4-ANDROSTADIEN-3-ONE (4-chloro-17α-methyl-1,4-androstadien-17β-ol-3-one; 4-chlorometandienone; 'oral turinabol').

9-Chloro-11β-hydroxy-16β-methyl-17,21-bis(1-oxopropoxy)pregna-1,4-diene-3,20-dione *see* Beclometasone dipropionate.

3-Chloro-7-hydroxy-4-methylcoumarin bis(2-chloroethyl) phosphate *see* Haloxon.

6-Chloro-17-hydroxy-1α,2α-methylene-pregna-4,6-diene-3,20-dione *see* Cyproterone.

6-CHLORO-17α-HYDROXY-16-METHYL-ENEPREGNA-4,6-DIENE-3,20-DIONE ACETATE ('chlorsuperlutin').

6-CHLORO-17α-HYDROXY-16-METH-YLENEPREGNA-4,6-DIENE-3,20-DIONE ACETATE WITH MESTRA-NOL ('biogest', 'sterolibrin').

2-Chloro-5-[4-hydroxy-3-methyl-2-(methylimino)thiazolidin-4-yl]benzene-sulfonamide *see* Tizolemide.

6-Chloro-17-hydroxy-16α-methylpregna-4,6-diene-3,20-dione *see* Clomegestone.

6-Chloro-17-hydroxy-19-norpregna-4,6-diene-3,20-dione *see* Amadinone.

21-Chloro-17-hydroxy-19-nor-17α-pregna-4,9-dien-20-yn-3-one *see* Ethynerone.

2-Chloro-5-(1-hydroxy-3-oxo-1-isoindolin-yl)benzenesulfonamide *see* Chlortalidone.

6-Chloro-17-hydroxypregna-1,4-diene-3,20-dione *see* Cismadinone.

6-Chloro-17-hydroxypregna-4,6-diene-3,20-dione *see* Chlormadinone.

6-Chloro-17α-hydroxypregna-1,4,6-triene-3,20-dione *see* Delmadinone.

6α-Chloro-17-hydroxyprogesterone *see* Hydromadinone.

1-(3-Chloro-2-hydroxypropyl)-2-methyl-5-nitroimidazole *see* Ornidazole.

7-Chloro-4-(4-hydroxy-3-pyrrolidin-1-yl-methylanilino)quinoline *see* Amopyroquine.

Chlorohydroxyquinoline *see* Cloxiquine.

2-Chloro-3-(2-imidazolin-2-ylamino)-4-methylthiophene *see* Tiamenidine.

4-Chloro-1-(2-imidazolin-2-ylmethyl)-naphthalene *see* Clonazoline.

p-Chloro-α-(2-imidazolin-2-yl)-α-pyrid-2-ylbenzyl alcohol *see* Dazadrol.

2-Chloro-N-(2-imidazolin-2-yl)-p-toluidine *see* Tolonidine.

3-Chloro-1-imidazol-1-yl-4-phenyliso-quinoline *see* Climiqualine.

Chloroimipramine *see* Clomipramine.

7-Chloro-4-indanol *see* Clorindanol.

Chloroiodoquine *see* Clioquinol.

5-Chloro-7-iodo-8-quinolinol *see* Clioquinol.

Chloro-IPC *see* Chlorpropham.

5'-Chloro-2-[p-[(5-isobutylpyrimidin-2-yl)sulfamoyl]phenyl]-o-acetaniside *see* Glidanile.

94

2-Chloro-*N*-isopropylacetanilide *see* Propachlor.

o-Chloro-α-isopropylaminomethylbenzyl alcohol *see* Clorprenaline.

p-Chloro-α-isopropylbenzyl nicotinate *see* Nicoclonate.

'Chlorol' *see* Dichloralphenazone.

(Chloromercuri)isobutylphenol *see* Mercurobutol.

(3-Chloromercuri-2-methoxypropyl)urea *see* Chlormerodrin.

Chloromerodrin *see* Chlormerodrin.

4-Chlorometandienone *see* 4-Chloro-17β-hydroxy-17-methyl-1,4-androstadien-3-one.

Chloromethapyrilene *see* Chloropyrilene.

Chloromethine *see* Chlormethine.

1-[*p*-[2-(5-Chloro-2-methoxybenzamido)-ethyl]benzenesulfonyl]-3-cyclohexyl-urea *see* Glibenclamide.

1-(5-Chloro-2-methoxybenzoyl)-3-[3-[4-(*m*-tolyl)piperazin-1-yl]propyl]urea *see* Ciltoprazine.

4-[*p*-[2-(5-Chloro-*N*-(*p*-methoxyphenyl)benz-amido]butyric acid *see* Clanobutin.

1-(3-Chloro-4-methoxyphenyl)-3,3-dimethylurea *see* Metoxuron.

4'-Chloro-5-methoxyvalerophenone (*E*)-*O*-(2-aminoethyl)oxime *see* Clovoxamine.

4-Chloro-17α-methylandrosta-1,4-dien-17β-ol-3-one *see* 4-Chloro-17β-hydroxy-17-methyl-1,4-androstadien-3-one.

7-Chloro-2-methylamino-5-phenyl-3H-1,4-benzodiazepine 4-oxide *see* Chlor-diazepoxide.

2-(3-Chloro-2-methylanilino)nicotinic acid *see* Clonixin.

p-[2-(5-Chloro-2-methylbenzamido)ethyl]-benzoic acid *see* Meglitinide.

2-(*p*-Chloro-α-methylbenzhydryloxy)-*N,N*-dimethylpropylamine *see* Meclox-amine.

2-[2-(*p*-Chloro-α-methylbenzhydryloxy)-ethyl]-1-methylpyrrolidine *see* Clemas-tine.

7-Chloro-3-methylbenzothiadiazine dioxide *see* Diazoxide.

5-Chloro-3-methylbenzo(b)thiophene-2-acetic acid *see* Tianafac.

(±)-6-Chloro-α-methylcarbazole-2-acetic acid *see* Carprofen.

3-Chloro-4-methylcoumarin-7-yl diethyl phosphate *see* Coroxon.

O-(3-Chloro-4-methylcoumarin-7-yl) *O,O*-diethyl phosphorothioate *see* Coumafos.

6-Chloro-1,2α-methylenepregna-4,6-dien-17α-ol-3,20-dione *see* Cyproterone.

6-Chloro-16-methylenepregna-4,6-dien-17α-ol-3,20-dione *see* 6-Chloro-17α-hydroxy-16-methylenepregna-4,6-diene-3,20-dione.

2-Chloro-6-methylergoline-8β-acetonitrile *see* Lergotrile.

2-Chloro-*N*-(1-methylethyl)-*N*-phenyl-acetamide *see* Propachlor.

2-Chloro-5-[(2-methylindolin-1-yl)-carbamoyl]benzenesulfonamide *see* Indapamide.

4-Chloro-*N*-(2-methylindol-1-yl)-3-sulfamoylbenzamide *see* Indapamide.

α-(Chloromethyl)-2-methyl-5-nitroimi-dazole-1-ethanol *see* Ornidazole.

4-Chloro-*N*-methyl-3-(methylsulfamoyl)-benzamide *see* Tiamizide.

3'-Chloro-α-[methyl(morpholinocarbon-ylmethyl)amino]-*o*-benzotoluidide *see* Fominoben.

3'-Chloro-2'-[[methyl(morpholinocarbon-ylmethyl)amino]methyl]benzanilide *see* Fominoben.

Chloromethyl 5-nitro-2-furyl ketone *see* Nifurmerone.

4-Chloro-1-methyl-5-nitroimidazole *see* Clomizole.

Chloromethyloxirane *see* Epichlorohydrin.

O-(3-Chloro-4-methyl-1-oxo-2H-1-benzo-pyran-7-yl) *O,O*-diethyl phosphoro-thioate *see* Coumafos.

2-Chloro-1-[3-[4-(2-(3-methyl-2-oxo-imidazolidin-1-yl)ethyl)piperazin-1-yl]-propyl]phenothiazine *see* Imiclopazine.

4-Chloro-3-methylphenol *see* Chlorocresol.

2-(4-CHLORO-2-METHYLPHENOXY)-ACETIC ACID (MCP; MCPA; 2-M-4-C; 'aprosone', 'cornox', 'dikotex', 'mephanac', 'metaxon', 'methoxone', 'weedex'). *See also* Chlorinated phenoxyacetic acid mixture.

4-(4-CHLORO-2-METHYLPHENOXY)-BUTYRIC ACID (MCBB; 4-MCB; 4-MCPB; 2,4-MCPB; 2M-4H-M; 'cantrol', 'thitrol'). *See also* Sodium 4-(4-chloro-2-methyl-phenoxy)butyrate.

2-(4-Chloro-2-methylphenoxy)propionic acid *see* Mecoprop.

7-Chloro-1-methyl-5-phenyl-1H-1,5-benzodiazepine-2,4(3H,5H)-dione *see* Clobazam.

p-Chloro-α-methyl-α-phenylbenzyl alcohol 2-(1-methylpyrrolidin-2-yl)-ethyl ether *see* Clemastine.

2-(*p*-Chloro-α-methyl-α-phenylbenzyl-oxy)-*N,N*-dimethylethylamine *see* Chlorphenoxamine.

2-(*p*-Chloro-α-methyl-α-phenylbenzyl-oxy)-*N,N*-dimethylpropylamine *see* Mecloxamine.

2-[2-(*p*-Chloro-α-methyl-α-phenylbenzyl-oxy)ethyl]-1-methylpyrrolidine *see* Clemastine.

2-(*p*-Chloro-α-methyl-α-phenylbenzyloxy)-triethylamine *see* Clofenetamine.

N'-(4-Chloro-2-methylphenyl)-*N,N*-dimethylformamidine *see* Chlorphenam-idine.

1-(3-Chloro-4-methylphenyl)-3,3-dimeth-ylurea *see* Chlorotoluron.

N-(3-Chloro-4-methylphenyl)-2-methyl-pentanamide *see* Pentanochlor.

N-(3-Chloro-4-methylphenyl)-2-methyl-valeramide *see* Pentanochlor.

trans-N-(6-Chloro-2-methylphenyl)-3-(1H-1-octahydropyrindin-1-yl)propionamide *see* Rodocaine.

8-Chloro-1-methyl-6-phenyl-4H-s-triazolo-(4,3-a)(1,4)benzodiazepine *see* Alprazolam.

8-Chloro-11-(4-methylpiperazin-1-yl)-5H-dibenzo(b,e)(1,4)diazepine *see* Clozapine.

2-Chloro-11-(4-methylpiperazin-1-yl)-dibenzo(b,f)(1,4)thiazepine *see* Clothiapine.

2-Chloro-11-(4-methylpiperazin-1-yl)-dibenz(b,f)(1,4)oxazepine *see* Loxapine.

2-Chloro-10-[3-(4-methylpiperazin-1-yl)-propyl]phenothiazine *see* Prochlorperazine.

9α-Chloro-16β-methylprednisolone *see* Beclometasone.

9-Chloro-16β-methylpregna-1,4-diene-11β,17,21-triol-3,20-dione *see* Beclometasone.

6-Chloro-16α-methylpregna-4,6-dien-17-ol-3,20-dione *see* Clomegestone.

6α-Chloro-16α-methylpregn-4-ene-3,20-dione *see* Clometerone.

6α-Chloro-16α-methylprogesterone *see* Clometerone.

2-Chloro-N-(1-methyl-2-propynyl)-acetanilide *see* Prynachlor.

4-Chloro-N′-methyl-N′-(tetrahydro-2-methylfurfuryl)-m-benzenedisulfonamide *see* Mefruside.

2-(2-Chloro-4-methylthien-3-ylamino)-2-imidazoline *see* Tiamenidine.

3-Chloro-α-methyl-4-(2-thienylcarbonyl)-benzeneacetic acid *see* Cliprofen.

2-Chloro-6-(2-morpholinoethylthio)-pyridine *see* Fopirtoline.

3-Chloro-4-[3-(4-morpholino)propoxy]-biphenyl *see* Chlordimorine.

'Chloronaftina' *see* Chlornaphazine.

4-Chloronandrolone *see* Norclostebol.

Chloronaphazine *see* Chlornaphazine.

Chloronaphthine *see* Chlornaphazine.

2-CHLORO-1,4-NAPHTHOQUINONE (antivitamin K₃).

2-(4-Chloro-1-naphthylmethyl)-2-imidazoline *see* Clonazoline.

'Chloronase' *see* Chlorpropamide.

CHLORONEB* (1,4-dichloro-2,5-dimethoxybenzene; 'demosan', 'tersan SP').

2-Chloro-4-nitrobenzamide *see* Aklomide.

2-(o-Chloro-α-nitromethylbenzylthio)-ethylamine *see* Nitralamine.

Chloronitromycin *see* Chloramphenicol.

2-CHLORO-4-NITROPHENOL ('nitrofungin').

O-(2-Chloro-4-nitrophenyl) O,O-dimethyl phosphorothioate *see* Dicapthon.

O-(3-Chloro-4-nitrophenyl) O,O-dimethyl phosphorothioate *see* Chlorothion.

O-(4-Chloro-3-nitrophenyl) O,O-dimethyl phosphorothioate *see* Phosnichlor.

6-Chloro-19-norpregna-4,6-diene-17-ol-3,20-dione *see* Amadinone.

21-Chloro-19-nor-17α-pregna-4,9-dien-20-yn-17-ol-3-one *see* Ethynerone.

4-Chloro-19-nortestosterone *see* Norclostebol.

trans-6′-Chloro-2,3,4,4a,5,6,7,7a-octahydro-1H-1-pyrindine-1-propiono-o-toluidide *see* Rodocaine.

4-[(5-Chloro-2-oxobenzothiazolin-3-yl)-acetyl]-1-piperazineethanol *see* Tiaramide.

1-[[(5-Chloro-2-oxobenzothiazolin-3-yl)-methyl]carbonyl]-4-(2-hydroxyethyl)-piperazine *see* Tiaramide.

4-Chloro-2-oxo-3(2H)-benzothiazoleacetic acid *see* Benazolin.

S-[(6-Chloro-2-oxobenzoxazol-3(2H)-yl)-methyl] O,O-diethyl phosphorodithioate *see* Phosalone.

5-CHLORO-6-OXO-2-NORBORNANE-CARBONITRILE O-(METHYLCARBAMOYL)OXIME (exo-3-chloro-endo-6-cyano-2-norbornanone O-(methylcarbamoyl)oxime; 'tranid').

Chloroperathiepine *see* Clorotepine.

CHLOROPHACINONE* (2-[(4′-chlorobiphenyl-1-yl)acetyl]-1H-indene-1,3(2H)-dione; 2-[(4-chlorophenyl)phenylacetyl]-1H-indene-1,3(2H)-dione; 2-(4′-chloroxenylacetyl)-1,3-indandione; 'caid', 'chloradione', 'drat', 'liphadione', 'quick', 'ratindan 3', 'raviac').

5-[3-[N-(p-Chlorophenacyl)methylamino]-propyl]-10,11-dihydro-5H-dibenz(b,f)-azepine *see* Lopramine.

Chlorophenarsine *see* Dichlorophenarsine.

Chlorophene *see* Clorofene.

Chlorophenesin *see* Chlorphenesin.

1-(p-Chlorophenethyl)-1,2,3,4-tetrahydro-6,7-dimethoxy-2-methylisoquinoline *see* Metofoline.

3-Chloro-N-phenethylpropionamide *see* Fenaclon.

Chlorophenindione *see* Clorindione.

Chlorpheniramine *see* Chlorpheniramine.

Chlorophenothane *see* DDT.

2(1H)-[2-[(2-Chlorophenothiazin-10-yl)-carbonyl]ethyl]hexahydropyrrolo-(1,2-a)pyrazine *see* Azaclorine.

2-Chlorophenothiazin-10-yl 2-diethylaminoethyl ketone *see* Chloracyzine.

2-Chlorophenothiazin-10-yl 2-dimethylaminoethyl ketone *see* Cloracizin.

2-Chlorophenothiazin-2-yl 2-(hexahydropyrrolo(1,2-a)pyrazin-2(1H)-yl)ethyl ketone *see* Azaclorine.

1-[3-(2-Chlorophenothiazin-10-yl)propyl]-4-(dihydro-2(3H)-oxofuran-3-yl)-4-hydroxypiperidine *see* Furomazine.

3-[1-[3-(2-Chlorophenothiazin-10-yl)-propyl]-4-hydroxypiperid-4-yl]dihydro-2(3H)-furanone *see* Furomazine.

1-[2-[4-[3-(2-Chlorophenothiazin-10-yl)-propyl]piperazin-1-yl]ethyl]-3-methyl-2-imidazolidinone *see* Imiclopazine.

2-[4-[3-(2-Chlorophenothiazin-10-yl)-propyl]piperazin-1-yl]ethyl 3,4,5-trimethoxybenzoate *see* Metofenazate.

8-[3-(2-Chlorophenothiazin-10-yl)propyl]-

1-thia-4,6-diazaspiro(4.8)decan-3-one *see* Spiclomazine.

1-[3-(2-Chlorophenothiazin-10-yl)propyl]-4-[2-(3,4,5-trimethoxybenzoyloxy)-ethyl]piperazine *see* Metofenazate.

Chlorophenoxamide *see* Clefamide.

2-(p-CHLOROPHENOXY)ACETIC ACID (4-CP; 4-CPA; 4-HFU; 'tomatotone').

p-Chlorophenoxyacetic acid amphetamine salt *see* Amphetamine *p*-chlorophenoxyacetate.

p-Chlorophenoxyacetic acid deanol ester *see* Meclofenoxate.

p-Chlorophenoxyacetic acid 2-isopropylhydrazide *see* Iproclozide.

p-Chlorophenoxyacetic acid metformin salt *see* Metformin *p*-chlorophenoxyacetate.

p-Chlorophenoxyacetylcholine iodide *see* Meclofenoxate methiodide.

1-(p-Chlorophenoxyacetyl)-2-isopropylhydrazine *see* Iproclozide.

1-(p-Chlorophenoxyacetyl)-4-piperonylpiperazine *see* Fipexide.

2-(p-Chlorophenoxy)-N-(2-diethylaminoethyl)acetamide *see* Clofexamide.

[2-(p-Chlorophenoxy)ethyl]dodecyldimethylammonium bromide *see* Dodeclonium bromide.

7-[[4-(m-Chlorophenoxy)-3-hydroxy-1-butenyl]-3,5-dihydroxycyclopentyl]-5-heptenoic acid *see* Cloprostenol.

3-(p-Chlorophenoxy)-2-hydroxypropyl carbamate *see* Chlorphenesin carbamate.

α-(p-Chlorophenoxy)isobutyric acid *see* Clofibric acid.

α-(p-Chlorophenoxy)isobutyric acid ethyl ester *see* Clofibrate.

1-(p-Chlorophenoxymethyl)-3,4-dihydroisoquinoline *see* Famotine.

6-[2-[2-(p-Chlorophenoxy)-2-methylpropionamido]-2-phenylacetamido]-penicillanic acid *see* Fibracillin.

2-(p-Chlorophenoxy)-2-methylpropionic acid *see* Clofibric acid.

2-[2-(p-Chlorophenoxy)-2-methylpropionoxy]ethyl nicotinate *see* Etofibrate.

1-(p-Chlorophenoxymethyl)-1,2,3,4-tetrahydro-6,7-isoquinolinediol *see* Clofeverine.

2-[p-(p-Chlorophenoxy)phenoxy]propionic acid *see* Fenofibric acid.

1-[p-(p-Chlorophenoxy)phenyl]-3,3-dimethylurea *see* Chloroxuron.

3-(p-Chlorophenoxy)-1,2-propanediol *see* Chlorphenesin.

2-(3-Chlorophenoxy)propionic acid *see* Cloprop.

1-(2-Chloro-2-phenylacetyl)urea *see* Chlorphenacemide.

3-(p-Chlorophenyl)alanine *see* Fenclonine.

O-[4-[(4-Chlorophenyl)azo]phenyl] O,O-dimethyl phosphorothioate *see* Azothoate.

4-Chlorophenyl benzenesulfonate *see* Fenson.

1-[α-(o-Chlorophenyl)benzhydryl]imidazole *see* Clotrimazole.

α-(p-Chlorophenyl)-2-benzofuranmethanol *see* Cloridarol.

2-[2-(p-Chlorophenyl)benzoxazol-5-yl]-propionic acid *see* Benoxaprofen.

1-(p-Chloro-α-phenylbenzyl)-4-cinnamylpiperazine *see* Clocinizine.

1-[α-(p-Chlorophenyl)benzyl]-4-m-methylbenzyl)piperazine *see* Meclozine.

1-[α-(p-Chlorophenyl)benzyl]-4-methylpiperazine *see* Chlorcyclizine.

1-[2-(o-Chloro-α-phenylbenzyloxy)ethyl]-4-(o-methylbenzyl)piperazine *see* Chlorbenzoxamine.

4-[2-(p-Chloro-α-phenylbenzyloxy)ethyl]-morpholine *see* Difencloxamine.

1-[2-(p-Chloro-α-phenylbenzyloxy)ethyl]-piperidine *see* Cloperastine.

3-(p-Chloro-α-phenylbenzyloxy)-1-methylpyrrolidine *see* Pyroxamine.

3-(p-Chloro-α-phenylbenzyloxy)tropane *see* Clobenztropine.

2-[2-[2-[4-(p-Chloro-α-phenylbenzyl)-piperazin-1-yl]ethoxy]ethoxy]ethanol *see* Etodroxizine.

1-[2-(o-Chloro-α-phenylbenzylthio)ethyl]-4-(o-methylbenzyl)piperazine *see* Bentipimine.

p-Chlorophenyl besilate *see* Fenson.

3-Chlorophenylcarbamic acid 1-methylethyl ester *see* Chlorpropham.

[4-(m-CHLOROPHENYLCARBAMOYLOXY)-2-BUTYNYL]TRIMETHYLAMMONIUM CHLORIDE ((4-hydroxy-2-butynyl)trimethylammonium chloride *m*-chlorophenylcarbamate; McN-A-343).

p-Chlorophenyl p-chlorobenzenesulfonate *see* Chlorfenson.

p-Chlorophenyl closilate *see* Chlorfenson.

4-Chloro-α-phenyl-o-cresol *see* Clorofene.

3-(p-Chlorophenyl)-1-cyanomethyl-4-iminoimidazolidin-2-one *see* Nimazone.

1-(p-Chlorophenylcyclohexyl) 2-diethylaminoethyl ether *see* Clofenciclan.

2-[1-(p-Chlorophenyl)cyclohexyloxy]-triethylamine *see* Clofenciclan.

1-(p-Chlorophenyl)-1,2-cyclopropanedicarboximide *see* Ciproximide.

1-(p-Chlorophenyl)-1-(2-diethylaminoethoxy)cyclohexane *see* Clofenciclan.

S-(p-Chlorophenyl) diethylcarbamothioate *see* Benthiocarb.

5-(p-Chlorophenyl)-2,3-dihydro-5-hydroxy-5H-imidazo(2,1-a)isoindole *see* Mazindol.

5-(p-Chlorophenyl)-2,5-dihydro-3H-imidazo(2,1-a)isoindol-5-ol *see* Mazindol.

5-(o-Chlorophenyl)-1,3-dihydro-7-nitro-2H-1,4-benzodiazepin-2-one *see* Clonazepam.

1-(o-Chlorophenyl)-4-(3,4-dimethoxyphenethyl)piperazine *see* Mefeclorazine.

1-(p-Chlorophenyl)-4-dimethylamino-2,3-dimethyl-2-butanol *see* Clobutinol.

1-(m-Chlorophenyl)-3-(2-dimethylaminoethyl)-2-imidazolidinone *see* Imidoline.

1-(*o*-**Chlorophenyl**)-3-**dimethylamino-1-
phenyl-1-propanol** *see* Clofedanol.
N-(*p*-**Chlorophenyl**)-*N*,*N*-**dimethylcarb-
amimidic acid ethyl ester** *see* Trimeturon.
4-[4-(*p*-**Chlorophenyl**)-4-**dimethylcarba-
moylpiperid-1-yl**]-4'-**fluorobutyro-
phenone** *see* Amiperone.
1-(3-**Chlorophenyl**)-2-[(1,1-**dimethyl-
ethyl**)**amino**]-1-**propanone** *see*
Bupropion.
O-(*m*-**CHLOROPHENYL**) *O*,*O*-**DIMETHYL
PHOSPHOROTHIOATE** ('neothiate').
1-(*p*-**Chlorophenyl**)-3,3-**dimethylpseudo-
urea** *O*-**methyl derivative** *see* Trimeturon.
3-(*p*-**Chlorophenyl**)-*N*,*N*-**dimethyl-3-pyrid-
2-ylpropylamine** *see* Chlorpheniramine.
1-(*p*-**Chlorophenyl**)-2,5-**dimethylpyrrole-
3-acetic acid** *see* Clopirac.
1-(*p*-**Chlorophenyl**)-3,3-**dimethylurea** *see*
Monuron.
N-(*p*-**Chlorophenyl**)-2,2-**dimethylvaler-
imide** *see* Monalide.
5-(*o*-**Chlorophenyl**)-7-**ethyl-1,3-dihydro-1-
methyl-2H-thieno(2,3-e)-1,4-diazepin-2-
one** *see* Clotiazepam.
4-(*p*-**Chlorophenyl**)-1-[3-(*p*-**fluorobenzoyl**)-
propyl]-*N*,*N*-**dimethylisonipecotamide**
see Amiperone.
4-(*p*-**Chlorophenyl**)-1-[3-(*p*-**fluorobenzoyl**)-
propyl]-4-**piperidinol** *see* Haloperidol.
4-[4-(*p*-**Chlorophenyl**)-4'-**fluoro-4-hydroxy-
piperid-1-yl**]**butyrophenone** *see* Haloperidol.
β-(4-**Chlorophenyl**)**GABA** *see* Baclofen.
1,1'-(*p*-**Chlorophenylguanidinoform-
imidoyl**)**bispiperazine** *see* Picloxydine.
2-(*p*-**Chlorophenyl**)-1,3,4,6,7,11b-**hexa-
hydro-9,10-dimethoxy-2H-benzo(a)-
quinolizine** *see* Quillifoline.
4-(*p*-**Chlorophenyl**)-4-**hydroxy-*N*,*N*-
dimethyl-α,α-diphenyl-1-piperidine-
butyramide** *see* Loperamide.
2-[(*p*-**Chlorophenyl**)**hydroxymethyl**]-
benzofuran *see* Cloridarol.
4-[4-(*p*-**Chlorophenyl**)-4-**hydroxypiper-
idino**]-*N*,*N*-**dimethyl-2,2-diphenyl-
butyramide** *see* Loperamide.
4-(*p*-**Chrophenyl**)-3-**hydroxy-*N*,*N*,2,3-
tetramethyl-1-butylamine** *see* Clobutinol.
α-(*p*-**Chlorophenyl**)-α-(2-**imidazolin-2-yl**)-
2-**pyridinemethanol** *see* Dazadrol.
(*o*-**Chlorophenyl**)**imidazol-1-yldiphenyl-
methane** *see* Clotrimazole.
1-(*p*-**Chlorophenyl**)-2-**imino-3-methyl-4-
imidazolidinone** *see* Clazolimine.
3-(*p*-**Chlorophenyl**)-4-**imino-2-oxo-1-
imidazolidineacetonitrile** *see* Nimazone.
2-(*p*-**Chlorophenyl**)-1,3-**indandione** *see*
Clorindione.
1-(*o*-**Chlorophenyl**)-2-**isopropylamino-
ethanol** *see* Clorprenaline.
(*p*-**Chlorophenyl**)**isopropylbiguanide** *see*
Proguanil.
1-(3-**Chloro-4-phenylisoquinolin-1-yl**)-
imidazole *see* Climiqualine.
1-(*p*-**Chlorophenyl**)-3-**methoxy-3-methyl-**

urea *see* Monolinuron.
2-(*o*-**Chlorophenyl**)-2-**methylaminocyclo-
hexanone** *see* Ketamine.
2-(*p*-**Chlorophenyl**)-α-**methyl-5-benz-
oxazoleacetic acid** *see* Benoxaprofen.
2-(*m*-**Chlorophenyl**)-3-**methyl-2,3-butane-
diol** *see* Metaglycodol.
2-(*p*-**Chlorophenyl**)-3-**methyl-2,3-butane-
diol** *see* Phenaglycodol.
7-[3-(*o*-**Chlorophenyl**)-5-**methylisoxazole-
4-carboxamido**]**cephalosporanic acid**
see Cefoxazole.
7-[3-(*o*-**Chlorophenyl**)-5-**methylisoxazole-
4-carboxamido**]-3-(**hydroxymethyl**)-2-
cephem-2-carboxylic acid acetate *see*
Cefoxazole.
[3-(*o*-**Chlorophenyl**)-5-**methylisoxazol-4-
yl**]**penicillin** *see* Cloxacillin.
1-(*p*-**Chlorophenyl**)-3-**methyl-3-(1-methyl-
2-propynyl**)**urea** *see* Buturon.
2-(*p*-**Chlorophenyl**)-4-**methyl-2,4-pentane-
diol** *see* Fenpentadiol.
2-[(*p*-**Chlorophenyl**)-α-**methyl-α-phenyl-
methoxy**]**propyldimethylamine** *see*
Mecloxamine.
1-(*o*-**Chlorophenyl**)-4-[2-(1-**methylpyrazol-
4-yl**)**ethyl**]**piperazine** *see* Enpiprazole.
1-(*m*-**Chlorophenyl**)-4-[2-(5-**methyl-
pyrazol-3-yl**)**ethyl**]**piperazine** *see*
Mepiprazole.
*N*¹-[1-(*m*-**Chlorophenyl**)-3-**methylpyrazol-
5-yl**]**sulfanilamide** *see* Sulfaclorazole.
3-(*o*-**Chlorophenyl**)-2-**methyl-4-quinazol-
inone** *see* Mecloqualone.
4-[5-(*o*-**Chlorophenyl**)-1,2,4-**oxadiazol-3-
yl**]**pyridine** *see* Pifexole.
3-[1-(4-**Chlorophenyl**)-3-**oxobutyl**]-4-
hydroxy-2H-1-benzopyran-2-one *see*
Coumachlor.
α-[*p*-(*p*-**Chlorophenyl**)**phenoxy**]**isobutyric
acid methyl ester** *see* Methyl clofenapate.
[2-*p*-(*p*-**Chlorophenyl**)**phenoxy**]-2-**methylpropionic acid methyl ester** *see* Methyl
clofenapate.
2-[(4-**Chlorophenyl**)**phenylacetyl**]-1H-
indene-1,3(2H)-dione *see* Chlorophacinone.
2-[1-(*p*-**Chlorophenyl**)-1-**phenylethoxy**]-
N,*N*-**dimethylethylamine** *see* Chlorphenoxamine.
N-[2-[1-(*p*-**Chlorophenyl**)-1-**phenylethoxy**]-
ethyl]**dimethylamine** *see* Chlorphenoxamine.
2-[2-[1-(*p*-**Chlorophenyl**)-1-**phenylethoxy**]-
ethyl]-1-**methylpyrrolidine** *see* Clemastine.
1-[(4-**Chlorophenyl**)**phenylmethyl**]-4-(3-
methylbenzyl)**piperazine** *see* Meclozine.
3-(*p*-**Chlorophenyl**)-1-**phenylpyrazole-4-
acetic acid** *see* Lonazolac.
1-(*p*-**Chlorophenyl**)-2-**phenyl-4-pyrrolid-1-
yl-2-butene** *see* Pyrrobutamine.
4-(*p*-**Chlorophenyl**)-2-**phenyl-5-thiazole-
acetic acid** *see* Fentiazac.
3-[3-[4-(*m*-**Chlorophenyl**)**piperazin-1-yl**]-
propyl]**quinazoline(1H,3H)-2,4-dione**
see Cloperidone.

2-[3-[4-(*m*-Chlorophenyl)piperazin-1-yl]-propyl]-*s*-triazolo(4,3-a)pyridin-3(2H)-one *see* Trazodone.
1-(*p*-CHLOROPHENYL)-1-PROPANOL (*p*-chloro-α-ethylbenzyl alcohol).
α-(*p*-Chlorophenyl)-α-pyrid-2-yl-2-imidazoline-2-methanol *see* Dazadrol.
5-(*o*-Chlorophenyl)-3-pyrid-4-yl-1,2,4-oxadiazole *see* Pifexole.
4-(4-*m*-Chlorophenyl-4-pyrrolidin-amidopiperid-1-yl)-4′-fluorobutyro-phenone *see* Haloperidide.
2-[*p*-(β-Chloro-α-phenylstyryl)phenoxy]-triethylamine *see* Clomifene.
1-(*p*-Chlorophenylsulfonyl)-3-(hexahydro-1H-azepin-1-yl)urea *see* Glypinamide.
1-(*p*-Chlorophenylsulfonyl)-3-propylurea *see* Chlorpropamide.
2-(*p*-Chlorophenyl)tetrahydro-3-methyl-4H-1,3-thiazin-4-one 1,1-dioxide *see* Chlormezanone.
10-(*m*-Chlorophenyl)-2,3,4,10-tetrahydro-pyrimido(1,2-a)indol-10-ol *see* Ciclaz-indol.
2-(*p*-Chlorophenyl)thiazol-4-ylacetic acid *see* Fenclozic acid.
S-[(*p*-Chlorophenylthio)methyl] *O,O*-di-ethyl phosphorodithioate *see* Carbo-fenotion.
S-[(*p*-Chlorophenylthio)methyl] *O,O*-di-methyl phosphorodithioate *see* Carbo-fenotion methyl.
2-[4-[(*p*-Chlorophenyl)thio]-3,5-xylyl]-*as*-triazine-3,5(2H,4H)-dione *see* Tiazuril.
(+)-2-[[α-(*p*-Chlorophenyl)-*p*-tolyl]oxy]-2-methylbutyric acid ethyl ester *see* Beclobrate.
8-Chloro-6-phenyl-4H-*s*-triazolo(4,3-a)-(1,4)benzodiazepine *see* Estazolam.
p-Chlorophenyl 2,4,5-trichlorophenyl sulfone *see* Tetradifon.
2-(*p*-Chlorophenyl)-2-(α,α,α-trifluoro-*m*-toloxy)acetic acid ester with *N*-(2-hydroxyethyl acetamide *see* Halofenate.
1-(*p*-Chlorophenyl)-3-valerimidoylurea *see* Carbantel.
Chlorophos (tr) *see* Metrifonate.
CHLOROPICRIN (trichloronitromethane; nitrochloroform; 'picfume').
2-Chloro-11-piperazin-1-yldibenz(b,f)-(1,4)oxazepine *see* Amoxapine.
CHLOROPREDNISONE*** (6α-chloro-17,21-dihydroxypregna-1,4-diene-3,11,20-trione; 6α-chloropregna-1,4-diene-17,21-diol-3,11,20-trione; 6α-chloroprednisone; chlorprednisone).
CHLOROPREDNISONE ACETATE* (chloroprednisone 21-acetate).
6-Chloropregna-4,6-diene-3β,17-diol-20-one *see* Clogestone.
6α-Chloropregna-1,4-diene-17,21-diol-3,11,20-trione *see* Chloroprednisone.
6α-Chloropregna-1,4-dien-17-ol-3,20-dione *see* Cismadinone.
6α-Chloropregna-4,6-dien-17-ol-3,20-dione *see* Chlormadinone.
6-Chloro-9β,10α-pregna-1,4,6-triene-3,20-

dione *see* Trengestone.
6-Chloropregna-1,4,6-triene-11β,17,21-triol-3,20-dione *see* Cloprednol.
CHLOROPROCAINE*** (2-diethylamino-ethyl 4-amino-2-chlorobenzoate; 'nesa-caine').
Chloropromazine *see* Chlorpromazine.
3-Chloro-1,2-propanediol *see* Chlorohydrin.
3-Chloro-1,2-propanediol dinitrate *see* Clonitrate.
Chloropropham *see* Chlorpropham.
Chloroprophenpyridamine *see* Chlor-pheniramine.
N-(3-Chloropropionyl)phenethylamine *see* Fenaclon.
N-(3-Chloropropyl)amphetamine *see* Mefenorex.
CHLOROPROPYLATE* (isopropyl 2,2-bis(*p*-chlorophenyl)glycolate; 1-methyl-ethyl 4-chloro-α-(4-chlorophenyl)-α-hydr-oxybenzeneacetate; isopropyl 4,4′-dichloro-benzilate; chlorpropylate; 'acaralate', 'rospin').
γ-Chloropropylene oxide *see* Epichloro-hydrin.
N-(3-Chloropropyl)-α-methylphenethyl-amine *see* Mefenorex.
5-(3-Chloropropyl)-4-methylthiazole *see* Cloprothiazole.
CHLOROPYRAMINE*** (*N*-(*p*-chloro-benzyl)-*N′,N′*-dimethyl-*N*-(2-pyridyl)-ethylenediamine; 2-[(*p*-chlorobenzyl)(2-dimethylaminoethyl)amino]pyridine; chlorpyramine; chlorotripelennamine; halopyramine; G-12114).
*N*¹-(6-Chloropyrazinyl)sulfanilamide *see* Sulfaclozine.
*N*¹-(6-Chloropyridazin-3-yl)sulfanilamide *see* Sulfachloropyridazine.
4-[3-(3-Chloro(10H)pyrido(3,2-b)(1,4)-benzothiazin-10-yl)propyl]-1-piper-azineëthanol *see* Cloxypendyl.
p-Chloro-α-pyrid-2-ylbenzyl 2-dimethyl-aminoethyl ether *see* Carbinoxamine; Rotoxamine.
1-(*p*-Chloro-α-pyrid-2-ylbenzyl)-4-[2-(2-hydroxyethoxy)ethyl]piperazine *see* Piclopastine.
4-(*p*-Chloro-α-pyrid-2-ylbenzylidene)-1-methylpyrimidine *see* Cycliramine.
2-(*p*-Chloro-α-pyrid-2-ylbenzyl)-2-imidazoline *see* Dazadrol.
2-[2-[4-(*p*-Chloro-α-pyrid-2-ylbenzyl)-piperazin-1-yl]ethoxy]ethanol *see* Piclopastine.
4-[2-(6-Chloropyrid-2-ylthio)ethyl]-morpholine *see* Fopirtoline.
CHLOROPYRILENE*** (*N*-(5-chloro-2-thenyl)-*N′,N′*-dimethyl-*N*-(2-pyridyl)-ethylenediamine; 2-[(5-chloro-2-thenyl)-(2-dimethylaminoethyl)amino]pyridine; chloromethapyrilene; chlorothenyl-pyramine).
CHLOROPYRILENE CITRATE (chloro-then).
3-Chloro-4-(3-pyrrolin-1-yl)hydratropic acid *see* Pirprofen.

2-[3-Chloro-4-(3-pyrrolin-1-yl)phenyl]
propionic acid *see* Pirprofen.
CHLOROQUINE*** (7-chloro-4-(4-diethyl-
amino-1-methylbutylamino)quinoline;
chlorochin; quingamine; RP-3377; W-7618;
WIN-244; 'artrochin', 'delagil', 'gontochin', 'tanakan').
CHLOROQUINE DIGENTISATE
('quinercyl').
Chloroquine di(8-hydroxy-7-iodo-5-
quinolinesulfonate *see* Cloquinate.
Chloroquine di(7-iodo-8-quinolinol-5-
sulfonate) *see* Cloquinate.
CHLOROQUINE DIPHOSPHATE
(SN-7618; 'aralen', 'avloclor', 'bemaphate',
'resochin', 'resoquine', 'sanoquin').
See also Broxyquinoline with broxaldine
& chloroquine diphosphate; Clioquinol
with chloroquine diphosphate & tetracycline; Cloquinate with chloroquine
diphosphate & diiodohydroxyquin.
CHLOROQUINE DIPHOSPHATE WITH
GLYCOBIARSOL ('neoviacept').
CHLOROQUINE SILICATE ('resochin S').
CHLOROQUINE SULFATE ('nivaquine',
'nivaquine B').
CHLOROQUINE SULFATE WITH
DIIODOHYDROXYQUIN ('nivembin').
Chloroquinol *see* Haloquinols.
5-Chloro-8-quinolinol *see* Cloxiquine.
4-(7-Chloroquinolin-4-ylamino)-*N*-ethyl-
N-(2-hydroxyethyl)-4-methyl-1-butyl-
amine *see* Hydroxychloroquine.
2-[[4-(7-Chloroquinolin-4-yl)amino]-
pentylamino]ethanol *see* Cletoquine.
4-(7-Chloroquinolin-4-ylamino)-α-pyrrol-
idin-1-yl-*o*-cresol *see* Amopyroquine.
N-(7-Chloro-4-quinolyl)anthranilic acid
2,3-dihydroxypropyl ester *see*
Glafenine.
2-Chloro-9-(quinuclidin-3-ylmethylene)-
thioxanthene *see* Nuclotixene.
'Chloros' *see* Sodium hypochlorite.
5-Chlorosalicylic acid 4-chloroanilide
see 4′,5-Dichlorosalicylanilide.
CHLOROSERPIDINE*** (10-chloro-11-
demethoxyreserpine; 10-chlorodeserpidine).
6-Chloro-9-(1-D-sorbityl)isoalloxazine
see Flavotine.
N-Chlorosuccinimide *see* Succinchlorimide.
4-Chloro-3-sulfamoylbenzamide *see*
Sulclamide.
1-(4-Chloro-3-sulfamoylbenzamido)-2,6-
dimethylpiperidine *see* Clopamide.
1-(4-Chloro-3-sulfamoylbenzamido)-2-
methylindoline *see* Indapamide.
2-[[*N*-(4-Chloro-3-sulfamoylbenzene-
sulfonyl)-*N*-methylamino]methyl]-
2-methyltetrahydrofuran *see* Mefruside.
4-Chloro-3-sulfamoylbenzoic acid 2,2-
dimethylhydrazide *see* Alipamide.
6-Chloro-7-sulfamoylbenzothiadiazine
dioxide *see* Chlorothiazide.
3-(4-Chloro-3-sulfamoylphenyl)-3-
hydroxy-1-isoindolinone *see* Chlortalidone.
4-(4-Chloro-3-sulfamoylphenyl)-4-

hydroxy-3-methyl-2-(methylimino)-
thiazolidine *see* Tizolemide.
3-(4-Chloro-2-sulfamoylphenyl)-3-hydr-
oxyphthalimidine *see* Chlortalidone.
N-(2-Chloro-4-sulfamoylphenyl)-2-
phenylsuccinimide *see* Suclofenide.
4-Chloro-5-sulfamoyl-2′,6′-salicyloxyl-
idide *see* Xipamide.
2-[[3-Chloro-4-sulfamoyl-6-(1H-tetrazol-5-
yl)anilino]methyl]thiophene *see* Azosemide.
5-[4-Chloro-5-sulfamoyl-2-(2-thenylam-
ino)phenyl]-1H-tetrazole *see* Azosemide.
4-Chlorotestosterone *see* Clostebol.
Chlorotetracycline *see* Chlortetracycline.
4′-Chloro-1,2,3,4-tetrahydro-1,3-dioxo-4-
isoquinolinecarboxanilide *see* Tesicam.
8-Chloro-1,2,3,4-tetrahydro-5-methoxy-
N,*N*-dimethyl-1-naphthylamine *see*
Lometraline.
2-Chloro-5,9,10,14b-tetrahydro-5-methyl-
isoquino(2,1-d)(1,4)benzodiazepin-
6(7H)-one *see* Clazolam.
8-Chloro-2,3,4,5-tetrahydro-2-methyl-5-
[2-(6-methylpyrid-3-yl)ethyl]-1H-pyri-
do(4,3-b)indole *see* Dorastine.
7-Chloro-1,2,3,4-tetrahydro-2-methyl-4-
oxo-3-*o*-tolyl-6-quinazolinesulfonamide
see Metolazone.
10-Chloro-2,3,7,11β-tetrahydro-2-methyl-
11b-phenyloxazolo(3,2-d)(1,4)benzo-
diazepin-6(5H)-one *see* Oxazolam.
7-Chloro-1,2,3,4-tetrahydro-4-oxo-2-
phenyl-6-quinazolinesulfonamide *see*
Fenquizone.
7-Chloro-1,2,3,4-tetrahydro-4-oxo-2-
phenyl-6-sulfamoylquinazoline *see*
Fenquizone.
Chlorotetrahydroxy[(2-hydroxy-5-oxo-
2-imidazolin-4-yl)ureato]dialuminium
see Alcloxa.
2-Chloro-5-(1H-tetrazol-5-yl)-*N*⁴-2-thenyl-
sulfanilamide *see* Azosemide.
CHLOROTHALONIL* (2,4,5,6-tetrachloro-
1,3-benzenedicarbonitrile; 1,3,4,5-tetra-
chloro-2,6-dicyanobenzene; 1,3,4,5-tetra-
chloro-2,6-dinitrilobenzene; tetrachloroisophthalonitrile; TPN; 'bravo', 'daconil
2787', 'exotherm termul', 'termil').
Chlorothen* *see* Chloropyrilene.
'Chlorothene' *see* 1,1,1-Trichloroethane.
3-Chloro-4-(2-thenoyl)hydratropic acid
see Cliprofen.
2-[(5-Chloro-2-thenyl)(2-dimethylamino-
ethyl)amino]pyridine *see* Chloropyrilene.
Chlorothenylpyramine *see* Chloropyrilene.
8-Chlorotheophyllinate(s) *see* Teoclate(s).
CHLOROTHIAZIDE*** (6-chloro-2H-
1,2,4-benzothiadiazine-7-sulfonamide
1,1-dioxide; 6-chloro-7-sulfamoyl-1,2,4-
benzothiadiazine 1,1-dioxide; chloro-
thiazine; 'alurene', 'chlortride', 'chlotride',
'clotride', 'diuril', 'diurilix', 'minizil',
'neodema', 'salisan', 'saluretil', 'saluric',
'tonuron', 'yadalan').
CHLOROTHIAZIDE SODIUM ('lyovac
diuril').

2-[3-Chloro-4-(thien-2-ylcarbonyl)-phenyl]propionic acid see Cliprofen.
CHLOROTHION (tr) (*O*-(3-chloro-4-nitrophenyl) *O,O*-dimethyl phosphorothioate; 'chlorthion').
3-(2-Chlorothioxanthen-9-ylidene)-*N,N*-dimethylpropylamine see Chlorprothixene.
3-[(2-Chlorothioxanthen-9-ylidene)-methyl]quinuclidine see Nuclotixene.
4-[3-(2-Chlorothioxanthen-9-ylidene)-propyl]-*N*-methyl-1-piperazinepropionamide see Clotixamide.
4-[3-(2-Chlorothioxanthen-9-ylidene)-propyl]-1-piperazineëthanol see Clopenthixol.
4-[3-(2-Chlorothioxanthen-9-yl)propyl]-1-piperazinepropanol see Xanthiol.
5-Chlorotoluene-2,4-disulfonamide see Disulfamide.
2-(2-Chloro-*p*-toluidino)-2-imidazoline see Tolonidine.
2-(3-Chloro-*o*-toluidino)nicotinic acid see Clonixin.
2-(3-Chloro-*o*-toluidino)nicotinic acid 2,3-dihydroxypropyl ester see Clonixeril.
4-(2-Chloro-*m*-toluidino)thiophene-3-carboxylic acid hydroxymethyl ester acetate see Aclantate.
CHLOROTOLURON* (1-(3-chloro-4-methylphenyl)-3,3-dimethylurea; 1-(*m*-chloro-*p*-tolyl)-3,3-dimethylurea; chlortoluron; 'dicuran').
N-(3-chloro-*o*-tolyl)anthranilic acid see Tolfenamic acid.
trans-1-[2-[*N*-(6-Chloro-*o*-tolyl)carboxamido]ethyl]octahydro-1H-1-pyrindine see Rodocaine.
N′-(4-Chloro-*o*-tolyl)-*N,N*-dimethylformamidine see Chlorphenamidine.
1-(3-Chloro-*p*-tolyl)-4-[6-[*p*-(1,1-dimethylpropyl)phenoxy]hexyl]piperazine see Teroxalene.
1-(*m*-Chloro-*p*-tolyl)-3,3-dimethylurea see Chlorotoluron.
4-Chloro-*o*-tolyldithioimidocarbonic acid cyclic methylene ester see Nimidane.
CHLOROTRIANISENE* *** (1-chloro-1,2,2-tris(*p*-methoxyphenyl)ethylene; α-chloro-4,4′-dimethoxy-α′-(*p*-methoxyphenyl)-stilbene; tri-*p*-anisylchloroethylene; chlortrianisoestrol; NSC-10108; 'merbentul', 'metace', 'tace').
6-Chloro-3-trichloromethyl-3,4-dihydro-7-sulfamoylbenzothiadiazine dioxide see Teclothiazide.
[2-Chloro-1-(2,4,5-trichlorophenyl)vinyl] dimethyl phosphate see Stirofos.
6-Chloro-*N,N′,N′*-triethyl-1,3,5-triazine-2,4-diamine see Trietazine.
1-Chloro-2,2,2-trifluoroethyl difluoromethyl ether see Isoflurane.
2-Chloro-1,1,2-trifluoroethyl difluoromethyl ether see Enflurane.
7-Chloro-1-(2,2,2-trifluoroethyl)-1,3-dihydro-5-phenyl-2H-1,4-benzodiazepin-2-one see Halazepam.

6-Chloro-3-[(2,2,2-trifluoroethyl)thio-methyl]-3,4-dihydro-2H-1,2,4-benzo-thiadiazine-7-sulfonamide 1,1-dioxide see Epitizide.
6-Chloro-3-[(2,2,2-trifluoroethyl)thio-methyl]-3,4-dihydro-2-methyl-7-sulfamoylbenzothiadiazine dioxide see Polythiazide.
6-Chloro-3-[(2,2,2-trifluoroethyl)thio-methyl]-3,4-dihydro-7-sulfamoyl benzothiadiazine dioxide see Epitizide.
4-(4-Chloro-3-trifluoromethylphenyl)-1-[3-(*p*-fluorobenzoyl)propyl]piperidin-4-ol see Clofluperol.
4-[4-(4-Chloro-3-trifluoromethylphenyl)-4-hydroxypiperid-1-yl]-*N,N*-dimethyl-2,2-diphenylbutyramide see Fluperamide.
4-[4-(4-Chloro-3-trifluoromethylphenyl)-4-hydroxypiperid-1-yl]-4′-fluorobutyrophenone see Clofluperol.
4-(4-Chloro-α,α,α-trifluoro-*m*-tolyl)-1-[4,4-bis(*p*-fluorophenyl)butyl]-4-piperidinol see Penfluridol.
4-(4-Chloro-α,α,α-trifluoro-*m*-tolyl)-4-hydroxy-*N,N*-dimethyl-α,α-diphenyl-1-piperidinebutyramide see Fluperamide.
4-[4-(*p*-Chloro-α,α,α-trifluoro-*m*-tolyl)-4-hydroxypiperid-1-yl]-4′-fluorobutyrophenone see Clofluperol.
9-Chloro-11β,17,21-trihydroxy-16β-methylpregna-1,4-diene-3,20-dione see Beclametasone.
6-Chloro-11β,17,21-trihydroxypregna-1,4,6-triene-3,20-dione see Cloprednol.
2-Chloro-10-[3-[4-(2-(3,4,5-trimethoxy-benzoyloxy)ethyl)piperazin-1-yl]-propyl]phenothiazine see Metofenazate.
7-Chloro-4,6,2′-trimethoxy-6′-methylgris-2′-ene-3,4′-dione see Griseofulvin.
7-Chloro-2′,4,6-trimethoxy-6′-methyl-spiro(benzofuran-2(3H),1′-(2)-cyclo-hexene)-3,4-dione see Griseofulvin.
2-Chloro-*N,N,N*-trimethylethanamium chloride see Chlormequat.
2-Chloro-*N,N*,6-trimethyl-4-pyrimidin-amine see Crimidine.
Chlorotripelennamine see Chloropyramine.
Chlorotriphenylstannane see Fentin chloride.
1-(*o*-Chlorotrityl)imidazole see Clotrimazole.
(2-Chlorovinyl)dichloroarsine see Lewisite.
β-Chlorovinyl ethynyl carbinol see Ethchlorvynol.
'Chlorox' see Sodium hypochlorite.
2-(4′-Chloroxenylacetyl)-1,3-indandione see Chlorophacinone.
Chloroxine see Halquinols.
CHLOROXURON* (1-[*p*-chlorophenoxy-phenyl)-3,3-dimethylurea; chloroxy-fenidim; 'tenoran').
Chloroxyfenidim see Chloroxuron.
CHLOROXYLENOL* ** (4-chloro-3,5-xylenol; 4-chloro-3,5-dimethylphenol; *p*-chloro-*m*-xylenol; PCMX).
6-Chloro-3,4-xylyl methylcarbamate see Carbanolate.

'Chlorpactin' *see* Monoxychlorosene.
'Chlorparacide' *see* Chlorbenside.
CHLORPENTAZIDE (1-(*p*-chlorobenzene-sulfonyl)-3-piperid-1-ylurea; 4-(*p*-chloro-benzenesulfonyl)-1,1-pentamethylenesemi-carbazide; HB-113).
Chlorpenthixol *see* Clopenthixol.
Chlorperazine *see* Prochlorperazine.
Chlorperphenazine *see* Perphenazine.
Chlorperphenthixene *see* Clopenthixol.
Chlorphedianol* *see* Clofedanol.
Chlorphen (tr) *see* Campheclor.
CHLORPHENACEMIDE (1-(2-chloro-2-phenylacetyl)urea; 'comitiadon').
CHLORPHENACYL (tr) (2-[*p*-[bis(2-chloroethyl)amino]phenyl]acetic acid; khlorfenatsil; NSC-72964).
Chlorphenacyl cholesteryl ester *see* Phenesterin.
Chlorphenacyl estradiol diester *see* Estradiol mustard.
CHLORPHENAMIDINE* (*N'*-(4-chloro-*o*-tolyl)-*N,N*-dimethylformamidine; *N'*-(4-chloro-2-methylphenyl)-*N,N*-dimethyl-methanimidamide; chlorphenamidine hydrochloride; chlordimeform; chloro-dimeform; C-8514; 'fundal', 'galecron').
CHLORPHENAMIDINE PLUS FORMETANATE ('fundal forte').
Chlorphenamine* *see* Chlorpheniramine.
Chlorphenarsine *see* Dichlorophenarsine.
Chlorphencyclan *see* Clofenciclan.
CHLORPHENESIN** (3-(*p*-chlorophenoxy)-1,2-propanediol; glyceryl *p*-chlorophenyl ether; 'adermykon', 'mycil').
CHLORPHENESIN CARBAMATE*
(3-(*p*-chlorophenoxy)-2-hydroxypropyl carbamate; U-19646; 'maolate').
Chlorphenethanum *see* DDT.
CHLORPHENIRAMINE* (3-(*p*-chloro-phenyl)-*N,N*-dimethyl-3-pyrid-2-ylpropyl-amine; 2-[*p*-chloro-α-(2-dimethylamino-ethyl)benzyl]pyridine; chlorprophen-pyridamine; chlorphenamine; chlorhistapyr-idamine).
CHLORPHENIRAMINE MALEATE
('allergisan', 'chlortrimeton').
See also Dexchlorpheniramine; Carbazo-chrome sodium sulfonate with chlorphen-iramine maleate; Pseudoephedrine with chlorpheniramine maleate.
Chlorphenisate *see* Clofibrate.
CHLORPHENOCTIUM AMSONATE*
((2,4-dichlorophenoxymethyl)dimethyl-octylammonium salt of 4,4'-diamino-stilbene-2,2'-disulfonic acid).
Chlorphenothane *see* DDT.
Chlorphenoxamide *see* Clefamide.
CHLORPHENOXAMINE* 2-[1-(*p*-chloro-phenyl)-1-phenylethoxy]-*N,N*-dimethyl-ethylamine; *N*-[2-[1-(*p*-chlorophenyl)-1-phenylethoxy]ethyl]dimethylamine; 2-(*p*-chloro-α-methyl-α-phenylbenzyloxy)-*N,N*-dimethylethylamine; 1-(*p*-chlorophenyl)-1-phenylethyl 2-dimethylaminoethyl ether; *p*-chloro-α-methyldiphenhydramine; chlor-phenoxamine hydrochloride; 'clorevan',

'contristamine', 'histol', 'phenoxene', 'phenoxine', 'systral').
CHLORPHENOXAMINE TEOCLATE
(chlorphenoxamine 8-chlorotheophyl-linate; chlorphenoxamine theoclate; 'rodavan').
CHLORPHENTERMINE* (*p*-chloro-α,α-dimethylphenethylamine; 2-(*p*-chlorobenz-yl)-2-propylamine; 1-(*p*-chlorophenyl)-2-methyl-2-propylamine; S-62; WX-2462; 'avicol', 'avipron', 'desopimon', 'lucofen', 'presate').
Chlorphthalidone *see* Chlortalidone.
Chlorpiprazine *see* Perphenazine.
Chlorpiprozine *see* Perphenazine.
Chlorprednisone *see* Chloroprednisone.
Chlorprenaline *see* Clorprenaline.
CHLORPROETHAZINE* (2-chloro-10-(3-diethylaminopropyl)phenothiazine; RP-4909; 'neuriplège').
CHLORPROGUANIL* (1-(3,4-dichloro-phenyl)-5-isopropylbiguanide; M-5943; 'lapudrine').
CHLORPROHEPTADIENE (3-chloro-5-(3-dimethylaminopropylidene)-10,11-dihydro(5H)dibenzo(a,d)cycloheptene; chloroamitriptyline).
CHLORPROHEPTATRIENE (3-chloro-5-(3-dimethylaminopropylidene)(5H)-dibenzo(a,d)cycloheptene).
CHLORPROMAZINE* (2-chloro-10-(3-dimethylaminopropyl)phenothiazine; aminasin; aminazine; chloropromazine; chlorpromazine hydrochloride; clordelazin; HL-5746; RP-4560; SKF-2601-A; aminosine; cloropromazine; klorproma-zine).
See also Amobarbital with chlorpromazine.
CHLORPROMAZINE SULFOXIDE
(opromazine; 'secotil').
CHLORPROPAMIDE* (1-(*p*-chlorobenz-enesulfonyl)-3-propylurea; 1-(*p*-chloro-phenylsulfonyl)-3-propylurea; P-607; 'catanil', 'chloronase', 'diabetasi', 'dia-betoral', 'diabinese', 'disparolene', 'eubetin', 'melitase', 'prodiaben').
CHLORPROPAMIDE WITH METFOR-MIN ('diabiformine', 'diabiphage').
CHLORPROPHAM* (isopropyl *m*-chlor-carbanilate; isopropyl *N*-(*m*-chlorophenyl)-carbamate; 1-methylethyl 3-chlorophenyl-carbamate; chlorpropham; chloropropham; chloro-IPC; klor-IFK; CIPC; 'metoxon').
Chlorprophenpyridamine *see* Chlorphenir-amine.
Chlorpropylate *see* Chloropropylate.
CHLORPROTHIXENE* (*trans* isomer of 3-(2-chlorothioxanthen-9-ylidene)-*N,N*-dimethylpropylamine; *trans*-2-chloro-*N,N*-dimethylthioxanthene-Δ-9,γ-propylamine; 2-chloro-10-(3-dimethylaminopropylidene)-thioxanthene; chlorprothixene hydrochlor-ide; N-7714; Ro-4-0403; 'taractan', 'tarasan', 'truxal').
Chlorpyramine *see* Chloropyramine.
CHLORPYRIFOS* (*O,O*-diethyl *O*-(3,5,6-trichloropyrid-2-yl) phosphorothioate;

3,5,6-trichloro-2-[(diethoxyphosphino-thioyl)oxy]pyridine; Dowco 179; OMS-971; 'dursban').

CHLORPYRIFOS-METHYL* (*O,O*-dimethyl *O*-(3,5,6-trichloropyrid-2-yl) phosphorothioate; Dowco 214; trichlormethylphos).

CHLORQUINALDOL*** (5,7-dichloro-2-methyl-8-quinolinol; dichlorohydroxy-quinaldine; dichloroxyquinaldine; 'gynosterosan', 'siogen', 'siosteran', 'sterosan', 'steroxin').

CHLORQUINALDOL WITH HALQUINOLS ('dignoquine').

Chlorquinol* *see* Halquinols.

CHLORQUINOX* (5,6,7,8-tetrachloro-quinoxaline; 'lucel').

'Chlorsuccillin' *see* Suxamethonium chloride.

Chlorsudimeprylum *see* Clopamide.

'Chlorsulphacide' *see* Chlorbenside.

Chlorsulthiadil *see* Hydrochlorothiazide.

'Chlorsuperlutin' *see* 6-Chloro-17α-hydroxy-16-methylenepregna-4,6-diene-3,20-dione.

CHLORTALIDONE*** (2-chloro-5-(1-hydroxy-3-oxo-1-isoindolinyl)benzene-sulfonamide; 3-(4-chloro-3-sulfamoyl-phenyl)-3-hydroxyphthalimidine; 3-(4-chloro-3-sulfamoylphenyl)-3-hydroxy-isoindolin-1-one; chlorphthalidone; chlorthalidone; clortalidone; phthalamudine; G-33182; 'hygroton', 'igroton').
See also Clonidine with chlortalidone; Reserpine with chlortalidone.

'Chlorten' *see* Campheclor.

CHLORTETRACYCLINE*** (7-chloro-4-dimethylamino-1,4,4a,5,5a,6,11,12a-octa-hydro-3,6,10,12,12a-pentahydroxy-6-methyl-1,11-dioxonaphthacene-2-carbox-amide; biomitsin; biomycin; biovetin; biovit-40; A-377; NSC-13252; 'acronize', 'aureocina', 'aureomycin', 'chrysomykine', 'duomycin').

CHLORTETRACYCLINE WITH α-AMYLASE ('amycycline').
See also Tetracycline with chlortetracycline and demeclocycline.

CHLORTHAL* (2,3,5,6-tetrachloro-1,4-benzenedicarboxylic acid; 2,3,5,6-tetra-chloroterephthalic acid).

CHLORTHAL-DIMETHYL* (dimethyl tetrachloroterephthalate; DCPA; 'dacthal').

Chlorthalidone* *see* Chlortalidone.

CHLORTHENOXAZINE*** (2-(2-chloro-ethyl)-2,3-dihydro-4-oxo-1,3-benzoxazine; 2-(2-chloroethyl)-2,3-dihydro-4H-1,3-benzoxazin-4-one; Ap-67; 'valmorin', 'valtorin').

CHLORTHIAMID* (2,6-dichlorothiobenz-amide; 2,6-dichlorobenzenecarbothi-amide; 'prefix').

Chlorthiazide *see* Chlorothiazide.

'Chlorthion' *see* Chlorothion.

CHLORTHIOPHOS* (*O*-[2,5-dichloro-4-(methylthio)phenyl] *O,O*-diethyl phos-phorothioate; CELA S-2957; S-2957).

Chlortoluron *see* Chlorotoluron.

'Chlortran' *see* Chlorbutol.

Chlortrianisoestrol* *see* Chlorotrianisene.

'Chlortride' *see* Chlorothiazide.

'Chlortrimeton' *see* Chlorpheniramine.

Chlorvalamide *see* Monalide.

Chlorxylam *see* Carbanolate.

'Chloryl' *see* Chloroethane.

CHLORZOXAZONE*** (5-chloro-2-benz-oxazolinone; 5-chloro-(2H)2-benzoxazo-lone; 'paraflex').

Chlosudimeprimylum *see* Clopamide.

'Chlotaon' *see* Chloramphenicol with oleandomycin.

'Chlotride' *see* Chlorothiazide.

'Chloxyl' *see* 1,4-Bis(trichloromethyl)benzene.

'Chobile' *see* Cholic acid.

'Choisine' *see* Piperazine dithiocarbamate.

'Choladine' *see* Iopanoic acid.

Cholaic acid *see* Taurocholic acid.

Cholalic acid *see* Cholic acid.

CHOLANIC ACID (17β-(3-carboxy-1-methylpropyl)etiocholanone; 5β-cholan-24-oic acid; 5β-cholanic acid; ursocholanic acid).

'Cholebrine' *see* Iocetamic acid.

Cholecalciferol* *see* Colecalciferol.

CHOLECYSTOKININ-PANCREOZYMIN (pancreozymin; 'cecekin').

'Choledyl' *see* Choline theophyllinate.

'Cholegyl' *see* Choline theophyllinate.

Choleic acid *see* Deoxycholic acid.

'Cholergol' *see* Choline orotate.

'Cholesolvin' *see* Simfibrate.

CHOLEST-5-ENE-3β,24-DIOL (24-hydr-oxycholesterol; cerebrostenediol; cerebro-sterol).

Cholest-5-en-3β-ol *see* Cholesterol.

CHOLEST-5-EN-24-OL-3-ONE (cerebro-stenolone).

Cholesterin *see* Cholesterol.

CHOLESTEROL (cholest-5-en-3β-ol; 5,6-cholesten-3-ol; NSC-8798; 'dythol').

Cholesteryl *p*-[bis(2-chloroethyl)amino]-phenylacetate *see* Phenesterin.

Cholestyramine* *see* Colestyramine.

CHOLIC ACID (3α,7α,12α-trihydroxy-5β-cholanic acid; cholalic acid; NSC-6135; 'chobile', 'colalin', 'felagol').

CHOLINE ((2-hydroxyethyl)trimethylammo-nium hydroxide; amanitine; bilineurine; bursine; fagine; gossypine; luridine; sincaline; vidine).

Choline acetate *see* Acetylcholine.

Choline benzilate *see* Metocinium iodide.

CHOLINE BORATE ('enzytol').

Choline bromide hexamethylenedicar-bamate *see* Hexcarbacholine bromide.

Choline carbamate *see* Carbachol.

CHOLINE CHLORIDE*** ((2-hydroxy-ethyl)trimethylammonium chloride; 'bio-choline', 'biocolina', 'hepacholine', 'lipotril').

CHOLINE CITRATE (choline dihydrogen citrate salt; 'cholinvel', 'chothyn', 'cirrco-lina', 'citracholin', 'delichol', 'neuro-tropan').

Choline cytidine 5'-pyrophosphate ester

see Citicholine.

Choline dihydrogen citrate *see* Choline citrate.

CHOLINE GLUCONATE*** ((2-hydroxy-ethyl)trimethylammonium D-gluconate).

Choline iodide benzilate *see* Metocinium iodide.

Choline iodide dimethylpipecolate methiodide *see* Dimecolonium iodide.

Choline iodide 1,1-dimethylpyrrolidinium iodide 2-carboxylate *see* Trepirium iodide.

Choline mesilate *see* Mesylcholine.

Choline methanesulfonate *see* Mesylcholine.

Choline nitrate *see* Nitricholine.

CHOLINE OROTATE ('cholergol').

'Cholinergol' *see* Carbachol.

CHOLINE SALICYLATE*** (choline salt of salicylic acid; 'actasal', 'arthropan', 'cholisate', 'mundisal').

Choline salicylate magnesium sulfate complex *see* Salcolex.

CHOLINE STEARATE ('chomelan').

Choline suberate *see* Dicholine suberate.

CHOLINE THEOPHYLLINATE*** (oxtriphylline; cholinophylline; oxtri-methylline; theophylline cholinate; 'ascorphylline', 'choledyl', 'cholegyl', 'dilasmyl', 'filoral', 'soliphylline', 'teokolin', 'theoxylline').

Choline thioglycolate *see* Thioglycolcholine.

Choline triethyl analog *see* Triethyl(2-hydroxyethyl)ammonium chloride.

Choline urocanoate *see* Murexine.

Choline xylyl ether bromide *see* Xylocholine.

Cholinophylline *see* Choline theophyllinate.

'Cholinvel' *see* Choline citrate.

'Choliopan' *see* Butropium bromide.

'Cholisate' *see* Choline salicylate.

Chologon (tr) *see* Dehydrocholic acid.

'Cholografin' *see* Adipiodone.

'Choloplant' *see* Ox bile.

'Cholospect' *see* Adipiodone.

'Choloxon' *see* Dextrothyroxine sodium.

Cholylglycine *see* Glycocholic acid.

Cholyltaurine *see* Taurocholic acid.

'Chomelan' *see* Choline stearate.

Chondodendrine *see* Bebeerine.

Chondrodendrine *see* Bebeerine.

Chondrodendron tomentosum extract *see* Tubocurarine.

CHONDROITINASE (chondroitin sulfatase; 'thiomucase').

See also Chymotrypsin with chondroitinase.

Chondroitin sulfatase *see* Chondroitinase.

Chondroitinsulfuric acid-B *see* β-Heparin.

Chondrosamine *see* Galactosamine.

'Chonex' *see* Dehydrocholic acid.

Chopramine *see* Lofepramine.

CHORIONIC GONADOTROPHIN*** (human chorionic gonadotrophin; HCG; pregnancy urine extract containing chiefly LH activity with little FSH activity).

'Choryl' *see* Carbachol.

'Chothyn' *see* Choline citrate.

CHQ *see* Haloquinols.

CHROMAN (3,4-dihydro-1,2H-benzopyran).

'Chromaphon' *see* Coumithoate.

Chromatophore-expanding factor *see* Intermedin.

Chromene *see* Benzopyran.

2H-Chromen-2-one *see* Coumarin.

'Chromitope sodium' *see* Sodium chromate (^{51}Cr).

Chromium sesquioxide *see* Dichromium trioxide.

CHROMOCARB*** (4-oxo-4H-1-benzo-pyran-2-carboxylic acid; chromone-2-carboxylic acid; LP-1; atremon).

'Chromocor' *see* Flavone.

CHROMOMYCIN ('toyomycin').

CHROMOMYCIN A₃ (NSC-58514).

Chromonar* *see* Carbocromen.

CHROMONE (4H-1-benzopyran-4-one; γ-benzopyrone).

Chromone-2-carboxylic acid *see* Chromo-carb.

'Chromosmon' *see* Methylene blue.

CHROMOTROPIC ACID (1,8-naphthalene-diol-3,6-disulfonic acid; 4,5-dihydroxy-2,7-naphthalenedisulfonic acid).

CHRYSANTHEMIC ACID (3-(2-methyl-1-propenyl)cyclopropanecarboxylic acid; chrysanthemummonocarboxylic acid; chrysanthemumic acid).

See also Allethrin; Bioallethrin; Bio-resmethrin; Cinerin; Cisresmethrin; Cyclethrin; Dimethrin; Prothrin; Pyres-methrin; Pyrethrin; Resmethrin; Tetra-methrin.

CHRYSANTHEMUMDICARBOXYLIC ACID (3-(2-carboxypropenyl)-2,2-dimethylcyclopropanecarboxylic acid; 3-carboxy-α,2,2-trimethylcyclopropane-acrylic acid).

See also Cinerin II; Pyrethrin II.

Chrysanthemumic acid *see* Chrysanthemic acid.

Chrysanthemummonocarboxylic acid *see* Chrysanthemic acid.

CHRYSAROBIN* (amorphous extract of *Andira aroba*; Goa powder).

Chrysatropic acid *see* Scopoletin.

Chrysazin *see* Dantron.

Chrysazin-3-carboxylic acid *see* Rhein.

Chrysin (5,7-dihydroxyflavone).

CHRYSOIDINE (2,4-diaminoazobenzene; 4-phenylazo-*m*-phenylenediamine).

CHRYSOIDINE-CITRATE COMPLEX ('azohel', 'azoangin').

CHRYSOIDINE DIHYDROIODIDE ('azoiodine', 'azojod').

CHRYSOIDINE MONOTHIOCYANATE ('azorhodan', 'dairin').

'Chrysomykine' *see* Chlortetracycline.

'Chryson' *see* Resmethrin.

CHRYSOPHANIC ACID (4,5-dihydroxy-2-methylanthraquinone; 1,8-dihydroxy-3-methylanthraquinone; methylchrysazin; chrysophanol; 'rumicin').

See also Bismuth chrysophanate.

Chrysophanol *see* Chrysophanic acid.

'**Chymolase**' *see* Chymotrypsin.
CHYMOPAPAIN**** (BAX-1526; 'discase').
Chymopsin (tr) *see* Chymotrypsin with trypsin.
'**Chymotest**' *see* Chymotrypsin.
CHYMOTRYPSIN*** (α-chymotrypsin; 'alphintren', 'aphlozyme', 'avazym', 'catarase', 'chymolase', 'chymotest', 'chymo-trypure', 'chytryp', 'enzeon', 'lyochym', 'quimar', 'quimotrase', 'trypchymase', 'zonulysin').
CHYMOTRYPSIN WITH CHONDRO-ITINASE ('alphamucase').
CHYMOTRYPSIN WITH TRYPSIN (chymopsin; 'brinastase', 'fortivenat').
'**Chymo-trypure**' *see* Chymotrypsin.
'**Chytryp**' *see* Chymotrypsin.
CI-072 *see* 2-(2-Benzylphenoxy)triethylamine.
CI-69 *see* Toluidine red.
CI-92 *see* Anazolene sodium.
CI-100 *see* Sulfadiasulfone sodium.
CI-301 *see* Bialamicol.
CI-336 *see* Carbocloral.
CI-366 *see* Ethosuximide.
CI-379 *see* Benzilonium bromide.
CI-395 *see* Phencyclidine.
CI-403-A *see* Pararosaniline embonate.
CI-406 *see* Oxymetholone.
CI-416 *see* Triclofenol piperazine.
CI-419 *see* Fenimide.
CI-427 *see* Prodilidine.
CI-433 *see* Clamoxyquin.
CI-440 *see* Flufenamic acid.
CI-456 *see* Tiamizide.
CI-501 *see* Cycloguanil embonate.
CI-505 *see* Dibutadiamin.
CI-515 *see* Guanoxyfen.
CI-546 *see* Alipamide.
CI-556 *see* Acedapsone.
CI-564 *see* Cycloguanil embonate with acedapsone.
CI-572 *see* Profadol.
CI-581 *see* Ketamine.
CI-583 *see* Meclofenamic acid.
CI-634 *see* Tiletamine.
CI-636 *see* Sulfacitine.
CI-662 *see* Brilliant green.
CI-673 *see* Vidarabine.
CI-683 *see* Ripazepam.
CI-686 *see* Trebenzomine.
CI-718 *see* Bentazepam.
CI-922 *see* Methylene blue.
CI-925 *see* Tolonium.
CI-14700 *see* Ponceau SX.
CI-14720 *see* Carmoisine.
CI-15970 *see* Orange RN.
CI-64976 *see* Zilantel.
'**Cianatil**' *see* Cyamemazine.
CIAPILOME** (*N*-(5-cyano-4-oxo-1(4H)-pyrimidinyl)acetamide; 1-acetamido-5-cyanopyrimidin-4-one).
'**Ciatyl**' *see* Clopenthixol.
'**Cibalgin**' *see* Aminophenazone with allobarbital.
'**Cibazole**' *see* Sulfathiazole.
CICARPERONE*** (4'-fluoro-4-(octahydro-4-hydroxy-1(2H)-quinolyl)butyrophenone

carbamate ester; 4-carbamoyloxy-1-[3-(*p*-fluorobenzoyl)propyl]octahydro-quinoline; 4-carbamoyloxy-1-(4-(*p*-fluorophenyl)-4-oxobutyl)decahydro-quinoline; L-7810).
CICLACILLIN** (6-(1-aminocyclohexane-carboxamido)penicillanic acid; (1-amino-cyclohexyl)penicillin; cyclacillin; Wy-4508; 'ultracillin', 'wypicil').
CICLACTATE*** (3,3,5-trimethylcyclo-hexyl lactate).
CICLAFRINE*** (*m*-(1-oxa-4-azaspiro(4,6)-undec-2-yl)phenol; Gö3026A; W43026A).
CICLAZINDOL* (10-(*m*-chlorophenyl)-2,3,4,10-tetrahydropyrimido(1,2-a)indol-10-ol; ciclazindol hydrochloride; Wy-23409).
CICLIOMENOL*** (2-cyclohexyl-4-iodo-3,5-xylenol).
Ciclobarbital *see* Hexobarbital.
CICLOBENDAZOLE** (methyl 5-cyclo-propylcarbonyl)-2-benzimidazolecarba-mate).
CICLOFENAZINE*** (10-[3-(4-cyclopropyl-piperazin-1-yl)propyl]-2-trifluoromethyl-phenothiazine; cyclophenazine; cyclo-phenazine hydrochloride; L-60284).
CICLONICATE*** (*trans*-3,3,5-trimethyl-cyclohexyl nicotinate).
CICLONIUM BROMIDE*** (2-(1-nor-bornen-5-yl-1-phenylethoxy)triethylamine methobromide; diethylmethyl[2-(α-methyl-α-5-norbornen-2-ylbenzyloxy)-ethyl]ammonium bromide; 2-[1-((2.2.1)-bicyclohept-2-en-5-yl-1-phenylethoxy)-ethyl]diethylmethylammonium bromide; 2-diethylaminoethyl α-methyl-2,5-endo-methylene-1,2,5,6-tetrahydrobenzhydryl ether methobromide; Astra-3746; 'adamon').
CICLOPIROX*** (6-cyclohexyl-1-hydroxy-4-methylpyridin-2(1H)-one; 6-cyclohexyl-1-hydroxy-4-methyl-2-pyridone; 'batrafen').
CICLOPRAMINE*** (2,3,7,8-tetrahydro-3-methylamino-1H-quino(1,8-ab)(1)-benzazepine).
CICLOPROFEN*** (α-methylfluorene-2-acetic acid; 2-fluoren-2-ylpropionic acid; SQ-20824).
CICLOTATE(S)** (4-methylbicyclo(2.2.2)-oct-2-ene-1-carboxylate(s)).
CICLOXILIC ACID*** (*cis*-2-hydroxy-2-phenylcyclohexanecarboxylic acid).
CICLOXOLONE*** (3β-(*cis*-2-carboxy-cyclohexylcarbonyloxy)-11-oxoolean-12-en-30-oic acid; 3β-hydroxy-11-oxoolean-12-en-30-oic acid hydrogen *cis*-1,2-cyclohexanedicarboxylate).
CICLOXONE DISODIUM (cicloxolone disodium salt; BX-363A).
CICORTONIDE*** (3-(2-chloroethoxy)-9-fluoro-11β,16α,17,21-tetrahydroxy-20-oxopregna-3,5-diene-6-carbonitrile cyclic 16,17-acetal with acetone 21-acetate; 3-(2-chloroethoxy)-6-cyano-9-fluoropregna-3,5-diene-11β,16α,17,21-tetrol-20-one

105

16,17-acetonide 21-acetate).

CICROTOIC ACID*** (β-methylcyclohexaneacrylic acid; 3-cyclohexyl-3-methyl-
acrylic acid; 3-cyclohexylcrotonic acid).

Cicutine see Coniine.

'Cidal' see Hexachlorophene and Triclosan.

'Cidermex' see Triamcinolone acetonide
with neomycin.

'Cidex' see Glutaral.

'Cidial' see Phenthoate.

'Cidomycin' see Gentamicin.

CIDOXEPIN*** (cis-11-(3-dimethylamino-
propylidene)dibenz(b,e)oxepin; N,N-di-
methyldibenz(b,e)oxepin-cis-Δ¹¹(6H),γ
propylamine; cidoxepin hydrochloride;
P-4599).

'Ciergin' see Mobecarb with pibecarb.

'Cifoform' see Clioquinol.

'Cignaethyl' see Dithranol.

'Cignolin' see Dithranol.

'Cigthranol' see Dithranol.

CIHEPTOLANE** (10,11-dihydro-N,N-
dimethylspiro[5H-dibenzo(a,d)cyclo-
heptene-5,2'-(1,3)dioxolane]-4'-methyl-
amine; 4'-(dimethylaminomethyl)-1,11-
dihydrospiro[5H-dibenzo(a,d)cycloheptene-
5,2'-(1,3)dioxolane]).

Cilag-61 see Hexamethylolmelamine.

'Cillenta' see Benzathine penicillin.

'Cillimycin' see Lincomycin.

'Ciloprine' see Acediasulfone.

CILTOPRAZINE*** (1-(5-chloro-2-meth-
oxybenzoyl)-3-[3-[4-(m-tolyl)piperazin-1-
yl]propyl]urea).

'Ciluan' see Captafol plus pyridinitril.

'Cimedone' see Solasulfone.

CIMEMOXIN*** (1-(cyclohexylmethyl)-
hydrazine).

CIMEPANOL** (α-isopropylcyclohexane-
methanol; 1-cyclohexyl-2-methyl-1-
propanol).

CIMÉTIDINE*** (1-cyano-2-methyl-3-
[2-[[(5-methylimidazol-4-yl)methyl]thio]-
ethyl]guanidine; 4-[[[2-(3-cyano-2-methyl-
guanidin-1-yl)ethyl]thio]methyl]-5-methyl-
imidazole; 1-methyl-3-[2-(5-methylimi-
dazol-4-ylmethylthio)ethyl]guanidine-2-
carbonitrile; SK&F-92334).

'Cimlac' see Aminoacridine.

CINAMETIC ACID*** (4-(2-hydroxy-
ethoxy)-3-methoxycinnamic acid; ANP-
3401; 'transoddi').

CINANSERIN*** (2'-(3-dimethylamino-
propylthio)cinnamanilide; cinanserin
hydrochloride; SQ-10643).

Cincaine see Cinchocaine.

CINCHOCAINE*** (2-butoxy-N-(2-diethyl-
aminoethyl)cinchoninamide; cinchocaine
hydrochloride; cincaine; dibucaine;
quinocaine; sovcaine; sovkain; tricaine).

CINCHOL (cupreol; quebrachol; rhamnol).

CINCHONIDINE (stereoisomer of cinchonine; cinchovatine; α-quinidine).

CINCHONINE (α-(4-quinolyl)-5-vinyl-2-
quinuclidinemethanol).

CINCHONINIC ACID (4-quinoline-
carboxylic acid).

CINCHOPHEN*** (2-phenylcinchoninic
acid; aciphenochinolin; amoniphan;
quinophan).

Cinchovatin see Cinchonidine.

'Cinecol' see 2-Chloroethanol.

Cineol see Cineole.

CINEOLE (1,3,3-trimethyl-2-oxabicyclo-
(2.2.2)octane; eucalyptole).

Cinepazate see Cinepazet.

CINEPAZET** (ethyl 4-(3,4,5-trimethoxy-
cinnamoyl)piperazin-1-ylacetate; ethyl
cinepazate; cinepazate; MD-6753;
'vascoril').

Cinepazic acid ethyl ester see Cinepazet.

CINEPAZIDE*** (1-pyrrolidin-1-ylcarbonyl-
methyl)-4-(3,4,5-trimethoxycinnamoyl)-
piperazine).

CINEPAZIDE MALEATE (MD-67350;
'vasodistal').

CINERIN I (3-(2-butenyl)-2-methyl-4-oxo-
2-cyclopenten-2-yl chrysanthemate; 2-(2-
butenyl)-4-hydroxy-3-methyl-2-cyclopenten-
1-one ester with 2,2-dimethyl-3-(2-methyl-
propenyl)cyclopropanecarboxylic acid).

CINERIN II (3-[3-(2-butenyl)-2-methyl-
4-oxo-2-cyclopenten-1-yl] 1-methyl
chrysanthemumdicarboxylate; 2-(2-
butenyl)-4-hydroxy-3-methyl-2-
cyclopenten-1-one ester with monomethyl
ester of chrysanthemumdicarboxylic acid).

CINERUBIN A (NSC-18334).

CINFENINE** ((E)-N-(2-diphenylmethoxy-
ethyl)-N-methylcinnamylamine; N-(2-
benzhydryloxyethyl)-N-methylcinnamyl-
amine).

CINGESTOL*** (19-nor-17α-pregn-5-en-
20-yn-17-ol; 17α-ethynyl-5-estren-17-ol).

CINMETACIN*** (1-cinnamoyl-5-methoxy-
2-methylindole-3-acetic acid).

CINNACAINE (3-diethylamino-1-propanol
cinnamate hydrochloride; 'apothesine').

CINNAMAVERINE*** (2-diethylamino-
ethyl-2,3-diphenylacrylate; 2-diethyl-
aminoethyl 2-phenylcinnamate).

CINNAMEDRINE*** (α-[(1-cinnamyl-
methylamino)ethyl]benzyl alcohol; 2-
(cinnamylmethylamino)-1-phenyl-1-
propanol; N-cinnamyl-β-hydroxy-N,α-
dimethylphenethylamine; 'midol').

CINNAMEIN (benzyl cinnamate).

Cinnamene see Styrene.

CINNAMIC ACID (3-phenylacrylic acid;
β-phenylacrylic acid; 3-phenylpropenoic
acid).

Cinnamol see Styrene.

**1-Cinnamoyl-5-methoxy-2-methylindole-
3-acetic acid** see Cinmetacin.

**Cinnamyl 3β-acetoxy-11-oxoolean-12-
en-30-oate** see Cinoxolone.

CINNAMYL ALCOHOL (3-phenyl-2-
propen-1-ol; phenylallyl alcohol; styrone).

**1-Cinnamyl-4-(p,p'-difluorobenzhydryl)-
piperazine** see Flunarizine.

**N-Cinnamyl-N,α-dimethyl-β-hydroxy-
phenethylamine** see Cinnamedrine.

**1'-Cinnamyl-2,6-dioxo-3-phenyl-3,4'-
bipiperidine** see Cinperene.

106

1-Cinnamyl-4-(2,6-dioxo-3-phenyl-piperid-3-yl)piperidine see Cinperene.
1-Cinnamyl-4-(diphenylmethyl)piperazine see Cinnarizine.
α-[(1-Cinnamylmethylamino)ethyl]-benzyl alcohol see Cinnamedrine.
2-(Cinnamylmethylamino)-1-phenyl-1-propanol see Cinnamedrine.
Cinnamyl methyl ketone see Benzylidene-acetone.
p-Cinnamylphenol see Obtusastyrene.
3-[2-[(4-Cinnamylpiperazin-1-yl)methyl]-benzimidazol-1-yl]propiophenone see Cinprazole.
2-(1-Cinnamylpiperid-4-yl)-2-phenyl-glutarimide see Cinperene.
3-Cinnamyl-8-propionyl-3,8-diazabicyclo-(3.2.1)octane see Azaprocin.
Cinnarazine see Cinnarizine.
CINNARIZINE*** (trans-1-cinnamyl-4-diphenylmethylpiperazine; 1-benzhydryl-4-trans-cinnamylpiperazine; 1-cinnamyl-4-(diphenylmethyl)piperazine; cinnarazine; cinnarizine hydrochloride; MD-516; R-516; R-1575; 'cinnipirine', 'dimitronal', 'midronal', 'mitronal', 'stugeron').
CINNARIZINE WITH HEPTAMINOL THEOPHYLLINEACETATE (MD-1035; 'sureptil').
'Cinnipirine' see Cinnarizine.
CINNOFURADIONE*** (4-tetrahydro-furfuryl-1,2-benzo(c)cinnolino-3,5-pyrazolinedione; 2-tetrahydrofurfuryl-1H-benzo(c)pyrazolo(1,2-a)cinnoline-1,3(2H)-dione).
CINNOLINE (1,2-benzodiazine).
CINNOPENTAZONE*** (2-pentyl-6-phenyl-1H-pyrazolo(1,2-a)cinnoline-1,3-(2H)dione).
Cinnopropazone see Azapropazone.
CINOCTRAMIDE** (octahydro-1-(3,4,5-trimethoxycinnamoyl)azocine).
'Cinopenil' see Meticillin.
CINOXACIN*** (1-ethyl-1,4-dihydro-4-oxo(1,3)dioxolo(4,5-g)cinnoline-3-carboxylic acid; 1-ethyl-4-oxo(1,3)dioxolo-(4,5-g)cinnoline-3-carboxylic acid; azolinic acid).
CINOXATE*** (2-ethoxyethyl p-methoxy-cinnamate).
CINOXOLONE*** (cinnamyl 3β-acetoxy-11-oxoolean-12-en-30-oate; cinnamyl 3β-hydroxy-11-oxolean-12-en-30-ate acetate; BX-311).
CINPERENE** (2-(1-cinnamylpiperid-4-yl)-2-phenylglutarimide; 1-cinnamyl-4-(2,6-dioxo-3-phenylpiperid-3-yl)piperidine; 1'-cinnamyl-2,6-dioxo-3-phenyl-3,4'-bipiperidine; R-5046).
CINPRAZOLE** (3-[2-[(4-cinnamyl-piperazin-1-yl)methyl]benzimidazol-1-yl]-propiophenone; 1-[[1-(2-benzoylethyl)-benzimidazol-2-yl]methyl]-4-cinnamyl-piperazine; 1-(2-benzoylethyl)-2-[(4-cinnamylpiperazin-1-yl)methyl]benzimid-azole).
CINPROPAZIDE** (N-(isopropyl)-4-

(3,4,5-trimethoxycinnamoyl)-1-piper-azineacetamide; 1-(isopropylcarbamoyl-methyl)-4-(3,4,5-trimethoxycinnamoyl)-piperazine).
CINTRAMIDE*** (3,4,5-trimethoxycinna-mamide; cintriamide).
Cintriamide* see Cintramide.
'Ciodrin' see Crotoxyphos.
CIPC see Chlorpropham.
CIPIONATE(S)** (3-cyclopentanepropion-ate(s); cypionate(s)).
See also Estradiol cipionate; Nandrolone cipionate; Oxabolone cipionate; Testosterone cipionate.
CIPROQUINATE*** (ethyl 6,7-bis(cyclo-propylmethoxy)-4-hydroxy-3-quinoline-carboxylate; cyproquinidate; cyproquinate; Su-18137; 'coxytrol').
CIPROXIMIDE*** (1-(p-chlorophenyl)-1,2-cyclopropanedicarboximide; cyprox-imide; CL-53415).
'Circladin' see Bromindione.
'Circupon' see Etilefrine.
CIROLEMYCIN*** (antibiotic from Str. bellus var. cirolerosis).
'Cirrasol OD' see Cetrimonium.
'Cirrcolina' see Choline citrate.
'Cirtonal' see Magnesium thiosulfate.
Cisclomifene see Enclomifene.
Cisclomiphene* see Enclomifene.
CISMADINONE*** (6α-chloropregna-1,4-diene-3,20-dione-17-ol; 6α-chloro-17-hydroxypregna-1,4-diene-3,20-dione).
CISMADINONE ACETATE* (cismadinone 17-acetate).
CISMETHRIN* (cis-(+)-5-benzylfuran-3-ylmethyl 2,2-dimethyl-3-(2-methyl-1-propenyl)cyclopropanecarboxylate; cis-(+)-resmethrin; NRDC-119; OMS-1800; RU-12063).
See also Bioresmethrin; Resmethrin.
'Cistobil' see Iopanoic acid.
'Citanest' see Prilocaine.
'Citarin' see Racemorphan and Sodium anhydromethylenecitrate and Tetramisole.
CITENAMIDE*** (5H-dibenzo(a,d)cyclo-heptene-5-carboxamide).
CITENAZONE*** (5-formyl-2-thiophene-carbonitrile thiosemicarbazone; 5-cyano-2-thiophenecarboxaldehyde thiosemicarba-zone; HOE-105).
'Citexal' see Methaqualone.
'Cithrol' see under Macrogols.
CITICOLINE** (choline cytidine 5'-pyro-phosphate ester; cytidine diphosphate choline; cyticholine; CDP-choline; 'ensign', 'nicholin').
CITIOLONE** (N-(tetrahydro-2-oxothien-3-yl)acetamide; 'thioxidrene').
'Citocillin' see Hydroxyprocaine-penicillin.
'Citracholin' see Choline citrate.
CITRACHONIC ACID (methylmaleic acid).
'Citramin' see Methenamine anhydromethyl-enecitrate.
'Citrazon' see Benzoximate.
Citrex (tr) see Dodine.
CITRIC ACID (2-hydroxy-1,2,3-propanetri-

carboxylic acid; 2-hydroxytricarballylic acid; 'renacidin').
CITRIN (eriodictyol glucoside).
CITRININ (4,6-dihydro-8-hydroxy-3,4,5-trimethyl-6-oxo-3H-2-benzopyran-7-carboxylic acid; antibiotic from *Penicillium citrinum*).
CITRODISALYL (methylenecitrodisalicylic acid; 'novaspirine', 'salicitrin').
'Citroformin' *see* Methenamine anhydromethylenecitrate.
'Citrohexal' *see* Methenamine anhydromethylenecitrate.
Citrohexamine *see* Methenamine anhydromethylenecitrate.
'Citrola' *see* Dimethyl phthalate.
'Citromint' *see* Paraformaldehyde.
CITROPTEN (5,7-dimethoxycoumarin; limet(t)in).
Citrovorum factor *see* Calcium folinate.
'Citrullamon' *see* Phenytoin.
CITRULLINE (5-ureidonorvaline).
CL-68 *see* Clocortolone pivalate.
CL-369 *see* Ketamine.
CL-473 *see* Mefenamic acid.
CL-639-C *see* Dioxadrol.
CL-911-C *see* Dexoxadrol.
CL-912-C *see* Levoxadrol.
CL-1388R *see* Guanadrel.
CL-1848C *see* Etoxadrol.
CL-2422 *see* Guancidine.
CL-8490 *see* Methazolamide.
CL-10304 *see* Aminocaproic acid.
CL-11366 *see* Benzolamide.
CL-13439 *see* Sulfamethoxypyridazine.
CL-13900 *see* Puromycin.
CL-14377 *see* Methotrexate.
CL-16536 *see* Puromycin.
CL-19823 *see* Triamcinolone.
CL-25477 *see* Azatepa.
CL-26193 *see* Simtrazene.
CL-27071 *see* Descinolone acetonide.
CL-34433 *see* Triamcinolone hexacetonide.
CL-36467 *see* Levomepromazine.
CL-39743 *see* Levomepromazine.
CL-39808 *see* Tozalinone.
CL-40881 *see* Ethambutol.
CL-48156 *see* Imidoline.
CL-53381 *see* Triamcinolone acetonide sodium phosphate.
CL-53415 *see* Ciproximide.
CL-54131 *see* Piperamide maleate.
CL-54998 *see* Brocresine.
CL-61965 *see* Triamcinolone acetonide sodium phosphate.
CL-62362 *see* Loxapine.
CL-65205 *see* Boxidine.
CL-65336 *see* Tranexamic acid.
CL-65562 *see* Triflocin.
CL-67772 *see* Amoxapine.
CL-69112 *see* Roletamide.
CL-71563 *see* Loxapine succinate.
CL-82204 *see* Fenbufen.
CL-84633 *see* Nimidane.
CL-106359 *see* Triamcinolone acetonide sodium phosphate.
'Clafen' *see* Cyclophosphamide.

CLAMIDOXIC ACID*** (3,4-dichloro-α-phenoxyhippuric acid; 2-(3,4-dichloro-benzamido)-2-phenoxyacetic acid; SNR-1804).
'Clamil' *see* Tolboxane.
'Clamoxyl' *see* Amoxicillin.
Clamoxyquin* *see* Clamoxyquine.
CLAMOXYQUINE*** (5-chloro-7-(3-diethylaminopropylaminomethyl)-8-quinolinol clamoxyquin trihydrochloride; CI-433; PAA-3854).
Clam poison *see* Saxitoxin.
CLANOBUTIN*** (4-[p-chloro-N-(p-methoxyphenyl)benzamido]butyric acid).
CLANTIFEN** (4-(2,6-dichloroanilino)-3-thiophenecarboxylic acid).
'Clarin' *see* Heparin potassium.
'Clarmil' *see* Tolboxane.
'Claviton' *see* Tridihexethyl iodide.
CLAZOLAM*** ((+)-2-chloro-5,9,10,14b-tetrahydro-5-methylisoquino(2,1-d)(1,4)-benzodiazepin-6(7H)-one).
CLAZOLIMINE*** (1-(p-chlorophenyl)-2-imino-3-methyl-4-imidazolidinone).
CLEBOPRIDE*** (4-amino-N-(1-benzyl-piperid-4-yl)-5-chloro-o-anisamide; 4-(4-amino-5-chloro-2-methoxybenzamido)-1-benzylpiperidine).
CLEFAMIDE*** (2,2-dichloro-N-(2-hydroxyethyl)-N-[p-(p-nitrophenoxy)benzyl]acetamide; chlorophenoxamide; 'mebinol').
CLEMASTINE*** ((+)-2-[2-(p-chloro-α-methyl-α-phenylbenzyloxy)ethyl]-1-methyl-pyrrolidine; 2-[2-(p-chloro-α-methylbenz-hydryloxy)ethyl]-1-methylpyrrolidine; 2-[2-[1-(p-chlorophenyl)-1-phenylethoxy]ethyl]-1-methylpyrrolidine; meclastine; mecloprodine; 'agasten').
CLEMASTINE FUMARATE (meclastine fumarate; HS-592; 'tavegil').
CLEMIZOLE*** (1-(p-chlorobenzyl)-2-(1-pyrrolidinylmethyl)benzimidazole; clemizole hydrochloride; 'allercur').
CLEMIZOLE PENICILLIN*** (penicillin G with clemizole; 'depocural', 'lergopenin', 'megacillin', 'neo-penyl').
CLENBUTEROL*** (4-amino-α-(tert-butyl-aminomethyl)-3,5-dichlorobenzyl alcohol; 1-(4-amino-3,5-dichlorophenyl)-2-tert-butylaminoethanol; NAB-365).
'Clenil' *see* Beclometasone dipropionate.
CLENPIRIN** (1-butyl-2-(3,4-dichloro-phenylimino)pyrrolidine).
'Cleocin' *see* Clindamycin.
'Cleosin' *see* Clindamycin.
'Cleregil' *see* Deanol aceglumate.
CLETOQUINE*** (7-chloro-4-[4-(2-hydroxyethylamino)-1-methylbutylamino]quinoline; 2-[[4-(7-chloroquinolin-4-yl)-amino]pentylamino]ethanol).
CLIBUCAINE*** (2',4'-dichloro-3-piperid-1-ylbutyranilide).
CLIDINIUM BROMIDE*** (3-hydroxy-1-methylquinuclidinium bromide benzilate; Ro-2-3773; 'libraxin', 'marplan bromide', 'quarzan').
See also Bromazepam with clidinium

bromide; Chlordiazepoxide with clidinium bromide.

CLIMIQUALINE*** (3-chloro-1-imidazol-1-yl)-4-phenylisoquinoline; 1-(3-chloro-4-phenylisoquinolin-1-yl)imidazole).

CLINDAMYCIN*** (methyl 7-chloro-6,7,8-trideoxy-6-(*trans*-1-methyl-4-propyl-L-2-pyrrolidinecarboxamido)-1-thio-L-*threo*-α-D-*galacto*-octopyranoside; 7(S)-chloro-7-deoxylincomycin; clinimycin; U-21251; 'cleocin', 'cleosin', 'dalacin C', 'sobelin').

Clindamycin hexadecanoate *see* Clindamycin palmitate.

CLINDAMYCIN PALMITATE (U-25179 E).

CLINDAMYCIN PHOSPHATE* (U-28508).

'Clinibolin' *see* Nandrolone laurate.

Clinimycin *see* Clindamycin.

'Clinimycin' *see* Oxytetracycline.

'Clinium' *see* Lidoflazine.

CLINOLAMIDE** (*N*-cyclohexyllinoleamide; linolexamide; CHLA; AC-32).

'Clinovir' *see* Medroxyprogesterone acetate.

CLIOQUINOL** (5-chloro-7-iodo-8-quinolinol; iodochlorhydroxyquin; iodochlorhydroxyquinoline; quiniodochlor; quinoform; chinoform; chloriodoquine; 'achloquin', 'amebil', 'amoenol', 'bactol', 'barquinol', 'cifoform', 'cliquinol', 'eczecidin', 'enterokin', 'enteroquinol', 'entero-septol', 'enterovioform', 'enterozol', 'hi-enterol', 'iodoenterol', 'nioform', 'quinamibicide', 'rometin', 'vioform').

CLIOQUINOL WITH CHLOROQUINE DIPHOSPHATE & TETRACYCLINE ('tequinopil').

CLIOQUINOL WITH A MACROGOL ('dysenterol').

CLIOQUINOL WITH PHANQUINONE & OXYPHENONIUM BROMIDE ('mexaform').

CLIOXANIDE*** (4'-chloro-3,5-diiodosalicylanilide acetate; 2-acetoxy-4'-chloro-3,5-diiodobenzanilide; SYD-230; 'tremerad').

CLIPROFEN*** (3-chloro-α-methyl-4-(2-thienylcarbonyl)benzeneacetic acid; 3-chloro-4-(2-thenoyl)hydratropic acid; 2-[4-(1-carboxyethyl)-2-chlorobenzoyl]-thiophene; 2-[3-chloro-4-(thien-2-yl-carbonyl)phenyl]propionic acid; 4-(1-carboxyethyl)-2-chlorophenyl 2-thenyl ketone; R-25160).

'Cliquinol' *see* Clioquinol.

'Cliradon' *see* Ketobemidone.

'Clistin' *see* Carbinoxamine.

'Clitizina' *see* Menazone.

CLOBAZAM*** (7-chloro-1-methyl-5-phenyl-1H-1,5-benzodiazepine-2,4(4H,5H)-dione; chlorepin; clorepin; Hr-376; HR-4723; LM-2717; RU-4723; 'urbanyl').

'Clobber' *see* Cypromid.

Clobenfurol *see* Cloridarol.

Clobenmetamide *see* Fominoben.

CLOBENOSIDE*** (ethyl 5,6-bis-*O*-(*p*-chlorobenzyl)-3-*O*-propyl-D-glucofuranoside).

CLOBENZEPAM*** (7-chloro-10-(2-di-methylaminoethyl)-5,10-dihydro-11H-dibenzo(b,e)(1,4)diazepin-11-one; clobenzepam hydrochloride; 'tarpane').

CLOBENZOREX*** ((+)-*N*-(*o*-chloro-benzyl)-α-methylphenethylamine; (+)-*N*-(*o*-chlorobenzyl)amphetamine; *N*-(*o*-chlorobenzyl)dexamphetamine; 'dinintel').

CLOBENZTROPINE*** (3-(*p*-chlorobenz-hydryloxy)tropane; 3-(*p*-chloro-α-phenyl-benzyloxy)tropane; tropine 4-chlorobenz-hydryl ether; chlorobenztropine; clobenz-tropine hydrochloride; FC-1; SL-6057).

CLOBENZTROPINE METHOBROMIDE (SL-6058).

CLOBETASOL*** (21-chloro-9α-fluoro-11β,17α-dihydroxy-16β-methylpregna-1,4-diene-3,20-dione).

CLOBETASOL 17-PROPIONATE (GR2/925; 'dermovate').

CLOBETASONE*** (21-chloro-9α-fluoro-17α-hydroxy-16β-methylpregna-1,4-diene-3,11,20-trione).

CLOBETASONE 17-BUTYRATE (GR2/1214).

CLOBUTINOL*** (*p*-chloro-α-(2-dimethyl-amino-1-methylethyl)-α-methylphenethyl alcohol; 4-(*p*-chlorophenyl)-3-hydroxy-*N*,*N*,2,3-tetramethyl-1-butylamine; 1-(*p*-chlorophenyl)-4-dimethylamino-2,3-di-methyl-2-butanol; KAT-256; 'silomat'). †

CLOCANFAMIDE*** (*p*-chloro-*N*-(2-hydr-oxyethyl)-*N*-(3-methylnorborn-2-ylmethyl)-benzamide; 2-[(*p*-chloro-*N*-(2-hydroxy-ethylbenzamido)methyl]-3-methyl-norbornane; *N*-(*p*-chlorobenzoyl)-*N*-(2-hydroxyethyl)-3-methyl-2-norbornane-methylamine; chlorocamphamide; chloro-canfamide; clorocanfamide).

CLOCAPRAMINE*** (5-[3-(4-carbamoyl-4-piperid-1-ylpiperid-1-yl)-propyl]-3-chloro-10,11-dihydro-5H-dibenz(b,f)-azepine; 1'-[3-(3-chloro-10,11-dihydro-5H-dibenz(b,f)azepin-5-yl)propyl]-[1,4'-bipiperidine]-4'-carboxamide; Y-4153).

Clochinate* *see* Cloquinate.

CLOCIGUANIL*** (4,6-diamino-1-(3,4-dichlorobenzyloxy)-1,2-dihydro-2,2-ethyl-*s*-triazine; BRL-50216).

CLOCINIZINE*** (1-(*p*-chlorobenzhydryl)-4-cinnamylpiperazine; 1-(*p*-chloro-α-phenylbenzyl)-4-cinnamylpiperazine).

CLOCORTOLONE*** (9-chloro-6α-fluoro-16α-methylpregna-1,4-diene-11β,21-diol-3,20-dione; 9-chloro-6α-fluoro-11β,21-dihydroxy-16α-methylpregna-1,4-diene-3,20-dione).

CLOCORTOLONE ACETATE* (clocor-tolone 21-acetate; SH-818).

CLOCORTOLONE PIVALATE* (clocor-tolone 21-pivalate; clocortolone trimethyl-acetate; CL-68; 'purantix').

Clocortolone trimethylacetate *see* Clocortolone pivalate.

CLOCOUMAROL** (3-[*p*-(2-chloroethyl)-α-propylbenzyl]-4-hydroxycoumarin; 3-[1-[*p*-(2-chloroethyl)phenyl]butyl]-4-hydroxycoumarin; DB-112).

CLODACAINE*** (2'-chloro-2-[(2-diethyl-aminoethyl)ethylamino]acetanilide).
CLODANOLENE** (1-[[5-(3,4-dichloro-phenyl)furfurylidene]amino]hydantoin).
Clodantocide* *see* Clodantoin.
CLODANTOIN*** (5-(1-ethylpentyl)-3-(trichloromethylthio)hydantoin; chlordan-toin; clodantocide; 'sporostacin').
CLODAZON** (5-chloro-1-(3-dimethyl-aminopropyl)-3-phenyl-2-benzimidazol-inone; AW-142446).
CLOFAZIMINE*** (3-(*p*-chloroanilino)-10-(*p*-chlorophenyl)-2,10-dihydro-2-iso-propyliminophenazine; B-663; G-30320; 'lamprene').
CLOFEDANOL*** (2-chloro-α-(2-dimethyl-aminoethyl)benzhydrol; 1-(*o*-chlorophenyl)-3-dimethylamino-1-phenyl-1-propanol; chlophedianol; chlorphedianol; clofedanol hydrochloride; Bayer-186; SK-74; SL-501; 'baltix', 'detigon', 'refugal', 'ulo').
CLOFEDANOL NOSCAPINE SUCCINATE (double succinate of clofedanol and noscapine; 'H-dulapine').
CLOFENAMIC ACID*** (*N*-(2,3-dichloro-phenyl)anthranilic acid).
CLOFENAMIDE*** (4-chloro-1,3-benzene-disulfonamide; *p*-chloro-*m*-benzenedi-sulfonamide; monochlorphenamide; 'aquedux', 'haflutan', 'salco', 'salzen', 'soluran').
Clofenapate *see* Methyl clofenapate.
CLOFENCICLAN*** (2-[1-(*p*-chlorophenyl)-cyclohexyloxy]-*N*,*N*-diethylethylamine; 2-[1-(*p*-chlorophenyl)cyclohexyloxy]tri-ethylamine; 1-(*p*-chlorophenyl)cyclohexyl 2-diethylaminoethyl ether; 1-(*p*-chloro-phenyl)-1-(2-diethylaminoethoxy)cyclo-hexane; chlorphencyclan; chlorphencyclan hydrochloride; KSW-786; 'veritan').
CLOFENETAMINE*** (2-chloro-α-methyl-α-phenylbenzyloxy)triethylamine; 2-(*p*-chloro-α-methylbenzhydryloxy)tri-ethylamine; 'keithon').
Clofenotane*** *see* DDT.
Clofenoxine *see* Meclofenoxate.
CLOFENOXYDE** (4',4'''-oxybis(2-chloro-acetophenone)).
CLOFENVINFOS*** (2-chloro-1-(2,4-di-chlorophenyl)vinyl diethyl phosphate; chlorfenvinphos; ENT-24969; GC-4072; SD-7859; 'birlane', 'sapecron', 'supona').
CLOFEVERINE** (1-(*p*-chlorophenoxy-methyl)-1,2,3,4-tetrahydro-6,7-isoquino-linediol; 1-(*p*-chlorophenoxymethyl)-1,2,3,4-tetrahydro-6,7-dihydroxy-quinoline).
CLOFEXAMIDE*** (2-(*p*-chlorophenoxy)-*N*-(2-diethylaminoethyl)acetamide).
CLOFEZONE*** (equimolecular combi-nation of clofexamide and phenylbutazone; 'perclusone').
CLOFIBRATE*** (ethyl α-(*p*-chlorophen-oxy)isobutyrate; ethyl 2-(*p*-chlorophen-oxy)-2-methylpropionate; chlorphenisate; klofibrat; AY-61123; ICI-28257; CPIB; 'aterosol', 'atherolip', 'atheropront',

'atromidin', 'atromid-S', 'clofipront', 'lipavlon', 'liprinal', 'miscleron', 'neo-atromidin', 'recolip', 'regadrin', 'regelan', 'skleromexe', 'tripavlon').
CLOFIBRATE WITH ANDROSTERONE ('atromid').
CLOFIBRIC ACID*** (2-(*p*-chlorophenoxy)-2-methylpropionic acid; α-(*p*-chloro-phenoxy)isobutyric acid).
See also Aluminium clofibrate; Calcium clofibrate; Clofibrate; Clofibride; Etofi-brate; Magnesium clofib ate; Nicofibrate; Picafibrate; Serfibrate; Simfibrate; Sito-fibrate; Tiafibrate; Tocofibrate; Xanti-fibrate.
CLOFIBRIDE*** (clofibric acid ester of 4-hydroxy-*N*,*N*-dimethylbutyramide; 3-(dimethylcarbamoylpropyl) clofibrate; Mg-46; 'lipenan').
Cloflucarban* *see* Halocarban.
CLOFLUPEROL*** (4-(4-chloro-3-tri-fluoromethylphenyl)-1-[3-(*p*-fluorobenz-oyl)propyl]piperidin-4-ol; 4-[4-(4-chloro-3-trifluoromethylphenyl)-4-hydroxypiperid-1-yl]-4'-fluorobutyrophenone; 4-[4-(*p*-chloro-α,α,α-trifluoro-*m*-tolyl)-4-hydroxy-piperid-1-yl]-4'-fluorobutyrophenone; seperidol; R-9298).
CLOFOREX*** (ethyl *N*-(*p*-chloro-α,α-di-methylphenethyl)carbamate; ethyl *N*-[2-(*p*-chlorophenyl)-1,1-dimethylethyl]-carbamate; ethyl *N*-[2-(*p*-chlorobenzyl)-prop-2-yl]carbamate; D-237; 'avicol SL', 'vidipon').
CLOGESTONE*** (6-chloro-3β,17-dihydr-oxypregna-4,6-dien-20-one; 6-chloro-pregna-4,6-diene-3β,17-diol-20-one).
CLOGESTONE ACETATE* (clogestone diacetate; AY-11440).
CLOGUANAMIL*** (1-amidino-3-(3-chloro-4-cyanophenyl)urea; 1-[*N*-(3-chloro-4-cyanophenyl)carbamoyl]guan-idine; cloguanamile; BW-57C65).
Cloguanamile* *see* Cloguanamil.
CLOMACRAN*** (2-chloro-9-(3-dimethyl-aminopropyl)acridan; 3-(2-chloro-9,10-dihydroacridin-9-yl)-*N*,*N*-dimethylpropyl-amine; clomacran phosphate; SK&F-14336).
'Clomag' *see* Magnesium clofibrate.
CLOMEGESTONE*** (6-chloro-17-hydr-oxy-16α-methylpregna-4,6-diene-3,20-dione; 6-chloro-16α-methylpregna-4,6-diene-17-ol-3,20-dione; 16α-methylchlor-madinone).
Clometacillin (tr) *see* Clometocillin.
CLOMETACIN*** (3-(*p*-chlorobenzoyl)-6-methoxy-2-methylindole-1-acetic acid; 'duperan').
CLOMETERONE*** (6α-chloro-16α-meth-ylpregn-4-ene-3,20-dione; 6α-chloro-16α-methylprogesterone; clometherone; L-38000).
Clometherone* *see* Clometerone.
CLOMETHIAZOLE*** (5-(2-chloroethyl)-4-methylthiazole; chlorethiazole; chlor-methiazole; hemithiamine).

CLOMETHIAZOLE EDISILATE
(clomethiazole ethanedisulfonate; clomethiazole edisylate; 'distaneurine', 'distrapax', 'hemineurine', 'heminevrine', 'SCTZ').
CLOMETOCILLIN*** (3,4-dichloro-α-methoxybenzylpenicillin; 6-[2-(3,4-dichlorophenyl)-2-methoxyacetamido]-penicillanic acid; clometacillin; clometocillin potassium; 'rixapen').
'Clomid' see Clomifene citrate.
CLOMIFENE*** (2-[p-(β-chloro-α-phenyl-styryl)phenoxy]triethylamine; 2-chloro-1-[p-(2-diethylaminoethoxy)phenyl]-1,2-diphenyl-ethylene; α-chloro-α'-[p-(2-diethylaminoethoxy)phenyl]stilbene; 2-[p-(2-chloro-1,2-diphenylvinyl)phenoxy]-triethylamine; chloramiphene; clomiphene; 'clostilbegyt').
See also Enclomifene; Zuclomifene.
CLOMIFENE CITRATE (MRL-41; 'clomid', 'dyneric', 'gravosan').
CLOMINOREX*** (2-amino-5-(p-chlorophenyl)-2-oxazoline; McN-1107).
Clomiphene* see Clomifene.
CLOMIPRAMINE*** (3-chloro-5-(3-di-methylaminopropyl)-10,11-dihydro-5H-dibenz(b,f)azepine; chlorimipramine; chloroimipramine; monochlor-imipramine; clomipramine hydrochloride; G-34586; 'anafranil').
CLOMIZOLE (tr) (4-chloro-1-methyl-5-nitroimidazole).
CLOMOCYCLINE*** (N^2-(hydroxymethyl)-chlortetracycline; methylolchlortetra-cycline; 'megachlor').
CLONAZEPAM*** (5-(o-chlorophenyl)-1,3-dihydro-7-nitro-2H-1,4-benzodiazepin-2-one; LA-6; Ro 5-4023; 'rivotril').
CLONAZOLINE*** (2-(4-chloro-1-naphth-ylmethyl)-2-imidazoline; 4-chloro-1-(2-imidazolin-2-ylmethyl)naphthalene).
CLONIDINE*** (2-(2,6-dichloroanilino)-2-imidazoline; 2-(2,6-dichlorophenyl-amino)-2-imidazoline; clonidine hydro-chloride; chlornidine; DCAI; St-155; 'catapres', 'catapresan', 'dixarit', 'haemiton', 'hemiton', 'isoglaucon', 'namestin').
CLONIDINE WITH CHLORTALIDONE
('combipresan').
CLONITAZENE*** (2-(p-chlorobenzyl)-1-(2-diethylaminoethyl)-5-nitrobenz-imidazole; C-193901).
CLONITRALIDE (niclosamide ethanol-amine salt; Bayer 73; 'bayluscide').
CLONITRATE*** (3-chloro-1,2-propanediol dinitrate; chlorhydrin dinitrate; 'dylate').
CLONIXERIL*** (2,3-dihydroxypropyl 2-(3-chloro-o-toluidino)nicotinate; clonixin dihydroxypropyl ester; Sch-12707).
CLONIXIN** (2-(3-chloro-o-toluidino)-nicotinic acid; 2-(3-chloro-2-methyl-anilino)nicotinic acid; Sch-10304).
Clonixin dihydroxypropyl ester see Clonixeril.
'Clont' see Metronidazole.
CLOPAMIDE*** (4-chloro-N-(cis-2,6-di-methylpiperid-1-yl)-3-sulfamoylbenzamide; 1-(4-chloro-3-sulfamoylbenzamido)-2,6-dimethylpiperidine; chlosudimeprimyl; DT-327; 'adurix', 'aquex', 'brinaldix').
See also Reserpine with clopamide and dihydroergocristine.
CLOPENTHIXOL*** (4-[3-(2-chlorothio-xanthen-9-ylidene)propyl]-1-piperazine-ethanol; 2-chloro-9-[3-[4-(2-hydroxyethyl)-piperazin-1-yl]propylidene]thioxanthene; chlorphenthixol; chlorperphenthixene; 'ciatyl', 'sordinol').
CLOPERASTINE** (1-[2-(p-chloro-α-phenylbenzyloxy)ethyl]piperidine; 1-[2-(p-chlorobenzhydryloxy)ethyl]piperidine; HT-11).
CLOPERIDONE*** (3-[3-[4-(m-chloro-phenyl)piperazin-1-yl]propyl]-2,4-(1H,3H)-quinazolinedione; cloperidone hydrochloride; MA-1337).
'Clophen' see Polychlorinated biphenyl mixture.
CLOPIDOL*** (3,5-dichloro-2,6-dimethyl-pyridin-4-ol; meticlorpindol; 'coyden').
CLOPIMOZIDE*** (1-[1-[4,4-bis(p-fluoro-phenyl)butyl]piperid-4-yl]-5-chlorobenz-imidazolin-2-one; 1-[4,4-bis(p-fluoro-phenyl)butyl]-4-(5-chloro-2-oxobenz-imidazolin-1-yl)piperidine).
CLOPIRAC** (1-(p-chlorophenyl)-2,5-dimethylpyrrole-3-acetic acid; BRL-13856; CP 172-AP; 'clopiran').
'Clopiran' see Clopirac.
CLOPONONE*** (DL-(3,4'-dichloro-2,2-dichloroacetamido)propiophenone; N-(p-chloro-α-chloromethylphenacyl)-2,2-dichloroacetamide; N-[2-chloro-1-(p-chlorobenzyl)ethyl]-2,2-dichloroacetamide; (±)-2,2-dichloro-N-(p-chloro-α-chloro-methylphenacyl)acetamide; 'golaval').
CLOPONONE WITH MYRALACT
('ginetris').
CLOPREDNOL** (6-chloro-11β,17,21-trihydroxypregna-1,4,6-triene-3,20-dione; 6-chloropregna-1,4,6-triene-11β,17,21-triol-3,20-dione; RS-4691).
CLOPROP* (2-(3-chlorophenoxy)propionic acid; 'frutone CPA').
CLOPROSTENOL*** ((±)-(Z)-7-[(1R*, 2R*,3R*,5S*)-2-[(E)-(3R*)-4-(m-chloro-phenoxy)-3-hydroxy-1-butenyl]-3,5-dihydr-oxycyclopentyl]-5-heptenoic acid).
CLOPROTHIAZOLE** (5-(3-chloropropyl)-4-methylthiazole).
CLOQUINATE*** (chloroquine di(7-iodo-8-quinolinol-5-sulfonate); chloroquine di(8-hydroxy-7-iodo-5-quinolinesulfonate); chlochinate).
CLOQUINATE WITH CHLOROQUINE DIPHOSPHATE & DIIODOHYDR-OXYQUIN ('resotren').
CLOQUINOZINE*** (3-(p-chlorobenzyl)-octahydroquinolizine; 3-(p-chlorobenzyl)-quinolizidine).
CLOQUINOZINE TARTRATE (QB-1).
Clor.... See also Chlor....
CLORACETADOL*** (β,β,β-trichloro-α-hydroxy-p-acetophenetidide; 1-(p-acet-

111

amidophenoxy)-2,2,2-trichloroethanol; *p*-(3,3,3-trichloro-1-hydroxyethoxy)-acetanilide).
CLORACIZIN (tr) (2-chloro-10-(3-dimethylaminopropionyl)phenothiazine; 2-chlorophenothiazin-10-yl 2-dimethylaminoethyl ketone; chloracizin).
Cloral betaine*** *see* Chloral betaine.
Cloramfenicol pantotenate complex*** *see* Chloramphenicol pantothenate complex.
'Cloramin' *see* Chlormethine.
CLORAZEPIC ACID* (2-chloro-2,3-dihydro-2,2-dihydroxy-5-phenyl-1H-1,4-benzodiazepine-3-carboxylic acid). *See also* Dipotassium clorazepate.
Clordelazine *see* Chlorpromazine.
'Clordion' *see* Chlormadinone.
Clorepin *see* Clobazam.
Cloresolone *see* Clorexolone.
CLORETATE*** (bis(2,2,2-trichloroethyl) carbonate; clorethate; SK&F-12866; 'clorets').
Clorethate* *see* Cloretate.
'Clorets' *see* Cloretate.
'Clorevan' *see* Chlorphenoxamine.
CLOREXOLONE** (5-chloro-2-cyclohexyl-6-sulfamoylisoindolin-1-one; 6-chloro-2-cyclohexyl-3-oxo-5-isoindolinesulfonamide; 5-chloro-2-cyclohexyl-6-sulfamoylphthalimidine; cloresolone; M&B-8430; 'flonatril', 'klorex', 'nefrolan').
CLORGILINE*** (*N*-[3-(2,4-dichlorophenoxy)propyl]-*N*-methylprop-2-ynylamine; clorgyline; M&B-9302).
Clorgyline* *see* Clorgiline.
CLORIDAROL*** (α-(*p*-chlorophenyl)-2-benzofuranmethanol; 2-[(*p*-chlorophenyl)-hydroxymethyl]benzofuran; α-benzofuran-2-yl-*p*-chlorobenzyl alcohol; 2-benzofuryl *p*-chlorophenyl carbinol; clobenfurol).
CLORIDAROL HEMISUCCINATE ('menacor').
CLORINDANIC ACID*** (7-chloro-4-hydroxy-5-indancarboxylic acid; 7-chloro-4-indanol-5-carboxylic acid; clorindanol-5-carboxylic acid; CHIA).
CLORINDANOL*** (7-chloro-4-indanol; 7-chloro-4-hydroxyindan; chlorindanol; 'lanesta').
CLORINDANOL WITH LAURETH 9 ('lanettes').
CLORINDIONE*** (2-(*p*-chlorophenyl)-1,3-indandione; chlophenadion; chlorophenindione; G-25766; 'indalitan').
CLORMECAINE*** (2-dimethylaminoethyl 3-amino-4-chlorobenzoate ester; deanol 3-amino-4-chlorobenzoate).
Clorocanfamide *see* Clocanfamide.
CLOROFENE** (2-benzyl-4-chlorophenol; 5-chloro-2-hydroxydiphenylmethane; 4-chloro-α-phenyl-*o*-cresol; chlorophene; septihene; 'santophen-1', 'ultraphen').
Cloronaftina *see* Chlornaphazine.
Clorophene* *see* Clorofene.
Cloropromazina *see* Chlorpromazine.
CLOROQUALONE** (3-(2,6-dichlorophenyl)-2-ethylquinazolin-4(3H)one).

CLOROTEPINE** (1-(8-chloro-10,11-dihydrodibenzo(b,f)thiepin-10-yl)-4-methylpiperazine; 8-chloro-10,11-dihydro-10-(4-methylpiperazin-1-yl)dibenzo(b,f)-thiepine; chloroperathiepine; octoclothepin; 'clotepin').
'Clorpactin' *see* Oxychlorosene.
CLORPRENALINE*** (2-chloro-α-iso-propylaminomethylbenzyl alcohol; 1-(2-chlorophenyl)-2-isopropylaminoethanol; chlorprenaline; clorprenaline hydrochloride; isoprophenamine; L-20025).
Clortalidone *see* Chlortalidone.
CLORTERMINE*** (*o*-chloro-α,α-dimethylphenethylamine).
'Clortran' *see* Chlorbutol.
CLOSILATE(S)** (*p*-chlorobenzene-sulfonate(s); closylate(s)). *See also* *p*-Chlorophenyl closilate; Thenium closilate.
'Closina' *see* Cycloserine.
CLOSIRAMINE*** (8-chloro-11-(2-dimethylaminoethyl)-6,11-dihydro-5H-benzo(5,6)-cyclohepta(1,2-b)pyridine).
CLOSIRAMINE ACETURATE* (closir-amine compound with *N*-acetylglycine; Sch-12169).
Clospirazine *see* Spiclomazine.
CLOSTEBOL*** (4-chloro-17β-hydroxyan-drost-4-en-3-one; 4-chlorotestosterone).
CLOSTEBOL ACETATE ('macrobin', 'steranabol', 'turinabol').
CLOSTEBOL ACETATE WITH NEO-MYCIN ('trofodermin', 'trophodermin').
'Clostilbegyt' *see* Clomifene.
Closudimeprimyl *see* Clopamide.
Closylate(s)* *see* Closilate(s).
'Clotam' *see* Tolfenamic acid.
'Clotepin' *see* Clorotepine.
Clothiapine* *see* Clotiapine.
Clothixamide* *see* Clotixamide.
CLOTIAPINE*** (2-chloro-11-(4-methyl-piperazin-1-yl)dibenzo(b,f)(1,4)thiazepine; clothiapine; HF-2159; 'entumine', 'etumine').
CLOTIAZEPAM** (5-(*o*-chlorophenyl)-7-ethyl-1,3-dihydro-1-methyl-2H-thieno-(2,3-e)(1,4)diazepin-2-one; Y-6047).
CLOTIOXONE*** (2-phenyl-4-(trichloro-methylthio)-△²-1,3,4-oxadiazolin-5-one).
CLOTIXAMIDE*** (4-[3-(2-chlorothioxan-then-9-ylidene)propyl]-*N*-methyl-1-piper-azinepropionamide; chlothixamide).
CLOTIXAMIDE MALEATE (clotixamide dimaleate; chlothixamide maleate; P-4385B).
'Clotride' *see* Chlorothiazide.
CLOTRIMAZOLE*** (1-[α-(*o*-chlorophen-yl)benzhydryl]imidazole; 1-(*o*-chloro-α,α-diphenylbenzyl)imidazole; (*o*-chlorophen-yl)imidazol-1-yldiphenylmethane; 1-(*o*-chlorotrityl)imidazole; Bay b-5097; FB b-5097; 'canesten', 'kanesten', 'myco-sporin').
CLOVOXAMINE** (4'-chloro-5-methoxy-valerophenone (*E*)-*O*-(2-aminoethyl)-oxime).

CLOXACILLIN*** (6-[3-(*o*-chlorophenyl)-
5-methylisoxazol-4-ylcarboxamido]penicil-
lanic acid; 3-(*o*-chlorophenyl)-5-methyl-
isoxazol-4-ylpenicillin; cloxacillin sodium
salt; sodium cloxacillin; BRL-1621; P-25;
'cloxypen', 'ekvacillin', 'gelstaph', 'orbenin',
'penstapho N', 'syntarpin 201', 'tegopen'). †
See also Ampicillin with cloxacillin.

CLOXACILLIN WITH HETACILLIN
('heclox', 'versaclox').

'Cloxamp' *see* Ampicillin with cloxacillin.

CLOXAZOLAM*** (10-chloro-11b-(*o*-
chlorophenyl)-2,3,7,11b-tetrahydrooxazolo-
(3,2-d)benzodiazepin-6(5H)-one;
'sepazon').

CLOXESTRADIOL*** (17β-(2,2,2-tri-
chloro-1-hydroxyethoxy)estra-1,3,5(10)-
trien-3-ol; 3-hydroxy-17β-(2,2,2-trichloro-
1-hydroxyethoxy)estra-1,3,5(10)-triene;
estradiol 17-trichlorohydroxyethyl ether).

CLOXESTRADIOL ACETATE* (cloxestradiol diacetate; 'genovul').

Cloxifenol *see* Triclosan.

CLOXIQUINE** (5-chloro-8-quinolinol;
cloxyquin; chlorhydroxyquinoline;
'chlorisept', 'dermofungine A').
See also Halquinols.

CLOXIQUINE ACETATE (chloracetoxyquinoline; cloxiquine acetate ester;
8-acetoxy-5-chloroquinoline).

CLOXOTESTOSTERONE*** 17β-(2,2,2-
trichloro-1-hydroxyethoxy)estra-1,3,5(10)-
trien-3-ol; 17β-(2,2,2-trichloro-1-hydroxy-
ethoxy)androst-4-en-3-one; testosterone
trichlorohydroxyethyl ether).

CLOXOTESTOSTERONE ACETATE*
('caprosem').

'Cloxypen' *see* Cloxacillin.

CLOXYPENDYL** (4-[3-(3-chloro(10H)-
pyrido(3,2-b)(1,4)benzothiazin-10-yl)-
propyl]-1-piperazineëthanol; 3-chloro-10-
[3-[4-(2-hydroxyethyl)piperazin-1-yl]-
propyl]-1-azaphenothiazine; D-1262).

Cloxyquin* *see* Cloxiquine.

CLOZAPINE*** (8-chloro-11-(4-methyl-
piperazin-1-yl)-5H-dibenzo(b,e)(1,4)-
diazepine; LX-100-129; W-108/HF-1854;
'leponex').

CLY-503 *see* Simfibrate.

'Clysodrast' *see* Bisacodyl tannex.

CMP *see* Cytidylic acid.

CMPP *see* Mecoprop.

CMU *see* Monuron.

C.N. *see* 2-Chloroacetophenone.

CN-155 *see* Quinocide.

CN-55945 *see* Nitromifene.

'Coalgan' *see* Calcium alginate.

'Cobadex' *see* Hydrocortisone.

Cobalamins *see* Aquocobalamin; Cyanocobalamin; Hydroxocobalamin; Nitro-
cobalamin.

Coballamine *see* Cyanocobalamin.

'Cobalion' *see* Cobamamide.

COBAMAMIDE** (inner salt of *Co*(5'-
deoxyadenosine-5') derivative of 3'-ester of
cobinamide phosphate with 5,6-dimethyl-
1,α-D-ribofuranosylbenzimidazole; 9-(5'-*Co*-

5'-deoxy-β-D-ribofuranosyl)adenine derivative of α-(5,6-dimethylbenzimidazolyl)-
cobamide; adenosylcobamide; coenzyme
B_{12}; 5'-deoxyadenosylcobamide; 5,6-dimeth-
ylbenzimidazole cobamide coenzyme;
dibencocid; dibencozide; dibencozamide;
dimebencozamide; 'cobalion', 'cobazymase',
'dibencozan', 'heraclene', 'indusil T',
'trofozim', 'trophozym', 'xobaline').

Cobamine *see* Cyanocobalamin.

'Coban' *see* Monensin.

'Cobantril' *see* Pyrantel embonate.

'Cobazymase' *see* Cobamamide.

Cobeminum *see* Cyanocobalamin.

'Coben' *see* Picoperine.

'Cobex' *see* Dinitramine.

COBH *see* Benquinox.

Cobinamide *Co*-methyl derivative hydroxide dihydrogen phosphate (ester),
inner salt 3'-ester with 5,6-dimethyl-1-
α-D-ribofuranosylbenzimidazole *see*
Mecobalamin.

COBRA VENOM* ('cobrotoxin', 'cobroxin',
'nyloxin').

'Cobrentin' *see* Benzatropine mesilate.

'Cobrotoxin' *see* Cobra venom.

'Cobroxin' *see* Cobra venom.

COCAINE (L-ecgonine 3-benzoate 2-methyl
ester; erythroxylin).

COCARBOXYLASE*** (thiamine pyrophosphate).

'Cocciden' *see* Beclotiamine.

Cocculin *see* Picrotoxin.

Coculine *see* Sinomenine.

CODACTIDE** (1-D-serine-17-L-lysine-18-L-
lysinamide-α$^{1-18}$-corticotrophin; Ba-41795;
C-41795-Ba).

Codecarboxylase *see* Pyridoxal phosphate.

Codehydrogenase I *see* Nadide.

Codehydrogenase II *see* Nadide phosphate.

CODEINE (morphine monomethyl ether;
methylmorphine; codeine phosphate;
'bronchodine').

β-Codeine *see* Neopine.

CODEINE METHYL BROMIDE (codeine
methobromide; 'eucodan', 'tecodin',
'thekodin').

'Codelsol' *see* Prednisolone phosphate.

Codethyline *see* Ethylmorphine.

'Codhydrine' *see* Dihydrocodeine.

'Codinovo' *see* Hydrocodone.

Cod-liver oil fatty acids, sodium salts
see Sodium morrhuate.

CODOXIME*** (dihydrocodeinone
O-carboxymethyloxime; hydrocodone
O-carboxymethyloxime).

Coenzyme I *see* Nadide.

Coenzyme II *see* Nadide phosphate.

Coenzyme B_{12} *see* Cobamamide.

Coenzyme Q *see* Ubiquinone.

Coenzyme R *see* Biotin.

'Cofacodide' *see* Hydrocodone.

'Cofadicon' *see* Thebacon.

'Cofalaudid' *see* Hydromorphone.

'Coffearine' *see* Trigonelline.

Coffein *see* Caffeine.

COFISATIN*** (3,3-bis(*p*-hydroxyphenyl)-

2-indolinone 3,7,12-trioxo-5β-cholan-24-oic acid diester; oxyphenisatin bis(dehydrocholate); dehydrocholic acid diester with oxyphenisatin).

'Coflavinase' *see* Flavin mononucleotide.
'Cogentin' *see* Benzatropine mesilate.
'Cogesic' *see* Prodilidine.
'Cohydrin' *see* Dihydrocodeine.
'Colace' *see* Sodium dioctyl sulfosuccinate.
'Col-Al' *see* Aluminium phosphosulfate.
'Colalin' *see* Cholic acid.
Colamine *see* Ethanolamine.
Colaspase* *see* L-Asparaginase.
'Colcemid' *see* Demecolcine.
Colchamine *see* Demecolcine.
COLCHICINE (7-acetamido-6,7-dihydro-1,2,3,10-tetramethoxybenzo(a)heptalen-9(5H)-one; NSC-757).
'Colebenz' *see* Benzyl benzoate.
'Colebrina' *see* Iocetamic acid.
COLECALCIFEROL*** (9,10-secocholesta-5,7,10(19)-trien-3-ol; activated 7-dehydrocholesterol; cholecalciferol; natural vitamin D; vitamin D₃).
'Colectril' *see* Amiloride.
'Colesterinex' *see* Pyridinedimethanol bis-(methylcarbamate).
'Colestid' *see* Colestipol.
COLESTIPOL*** (tetraethylenepentamine polymer with 1-chloro-2,3-epoxypropane; tetraethylenepentamine polymer with epichlorohydrin; polyethylenepolyamine polymer with (chloromethyl)oxirane; polyethylenepolyamine polymer with 1-chloro-2,3-epoxypropane; colestipol hydrochloride; U-26597-A; 'colestid').
COLESTYRAMINE*** (a styryldivinyl-benzene copolymer containing quaternary ammonium groups; cholestyramine; MK-135; 'cuemid', 'quantalan', 'quemid', 'questran').
COLFENAMATE*** (N-(α,α,α-trifluoro-m-tolyl)anthranilic acid ester with glycolamide; flufenamic acid ester with glycolamide).
'Colferit' *see* Acetylsalicylic acid.
'Colidon' *see* Povidone.
'Colidosan' *see* Sodium ricinoleate.
COLIMECYCLINE*** (reaction product of 1 mol. colistin with 3 mol. tetracycline in presence of formaldehyde; N,N′,N″-tris[[4-(dimethylamino)-1,4,4a,5,5a,6,11,12a-octahydro-3,5,6,10,12,12a-hexahydr-oxy-6-methyl-1,11-dioxo-2-naphthacene-carboxamido]methyl]polymyxin E).
Colimycin (tr) *see* Neomycin.
'Colimycin' *see* Colistin.
Colistimethate sodium* *see* Colistin mesilate.
COLISTIN** (antibiotic from *Bac. polymyxa* var. *colistinus*; colistin sulfate; polymyxin E; W-1929; 'belcomycin', 'colimycin-CS', 'colomycin', 'coly-mycin', 'multimycin').
See also Penicillin with colistin.
COLISTIN MESILATE (colistimethate sodium; colistin methanesulfonate; colistin sodium methanesulfonate; colistin mesylate;

'colimycin-CM', 'colomycin', 'coly-mycin injectable', 'methacolimycin').
Colistin methanesulfonate *see* Colistin mesilate.
Colistin tetracycline compound *see* Colimecycline.
COLITOSE (3-deoxy-L-fucose).
D-Colitose *see* Abequose.
Colloidal radiogold *see* Gold (¹⁹⁸Au) colloidal.
Collongite *see* Phosgene.
'Collosol calcium' *see* Calcium oleate.
'Colofac' *see* Mebeverine.
'Colomenthol' *see* Menglytate.
'Colomycin' *see* Colistin.
'Colpotrophin' *see* Promestriene.
'Colprone' *see* Medrogestone.
'Coltromyl' *see* Thiocolchicoside.
'Coly-mycin' *see* Colistin.
'Combantrin' *see* Pyrantel embonate.
'Combelen' *see* Propiomazine.
'Combetin' *see* Strophanthin.
'Combiflex' *see* Indometacin arginine salt.
'Combipresan' *see* Clonidine with chlortalidone.
'Comitiadon' *see* Chlorphenacemide.
'Compazine' *see* Prochlorperazine.
'Compenamine' *see* Ephenamine penicillin.
'Complamex' *see* Xantinol nicotinate.
'Complamin' *see* Xantinol nicotinate.
'Complexic acid' *see* Edetic acid.
'Complexon' *see* Trisodium edetate.
'Complexon IV' *see* 1,2-Diaminocyclohex-anetetraacetic acid.
'Compocillin' *see* Hydrabamine penicillin.
COMPOUND 48/80 (formaldehyde condensation product of p-methoxy-N-methyl-phenethylamine; formaldehyde condensation product of N-methylhomoanisyl-amine; BW-48180).
'Conadil' *see* Sultiame.
'Concentrin' *see* Escin.
'Conceptrol' *see* Nonoxinol.
Conchinine *see* Quinidine.
'Concordin' *see* Protriptyline.
'Concurat' *see* Tetramisole.
'Conditio' *see* Potassium magnesium aspartate.
Conessi bark *see* Kurchi.
CONESSINE*** (3β-dimethylaminocon-5-ene; neriine; roquessine; wrightine).
'Confortid' *see* Indometacin.
Congo blue *see* Trypan blue.
CONGOCIDINE (3-[4-(4-guanidinoacet-amido-1-methyl-2-pyrrolecarboxamido)-1-methyl-2-pyrrolecarboxamido]propion-amide; T-1384; 'netropsin', 'sinanomycin').
CONGO RED (4,4′-biphenylylbisazo(1-naphthylamine-4-sulfonic acid sodium salt); di-Na salt of 4,4′-bis(1-amino-4-sulfo-naphth-2-ylazo)biphenyl; direct red).
Conicine *see* Coniine.
CONIINE (2-propylpiperidine; cicutine; conicine).
CONJUGATED ESTROGENS, EQUINE (estrogen sulfate; 'dagynil', 'menest', 'premarin', 'presomen', 'SK-estrogens',

'transannon').

CONJUGATED ESTROGENS WITH OXAZEPAM ('ovaribran').

'**Conlumin**' *see* Norethisterone with mestranol.

CONOPHARYNGINE (18-carbomethoxy-12,13-dimethoxyibogamine; methyl 12,13-dimethoxyibogamine-18-carboxylate).

'**Conotrane**' *see* Hydrargaphen.

'**Conovid**' *see* Noretynodrel with mestranol.

Conquinine *see* Quinidine.

'**Conray**' *see* Iotalamic acid.

'**Conray 30**' *see* Meglumine iotalamate.

'**Conray 60**' *see* Meglumine iotalamate.

'**Conray 70**' *see* Meglumine iotalamate with sodium iotalamate.

'**Conray 80**' *see* Sodium iotalamate.

'**Conray-FL**' *see* Meglumine iotalamate.

'**Conservasept**' *see* Propham.

'**Constaphyl**' *see* Dicloxacillin.

'**Continuin**' *see* Etynodiol diacetate.

'**Contradol**' *see* Carbromal with APC.

'**Contramine**' *see* Brocresine.

'**Contrapar**' *see* Gloxazone.

'**Contrathion**' *see* Pralidoxime mesilate.

'**Contravul**' *see* Sultiame.

'**Contrical**' *see* Aprotinin.

'**Contristamine**' *see* Chlorphenoxamine.

'**Contrix 28**' *see* Meglumine iotalamate.

'**Contrykal**' *see* Aprotinin.

'**Contusol**' *see* Heparin.

'**Convallan**' *see* Convallaria glycosides.

CONVALLARIA GLYCOSIDES (convallatoxin; corglycon; 'convallan', 'convallaton').

'**Convallaton**' *see* Convallaria glycosides.

Convallatoxol *see* Strophanthidol rhamnoside.

'**Convenil**' *see* Butetamate.

'**Convulex**' *see* Sodium valproate.

'**Coomassie blue**' *see* Anazolene sodium.

'**Co-Ord**' *see* Albutoin.

COPARAFFINATE* (paraffinic ointment base; 'iso-par').

Copper etc.... *See also* Cupric etc....

Copper salicylate *see* Salicylic acid copper complex.

Copper undecenate *see under* Undecenoic acid.

'**Coprol**' *see* Sodium dioctyl sulfosuccinate.

'**Coprolax**' *see* Sodium dioctyl sulfosuccinate.

COPROSTANE (pseudocholestane).

Coprostanol *see* Coprosterol.

COPROSTEROL (coprostanol; stercorin).

'**Co-ral**' *see* Coumafos.

Corazol (tr) *see* Pentetrazole.

CORBADRINE** (α-(1-aminoethyl)-3,4-dihydroxybenzyl alcohol; α-(1-aminoethyl)protocatechuyl alcohol; 3,4-dihydroxynorephedrine; α-methylnoradrenaline; homoarterenol; isoadrenaline; nordefrin).

(−)-**CORBADRINE** (levonordefrin; 'neocobefrin').

Corconium (tr) *see* Dicholine suberate.

'**Cordabromin**' *see* Protheobromine.

'**Cordalin**' *see* Etofylline.

'**Cordarone**' *see* Amiodarone.

Cordiamin (tr) *see* Nikethamide.

Cordianin *see* Allantoin.

'**Cordilan**' *see* Lanatosides.

'**Cordilox**' *see* Verapamil.

'**Cordoxene**' *see* Fenalcomine.

'**Cordran**' *see* Fludroxycortide.

CORDYCEPIN (3'-deoxyadenosine; adenine 3-deoxyriboside).

'**Coretal**' *see* Oxprenolol.

'**Corflazine**' *see* Lidoflazine.

'**Corglycon**' *see* Convallaria.

'**Coriban**' *see* Diamfenetide.

Cori ester *see* Glucose 1-phosphate.

Corkonium (tr) *see* Dicholine suberate.

'**Corlan**' *see* Hydrocortisone sodium succinate.

'**Cormelian**' *see* Dilazep.

'**Cormelian digotab**' *see* β-Acetyldigoxin with dilazep.

CORMETASONE** (6,6,9-trifluoro-11β,17,21-trihydroxy-16α-methylpregna-1,4-diene-3,20-dione; 6,6,9-trifluoro-16α-methylpregna-1,4-diene-11β,17,21-triol-3,20-dione; 6,6,9-trifluoro-16α-methylprednisolone; cormethasone).

CORMETASONE ACETATE (cormetasone 21-acetate; cormethasone acetate; RS-3694R).

Cormethasone* *see* Cormetasone.

'**Cornocentin**' *see* Ergometrine.

'**Cornox**' *see* (4-Chloro-2-methylphenoxy)-acetic acid.

'**Cornox CWK**' *see* Benazolin.

'**Cornox RK**' *see* Dichlorprop.

Corn sugar *see* Glucose.

'**Corodenin**' *see* Sodium actinoquinol.

Coronamide *see* Carinamide.

'**Corontin**' *see* Prenylamine.

COROXON ((3-chloro-4-methylcoumarin-7-yl) diethyl phosphate).

'**Corozate**' *see* Ziram.

'**Cortenil**' *see* Desoxycortone.

'**Cortexilar**' *see* Flumetasone.

Cortexolone *see* Cortodoxone.

Cortexone *see* Desoxycortone.

'**Corthion**' *see* Parathion.

'**Corticoderm**' *see* Fluprednidene acetate.

CORTICOSTERONE (pregn-4-ene-11β,21-diol-3,20-dione; 11β,21-dihydroxypregn-4-ene-3,20-dione; Kendall's compound B; Reichstein's substance H; NSC-9705).

Corticotrophin** *see* ACTH.

α^{1-28}-**Corticotrophin (human)** *see* Tosactide.

Corticotropin* *see* ACTH.

'**Cortiphenicol**' *see* Chloramphenicol with prednisone.

'**Cortiron**' *see* Desoxycortone.

CORTISONE*** (pregn-4-ene-17α,21-diol-3,11,20-trione; 11-dehydro-17-hydroxycorticosterone; 17α,21-dihydroxypregn-4-ene-3,11,20-trione; Kendall's compound E; Reichstein's substance Fa; Wintersteiner's compound F; NSC-9703).

CORTISUZOL** (11β,17,21-trihydroxy-6,16α-dimethyl-2'-phenyl-2'H-pregna-2,4,6-trieno(3,2-c)pyrazol-2-one 21-(m-sulfobenzoate)).

CORTIVAZOL** (11β,17,21-trihydroxy-

6,16α-dimethyl-2'-phenyl-2'H-pregna-2,4,6-trieno(3,2-c)pyrazol-20-one 21-acetate; Ref-185).

CORTODOXONE** (pregn-4-ene-17,21-diol-3,20-dione; 17,21-dihydroxyprogesterone; 11-deoxy-17-hydroxycorticosterone; 17,21-dihydroxypregn-4-ene-3,20-dione; 11-deoxycortisone; Reichstein's substance S; cortexolone; SK&F-3050).

CORTOL (α-cortol; pregnane-3α,11β,17α,20α,21-pentol).

α-Cortol *see* Cortol.

β-CORTOL (pregnane-3α,11β,17α,20β,21-pentol).

CORTOLONE (α-cortolone; pregnan-11-one-3α,17α,20α,21-tetrol).

α-Cortolone *see* Cortolone.

β-CORTOLONE (pregnan-11-one-3α,17α,20β,21-tetrol).

'Cortrosyn' *see* Tetracosactide.

'Corva-C' *see* Oxedrine ascorbate.

'Corvasymton' *see* Oxedrine.

'Corverum' *see* Diniprofylline with phenobarbital.

'Coryfin' *see* Menglytate.

Corynine *see* Yohimbine.

'Cosaldon' *see* Pentifylline with nicotinic acid.

'Cosban' *see* 3,5-Xylyl methylcarbamate.

'Coscopine' *see* Noscapine.

'Coscotabs' *see* Noscapine.

'Cosmegan' *see* Dactinomycin.

'Cosmegen' *see* Dactinomycin.

Cosyntropin* *see* Tetracosactide.

COTARNINE CHLORIDE ('stypticin').

COTARNINE-FERRIC CHLORIDE DOUBLE SALT ('cotargin').

COTARNINE PHTHALATE ('styptol').

'Cotazym' *see* Pancrelipase.

'Cothera' *see* Dimethoxanate.

COTININE*** ((−)-1-methyl-2-oxo-5-pyrid-3-yl-pyrrolidine; (−)-1-methyl-5-pyrid-3-yl-2-pyrrolidinone).

COTININE FUMARATE* (cotinine compound (2:1) with fumaric acid; 'scotine').

'Cotofor' *see* Dipropetryn.

'Cotoran' *see* Fluometuron.

'Cotrane' *see* Dimethoxanate.

CO-TRIMOXAZOLE* (sulfamethoxazole with trimethoprim; Ro 6-2580/11; 'abacin', 'abactrim', 'bactrim', 'biseptol', 'espectrin', 'eusaprim', 'septa', 'septran', 'septrim', 'sulfotrim', 'sulprim', 'sumetrolim', 'trib').

COTRIPTYLINE*** (3-(10,11-dihydro-5H-dibenzo(a,d)cyclohepten-5-ylidene)-1-dimethylamino-2-propanone; 5-[3-(dimethylamino)-2-oxopropylidene]-10,11-dihydro-5H-dibenzo(a,d)cycloheptene.

COUMACHLOR (3-[2-acetyl-1-(p-chlorophenyl)ethyl]-4-hydroxycoumarin; 3-(α-acetonyl-p-chlorobenzyl)-4-hydroxycoumarin; 3-[1-(4-chlorophenyl)-3-oxobutyl]-4-hydroxy-2H-1-benzopyran-2-one; 'ratilan', 'tomorin').

'Coumadin' *see* Warfarin.

Coumafene *see* Warfarin.

COUMAFOS*** (O-(3-chloro-4-methyl-coumarin-7-yl) O,O-diethyl phosphorothioate; coumaphos; Bayer-21/199; 'asuntol', 'co-ral', 'muscatox', 'resitox').

COUMAFURYL* (3-(2-acetyl-1-furan-2-ylethyl)-4-hydroxycoumarin; 3-(α-acetonylfurfuryl)-4-hydroxycoumarin; 3-(1-furan-2-yl-3-oxobutyl)-4-hydroxy-2H-1-benzo-pyran-2-one; fumarin; furmarin; tomarin).

COUMAFURYL SODIUM ('fumasol').

COUMAMYCIN** (5-methylpyrrole-2-carboxylic acid diester with 3,3'-[(3-methyl-pyrrole-2,4-diyl)bis(carbonylimino)]bis-[4-hydroxy-8-methyl-7-[(tetrahydro-3,4-dihydroxy-5-methoxy-6,6-dimethylpyran-2-yl)oxy]coumarin]; coumermycin; cumamycin).

Coumaphos* *see* Coumafos.

Coumaran-3-one-2-spiro-1'-(cyclohex-2'-en-4'-one) *see* Gris-2'-ene-3,4'-dione.

o-Coumaric acid *see* trans-o-Hydroxy-cinnamic acid.

p-Coumaric acid *see* p-Hydroxycinnamic acid.

COUMARILIC ACID (2-benzofurancarb-oxylic acid; coumarylic acid).

COUMARIN (benzo-α-pyrone; (2H)-1-benzopyran-2-one; (2H)chromen-2-one; cis-o-hydroxycinnamic acid lactone; o-coumaric acid lactone; coumarinic anhydride; cumarin; Tonka bean camphor). *See also* Melilotus officinalis.

Coumarinic acid *see* cis-o-Hydroxycinnamic acid.

Coumarinic acid lactone *see* Coumarin.

Coumarinic anhydride *see* Coumarin.

Coumarone *see* Benzofuran.

Coumarylic acid *see* Coumarilic acid.

COUMATETRALYL* (4-hydroxy-3-(1,2,3,4-tetrahydronaphth-1-yl)coumarin; 'racumin').

COUMAZOLINE*** (2-(2-ethylbenzofuran-3-ylmethyl)-2-imidazoline; 2-ethyl-3-(2-imidazolin-2-ylmethyl)benzofuran).

Coumermycin* *see* Coumamycin.

COUMESTROL (2-(2,4-dihydroxyphenyl) 6-hydroxy-3-benzofurancarboxylic acid δ-lactone).

COUMETAROL*** (3,3'-(2-methoxyethyl-idene)bis(4-hydroxycoumarin); cumetarol; cumethoxethan; cumetharol; 'dicumoxane', 'dicoumoxyl').

COUMITHOATE* (O,O-diethyl O-(7,8,9,10-tetrahydro-6-oxo-6H-dibenzo(bd)pyran-3-yl) phosphorothioate; O,O-diethyl O-(3,4-tetramethylenecoumarin-7-yl) phosphorothioate; 3-[(diethoxyphosphino-thioyl)oxy]-6-oxo-6H-dibenzo(bd)pyran; 'chromaphon', 'dition').

'Covalan' *see* Folescutol.

'Covatin' *see* Captodiame.

'Covatix' *see* Captodiame.

'Covicone' *see* Dimeticone.

'Coxytrol' *see* Ciproquinate.

'Coyden' *see* Clopidol.

Cozymase *see* Nadide.

'Cozyme' *see* Dexpanthenol.

CP-73 *see* Norclostebol acetate.

CP 172-AP see Clopirac.
CP-271B see Talampicillin.
CP-1044-J3 see Bufexamac.
CP-10188 see Fenclonine.
CP-10308-8 see Quinprenaline.
CP-10423-16 see Pyrantel embonate.
CP-10423-18 see Pyrantel tartrate.
CP-11332-1 see Quinazosin.
CP-12299-1 see Prazosin.
CP-12521-1 see Piquizil.
CP-12574 see Tinidazole.
CP-14185-1 see Hoquizil.
CP-14445 see Oxantel.
CP-14445-16 see Oxantel embonate.
CP-15464 see Carindacillin.
CP-15467-61 see Lithium carbonate.
CP-15639-2 see Carbencillin.
CP-15973 see Sudoxicam.
CP-18524 see Tibric acid.
CP-22665 see Flumizole.
CP-24314-1 see Pirbuterol.
CP-25673 see Tiazuril.
CP-28720 see Glipizide.
4-CPA see p-Chlorophenoxyacetic acid.
CPAS see Chlorfenethol.
CPBS see Fenson.
CPCBS see Chlorfenson.
CPIB see Clofibrate.
'C-quens' see Chlormadinone acetate with
  mestranol.
CR see Dibenz(b,f)(1,4)oxazine.
CR-242 see Proglumide.
CR-242-B see Proglumide with scopolamine
  butyl bromide.
CR-1639 see Dinocap.
'Crab-E-rad' see Disodium methanearsonate.
'Crabgrass killer' see Disodium methane-
  arsonate.
'Crasnitin' see L-Asparaginase.
CRD-401 see Diltiazem.
Cream of tartar see Potassium hydrogen
  tartrate.
CREATINE (methylguanidoacetic acid;
  methylglycocyamine; N-guanyl-N-methyl-
  glycine).
CREATINEPHOSPHORIC ACID (phos-
  phagen; phosphocreatine).
CREATININE (2-imino-1-methyl-4-imid-
  azolinone; 1-methylglycocyamidine;
  1-methylhydantoin-1-imide).
CREATINOLFOSFATE*** (1-(2-hydroxy-
  ethyl)-1-methylguanidine dihydrogen
  phosphate ester; 'aplodan').
'Creosalol' see p-Cresyl salicylate.
CREOSOL (2-methoxy-4-methylphenol;
  4-methylguaiacol; 2-methoxy-p-cresol).
'Cresatin' see m-Cresyl acetate.
'Crescormon' see Human growth hormone.
'Cresival' see Calcium cresolsulfonate.
CRESOL(S) (cresylic acid; methylphenol(s);
  hydroxytoluene(s)).
  See also below and Tricresol; Tricresyl
  phosphate.
m-CRESOL (3-methylphenol).
  See also m-Cresyl acetate.
o-CRESOL (2-methylphenol).
p-CRESOL (4-methylphenol).

See also p-Cresyl salicylate.
Cresolsulfonic acid(s) see below and Calcium
  cresolsulfonate.
m-Cresolsulfonic acid formaldehyde
  condensation product see Methylenedi-
  (m-cresolsulfonic acid)polymer.
'Cresopyrine' see Acetylcresotic acid.
CRESOTAMIDE** (2,3-cresotamide; 2-
  hydroxy-3-methylbenzamide; 3-methyl-
  salicylamide; ar-methylsalicylamide).
  See also Proxifezone with cresotamide.
2,3-Cresotic acid see Hydroxytoluic acid.
2,5-CRESOTIC ACID (2-hydroxy-5-methyl-
  benzoic acid; p-cresotic acid; p-cresotinic
  acid; 6-hydroxy-m-toluic acid; p-homo-
  salicylic acid).
Cresotinic acid see Cresotic acid.
o-Cresotinic acid see Hydroxytoluic acid.
Cresoxydiol see Mephenesin.
'Crestomicina' see Paromomycin.
m-CRESYL ACETATE (acetylmetacresol;
  metacresylacetate; m-tolyl acetate;
  'cresatin', 'kresatin').
o-Cresyl glyceryl ether see Mephenesin.
Cresylic acid see Cresol(s).
p-CRESYL SALICYLATE ('creosalol').
'Crillin' see Pentapiperium metilsulfate.
'Crill(s)' see Polysorbate(s).
CRIMIDINE* (2-chloro-4-dimethylamino-6-
  methylpyrimidine; 2-chloro-N,N,6-tri-
  methyl-4-pyrimidinamine; 'castrix').
'Crisalbine' see Sodium aurotiosulfate.
'Cristerona' see Androstanolone.
Croceine orange see Orange RN.
'Crodimyl' see Methylchromone.
CROFILCON A* (2,3-dihydroxypropyl
  2-methyl-2-propenoate polymer with
  methyl 2-methyl-2-propenoate; 2,3-
  dihydroxypropyl methacrylate polymer
  with methyl methacrylate; CS-151).
'Crolax' see Sodium dioctyl sulfosuccinate.
CROMACATE(S)** (6-hydroxy-4-methyl-
  coumarin-7-yloxy)acetate(s)).
'Cromadrenal' see Carbazochrome.
CROMESILATE(S)** ((6,7-dihydroxy-
  coumarin-7-yl)methanesulfonate(s)).
'Cromoci' see Cytochrome c.
'Cromoformin' see Phenformin.
CROMOGLICIC ACID*** (1,3-bis(2-carb-
  oxy-4-oxochromen-5-yloxy)propan-2-ol;
  5,5'-(2-hydroxytrimethylenedioxy)bis(4-
  oxo-4H-1-benzopyran-2-carboxylic acid);
  4-oxo-4H-1-benzopyran-2-carboxylic acid
  5,5'-diether (1,3) with glycerol; 1,3-bis(2-
  carboxy-4-oxobenzopyran-5-yloxy)-2-
  propanol; cromoglycic acid).
Cromoglicic acid disodium salt see
  Disodium cromoglicate.
Cromoglycic acid* see Cromoglicic acid.
Cromolyn sodium* see Disodium cromoglicate.
'Cromosil' see Carbazochrome.
'Cronolone' see Flugestone acetate.
CROPROPAMIDE* (N-[α-(N-crotonoyl-N-
  propylamino)butyryl]dimethylamine;
  2-crotonoylpropylamino-N,N-dimethyl-
  butyramide).

117

See also Prethcamide.
CROSS-LINKED DEXTRAN ('sephadex').
'Crotalin' *see* Rattlesnake venom.
CROTAMITON*** (N-ethyl-o-crotono-
toluidide; N-ethyl-N-o-tolylcrotonamide;
'eurax', 'euraxil').
CROTETHAMIDE* (N-[α-(N-crotonoyl-N-
ethylamino)butyryl]dimethylamine;
2-crotonoylethylamino-N,N-dimethyl-
butyramide).
See also Prethcamide.
CROTONAMIDE (2-butenamide; ethylideneacetamide).
Croton-chloral hydrate *see* Butylchloral
hydrate.
CROTONIAZIDE*** (2-(2-butenylidene)-1-
isonicotinoylhydrazine; butenylideneisoniazid; isonicotinic acid 2-butenylidene·
hydrazide).
CROTONIC ACID (*trans*-2-butenoic acid;
3-methylacrylic acid; β-methylacrylic
acid).
**Crotonic acid 2,6-dinitro-4-octylphenyl
ester** *see* Dinocap.
Crotonolic acid *see* Tiglic acid.
CROTONOYLCARBUTAMIDE (N⁴-
crotonoylcarbutamide; 'crotulin').
**(Crotonoylethylamino)dimethylbutyr-
amide** *see* Crotethamide.
**(Crotonoylpropylamino)dimethylbutyr-
amide** *see* Cropropamide.
'Crotothane' *see* Dinocap.
CROTOXYPHOS* (1-phenylethyl 3-(dimethoxyphosphinyloxy)-2-butenoate;
3-(dimethoxyphosphinyloxy)crotonic acid
α-methylbenzyl ester; α-methylbenzyl
3-hydroxycrotonate dimethyl phosphate;
'ciodrin', 'cyodrin').
'Crotulin' *see* Crotonoylcarbutamide.
Crotylethylbarbituric acid *see* Barotal.
'Croysulfone' *see* Dapsone.
CRUFOMATE*** (4-*tert*-butyl-2-chloro-
phenyl methyl methylphosphoramidate;
2-chloro-4-(1,1-dimethylethyl)phenyl
methyl methylphosphoramidate; 'ruelene').
'Crylene' *see* Pentapiperium metilsulfate.
CRYOFLUORANE*** (1,2-dichloro-1,1,2,2-
tetrafluoroethane; chlorfluoran; 'arcton-33',
'freon-114', 'frigen-114', 'frigiderm',
'pharmaethyl 144').
'Cryogenin' *see* Phenicarbazide.
CRYPTENAMINE TARTRATE*
('unitensen').
'Cryptocillin' *see* Oxacillin.
Crystallinic acid *see* Novobiocin.
CRYSTAL VIOLET* (p,p',p''-tris(dimethyl-
amino)triphenylmethane chloride; aniline
violet; hexamethylpararosaniline hydro-
chloride; methylrosaniline chloride;
gentian violet; hexamethyl violet).
See also Methyl violet.
'Crystocillin' *see* Oxacillin.
'Cristodigin' *see* Digitoxin.
'Crystoids' *see* Hexylresorcinol.
'Crystural' *see* Etoxazene.
C.S. *see* o-Chlorobenzylidenemalononitrile.
CS-310 *see* Carboquone.

CS-359 *see* Bucumolol.
CS-370 *see* Oxazolam.
CS-1507 *see* Drostanolone propionate.
CSAG-144 *see* Mebeverine.
CT-871 *see* Bialamicol.
CT-1341 *see* Alfadolone acetate with
alfaxalone.
CTAB *see* Cetrimonium.
'C-total' *see* Mobecarb with pibecarb.
CTR-6110 *see* Nitrodan.
'C-tre' *see* Capobenic acid.
CTS *see* Sodium cysteinethiosulfonate.
'Cuemid' *see* Colestyramine.
CULARINE (7-methoxy-8-(p-methoxy-
phenoxy)-2-methylisoquinoline).
CUMALDEHYDE (p-isopropylbenz-
aldehyde).
Cumaldehyde thiosemicarbazone *see*
Cutizone.
Cumamycin* *see* Coumamycin.
'Cumarene' *see* Dicoumarol.
Cumarin *see* Coumarin.
'Cumarina' *see* Warfarin.
'Cumertilin' *see* Mercumatilin sodium.
Cumetarol* *see* Coumetarol.
Cumetharol* *see* Coumetarol.
Cumethoxethan *see* Coumetarol.
Cumic acid *see* p-Isopropylbenzoic acid.
'Cumid' *see* Dicoumarol.
'Cumopyran' *see* Cyclocoumarol.
'Cumopyrin' *see* Cyclocoumarol.
'Cunate' *see under* Undecenoic acid.
'Cupradyl' *see* Allocupreide.
'Cupralene' *see* Allocupreide.
'Cupralyl' *see* Allocupreide.
'Cupramate' *see* Cupric dimethyldithio-
carbamate.
**CUPRAMMONIUM DODECYL
SULFONATE** (cuprammonium lauryl
sulfonate; 'laurycuivre').
CUPREINE (6-hydroxycinchonine;
6-demethylquinine; 'ultraquinine').
'Cuprelon' *see* Allocupreide.
Cupreol *see* Cinchol.
'Cupri-aseptol' *see* Cupric phenolsulfonate.
CUPRIC CHLORIDE (basic cupric chloride;
'bilitox').
**CUPRIC DIMETHYLDITHIOCARBAM-
ATE** ('cupramate').
CUPRIC MORRHUATE (cupric salts of
cod-liver oil fatty acids; 'gadusan').
CUPRIC 2-PHENOLSULFONATE
(2-phenolsulfonic acid cupric salt; cupric
sulfocarbolate; 'cupri-aseptol').
Cupric sulfocarbolate *see* Cupric 2-phenol-
sulfonate.
'Cuprimine' *see* Penicillamine.
'Cuprimyl' *see* Cuproxolin.
CUPRIMYXIN** (bis(6-methoxy-1-phen-
azinol-5,10-dioxidato-O^1,O^{16})copper;
Ro 7-4488/1; 'unitop').
'Cuprion' *see* Allocupreide.
Cuproallylthiourea-m-benzoic acid *see*
Allocupreide.
CUPROXOLIN (cupric bis(8-hydroxy-
quinoline) di(diethylammonium sulfonate);
cuproxyquinoline diethylamine disulfonate;

'cuprimyl', 'dicupreine').
Curaçaolin see Barbaloin.
'Curaglymol' see Hexachlorophene.
'Curam' see Decamethonium bromide.
'Curamil' see Pyrazophos.
'Curantyl' see Dipyridamole.
Curare see Tubocurarine.
Curarexine methylsulfate see Laudexium metilsulfate.
Curarexium methylsulfate see Laudexium metilsulfate.
'Curatin' see Doxepin.
Curling factor see Griseofulvin.
'Cutheparin' see Magnesium heparinate.
'Cutilene' see Mesulfen.
'Cutisan' see Triclocarban.
Cutisone see Cutizone.
CUTIZONE (tr) (cumaldehyde thiosemicarbazone; *p*-isopropylbenzaldehyde thiosemicarbazone; cutisone; kutizon; SHCH-58).
CV-58903 see Xenazoic acid.
CVMP see Stirofos.
CY-116 see Aminocaproic acid.
CYACETACIDE* (cyanatoacetic acid hydrazide; cyanoacetic acid hydrazide; cyanacetohydrazide; cyanacetylhydrazide; cyanoacetohydrazide; cyacetazide; cyanazide; cyanizide; cyanoethydrazide; AB-42; 'armazal', 'cyaceticid', 'dictyzide', 'helmox', 'hidacian', 'leandin', 'neohydrazid', 'reacid', 'reazide').
Cyacetazide* see Cyacetacide.
'Cyaceticid' see Cyacetacide.
CYAMEMAZINE** (10-(3-dimethylamino-2-methylpropyl)phenothiazine-2-carbonitrile; 2-cyano-10-(3-dimethylamino-2-methylpropyl)phenothiazine; cyamepromazine; RP-7204; 'cianatil', 'tercian').
Cyamepromazine* see Cyamemazine.
2-Cyanacetamidocephalosporanic acid see Cefacetrile.
Cyanacetic acid see Cyanatoacetic acid.
Cyanacetohydrazide* see Cyacetacide.
Cyanacetylhydrazide see Cyacetacide.
CYANATOACETIC ACID (cyanacetic acid; cyanoacetic acid; malonic mononitrile; malononitrile).
Cyanatoacetic acid hydrazide see Cyacetacide.
Cyanazide see Cyacetacide.
CYANAZINE* (2-chloro-4-ethylamino-6-(1-cyano-1-methylethylamino)-*s*-triazine; 2-[[4-chloro-6-(ethylamino)-1,3,5-triazin-2-yl]amino]-2-methylpropionitrile; SD-15418; WL-19805; 'bladex', 'fortrol', 'radikill').
Cyanizide see Cyacetacide.
7-(2-Cyanoacetamido)cephalosporanic acid see Cefacetrile.
7-(2-Cyanoacetamido)-3-(hydroxymethyl)-2-cephem-2-carboxylic acid see Cefacetrile.
Cyanoacetic acid see Cyanatoacetic acid.
Cyanoacetohydrazide see Cyacetacide.
2-Cyanoacrylic acid esters see Bucrilate; Enbucrilate; Flucrilate; Mecrilate; Ocrilate.

Cyanobenzene see Benzonitrile.
N-(α-Cyanobenzyl)amphetamine see Amphetaminil.
O-(α-Cyanobenzylimino) O,O-diethyl phosphorothioate see Phoxim.
CYANOCOBALAMIN** (5,6-dimethylbenzimidazolylcobamide cyanide; 5,6-dimethylbenzimidazole cyanocobamide; aquocobinamide cyanide; cobamin; cobalamin; coballamine; cobeminum; cycobemin; CN-cobalamin; extrinsic factor; LLD factor; vitamin B_{12}).
CYANOCOBALAMIN (^{57}Co) (radiocyanocobalamin; 'racobalamin-57').
CYANOCOBALAMIN (^{58}Co)*** (radiocyanocobalamin).
CYANOCOBALAMIN (^{60}Co) (radiocyanocobalamin; radiocycobemin).
2-Cyano-10-(3-dimethylamino-2-methylpropyl)phenothiazine see Cyamemazine.
1-Cyano-3-(1,1-dimethylpropyl)guanidine see Guancidine.
4-[2-[(5-Cyano-5,5-diphenylpentyl)methylamino]ethyl]-4-methylmorpholinium chloride methochloride see Pentacynium chloride.
N-(5-Cyano-5,5-diphenylpentyl)-N,N,N'-trimethylethyl-1-ammonium-2-morpholinium chloride see Pentacynium chloride.
1-(2-Cyano-3,3-diphenylpropyl)-4-(2-oxo-3-propionylbenzimidazolin-1-yl)piperidine see Bezitramide.
1-(3-Cyano-3,3-diphenylpropyl)-4-phenylisonipecotic acid see Difenoxin.
N-[[1-(3-Cyano-3,3-diphenylpropyl)-4-phenylisonipecotoyl]oxy]succinimide see Difenoximide.
1-(3-Cyano-3,3-diphenylpropyl)-4-phenylpiperidine-4-carboxylic acid see Difenoxin.
1-(3-Cyano-3,3-diphenylpropyl)-4-piperid-1-ylisonipecotamide see Piritramide.
1-[1-(3-Cyano-3,3-diphenylpropyl)piperid-4-yl]-3-propionyl-2-benzimidazolinone see Bezitramide.
Cyanoethane see Propionitrile.
Cyanoethydrazide see Cyacetacide.
N-(2-Cyanoethyl)amphetamine see Fenproporex.
Cyanoethylene see Acrylonitrile.
2-Cyanoethyl N-[[(methylamino)carbonyl]oxy]ethanimidothioate see Thiocarboxim.
2-Cyanoethyl N-(methylcarbamoyloxy)acetimidothioate see Thiocarboxim.
CYANOFENPHOS* (O-(4-cyanophenyl) O-ethyl phenylphosphonothioate; CYP; S-4087; 'surecide').
Cyanoferrates (II) see Ferrocyanides.
Cyanoferrates (III) see Ferricyanides.
Cyanoformic acid methyl ester see Methyl cyanoformate.
2-Cyano-10-[3-(4-hydroxypiperid-1-yl)propyl]phenothiazine see Periciazine.
2α-Cyano-17β-hydroxy-4,4,17-trimethylandrost-5-en-3-one see Cyanoketone.

119

4-Cyano-2-iodo-6-nitrophenol *see* Nitroxinil.
CYANOKETONE (2α-cyano-4,4,17α-tri-
methylandrost-4-en-17β-ol-3-one; 2α-
cyano-17β-hydroxy-4,4,17-trimethyl-
androst-5-en-3-one; WIN-19578).
**4-[[[2-(3-Cyano-2-methylguanidin-1-yl)-
ethyl]thio]methyl]-5-methylimidazole**
see Cimetidine.
**1-Cyano-2-methyl-3-[2-[[(5-methyl-
imidazol-4-yl)methyl]thio]ethyl]-
guanidine** *see* Cimetidine.
**2-Cyano-10-[3-(4-methylpiperazin-1-yl)-
propyl]phenothiazine** *see* Cyanperazine.
Cyanomycin *see* Pyocyanine.
**N-(5-Cyano-4-oxo-1(4H)-pyrimidinyl)-
acetamide** *see* Ciapilome.
1-Cyano-3-*tert*-pentylguanidine *see*
Guancidine.
**O-(p-Cyanophenyl) O,O-dimethyl phos-
phorothioate** *see* Cyanophos.
**O-(p-Cyanophenyl) O-ethyl phenylphos-
phonothioate** *see* Cyanofenphos.
CYANOPHOS* (O-(p-cyanophenyl) O,O-
dimethyl phosphorothioate; CYAP;
'cyanox').
N'-Cyanosulfanilamide *see* Sulcymide.
**5-Cyano-2-thiophenecarboxaldehyde
thiosemicarbazone** *see* Citenazone.
**2-Cyano-4,4,17-trimethylandrost-5-en-
17β-ol-3-one** *see* Cyanoketone.
'Cyanox' *see* Cyanophos.
CYANPERAZINE (2-cyano-10-[3-(4-
methylpiperazin-1-yl)propyl]phenothiazine
dihydrochloride).
'Cyantin' *see* Nitrofurantoin.
CYANURIC ACID (2,4,6-trihydroxy-s-
triazine; *sym*-triazinetriol; tricyanic acid;
trihydroxycyanidine).
Cyanurotriamide *see* Melamine.
CYAP *see* Cyanophos.
CYCASIN (methylazoxymethanol glucoside).
Cyclacillin* *see* Ciclacillin.
'Cycladiene' *see* Dienestrol.
'Cyclaine' *see* Hexylcaine.
Cyclamate *see* Calcium cyclamate; Sodium
cyclamate.
CYCLAMIC ACID* (N-cyclohexylsulfamic
acid; cyclohexanesulfamic acid; 'hexamic
acid').
See also Aminophenazone cyclamate,
Calcium cyclamate; 1-(3-Phenylpropoxy)-
guanidine cyclamate; Sodium cyclamate;
Tetracycline cyclamate.
Cyclamide (tr) *see* Glycyclamide.
Cyclamidomycin *see* Desdanine.
'Cyclamycin' *see* Troleandomycin.
'Cyclan' *see* Calcium cyclamate.
CYCLANDELATE* (3,3,5-trimethyl-
cyclohexyl mandelate; 3,3,5-trimethyl-
cyclohexanol α-phenyl-α-hydroxyacetate;
cyclomandol; BS-572; 'cyclospasmol',
'spasmocyclone').
CYCLARBAMATE* (1,1-bis(phenylcarbamoyloxymethyl)cyclopentane; 1,1-cyclo-
pentanedimethanol dicarbanilate; 1,1-bis-
(hydroxymethyl)cyclopentane dicarbanilate; N,N'-diphenyldicarbamate of 1,1-

dimethylolcyclopentane; cyclopentylidenedimethanol dicarbanilate; 'camalon',
'casmalon').
Cyclazenin *see* Guanacline.
CYCLAZOCINE* (3-(cyclopropylmethyl)-
1,2,3,4,5,6-hexahydro-6,11-dimethyl-2,6-
methano-3-benzazocin-8-ol; 2-cyclopropyl-
methyl-2'-hydroxy-5,9-dimethyl-6,7-benzo-
morphan).
CYCLAZODONE* (2-cyclopropylamino-
5-phenyl-2-oxazolin-4-one; LD-3695).
CYCLETHRIN* (3-(2-cyclopenten-1-yl)-2-
methyl-4-oxo-2-cyclopenten-1-yl 2,2-
dimethyl-3-(2-methyl-1-propenyl)-
cyclopropanecarboxylate).
CYCLEXANONE (2-cyclopenten-1-yl-2-
(2-morpholinoethyl)cyclopentanone;
'exopon').
Cyclic AMP *see* Adenosine 3',5'-phosphate.
**Cyclic methylene (4-chloro-o-tolyl)-
dithioimidocarbonate** *see* Nimidane.
'Cyclipen' *see* Penimepicycline.
CYCLIRAMINE* (4-(p-chloro-α-pyrid-2-
ylbenzylidene)-1-methylpiperidine; cycliramine maleate; 'prolergic').
CYCLIZINE* ((±)-1-(diphenylmethyl)-4-
methylpiperazine; 1-benzhydryl-4-methyl-
piperazine; cyclizine dihydrochloride;
BW-47-83).
See also Dipipanone with cyclizine.
2,2'-Cyclo-1-β-D-arabinofuranosylcytosine
see Ancitabine.
2,2'-Cyclo-ara C *see* Ancitabine.
CYCLOATE (S-ethyl cyclohexylethyl-
carbamothioate; 'ro-neet').
CYCLOBARBITAL* (5-(1-cyclohexen-1-
yl)-5-ethylbarbituric acid; cyclobarbitone;
cyclohexemal; ethylhexabital; hexemal;
tetrahydrophenobarbital; cyclobarbital
calcium).
CYCLOBENZAPRINE* (5-(3-dimethyl-
aminopropylidene)dibenzo(a,e)cyclo-
heptatriene; [3-(5H-dibenzo(a,d)cyclo-
hepten-5-ylidene)propyl]dimethylamine;
MK-130; RP-9715).
CYCLOBUTOIC ACID (3-cyclohexyl-
3-hydroxy-3-methylpropionic acid; 3-cyclo-
hexyl-3-hydroxybutyric acid; β-hydroxy-
β-methylcyclohexanepropionic acid).
**2-Cyclobutylamino-1-(3,4-dihydroxy-
phenyl)ethanol** *see* Norbudrine.
**α-Cyclobutylaminomethyl-3,4-dihydroxy-
benzyl alcohol** *see* Norbudrine.
**17-Cyclobutylmethyl-4,5a-epoxymorphi-
nan-3,6a,14-triol** *see* Nalbuphine.
**17-(Cyclobutylmethyl)morphinan-3,14-
diol** *see* Butorphanol.
**12-Cyclobutylmethyl-7,7a,8,9-tetrahydro-
3,7a-dihydroxy-6H-8,9c-iminoethano-
phenanthro(4,5-bcd)furan-5(4aH)-ol**
see Nalbuphine.
N-Cyclobutylnoradrenaline *see* Norbudrine.
CYCLOBUTYROL* (α-ethyl-1-hydroxy-
cyclohexaneacetic acid; 2-(1-hydroxy-
cyclohexyl)butyric acid).
CYCLOBUTYROL SODIUM (sodium
α-ethyl-1-hydroxycyclohexaneacetate;

sodium 2-(1-hydroxycyclohexyl)butyrate, 'hebucol').

'Cyclocaine' *see* Isobutylcaine.

'Cyclocapron' *see* Tranexamic acid.

CYCLOCOUMAROL* (3,4-dihydro-2-methoxy-2-methyl-4-phenylpyrano(3,2-c)-(1)benzopyran-5-one; Link's compound 63; BL-5; 'cumopyran', 'cumopyrin', 'methanopyranorin', 'methopyranorin').

2,2′-Cyclocytarabine *see* Ancitabine.

Cyclocytidine *see* Ancitabine.

Cyclocytidine acetate *see* Ancitabine acetate.

'Cyclodan' *see* Endosulfan.

CYCLOFENIL** (4,4′-(cyclohexylidenemethylene)diphenol diacetate ester; 4,4′-diacetoxybenzhydrylidenecyclohexane; bis(*p*-acetoxyphenyl)cyclohexylidenemethane; F-6066; H-3452; ICI-48213; 'fertodur', 'ondogyne', 'ondomid', 'sexovid').

'Cycloform' *see* Isobutylcaine.

'Cyclogesin' *see* Isobutylcaine.

'Cyclogol' *see* Cetomacrogols.

CYCLOGUANIL EMBONATE*** (4,6-diamino-1-(*p*-chlorophenyl) 1,2-dihydro-2,2-dimethyl-*s*-triazine compound (2:1) with 4,4′-methylenebis(3-hydroxy-2-naphthoic acid); cycloguanil pamoate; chlorguanide triazine pamoate; chlorazine; CI-501; DHT; PAM-MR-807-23a; 'camolar').

CYCLOGUANIL EMBONATE WITH ACEDAPSONE (CI-564; 'dapolar').

Cycloguanil pamoate* *see* Cycloguanil embonate.

'Cyclogyl' *see* Cyclopentolate.

2,4,6-Cycloheptatrien-2-ol-1-one *see* Tropolone.

5-Cyclohepten-1-yl-5-ethylbarbituric acid *see* Heptabarb.

1-Cycloheptyl-3-(*p*-toluenesulfonyl)urea *see* Heptolamide.

2,5-Cyclohexadiene-1,4-dione *see* *p*-Benzoquinone.

2,5-Cyclohexadiene-1-ol-4-one-sulfonic acid diethylamine salt *see* Etamsylate.

CYCLOHEXANE (hexahydrobenzene; hexamethylene; hexanaphthene).

Cyclohexanecarbamic acid 1,1-diphenyl-2-propynyl ester *see* Enpromate.

Cyclohexanehexol *see* Inositol.

Cyclohexanehexol hexaphosphate *see* Phytic acid.

Cyclohexanepentol *see* Quercitol.

Cyclohexanepropionic acid 2-dimethylaminoethyl ester *see* Cyprodenate.

Cyclohexanesulfamic acid *see* Cyclamic acid.

Cyclohexemal* *see* Cyclobarbital.

5-(1-Cyclohexen-1-yl)-1,3-dihydro-1-methyl-7-nitro-2H-1,4-benzodiazepin-2-one *see* Menitrazepam.

5-Cyclohexen-1-yl-1,5-dimethylbarbituric acid *see* Hexobarbital.

5-Cyclohexen-1-yl-5-ethylbarbituric acid *see* Cyclobarbital.

(*R*)-3-Cyclohexenylglyoxylic acid *see*

Ketomycin.

(*p*-(1-Cyclohexen-1-yl)hydratropic acid *see* Tetriprofen.

N-[*p*-[[3-(3-Cyclohexen-1-yl)-2-iminoimidazolidin-1-yl]sulfonyl]phenethyl]butyramide *see* Glibutimine.

5-Cyclohexen-1-yl-5-methylbarbituric acid *see* Norhexobarbital.

17*β*-Cyclohexen-1-yloxyestra-1,3,5(10)-trien-3-ol propionate *see* Orestrate.

2-(*p*-(Cyclohexen-1-yl)phenyl)propionic acid *see* Tetriprofen.

1-(3-Cyclohexen-1-yl-3-phenylpropyl)-1-methylpiperidinium methylsulfate *see* Fenclexonium metilsulfate.

CYCLOHEXIMIDE* (3-[2-(3,5-dimethyl-2-oxocyclohexyl)-2-hydroxyethyl]glutarimide; NSC-185; U-4527; 'actidione', 'naramycin').

Cyclohexitol *see* Inositol.

N-[2-[4-[[[(Cyclohexylamino)carbonyl]amino]sulfonyl]phenyl]ethyl]-5-methylpyrazine-2-carboxamide *see* Glipizide.

2-Cyclohexylamino-1-methylethyl benzoate *see* Hexylcaine.

1-Cyclohexylamino-2-propyl benzoate *see* Hexylcaine.

2-(α-Cyclohexylbenzyl)-N,N,N′,N′-tetraethyl-1,3-propanediamine *see* Phenetamine.

2-(Cyclohexylcarbonyl)-1,3,4,6,7,11b-hexahydro-2H-pyrazino(2,1-a)isoquinolin-4-one *see* Praziquantel.

1-(Cyclohexylcarbonyl)-4-methylpiperazine *see* Pexantel.

3-Cyclohexylcrotonic acid *see* Cicrotoic acid.

1-Cyclohexylcyclohexanecarboxylic acid *see* (Bicyclohexyl)-1-carboxylic acid.

N-Cyclohexyl-N′,N″-diethylenephosphorothioic triamide *see* Hexaphosphamide.

1-Cyclohexyl-3-[*p*-[2-(3,4-dihydro-7-methoxy-4,4-dimethyl-1,3-dioxo-2(1H)isoquinolinyl)ethyl]benzenesulfonyl]urea *see* Gliquidone.

1-Cyclohexyl-3-dimethylamino-1-phenyl-1-propanol ethiodide *see* Tridihexethyl iodide.

3-Cyclohexyl-N,N-dimethyl-3-phenylpropylamine *see* Gamfexine.

2-Cyclohexyl-4,6-dinitrophenol *see* Dinex.

Cyclohexylethylcarbamothioic acid S-ethyl ester *see* Cycloate.

1-Cyclohexyl-3-[*p*-[2-(1-ethyl-4-isopentyloxy-3-methyl-1H-pyrazolo(3,4-b)pyridine-5-carboxamido)ethyl]benzenesulfonyl]urea *see* Glicaramide.

Cyclohexyl 4-[3-(*p*-fluorobenzoyl)propyl]-1-piperazinecarboxylate *see* Fenaperone.

2-Cyclohexyl-N-hexylethylamine *see* Hecylamine.

(*p*-Cyclohexylhydratropic acid *see* Hexaprofen.

3-Cyclohexyl-3-hydroxybutyric acid *see* Cyclobutoic acid.

4-Cyclohexyl-2-hydroxybutyric acid *see*

α-Hydroxycyclohexanebutyric acid.
6-Cyclohexyl-1-hydroxy-4-methylpyridin-2(1H)-one *see* Ciclopirox.
4-(β-Cyclohexyl-β-hydroxyphenethyl)-1,1-dimethylpiperazinium methylsulfate *see* Hexocyclium metilsulfate.
(3-Cyclohexyl-3-hydroxy-3-phenylpropyl)-trimethylammonium iodide *see* Tridihexethyl iodide.
4,4′-(Cyclohexylidenemethylene)diphenol diacetate *see* Cyclofenil.
1-Cyclohexyl-3-indan-5-ylsulfonylurea *see* Glyhexamide.
2-Cyclohexyl-4-iodo-3,5-xylenol *see* Cicliomenol.
N-Cyclohexyllinoleamide *see* Clinolamide.
Cyclohexylmandelic acid *see* α-Phenyl-cyclohexaneglycolic acid.
3-Cyclohexyl-3-methylacrylic acid *see* Cicrotoic acid.
1-Cyclohexyl-2-methylaminopropyl 5-ethyl-5-phenylbarbiturate *see* Barbexaclone.
1-(Cyclohexylmethyl)hydrazine *see* Cimemoxin.
Cyclohexyl 4-methylpiperazin-1-yl ketone *see* Pexantel.
1-Cyclohexylmethylpiperidine *see* Leptacline.
1-Cyclohexyl-2-methyl-1-propanol *see* Cimepanol.
1-Cyclohexyl-N-methyl-2-propylamine *see* Propylhexedrine.
1-Cyclohexyl-3-[p-[2-(5-methylpyrazine-2-carboxamido)ethyl]benzenesulfonyl]-urea *see* Glipizide.
1-Cyclohexyl-3-[[p-[2-(5-methylpyrazine-2-carboxamido)ethyl]phenyl]sulfonyl]-urea *see* Glipizide.
1-Cyclohexyl-3-(p-methylthiobenzene-sulfonyl)urea *see* Thiohexamide.
2-(8-Cyclohexyloctyl)-3-hydroxy-1,4-naphthoquinone *see* Menoctone.
p-Cyclohexyloxybenzoic acid methyl-piperidylpropyl ester *see* Cyclomethycaine.
4-[(4-Cyclohexyloxycarbonyl)piperazin-1-yl]-4′-fluorobutyrophenone *see* Fenaperone.
1-(o-Cyclohexylphenoxy)-3-isopropyl-amino-2-propanol *see* Exaprolol.
1-(2-Cyclohexyl-2-phenyl-1,3-dioxolan-4-ylmethyl)-1-methylpiperidinium iodide *see* Oxapium iodide.
α-Cyclohexyl-α-phenyl-1-piperidine-propanol *see* Trihexyphenidyl.
2-(p-Cyclohexylphenyl)propionic acid *see* Hexaprofen.
α-Cyclohexyl-α-phenyl-1-pyrrolidine-propanol *see* Tricyclamol.
1-Cyclohexylpropyl carbamate *see* Procymate.
N-Cyclohexylsulfamic acid *see* Cyclamic acid.
α-Cyclohexyl-3-thiopheneacetic acid 2-(hexahydro-1H-azepin-1-yl)ethyl ester *see* Cetiedil.

1-Cyclohexyl-3-p-toluenesulfonylurea *see* Glycyclamide.
2-Cyclohexyl-3,5-xylenol *see* Cyclomenol.
'Cyclokapron' *see* Tranexamic acid.
CYCLOLEUCINE (1-aminocyclopentane-carboxylic acid; CB-1639; NSC-1026).
Cyclomandol *see* Cyclandelate.
CYCLOMENOL*** (2-cyclohexyl-3,5-xylenol; 2-cyclohexyl-3,5-dimethylphenol).
CYCLOMETHONE (cyclooctadecane-1,10-bis(trimethyl ammonium iodide); Lü-274).
CYCLOMETHYCAINE*** (3-(2-methyl-piperid-1-ylpropyl) p-cyclohexyloxybenzo-ate sulfate; 'surfacaine', 'surfathesin', 'topocaine').
'Cyclon A' *see* Methyl cyanoformate.
Cyclonamine* *see* Etamsylate.
Cyclooctadecane-1,10-bis(trimethyl-ammonium iodide) *see* Cyclomethone.
CYCLOOCTYLAMINE (SK&F-23880A).
1-Cyclooctyl-3,3-dimethylurea *see* Cycluron.
1-Cyclooctyl-3-p-toluenesulfonylurea *see* Glyoctamide.
Cyclo-oxapentamethylenebiguanide *see* Moroxydine.
'Cyclopal' *see* Cyclopentobarbital.
'Cyclopen' *see* Cyclopentobarbital.
Cyclopentacycloheptene *see* Azulene.
Cyclopentadrin *see* Cyclopentamine.
CYCLOPENTAMINE*** (N,α-dimethyl-cyclopentaneëthylamine; 1-cyclopentyl-N-methylisopropylamine; 1-cyclopentyl-2-methylaminopropane; cyclopentadrin; cyclopentamine hydrochloride).
Cyclopentaneacetic acid dimethylamino-ethyl ester *see* Cyclopentolate.
1,1-Cyclopentanedimethanol dicarbanil-ate *see* Cyclarbamate.
3-Cyclopentanepropionic acid, esters and salts *see* Cipionate(s).
Cyclopentanone 2α,3α-epithio-5α-androstan-17β-yl methyl acetal *see* Mepitiostane.
2-Cyclopentene-2,3-diol *see* Reductic acid.
11-(2-Cyclopenten-1-yl)undecanoic acid *see* Hydnocarpic acid.
3-(2-Cyclopenten-1-yl)-2-methyl-4-oxo-2-cyclopenten-1-yl 2,2-dimethyl-3-(2-methyl-1-propenyl)cyclopropane-carboxylate *see* Cyclethrin.
2-Cyclopenten-1-yl-2-(2-morpholinoethyl)-cyclopentanone *see* Cyclexanone.
17β-Cyclopenten-1-yloxyandrosta-1,4-dien-3-one *see* Quinbolone.
CYCLOPENTHIAZIDE*** (6-chloro-3-cyclopentylmethyl-3,4-dihydro-7-sulfamoyl-(2H)1,2,4-benzothiadiazine 1,1-dioxide; Su-8341; 'navidrex', 'navidrix').
CYCLOPENTOBARBITAL (5-allyl-5-(2-cyclopenten-1-yl)barbituric acid; 'cyclopal', 'cyclopen', 'cyclopal', 'dormisan').
CYCLOPENTOLATE* (2-dimethylamino-ethyl 1-hydroxy-α-phenylcyclopentane acetate; deanol 1-hydroxy-α-phenyl-cyclopentaneacetate; cyclopentolate hydro-chloride; GT-75; 'cyclogyl', 'cyplegin',

'mydrilate', 'zyklolat').

1-Cyclopentyl-3-[[p-[2-(o-anisamido)-ethyl]phenyl]sulfonyl]urea *see* Glipentide.

Cyclopentylidenedimethanol dicarbanilate *see* Cyclarbamate.

N-**CYCLOPENTYLLYSERGAMIDE** (lysergic acid cyclopentylamide; 'cepentyl').

1-Cyclopentyl-3-[p-[2-(o-methoxy-benzamido)ethyl]benzenesulfonyl]-urea *see* Glipentide.

3-Cyclopentyloxy-16α,17-dihydroxy-19-nor-17α-pregna-1,3,5(10)-trien-20-yne *see* Nilestriol.

3-Cyclopentyloxyestratriene-16α,17β-diol *see* Quinestradiol.

3-Cyclopentyloxy-17α-ethynylestra-1,3,5(10)-trien-17β-ol *see* Quinestrol.

3-Cyclopentyloxy-17-methylandrosta-3,5-dien-17β-ol *see* Penmesterol.

3-Cyclopentyloxy-19-nor-17α-pregna-3,5-dien-20-yn-17-ol *see* Quingestanol.

3-Cyclopentyloxy-19-nor-17α-pregna-1,3,5(10)-trien-20-yne-16α,17-diol *see* Nilestriol.

3-Cyclopentyloxy-19-nor-17α-pregna-1,3,5(10)-trien-20-yn-17β-ol *see* Quinestrol.

3-Cyclopentyloxypregna-3,5-dien-17-ol-20-one *see* Pentagestrone.

3-Cyclopentyloxypregna-3,5-dien-20-one *see* Quingestrone.

1-Cyclopentyl-1-phenyl-3-piperid-1-yl-1-propanol *see* Cycrimine.

17β-(3-Cyclopentylpropionoxy)-4-hydroxyestr-4-en-3-one *see* Oxabolone cipionate.

1-Cyclopentyl-3-p-toluenesulfonylurea *see* Tolpentamide.

Cyclophenazine*** *see* Ciclofenazine.

CYCLOPHOSPHAMIDE********* (2-[bis(2-chloroethyl)amino]tetrahydro-2H-1,3,2-oxazaphosphorine 2-oxide; 2-[bis(2-chloroethyl)amino](2H)-1,3,2-oxazaphosphorinane 2-oxide; intramolecular ester of *N,N*-bis-(2-chloroethyl)-*N'*-(3-hydroxypropyl)-phosphorodiamidic acid; cyclic *N',O*-propylene ester of *N,N*-bis(2-chloroethyl) phosphorodiamidic acid; 2-[bis(2-chloroethyl)amino]-1-oxa-3-aza-2-phosphacyclohexane 2-oxide; B-518; NSC-26271; 'clafen', 'cytoxan', 'endoxan', 'endoxana', 'enduxan', 'genoxal', 'lostinil', 'procytox', 'semdoxan', 'sendoxan').

3,5-Cyclopregnan-6β-ol-20-one *see* Cyclopregnol.

CYCLOPREGNOL********* (3,5-cyclopregnan-6β-ol-20-one; 6β-hydroxy-3,5-cyclopregnan-20-one; 'neurosterone').

CYCLOPROPANE********* (trimethylene).

2-Cyclopropylamino-5-phenyl-2-oxazolin-4-one *see* Cyclazodone.

5-Cyclopropylcarbonyl-2-benzimidazole-carbamic acid methyl ester *see* Ciclobendazole.

22-Cyclopropyl-7α((R)-1-hydroxy-1-methylpropyl)-6,14-endo-ethenotetra-hydrothebaine *see* Homprenorphine.

N-**Cyclopropyl-3-hydroxymorphinan** *see* Cyclorphan.

21-Cyclopropyl-7α-((S)-1-hydroxy-1,2,2-trimethylpropyl)-6,14-endo-ethano-6,7,8,14-tetrahydrooripavine *see* Buprenorphine.

α-Cyclopropyl-α-(p-methoxyphenyl)-5-pyrimidinemethanol *see* Ancymidol.

17-(Cyclopropylmethyl)-3,4-dihydroxy-morphinan *see* Oxilorphan.

3-Cyclopropylmethyl-6,11-dimethyl-6,7-benzomorphan-8-ol *see* Cyclazocine.

3-Cyclopropylmethyl-6,11-dimethyl-2,6-methano-6,7-benzomorphan *see* Volazocine.

17-Cyclopropylmethyl-3,5α-epoxy-3,14-dihydroxymorphinan-6-one *see* Naltrexone.

3-Cyclopropylmethyl-6-ethyl-1,2,3,4,5,6-hexahydro-11,11-dimethyl-2,6-methano-3-benzazocin-8-ol *see* Gemazocine.

3-Cyclopropylmethyl-1,2,3,4,5,6-hexa-hydro-6,11-dimethyl-2,6-methano-3-benzazocine *see* Volazocine.

3-Cyclopropylmethyl-1,2,3,4,5,6-hexa-hydro-6,11-dimethyl-2,6-methano-3-benzazocin-8-ol *see* Cyclazocine.

2-Cyclopropylmethyl-2'-hydroxy-5,9-dimethyl-6,7-benzomorphan *see* Cyclazocine.

N-**Cyclopropylmethyl-7α-(1(R)-hydroxy-1-methylpropyl)-6,14-endo-ethenotetra-hydronorthebaine** *see* Homprenorphine.

N-**Cyclopropylmethyl-3-hydroxymorphi-nan** *see* Cyclorphan.

N-**Cyclopropylmethyl-7α-(1-hydroxy-1-methylethyl)-O⁶-methyldihydro-endo-ethanonormorphine** *see* Diprenorphine.

N-**Cyclopropylmethyl-19-methylnorvinol** *see* Cyprenorphine.

17-(Cyclopropylmethyl)morphinan-3,14-diol *see* Oxilorphan.

14-Cyclopropylmethyloctahydro(5,11b)-iminoethano(11bH)benzo(a)carbazole *see* Carbazocine.

3-(Cyclopropylmethyl)-3,4,5,6-tetrahydro-8-hydroxy-6,11-dimethyl-2,6-methano-3-benzazocin-1(2H)-one *see* Ketazocine.

N-**Cyclopropylmethyl-6,7,8,14-tetrahydro-7α-(1-hydroxy-1-methylethyl)-6,14-endo-ethenonororipavine** *see* Cyprenorphine.

1-(o-Cyclopropylphenoxy)-3-isopropyl-amino-2-propanol *see* Procinolol.

10-[3-(4-Cyclopropylpiperazin-1-yl)-propyl]-2-trifluoromethylphenothiazine *see* Ciclofenazine.

CYCLOPYRRONIUM BROMIDE********* (1-ethyl-3-hydroxy-1-methylpyrrolidinium bromide α-cyclopentylphenylacetate).

CYCLOQUINE (tr) (4-[3,5-bis(2-diethyl-aminoethyl)-4-hydroxyanilino]-7-chloro-quinoline).

CYCLORPHAN*** (*N*-cyclopropylmethyl-3-hydroxymorphinan).

'Cycloryl' *see* Sodium dodecyl sulfate.

CYCLOSERINE********* (D-4-amino-3-isoxazolidinone; oxamycin; MK-65; PA-94; 'closina', 'farmiserina', 'orientomycin', 'seromycin', 'trisomycin').

'Cyclospasmol' see Cyclandelate *and* Drofenine.

CYCLOTHIAZIDE*** (6-chloro-3,4-dihydro-3-(5-norbornen-2-yl)-7-sulfamoyl-(2H)-1,2,4-benzothiadiazine 1,1-dioxide; 3-(bicyclo[2.2.1]hept-5-en-2-yl)-6-chloro-3,4-dihydro-7-sulfamoyl(2H)-1,2,4-benzo-thiadiazine 1,1-dioxide; L-35483; Mdi-193; 'anhydron', 'doburil').

Cyclouron see Cycluron.

CYCLOVALONE*** (2,6-divanillylidene-cyclohexanone; 'beveno', 'cycvalone', 'divanil', 'divanon', 'flavugal', 'vanidene', 'vanilone,').

Cyclo-(L-valyl-L-ornithyl-L-leucyl-D-phenylalanyl-L-propyl-L-valyl-L-ornithyl-L-leucyl-D-phenylalanyl-L-propyl) see Gramicidin S.

Cyclozanin* see Guanacline.

CYCLURON* (1-cyclooctyl-3,3-dimethyl-urea; cyclouron; OMU).
See also Chlorbufam plus cycluron.

'Cycocel' see Chlormequat.

CYCOTIAMINE*** (N-(4-amino-2-methyl-pyrimidin-5-ylmethyl)-N-[1-(2-oxo-1,3-oxathian-4-ylidene)ethyl]formamide).

CYCRIMINE*** (α-cyclopentyl-α-phenyl-1-piperidinepropanol; 1-cyclopentyl-1-phenyl-3-piperid-1-yl-1-propanol; cycrimine hydrochloride; 'pagitane').

'Cycvalon' see Cyclovalone.

'Cydril' see Levamfetamine succinate.

'Cygon' see Dimethoate.

CYHEPTAMIDE*** (10,11-dihydro(5H)-dibenzo(a,d)cycloheptene-5-carboxamide; AY-8682; BS-7029; ICI-51426).

CYHEPTROPINE*** (tropine 10,11-dihydro-(5H)dibenzo(a,d)cycloheptene-5-carboxylate).

CYHEXATIN* (tricyclohexylhydroxy-stannane; 'plictran').

'Cylan' see Cyclamate *and* Phosfolan.

'Cylert' see Pemoline with magnesium hydroxide.

'Cylopal' see Cyclopentobarbital.

Cymarin see Strophanthin.

Cymarol see Strophanthidol cymaroside.

'Cymbi' see Ampicillin.

CYMENE(S) (isopropyltoluene(s)).

p-**Cymene-2,5-diol** see Thymohydroquinone.

p-**Cymene-2,5-dione** see Thymoquinone.

3-*p*-**Cymenol** see Thymol.

'Cymetox' see Demephion-O plus demephion-S.

'Cymidon' see Ketobemidone.

CYN see Cynarine.

CYNARINE*** (1,4-dicaffeylquinic acid; 3,4-dihydroxycinnamic acid 1-carboxy-4,5-dihydroxy-1,3-cyclohexylene ester; CYN; 'anghirol', 'cynarix', 'listrochol').

'Cynem' see Thionazin.

'Cynkotox' see Zineb.

'Cynomel' see Liothyronine sodium.

'Cyodrin' see Crotoxyphos.

'Cyolane' see Phosfolan.

CYP see Cyanofenphos.

CYPENAMINE*** (2-phenylcyclopentyl-amine).

Cypionate(s)* see Cipionate(s).

'Cyplegin' see Cyclopentolate.

CYPRAZEPAM*** (7-chloro-2-[(cyclo-propylmethyl)amino]-5-phenyl-3H-1,4-benzodiazepine 4-oxide; W-3623).

CYPRENORPHINE*** (N-cyclopropyl-methyl-6,7,8,14-tetrahydro-7α-(1-hydroxy-1-methylethyl)-6,14-endo-ethenonorori-pavine; 12-cyclopropylmethyl-1,2,3,3a,8,9-hexahydro-5-hydroxy-2α-(1-hydroxy-1-methylethyl)-3-methoxy-3,9a-etheno-9,9b-iminoethanophenanthro(4,5-bcd)furan; N-cyclopropylmethyl-7,8-dihydro-7α-(1-hydroxy-1-methylethyl)-O⁶-methyl-6,14-endoethenonormorphine; N-cyclo-propylmethyl-7α-(1-hydroxy-1-methyl-ethyl)-6,14-endo-ethenotetrahydroooripavine; N-cyclopropylmethyl-19-methylnorvinol; M-285).

'Cyprex' see Dodine.

Cyprodemanol* see Cyprodenate.

CYPRODENATE*** (2-dimethylamino-ethyl cyclohexanepropionate; deanol cyclohexanepropionate; cyprodemanol; 'actebral').

CYPRODENATE MALEATE (LB-125).

CYPROHEPTADINE*** (4-(5-dibenzo(a,d)-cyclohepten-5-ylidene)-1-methylpiperidine; cyproheptadine hydrochloride; 'nuran', 'periactin', 'periactinol', 'peritol').

CYPROLIDOL*** (diphenyl(2-pyrid-4-yl-cyclopropyl)methanol; α,α-diphenyl-2-pyrid-4-ylcyclopropanemethanol; α-(2-pyrid-4-ylcyclopropyl)benzhydrol; cyprolidol hydrochloride; IN-1060).

CYPROMID* (N-(3,4-dichlorophenyl)-cyclopropanecarboxamide; 3,4-dichloro-N-(cyclopropylcarbonyl)aniline; 'clobber').

'Cypromin' see Rolicyprine.

Cyproquinate* see Ciproquinate.

CYPROTERONE*** (6-chloro-17α-hydroxy-1α,2α-methylenepregna-4,6-diene-3,20-dione; 6-chloro-1,2α-methylenepregna-4,6-diene-17α-ol-3,20-dione; methylene-chlormadinone; SH-714).

CYPROTERONE ACETATE ('androcur', 'sinovir').

Cyproximide* see Ciproximide.

CYSTAFOS (tr) (2-aminoethyl sodium thio-phosphate; mercaptamine S-phosphate; sodium 2-aminoethylthio phosphate; cystaphos).

'Cystamin' see Methenamine.

CYSTAMINE (2,2'-dithiobisethylamine; decarboxylated cystine; cystinamine; L-1591).

'Cystamine' see Hexamine.

Cystaphos see Cystafos.

CYSTATHIONINE (2-amino-4-(2-amino-2-carboxyethylthio)butyric acid).

Cysteamine see Mercaptamine.

CYSTEIC ACID (3-sulfoalanine).

Cysteinamine see Mercaptamine.

124

CYSTEINE (3-mercaptoalanine; 2-amino-3-mercaptopropionic acid; NSC-8746; cysteine hydrochloride; 'cysthion').
See also Acetylhomocysteine thiolactone with cysteine.

Cysteinethiosulfonate *see* Sodium cysteine-thiosulfonate.

'Cysthion' *see* Cysteine.

Cystinamine *see* Cystamine.

CYSTINE (β,β'-dithiodialanine; dicysteine; 'nephrin').

'Cystogen' *see* Methenamine.

'Cystografin' *see* Meglumine diatrizoate with sodium diatrizoate.

CYTARABINE*** (4-amino-1-arabino-furanosyl-1,2-dihydro-2-pyrimidinone; 1-β-D-arabinofuranosylcytosine; cytosine arabinoside; cytarabine hydrochloride; ara-C; ara-cytidine; AC-1075; NSC-63878; U-19920-A; 'alexan', 'aracytine', 'cytosar').

Cytarabine 5'-(1-adamantanecarboxylate) *see* Adamantoylcytarabine.

CYTARABINE 5'-PHOSPHATE (arabino-furanosylcytosine monophosphate; ara-CMP).

'Cytellin' *see* Sitosterol(s).

'Cytembena' *see* Bromebric acid.

CYTHIOATE (*O,O*-dimethyl *O*-(*p*-sulfamoyl-phenyl) phosphorothioate; 'proban').

Cyticholine *see* Citicoline.

CYTIDINE (cytosine riboside).

Cytidine diphosphate choline *see* Citicoline.

Cytidinephosphoric acid *see* Cytidylic acid.

CYTIDYLIC ACID (cytidinephosphoric acid; cytosylic acid; CMP).

CYTISINE (baptitoxine; cytiton; laburnine; sophorine; ulexine).

Cytiton (tr) *see* Cytisine.

CYTOCHROME c (hematin-protein; myo-hematin; 'cromoci', 'cyto-Mack', 'landrax').

'Cytoflav' *see* Flavin mononucleotide.

'Cytofol' *see* Folic acid.

'Cytogran' *see* Buthiopurine.

'Cytoleukon' *see* Busulfan.

'Cyto-Mack' *see* Cytochrome c.

'Cytomel' *see* Liothyronine sodium.

'Cytonal' *see* Fosfestrol.

'Cytosar' *see* Cytarabine.

CYTOSINE (4-amino-2(1H)-pyrimidinone).

Cytosine arabinoside *see* Cytarabine.

Cytosine riboside *see* Cytidine.

Cytosylic acid *see* Cytidylic acid.

'Cytoval' *see* Bromebric acid.

'Cytoxan' *see* Cyclophosphamide.

'Cytrol' *see* Amitrole.

'Cytrolane' *see* Mephosfolan.

D

2,4-D *see* Dichlorophenoxyacetic acid.

D-6 *see* Dicholine suberate.

D-15-14 *see* Octamoxin.

D-25 *see* Fenticlor.

D-26 *see* Bithionol.

D-40 *see* Iodoxyl.

D-40TA *see* Estazolam.

D-41 *see* Tromantadine.

D-47 *see* Sulbentine.

D-50 *see* Pyrazinamide.

D-109 *see* Hexylcaine.

D-138 *see* Norgestimate.

D-201 *see* Isothipendyl.

D-206 *see* Prothipendyl.

D-237 *see* Cloforex.

D-254 *see* Pipazetate.

D-365 *see* Verapamil.

D-563 *see* Oxyfedrine.

D-753 *see* Carboxin.

D-860 *see* Tolbutamide.

D-1201 *see* Prothrin.

D-1262 *see* Cloxypendyl.

D-1593 *see* Tiamizide.

D-1721 *see* Alipamide.

DA-369 *see* Tripyraphene.

DA-398 *see* Epirizole.

DA-708 *see* Teflurane.

DA-808 *see* Nafcaproic acid.

DA-893 *see* Roflurane.

DA-914 *see* Nafiverine.

DA-992 *see* Naftypramide.

DA-1128 *see* Meprophenidol.

DA-1773 *see* Sodium picosulfate.

DA-1813 *see* Pantothenyl trifarnesylacetate.

DA-2370 *see* Feprazone.

'Daartil' *see* Normethadone.

DABI *see* 1-(4-Dimethylaminobenzylidene)-indene.

'Dabical' *see* Calcium clofibrate.

DACARBAZINE*** (1-(4-carboxamidoimi-dazol-5-yl)-3,3-dimethyltriazene; 5-(3,3-dimethyl-1-triazeno)imidazole-4-carbox-amide; DIC; DTIC; DTIC-Dome; NSC-45388).

'Daconil 2787' *see* Chlorothalonil.

'Dactarin' *see* Miconazole.

'Dacthal' *see* Chlorthal-dimethyl.

'Dactil' *see* Piperidolate.

DACTINOMYCIN*** (actinomycin D; meractinomycin; NSC-3053; 'cosmegan', 'cosmegen').

DACTYLIFERIC ACID (3-*O*-caffeoylshiki-mic acid).

DACURONIUM BROMIDE*** (2β,16β-

dipiperid-1-yl-5α-androstane-3α,17β-diol 3-acetate dimethobromide; (3α,17β-dihydroxy-5α-androstan-2β,16β-ylene)bis (1-methylpiperidinium bromide) 3-acetate).

DAD see Dianhydrogalactitol.

DADDS see Acedapsone.

DADPS see Dapsone.

DAEP see 2-Acetamidoethyl dimethyl phosphorodithioate.

DAES see Diethylstilbestrol.

Daftazol(tr) see Amiphenazole.

'Dagenan' see Sulfapyridine.

'Dagicide' see Lindane.

'Dagralax' see Dantron.

'Dagynil' see Conjugated estrogens.

Dahlin see Inulin.

DAIDZEIN (4',7'-dihydroxyisoflavone).

DAIDZIN (daidzein 7-glucoside).

'Daimeton' see Sulfamonomethoxine.

'Daktarin' see Miconazole.

'Dalacin C' see Clindamycin.

DALANATED INSULIN** (insulin derivative obtained by removal of C-terminal alanine from B-chain; dealanated insulin; SN-44).

DALAPON* (2,2-dichloropropionic acid).

DALAPON SODIUM* (sodium 2,2-dichloropropionate; 'dowpon', 'radapon').

Dalapon trichlorophenoxyethyl ester see Erbon.

DALBERGIN (6-hydroxy-7-methoxy-4-phenyl-2H-1-benzopyran-2-one; 6-hydroxy-7-methoxy-4-phenylcoumarin).

DALEDALIN*** (3-methyl-3-(3-methylaminopropyl)-1-phenylindoline; UK-3557).

'Dalf' see Parathion-methyl.

'Dalmadorm' see Flurazepam.

'Dalmane' see Flurazepam.

'Dalnate' see Tolindate.

'Dalysep' see Sulfalene.

'Dalzic' see Practolol.

DAM see Diacetyl monoxime.

DAMASCENINE (methyl 3-methoxy-2-methylaminobenzoate; methyl 3-methoxy-N-methylanthranilate; methyldamascenine; nigelline).

Dambose see Inositol.

'D-amfetasul' see Dexamphetamine.

DAMINOZIDE* (butanedioic acid mono-2,2-dimethylhydrazide; succinic acid dimethylhydrazide; 'alar', 'B-nine').

DAMOTEPINE** (N,N-dimethyldibenzo-(b,f)thiepin-10-methylamine; 10-dimethylaminomethyldibenzo(b,f)thiepin; GP-41299).

DANAZOL** (17α-pregna-2,4-dien-20-yno-(2,3-d)isoxazol-17-ol; WIN-17757; 'danol').

'Daneral' see Pheniramine.

DANITRACEN** (9,10-dihydro-10-(1-methylpiperid-4-ylidene)-9-anthrol; 4-(9,10-dihydro-9-hydroxyanthr-10-ylidene)-1-methylpiperidine).

'Dano' see Amitriptyline N-oxide.

'Danol' see Danazol.

DANT see Alcuronium.

Danthron* see Dantron.

'Dantrium' see Dantrolene.

DANTROLENE*** (1-[5-(p-nitrophenyl)-furfurylideneamino]hydantoin; dantrolene sodium; F-368; F-440; 'dantrium').

DANTRON** (1,8-dihydroxyanthraquinone; anthrapurol; antrapurol; chrysazin; danthron; dianthone; 'altan', cavolax', 'dagralax', 'diaquone', 'dorbane', 'istin', 'istizin', 'laxanthrene', 'zwitsalax').

DANTRON WITH CALCIUM DIOCTYL SULFOSUCCINATE ('dioxidan').

DANTRON WITH POLOXALKOL ('dorbanex').

'Daonil' see Glibenclamide.

'Dapanone' see Phenisonone.

'Dapolar' see Cycloguanil embonate with acedapsone.

'Dapotum' see Fluphenazine enantate.

'Dapotum D' see Fluphenazine decanoate.

DAPSONE*** (4,4'-diaminodiphenyl sulfone; p,p'-sulfodianiline; diaphenylsulfone; diphenason; DADPS; DDS; sulphone-mère; bis(4-aminophenyl) sulfone; 'avlosulfone', 'croysulfone', 'diatox', 'diphone', 'disulone', 'dubronax', 'dumitone', 'eporal', 'novophone', 'sulfadione', 'udolac').

DAPSONEDISULFONIC ACID DISODIUM SALT (M-2196; 'avlosulfone EOS').

DAPT see Amiphenazole.

'Daptazole' see Amiphenazole.

'Daquin' see Chlorazanil.

'Daramin' see Saccharin.

'Daranide' see Diclofenamide.

Daraprim* see Pyrimethamine.

'Darbid' see Isopropamide.

'Darcil' see Pheneticillin.

'Darebon' see Reserpine with chlortalidone.

'Darenthin' see Bretylium tosilate.

'Daricon' see Oxyphencyclimine.

'Daritran' see Meprobamate with oxyphencyclimine.

'Darkinal' see Batroxobin plus heparin.

'Darovermex' see Piperazine adipate.

'Darstine' see Piperphenamine.

'Dartal' see Thiopropazate.

'Dartalan' see Thiopropazate.

'Dartan' see Thiopropazate.

'Darvisul' see Phenolsulfazole.

'Darvon' see Dextropropoxyphene.

'Darvon-N' see Dextropropoxyphene napsilate.

'Dasanil' see Fensulfothion.

DATC see Diallate and Tiocarlide.

DATISCETIN (2',3,5,7-tetrahydroxyflavone).

DATISCIN (datiscetin rutoside; datiscoside).

DATISCIN (datiscetin rutoside; datiscoside).

Datura stramonium see Stramonium.

Daturine see Hyoscyamine.

Dau ET-14 (tr) see Fenclofos.

Dau ET-57 (tr) see Fenclofos.

'Daunoblastin' see Daunorubicin.

Daunomycin see Daunorubicin.

DAUNORUBICIN** (antibiotic from Str. peuceticus or Str. caerulorubidus; (1S,3S)-3-acetyl-1,2,3,4,6,11-hexahydro-3,5,12-trihydroxy-10-methoxy-6,11-dioxo-1-naphthacenyl 3-amino-2,3,6-trideoxy-α-L-lyxo-hexopyranoside; daunomycin; rubido-

126

mycin; NSC-82151; NSC-83142; RP-13057; 'cerubidin', 'daunoblastin', 'ondena').

DAUNORUBICIN BENZOYLHYDRA-ZONE (RP-22950; rubidazone).

DAUNORUBICIN OXIME (daunomycin 3-oxime; NSC-143491).

DAUNORUBICIN SEMICARBAZONE (daunomycin 3-semicarbazone; NSC-143114).

DAUNOSAMINYLDAUNORUBICIN (daunosaminyldaunomycin; NSC-140781).

'Davosine' *see* Sulfamethoxypyridazine.

'Daxid' *see* Xanthiol.

DAZADROL*** (α-(*p*-chlorophenyl)-α-2-imidazolin-2-yl-2-pyridinemethanol; α-(*p*-chlorophenyl)-α-pyrid-2-yl-2-imidazoline-2-methanol; *p*-chloro-α-2-imidazolin-2-yl-benzyl alcohol; 2-(*p*-chloro-α-hydroxy-α-pyrid-2-ylbenzyl)-2-imidazoline).

DAZADROL MALEATE* (dazadrol maleate (1:1) salt).

DAZOMET* (tetrahydro-3,5-dimethyl-2H-1,3,5-thiadiazine-2-thione; DMTT; thiazon; tiazon; 'basamid', 'mylone').

2,4-DB* *see* 4-(2,4-Dichlorophenoxy)butyric acid.

DB-112 *see* Clocoumarol.

DB-136 *see* Furidarone.

DB-139 *see* Pyrazinobutazone.

DB-2041 *see* Meglumine iocarmate.

DBD *see* Azinphos-methyl *and* Mitolactol.

DBED *see* Benzathine.

'DBI' *see* Phenformin.

DBM *see* Mitobronitol.

DBMA *see* Dibemethine.

DBP *see* Dibutyl phthalate.

DBPC *see* Butylated hydroxytoluene.

'DB-retard' *see* Phenformin.

'DBS' *see* Dibromsalicil.

DBV *see* Buformin.

DCA *see* Desoxycortone acetate.

DCAI *see* Clonidine.

'DC antifoam' *see* Dimeticone.

DCBAG *see* Guanabenz.

DCDE *see* Diponium bromide.

2,3-DCDT *see* Diallate.

DCET *see* Cetotiamine.

DCF *see* Mefechlorazine.

DCI (3,4-dichloro-α-(isopropylaminoethyl)-benzyl alcohol; 1-(3,4-dichlorophenyl)-2-isopropylaminoethanol; dichlorodideoxy-isoprenaline; dichlorisoprenaline; dichloroisoproterenol; L-20522).

DCMO *see* Carboxin.

DCMOD *see* Carboxin dioxide.

DCMU *see* Diuron.

DCP *see* Amiloride.

DCPA *see* Chlorthal-dimethyl.

DCPC *see* Chlorfenethol.

DCPE *see* Chlorfenethol.

DCPM *see* Bis(*p*-chlorophenoxy)methane.

DCR-515 *see* Reserpine with clopamide and dihydroergocristine.

D & C red No. 10 *see* Carmoisine.

D & C red No. 35 *see* Toluidine red.

DCS-90 *see* Dihydroergocristine.

DD-234 *see* Scopolamine methyl methosulfate.

DDAVP *see* Desmopressin.

DDD (1,1-dichloro-2,2-bis(*p*-chlorophenyl)-ethane; 1,1'-(2,2-dichloroethylene)bis(4-chlorobenzene); *p,p'*-DDD; TDE; 'rhothane').

o,p'-**DDD** *see* Mitotane.

p,p'-**DDD** *see* DDD.

DDDM *see* Dichlorophen.

DDE (1,1-dichloro-2,2-bis(*p*-chlorophenyl)-ethylene; 1,1'-dichloroethylidenebis-(4-chlorobenzene); *p,p'*-DDE).

p,p'-**DDE** *see* DDE.

DDGA *see* Dodine.

DDM *see* Dichlorophen.

DDMP *see* Metodiclorofen.

DDS *see* Dapsone.

DDT* (1,1,1-trichloro-2,2-bis(*p*-chloro-phenyl)ethane; 1,1'-(2,2,2-trichloroethyl-ene)bis(4-chlorobenzene; *p,p'*-DDT; chlorophenothane; chlorphenothane; clofenotane; chlorphenethanum; dico-phane; gesarol; parachlorocide; penta-chlorin; penticidum; benzochloryl', 'detane', 'dodat', 'esoderm', 'estonate', 'gesapon', 'gesarex', 'neocide', 'neocidol', 'suleo', 'trichomon').

See also Lindane with DDT.

DDT WITH LINDANE & METHOXY-CHLOR ('tritox').

o,p'-**DDT** (2,2,2-trichloro-1-(*o*-chlorophenyl)-1-(*p*-chlorophenyl)ethane; 1-chloro-2-[2,2,2-trichloro-1-(4-chlorophenyl)ethyl]-benzene).

p,p'-**DDT** *see* DDT.

DDVF (tr) *see* Dichlorvos.

DDVP *see* Dichlorvos.

Deacetyldigilanide C *see* Deslanoside.

Deacetyllanatoside C *see* Deslanoside.

N-**Deacetyl-*N*-methylcolchicine** *see* Demecolcine.

N-**DEACETYLTHIOCOLCHICINE** (NCS-9170; R-261-P; 'thiocolciran').

Deacetylvinblastine dimethylglycinate *see* Vinglycinate.

Dealanated-insulin *see* Dalanated insulin.

1-Deamino-8-D-arginine vasopressin *see* Desmopressin.

1-DEAMINO-2-ISOLEUCINE OXYTOCIN (1-(3-mercaptopropionic acid)-2-isoleucine oxytocin).

Deaminooxytocin *see* Demoxytocin.

'Deaner' *see* Deanol *p*-acetamidobenzoate.

DEANOL* (2-dimethylaminoethanol; DMAE; 'dimaestad', 'recrein').

DEANOL ACEGLUMATE** (dimethyl-aminoethyl hydrogen *N*-acetylglutamate; demanol aceglumate; 'cleregil', 'risatarun').

DEANOL *p*-ACETAMIDOBENZOATE ('cervoxan', 'deaner', 'diforene').

DEANOL BENZILATE (2-dimethylamino-ethyl benzilate; benzacine; 'diphemin', 'labotropine').

Deanol 2-(*p*-biphenylyl)butyrate salt *see* Namoxyrate.

DEANOL BITARTRATE ('atrol',

'stimulest').

Deanol esters *see above and* Amindocate; Botiacrine; Clormecaine; Cyclopentolate; Cyprodenate; Denaverine; Dicarfen; Dimenoxadol; Hydroxytetracaine; Indocate; Meclofenoxate; Tetracaine.

DEANOL HEMISUCCINATE (S-167; 'tonibral').

DEANOL PHOSPHATE (phosphoryl-dimethylaminoethanol; 'panclar', 'panklar').

DEANOL PROPYNYLOXYBENZILATE (2-dimethylaminoethyl propynyloxy-benzilate; deanol propynyloxyphenyl-mandelate; propinox; 'sertal').

Deanol propynyloxyphenylmandelate *see* Deanol propynyloxybenzilate.

DEANOL PYROGLUTAMATE (deanol 2-pyrrolidone-5-carboxylate; 2-dimethyl-aminoethyl 5-oxopyrrolidine-2-carboxylate).

DEANOL PYROGLUTAMATE WITH HEPTAMINOL ('debrumyl').

Deanol 2-pyrrolidone-5-carboxylate *see* Deanol pyroglutamate.

Deanol warfarin compound *see* Warfarin-deanol.

Deanol xenbucin salt *see* Namoxyrate.

'Deanxit' *see* Flupentixol with melitracen.

7-DEAZAADENOSINE (4-amino-7H-pyrrolo(2,3-d)pyrimidine riboside; 'tuber-cidin').

DEAZAAMINOPTERIN (N-[p-[2,4-diaminoquinazolin-6-ylmethyl]amino]-benzoyl]glutamic acid; NSC-529860).

'Deazin' *see* Bromelains.

'Debecylina' *see* Benzathine penicillin.

'Debendrin' *see* Diphenhydramine.

'Debetrol' *see* Dextrothyroxine sodium.

'Debilon' *see* 9-Hydroxy-1(10)-aristolen-2-one.

'Debinyl' *see* Phenformin.

'Debridat' *see* Trimebutine maleate.

'Debrisan' *see* Dextranomer.

Debrisochin* *see* Debrisoquine.

DEBRISOQUINE* (3,4-dihydro-2(1H)-iso-quinolinecarboxamidine; debrisoquin sulfate; 2-amidino-1,2,3,4-tetrahydroiso-quinoline; debrisochin; Ro-5-3307/B1; isocaramidine sulfate; 'declinax').

'Debrumyl' *see* Deanol pyroglutamate with heptaminol.

1,1',2,2',3,3',4,4',5,5'-Decachlorobi[2,4-cyclopentadien-1-yl] *see* Dienochlor.

Decachlorooctahydro-1,3,4-metheno-2H-cyclobuta(cd)pentalen-2-one *see* Chlor-decone.

Decachloropentacyclodecan-4-one *see* Chlordecone.

DECADONIUM IODIDE (tr) (decameth-ylene-1,10-bis(adamant-1-yldimethyl-ammonium iodide).

'Decadron' *see* Dexamethasone.

'Deca-durabolin' *see* Nandrolone decanoate.

Decahydro-2-hydroxy-2,4b-dimethyl-7-oxo-1-phenanthrenepropionic acid δ-lactone *see* Testolactone.

1,2,3,4,4aβ,5,6,6a,11bβ,13bβ-Decahydro-

4,4,6aβ,9-tetramethyl-13H-benzo(a)-furo(2,3,4-mn)-xanthen-11-ol *see* Siccanin.

3,4,5,6,7,8,9,10,11,12-Decahydro-7,14,16-trihydroxy-3-methyl-1H-2-benzoxa-cyclotetradecin-1-one
(3S,7R)- *see* Zeranol.
(3S,7S)- *see* Taleranol.

'Decalcinor' *see* Disodium edetate.

DECAMETHONIUM BROMIDE* (or **IODIDE**) (decamethylene-1,10-bis[tri-methylammonium bromide (or iodide)]; C 10).

Decamethylene-1,10-bis(adamant-1-yldi-methylammonium iodide) *see* Deca-donium iodide.

1,1'-Decamethylenebis(4-aminoquinal-dinium acetate) *see* Dequalinium acetate.

1,1'-Decamethylenebis(4-aminoquinal-dinium chloride) *see* Dequalinium chloride.

Decamethylenebis(m-dimethylamino-phenyl-N-methylcarbamate) dimetho-bromide *see* Demecarium bromide.

Decamethylenebis[dimethyl(2-thymyl-oxyethyl)ammonium bromide] *see* Deditonium bromide.

Decamethylenebis(methylcarbamic acid) ester with (m-hydroxyphenyl)trimethyl-ammonium bromide *see* Demecarium bromide.

2,2'-Decamethylenebis(1,2,3,4-tetrahydro-6,7-dimethoxy-1-veratrylisoquino-linium methylsulfate) *see* Laudexium metilsulfate.

Decamethylenebis(trimethylammonium bromide) *see* Decamethonium bromide.

4,4'-Decamethylenediiminodiquinaldine *see* Quindecamine.

2,2'-(Decamethylenedithio)diethanol *see* Tiadenol.

2,2'-(Decamethylenedithio)diethanol bis(clofibrate) *see* Tiafibrate.

Decanedioic acid *see* Sebacic acid.

DECANOIC ACID (capric acid; decylic acid).

'Decapryn' *see* Doxylamine succinate.

Decarboxycysteine *see* Mercaptamine.

Decarboxycystine *see* Cystamine.

'Decaserpyl' *see* Methoserpidine.

'Decasone' *see* Dexamethasone.

Decaspiride *see* Fenspiride.

'Deccox' *see* Decoquinate.

DECENOIC ACID (decylenic acid).

'Decentan' *see* Perphenazine.

'Decilderm' *see under* Undecenoic acid.

DECIMEMIDE* (4-decyloxy-3,5-di-methoxybenzamide).

DECITROPINE* (3α-(5H-dibenzo(a,d)-cyclohepten-5-yloxy)tropane).

'Declid' *see under* Undecenoic acid.

'Declinax' *see* Debrisoquine.

'Declomycin' *see* Demeclocycline.

DECLOXIZINE* (2-[2-(4-diphenylmethyl-piperazin-1-yl)ethoxy]ethanol; 1-(diphenyl-methyl)-4-[2-(2-hydroxyethoxy)ethyl]-piperazine; 1-benzhydryl-4-[2-(2-hydroxy-ethoxy)ethyl]piperazine; UCB-1402).

'**Decoderm**' *see* Fluprednidene acetate.
'**Decofilina**' *see* Etamiphylline dehydro-
cholate.
'**Deconamine**' *see* Pseudoephedrine with
chlorpheniramine maleate.
DECOQUINATE*** (ethyl 6-decyloxy-7-
ethoxy-4-hydroxyquinoline-3-carboxylate;
HC-1528; M&B-15497; 'deccox').
'**Decortilen**' *see* Prednylidene.
DECTAFLUR*** (9-octadecenylamine
hydrofluoride; SK&F-38094).
'**Dectancyl**' *see* Dexamethasone.
'**Decupryl**' *see under* Undecenoic acid.
Decylenic acid *see* Decenoic acid.
Decylic acid *see* Decanoic acid.
'**Decylon**' *see under* Undecenoic acid.
4-Decyloxy-3,5-dimethoxybenzamide *see*
Decimemide.
**6-Decyloxy-7-ethoxy-4-hydroxyquinoline-
3-carboxylic acid ethyl ester** *see*
Decoquinate.
'**Dedetane**' *see* DDT.
'**Dedevap**' *see* Dichlorvos.
Dediton* *see* Deditonium bromide.
DEDITONIUM BROMIDE*** (decamethyl-
enebis[dimethyl(2-thymyloxyethyl)-
ammonium bromide]; dediton).
Deet *see* Diethyltoluamide.
DEF *see* Tributyl phosphorotrithioate.
'**Defekton**' *see* Carpipramine.
'**Defencin**' *see* Isoxsuprine.
DEFEROXAMINE** (30-amino-3,14,25-
trihydroxy-3,9,14,20,25-pentaazatriacon-
tane-2,10,13,21,24-pentaone; *N*-[5-[3-[(5-
aminopentyl)hydroxycarbamoyl]propion-
amido]pentyl]-3-[[5-(*N*-hydroxyacet-
amido)pentyl]carbamoyl]propionohydrox-
amic acid; desferrioxamine; deferoxamine
hydrochloride; Ba-29837; 'desferal').
DEFEROXAMINE MESILATE (deferox-
amine methanesulfonate; deferoxamine
mesylate; Ba-33112; DFOM; 'desferol').
'**Defibrase**' *see* Batroxobin.
'**Defilin**' *see* Sodium dioctyl sulfosuccinate.
'**Deflamene**' *see* Formocortal.
'**Deflamon**' *see* Metronidazole with lysozyme.
'**Defluina**' *see* Raubasine with dihydro-
ergocristine mesilate.
DEFOSFAMIDE*** (2-chloroethyl ester of
N,*N*-bis(2-chloroethyl)-*N*'-(3-hydroxy-
propyl)phosphorodiamidic acid; 'mitarson').
'**Degalol**' *see* Deoxycholic acid.
DEGLYCYRRHIZINIZED LIQUORICE
('caved S', 'cedona', 'rucedal').
'**Degranol**' *see* Mannomustine.
'**Degripol**' *see* Propyphenazone.
'**Dehacodin**' *see* Dihydrocodeine.
'**Dehydranone**' *see* Dehydroacetic acid.
'**Dehydrasal**' *see* Diethylaminoethanol.
DEHYDROACETIC ACID (3-acetyl-6-
methyl(2H)pyran-2,4(3H)-dione;
2-acetyl-5-hydroxy-3-oxo-4-hexenoic acid
δ-lactone; methylacetopyronone; DHA;
'dehydranone').
Dehydrobenzperidol *see* Droperidol.
7-DEHYDROCHOLESTEROL (cholesta-
5,7-dien-3-ol; provitamin D3).

See also Colecalciferol.
24-Dehydrocholesterol *see* Desmosterol.
DEHYDROCHOLIC ACID*** (3,7,12-tri-
oxocholanic acid; 3,7,12-triketocholanic
acid and/or its sodium salt; chologon).
Dehydrocholic acid oxyphenisatin ester
see Cofisatin.
11-DEHYDROCORTICOSTERONE
(4-pregnen-21-ol-3,11,20-trione; 17-(2-
hydroxy-1-oxoethyl)-4-androsten-3,11-
dione; Kendall's compound A; NSC-9702).
Dehydrocortisol *see* Prednisolone.
2,2'-Dehydrodimorphine *see* Pseudomorphine.
DEHYDROEMETINE*** (3-ethyl-1,6,7,11b-
tetrahydro-9,10-dimethoxy-2-(1,2,3,4-tetra-
hydro-6,7-dimethoxy-1-isoquinolyl)methyl-
4H-benzo(a)quinolizine; 2,3-dehydro-
emetine; dehydroemetine hydrochloride;
DHE; BT-436; Ro-9334; 'mebadin').
Dehydroepiandrosterone *see* Prasterone.
11-Dehydro-17-hydroxycorticosterone *see*
Cortisone.
**6-Dehydro-17α-hydroxy-16-methylene-
progesterone** *see* 17α-Hydroxy-16-methyl-
enepregna-4,6-diene-3,20-dione.
Dehydroimipramine *see* Depramine.
5,6-Dehydroisoandrosterone *see* Prasterone.
Dehydropempidine *see* Dropempine.
6-Dehydro-9β,10α-progesterone *see*
Dydrogesterone.
3-DEHYDRORETINOL (vitamin A2).
6-Dehydroretroprogesterone *see* Dydro-
gesterone.
Dehydrostilbestrol *see* Dienestrol.
'**Dekadin**' *see* Dequalinium.
'**Dekelmin**' *see* Metyridine.
'**Dekrysil**' *see* Dinitro-o-cresol.
'**Deladroxate**' *see* Algestone acetofenide with
estradiol enantate.
'**Deladumone**' *see* Estradiol valerate with
testosterone enantate.
'**Delagil**' *see* Chloroquine diphosphate.
'**Delalutin**' *see* Hydroxyprogesterone.
'**Delan**' *see* Dithianon.
'**Delassine veride**' *see* Potassium magnesuim
aspartate.
'**Delatestryl**' *see* Testosterone enantate.
'**Delcaine**' *see* Pseudococaine.
'**Delegol**' *see* o-Benzylphenol.
'**Delesan**' *see* Dimeticone.
'**Delestren**' *see* Estradiol undecylate.
'**Delestrogen**' *see* Estradiol valerate.
'**Delfen**' *see* Nonoxinol 9.
DELFANTRINE*** (*N*',*N*'-dimethyl-3-(4-
methylpiperazin-1-ylcarbonyl)sulfanil-
amide).
'**Delichol**' *see* Choline citrate.
'**Delicia**' *see* Aluminium phosphide.
'**Delinal**' *see* Oxyclipine.
DELMADINONE*** (6-chloro-17α-hydroxy-
pregna-1,4,6-triene-3,20-dione; △1-chlor-
madinone).
DELMADINONE ACETATE (RS-1301;
'estrex').
'**Delmeson**' *see* Fluorometholone.
'**Delnav**' *see* Dioxation.

129

'Deloxadrate' see Algestone acetofenide.
m-Delphene see Diethyl-toluamide.
'Delphicort' see Triamcinolone.
'Delpregnen' see Megestrol acetate with mestranol.
'Delprosyn' see Propicillin.
'Delta-asverin' see Tipepidine.
'Delta-butazolidine' see Phenylbutazone with prednisone.
Deltacortisone see Prednisone.
Delta-E see Prednisone.
'Delta-elmedal' see Phenylbutazone with prednisolone.
Delta-F see Prednisolone.
'Deltafluorene' see Dexamethasone.
Deltahydrocortisone see Prednisolone.
'Deltamide' see Diethyl-toluamide.
'Deltamin' see Metformin.
'Deltamine' see Pemoline.
'Deltan Berna' see Dimethyl sulfoxide.
'Deltoin' see Metetoin.
'Deltyl' see Barbipyrine.
'Deluteval' see Estradiol valerate with progesterone hexanoate.
'Delvex' see Dithiazanine.
'Delvinal' see Vinbarbital.
'Delysid' see Lysergide.
'Dema' see Chlormethine.
'Demalon' see 1α,17α-Dimethylandrostan-17β-ol-3-one.
Demanol aceglumate* see Deanol aceglumate.
'Demazin' see Pseudoephedrine with chlorpheniramine maleate.
DEMECARIUM BROMIDE*** ((m-hydroxyphenyl)trimethylammonium bromide. decamethylenebis(methylcarbamate) ester; decamethylenebis(m-dimethylaminophenyl-N-methylcarbamate) dimethobromide; demecastigmine; BC-48-Br; 'humorsol', 'tosmilen').
Demecastigmine' see Demecarium.
DEMECLOCYCLINE*** (7-chloro-6-demethyltetracycline; demethylchlortetracycline; demeclocycline hydrochloride; DMCT; 'declomycin', 'ledermycin', 'mexocine').
DEMECLOCYCLINE WITH TRIAMCINOLONE ('ledermix').
See also Tetracycline with chlortetracycline and demeclocycline.
DEMECOLCINE*** (N-deacetyl-N-methylcolchicine; colchamine; omain; Reichstein's substance F; Santavy's substance F; C-12669/A; NSC-3096; 'colcemid').
DEMECYCLINE*** (4-dimethylamino-1,4,4a,5,5a,6,11,12a-octahydro-3,6,10, 12,12a-pentahydroxy-1,11-dioxo-2-naphthacenecarboxamide; demethyltetracycline).
DEMEFOX (N,N,N',N'-tetramethylphosphorodiamidic fluoride).
DEMEGESTONE*** (17-methyl-19-norpregna-4,9-diene-3,20-dione; 17α-methyl-Δ⁹-19-norprogesterone; 19-demethyl-17α-methylpregna-4,9-diene-3,20-dione; R-2453; 'lutionex').

DEMELVERINE*** (N-methyldiphenethylamine).
Demephion see Demephion-O plus demephion-S.
DEMEPHION-O* (O,O-dimethyl O-[2-(methylthio)ethyl] phosphorothioate).
DEMEPHION-S (O,O-dimethyl S-[2-(methylthio)ethyl] phosphorothioate; M-82; methyl demeton methyl; 'tinox').
DEMEPHION-O PLUS DEMEPHION-S (demephion; 'atlasetox', 'cymetox').
'Demerol' see Pethidine.
Demethyl.... See also Desmethyl....
Demethylchlortetracycline* see Demeclocycline.
6-Demethyl-6-deoxy-7-dimethylaminotetracycline see Minocycline.
6-Demethyl-6-deoxy-7-nitrotetracycline see Nitrocycline.
6-Demethyl-6-deoxytetracycline see Sancycline.
DEMETHYLDIAZEPAM (7-chloro-1,3-dihydro-5-phenyl-1,4-benzodiazepin-2-one; N-demethyldiazepam; A-101; 'madar')'
Demethyldiazepam oxide see Demoxepam.
Demethyldopan see Oramustine.
4'-Demethylepipodophyllotoxin 9-(4,6-O-ethylidene)-β-D-glucopyranoside see Etoposide.
4'-Demethylepipodophyllotoxin 9-(4,6-O-2-thenylidene)-β-D-glucopyranoside see Teniposide.
19-Demethyl-17α-methylpregna-4,9-diene-3,20-dione see Demegestone.
N-Demethylorphenadrine see Tofenacin.
Demethylpapaverine see Papaveroline.
4'-Demethyltangeretin see 4'-Hydroxy-5,6,7,8-tetramethoxyflavone.
Demethyltetracycline see Demecycline.
Demeton see Demeton-O plus demeton-S.
Demeton-methyl see Demeton-O-methyl plus demeton-S-methyl.
DEMETON-O* (O,O-diethyl O-[2-(ethylthio)ethyl] phosphorothioate; mercaptophossystox; merkaptofos; thionosystox).
DEMETON-O PLUS DEMETON-S (demeton; diethyl ethylthioglycol thiophosphate; Bayer 8196; E-1059; mercaptophas; 'systox', 'vnuran').
DEMETON-O-METHYL* (O-[2-(ethylthio)ethyl] O,O-dimethyl phosphorothioate; methyl-mercaptophos; metil-merkaptofos).
DEMETON-O-METHYL PLUS DEMETON-S-METHYL (demetonmethyl; methyl-demeton; methylsystox; 'metaisosystox', 'metasystox').
DEMETON-S* (O,O-diethyl S-[2-(ethylthio)ethyl] phosphorothioate; isosystox; isodemeton; merkaptofos tiolovyj; thiolosystox; thiolsystox).
See also Demeton-O plus demeton-S.
DEMETON-S-METHYL* (S-[2-(ethylthio)ethyl] O,O-dimethyl phosphorothioate; isodemeton methyl; methylisodemeton; methylisosystox; metilmerkaptofos tiolovyj; 'metaisosystox(i)', 'metasystox(i)').

130

See also Demeton-O-methyl plus demeton-S-methyl.

DEMETON-S-METHYLSULFON* (*S*-[2-(ethylsulfonyl)ethyl] *O,O*-dimethyl phosphorothioate; demeton-S-methyl-sulfone; dioxy-demeton-S-methyl; methyl-isosystoxsulfon; 'metaisosystox sulfon').

Demeton-S-methylsulfoxide
see Oxydemeton-methyl.

Demeton-S-methylsulphone *see* Demeton-S-methylsulfon.

'**Demetrim**' *see* Prazepam.

'**Demetrin**' *see* Prazepam.

'**Demidone**' *see* Hydroxypethidine.

'**Demigran**' *see* Flumedroxone acetate.

'**Demosan**' *see* Chloroneb.

'**Demotil**' *see* Diphemanil metilsulfate.

DEMOXEPAM*** (7-chloro-1,3-dihydro-5-phenyl-2H-1,4-benzodiazepin-2-one 4-oxide; demethyldiazepam oxide; Ro 5-2092).

DEMOXYTOCIN*** (deaminooxytocin; 1-(3-mercaptopropionic acid) oxytocin; ODA-914; 'sandopart').

'**Demulen**' *see* Etynodiol diacetate with ethinylestradiol.

'**Demycin**' *see* Buclosamide.

DENA *see* Diethylnitrosamine.

Denaton* *see* Denatonium.

DENATONIUM BENZOATE*** (benzyl-diethyl(2,6-xylylcarbamoylmethyl)ammo-nium benzoate; benzyldiethyl(hydroxy-methyl)ammonium benzoate 2,6-xylyl-carbamate; denaton; THS-839; 'bitrex').

DENAVERINE*** (2-dimethylaminoethyl 2-(2-ethylbutoxy)-2,2-diphenylacetate; deanol 2-(2-ethylbutoxy)-2,2-diphenyl-acetate; denaverine hydrochloride; X-60; 'spasmalgan').

'**Dendrid**' *see* Idoxuridine.

'**Denka antisprout**' *see* Propham.

DENPIDAZONE*** (4-butyl-1,2-dihydro-5-hydroxy-1,2-diphenyl-3,6-pyridazinedione).

'**Dentromin**' *see* Pemoline.

'**Deosan**' *see* Sodium hypochlorite.

1-De(5-oxo-L-proline)-2-de-L-glutamine-5-L-methioninecaerulein *see* Sincalide.

Deoxy.... *See also* Desoxy.

3′-Deoxyadenosine *see* Cordycepin.

5-Deoxyadenosylcobamide *see* Cobamam-ide.

DEOXYCHOLIC ACID (3α,12α-dihydroxy-cholanic acid; choleic acid; deoxycholic acid), and/or its sodium salt ('delagol', 'droxolan').

11-Deoxycortisone *see* Cortodoxone.

Deoxycortone* *see* Desoxycortone.

6-Deoxy-6-demethyl-6-methylene-5-oxy-tetracycline *see* Metacycline.

17-Deoxydexamethasone *see* Desoximeta-sone.

12-Deoxyerythromycin *see* Berythromycin.

21-Deoxy-F-4 *see* Descinolone.

3-Deoxy-D-fumaric acid *see* Abequose.

3-Deoxy-L-fumaric acid *see* Colitose.

3-Deoxy-17α-hydroxy-6α-methylprogest-erone *see* Anagestone.

6-Deoxy-5-hydroxytetracycline *see* Doxycycline.

3-[6-(*O*-6-Deoxy-α-L-mannopyranosyl)-β-D-glucopyranosyloxy]-3′,4′,5,7-tetra-hydroxyflavylium chloride *see* Kera-cyanin.

1-Deoxy-1-methylamino-D-glucitol *see* Meglumine.

2-Deoxy-2-(3-methyl-3-nitrosoureido)-D-glucopyranose *see* Streptozocin.

21-Deoxy-21-(4-methylpiperazin-1-yl)-prednisolone *see* Mazipredone.

6-Deoxyoxytetracycline *see* Doxycycline.

2-Deoxyphenytoin *see* Doxenitoin.

21-Deoxyprednisolone *see* Deprodone.

DEOXYPYRIDOXINE (4,6-dimethyl-5-hydroxy-3-pyridinemethanol; 4-desoxy-pyridoxine).

Deoxyribonuclease(s) *see* Pancreatic dornase; Streptodornase.

2-Deoxy-2-(tetracyclinylmethylamino)-β-D-glucopyranose *see* Meglucycline.

21-Deoxytriamcinolone *see* Descinolone.

2′-Deoxy-5-trifluoromethyluridine *see* Trifluorothymidine.

14-Deoxyvincaminic acid 2-hydroxy-propyl ester *see* Vinpoline.

2,4-DEP (2-(2,4-dichlorophenoxy)ethanol phosphite (3:1); 'falone').

'**Depakene**' *see* Sodium valproate.

'**Depakine**' *see* Sodium valproate.

'**Depamide**' *see* 2-Propylvaleramide.

'**Depasan**' *see* Sparteine.

'**Depepsen**' *see* Sodium amylosulfate.

'**Depersolon**' *see* Mazipredone.

Dephosphamide* *see* Defosfamide.

'**Depigman**' *see* Monobenzone.

'**Depixol**' *see* Flupentixol decanoate.

'**Depleil**' *see* Teclothiazide.

'**Deplet**' *see* Teclothiazide.

'**Depo-clinovir**' *see* Medroxyprogesterone acetate.

'**Depocural**' *see* Clemizole penicillin.

'**Depo-estradiol**' *see* Estradiol cipionate.

'**Depoestromon**' *see* Dianisylhexene.

'**Depofemin**' *see* Estradiol cipionate.

'**Depo-medrol**' *see* Methylprednisolone.

'**Depro-medrone**' *see* Methylprednisolone.

'**Depo-nortestonate**' *see* Nandrolone cipionate.

'**Depo-prodasone**' *see* Medroxyprogesterone acetate.

Depoprogesterone *see* Medroxyprogesterone acetate.

'**Depo-provera**' *see* Medroxyprogesterone acetate.

'**Deposiston**' *see* Ethinylestradiol 3-iso-propylsulfonate.

'**Depostat**' *see* Gestonorone caproate.

'**Deposteron**' *see* Testosterone undecenate.

'**Depot-oestromenine**' *see* Dianisyl-hexene.

'**Depot-ostromon**' *see* Dianisylhexene.

'**Depovernil**' *see* Sulfamethoxypyridazine.

'**Depovirin**' *see* Testosterone cipionate.

DEPRAMINE** (5-(3-dimethylamino-propyl)-5H-dibenz(b,f)azepine; dehydroimipramine).

'Deprelin' see Succinonitrile.
'Deprenon' see Acetergamine tartrate.
'Depressan' see Dihydralazine dimesilate.
'Deprex' see Dibenzepin.
'Depridol' see Droperidol.
'Deprinol' see Imipramine.
DEPRODONE** (11β,17α-dihydroxy-pregna-1,4-diene-3,20-dione; pregna-1,4-diene-11β,17α-diol-3,20-dione; 21-deoxy-prednisolone; desolone).
DEPRODONE PROPIONATE (deprodone 17-propionate; RD-20000).
'Deprol' see Meprobamate with benactyzine.
'Depronal' see Dextropropoxyphene.
'Depropanex' see Kallidogenase.
DEPROSTIL*** ((1R,2S)-2-(3-hydroxy-3-methyloctyl)-5-oxocyclopentaneheptanoic acid; 15-hydroxy-15-methyl-9-oxoprostan-1-oic acid; AY-22469).
'Depsococaine' see Pseudococaine.
DEPTROPINE*** (3-(10,11-dihydro(5H)-dibenzo(a,d)cyclohepten-5-yloxy)tropane dihydrogen citrate; dibenzheptropine citrate; BS-6987; 'brontina', 'brontine').
DEPTROPINE METHOBROMIDE (or **METHIODIDE**) (N-methyldeptropine; BS-7020A).
'Dequadin' see Dequalinium.
DEQUALINIUM ACETATE ('salvicyclin').
DEQUALINIUM CHLORIDE*** (1,1'-decamethylenebis(4-aminoquinaldinium chloride); dequalon; BAQD-10; 'dekadin', 'dequadin', 'dequavagyn', 'gargilon', 'sorot', 'voxifral').
Dequalon* see Dequalinium chloride.
'Dequavagyn' see Dequalinium chloride.
'Deracil' see Thiouracil.
'Dereuma' see Aminophenazone with aminochlorthenoxazine.
'Derfon' see Amfepramone.
'Deripen' see Ampicillin.
'Dermafos' see Fenclofos.
'Dermalar' see Fluocinolone acetonide.
'Dermanirol' see Tretinoin.
'Dermatol' see Bismuth gallate.
'Dermofungine-A' see Cloxiquine.
'Dermofungine-B' see Dichlorobenzo-dodecinium.
'Dermol' see Bismuth chrysophanate.
'Dermonistat' see Miconazole.
'Dermovate' see Clobetasol propionate.
'Dermoxin' see Tolnaftate.
'Deronil' see Dexamethasone.
'DES' see Diethylstilbestrol.
2,4-DES see Disul.
'Desacé' see Deslanoside.
Desacetyl.... see Deacetyl....
'Desaci' see Deslanoside.
Desaglybuzole* see Glybuzole.
'Desalfa' see Dexamethasone isonicotinate.
4-Desamino-4-hydroxythiamine see Oxythiamine.
DESASPIDIN*** (3'-(5-butyryl-2,4-dihydroxy-3,3-dimethyl-6-oxo-1,4-cyclohexadien-1-ylmethyl)-2',6'-dihydroxy-4'-methoxybutyrophenone; phlorobutyro-

phenone 4-methyl ether).
Deschlorbiomycin see Tetracycline.
DESCINOLONE*** (9-fluoro-11β,16α,17-trihydroxypregna-1,4-diene-3,20-dione; 9-fluoropregna-1,4-diene-3,20-dione-11β,16α,17-triol; 21-deoxytriamcinolone; 21-deoxy-F-4).
DESCINOLONE ACETONIDE** (descinolone cyclic 16,17-acetal with acetone; CL-27071).
'Desclidium' see Viquidil.
'Descresept' see Aristolochic acid.
DESDANINE (trans-3-(1-pyrrolin-3-yl)-acrylamide; cyclamidomycin; pyr-acrimycin A).
'Desenex' see under Undecenoic acid.
'Desenovis' see Xenyhexenic acid.
'Deseril' see Methysergide.
'Desernil' see Methysergide.
'Deserol' see Bromazine.
'Deseronil' see Dexamethasone acetate.
DESERPIDINE*** (11-demethoxyreserpine; trimethoxybenzoate of methyl 11-desmethoxyreserpate; canescine; 'harmonyl', 'raunormine', 'recanescine').
'Desferal' see Deferoxamine.
'Desferol' see Deferoxamine.
Desferrioxamine* see Deferoxamine mesilate.
Desfluorotriamcinolone acetonide see Desonide.
Desglucolanatoside C see Acetyldigoxin.
'Desibyl' see Ox bile.
DESIPRAMINE*** (10,11-dihydro-5-(3-methylaminopropyl)-dibenz(b,f)-azepine; desmethylimipramine; desipramine hydrochloride; norimipramine; DMI; EX-4355; G-35020; JB-8181; 'norpramine', 'pentrofane', 'pertofran', 'pertofrina').
Desitriptyline see Nortriptyline.
'Desivon' see Benzalkonium.
DESLANOSIDE*** (deacetyllanatoside C; deacetyldigilanide C; purpurea glycoside C; 'cedilanid D', 'desacé', 'desaci').
Desmeth.... See also Demeth....
11-Desmethoxy-10-methoxyreserpine see Methoserpidine.
11-Desmethoxyreserpine see Deserpidine.
Desmethylamitriptyline see Nortriptyline.
DESMETHYLBACIMETHRIN (5-hydroxymethylcytosine).
N-Desmethylcodeine see Norcodeine.
Desmethyldopan see Uracil mustard.
Desmethylimipramine see Desipramine.
DESMETHYLMORAMIDE*** (1-(4-morpholino-2,2-diphenylbutyryl)pyrrolidine).
N-Desmethylmorphine see Normorphine.
Desmethylpipazuroylguanidine see Amiloride.
Desmethylprothiadene see Northiadene.
8-Desmethylpseudotropine see Norpseudo-tropine.
Desmethyltetracycline see Demecycline.
'Desmodure-15' see Naphthalene diiso-cyanate.

132

'Desmodur T' *see* Toluylene diisocyanate.
'Desmoid' *see* Methylene blue.
DESMOPRESSIN*** (1-deamino-8-D-arginine-vasopressin; 1-(3-mercaptopropionic acid)-8-D-arginine vasopressin; DDAVP; 'adiuretin').
DESMOPRESSIN DIACETATE ('desurin', 'minirin', 'minurin').
DESMOSTEROL (24-dehydrocholesterol).
'Desogen' *see* Dofamium chloride *and* Toloconium chloride.
Desolone *see* Deprodone.
'Desomidine' *see* Hexamidine.
DESOMORPHINE*** (dihydrodeoxymorphine; 4,5-epoxy-3-hydroxy-*N*-methylmorphinan; 'permonid').
DESONIDE** (11β,16α,17,21-tetrahydroxypregna-1,4-diene-3,20-dione cyclic 16,17-acetal with acetone; 11β,21-dihydroxy-16α,17α-isopropylidenedioxypregna-1,4-diene-3,20-dione; 16α-hydroxyprednisolone 16,17-acetonide; prednacinolone acetonide; desfluorotriamcinolone acetonide; 'reticus', 'tridesilon', 'tridesonit').
'Desopimon' *see* Chlorphentermine.
DESOXIMETASONE*** (9-fluoro-11β,21-dihydroxy-16α-methylpregna-1,4-diene-3,20-dione; 9-fluoro-16α-methylpregna-1,4-diene-11β,21-diol-3,20-dione; 9α fluoro-16α-methyl-17-deoxyprednisolone; 17-deoxydexamethasone; desoxymethasone; A-41304; 'topicorte', 'topisolone').
Desoxy.... *See also* Deoxy....
Desoxyalizarin *see* Anthrarobin.
DESOXYBENZOIN (benzyl phenyl ketone; α-phenylacetophenone).
11-Desoxycorticosterone *see* Desoxycortone.
11-Desoxycortisone *see* Cortodoxone.
DESOXYCORTONE*** (21-hydroxy-4-pregnene-3,20-dione; 11-desoxycorticosterone; compound A; deoxycortone; DOC; Reichstein's substance Q; Kendall's dioxy compound B; NSC-11319; cortexone; 4-pregnen-21-ol-3,20-dione; desoxycortone acetate).
See also Nandrolone phenpropionate with desoxycortone phenpropionate.
DESOXYCORTONE ACETATE ('doca').
Desoxyephedrine *see* Methamphetamine.
2′-Desoxy-5-fluorouridine *see* Floxuridine.
D-Desoxyfucose *see* Abequose.
L-Desoxyfucose *see* Colitose.
Desoxyhexahydroephedrine *see* Propylhexedrine.
11-Desoxy-17-hydroxycorticosterone *see* Cortodoxone.
2′-Desoxy-5-iodouridine *see* Idoxuridine.
Desoxymethasone *see* Desoximetasone.
Desoxynorephedrine *see* Amphetamine.
3-Desoxy-19-nortestosterone *see* Allylestrenol.
6-Desoxy-5-oxytetracycline *see* Doxycycline.
Desoxyphenobarbital *see* Primidone.
'Dessin' *see* Dinobuton.
DESTHIOBIOTIN (5-methyl-2-oxo-4-imidazolidinehexanoic acid; dethiobiotin;

NSC-3085).
N-**Desulfo-*N*-(2-sulfobenzoyl)heparin** *see* o-Sulfobenzheparide.
'Desuric' *see* Benzbromarone.
'Desurin' *see* Desmopressin diacetate.
DESYLAMINE (α-phenylphenacylamine; 2-amino-2-phenylacetophenone; α-amino-desoxybenzoin).
DET *see* Diethyltoluamide.
m-**DET** *see* Diethyltoluamide.
DETA *see* Diethyltoluamide.
DETAJMIUM BITARTRATE** (4-[3-(diethylamino)-2-hydroxypropyl]-ajmalinium hydrogen tartrate monohydrate).
'Detal' *see* Dinitro-o-cresol.
'Detamide' *see* Diethyl-*m*-toluamide.
DETANOSAL** (2-diethylaminoethyl salicylate).
'Deteclo' *see* Tetracycline with chlortetracycline and demeclocycline.
DETERENOL***((±)-*p*-hydroxy-α-(isopropylaminomethyl)benzyl alcohol; (±)-1-(*p*-hydroxyphenyl)-2-isopropylaminobenzyl alcohol; AL-842).
DETF *see* Metrifonate.
Dethiobiotin *see* Desthiobiotin.
Dethylandiamine *see* Thenyldiamine.
'Dethyrone' *see* Dextrothyroxine sodium.
'Detigon' *see* Clofedanol.
DETRALFATE*** (dextran sulfate sodium salt aluminium complex; APD).
DETROTHYRONINE*** (D-3-[4-(4-hydroxy-3-iodophenoxy)-3,5-diiodophenyl]-alanine).
'Detrovel' *see* 2-(4-Allyl-2-methoxyphenoxy)-*N*,*N*-diethylacetamide.
'Deturgylone' *see* Prednazoline.
'Develin' *see* Dextropropoxyphene.
'Devincan' *see* Vincamine.
'Devoran' *see* Lindane.
'Devrinol' *see* Napropamide.
'Dexabolin' *see* Dexamethasone with ethylestrenol.
'Dexacillin' *see* Epicillin.
'Dexa-cortancyl' *see* Dexamethasone acetate.
'Dexa-cortisyl' *see* Dexamethasone.
'Dexambutol' *see* (+)-Ethambutol.
'Dexameth' *see* Dexamethasone.
DEXAMETHASONE*** (9α-fluoro-11β,17α,21-trihydroxy-16α-methyl-1,4-pregnadiene-3,20-dione; △¹-dehydro-9α-fluoro-16α-methylhydrocortisone; 9α-fluoro-16α-methylprednisolone; 9α-fluoro-16α-methyl-1,4-pregnadiene-11β,17α,21-triol-3,20-dione; dexadecadrol; dexamethasone disodium phosphate; dexamethasone sulfate; NSC-34521; MK-125; 'decadron', 'deltafluorene', 'dexa-cortisyl', 'dexameth', 'dexascheroson', 'dextelan', 'fissancort', 'gammacorten', 'hexadrol', 'lammacorten', 'maidex', 'millicorten', 'oradexon').
DEXAMETHASONE ACETATE ('dectancyl', 'deronil', 'deseronil', 'dexacortancyl', 'fortecortin').

DEXAMETHASONE WITH BENZYL NICOTINATE ('rheumasit').
DEXAMETHASONE WITH ETHYL-ESTRENOL ('dexabolin').
DEXAMETHASONE WITH INDO-METACIN (C-209; 'inflacine').
DEXAMETHASONE 21-ISONICOTINATE (dexamethasone 4-pyridinecarboxylate; HE-111; 'auxiloson', 'auxisone', 'desalfa', 'voren').
DEXAMETHASONE PIVALATE (dexamethasone trimethylacetate; 'opticortenol').
DEXAMETHASONE PIVALATE WITH PHENYLMERCURIC BORATE (Z-1141C; 'exosterol').
DEXAMETHASONE PIVALATE WITH PREDNISOLONE ('opticortenol-S').
Dexamethasone 4-pyridinecarboxylate see Dexamethasone isonicotinate.
DEXAMETHASONE SODIUM m-SULFOBENZOATE ('dexa-sol', 'hubersona').
DEXAMETHASONE SUCCINATE (dexamethasone hydrogen succinate; 'betafluorene').
Dexamethasone trimethylacetate see Dexamethasone pivalate.
DEXAMISOLE** (($+$)-2,3,5,6-tetrahydro-6-phenylimidazo(2,1-b)thiazole).
See also Levamisole; Tetramisole.
DEXAMPHETAMINE** (($+$)-amphetamine; ($+$)-α-methylphenethylamine; dextroamphetamine; ($+$)-β-phenyliso-propylamine; dexamphetamine sulfate).
DEXAMPHETAMINE WITH AMOBARBITAL ('dexamyl').
'Dexamyl' see Dexamphetamine with amobarbital.
'Dexascheroson' see Dexamethasone.
'Dexa-sol' see Dexamethasone sodium sulfobenzoate.
Dexbenzetimide see Dexetimide.
DEXBROMPHENIRAMINE*** (($+$)-2-[p-bromo-α-(2-dimethylaminoethyl)benzyl]-pyridine; ($+$)-3-(p-bromophenyl)-N,N-dimethyl-3-pyrid-2-ylpropylamine).
DEXBROMPHENIRAMINE MALEATE* ('disomer').
See also Brompheniramine.
DEXCHLORPHENIRAMINE*** (($+$)-2-[p-chloro-α-(2-dimethylaminoethyl)benzyl]-pyridine; ($+$)-3-(p-chlorophenyl)-N,N-dimethyl-2-pyrid-2-ylpropylamine).
DEXCHLORPHENIRAMINE MALEATE* ('polaramine').
See also Chlorpheniramine.
DEXCLAMOL*** (($+$)-2,3,4,4aβ,8,9,13bα, 14-octahydro-3α-isopropyl-1H-benzo-(6,7)cyclohepta(1,2,3-de)pyrido(2,1-a)-isoquinolin-3-ol).
'Dexedrine' see Dexamphetamine.
DEXETIMIDE** (($+$)-2-(1-benzylpiperid-4-yl)-2-phenylglutarimide; ($+$)-3-(1-benzyl-piperid-4-yl)-3-phenylpiperidine-2,6-dione; dexbenzetimide; R-16470; 'tremblex').
See also Benzetimide.
DEXIMAFEN*** (($+$)-2,3,5,6-tetrahydro-

5-phenyl-1H-imidazo(1,2-a)imidazole; deximafen hydrochloride; R-26333).
See also Imafen.
'Dexium' see Calcium dobesilate.
DEXIVACAINE*** (($+$)-1-methyl-2',6'-pipecoloxylidide; mepivacaine ($+$)-isomer).
Dexnorgestrel see Levonorgestrel.
'Dexol' see Sodium perborate.
'Dexon' see Polyglycolic acid.
DEXOXADROL*** (($+$)-2,2-diphenyl-4-piperid-2-yl-1,3-dioxolane; ($+$)-dioxadrol; ($+$)-2-(2,2-diphenyl-1,3-dioxolan-4-yl)-piperidine; CL-911-C; U-22559A; 'relane').
DEXPANTHENOL*** (D-($+$)-2,4-di-hydroxy-N-(3-hydroxypropyl)-3,3-di-methylbutyramide; 'bepanthen', 'cozyme', 'ilopan', 'motilyn').
See also Panthenol.
Dexphenmetrazine see Phenmetrazine.
DEXPROPRANOLOL*** (($+$)-1-iso-propylamino-3-naphth-1-yloxy-2-propanol; ($+$)-propranolol; dexpropranolol hydro-chloride; AY-20694; ICI-47319).
See also Propranolol.
DEXPROXIBUTENE*** (($+$)-3-dimethyl-aminomethyl-1,2-diphenyl-3-buten-2-ol propionate).
See also Proxibutene.
'Dextelan' see Dexamethasone.
DEXTILIDINE** (($+$)-ethyl trans-2-di-methylamino-1-phenyl-3-cyclohexene-1-carboxylate).
See also Tilidine.
'Dextim' see Methamphetamine.
Dextramycin (tr) see ($+$)-Chloram-phenicol.
DEXTRAN*** (polysaccharide formed by Leuconostoc mesenteriodides; gemodex; PVTD; polyglucin; sinkol; 'dextraven', 'expandex', 'gentran', 'intradex', 'lomodex', 'macrodex', 'macrose', 'onkotin', 'pharm-odex', 'plasmodex', 'plavolex').
See also Cross-linked dextran.
DEXTRAN 40* (low molecular weight dextran; reoisodex; reopoliglukin; 'fluidex', 'infukoll M-40', 'LMD', 'lomodex', 'rheomacrodex', 'rheotran').
DEXTRAN 70* ('gentran', 'macrodex').
Dextran 2-(diethylaminoethyl) 2-[(2-diethylaminoethyl)diethylammonio]-ethyl ether chloride, hydrochloride, epichlorohydrin cross-linked see Polidexide.
Dextran epichlorohydrin reaction products see Dextranomer; Polidexide.
DEXTRANOMER*** (reaction product of dextran with epichlorohydrin; dextran cross-linked with epichlorohydrin; 'debrisan').
DEXTRAN SULFATE ('dexulate', 'poly-ran').
Dextran sulfate sodium salt aluminium complex see Detralfate.
'Dextraven' see Dextran.
DEXTRIFERRON*** (iron-dextrin complex; 'astrafer', 'ferrigen').
Dextroamphetamine see Dexamphetamine.

134

Dextrococaine see Pseudococaine.
DEXTROFEMINE** ((+)-α-methyl-*N*-(1-methyl-2-phenoxyethyl)phenethylamine; *N*-(1-methyl-2-phenoxyethyl)dexamphetamine; (+)-*threo*-3,5-dimethyl-1,6-diphenyl-1-oxa-4-azahexane; CB-3697; 'dysmalgine').
See also Racefemine.
DEXTROMETHORPHAN** ((+)-*cis*-1,3,4,9,10,10a-hexahydro-6-methoxy-11-methyl-2H-10,4a-iminoethanophenanthrene; (+)-3-methoxy-*N*-methylmorphinan; dextromethorphan hydrobromide; Ro-1-5479; 'romilar', 'tussilan').
DEXTROMORAMIDE** ((+)-4-(2-methyl-4-oxo-3,3-diphenyl-4-pyrrolidin-1-ylbutyl)morpholine; (+)-1-(3-methyl-4-morpholino-2,2-diphenylbutyryl)pyrrolidine; pyrrolamidole; 'erracalma', 'narcolo').
DEXTROMORAMIDE BITARTRATE* (R-875; SKF-5137; 'dimorlin', 'jetrium', 'palfium', 'palphium').
Dextromycetin (tr) see D-Chloramphenicol.
'Dextrone' see Diquat.
Dextronic acid see Gluconic acid.
DEXTROPROPOXYPHENE** (α-(+)-4-dimethylamino-3-methyl-1,2-diphenyl-2-butanol propionate ester; α-(+)-*N*,*N*,2-trimethyl-3,4-diphenyl-3-propionoxy-1-butylamine; propoxyphene; dextropropoxyphene hydrochloride; (+)-propoxyphene hydrochloride; L-16298; 'abalgin', 'algaphan', 'antalvic', 'darvon', 'depronal', 'develin', 'dolorphen', 'doloxene', 'erantin').
Dextropropoxyphene compound with phenylbutazone see Proxifezone.
DEXTROPROPOXYPHENE NAPSILATE (dextropropoxyphene naphthalene-2-sulfonate; propoxyphene napsylate; S-9700; 'darvon-N').
DEXTROPROPOXYPHENE THEOBROMIN-1-YLACETATE (Z-867; 'lenigesal').
DEXTRORPHAN** ((+)-*cis*-1,3,4,9,10,10a-hexahydro-11-methyl-2H-10,4a-iminoethanophenanthren-6-ol; (+)-3-hydroxy-*N*-methylmorphinan; Ro-1-6794).
Dextrose see Glucose.
Dextrosulfenidol see Thiamphenicol.
DEXTROTHYROXINE SODIUM*** (D-3,5,3',5'-tetraiodothyronine sodium; D-[3-(4-hydroxy-3,5-diiodophenoxy)-3,5-diiodophenyl]alanine sodium salt; sodium dextrothyroxine; 'choloxin', 'choloxon', 'debetrol', 'dethyrone', 'dynothel').
'Dexulate' see Dextran sulfate.
'Dezentan' see Perphenazine.
DEZOCINE** ((−)-13β-amino-5,6,7,8,9,10,11α,12-octahydro-5α-methyl-5,11-methanobenzocyclodecen-3-ol).
DF-69 see Raubasine with dihydroergocristine mesilate.
DF-118 see Dihydrocodeine.
DFDT see 1,1,1-Trichloro-2,2-bis(*p*-fluorophenyl)ethane.

DFOM see Deferoxamine mesilate.
DFP see Dyflos.
'D₂H' see Proxibarbal.
DH-524 see Fenmetozole.
DH-581 see Probucol.
DHA see Prasterone.
'DHA' see Dehydroacetic acid.
'DHA 245' see Amiphenazole.
'DH-codeine' see Dihydrocodeine.
DHE see Dehydroemetine.
DHE-45 see Dihydroergotamine mesilate.
DHK-135 see Dihydroergocryptine.
DHO-180 see Dihydroergocornine.
'Diabesulf' see Carbutamide.
'Diabeta' see Glibenclamide.
'Diabetal' see Carbutamide.
'Diabetasi' see Chlorpropamide.
'Diabetol' see Tolbutamide.
'Diabetoral' see Chlorpropamide.
'Diabiformine' see Chlorpropamide with metformin.
'Diabinese' see Chlorpropamide.
'Diabiphage' see Chlorpropamide with metformin.
'Diaboral' see Glycyclamide.
'Diabtyl' see Batroxobin plus heparin.
'Diabuton' see Tolbutamide.
Diacarb (tr) see Acetazolamide.
Diacephine see Diamorphine.
DIACETAMATE*** (*p*-acetamidophenyl acetate; paracetamol acetate ester).
3,5-Diacetamido-2,4,6-triiodobenzoic acid see Diatrizoic acid.
α,5-Diacetamido-2,4,6-triiodo-*m*-toluic acid see Iodamide.
2,5-Diacetamidovaleric acid see Bisorcic.
DIACETAZOTOL (4''-(*o*-tolylazo)-*o*-diacetotoluidide; *N*,*N*-diacetyl-*o*-tolylazo-*o*-toluidine; diacetylaminoazotoluene; amidoazotoluene diacetate; 4-diacetylamino-2',3-diaminoazobenzene; periphermium; diacetotoluide; 'dimazon', 'epidon', 'opidon', 'pellidol').
DIACETIN (glyceryl diacetate).
DIACETONE ALCOHOL (4-hydroxy-4-methyl-2-pentanone; 'tyranton').
Diacetotoluide see Diacetazotol.
4,4'-Diacetoxybenzhydrylidenecyclohexane see Cyclofenil.
2,3-Diacetoxybenzoic acid see Dipyrocetyl.
18,20α-Diacetoxy-3β-(dimethylamino)-5α-pregnane see Stevaladil.
Diacetoxydiphenylisatin see Acetphenolisatin.
DIACETOXYSCIRPENOL (4,15-diacetoxyscirp-9-en-3-ol; anguidin; ANG-66).
Diacetyl see 2,3-Butanedione.
Diacetylaminozotoluene see Diacetazotol.
3-Diacetylamino-2,4,6-triiodobenzoic acid see Docetrizoic acid.
Diacetylcholine see Suxamethonium.
Diacetyldapsone see Acedapsone.
Diacetyldiaphenylsulfone see Acedapsone.
DIACETYLDIHYDROMORPHINE (dihydroheroin; paralaudin).
Diacetyldihydroxyphenylisatin see Acetphenolisatin.

135

Diacetyldiphenolisatin *see* Acetphenolisatin.
DIACETYL MONOXIME (2,3-butanedione monoxime; DAM; NSC-660).
Diacetylmorphine *see* Diamorphine.
N^2,N^5-**Diacetyl-L-ornithine** *see* Bisorcic.
Diacetylprotocatechuic acid *see* Dipyrocetyl.
1α,7α-**Diacetylthio-17-methylandrost-4-en-17b-ol-3-one** *see* Tiomesterone.
'**Diacid**' *see* Carbromal.
'**Diacromone**' *see* Methylchromone.
'**Di-ademil**' *see* Hydroflumethiazide.
Diadonium diiodide *see* Diadonium iodide.
DIADONIUM IODIDE (tr) ((3,8-dioxa-4,7-dioxodecamethylene-1,10)-bis(adamant-1-yldimethylammonium iodide); succinic acid bis[2-(N-adamant-1-yl-N-methylamino)ethyl] ester dimethiodide; bis[2-(N-adamant-1-yl-N-methylamino)ethyl] succinate dimethiodide; diadonium diiodide).
'**Diafen**' *see* Diphenylpyraline.
'**Diaflexol**' *see* Phenprobamate with acetylsalicylic acid.
'**Diaginol**' *see* Sodium acetrizoate.
'**Diagnex blue**' *see* Azuresin.
'**Diakarmon**' *see* Sorbitol.
'**Dial**' *see* Allobarbital.
'**Dialicor**' *see* Etafenone.
Dialifor* *see* Dialifos.
DIALIFOS* (S-[2-chloro-1-(1,3-dihydro-1,3-dioxo-2H-isoindol-2-yl)ethyl] O,O-diethyl phosphorodithioate; N-[2-chloro-1-[(diethoxyphosphinothioyl)thio]ethyl]phthalimide; dialifor; 'torak').
DIALLATE* (S-(2,3-dichloro-2-propenyl) bis(1-methylethyl)carbamothioate; di-allate; S-(2,3-dichloroallyl) diisopropylcarbamothioate; DATC; 2,3-DCDT; 'avadex', 'CFT').
Di-allate* *see* Diallate.
Diallylacetic acid *see* 2-Allyl-4-pentenoic acid.
2-**Diallylamino-4,6-diamino-s-triazine** *see* Diallylmelamine.
Diallylbarbital *see* Allobarbital.
5,5-**Diallylbarbituric acid** *see* Allobarbital.
5,5'-**Diallyl-α,α'-bis(diethylamino)-m,m'-bitolyl-4,4'-diol** *see* Bialamicol.
Diallylbis(diethylaminomethyl)biphenol *see* Bialamicol.
Diallylbisnortoxiferine *see* Alcuronium.
N,N-**Diallyl-2-chloroacetamide** *see* Allidochlor.
DIALLYLMELAMINE (2-diallylamino-4,6-diamino-s-triazine; U-7720).
Diallylmelamine N-**oxide** *see* Oxonazine.
Diallylnortoxiferine *see* Alcuronium.
Diallymal* *see* Allobarbital.
'**Dialose plus**' *see* Oxyphenisatin.
DIALURIC ACID (5-hydroxybarbituric acid; tartronylurea).
Diamantane *see* Adamantane.
'**Diamethine**' *see* Dimethyltubocurarine.
DIAMFENETIDE** (2,2'-bis(4-acetamidophenoxy)ethyl ether; β,β'-oxybis(p-acetophenetidide); oxybisphenacetin; oxybis(p-

ethoxyacetanilide); diamphenethide; 'coriban').
'**Diamicron**' *see* Gliclazide.
DIAMIDE (1,1'-azobis(N,N-dimethylformamide); bis(dimethylcarbamoyl-diimide; N,N,N',N'-tetramethylazoformamide; diazenedicarboxylic acid bis-(dimethylamide).
4,4'-**Diamidinodiphenoxypropane** *see* Propamidine.
4,4'-**Diamidinodiphenyl ether** *see* Phenamidine.
p,p'-**Diamidino-1,3-diphenyltriazene** *see* Diminazene.
'**Diamine blue**' *see* Trypan blue.
DIAMINE OXIDASE (histaminase; 'torantil', 'torantyl').
3,6-**Diaminoacridine** *see* Proflavine.
2,4-**Diaminoazobenzene** *see* Chrysoidine.
Diaminobenzpyrylum *see* Tripelennamine.
Diaminocaproic acid *see* Lysine.
2,6-**Diamino-3-carboguanidino-5-chloropyrazine** *see* Amiloride.
N^4-(2,4-**Diamino-6-carboxyphenylazo)-sulfanilamide** *see* Sulfachrysoidine.
4,6-**Diamino-1-(p-chlorophenyl)-1,2-dihydro-2,2-dimethyl-s-triazine** *see* Cycloguanil.
2,4-**Diamino-5-(p-chlorophenyl)-6-ethyl-pyrimidine** *see* Pyrimethamine.
2,4-**Diamino-5-(p-chlorophenyl)-9-methyl-1,3,5-triazaspiro(5.5)undeca-1,3-diene** *see* Spirazine.
N-(p-[(2,4-**Diamino-5-chloroquinazolin-6-ylmethyl)amino]benzoyl] aspartic acid** *see* Chlorasquin.
1,2-**DIAMINOCYCLOHEXANETETRA-ACETIC ACID** (chenta; 'complexon IV', 'komplexon IV').
4,6-**Diamino-1-(3,4-dichlorobenzyloxy)-1,2-dihydro-2,2-dimethyl-s-triazine** *see* Clociguanil.
2,4-**Diamino-5-(3,4-dichlorophenyl)-6-methylpyrimidine** *see* Metodiclorofen.
O-[2,6-**Diamino-2,6-dideoxy-α-D-glucopyranosyl-(1→4)]-O-[β-D-ribofuranosyl-(1→5)]-2-deoxystreptamine** *see* Ribostamycin.
O-[2,6-**Diamino-2,6-dideoxy-α,D-gluco-pyranosyl-(1→4)]-O-[β,D-xylofuranosyl-(1→5)]-N¹-(4-amino-2-hydroxybuty-ryl)-2-deoxystreptamine** *see* Butirosin.
O-(2,6-**Diamino-2,6-dideoxy-β-L-idopyr-anosyl-(1→3)-O-β-D-ribofuranosyl)-(1→5)-O-[2-amino-2-deoxy-α-D-gluco-pyranosyl)-(1→4)]-2-deoxystreptamine** *see* Paromomycin.
4,6-**Diamino-1,2-dihydro-2,2-dimethyl-1-[p-(methylthio)phenyl]-s-triazine** *see* Methiotrizamine.
3,3'-**Diamino-4,4'-dihydroxyarsenobenz-enemethylenesulfoxylic acid** *see* Neoarsphenamine.
2,4-**Diamino-5-(3,4-dimethoxybenzyl)-pyrimidine** *see* Diaveridine.
2,4-**Diamino-5-[3,5-dimethoxy-4-(2-methoxyethoxy)benzyl]pyrimidine** *see*

Tetroxoprim.

2,4-Diamino-5-(3,4-dimethoxy-6-methyl-benzyl)pyrimidine see Ormetoprim.

4,4'-Diaminodiphenylmethane see p,p'-Methylenedianiline.

4,4'-Diaminodiphenyl sulfone see Dapsone.

Diaminoethoxyacridine see Ethacridine.

Diaminoethoxyazobenzene see Etoxazene.

3,8-Diamino-5-ethyl-6-phenylphenanthridinium chloride see Ethidium chloride.

Diaminohexanoic acid see Lysine.

4,6-Diamino-2-hydroxy-1,3-cyclohexene 3,6'-diamino-3,6'-dideoxydi-α-D-glucoside see Kanamycin.

[[15-(3,6-Diamino-4-hydroxyhexanamido)-3-(hexahydro-2-iminopyrimidin-4-yl)-9,12-bis(hydroxymethyl)-2,5,8,11,14-pentaoxo-1,4,7,10,13-pentaazacyclohexadec-6-ylidene]methyl]-urea see Enviomycin.

3,8-Diamino-5-methyl-6-phenylphenanthridinium bromide see Dimidium.

N-[p-[(2,4-Diamino-5-methylquinazolin-6-ylmethyl)amino]benzoyl]-L-aspartic acid see Methasquin.

2,4-Diamino-4-(6-methylveratryl)pyrimidine see Ormetoprim.

2,4-DIAMINOPHENOL ('acrol', 'amidol', 'dianol').

2,6-Diamino-3-phenylazopyridine see Phenazopyridine.

Diaminophenylthiazole see Amiphenazole.

2,4-Diamino-6-piperid-1-ylpyrimidine 3-oxide see Minoxidil.

Di(aminopropyl)tetramethylenediamine see Spermine.

N-[p-[(2,4-Diaminoquinazolin-6-yl-methyl)-amino]benzoyl]aspartic acid see Quinaspar.

N-[p-[(2,4-Diaminoquinazolin-6-yl-methyl)-amino]benzoyl]glutamic acid see Deazaaminopterin.

4,4'-Diaminostilbene-2,2'-disulfonic acid see Amsonic acid.

4,4'-Diamino-2-sulfamoyldiphenyl sulfone see Sulfamoyldapsone.

3,5-Diamino-2-(p-sulfamoylphenylazo)-benzoic acid see Sulfachrysoidine.

O-(2,6-Diamino-2,3,4,6-tetradeoxy-α,D-glycerohex-4-enopyranosyl-(1→4)-O-(3-deoxy-4-C-methyl-3-methylamino-β,L-arabinopyranosyl)-(1→6))-2-deoxy-D-streptamine see Sisomicin.

O-2,6-Diamino-2,3,4,6-tetradeoxy-α-D-erythro-hexapyranosyl-(1→4)-O-[3-deoxy-4-C-methyl-3-(methylamino)-β-L-arabinopyranosyl-(1→6)]-2-deoxy-streptamine see Gentamicin.

Diaminotetrahydroxycyclohexane see Streptamine.

S-(4,6-Diamino-s-triazin-2-ylmethyl) O,O-dimethyl phosphorodithioate see Menazon.

3,5-Diamino-1,2,4-triazole see Guanazole.

2,4-Diamino-5-(3,4,5-trimethoxybenzyl)-pyrimidine see Trimethoprim.

Diaminovaleric acid see Ornithine.

2,4-Diamino-5-veratrylpyrimidine see Diaveridine.

DIAMOCAINE*** (1-(2-anilinoethyl)-4-(2-diethylaminoethoxy)-4-phenylpiperidine).

DIAMOCAINE CYCLAMATE* (diamocaine dicyclamate; R-10948).

Diamocaine dicyclamate see Diamocaine cyclamate.

Diamond Green G see Brilliant green.

DIAMORPHINE* (diacetylmorphine; 3,6-diacetylmorphine; acetomorphine; diacephine; diaphorin; heroin; morphacetin).

'Diamox' see Acetazolamide.

Diamphenethide* see Diamfenetide.

'Diampicicol' see Ampicillin guaiacyldiethylaminoacetate.

'Diamplicil' see Ampicillin with dicloxacillin.

DIAMPROMIDE*** (N-[2-(N-methylphenethylamino)propyl]propionanilide; diampromide sulfate).

'Diampron' see Amicarbalide isetionate.

Diamthazole see Dimazole.

'Dianabol' see Metandienone.

Dianat (tr) see Dicamba.

'Diandrone' see Prasterone.

Dianhydrodulcitol see Dianhydrogalactitol.

DIANHYDROGALACTITOL (1,2:5,6-dianhydrogalactitol; dianhydrodulcitol; DAD; NSC-132313).

1,4:3,6-Dianhydroiditol see Isoidide.

1,4:3,6-Dianhydromannitol see Isomannide.

1,4:3,6-Dianhydrosorbitol see Isosorbide.

'Dianil blue' see Trypan blue.

3,3'-Dianisolebis-4,4'-(3,5-diphenyltetrazolium chloride) see Tetrazolium blue.

DIANISYLHEXENE (α,α'-diethyl-4,4'-dimethoxystilbene; stilbestrol dimethyl ether; dimestrol; 3,4-dianisyl-4-hexene; 'depoestromon', 'depot-oestromenine', 'depot-oestromon', 'synthila').

DIANISYLNEOPENTANE (1,1-bis(p-methoxyphenyl)-2,2-dimethylpropane).

Dianisylphenetylguanidine see Guanicaine.

Dianisyltrichloroethane see Methoxychlor.

'Dianol' see Diaminophenol.

Dianthone see Dantron.

'Diantil' see Chlorbetamide.

Diapamide* see Tiamizide.

'Diaparene' see Methylbenzethonium.

Diaphenylsulfone see Dapsone.

'Diaphine' see Xenysalate.

Diaphorm see Diamorphine.

'Diapid' see Lypressin.

'Diaquone' see Dantron.

DIARBARONE*** (N-(2-diethylaminoethyl)-4-hydroxy-2-oxo-2H-1-benzopyran-3-carboxamide; N-(2-diethylaminoethyl)-4-hydroxy-2-oxo-2H-chromen-3-carboxamide; 'thrombossoine-heparin').

'Diarsed' see Diphenoxylate with atropine.

Diasatin see Acetphenolisatin.

'Diasone' see Aldesulfone.

'Diaspasmyl' see Propyromazine.

'Diasprin' see Succinylsalicylic acid.

Diastase* see Amylase.

'Diathesin' see Saligenin.

137

DIATHYMOSULFONE*** (bis[*p*-(4-hydroxy-2-methyl-5-isopropylphenylazo)-phenyl]sulfone; 4,4'-bis(*p*-isopropyl-*m*-cresylazo)diphenyl sulfone; di[4-(4-hydroxy-5-isopropyl-2-methylphenylazo)-phenyl]sulfone; 6,6'-[sulfonylbis(*p*-phenyleneazo)]dithymol; thymosulfone; timosulfon).

DIATHYMOSULFONE SILVER (silver sulfone; thymolated silver sulfone; J-51; 'diatox argentique').

'Diatox' *see* Dapsone.

'Diatox argentique' *see* Diathymosulfone silver.

DIATRIZOIC ACID* (3,5-diacetamido-2,4,6-triiodobenzoic acid; amidotrizoic acid; 'odiston').
See also Ethyl cartrizoate; Meglumine diatrizoate; Propyl docetrizoate; Sodium diatrizoate.

DIAVERIDINE*** (2,4-diamino-5-veratrylpyrimidine; 2,4-diamino-5-(3,4-dimethoxybenzyl)pyrimidine; BW-49-210.

DIAVERIDINE WITH SULFADIMETHOXINE ('mesulene').

22,25-DIAZACHOLESTANOL (17-[1-(2-dimethylaminoethyl)aminoethyl]androstanol; diazacholestanol dihydrochloride; SC-11952).

20,25-Diazacholesterol *see* Azacosterol.

Diazacycloheptane *see* Hexahydrodiazepine.

Diazacycloheptatriene *see* Diazepine.

Diazadamantanol *see* 5,7-Diphenyl-1,3-diazadamantan-6-ol.

Diazenedicarboxylic acid bis(dimethylamide) *see* Diamide.

DIAZEPAM*** (7-chloro-1,3-dihydro-1-methyl-5-phenyl-2H-1,4-benzodiazepin-2-one; methyldiazepinone; duxen; LA-111; Ro-5-2807; Wy-3467; 'apaurin', 'atensine', 'calmpose', 'cercine', 'faustan', 'fraustan', 'levium', 'noan', 'nocu', 'relanium', 'seduxen', 'stesolid', 'tensopam', 'vaelo', 'valium', 'vivol').
See also Phenytoin with diazepam.

DIAZEPINE (diazacycloheptatriene).

Diazil (tr) *see* Benactyzine.

1,2-Diazine *see* Pyridazine.

1,3-Diazine *see* Pyrimidine.

1,4-Diazine *see* Pyrazine.

Diazinon* *see* Dimpylate.

Diazoacetylserine *see* Azaserine.

4,4'-(Diazoamino)benzamidine *see* Diminazene.

DIAZOAMINOBENZENE (1,3-diphenyltriazene).

Diazo bleu* *see* Evans blue.

1,2-Diazole *see* Pyrazole.

1,3-Diazole *see* Imidazole.

'Diazolina' *see* Morinamide.

Diazoline *see* Mebhydrolin.

Diazomycins *see* Ambomycin; Azotomycin; Duazomycin.

'Diazon' *see* Aldesulfone.

6-Diazo-5-oxonorleucine *see* DON.

DIAZOXIDE*** (7-chloro-3-methyl-2H-1,2,4-benzothiadiazine 1,1-dioxide; SRG-

95213; 'eudemine', 'hyperstat', 'hypertonal', 'mutabase', 'proglicem').

DIAZOXON (diethyl (2-isopropyl-6-methylpyrimidin-4-yl) phosphate; diethyl [6-methyl-2-(1-methylethyl)pyrimidin-4-yl] phosphate; 4-(diethoxyphosphinyloxy)-2-isopropyl-6-methylpyrimidine).

Dibazole (tr) *see* Bendazol.

'Dibein' *see* Phenformin.

DIBEKACIN*** (*O*-3-amino-3-deoxy-α-D-glucopyranosyl-(1→4)-*O*-[2,6-diamino-2,3,4,6-tetradeoxy-α-D-*erythro*-hexopyranosyl-(1→6)]-2-deoxy-L-streptamine; 3',4'-dideoxykanamycin B; DKB).

DIBEMETHINE*** (α-benzylphenethylamine; *N*,*N*-dibenzylmethylamine; dibenzylcarbinamine; 2-amino-1,3-diphenylpropane; diphenylisopropylamine; DBMA; L-566; 'revoxyl').

'Dibenal' *see* Sulfadiazine.

DIBENAMINE (*N*-(2-chloroethyl)dibenzylamine; sympatholytin).

'Dibencil' *see* Benzathine penicillin.

'Dibencillin' *see* Benzathine penicillin.

Dibencocid *see* Cobamamide.

Dibencozamide *see* Cobamamide.

'Dibencozan' *see* Cobamamide.

Dibencozide *see* Cobamamide.

'Dibenyline' *see* Phenoxybenzamine.

11H-Dibenz(b,e)azepine *see* Morphanthridine.

4-[3-(5H-Dibenz(b,f)azepin-5-yl)propyl]-hexahydro-1H-1,4-diazepine-1-ethanol *see* Homopipramol.

4-[3-(5H-Dibenz(b,f)azepin-5-yl)propyl]-1-(2-hydroxyethyl)homopiperazine *see* Homopipramol.

DIBENZEPIN*** (10-(2-dimethylaminoethyl)-5,10-dihydro-5-methyl-11H-dibenzo-(b,e)(1,4)diazepin-11-one; dibenzepin hydrochloride; HF-1927; 'deprex', 'ecatril', 'noveril').

Dibenzheptropine* *see* Deptropine.

Dibenzo(b,e)bicyclo(2.2.2)octadiene *see* 9,10-Ethanoanthracene.

Dibenzo(a,d)cyclohepta-1,4-diene *see* 10,11-Dihydro-5H-dibenzo(a,d)cycloheptene.

5H-Dibenzo(a,d)cycloheptene-5-carboxamide *see* Citenamide.

4-(5H-Dibenzo(a,d)cyclohepten-5-ylidene)-*N*,*N*-dimethyl-2-butynylamine *see* Intriptyline.

[3-(5H-Dibenzo(a,d)cyclohepten-5-ylidene)propyl]dimethylamine *see* Cyclobenzaprine.

3α-(5H-Dibenzo(a,d)cyclohepten-5-yloxy)tropane *see* Decitropine.

[3-(5H-Dibenzo(a,d)cyclohepten-5-yl)propyl]methylamine *see* Protriptyline.

DIBENZOFURAN (biphenylene oxide; diphenylene oxide).

Dibenzoparadiazine *see* Phenazine.

Dibenzoparathiazine *see* Phenothiazine.

Dibenzo-γ-pyran *see* 9-Xanthenone.

Dibenzopyrazine *see* Phenazine.

Dibenzo(b,e)pyridine *see* Acridine.
Dibenzo-γ-pyrone *see* 9-Xanthenone.
Dibenzopyrrole *see* Carbazole.
3-Dibenzo(b,e)thiepin-11(6H)-ylidene-1αH,5αH-tropane *see* Tropatepine.
DIBENZ(b,f)(1,4)OXAZEPINE (CR; EA-3547).
Dibenzoxine *see* Noxiptiline.
Dibenzoyl *see* Benzil.
Dibenzoyl disulfide *see* Bensulfene.
Dibenzoyl peroxide *see* Benzoyl peroxide.
Dibenzthion *see* Sulbentine.
1,3-Dibenzyldecahydro-2-oxoimidazo(4,5-c)thieno(1,2-a)thiolium 10-camphorsulfonate *see* Trimetaphan camsilate.
N,N′-Dibenzylethylenediamine *see* Benzathine.
'Dibenzyline' *see* Phenoxybenzamine.
3,4-(1,3-Dibenzyl-2-ketoimidazolido)-1,2-trimethylenethiophanium camphorsulfonate *see* Trimetaphan camsilate.
Dibenzylmethylamine *see* Dibemethine.
4,6-Dibenzyl-5-oxo-1-thia-4,6-diazatricyclo(6,3,0,0³,⁷)undecanium camphorsulfonate *see* Trimetaphan camsilate.
DIBENZYL SUCCINATE (dibenzyl ester of succinic acid; 'spasmine').
See also Benzyl succinate.
3,5-Dibenzyltetrahydro-1,3,5-thiadiazine-2-thione *see* Sulbentine.
(DIBENZYLTIN)-S,S′-BIS(ISOOCTYL THIOGLYCOLATE) ('ergoterm TGO').
'Dibestil' *see* Diethylstilbestrol dipropionate.
'Dibotin' *see* Phenformin.
'Dibrom' *see* Naled.
'Dibromdulcitol' *see* Mitolactol.
'Dibromin' *see* Dibromobarbituric acid.
Dibrominum *see* Dibromobarbituric acid.
5,5-DIBROMOBARBITURIC ACID (dibrominum; 'dibromin').
Dibromobehenic acid calcium salt *see* Calcium dibromobehenate.
4,4′-Dibromobenzilic acid isopropyl ester *see* Bromopropylate.
3,5-Dibromo-N-(p-bromobenzyl)salicylamide *see* Bensalan.
3,4′-Dibromo-5-chlorothiosalicylanilide acetate *see* Brotianide.
5,6β-Dibromo-5α-cholestan-3β-ol acetate *see* Acebrochol.
2′,4′-Dibromo-α-(cyclohexylmethylamino)-o-vanillotoluidide acetate *see* Brovanexine.
1,2-Dibromo-2,2-dichloroethyl dimethyl phosphate *see* Naled.
1,6-Dibromo-1,6-dideoxydulcitol *see* Mitolactol.
1,6-Dibromo-1,6-dideoxy-D-galactitol *see* Mitolactol.
1,6-Dibromo-1,6-dideoxy-D-mannitol *see* Mitobronitol.
Dibromodihydroxybenzil *see* Dibromsalicil.
Dibromodihydroxyquinoline *see* Broxyquinoline.
Dibromodulcitol *see* Mitolactol.
3,5-Dibromo-4-hydroxybenzaldehyde O-(2,4-dinitrophenyl)oxime *see* Bromofenoxim.
3,4′-Dibromo-6-hydroxybenzanilide *see* Dibromsalan.
3,5-Dibromo-4-hydroxybenzonitrile *see* Bromoxynil.
3,5-Dibromo-Nᵅ-(trans-4-hydroxycyclohexyl)toluene-α,2-diamine *see* Ambroxol.
2′,7-Dibromo-4-hydroxymercurifluorescein *see* Merbromin.
3,5-Dibromo-4-hydroxyphenyl 2-ethylbenzofuran-3-yl ketone *see* Benzbromarone.
2-[[(6,8-Dibromo-9H-indeno(2,1-d)-pyrimidin-9-ylidene)amino]oxy]-N-(2-dimethylaminoethyl)propionamide *see* Brindoxime.
N-[2-[[(6,8-Dibromo-9H-indeno(2,1-d)-pyrimidin-9-ylidene)amino]oxy]-propionyl]-N′,N′-dimethylethylenediamine *see* Brindoxime.
Dibromomannitol *see* Mitobronitol.
Dibromomethyldihydroxyquinoline *see* Broxaldine.
5,7-Dibromo-2-methyl-8-quinolinol *see* Broquinaldol.
6,8-Dibromo-9-oxo-9H-indeno(2,1-d)-pyrimidine O-[1-[[[(2-dimethylaminoethyl)amino]carbonyl]ethyl]oxime *see* Brindoxime.
2,2′-Dibromopropamidine *see* Dibrompropamidine.
Di(bromopropionyl)piperazine *see* Pipobroman.
'Dibromoquin' *see* Broxyquinoline.
5,7-Dibromo-8-quinolinol *see* Broxyquinoline.
3,5-Dibromosalicylanilide *see* Metabromsalan.
4′,5-Dibromosalicylanilide *see* Dibromsalan.
3,5-Dibromo-N-tetrahydrofurfurylsalicylamide *see* Fursalan.
3,5-Dibromo-3′-trifluoromethylsalicylanilide *see* Flusalan.
3,5-Dibromo-α,α,α-trifluorosalicylotoluidide *see* Flusalan.
DIBROMPROPAMIDINE*** (4,4′-(trimethylenedioxy)bis(3-bromobenzamidine); 1,3-bis(4-amidino-2-bromophenoxy)-propane; 2,2′-dibromopropamidine).
Dibrompropamidine diisethionate *see* Dibrompropamidine isetionate.
Dibrompropamidine isethionate* *see* Dibrompropamidine isetionate.
DIBROMPROPAMIDINE ISETIONATE*** (dibrompropamidine di(ethanol-2-sulfonate); dibrompropamidine diisethionate; dibrompropamidine isethionate; 'brolene', 'brulidene').
DIBROMSALAN** (3-bromo-6-hydroxybenz-p-bromanilide; 4′,5-dibromosalicylanilide; 3,4′-dibromo-6-hydroxybenzanilide; 'diaphene').
DIBROMSALAN WITH TRIBROMSALAN (ASC-4; 'hilomid', 'hitreman', 'mitenyl', 'temasept IV').
DIBROMSALICIL (5,5′-dibromo-2,2′-dihydroxybenzyl; dibromsalicyl; 'DBS', 'dibro-

sal', 'respectol').
Dibromsalicyl see Dibromsalicil.
'Dibrosal' see Dibromsalicil.
Dibucaine see Cinchocaine.
DIBUDINATE(S)** (2,6-di-*tert*-butyl-1,5-
naphthalenedisulfonate(s)).
See also Levopropoxyphene dibudinate.
'Dibuline' see Dibutoline.
Dibunate see Ethyl dibunate; Sodium
dibunate.
DIBUPROL*** (1,3-dihydroxy-2-propanol;
7-hydroxy-5,9-dioxatridecane).
DIBUPYRONE** (4-isobutylamino-2,6-di-
methyl-1-phenyl-3-pyrazolin-5-one sodium
methanesulfonate; 2,3-dimethyl-4-isobutyl-
amino-1-phenyl-3-pyrazolin-5-one sodium
methane sulfonate; sodium (antipyrinylisobutylamino)methanesulfonate; isobutylphenazone methanesulfonate; isobutylphenazone mesilate; 'melufin').
DIBUSADOL*** (*N*-(4-diethylaminobutyl)-
salicylamide acetate (ester)).
DIBUTADIAMIN (*N*-*tert*-butyl-1,4-butane-
diamine dihydrochloride; CI-505).
Dibutamide see Ambucetamide.
DIBUTOLINE (ethyl(2-hydroxyethyl)-
dimethylammonium sulfate dibutylcarbamate; 'dibuline').
1,3-Dibutoxy-2-propanol see Dibuprol.
'Dibutox' see Dinoseb.
**5-(2-Dibutylaminoethylamino)-3-phenyl-
1,2,4-oxadiazole** see Butalamine.
2-Dibutylamino-4′-methoxyacetanilide
see Ambucetamide.
3-Dibutylaminopropyl *p*-aminobenzoate
see Butocaine.
2,6-Di-*tert*-butyl-*p*-cresol see Butylated
hydroxytoluene.
N,*N*′-**Dibutyl-*N*,*N*′-dicarboxymorpholine-
ethylenediamine** see Dimorpholamine.
N,*N*-**Dibutyl-4-hexyloxy-1-naphthamidine**
see Bunamine.
**4-(3,5-Di-*tert*-butyl-4-hydroxyphenoxy)-3,5-
diiodohydrocinnamic acid** see Hinderin.
3,5-Di-*tert*-butyl-4-hydroxytoluene see
Butylated hydroxytoluene.
Di-*tert*-butylmethylphenol see Butylated
hydroxytoluene.
**2,6-Di-*tert*-butyl-4-methylphenyl methyl-
carbamate** see Terbucarb.
**2,6-Di-*tert*-butylnaphthalene-1,5-disulfonic
acid,** esters and salts see Dibudinate(s).
**3,7-Di-*tert*-butylnaphthalene-1,5-disulfonic
acid,** esters and salts see Bunapsilate(s).
**3,6-Di-*tert*-butylnaphthalene-1-sulfonic
acid,** esters and salts see Ethyl dibunate;
Sodium dibunate.
Dibutyl *p*-nitrophenyl phosphate see
Nibufin.
**Dibutylphosphinic acid *p*-nitrophenyl
ester** see *p*-Nitrophenyl dibutylphosphinate.
DIBUTYL PHTHALATE (butyl phthalate;
DBP).
DIBUTYL SUCCINATE ('tabutrex').
p-**Dibutylsulfamoylbenzoic acid** see
Butacid.
DIC see Dacarbazine.

1,3-Dicaffeylquinic acid see Cynarine.
Dicaine (tr) Tetracaine.
DICAMBA* (3,6-dichloro-2-methoxybenzoic
acid; dianat; 'banvel', 'mediben').
DICAMBA-METHYL (methyl 3,6-dichloro-
2-methoxybenzoate; disugran; 'racuza').
'Di-captan' see Dicapthon.
DICAPTHON* (*O*-(2-chloro-4-nitrophenyl)
O,*O*-dimethyl phosphorothioate; 'di-
captan', 'noltran').
Dicaptol (tr) see Dimercaprol.
Dicarbamoyldiimide see Azoformamide.
**3,3-Dicarbethoxy-*N*,*N*-diethyl-4-phenyl-
1-butylamine** see Diethyl 1-benzyl-
1-(2-diethylaminoethyl)malonate.
O,*S*-**Dicarbethoxythiamine** see Cetotiamine.
DICARBINE*** (2,3,4,4a,5,9b-hexahydro-
2,8-dimethyl-1H-pyrido(4,3-b)indole; 3,6-
dimethyl-1,2,3,4,4a,9a-hexahydro-γ-
carboline; carbidine).
DICARFEN*** (2-dimethylaminoethyl
diphenylcarbamate ester; deanol diphenyl-
carbamate).
'Dicarzol' see Formetanate.
'Dicertan' see Papaverine adenylate.
'Dicestal' see Dichlorophen.
DICHLOBENIL* (2,6-dichlorobenzonitrile;
'casoron 133').
DICHLOFENTHION* (*O*-(2,4-dichloro-
phenyl) *O*,*O*-diethyl phosphorothioate;
V-C 13; 'nemacide').
DICHLOFLUANID* (1,1-dichloro-*N*-[(dimethylamino)sulfonyl]-1-fluoro-*N*-phenyl-
methanesulfenamide; dichlorofluanide;
'elvaron', 'euparen').
DICHLONE* (2,3-dichloro-1,4-naphtho-
quinone; 2,3-dichloro-1,4-naphthalene-
dione; 'phygon').
DICHLORALPHENAZONE* (compound of
1 mol. phenazone and 2 mol. chloral
hydrate; dichloralantipyrine; 'bihypnal',
'chloral', 'dormuphar', 'duodorm',
'sominat', 'welldorm').
DICHLORAMINE (*N*,*N*-dichloro-*p*-
toluenesulfonamide; dichloramine T).
cis-**Dichlordiammine platinum (II)** see
cis-Platinum (II) diaminodichloride.
'Dichloren' see Chlormethine.
Dichloresul see Disul.
'Di-chloricide' see Dichlorobenzene.
DICHLORISONE*** (9α,11β-dichloro-1,4-
pregnadiene-17α,21-diol; 9α,11β-dichloro-
17α,21-dihydroxypregna-1,4-diene-
3,20-dione).
DICHLORISONE ACETATE* (dichlorisone
21-acetate; 'diloderm', 'disoderm').
Dichlorisoprenaline see DCI.
DICHLORMATE* (3,4-dichlorobenzyl
methylcarbamate; 'rowmate', 'sirmate').
DICHLORMEZANONE*** (2-(3,4-dichloro-
phenyl)-2,3,5,6-tetrahydro-3-methyl-4H-
1,3-thiazin-4-one, 1,1-dioxide; 2-(3,4-
dichlorophenyl)-3-methyl-4-metathiazanone
1,1-dioxide; WIN-12267).
**2-Dichloroacetamido-1-(*p*-acetylphenyl)-
1,3-propanediol** see Cetofenicol.
2-Dichloroacetamido-1-(*p*-methylsulfon-

ylphenyl)-1,3-propanediol *see* Thiamphenicol.

2-Dichloroacetamido-1-(*p*-nitrophenyl)-1,3-propanediol *see* Chloramphenicol.

(±)-*threo-N*-(2,2-Dichloroacetyl)-*β*-hydroxy-*α*-hydroxymethyl-*p*-methylsulfonylphenethylamine *see* Racefenicol.

2,2-Dichloro-*N*-[*p*-acetyl-*β*-hydroxy-*α*-(hydroxymethyl)phenethyl]acetamide *see* Cetofenicol.

S-(2,3-Dichloroallyl) diisopropylcarbamothioate *see* Diallate.

[2-(2,6-Dichloroanilino)ethyl]guanidine *see* Guanclofine.

2-(2,6-Dichloroanilino)-2-imidazoline *see* Clonidine.

2-(2,3-Dichloroanilino)nicotinic acid *see* Diclonixin.

o-(2,6-Dichloroanilino)phenylacetic acid *see* Diclofenac.

4-(2,6-Dichloroanilino)-3-thiophenecarboxylic acid *see* Clantifen.

N-[1-(3,4-Dichloroanilino)-2,2,2-trichloroethyl]formamide *see* Chloraniformethan.

2-(3,4-Dichlorobenzamido)phenoxyacetic acid *see* Clamidoxic acid.

p-DICHLOROBENZENE ('di-chloricide', 'paramoth'.

2,6-Dichlorobenzenecarbothiamide *see* Chlorthiamid.

4,4′-Dichlorobenzilic acid ethyl ester *see* Chlorobenzilate.

4,4′-Dichlorobenzilic acid isopropyl ester *see* Chloropropylate.

DICHLOROBENZODODECINIUM CHLORIDE ((3,4-dichlorobenzyl)-dodecyldimethylammonium chloride; 'dermofungine-B', 'riseptin').

2,6-Dichlorobenzonitrile *see* Dichlobenil.

S-(5,7-Dichlorobenzoxazol-2-ylmethyl) *O,O*-diethyl phosphorodithioate *see* Benoxafos.

2,4-DICHLOROBENZYL ALCOHOL ('dybenal', 'rapidosept').

(3,4-Dichlorobenzyl)dodecyldimethylammonium chloride *see* Dichlorobenzododecinium chloride.

1-(2,6-Dichlorobenzylideneamino)-guanidine *see* Guanabenz.

1-[(2,6-Dichlorobenzylidene)amino]-3-hydroxyguanidine *see* Guanoxabenz.

3,4-Dichlorobenzyl methylcarbamate *see* Dichlormate.

1,1-Dichloro-2,2-bis(*p*-chlorophenyl)-ethane *see* DDD.

1,1-Dichloro-2,2-bis(*p*-chlorophenyl)-ethanol *see* Hydroxy-DDD.

1,1-Dichloro-2,2-bis(*p*-chlorophenyl)-ethylene *see* DDE.

1,1-DICHLORO-2,2-BIS(*p*-ETHYLPHENYL)ETHANE (1,1′-(2,2′-dichloroethylene)bis(4-ethylbenzene); Q-137; 'perthane').

3,4-Dichlorocarbanilic acid methyl ester *see* Swep.

4,6-Dichloro-2-(*o*-chloroanilino)-*s*-triazine

see Anilazine.

1-(2,4-Dichloro-*β*-(*p*-chlorobenzyloxy)-phenethyl)imidazole *see* Econazole.

2,2-Dichloro-*N*-(*p*-chloro-*α*-chloromethylphenacyl)acetamide *see* Cloponone.

1,1-Dichloro-2-(*o*-chlorophenyl)-2-(*p*-chlorophenyl)ethane *see* Mitotane.

4,6-Dichloro-*N*-(2-chlorophenyl)-1,3,5-triazin-2-amine *see* Anilazine.

6,7-Dichloro-3-(3-cyclopenten-1-yl)-2H-1,2,4-benzothiadiazine 1,1-dioxide *see* Pazoxide.

3,4-Dichloro-*N*-(cyclopropylcarbonyl)-aniline *see* Cypromid.

2,10-Dichloro-12H-dibenzo(d,g)(1,3)-dioxocin-6-carboxylic acid methyl ester *see* Treloxinate.

3,4′-Dichloro-2-(2,2-dichloroacetamido)-propiophenone *see* Cloponone.

1-[2,4-Dichloro-*β*-[(2,4-dichlorobenzyl)-oxy]phenethyl]-3-(*p*-fluorophenacyl)-imidazolium chloride *see* Fludazonium chloride.

1-[2,4-Dichloro-*β*-(2,4-dichlorobenzyloxy)-phenethyl]imidazole *see* Miconazole.

1-[2,4-Dichloro-*β*-(2,6-dichlorobenzyloxy)-phenethyl]imidazole *see* Isoconazole.

1-[2,4-Dichloro-*β*-[(2,4-dichlorobenzyl)-oxy]phenethyl]-3-phenethylimidazolium chloride *see* Sepazonium chloride.

4,4′-Dichloro-*α*-dichloromethylbenzhydrol *see* Hydroxy-DDD.

Dichlorodideoxyisoprenaline *see* DCI.

3,5-Dichloro-*N*-(2-diethylaminoethyl)-*o*-anisamide *see* Diclometide.

3,5-Dichloro-*N*-(2-diethylaminoethyl)-2-methoxybenzamide *see* Diclometide.

9,11-Dichloro-6,21-difluoro-16,17-dihydroxypregna-1,4-diene-3,20-dione 16,17-acetonide *see* Tralonide.

2,2-Dichloro-1,1-difluoroethyl methyl ether *see* Methoxyflurane.

2,2-Dichloro-1,1-difluoroethyl methyl sulfide *see* Methioflurane.

DICHLORODIFLUOROMETHANE CFC-12; 'arcton-6', 'freon-12', 'frigen-12', 'gentron-12', 'halon', 'isoton-12').

Dichlorodifluoromethoxyethane *see* Methoxyflurane.

9,11-Dichloro-6,21-difluoropregna-1,4-diene-16,17-diol-3,20-dione 16,17-acetonide *see* Tralonide.

2,5-Dichloro-3,6-dihydroxy-*p*-benzoquinone *see* Chloranilic acid.

5,5′-Dichloro-2,2′-dihydroxy-3,3′-dinitro-biphenyl *see* Niclofolan.

Dichlorodihydroxydiphenylmethane *see* Dichlorophen.

Dichlorodihydroxydiphenyl sulfide *see* Fenticlor.

9*α*,11*β*-Dichloro-17*α*,21-dihydroxypregna-1,4-diene-3,20-dione *see* Dichlorisone.

1,4-Dichloro-2,5-dimethoxybenzene *see* Chloroneb.

2,4-Dichloro-10-(3-dimethylaminopropyl)-phenothiazine *see* Dichlorpromazine.

1,1-Dichloro-*N*-[(dimethylamino)sulfon-

141

yl]-1-fluoro-*N*-phenylmethanesulfen-amide *see* Dichlofluanid.
3,5-Dichloro-*N*-(1,1-dimethyl-2-propynyl)-benzamide *see* Propyzamide.
3,5-Dichloro-2,6-dimethylpyridin-4-ol *see* Clopidol.
4,4′-Dichloro-6,6′-dinitro-*o,o*-biphenol *see* Niclofolan.
5,5′-Dichloro-3,3′-dinitro-2,2′-biphenol *see* Niclofolan.
p,p′-Dichlorodiphenyl methyl carbinol *see* Chlorfenethol.
1,2-Dichloro-3,5-disulfamoylbenzene *see* Diclofenamide.
2,2-Dichloroethenyl dimethyl phosphate *see* Dichlorvos.
2,2-Dichloro-*N*-(2-ethoxyethyl)-*N*-[(*p*-nitrophenoxy)benzyl]acetamide *see* Etofamide.
2,3-Dichloro-4-(2-ethylacryloyl)phenoxy-acetic acid *see* Etacrynic acid.
1,1-DICHLOROETHYLENE (vinylidene chloride).
1,2-DICHLOROETHYLENE (ethylene chloride; Dutch liquid; 'brocide').
1,1′-(2,2-Dichloroethylene)bis(4-chlorobenzene) *see* DDD.
1,1′-(2,2′-Dichloroethylene)bis(4-ethyl-benzene) *see* 1,1-Dichloro-2,2-bis(*p*-ethyl-phenyl)ethane.
Dichlorofenidim *see* Diuron.
Dichlorofluanid *see* Dichlofluanid.
2,6-Dichloro-*N*-(2-guanidinoethyl)aniline *see* Guanclofine.
9α,11β-Dichloro-6α-fluoro-21-hydroxy-16α,17α-isopropylidenedioxypregna-1,4-diene-3,20-dione *see* Fluclorolone acetonide.
9α,11β-Dichloro-6α-fluoropregna-1,4-diene-16α,17α,21-triol-3,20-dione *see* Fluclorolone.
9α,11β-Dichloro-6α-fluoro-16α,17α,21-trihydroxypregna-1,4-diene-3,20-dione *see* Fluclorolone.
2,4′-Dichloro-4-(2-hydroxy-3,5-diiodo-benzamido)benzophenone *see* Salantel.
2,2-Dichloro-*N*-(2-hydroxyethyl)-*N*-[*p*-(*p*-nitrophenoxy)benzyl]acetamide *see* Clefamide.
threo-2,2-Dichloro-*N*-(β-hydroxy-α-hydroxymethyl-*p*-methylsulfonyl-phenethyl)acetamide *see* Racefenicol; Thiamphenicol.
2,2-Dichloro-*N*-(β-hydroxy-α-hydroxy-methyl-*p*-nitrophenyl)acetamide *see* Chloramphenicol.
2′,5-Dichloro-2-hydroxy-4′-nitrobenzanil-ide *see* Niclosamide.
Dichlorohydroxyquinaldine *see* Chlor-quinaldol.
Dichlorohydroxyquinoline *see* 5,7-Dichloro-8-quinolinol.
O-(2,5-Dichloro-4-iodophenyl) *O,O*-di-methyl phosphorothioate *see* Iodo-fenphos.
Dichloroisocyanuric acid *see* Troclosene.
3,4-Dichloro-α-(isopropylaminomethyl)-

benzyl alcohol *see* DCI.
Dichloroisoproterenol *see* DCI.
DICHLOROMETHANE (methylene chloride; 'solaesthin', 'solmethin').
3,6-Dichloro-2-methoxybenzoic acid *see* Dicamba.
3,4-Dichloro-α-methoxybenzylpenicillin *see* Clometocillin.
4,4′-Dichloro-α-methylbenzhydrol *see* Chlorfenethol.
2,3-Dichloro-4-(2-methylenebutyryl)-phenoxyacetic acid *see* Etacrynic acid.
Dichloromethylquinolinol *see* Chlor-quinaldol.
O-[2,5-Dichloro-4-(methylthio)phenyl] *O,O*-diethyl phosphorothioate *see* Chlor-thiophos.
3′,4′-DICHLORO-2-METHYLVALERAN-ILIDE (*N*-(3,4-dichlorophenyl)-2-methyl-valeramide; *N*-(3,4-dichlorophenyl)-2-methylpentanamide; 'karsil').
2,3-Dichloro-1,4-naphthoquinone *see* Dichlone.
2,6-Dichloro-4-nitroaniline *see* Dicloran.
2,4-Dichloro-4′-nitrodiphenyl ether *see* Nitrofen.
2,4-Dichloro-1-(*p*-nitrophenoxy)benzene *see* Nitrofen.
2′,5-Dichloro-4′-nitrosalicylanilide *see* Niclosamide.
DICHLOROPHEN*** (2,2′-methylenebis(4-chlorophenol); dichlorodihydroxydiphenyl-methane; bis(5-chloro-2-hydroxyphenyl)-methane; diphenthane-70; dichlosal; DDDM; DDM; 'anthipen', 'antiphen', 'dicestal', 'didroxane', 'G 4', 'gingivit', 'halenol', 'hyosan', 'preventol G-D', 'parabis', 'teniathane', 'teniatol').
DICHLOROPHENARSINE*** (2-amino-4-(dichloroarsino)phenol; 3-amino-4-hydr-oxyphenyldichloroarsine; arsphendi-chloride; chlorophenarsine; dichloro-phenarsine hydrochloride; dichlorphen-arsine; M-4000; RP-2591).
Dichlorophene *see* Dichlorophen.
DICHLOROPHENOBARBITAL (5-(3,5-dichlorophenyl)-5-ethylbarbituric acid).
2,4-DICHLOROPHENOXYACETIC ACID (2,4-D; 'dikonirit', 'pielik').
See also Butyl dichlorophenoxyacetate; Chlorinated phenoxyacetic acid mixture; Dimethylamine dichlorophenoxyacetate; Ioxynil plus (2,4-dichlorophenoxy)acetic acid.
4-(2,4-DICHLOROPHENOXY)BUTYRIC ACID (2,4-DB; 'embutox').
2-(2,4-Dichlorophenoxy)ethanol phosphite *see* 2,4-DEP.
1-[2-(2,6-Dichlorophenoxy)ethylamino]-guanidine *see* Guanochlor.
2-(2,4-Dichlorophenoxy)ethyl hydrogen sulfate *see* Disul.
2-[1-(2,6-Dichlorophenoxy)ethyl]-2-imidazoline *see* Lofexidine.
3,4-Dichloro-α-phenoxyhippuric acid *see* Clamidoxic acid.
2-(3,4-Dichlorophenoxymethyl)-2-

imidazoline *see* Fenmetozole.

2-(2,4-Dichlorophenoxy)phenylacetic acid *see* Fenclofenac.

(2,4-Dichlorophenoxy)propionic acid *see* Dichlorprop.

N-[3-(2,4-Dichlorophenoxy)propyl]-*N*-methylprop-2-ynylamine *see* Clorgiline.

2-(2,6-Dichlorophenylamino)-2-imidazoline *see* Clonidine.

N-(2,6-Dichlorophenyl)-*o*-aminophenylacetic acid *see* Diclofenac.

N-(2,3-Dichlorophenyl)anthranilic acid *see* Clofenamic acid.

2,4-Dichlorophenyl benzenesulfonate *see* Dichlorophenyl besilate.

DICHLOROPHENYL BESILATE (2,4-dichlorophenyl benzenesulfonate; 'genite').

N-(3,4-Dichlorophenyl)cyclopropanecarboxamide *see* Cypromid.

1-[2-(2,4-Dichlorophenyl)-2-(2,4-dichlorophenylmethoxy)ethyl]-1H-imidazole *see* Miconazole.

1-[2-(2,4-Dichlorophenyl)-2-(2,6-dichlorophenylmethoxy)ethyl]-1H-imidazole *see* Isoconazole.

O-(2,4-Dichlorophenyl) *O,O*-diethyl phosphorothioate *see* Dichlofenthion.

N-(3,4-Dichlorophenyl)-*N*-(dimethylaminocarbamoyl)-*p*-anisamide *see* Anisuron.

N-(3,4-Dichlorophenyl)-*N*-[(dimethylamino)carbonyl]benzamide *see* Phenobenzuron.

N-(3,4-Dichlorophenyl)-*N*-[(dimethylamino)carbonyl]-4-methoxybenzamide *see* Anisuron.

3-(3,5-Dichlorophenyl)-5,5-dimethyl-2,4-oxazolidinedione *see* Dichlozoline.

1-(3,4-Dichlorophenyl)-3,3-dimethylurea *see* Diuron.

N-(3,4-Dichlorophenyl)-*N*-[1-(ethoxycarbonyl)ethyl]benzamide *see* Benzoylprop-ethyl.

5-(3,5-Dichlorophenyl)-5-ethylbarbituric acid *see* Dichlorophenobarbital.

3-(2,6-Dichlorophenyl)-2-ethylquinazolin-4(3H)-one *see* Cloroqualone.

1-[[5-(3,4-Dichlorophenyl)furfurylidene]-amino]hydantoin *see* Clodanolene.

1-(3,4-Dichlorophenyl)-2-isopropylaminoethanol *see* DCI.

1-(3,4-Dichlorophenyl)-5-isopropylbiguanide *see* Chlorproguanil.

6-[2-(3,4-Dichlorophenyl)-2-methoxyacetamido]penicillanic acid *see* Clometocillin.

1-(3,4-Dichlorophenyl)-1-(*p*-methoxybenzoyl)-3,3-dimethylurea *see* Anisuron.

1-(3,4-Dichlorophenyl)-3-methoxy-3-methylurea *see* Linuron.

N-3,4-Dichlorophenyl-2-methylacrylamide *see* Chloranocryl.

2-[(2,6-Dichlorophenyl)methylene]-*N*-hydroxyhydrazinecarboximidamide *see* Guanoxabenz.

6-[3-(2,6-Dichlorophenyl)-5-methyl-4-isoxazolecarboxamido]penicillanic

acid *see* Dicloxacillin.

2-(3,4-Dichlorophenyl)-4-methyl-1,2,4-oxazolidine-3,5-dione *see* Chlormethazole.

N-(3,4-Dichlorophenyl)-2-methylpentanamide *see* 3′,4′-Dichloro-2-methylvaleranilide.

N-(3,4-Dichlorophenyl)-2-methyl-2-propenamide *see* Chloranocryl.

6-[[1-(2,6-Dichlorophenyl)-4-methylpyrazol-5-yl]carboxamido]penicillanic acid *see* Pirazocillin.

N-(3,4-Dichlorophenyl)-2-methylvaleramide *see* 3′,4′-Dichloro-2-methylvaleranilide.

α-(2,4-Dichlorophenyl)-α-phenyl-5-pyrimidinemethanol *see* Triarimol.

N-[3-[4-(2,5-Dichlorophenyl)piperazin-1-yl]propyl]acetamide *see* Acaprazine.

N-(3,4-Dichlorophenyl)propionamide *see* Propanil.

2,6-Dichloro-4-phenyl-3,5-pyridinedicarbonitrile *see* Pyridinitril.

2-(3,4-Dichlorophenyl)-2,3,5,6-tetrahydro-3-methyl-4H-1,3-thiazin-4-one 1,1-dioxide *see* Dichlormezanone.

S-[(2,5-Dichlorophenylthio)methyl] *O,O*-diethyl phosphorodithioate *see* Phenkapton.

2′,4′-Dichloro-3-piperid-1-ylbutyranilide *see* Clibucaine.

9α,11β-Dichloro-1,4-pregnadiene-17α,21-diol-3,20-dione *see* Dichlorisone.

Dichloropromazine *see* Dichlorpromazine.

Dichloroprop *see* Dichlorprop.

S-(2,3-Dichloro-2-propenyl) bis(1-methylethyl)carbamothioate *see* Diallate.

3′,4′-Dichloropropionanilide *see* Propanil.

2,2-Dichloropropionic acid *see* Dalapon.

2,2-Dichloropropionic acid trichlorophenoxyethyl ester *see* Erbon.

p,p′-Dichloro-α-pyrid-3-ylbenzhydrol *see* Parinol.

5,7-DICHLORO-8-QUINOLINOL (dichlorohydroxyquinoline; 'endiaton'). *See also* Halquinols.

4′,5-DICHLOROSALICYLANILIDE (5-chlorosalicylic acid 4-chloroanilide; 'arylid').

p-(*N,N*-Dichlorosulfamoyl)benzoic acid *see* Halazone.

Dichlorotetrafluoroethane *see* Cryoflurane.

2-[2,3-Dichloro-4-(2-thenoyl)phenoxy]-acetic acid *see* Tienilic acid.

2,6-Dichlorothiobenzamide *see* Chlorthiamid.

N,N-Dichloro-*p*-toluenesulfonamide *see* Dichloramine.

N-(2,6-Dichloro-*m*-tolyl)anthranilic acid *see* Meclofenamic acid.

3,5-Dichloro-*s*-triazine-2,4,6(1H,3H,5H)-trione *see* Troclosene.

4,4′-Dichloro-α-(trichloromethyl)benzhydrol *see* Dicofol.

4,5-Dichloro-2-(trifluoromethyl)-1H-benzimidazole *see* Chlorflurazole.

5,6-Dichloro-2-(trifluoromethyl)-1H-benzimidazole-1-carboxylic acid

phenyl ester see Fenazaflor.
4,4'-Dichloro-3-(trifluoromethyl)carbanilide see Halocarban.
2,2-Dichlorovinyl dimethyl phosphate see Dichlorvos.
2,2-Dichlorovinyl methyl octyl phosphate see Vincofos.
Dichlorovos see Dichlorvos.
DICHLOROXYLENOL*** (2,4-dichloro-3,5-xylenol; 2,4-dichloro-3,5-dimethylphenol; dichloro-m-xylenol).
Dichloroxyquinaldine see Chlorquinaldol.
Dichlorphenamide* see Diclofenamide.
Dichlorphenarsine see Dichlorophenarsine.
Dichlorphos see Dichlorvos.
DICHLORPROMAZINE (2,4-dichloro-10-(3-dimethylaminopropyl)phenothiazine; dichloropromazine).
DICHLORPROP* (2-(2,4-dichlorophenoxy)-propionic acid; 2,4-DP; dichloroprop; 'cornox RK').
'Dichlor-stapenor' see Dicloxacillin.
DICHLORVOS*** (2,2-dichlorovinyl dimethyl phosphate; 2,2-dichloroethenyl dimethyl phosphate; dichlorophos; dichlorphos; dichlorovos; DDVF; DDVP; SD-1750; 'atgard', 'canogard', 'dedevap', 'equigard', 'herkol', 'mutox', 'nogos', 'nuvan', 'task', 'tenac', 'vapona', 'vinylofos').
DICHLORVOS WITH CALCIUM 2,2-DICHLOROVINYL METHYL PHOSPHATE ('krecalvin').
Dichlorvos demethyl calcium salt see Calcium 2,2-dichlorovinyl methyl phosphate.
Dichlosal see Dichlorophen.
'Dichlotride' see Hydrochlorothiazide.
DICHLOZOLINE* (3-(3,5-dichlorophenyl)-5,5-dimethyl-2,4-oxazolidinedione; MW-274115; S-55009; 'solex')'
DICHOLINE SUBERATE (suberyldicholine; suberoylbis(choline); D-6; corconium; korkonium; subecholine).
DICHROMIUM TRIOXIDE* (chromium sesquioxide).
Dichystrol see Dihydrotachysterol.
'Dicinon' (tr) see Etamsylate.
'Diclocil' see Dicloxacillin.
'Dicloeta' see Dicloxacillin with hetacillin.
DICLOFENAC*** (o-(2,6-dichloroanilino)-phenylacetic acid; N-(2,6-dichlorophenyl)-o-aminophenylacetic acid).
DICLOFENAC SODIUM* (sodium o-(2,6-dichloroanilino)phenylacetate; GP-45840; 'voltaren', 'voltarol').
DICLOFENAMIDE*** (1,2-dichloro-3,5-disulfamoylbenzene; 4,5-dichloro-1,3-benzenedisulfonamide; dichlorphenamide; 'antidrase', 'daranide', 'oralcon', 'oratrol').
DICLOMETIDE*** (3,5-dichloro-N-(2-diethylaminoethyl)-o-anisamide; 3,5-dichloro-N-(2-diethylaminoethyl)-2-methoxybenzamide).
DICLONIXIN** (2-(2,3-dichloroanilino)-nicotinic acid).
DICLORALUREA** (1,3-bis(2,2,2-tri-

chloro-1-hydroxyethyl)urea).
DICLORAN* (2,6-dichloro-4-nitroaniline; 'allisan', 'botran').
'Diclotride' see Hydrochlorothiazide.
DICLOXACILLIN*** (6-[3-(2,6-dichlorophenyl)-5-methyl-4-isoxazolecarboxamido]-penicillanic acid; [3-(2,6-dichlorophenyl)-5-methylisoxazol-4-yl]penicillin; dicloxacillin sodium; sodium dicloxacillin; BRL-1702; P-1011; 'dichlor-stapenor', 'diclocil', 'dicloxypen', 'dynapen', 'maclicine', 'pathocil', 'stampen', 'veracillin'). †
See also Ampicillin with dicloxacillin.
DICLOXACILLIN WITH HETACILLIN ('dicloeta').
'Dicloxypen' see Dicloxacillin.
'Dico' see Hydrocodone.
'Dicodid' see Hydrocodone.
DICOFOL* (2,2,2-trichloro-1,1-bis(p-chlorophenyl)ethanol; 4,4'-dichloro-α-trichloromethylbenzhydrol; 4-chloro-α-(4-chlorophenyl)-α-trichloromethylbenzenemethanol; p-chloro-α-(p-chlorophenyl)-α-trichloromethylbenzyl alcohol; hydroxy-DDT; DTMC; 'kelthane', 'keltan').
Dicoline (tr) see Dicolinium iodide.
DICOLINIUM IODIDE*** (2-carboxy-1,1,6-trimethylpiperidinium iodide ester with diethyl(2-hydroxyethyl)methylammonium iodide; diethylaminoethyl ester dimethiodide of 1-methylpipecolic acid; diethyl(2-hydroxyethyl)methylammonium iodide methylpipecolate methiodide; dicoline).
'Diconal' see Dipipanone with cyclizine.
'Dicopal' see Prochlorperazine.
Dicophane see DDT.
Dicoumarin see Dicoumarol.
DICOUMAROL*** (3,3'-methylenebis(4-hydroxycoumarin); dicoumarin; bishydroxycoumarin; biscumarolum; 'anathrombase', 'cumarene', 'cumid', 'dicuman', 'dicumarol', 'dicumol', 'kumoran', 'melitoxin', 'temparin').
'Dicoumoxyl' see Coumetarol.
'Dicrotalin' see Rattlesnake venom.
DICROTOPHOS* (3-dimethylamino-1-methyl-3-oxo-1-propenyl dimethyl phosphate; [2-(dimethylcarbamoyl)-1-methylvinyl] dimethyl phosphate; [2-(dimethylcarboxamido)-1-methylvinyl] dimethyl phosphate; [1-(dimethylcarboxamido)-1-propen-2-yl] dimethyl phosphate; 3-(dimethoxyphosphinyloxy)-N,N-dimethyl-cis-crotonamide; 3-hydroxy-N,N-dimethyl-cis-crotonamide dimethyl phosphate; 'bidrin', 'carbicron', 'ektafos').
'Dicryl' see Chloranocryl.
'Dictyzide' see Cyacetacide.
'Dicumacyl' see Ethyl biscoumacetate.
'Dicuman' see Dicoumarol.
'Dicumarol' see Dicoumarol.
'Dicumol' see Dicoumarol.
'Dicumoxane' see Coumetarol.
'Dicupreine' see Cuproxolin.
'Dicuran' see Chlorotoluron.
'Dicusat' see Warfarin.

sym. **Dicyanoethane** *see* Succinonitrile.
2-(2,2-Dicyclohexylethyl)piperidine *see*
Perhexiline.
2-(2,2-Dicyclohexylvinyl)piperidine *see*
Hexadiline.
Dicyclomine* *see* Dicycloverine.
DICYCLOPENTADIENYLIRON (ferrocene).
**(2-Dicyclopentylacetoxyethyl)diethyloc-
tylammonium bromide** *see* Penoctonium
bromide.
**(2-Dicyclopentylacetoxyethyl)trimethyl-
ammonium bromide** *see* Diponium
bromide.
DICYCLOVERINE*** (2-diethylaminoethyl
ester of 1-cyclohexylcyclohexanecarboxylic
acid; 2-diethylaminoethyl (bicyclohexyl)-1-
carboxylate; dicyclomine; dicycloverine
hydrochloride; JL-998; M-33536; 'atumin',
'bentyl', 'bentylol', 'diocyl', 'esentil',
'kolantyl', 'merbentyl', 'wyovin').
'Dicynene' *see* Etamsylate.
'Dicynone' *see* Etamsylate.
Dicysteine *see* Cystine.
'Didakene' *see* Tetrachloroethylene.
'Didandin' *see* Diphenadione.
**9,10-Didehydro-*N*-[(*S*)-2-hydroxy-1-
methylethyl]-1,6-dimethylergoline-8β-
carboxamide** *see* Propisergide.
**3-(9,10-Didehydro-6-methylergolin-8a-yl)-
1,1-diethylurea** *see* Lisuride.
**2,10-Di(demethoxy)-2-glucosyloxy-10-
methylthiocolchicine** *see* Thiocolchicoside.
**1,4-Dideoxy-1,4-bis[(2-hydroxyethyl)-
amino]erythritol 1,4-dimethanesul-
fonate** *see* Ritrosulfan.
**3β-[(Dideoxy-β-D-*ribo*-hexopyranosyl-
(1→4)-O-2,6-dideoxy-β-D-*ribo*-hexopyra-
nosyl-(1→4)-2,6-dideoxy-β-D-*ribo*-
hexopyranosyl)oxy]-14,16β-dihydroxy-
5β-card-20(22)-enolide 3′,3″,3‴,4‴,16-
pentaformate** *see* Gitoformate.
3′,4′-Dideoxykanamycin B *see* Dibekacin.
'Didione' *see* Ethadione.
'Didrate' *see* Dihydrocodeine.
'Didrex' *see* Benzphetamine.
'Didropantin' *see* Dihydrostreptomycin.
Didropyridine *see* Pyrithyldione.
'Didrothenate' *see* Dihydrostreptomycin.
DIDROVALTRATE*** (3a,4,5,6-tetrahydro-
3,4-dihydroxyspiro(benzofuran-2(3H),2′-
oxirane)-6-methanol-6-acetate 3,4-diiso-
valerate; 1,4a,5,7a-tetrahydro-1,6-dihydro-
xyspiro(cyclopenta(c)pyran-7(6H),2′-
oxirane)-4-methanol 6-acetate 1,4-diiso-
valerate).
See also Valepotriate.
'Didroxane' *see* Dichlorophen.
'Diedi' *see* Diisopropylamine dichloroacetate.
DIELDRIN** (product containing 85% of
1,2,3,4,10,10-hexachloro-6,7-epoxy-
1,4,4a,5,6,7,8,8a-octahydro-1,4-*exo*-5,8-
endo-dimethanonaphthalene; 1aα,2β,
2aα,3β,6β,6aα,7β,7aα-3,4,5,6,9,9-
hexachloro-1a,2,2a,3,6,6a,7,7a-octahydro-
2,7:3,6-dimethanonaphth(2,3-b)oxirene;
HEOD; 'alvit-55', 'octalox').

See also Endrin.
Diemal* *see* Barbital.
DIENESTROL** (4,4′-diethylidenethylene
diphenol; α,α′-diethylidene-4,4′-dihydroxy-
bibenzyl; 3,4-bis(*p*-hydroxyphenyl)-2,4-
hexadiene; dehydrostilbestrol; dienoestrol;
dihydroxydiphenylhexadine; dienestrol
diacetate).
DIENOCHLOR* (1,1′,2,2′,3,3′,4,4′,5,5′-
decachlorobi[2,4-cyclopentadien-1-yl];
'pentac').
Dienoestrol* *see* Dienestrol.
**1,2:3,4-Diepoxybutane ethylenimine
polymer** *see* Polyetadene.
Diepoxypiperazine *see* Epoxypropylpiperazine.
**1,2:15,16-Diepoxy-4,7,10,13-tetraoxahexa-
decane** *see* Etoglucid.
'Diepropon' *see* Amfepramone.
Dietamfenazole *see* Ditazole.
DIETHADIONE*** (5,5-diethyldihydro-2H-
1,3-oxazine-2,4(3H)-dione; 5,5-diethyltetra-
hydro-1,3-oxazine-2,4-dione; dietroxine;
'dioxine', 'ledosten', 'toce').
Diethamphenazole *see* Ditazole.
DIETHANOLAMINE (2,2′-iminodiethanol;
diolamine).
DIETHAZINE** (10-(2-diethylaminoethyl)-
phenothiazine; dinezin; eazamine; RP-
2987).
DIETHAZINE ETHIODIDE ([2-(10-pheno-
thiazinyl)ethyl]triethylammonium iodide;
RP-3580).
Diethchinalphion *see* Quinalphos.
Diethion *see* Ethion.
'Diethoxin' *see* Parethoxycaine.
**1-(3,4-Diethoxybenzyl)-6,7-diethoxy-
isoquinoline** *see* Ethaverine.
**1-(3,4-Diethoxybenzylidene)-6,7-diethoxy-
1,2,3,4-tetrahydroisoquinoline** *see*
Drotaverine.
**1,3-Diethoxy-5-(2-diethylaminoethoxy)-
benzene** *see* Amifloverine.
DIETHOXYMETHANE (ethylal).
**1,3-Diethoxy-5-(2-morpholinoethoxy)-
benzene** *see* Floredil.
**4-[2-(3,5-Diethoxyphenoxy)ethyl]-
morpholine** *see* Floredil.
2-(3,5-Diethoxyphenoxy)triethylamine
see Amifloverine.
**α-[[(Diethoxyphosphinothioyl)oxy]-
imino]benzeneacetonitrile** *see* Phoxim.
**3-[(Diethoxyphosphinothioyl)oxy]-1-
phenyl-1H-1,2,4-triazole** *see* Phentriazophos.
**3-[(Diethoxyphosphinothioyl)oxy]-6-oxo-
6H-dibenzo(bd)pyran** *see* Coumithoate.
**2-[(Diethoxyphosphinothioyl)oxy]-
quinoxaline** *see* Quinalphos.
**[[[(Diethoxyphosphinothioyl)thio]-
acetyl]methyl]carbamic acid ethyl
ester** *see* Mecarbam.
**2-(Diethoxyphosphinylimino)-1,3-
dithiolane** *see* Phosfolan.
**4-(Diethoxyphosphinyloxy)-2-isopropyl-
6-methylpyrimidine** *see* Diazoxon.
[[2-(Diethoxyphosphinyl)thio]ethyl]-

145

dimethylamine see Amiton.

(2-Diethoxyphosphinylthioethyl)tri-methylammonium iodide see Ecothiopate iodide.

DIETHOXYPROPANOL (glycerol diethyl ether; 'diethyline').

4,4'-Diethoxythiocarbanilide see Etocarlide.

Diethyl aldehyde see Acetal.

Diethylamine cyclohexadien-1-ol-4-one-1-sulfonate see Etamsylate.

Diethylamine 2,5-dihydroxybenzene-sulfonate see Etamsylate.

2-(2-Diethylaminoacetamido)-*m*-toluic acid methyl ester see Tolycaine.

2-DIETHYLAMINOACETIC ACID (*N*,*N*-diethylglycine).

2-Diethylaminoacetic acid prednisolone ester see Prednisolamate.

2-Diethylaminoacetomesidide see Trimecaine.

10-(DIETHYLAMINOACETYL)PHENO-THIAZINE (difasin; difazin; diphasin; diphazin).

N-(4-Diethylaminobutyl)salicylamide acetate see Dibusadol.

4-Diethylamino-2-butynyl α-phenylcyclo-hexaneglycolate see Oxybutynin.

3-Diethylaminobutyranilide see Octacaine.

3-Diethylamino-1,2-dimethylpropyl *p*-aminobenzoate see Dimethocaine.

3-Diethylamino-1,2-dimethylpropyl *p*-butoxybenzoate ethiodide see Quateron.

3-Diethylamino-1,2-dimethylpropyl *p*-isobutoxybenzoate see Ganglefene.

6-Diethylamino-4,4-diphenyl-3-hexanone see Normethadone.

3-Diethylamino-1,1-dithien-2-ylbut-1-ene see Diethylthiambutene.

2-Diethylaminoethanethiol diphenyl-carbamate see Fencarbamide.

2-DIETHYLAMINOETHANOL ('dehydra-sal').

2-Diethylaminoethanol ribonucleate see Ribaminol.

2-(2-Diethylaminoethoxy)benzanilide see Salverine.

3-[4-(2-Diethylaminoethoxy)benzoyl]-2-ethylbenzofuran see Etabenzarone.

2-(2-Diethylaminoethoxy)diphenyl-methane see Etoloxamine.

6-(2-Diethylaminoethoxy)-2-dimethyl-aminobenzothiazole see Dimazole.

2-(2-Diethylaminoethoxy)ethyl 2-ethyl-2-phenylbutyrate see Oxeladin.

2-(2-Diethylaminoethoxy)ethyl phenothi-azine-10-carboxylate see Dimethoxanate.

2-(2-Diethylaminoethoxy)ethyl 2-phenyl-butyrate see Butamirate.

2-(2-Diethylaminoethoxy)ethyl 1-phenyl-cyclopentanecarboxylate see Pentoxy-verine.

2-(2-Diethylaminoethoxy)ethyl phenyl-ethylacetate see Butamirate.

2-(2-Diethylaminoethoxy)ethyl α-phenyl-1-piperidineacetate dimethiodide see Piprocurarium.

4-(2-Diethylaminoethoxy)-α-hydroxy-4'-methoxy-α-phenylbibenzyl see Ethamoxytriphetol.

4-(2-Diethylaminoethoxy)phenyl 2-ethyl-benzofuran-3-yl ketone see Etabenzarone.

1-[*p*-(2-Diethylaminoethoxy)phenyl]-2-(*p*-methoxyphenyl)-1-phenylethanol see Ethamoxytriphetol.

1-[*o*-[2-Diethylaminoethoxy)phenyl]-2-methyl-5-phenylpyrrole see Leiopyrrole.

2-(2-Diethylaminoethoxyphenyl)phen-ethyl ketone see Etafenone.

4-(2-Diethylaminoethoxy)phenyl phen-ethyl ketone see Dietifen.

2'-(2-Diethylaminoethoxy)-3-phenylpro-piophenone see Etafenone.

4'-(2-Diethylaminoethoxy)-3-phenylpro-piophenone see Dietifin.

α-[2-(2-Diethylaminoethoxy)phenyl]-toluene see Etoloxamine.

***p*-(2-Diethylaminoethoxy)stilbene ethiodide** see Stilonium iodide.

2-Diethylaminoethyl *p*-aminobenzoate see Procaine.

2-Diethylaminoethyl 3-amino-2-butoxy-benzoate see Metabutoxycaine.

2-Diethylaminoethyl 4-amino-2-butoxy-benzoate see Ambucaine.

2-Diethylaminoethyl 4-amino-3-butoxy-benzoate see Oxybuprocaine.

1-[[2-(Diethylamino)ethyl]amino]-3,4-dihydroisoquinoline see Iquindamine.

1-(2-Diethylaminoethylamino)-4-hydroxy-methylthioxanthone see Hycanthone.

2-Diethylaminoethylaminoisopentyl phenylacetate see Camylofin.

1-(2-Diethylaminoethylamino)-4-methyl-thioxanthen-9-one see Lucanthone.

2-Diethylaminoethyl 4-amino-1-naphtho-ate see Naphthocaine.

2-Diethylaminoethyl 3-amino-4-propoxy-benzoate see Proxymetacaine.

2-Diethylaminoethyl 4-amino-2-propoxy-benzoate see Propoxycaine.

2-Diethylaminoethyl *p*-aminosalicylate see Hydroxyprocaine.

2-Diethylaminoethyl *p*-aminothiolo-benzoate see Thiocaine.

2-Diethylaminoethyl benzilate see Ben-actyzine.

2-DIETHYLAMINOETHYL BENZOATE (bencaine).

3-(2-Diethylaminoethyl)-2H-1,3-benzoxa-zine-2,4(3H)-dione see Letimide.

2-Diethylaminoethyl 4-benzyl-1-piper-idinecarboxylate see Benrixate.

2-Diethylaminoethyl (bicyclohexyl)-1-carboxylate see Dicycloverine.

2-Diethylaminoethyl 2-(4-biphenylyl)-thiolobutyrate see Xenthiorate.

2-DIETHYLAMINOETHYL *p*-BUTYL-AMINOBENZOATE (T-caine; 'farmo-caine; 'pharmocaine', 'teecaine').

2-DIETHYLAMINOETHYL 4-BUTYL-AMINOSALICYLATE (S-567; 'broncho-caine', 'gynodal', 'wofacaine A').

2-Diethylaminoethyl 1-cyclohexylcyclo-

hexanecarboxylate see Dicycloverine.

2-Diethylaminoethyl di(azodibenzoate) *see* Azoprocaine.

S-(2-Diethylaminoethyl) O,O-diethyl phosphorothioate *see* Amiton.

2-Diethylaminoethyl 2-[3,5-diiodo-4-(3-iodo-4-methoxyphenoxy)phenyl]-acetate *see* Tyromedan.

2-Diethylaminoethyl 2,3-diphenylacrylate *see* Cinnamaverine.

2-Diethylaminoethyl 2,2-diphenylpropionate *see* Aprofene.

2-Diethylaminoethyl diphenylpropylacetate *see* Proadifen.

N-(2-Diethylaminoethyl)-S,S-diphenylsulfoximide *see* Suloxifin.

2-Diethylaminoethyl diphenylthiocarbamate *see* Fencarbamide.

2-Diethylaminoethyl diphenylthioloacetate *see* Tifen.

2-Diethylaminoethyl diphenylvalerate *see* Proadifen.

2-Diethylaminoethyl p-ethoxybenzoate *see* Parethoxycaine.

1-(2-Diethylaminoethyl)-2-(p-ethoxybenzyl)-5-nitrobenzimidazole *see* Etonitazene.

2-[2-(2-Diethylaminoethyl)ethylamino]-ethyl p-aminobenzoate *see* Amoxecaine.

5-(2-Diethylaminoethyl)-3-(α-ethylbenzyl)-1,2,4-oxadiazole *see* Proxazole.

N-(2-Diethylaminoethyl)-2-ethyl-2-phenylmalonamic acid ethyl ester *see* Fenalamide.

Diethylaminoethyl guaicyl ether *see* Guaiactamine.

2-Diethylaminoethyl 2-hydroxybiphenyl-3-carboxylate *see* Xenysalate.

N-(2-Diethylaminoethyl)-4-hydroxy-2-oxo-(2H)-1-benzopyran-3-carboxamide *see* Diarbarone.

N-(2-Diethylaminoethyl)-4-hydroxy-2-oxo-2H-chromen-3-carboxamide *see* Diarbarone.

4-(2-Diethylaminoethyl)-5-imino-3-phenyl-1,2,4-oxadiazoline *see* Imolamine.

2-Diethylaminoethyl p-isopropylbenzoate *see* Isopropylcaine.

1-(2-Diethylaminoethyl)-3-(p-methoxybenzyl)-2(1H)-quinoxalinone *see* Caroverine.

N-(2-Diethylaminoethyl)-2-methoxy-5-(methylsulfonyl)benzamide *see* Tiapride.

N-(2-Diethylaminoethyl)-2-(p-methoxyphenoxy)acetamide *see* Mefexamide.

3-(2-Diethylaminoethyl)-4-methylcoumarin-7-yloxyacetic acid ethyl ester *see* Carbocromen.

2-Diethylaminoethyl α-methyl-2,5-endomethylene-1,2,5,6-tetrahydrobenzhydryl ether methobromide *see* Ciclonium bromide.

2-Diethylaminoethyl 3-methyl-2-phenylvalerate methobromide *see* Valethamate.

2-Diethylaminoethyl 1-methylpipecolate dimethiodide *see* Dicoline.

N-(2-Diethylaminoethyl)-5-(methyl-

sulfonyl)-o-anisamide *see* Tiapride.

2-Diethylaminoethyl nicotinate *see* Nicametate.

2-Diethylaminoethyl p-nicotinoylaminobenzoate *see* Nicotinoylprocaine.

2-Diethylaminoethyl penicillin ester *see* Penethamate.

10-(2-Diethylaminoethyl)phenothiazine *see* Diethazine.

2-Diethylaminoethyl 2-phenylbutyrate *see* Butetamate.

2-Diethylaminoethyl 2-phenylcinnamate *see* Cinnamaverine.

2-Diethylaminoethyl α-phenylcyclohexaneacetate *see* Drofenine.

2-Diethylaminoethyl α-phenylcyclohexaneglycolate methobromide *see* Oxyphenonium bromide.

2-Diethylethyl 1-phenylcyclopentanecarboxylate *see* Pentoxyverine.

2-Diethylaminoethyl phenylethylacetate *see* Butetamate.

2-(2-Diethylaminoethyl)-2-phenylglutarimide *see* Phenglutarimide.

N-(2-Diethylaminoethyl)-2-phenylglycine isoamyl ester *see* Camylofin.

5-(2-Diethylaminoethyl)-3-phenyl-1,2,4-oxadiazole *see* Oxolamine.

2-Diethylaminoethyl α-phenyl-1-piperidineacetate *see* Bietamiverine.

5-(2-Diethylaminoethyl)-3-(1-phenylpropyl)-1,2,4-oxadiazole *see* Proxazole.

2-Diethylaminoethyl-3-phenylsalicylate *see* Xenysalate.

2-Diethylaminoethyl phenylthiopheneacetate *see* Thiphen.

2-Diethylaminoethyl 2-phenylvalerate *see* Propivane.

2-Diethylaminoethyl 2-quinuclidinecarboxylate dimethiodide *see* Dioquin.

1-(2-Diethylaminoethyl)reserpine *see* Bietaserpine.

N-(2-Diethylaminoethyl)salicylamide *see* Saletamide.

2-Diethylaminoethyl salicylate *see* Detanosal.

2-Diethylaminoethyl tetrahydro-α-(1-naphthylmethyl)-2-furanpropionate *see* Naftidrofuryl.

7-(2-Diethylaminoethyl)theophylline *see* Etamiphyllin.

[[2-(Diethylamino)ethyl]thio]acetic acid 8-ester with octahydro-5,8-dihydroxy-4,6,9,10-tetramethyl-6-vinyl-3a,9-propano-3aH-cyclopentacycloocten-1(4H)-one *see* Tiamulin.

2-Diethylaminoethyl 2-(trifluoromethyl)-phenothiazin-10-yl ketone *see* Fluacizine.

2-Diethylaminoethyl 9-xanthenecarboxylate methobromide *see* Methantheline.

2-Diethylaminoethyl o-xylylcyclopentanecarboxylate *see* Metcaraphen.

4-Diethylamino-2-(o-hydroxyphenyl)-2-phenylbutyric acid lactone *see* Amolanone.

4-(2-Diethylamino-2-hydroxypropyl)-ajmalinium hydrogen tartrate *see*

Detajmium bitartrate.

7-Diethylamino-4-hydroxy-6-propyl-3-quinolinecarboxylic acid methyl ester *see* Amquinate.

2-Diethylaminoisopropyl 2,2-diphenylacetate *see* Methyladiphenine.

2-DIETHYLAMINOMETHYL-1,4-BENZODIOXAN (F-883; 'prosympal').

α-**(Diethylaminomethyl)benzyl alcohol benzoate** *see* Elucaine.

2-(Diethylamino)-1-methylethyl *cis*-**1-hydroxy[bicyclohexyl]-2-carboxylate** *see* Rociverine.

6-Diethylaminomethyl-3-methylflavone *see* Flavamine.

O-**(2-Diethylamino-6-methylpyrimidin-4-yl)** *O,O*-**diethyl phosphorothioate** *see* Pirimphos ethyl.

O-**(2-Diethylamino-6-methylpyrimidin-4-yl)** *O,O*-**dimethyl phosphorothioate** *see* Pirimphos methyl.

4,6-Diethylamino-2-(methylthio)-*s*-triazine *see* Simetryn.

7-Diethylamino-5-methyl-*s*-triazolo-(1,5-a)pyrimidine *see* Trapidil.

3-Diethylaminopentyl *p*-**butoxybenzoate** *see* 3-Diethylamino-1,2-dimethylpropyl *p*-butoxybenzoate.

3-Diethylamino-1-phenyl-1-propanone *O*-**[[(4-methoxyphenyl)amino]-carbonyl]oxime** *see* Anidoxime.

3-Diethylamino-1-phenylpropyl benzoate *see* Propanocaine.

10-(3-Diethylaminopropionyl)-2-(trifluoromethyl)phenothiazine *see* Fluacizine.

2-Diethylaminopropiophenone *see* Amfepramone.

3-Diethylaminopropiophenone *O*-**[[(p-methoxyphenyl)amino]carbonyl]-oxime** *see* Anidoxime.

3-Diethylaminopropiophenone *O*-**(p-methoxyphenylcarbamoyl) oxime** *see* Anidoxime.

2-(Diethylamino)propyl benzilate *see* Metamizil.

3-Diethylaminopropyl cinnamate *see* Cinnacaine.

N-**(3-Diethylaminopropyl)-2,2-diphenylacetamide** *see* Aprenal.

3-Diethylaminopropyl 2,2-diphenylacetate methyl methosulfate *see* Mesfenal.

3-Diethylaminopropyl 2-ethoxy-2,2-diphenylacetate *see* Etpenal.

10-(Diethylaminopropyl)phenothiazine *see* Prophenamine.

3-Diethylaminopropyl 2-phenylbicyclo-(2.2.1)heptane-2-carboxylate *see* Bornaprine.

N-**(3-Diethylaminopropyl)-*N*-phenyl-2-indanamine** *see* Aprindine.

2-Diethylamino-2',4',6'-trimethylacetanilide *see* Trimecaine.

5,5-Diethylbarbituric acid *see* Barbital.

DIETHYL BENZYL(2-DIETHYLAMINO-ETHYL)MALONATE (3,3-dicarbethoxy-

N,N-diethyl-4-phenyl-1-butylamine; 'spasmocalm', 'spazmokalm').

Diethylbromacetylurea *see* Carbromal.

DIETHYLCARBAMAZINE*** (*N,N*-diethyl-4-methyl-1-piperazinecarboxamide; 1-(diethylcarbamoyl)-4-methylpiperazine dihydrogen citrate; ditrazin; RP-3799; L-84).

Diethylcarbamothioic acid *S*-**(p-chlorophenyl)ester** *see* Benthiocarb.

Diethylcarbamothioic acid *S*-**ethyl ester** *see* Ethiolate.

6-Diethylcarbamoyl-3-cyclohexene-1-carboxylic acid compound with 4-(2-dimethylaminoethylamino)-6-methoxyquinoline *see* Quinetalate.

1-[1-(Diethylcarbamoyl)ethoxy]naphthalene *see* Napropamide.

[4-[(Diethylcarbamoyl)methoxy]-3-methoxyphenyl]acetic acid propyl ester acetate *see* Propanidid.

1-(Diethylcarbamoyl)-4-methylpiperazine *see* Diethylcarbamazine.

N-**(Diethylcarbamoylmethyl)-3,4,5-trimethoxybenzamide** *see* Trimeglamide.

1-(Diethylcarbamoyl)-1,2,3,4,5,6,7,8-octahydro-6,6-dimethyl-8-oxo-3-phenyl-2-naphthoic acid *see* Fenaftic acid.

O,O-**Diethyl** *O*-**1,4-diazinyl phosphorothioate** *see* Thionazin.

5,5-Diethyldihydro-2H-1,3-oxazine-2,4-(3H)-dione *see* Diethadione.

α,α'-**Diethyl-4,4'-dihydroxybibenzyl** *see* Hexestrol.

α,α'-**Diethyl-4,4'-dihydroxy-3,3'-dimethylbibenzyl** *see* Methestrol.

N,N-**Diethyl-9,10-dimethoxy-2-hydroxy-hexahydrobenzo(a)quinolizine-3-carboxamide acetate** *see* Benzquinamide.

Diethyl [(dimethoxyphosphinothioyl)-thio]succinate *see* Malathion.

α,α'-**Diethyl-4,4'-dimethoxystilbene** *see* Dianisylhexene.

*N*³,*N*³-**Diethyl-2,4-dinitro-6-(trifluoromethyl)-*m*-phenylenediamine** *see* Dinitramine.

Diethyl dithiobis(thionoformate) *see* Dixanthogen.

S,S-**Diethyl 1,3-dithioisophthalate** *see* Ditophal.

Diethyl 1,3-dithiolan-2-ylidenephosphoramidate *see* Phosfolan.

Diethyldixanthogen *see* Dixanthogen.

N,N'-**Diethylenebis(*N,N*-diethylenephosphoric diamide)** *see* Dipin.

N,N'-**Diethylenebis(*N,N*'-diethylenephosphorothioic diamide)** *see* Thiodipin.

Diethylenebis(phenyltrimethylammonium iodide) *see* Paramyon.

Diethylenediamine *see* Piperazine.

4,4'-(1,2-Diethylene)di-*o*-cresol *see* Methestrol.

4,4'-(1,2-Diethylene)diphenol *see* Hexestrol.

DIETHYLENE GLYCOL (3-oxapentane-1,5-diol; 2,2'-oxydiethanol; diglycol).

Diethylene glycol monoethyl ether *see* 2-(2-Ethoxyethoxy)ethanol.

DIETHYLENE GLYCOL MONO-

148

LAURATE (diglycol laurate; 'glaurin').
Diethylene imidoxide *see* Morpholine.
Diethylene oximide *see* Morpholine.
DIETHYLENETRIAMINE (2,2'-diamino-
diethylamine; 3-azapentane-1,5-diamine).
Diethylenetriaminopentaacetic acid *see*
Pentetic acid.
2,6-Diethylenimino-4-chloropyrimidine
see Ethymidine.
Diethyl ether *see* Ether.
O,O-Diethyl *S*-[2-(ethylsulfinyl)ethyl]
phosphorodithioate *see* Oxydisulfoton.
O,O-Diethyl *S*-[(ethylthio)ethyl] phos-
phorodithioate *see* Disulfoton.
O,O-Diethyl *O*-[2-(ethylthio)ethyl] phos-
phorothioate *see* Demeton-O.
O,O-Diethyl *S*-[2-(ethylthio)ethyl] phos-
phorothioate *see* Demeton-S.
Diethyl ethylthioglycol thiophosphate *see*
Demeton-O plus demeton-S.
O,O-Diethyl *S*-(ethylthiomethyl) phosphorodithioate *see* Phorate.
N,N-Diethylglycine *see* 2-Diethylamino-
acetic acid.
13,17-Diethylgon-4-en-17-ol-3-one *see*
Norboletone.
6,11-Diethyl-1,2,3,4,5,6-hexahydro-3-
methyl-2,6-methano-3-benzazocin-8-ol
see Etazocine.
DIETHYLHEXALDECYLMETHYLAM-
MONIUM METHOSULFATE (cetyl-
diethylmethylammonium methosulfate;
'laboran').
Diethyl(3-hydroxybutyl)methylammo-
nium iodide 5-bromo-2-furoate *see*
Fubrogonium iodide.
Diethyl[2-(2-hydroxyethoxy)ethyl]-
methylammonium iodide ester with
1-(α-carboxybenzyl)-1-methylpiperi-
dinium iodide *see* Piprocurarium.
Diethyl(2-hydroxyethyl)methylammo-
nium bromide benzilate *see* Methylbenactyzium bromide.
Diethyl(2-hydroxyethyl)methylammo-
nium bromide α-phenylcyclohexaneglycolate *see* Oxyphenonium bromide.
Diethyl(2-hydroxyethyl)methylammo-
nium bromide α-phenyl-2-thiophene-
glycolate *see* Oxitefonium bromide.
Diethyl(2-hydroxyethyl)methylammo-
nium bromide 9-xanthenecarboxylate
see Methantheline bromide.
Diethyl(2-hydroxyethyl)methylammo-
nium iodide dimethylpipecolate
methiodide *see* Dicolinium iodide.
Diethyl(2-hydroxyethyl)octylammonium
bromide dicyclopentylacetate *see*
Penoctonium bromide.
α,α'-Diethyl-4-hydroxy-4-methoxystilbene
see Mestilbol.
5,7-Diethyl-2'-hydroxy-2-methyl-6,7-
benzomorphan *see* Etazocine.
Diethyl *N*-hydroxynaphthylimido
phosphate *see* Naftalofos.
N,N-Diethyl-β-hydroxyphenethylamine
benzoate *see* Elucaine.
Diethyl(3-hydroxypropyl)methylammo-

nium iodide 2,4-diphenyl-1,3-cyclo-
butanedicarboxylate *see* Truxicurium
iodide.
Diethylhydroxypyrrolidinium bromide
benzilate *see* Benzilonium bromide.
N,N'-Diethylimidazole-4,5-dicarboxamide
see Etimizole.
N,N-Diethyl-*N'*-indan-2-yl-*N'*-phenyl-
1,3-propanediamine *see* Aprindine.
'Diethyline' *see* Diethoxypropanol.
O,O-Diethyl *S*-(isopropylcarbamoyl-
methyl) phosphorodithioate *see* Pro-
thoate.
Diethyl (2-isopropyl-6-methylpyrimidin-
4-yl) phosphate *see* Diazoxon.
O,O-Diethyl *O*-(2-isopropyl-6-methyl-
pyrimidin-4-yl) phosphorothioate *see*
Dimpylate.
N,N-Diethylleucinyl *p*-aminobenzoate *see*
Leucinocaine.
N,N-Diethyllysergamide *see* Lysergide.
N-(β,β-Diethyl-*m*-methoxyphenyl)-4-
hydroxybutyramide *see* Embutramide.
N,N-Diethyl-2-(3-methoxy-4-propyl-
phenoxy)acetamide *see* Propinal.
5,5-Diethyl-1-methylbarbituric acid *see*
Metharbital.
N,N-Diethyl-1-methyl-3,3-dithien-2-
ylallylamine *see* Diethylthiambutene.
Diethyl (4-methyl-1,3-dithiolan-2-ylidene)-
phosphoramidate *see* Mephosfolan.
O,O-Diethyl *S*-[2-[(1-methylethyl)amino]-
2-oxoethyl] phosphorodithioate *see*
Prothoate.
3,3-Diethyl-1-(6-methylisoergolen-8-yl)-
urea *see* Lisuride.
Diethyl [(6-methyl-2-(1-methylethyl)-
pyrimidin-4-yl] phosphate *see* Diazoxon.
O,O-Diethyl *O*-[6-methyl-2-(1-methyl-
ethyl)pyrimidin-4-yl] phosphorothioate
see Dimpylate.
Diethylmethyl[2-(α-methyl-α-5-norbor-
nen-2-ylbenzyloxy)ethyl]ammonium
bromide *see* Ciclonium bromide.
Diethylmethyl[2-[[4-[*p*-(phenylthio)-
phenyl]3H-1,5-benzodiazepin-2-yl]thio]-
ethyl]ammonium iodide *see* Tibezonium iodide.
N,N-Diethyl-4-methyl-1-piperazine-
carboxamide *see* Diethylcarbamazine.
DIETHYL 3-METHYLPYRAZOL-5-YL
PHOSPHATE (parasoxon; parazoxon;
G-24483).
O,O-Diethyl *O*-(4-methylsulfinylphenyl)
phosphorothioate *see* Fensulfothion.
3,3-Diethyl-5-methyltetrahydropyridine-
dione *see* Ethypicone.
N,N'-Diethyl-6-(methylthio)-1,3,5-tria-
zine-2,4-diamine *see* Simetryn.
4,4'-(1,2-Diethyl-3-methyltrimethylene)-
diphenol *see* Benzestrol.
Diethyl naphthyloximido phosphate
see Naftalofos.
N,N-Diethyl-2-(naphth-1-yloxy)propion-
amide *see* Napropamide.
N,N-Diethylnicotinamide *see* Nikethamide.
O,O-Diethyl *O*-(α-nitrilobenzylimino)

149

phosphorothioate *see* Phoxim.
Diethyl (*p*-**nitrophenyl**) **phosphate** *see* Paraoxon.
O,O-**Diethyl** *O*-(*p*-**nitrophenyl**) **phosphorothioate** *see* Parathion.
DIETHYLNITROSAMINE (nitrosodiethylamine; DENA).
N,N-**DIETHYL-5-NORBORNENE**-*trans*-**2,3-DICARBOXAMIDE** ('endomid').
Diethylolthioglycine *see* Bis(2-hydroxyethyl)glycine.
5,5-Diethyl-1,3-oxazine-2,4-dione *see* Dietroxine.
O,O-**Diethyl** *S*-(**4-oxobenzotriazin-3-yl-methyl**) **phosphorodithioate** *see* Azinphosethyl.
2,2-DIETHYL-4-PENTENOIC AMIDE (2-allyl-2,2-diethylacetamide; 'novonal').
5,5-Diethyl-1-phenylbarbituric acid *see* Phetharbital.
Diethyl [**1,2-phenylenebis**(**iminocarbonothioyl**)]**bis**(**carbamate**) *see* Thiophanate.
Diethyl **4,4'**-*o*-**phenylenebis**(**3-thioallophanate**) *see* Thiophanate.
O,O-**Diethyl** *O*-(**1-phenyl-1H-1,2,4-triazol-3-yl**) **phosphorothioate** *see* Phentriazophos.
Diethylpropion* *see* Amfepramone.
O,O-**Diethyl** *O*-**pyrazinyl phosphorothioate** *see* Thionazin.
3,3-Diethyl-2,4(1H,3H)-pyridinedione *see* Pyrithyldione.
DIETHYL PYROCARBONATE ($C_6H_{10}O_5$; piref).
O,O-**Diethyl** *O*-**quinoxalin-2-yl phosphorothioate** *see* Quinalphos.
N,N-**Diethylrifamycin B amide** *see* Rifamide.
trans-α,α'-**Diethyl-4,4'-stilbenediol** *see* Diethylstilbestrol.
DIETHYLSTILBESTROL*** (*trans*-α,α'-diethyl-4,4'-stibenediol; *trans*-3,4-bis(*p*-hydroxyphenyl)-3-hexene; sinestrol; stilbestrol; stilboestrol; DAES; NSC-3070).
Diethylstilbestrol di(2-furoate) *see* Furostilbestrol.
Diethylstilbestrol dimethyl ether *see* Dianisylhexene.
Diethylstilbestrol dipalmitate *see* Stilpalmitate.
Diethylstilbestrol diphosphate *see* Fosfestrol.
Diethylstilbestrol furoate *see* Furostilbestrol.
Diethylstilbestrol monomethyl ether *see* Mestilbol.
p-**Diethylsulfamoylbenzoic acid** *see* Etebenecid.
5,5-Diethyltetrahydro-1,3-oxazine-2,4-dione *see* Diethadione.
O,O-**Diethyl** *O*-(**7,8,9,10-tetrahydro-6-oxo-6H-dibenzo(b,d)pyran-3-yl phosphorothioate** *see* Coumithoate.
1,8-Diethyl-1,3,4,9-tetrahydropyrano-(3,4-b)indole-1-acetic acid *see* Etodolic acid.

3,3-Diethyl-1,2,3,4-tetrahydropyridine-2,4-dione *see* Pyrithyldione.
O,O-**Diethyl** *O*-(**3,4-tetramethylene-coumarin-7-yl**) **phosphorothioate** *see* Coumithoate.
Diethylthiadicarbocyanine iodide *see* Dithiazanine.
DIETHYLTHIAMBUTENE*** (3-diethylamino-1,1-dithien-2-ylbut-1-ene; *N,N*-diethyl-1-methyl-3,3-dithien-2-ylallylamine; BW-191C49; 'themalon', 'theuralon').
5,5-Diethyl-2-thiobarbituric acid *see* Thiobarbital.
O,S-**DIETHYL THIOSULFITE** (ethios).
DIETHYLTOLUAMIDE* *N,N*-diethyl-*m*-toluamide; *m*-toluic acid diethylamide; *m*-delphene; *m*-DET; *N,N*-diethyl-3-methylbenzamide; deet; DET; DETA; BAS-3170F; 'autan', 'deltamide', 'metadelphene', 'off', 'tabard').
N^1-(**4,6-Diethyl-***s***-triazin-2-yl**)**sulfanilamide** *see* Sulfasymazine.
O,O-**Diethyl** *O*-(**3,5,6-trichloropyrid-2-yl**) **phosphorothioate** *see* Chlorpyrifos.
N^4,N^4-**Diethyl-**α,α,α-**trifluoro-3,5-dinitro-toluene-2,4-diamine** *see* Dinitramine.
9-(3,3-Diethylureido)-4,6,6a,7,8,9-hexahydro-7-methylindolo(4,3-f,g)quinoline *see* Lisuride.
N,N-**DIETHYLVALERAMIDE** (valeric acid diethylamide; 'valyl', 'xalyl').
N,N-**Diethylvanillamide** *see* Etamivan.
Diethylxanthogen *see* Dixanthogen.
Diethyxime (tr) *see* Dietixim.
DIETIFEN*** (4-(2-diethylaminoethoxy)-phenyl phenethyl ketone; 4'-(2-diethylaminoethoxy)-3-phenylpropiophenone).
DIETIXIM (tr) (*p*-bromobenzothiohydroxamic acid *S*-(2-diethylaminoethyl) ester; diethyxime).
'**Dietrol**' *see* Phendimetrazine.
Dietroxine *see* Diethadione.
'**Difacil**' *see* Adiphenine.
Difamizole *see* Difenamizole.
2-Difarnesyl-3-methyl-1,4-naphthoquinone *see* Farnoquinone.
Difasin (tr) *see* 10-(Diethylaminoacetyl)-phenothiazine *and* Promethazine.
Difazin (tr) *see* 10-(Dimethylaminoacetyl)-phenothiazine *and* Promethazine.
'**Difco-M**' *see* Phytohemagglutinin.
DIFEBARBAMATE*** (1,3-bis(3-butoxy-2-hydroxypropyl)phenobarbital dicarbamate ester).
DIFEMERINE*** (2-dimethylamino-2-methylpropyl benzilate ester).
DIFENAMIZOLE*** (5-(2-dimethylamino-propionamido)-1,3-diphenylpyrazole; 2-dimethylamino-*N*-(1,3-diphenylpyrazol-5-yl)propionamide; difamizole; diphenamizole; AP-14; 'pasalin').
Difenatsin (tr) *see* Diphenadione.
DIFENCLOXAZINE*** (4-[2-(*p*-chloro-α-phenylbenzyloxy)ethyl]morpholine; 4-[2-(*p*-chlorobenzhydryloxy)ethyl]morpholine; 'olympax').
DIFENIDOL** (α,α-diphenyl-1-piperidine-

butanol; 1,1-diphenyl-4-piperid-1-yl-1-
butanol; diphenidol; SK&F-478; 'vontrol').
Difenin (tr) *see* Phenytoin.
Difenoxilic acid *see* Difenoxin.
DIFENOXIMIDE*** (*N*-[[1-(3-cyano-3,3-
diphenylpropyl)-4-phenylisonipecotoyl]-
oxy]succinimide; 4-[(2,5-dioxopyrrolidin-
1-yloxy)carbonyl]-α,α,4-triphenyl-1-
piperidinebutanenitrile; SC-26100;
difenoximide hydrochloride;
DIFENOXIN*** (1-(3-cyano-3,3-diphenyl-
propyl)-4-phenylisonipecotic acid; 1-(3-
cyano-3,3-diphenylpropyl)-4-phenylpiperi-
dine-4-carboxylic acid; difenoxilic acid;
R-15403).
Difenoxin butyl ester *see* Butoxylate.
Difenoxin ethyl ester *see* Diphenoxylate.
Difenoxin 2-phenoxyethyl ester *see*
Fetoxilate.
Difenson *see* Chlorfenson.
Difesyl (tr) *see* Difezil.
DIFETARSONE*** (1,2-bis(*p*-arsonophenyl-
amino)ethane; *N*,*N*′-bis(*p*-arsonophenyl-
ethylenediamine; *N*,*N*′-ethylenediarsanilic
acid; difetarsone sodium; diphetarsone;
RP-47631; 'amebarsin', 'bemarsal',
'rodameb').
DIFEZIL (tr) ((3-acetyl-5-chloro-2-hydroxy-
benzyl)dimethyl(2-phenoxyethyl)ammon-
ium 3-hydroxy-2-naphthoate; difesyl;
diphesyl).
DIFLORASONE** (6α,9-difluoro-11β,17,21-
trihydroxy-16β-methylpregna-1,4-diene-
3,20-dione; 6α,9-difluoro-16β-methylpreg-
na-1,4-diene-11β,17,21-triol-3,20-dione;
6α,9-difluoro-16β-methylprednisolone).
DIFLORASONE DIACETATE (U-34865).
DIFLUANAZINE*** (1-(2-anilinoethyl)-4-
[4,4-bis(*p*-fluorophenyl)butyl]piperazine;
difluanine hydrochloride; McN-JR-7242-
11).
Difluanine* *see* Difluanazine.
DIFLUCORTOLONE*** (6α,9-difluoro-11β,
21-dihydroxy-16α-methylpregna-1,4-diene-
3,20-dione; 6α,9-difluoro-16α-methyl-
pregna-1,4-diene-11β,21-diol-3,20-dione;
6α,9-difluoro-16α-methyl-1-dehydrocorti-
costerone).
DIFLUCORTOLONE PIVALATE* (diflucortolone 21-pivalate; diflucortolone
2,2-dimethylpropionate).
DIFLUMIDONE*** (3′-benzoyl-1,1-difluoro-
methanesulfonanilide).
DIFLUMIDONE SODIUM* (BA-4164-8;
MBR-4164-8).
DIFLUNISAL*** (2′4′-difluoro-4-hydroxy-
3-biphenylcarboxylic acid; 5-(2,4-difluoro-
phenyl)salicylic acid).
2-(4,4′-Difluorobenzhydryloxy)ethylamine
see Flunamine.
**6α,9-Difluoro-11β,21-dihydroxy-16α-
methylpregna-1,4-diene-3,20-dione** *see*
Diflucortolone.
1,1-DIFLUOROETHANE (fluorocarbon
152a; FC-152a; 'genetron-152A').
**2′,4′-Difluoro-4-hydroxy-3-biphenyl-
carboxylic acid** *see* Diflunisal.

6α,9α-Difluoro-16α-hydroxyprednisolone
see Fluocinolone.
**6α,9-Difluoro-16α-methyl-1-dehydro-
corticosterone** *see* Diflucortolone.
6α,9α-Difluoro-16α-methylprednisolone
see Flumetasone.
6α,9-Difluoro-16β-methylprednisolone
see Diflorasone.
**6α,9-Difluoro-16α-methylpregna-1,4-diene-
11β,21-diol-3,20-dione** *see* Diflucortolone.
5-(2,4-Difluorophenyl)salicylic acid *see*
Diflunisal.
**6α,9α-Difluoro-1,4-pregnadiene-11β,16α,
17α,21-tetrol-3,20-dione** *see* Fluocinolone.
**6α,9α-Difluoro-16α-methylpregna-1,4-
diene-11β,17α,21-triol-3,20-dione** *see*
Flumetasone.
**6α,9-Difluoro-16β-methylpregna-1,4-diene-
11β,17,21-triol-3,20-dione** *see* Diflorasone.
**6α,9-Difluoroprednisolone 21-acetate 17-
butyrate** *see* Difluprednate.
Difluorotetrachloroethane *see* 1,1,2,2-
Tetrachloro-1,2-difluoroethane.
**6α,9α-Difluoro-11β,16α,17α,21-tetrahydr-
oxypregna-1,4-diene-3,20-dione** *see*
Fluocinolone.
**6α,9α-Difluoro-11β,17α,21-trihydroxy-16α-
methylpregna-1,4-diene-3,20-dione** *see*
Flumetasone.
**6α,9-Difluoro-11β,17,21-trihydroxy-16β-
methylpregna-1,4-diene-3,20-dione** *see*
Diflorasone.
**6α,9-Difluoro-11β,17,21-trihydroxypregna-
1,4-diene-3,20-dione 21-acetate 17-
butyrate** *see* Difluprednate.
DIFLUPREDNATE*** (6α,9-difluoro-11β,17,
21-trihydroxypregna-1,4-diene-3,20-dione
21-acetate 17-butyrate; 6α,9-difluoropred-
nisolone 21-acetate 17-butyrate).
'Diflupyl' *see* Dyflos.
Diflurophate* *see* Dyflos.
DIFO *see* Dimefox.
'Difolatan' *see* Captafol.
'Diforene' *see* Deanol acetamidobenzoate.
DIFTALONE** (phthalazino(2,3-b)phthala-
zine-5,12(7H,14H)-dione; L-5418; 'ala-
dione').
'Digacin' *see* Digoxin.
Digenic acid *see* Kainic acid.
'Digenin' *see* Kainic acid.
'Digilanid' *see* Lanatosides.
'Digilong' *see* Digitoxin.
'Digimed' *see* Lanatosides.
'Digimerck' *see* Digitoxin.
'Diginorgin' *see* Digitalin.
'Digipan' *see* Digitoxin.
'Digisidin' *see* Digitoxin.
DIGITALIN (mixture of amorphous glycosi-
des from digitalis; digitalinum verum;
'diginorgin').
Digitalin crystalline *see* Digitoxin.
'Digitaline' *see* Digitoxin.
Ψ-Digitonin *see under* Gitalin.
DIGITOXIGENIN HEMISUCCINATE
(AY-17611).
DIGITOXIN*** (3β,14-dihydroxy-5β-card-
20(22)-enolide 3-tridigitoxoside; crystalline

digitalin; digitoxoside; 'cardigin', 'crysto-digin', 'digimerck', 'digilong', 'digipan', 'digisidin', 'digitaline Nativelle', 'ditaven', 'foxalin', 'glucodigin', 'purodigin', 'purpurid', 'unidigin').
Ψ-Digitoxin *see* Gitoxin.
Digitoxoside *see* Digitoxin.
'Diglanex' *see* Lanatosides.
DIGLYCOCOLL HYDRIODIDE IODINE* ('bursoline').
Diglycol *see* Diethylene glycol.
DIGLYCOLIC ACID (2,2'-oxydiacetic acid).
Diglycolic acid bis(3-carboxy-2,4,6-tri-iodoanilide) *see* Ioglycamic acid.
Diglycol laurate *see* Diethyleneglycol mono-laurate.
N,N'-Diglycoloyldi(3-carboxy-2,4,6-triiodoaniline) *see* Ioglycamic acid.
3,3'-(Diglycoloyldiimino)bis(2,4,6-triiodobenzoic acid) *see* Ioglycamic acid.
DIGOXIN*** (3β,12,14-trihydroxy-5β-card-20(22)-enolide 3-tridigitoxoside; 12-hydroxydigitoxin; 'digacin', 'lanicor', 'lanoxin').
'Dignoquine' *see* Chlorquinaldol with halquinols.
Diguanide *see* Biguanide.
Diguanidiotetrahydroxycyclohexane *see* Streptidine.
N-(4-Diguanidopiperazin-1-ylmethyl)-tetracycline *see* Guamecycline.
Diguanyl *see* Proguanil.
Diguanyldiazoaminobenzene *see* Diminazene.
1,3-Diguanyl-4-lauryloxybenzene *see* Lauroguadine.
Dihexiverine *see* Dihexyverine.
Dihexyl sodium sulfosuccinate *see* Sodium dihexyl sulfosuccinate.
DIHEXYVERINE*** (2-(1-piperidyl)ethyl ester of 1-cyclohexylcyclohexanecarboxylic acid; 2-piperid-1-ylethyl bicyclohexyl-1-carboxylate; dihexiverine; JL-1078; 'metaspas', 'spasmodex').
'Dihydergot' *see* Dihydroergotamine mesilate.
2,4-Dihydracryloylpiperazine dimesilate *see* Piposulfan.
'Dihydral' *see* Dihydrotachysterol.
DIHYDRALAZINE*** (1,4-dihydrazino-phthalazine; C-7441; 'nepresol').
DIHYDRALAZINE DIMESILATE (dihydralazine bis(methanesulfonate); dihydralazine dimesylate; 'depressan').
Dihydrazinophthalazine *see* Dihydralazine.
'Dihydrin' *see* Dihydrocodeine.
Dihydroampicillin *see* Epicillin.
Dihydrobaikiaine *see* Pipecolic acid.
4-(9,10-Dihydro-4H-benzo(4,5)cyclohepta-(1,2-b)thien-4-ylidene)-1-methyl-piperidine *see* Pizotifen.
3,4-Dihydro-1,2H-benzopyran *see* Chroman.
3,4-Dihydro-2,1H-benzopyran *see* Iso-chroman.
3,4-Dihydro-1,2H-benzothiopyran *see* Thiochroman.
3,4-Dihydro-2H-1,3-benzoxazine-2,4-dione

see Carsalam.
Dihydrobenzthiazide *see* Hydrobentizide.
Dihydrochlorothiazide *see* Hydrochloro-thiazide.
DIHYDROCODEINE*** (4,5-epoxy-6-hydroxy-3-methoxy-N-methylmorphinan; 5,6,7,7a,8,9-hexahydro-3-methoxy-10-methyl-4aH-8,9c-iminoethanophenanthro-(4,5-bcd)furan-5-ol; 7,8-dihydrocodeine; hydrocodeine; dihydrocodeine bitartrate or phosphate; DF-118; 'codhydrin', 'cohydrin', 'DH-codeine', 'dehacodin', 'didrate', 'dihydrin', 'dihydroneopine', 'hydrocodin', 'nadeine', 'novicodin', 'paracodin', 'parzone', 'rapacodin').
Dihydrocodeine 6-nicotinate *see* Nicodi-codine.
Dihydrocodeinone *see* Hydrocodone.
Dihydrocodeinone enol acetate *see* Thebacon.
Dihydrocupreine *see* Hydrocupreine.
Dihydrodesoxymorphine *see* Desomorphine.
9,10-Dihydro(8a,10a)diazoniaphenan-threne dibromide *see* Diquat.
10,11-DIHYDRO-5H-DIBENZ(b,f)-AZEPINE (2,2'-iminobibenzyl; iminodi-benzyl).
3-(10,11-Dihydro-5H-dibenz(b,f)azepin-5-yl)quinuclidine *see* Quinupramine.
10,11-DIHYDRO-5H-DIBENZO(a,d)-CYCLOHEPTENE (dibenzo(a,d)cyclo-hepta-1,4-diene).
10,11-Dihydro-5H-dibenzo(a,d)cyclo-hepten-5-one O-(2-dimethylamino-ethyl)oxime *see* Noxiptiline.
3-(10,11-Dihydro-5H-dibenzo(a,d)cyclo-hepten-5-ylidene)-1-dimethylamino-2-propanone *see* Cotriptyline.
3-(10,11-Dihydro-5H-dibenzo(a,d)cyclo-hepten-5-ylidene)-1-ethyl-2-methyl-pyrrolidine *see* Piroheptine.
3-(10,11-Dihydro-5H-dibenzo(a,d)cyclo-hepten-5-yl)-2-methylpropyldiethyl-amine *see* Butriptyline.
2-(10,11-Dihydro-5H-dibenzo(a,d)cyclo-hepten-5-yloxy)-N,N-dimethylacet-amide *see* Oxitriptyline.
10,11-DIHYDRODIBENZO(b,f)(1,4)-THIAZEPINE (1-aza-4-thia-2,3:5,6-diben-zocycloheptadiene; homophenothiazine).
Dihydrodiethylstilbestrol *see* Hexestrol.
3α,4-Dihydro-3,4-dihydroxyspiro(benzo-furan-2(3H),2'-oxirane)-6-methanol 6-acetate 3,4-diisovalerate *see* Valtrate.
1,7a-Dihydro-1,6-dihydroxyspiro(cyclo-penta(c)pyran-7(6H),2'-oxirane)-4-methanol 4-acetate 1,6-diisovalerate *see* Valtrate.
1,7a-Dihydro-1,6-dihydroxyspiro-(cyclopenta(c)pyran-7(6H),2'-oxirane)-4-methanol 4-acetate 1(or 6)-iso-valerate 6(or 1)-(3-hydroxy-3-methyl-butyrate)-acetate *see* Acevaltrate.
8,9-Dihydro-4,11-dimethoxy-9-methylene-5-oxospiro[5H-furo(3',2':6,7)(1)benzo-pyrano(3,2-c)pyridine-7(6H),1'-piperi-dinium] chloride *see* Azaspirium chloride.

2,3-Dihydro-2,2-dimethylbenzofuran-7-yl methylcarbamate *see* Carbofuran.
10,11-Dihydro-*N*,*N*-dimethyl-5H-dibenzo-(a,d)cycloheptene-△5,γ-propylamine *see* Amitriptyline.
9,10-Dihydro-10,10-dimethyl-9-(3-dimethylaminopropylidene)anthracene *see* Melitracen.
1,4-Dihydro-2,6-dimethyl-4-(2-nitrophenyl)pyridine-3,5-dicarboxylic acid dimethyl ester *see* Nifedipine.
2,3-Dihydro-4,6-dimethylpyridazin-3-one *see* Cetohexazine.
10,11-Dihydro-*N*,*N*-dimethylspiro(5H-dibenzo(a,d)cycloheptene-5,2′-(1,3)-dioxolane)-4′-methylamine *see* Ciheptolane.
Dihydro-*m*-dioxin *see* 1,3-Dioxane.
S-[(1,3-Dihydro-1,3-dioxo-2H-isoindol-2-yl)methyl] *O,O*-dimethyl phosphorodithioate *see* Phosmet.
5,10-Dihydro-5,10-dioxonaphtho(2,3-b)-1,4-dithiin-2,3-dicarbonitrile *see* Dithianon.
6,7-Dihydrodipyrido[1,2-a: 2′,1′-c]-pyrazinediium dibromide *see* Diquat.
Dihydro-E-73 *see* Acetoxydihydrocycloheximide.
DIHYDROERGOCORNINE (DHO-180).
DIHYDROERGOCRISTINE (DCS-90; 'ergotren').
See also Raubasine with dihydroergocristine mesilate; Reserpine with clopamide and dihydroergocristine.
DIHYDROERGOCRYPTINE (DHK-135).
DIHYDROERGOTAMINE MESILATE*** (dihydroergotamine methanesulfonate; DHE-45; 'dihydergot', 'orstanon').
DIHYDROERGOTOXINE (mixture of dihydroergocornine, dihydroergocristine and dihydroergocryptine as methanesulfonates; dihydroergotoxine mesilate; redergam; CCK-179; 'hydergin', 'optamine').
DIHYDROERGOTOXINE WITH LEUCINOCAINE MESILATE ('bivelin').
DIHYDROERGOTOXINE WITH THIORIDAZINE ('visergil').
DIHYDROERGOTOXINE ESILATE WITH PAPAVERINE ('progeril', 'progeryl').
1-(9,10-Dihydro-9,10-ethanoanthryl)-4-methylpiperazine *see* Trazitiline.
Dihydroethaverine *see* Drotaverine.
Dihydroflumethiazide *see* Hydroflumethiazide.
Dihydrofolliculin *see* Estradiol.
Dihydrofucosterol *see* Sitosterol.
Dihydroheroin *see* Diacetyldihydromorphine.
4-(9,10-Dihydro-9-hydroxyanthr-10-ylidene)-1-methylpiperidine *see* Danitracen.
Dihydrohydroxycodeinone *see* Oxycodone.
1,2-Dihydro-1-hydroxyimino-4-(2-dimethylaminoethoxy)phthalazine *see* Taloximine.
5,6-Dihydro-1-(2-hydroxy-3-isopropylaminopropoxy)naphthalene *see* Idropranolol.

7,8-Dihydro-14-hydroxy-*N*-(3-methyl-2-butenyl)normorphinone *see* Nalmexone.
7,8-Dihydro-1-hydroxymorphine *see* Hydromorphinol.
6,7-Dihydro-17-hydroxy-3-oxo-3′H-cyclopropa(6,7)-17α-pregna-4,6-diene-21-carboxylic acid potassium salt *see* Prorenoate potassium.
10,11-Dihydro-10-[4-(3-hydroxypropyl)-piperazin-1-yl]-8-(methylthio)dibenzo-(b,f)thiepin *see* Oxyprothepine.
Dihydro-14-hydroxy-6β-thebainol 4-methyl ether *see* Oxymethebanol.
2,3-Dihydroindene *see* Indan.
N-(2,3-Dihydro-1H-inden-2-yl)-*N′*,*N′*-diethyl-*N*-phenyl-1,3-propanediamine *see* Aprindine.
1,3-Dihydroisobenzofuran *see* Phthalan.
3,4-Dihydro-3(1H)-isoquinolinecarboxamidine *see* Debrisoquin.
DIHYDROLYSERGAMINE (8β-aminomethyl-6-methyl-10a-ergoline).
'Dihydromenformon' *see* Estradiol.
5,6-Dihydro-4-methoxy-6-(3,4-methylenedioxystyryl)-2-pyrone *see* Methysticin.
1,3-Dihydro-1-(methoxymethyl)-7-nitro-5-phenyl-2H-1,4-benzodiazepin-2-one *see* Motrazepam.
4,9-Dihydro-7-methoxy-1-methyl(3H)-pyrido(3,4b)indole *see* Harmaline.
3,4-Dihydro-1-(*p*-methoxyphenoxymethyl)isoquinoline *see* Memotine.
1-[2-[*p*-(3,4-Dihydro-6-methoxy-2-phenyl-naphth-1-yl)phenoxy]ethyl]pyrrolidine *see* Nafoxidine.
5,6-Dihydro-4-methoxy-6-styryl-2-pyrone *see* Kavain.
3,12-Dihydro-6-methoxy-3,3,12-trimethyl-7H-pyrano(2,3-c)acridin-7-one *see* Acronine.
5,6-Dihydro-5-(3-methylaminopropyl)-11H-dibenz(b,e)azepine *see* Mezepine.
10,11-Dihydro-5-(3-methylaminopropyl)-5H-dibenz(b,f)azepine *see* Desipramine.
Dihydro-6-(3-methylaminopropylidene)-dibenzo(a,e)cyclopropa(c)cycloheptene *see* Octriptyline.
Dihydro-*N*-methyldibenzo(a,e)cyclopropa(c)cyclohepten-△6(1H),γ-propyl-amine *see* Octriptyline.
N-[3-(6,11-Dihydro-6-methyl-5,5-dioxido-dibenzo(1,2,5)thiadiazepin-11-yl)-propyl]-*N*,α-dimethylphenethylamine *see* Pretiadil.
N-[3-(6,11-Dihydro-6-methyl-5,5-dioxi-dodibenzo(1,2,5-thiadiazepin-11-yl)-propyl]-*N*-methylamphetamine *see* Pretiadil.
5,6-Dihydro-1-methyl-5,6-dioxo-3-indolinesulfonic acid 5-semicarbazone sodium salt *see* Carbazochrome sodium sulfonate.
(2,5-Dihydro-5-methyl-2-furan)glycine *see* Furanomycin.
5,6-Dihydro-1-methylindoxyl *see* Adrenolutin.
10,11-Dihydro-5-methyl-10-(methyl-

amino)-5H-dibenz(b,f)azepine *see* Metapramine.

6,11-Dihydro-6-methyl-11[3-[methyl(α-methylphenethyl)amino]propyl]dibenzo(1,2,5)iadiazepine 5,5-dioxide *see* Pretiacil.

7,8-Dihydro-O^3-methyl-O^6-nicotinoylmorphine *see* Nicodicodine.

1,3-Dihydro-1-methyl-7-nitro-5-phenyl-2H-1,4-benzodiazepin-2-one *see* Nimetazepam.

3,6-Dihydro-1(2H)-(2-(3-methyl-2-oxo-oxazolidin-5-yl)ethyl)-4-phenylpyridine *see* Fenpipalone.

5,6-Dihydro-2-methyl-N-phenyl-1,4-oxathiin-3-carboxamide *see* Carboxin.

5,11-Dihydro-11-[(4-methylpiperazin-1-yl)acetyl]-6H-pyrido(2,3-b)(1,4)benzodiazepin-2-one *see* Pirenzepine.

10,11-Dihydro-10-(4-methylpiperazin-1-yl)benzo(b,f)thiepin *see* Perathiepine.

9,10-Dihydro-9-(4-methylpiperazin-1-yl)-9,10-ethanoanthracene *see* Trazitiline.

10,11-Dihydro-10-(4-methylpiperazin-1-yl)-8-(methylthio)dibenzo(b,f)thiepin *see* Metitepine.

9,10-Dihydro-10-(1-methylpiperid-4-ylidene)-9-anthrol *see* Danitracen.

6,11-Dihydro-11-(1-methylpiperid-4-ylidene)-5H-benzo(5,6)cyclohepta(1,2-b)pyridine *see* Azatadine.

9,10-Dihydro-4-(1-methylpiperid-4-ylidene)-4H-benzo(4,5)cyclohepta(1,2-b)-thiophene *see* Pizotifen.

4,9-Dihydro-4-(1-methylpiperid-4-ylidene)-10H-benzo(4,5)cyclohepta-(1,2-b)thiophen-10-one *see* Ketotifen.

6,11-Dihydro-11-(1-methylpiperid-4-ylidene)dibenzo(b,e)thiepin *see* Perithiadene.

1-[2-(3,6-Dihydro-4-methyl-1(2H)-pyridyl)ethyl]guanidine *see* Guanacline.

4,5α-Dihydro-2α-methyltestosterone *see* Drostanolone.

1-[10,11-Dihydro-8-(methylthio)dibenzo-(b,f)thiepin-10-yl]-4-methylpiperazine *see* Metitepine.

6,11-Dihydro-6-methyl-11-(1αH,5αH-tropan-3α-yloxy)dibenzo(c,f)(1,2)-thiazepine *see* Zepastine.

Dihydromorphine *see* Paramorphan.
Dihydromorphinone *see* Hydromorphone.
2,3-Dihydro-1-(morpholinoacety)-3-phenyl-4(1H)-quinazolinone *see* Moquizone.

1-(5,6-Dihydronaphth-2-yloxy)-3-iso-propylamino-2-propanol *see* Idropranolol.
'Dihydroneopine' *see* Dihydrocodeine.
Dihydronorguaiaretic acid *see* Nordihydroguaiaretic acid.
Dihydronovobiocin tetracycline compound *see* Tetracycline dihydronovobiocin sodium phytate.

1,3-Dihydro-3-oxo-1-isobenzofuranyl 6-[(aminophenylacetyl)amino]-penicillanate *see* Talampicillin.

1-[[(5,11-Dihydro-6-oxo-6H-pyrido(2,3-b)-(1,4)benzodiazepin-11-yl)carbonyl]-methyl]-4-methylpiperazine *see* Pirenzepine.

5,11-Dihydro-6-oxo-6H-pyrido(2,3-b)(1,4)-benzodiazepin-11-yl 4-methylpiperazin-1-ylmethyl ketone *see* Pirenzepine.

3,4-Dihydro-3-pentyl-6-trifluoromethyl-2H-1,2,4-benzothiadiazine-7-sulfonamide 1,1-dioxide *see* Penflutizide.
'Dihydroperparin' *see* Drotaverine.

1,3-Dihydro-1-(1-(2-phenoxyethyl)-piperid-4-yl)-2H-benzimidazol-2-one *see* Oxiperomide.

5-(4,5-Dihydro-2-phenyl-3H-benz(e)indol-3-yl)salicylic acid *see* Fendosal.

3,4-Dihydro-2-phenyl-2H-1-benzopyran *see* Flavan.

5,6-Dihydro-6-phenylimidazo(2,1-b)-thiazole *see* Antafenite.

5-[2-(3,6-Dihydro-4-phenyl-1(2H)-pyridyl)-ethyl]-3-methyl-2-oxazolidinone *see* Fenpipalone.

2,3-Dihydro-1,4-phthalazinedione *see* Phthalhydrazide.

Dihydropropranolol *see* Idropranolol.
Dihydroprothiadene *see* Hydrothiadene.
Dihydropyridinium *see* Pyrithyldione.
2,3-Dihydroquercetin *see* Taxifolin.
10,11-Dihydro-5-quinuclidin-3-yl-5H-dibenz(b,f)azepine *see* Quinupramine.
2,3-Dihydrospiro(naphthalene-1(4H),3'-piperidine)-2',4,6'-trione *see* Alonimid.
Dihydrostigmasterol *see* Sitosterol.
Dihydrostilbestrol *see* Hexestrol.
DIHYDROSTREPTOMYCIN* (2,4-diguanidino-3,5,6-trihydroxycyclohexyl-5-deoxy-2-O-(2-deoxy-2-methylamino-α-L-glucopyranosyl)-3-hydroxymethyl-β-L-*lyxo*-pentano furanoside).
See also Streptoduocin.
DIHYDROSTREPTOMYCIN AMINO-SALICYLATE (dihydrostreptomycin 4-aminosalicylate salt; dihydrostreptomycin PAS salt; 'pasomycin').
DIHYDROSTREPTOMYCIN PANTO-THENATE ('didropantine', 'didrothenate', 'enterastrept').
DIHYDROSTREPTOMYCIN WITH PROCAINE PENICILLIN ('mixtencillin').
DIHYDROSTREPTOMYCIN TRISNICO-TINOYLHYDRAZONE PYRUVATE ('streptotibine').
DIHYDROTACHYSTEROL* (9,10-*seco*-ergosta-5,7,22-trien-3β-ol; 24-methyl-9,10-*seco*-cholesta-5,7,22-trien-3β-ol; dichystrol; 'AT 10', 'antitanil', 'calcamine', 'dihydral', 'dygratal', 'hytacherol', 'hytakerol', 'manipal', 'parterol', 'tachystin', 'tachystol').
Dihydrotestosterone *see* Androstanolone.
5α-Dihydrotestosterone *see* Androstanolone.
Dihydrotheelin *see* Estradiol.
5,6-Dihydro-6-thien-2-ylimidazo(2,1-b)-thiazole *see* Antenite.
3,4-Dihydro-6-trifluoromethyl-2H-1,2,4-benzothiadiazine 1,1-dioxide *see* Hydroflumethiazide.

10,11-Dihydro-N,N,β-trimethyl-5H-dibenzo(a,d)cycloheptene-5-propylamine *see* Butryptyline.

1,3-Dihydro-$N,3,3$-trimethyl-1-phenylbenzo(c)thiophene-1-propylamine *see* Talsupram.

Dihydrovitamin K₁ *see* Phytonadiol.

Dihydroxyacetaldehyde *see* Glyoxal.

DIHYDROXYACETONE (1,3-dihydroxy-2-propanone).

Dihydroxyacetophenone(s) *see* Quinacetophenone; Resacetophenone.

Dihydroxy aluminium aminoacetate* *see* Aluminium glycinate.

($3\alpha,17\beta$-Dihydroxy-5α-androstan-$2\beta,16\beta$-ylene)bis(1-methylpiperidinium bromide) 3-acetate *see* Dacuronium bromide.

($3\alpha,17\beta$-Dihydroxy-5α-androstan-$2\beta,16\beta$-ylene)bis(1-methylpiperidinium bromide) 3,17-diacetate *see* Pancuronium bromide.

1,4-Dihydroxyanthraquinone *see* Quinizarine.

1,8-Dihydroxyanthraquinone *see* Dantron.

4,5-Dihydroxyanthraquinone-2-carboxylic acid *see* Rhein.

10,11-Dihydroxyaporphine *see* Apomorphine.

m-Dihydroxybenzene *see* Resorcinol.

o-Dihydroxybenzene *see* Pyrocatechol.

p-Dihydroxybenzene *see* Hydroquinone.

2,5-Dihydroxybenzenesulfonic acid calcium salt *see* Calcium dobesilate.

2,5-Dihydroxybenzenesulfonic acid diethylamine salt *see* Etamsylate.

2,2'-Dihydroxybenzil *see* Salicil.

Dihydroxybenzoic acids *see* Gentisic acid; Protocatechuic acid; Pyrocatechuic acid; Resorcylic acids.

2,3-Dihydroxybenzoic acid diacetate *see* Dipyrocetyl.

2-(3,4-Dihydroxybenzyl)-2-hydrazinopropionic acid *see* Carbidopa.

1-(3,4-Dihydroxybenzyl)-6,7-isoquinolinediol *see* Papaveroline.

5,5'-Dihydroxy-5,5'-bibarbituric acid *see* Alloxantin.

$3\beta,14\beta$-Dihydroxybufa-4,20,22-trienolide 3-rhamnoglucoside *see* Scillarenin A.

3,14-Dihydroxybufa-4,20,22-trienolide 3-rhamnoside *see* Proscillaridin.

D-DIHYDROXYBUSULFAN (D-threityl 1,4-dimesilate; D-threitol 1,4-dimethanesulfonate; D-*threo*-1,2,3,4-butanetetrol 1,4-bis(methanesulfonate) ester; NSC-39068).

L-Dihydroxybusulfan *see* Treosulfan.

$3\beta,14\beta$-Dihydroxy-5β-card-20(22)-enolide 3-(4'''-acetyltridigitoxoside) *see* Acetyldigitoxin.

$3\beta,14\beta$-Dihydroxy-5β-card-20(22)-enolide 3-tridigitoxoside *see* Digitoxin.

3,6-Dihydroxycholanic acid *see* Hyodeoxycholic acid.

3,7-Dihydroxycholanic acid *see* Chenodeoxycholic acid.

3,12-Dihydroxycholanic acid *see* Deoxycholic acid.

3,4-Dihydroxycinnamic acid 1-carboxy-4,5-dihydroxy-1,3-cyclohexylene ester *see* Cynarine.

5,6-Dihydroxycoumarin *see* Citropten.

6,7-Dihydroxycoumarin *see* Esculetin.

6,7-Dihydroxycoumarin-7-ylmethanesulfonic acid, esters and salts *see* Cromesilate(s).

6,7-Dihydroxy-1-(3,4-dihydroxybenzyl)-isoquinoline *see* Papaveroline.

2,9-Dihydroxy-1,10-dimethoxy-6-methyl-4H-dibenzo(de,g)quinoline *see* Boldine.

$6\beta,14$-Dihydroxy-3,4-dimethoxy-17-methylmorphinan *see* Drotebanol.

D-(+)-4-(2,4-Dihydroxy-3,3-dimethylbutyramido)butyric acid *see* Hopantenic acid.

2,4-Dihydroxy-3,3-dimethylbutyric acid *see* Pantoic acid.

N-(2,4-Dihydroxy-3,3-dimethylbutyryl)-β-alanine *see* Pantothenic acid.

2-[(2,4-Dihydroxy-3,3-dimethylbutyryl)-amino]ethanesulfonic acid *see* Pantoyltaurine.

3,5-Dihydroxy-6,6-dimethyl-2,4-cyclohexadien-1-one *see* Filixic acid.

3,6-Dihydroxy-6,N-dimethyl-4,5-epoxymorphinan *see* Methyldihydromorphine.

2,5-DIHYDROXY-3,6-DIPHENYL-p-BENZOQUINONE (polyporic acid; polyporin; NSC-44175).

Dihydroxydiphenylhexadine *see* Dienestrol.

2,2'-Dihydroxy-N-(4,5-diphenyloxazol-2-yl)diethylamine *see* Ditazole.

1,16-Dihydroxy-3,14-dithiahexadecane *see* Tiadenol.

4,17β-Dihydroxyestr-4-en-3-one 17-cyclopentanepropionate *see* Oxabolone cipionate.

Dihydroxyestrin *see* Estradiol.

Dihydroxyhexachlorodiphenylmethane *see* Hexachlorophene.

4,7-Dihydroxy-3-[4-hydroxy-3-(3-methyl-2-butenyl)benzamido]-8-methylcoumarin glucoside *see* Novobiocin.

7-[3,5-Dihydroxy-2-(3-hydroxy-3-methyl-1-octenyl)cyclopentyl]-4,5-heptadienoic acid methyl ester *see* Prostalene.

3,5-Dihydroxy-α-(p-hydroxy-α-methylphenethylaminomethyl)benzyl alcohol *see* Fenoterol.

7-[$3\alpha,5\alpha$-Dihydroxy-2β-[3(S)-hydroxy-*trans*-oct-1-enyl]cyclopent-1-yl]-*cis*-hept-5-enoic acid *see* Dinoprost.

Dihydroxy-[(2-hydroxy-5-oxo-2-imidazolin-4-yl)ureato]aluminium *see* Aldioxa.

5,7-Dihydroxy-2-(p-hydroxyphenyl)-chromone *see* Apigenin.

3,5-Dihydroxy-α-[[-2-(p-hydroxyphenyl)-1-methylethyl]aminomethyl]benzyl alcohol *see* Fenoterol.

2,3-Dihydroxy-N-[3-(p-hydroxyphenyl)-1-methylpropyl]phenethylamine *see* Dobutamine.

155

2,4-Dihydroxy-*N*-(3-hydroxypropyl)-3,3-dimethylbutyramide *see* Dexpanthenol; Panthenol.

[3,5-Dihydroxy-2-[3-hydroxy-4-[(α,α,α-trifluoro-*m*-tolyl)oxy]-1-butenyl]cyclopentyl]-5-heptenoic acid *see* Fluprostenol.

5,5′-Dihydroxyhydurilic acid *see* Alloxantin.

4′,7-Dihydroxyisoflavone *see* Daidzein.

3,4-Dihydroxy-α-isopropylaminomethylbenzyl alcohol *see* Isoprenaline.

3,5-Dihydroxy-α-isopropylaminomethylbenzyl alcohol *see* Orciprenaline.

3′,4′-Dihydroxy-2-isopropylaminopropiophenone *see* Phenisonone.

3,4-Dihydroxy-α-(1-isopropylaminopropyl)benzyl alcohol *see* Isoetarine.

11β,21-Dihydroxy-16α,17α-isopropylidenedioxypregna-1,4-diene-3,20-dione *see* Desonide.

5,6-Dihydro-2-(2,6-xylidino)-4H-1,3-thiazine *see* Xylazine.

Dihydroxymalonic acid *see* Mesoxalic acid.

2,2′-Dihydroxy-4-methoxybenzophenone *see* Dioxybenzone.

16α,17α-Dihydroxy-3-methoxyestra-1,3,5-(10)-triene *see* Epimestrol.

2′,6′-Dihydroxy-4′-methoxy-3′-methylbutyrophenone *see* Aspidinol.

3,17-Dihydroxy-11β-methoxy-19-nor-17α-pregna-1,3,5(10)-trien-20-yne *see* Moxestrol.

3,4-Dihydroxy-α-[4-(*o*-methoxyphenyl)piperazin-1-ylmethyl]benzyl alcohol *see* Pipratecol.

3′,4′-Dihydroxy-2-methylaminoacetophenone *see* Adrenalone.

3,4-Dihydroxy-α-methylaminomethylbenzyl alcohol *see* Epinephrine.

18,20-Dihydroxy-3β-methylaminopregn-5-ene *see* Paravallarinol.

4,17β-Dihydroxy-17-methylandrosta-1,4-dien-3-one *see* Enestebol.

4,5-Dihydroxy-2-methylanthraquinone *see* Chrysophanic acid.

6,7-Dihydroxy-4-methylcoumarin bis(hydrogen sulfate) *see* Sulmarin.

10,11-Dihydroxy-6-methyl-4H-dibenzo-(de,g)quinoline *see* Apomorphine.

DI(HYDROXYMETHYL)FURALAZINE (3-[bis(hydroxymethyl)amino]-6-[2-(5-nitro-2-furyl)vinyl]-1,2,4-triazine; dihydroxymethylfuratrizine; 3-[bis(hydroxymethyl)amino]-6-[2-(5-nitro-2-furyl)ethenyl]-1,2,4-triazine; SD-100-2; 'panfuran S').

Dihydroxymethylfuratrizine *see* Di(hydroxymethyl)furalazine.

5,6-Dihydroxy-1-methylindoxyl *see* Adrenolutin.

Di[4-(4-hydroxy-2-methyl-5-isopropylphenylazo)phenyl] sulfone *see* Diathymosulfone.

3,4-Dihydroxy-α-[(α-methyl-3,4-methylenedioxyphenethylamino)methyl]benzyl alcohol *see* Protokylol.

11α,17β-Dihydroxy-17-methyl-3-oxoan-

drosta-1,4-diene-2-carboxaldehyde *see* Formebolone.

9,11-Dihydroxy-8-methyl-5-oxotetrahydro(1H)pyrrolo(2,1-c) (1,4)benzodiazepine-2-acrylamide *see* Antramycin.

3,4-Dihydroxy-α-methylphenylalanine *see* Methyldopa.

3,4-DIHYDROXY-3-METHYL-4-PHENYL-1-BUTYNE (Kö-339; 'centalun').

11β,17-Dihydroxy-21-(4-methyl-piperazin-1-yl)pregna-1,4-diene-3,20-dione *see* Mazipredone.

17,12-Dihydroxy-16β-methylpregna-1,4-diene-3,11,20-trione *see* Meprednisone.

Dihydroxy(6-methyl-8-quinolinolato)bismuth *see* Mebiquine.

3,5-Dihydroxy-3-methylvaleric acid *see* Mevalonic acid.

6,7-Dihydroxy-4-morpholinomethylcoumarin *see* Folescutol.

4,5-Dihydroxy-2,7-naphthalenedisulfonic acid *see* Chromotropic acid.

2,6-Dihydroxy-3-nitro-3′,5′-bis(trifluoromethyl)benzanilide diacetate *see* Flurantel.

3,4-Dihydroxynorephedrine *see* Corbadrine.

11α,15-Dihydroxy-9-oxo-5-*cis*-13-*trans*-prostadienoic acid *see* Dinoprostone.

3,4-Dihydroxyphenanthrene *see* Morphol.

3,4-Dihydroxyphenethylamine *see* Dopamine.

β,4-Dihydroxyphenethylamine *see* Octopamine.

N-(3,4-Dihydroxyphenethyl)-1-adamantanecarboxylic acid *see* Dopamantine.

2,5-Dihydroxyphenylacetic acid *see* Homogentisic acid.

3,4-Dihydroxyphenylacetic acid *see* Homoprotocatechuic acid.

3-(3,4-Dihydroxyphenyl)alanine *see* Dopa.

1-(3,4-Dihydroxyphenyl)-2-ethylamino-1-propanol *see* Dioxethedrin.

N-[2-(2,3-Dihydroxyphenyl)ethyl]-4-(*p*-hydroxyphenyl)-2-butylamine *see* Dobutamine.

Dihydroxyphenylhexane *see* Hexylresorcinol.

2-(2,4-Dihydroxyphenyl)-6-hydroxy-3-benzofurancarboxylic acid δ-lactone *see* Coumestrol.

7-[2[2-(3,4-Dihydroxyphenyl)-2-hydroxyethylamino]ethyl]theophylline *see* Theodrenaline.

N-[2-(3,5-Dihydroxyphenyl)-2-hydroxyethyl]-*p*-hydroxyamphetamine *see* Fenoterol.

1-[2-(3,4-Dihydroxyphenyl)-2-hydroxyethyl]-4-(*o*-methoxyphenyl)piperazine *see* Pipratecol.

1-(3,5-Dihydroxyphenyl)-1-hydroxy-2-[(*p*-hydroxyphenyl)isopropylamino]ethane *see* Fenoterol.

1-(3,4-Dihydroxyphenyl)-2-isopropylamino-1-butanol *see* Isoetharine.

Dihydroxyphenylmethenylbenzyl alcohol *see* Phenolphthalol.

α-(3,4-Dihydroxyphenyl)-4-(2-methoxy-

156

phenyl)-1-piperazineethanol *see* Pipratecol.

3-(3,4-Dihydroxyphenyl)-2-methylalanine *see* Methyldopa.

α-(3,4-Dihydroxyphenyl)-2-piperidinemethanol *see* Rimiterol.

2-(3,4-DIHYDROXYPHENYL)VALERAMIDE (2-(3,4-dihydroxyphenyl)-2-propylacetamide; 2-propyldopacetamide; H-22/54).

erythro-**3,4-Dihydroxy-α-piperid-2-ylbenzyl alcohol** *see* Rimiterol.

11α,17α-Dihydroxypregna-1,4-diene-3,20-dione *see* Deprodone.

17α,21-Dihydroxypregna-1,4-diene-3,11,20-trione *see* Prednisone.

3α,21-Dihydroxy-5α-pregnane-11,20-dione *see* Alfadolone.

16α,17-Dihydroxypregn-4-ene-3,20-dione *see* Algestone.

17,21-Dihydroxypregn-4-ene-3,20-dione *see* Cortodoxone.

11β,21-Dihydroxypregn-4-ene-3,20-dione *see* Corticosterone.

14,17-Dihydroxypregn-4-ene-3,20-dione cyclic acetal with propionaldehyde *see* Proligestone.

11β,21-Dihydroxypregn-4-ene-3,18,20-trione *see* Aldosterone.

17α,21-Dihydroxypregn-4-ene-3,11,20-trione *see* Cortisone.

16α,17-Dihydroxyprogesterone *see* Algestone.

17,21-Dihydroxyprogesterone *see* Cortodoxone.

14,17-Dihydroxyprogesterone cyclic acetal with propionaldehyde *see* Proligestone.

2,3-Dihydroxypropanal *see* Glyceraldehyde.

1,3-Dihydroxy-2-propanone *see* Dihydroxyacetone.

2,3-Dihydroxypropionaldehyde *see* Glyceraldehyde.

2,3-Dihydroxypropyl *N*-(7-chloroquinolin-4-yl)anthranilate *see* Glafenine.

2,3-Dihydroxypropyl 2-(3-chloro-*o*-toluidino)nicotinate *see* Clonixeril.

1-(2,3-Dihydroxypropyl)-3,5-diiodo-4-pyridone *see* Iopydol.

2,3-Dihydroxypropyl methacrylate polymer with methyl methacrylate *see* Crofilcon A.

3-(2,3-Dihydroxypropyl)-2-methyl-4-(3H)-quinazolinone *see* Diproqualone.

1-(2,3-Dihydroxypropyl)-4-phenyl-piperazine *see* Dropropizine.

7-(2,3-Dihydroxypropyl)theophylline *see* Diprophylline.

7-(2,3-Dihydroxypropyl)theophylline bis-(nicotinate ester) *see* Diniprophylline.

2,3-Dihydroxypropyl *N*-(8-trifluoromethylquinolin-4-yl)anthranilate *see* Floctafenine.

(Dihydroxypropyl)trimethylammonium iodide formal *see* Oxapropanium.

Dihydroxyprotocatechuylisoquinoline *see* Papaveroline.

4,8-Dihydroxyquinaldic acid *see* Xanthurenic acid.

2,3-Dihydroxysuccinic acid *see* Tartaric acid.

3,5-Dihydroxytoluene *see* Orcinol.

2,5-Dihydroxy-α-toluic acid *see* Homogentisic acid.

Dihydroxytrimethoxyfuchsone *see* Rubrophen.

6-(6,10-Dihydroxyundecyl)-β-resorcylic acid lactone *see* Zeranol.

DIHYPRYLONE* (3,3-diethyl-2,4-piperidinedione; piperidione; Nu-1510; 'sedilan', 'sedulon').

3,3'-Di-2-imidazolin-2-ylcarbanilide *see* Imidocarb.

Diindogen *see* Indigotin.

Diiodobrassidic acid ethyl ester *see* Iodobrassid.

Diiododithymol *see* Dithymol diiodide.

DIIODOHYDROXYQUIN* (5,7-diiodo-8-quinolinol; diiodohydroxyquinoline; diodoxyquinoline; iodoxine; SS-578). *See also* Chloroquine sulfate with diiodohydroxyquin; Cloquinate with chloroquine diphosphate & diiodohydroxyquin.

DIIODOHYDROXYQUIN WITH TETRACYCLINE ('diocyclin').

DIIODOHYDROXYQUIN GLYCOLYLARSANILATE ('triamar').

Diiodohydroxyquinoline*** *see* Diiodohydroxyquin.

3,5-Diiodo-4-(3-iodo-4-methoxyphenoxy)-phenylacetic acid *see* Tyromedan.

Diiodomethanesulfonic acid *see* Dimethiodal.

3,5-Diiodo-1-methylchelidamic acid sodium salt *see* Iodoxyl.

2,6-Diiodo-4-nitrophenol *see* Disophenol.

3,5-Diiodo-4-oxo-1-pyridineacetic acid salts *see* Diodone; Iodopyridone; Propyliodone.

2,6-DIIODO-1-PHENOL-4-SULFONIC ACID (3,5-diiodo-*p*-phenolsulfonic acid; soziodic acid; sozoiodolic acid; 'diiozol', 'iodozol', 'optojod', 'renopac', 'rolinex', 'soziodol', 'sziodol').

3,5-Diiodo-*p*-phenolsulfonic acid *see* 2,6-Diiodo-1-phenol-4-sulfonic acid.

3,5-Diiodo-α-phenylphloretic acid *see* Pheniodol.

3,5-Diiodo-4-pyridone *see* Iopydone.

'Diiodoquin' *see* Diiodohydroxyquin.

5,7-Diiodo-8-quinolinol *see* Diiodohydroxyquin.

Diiodostearic acid ethyl ester *see* Iodetryl.

3,5-DIIODOTYROSINE (3-(4-hydroxy-3,5-diiodophenyl)alanine; iodogorgoic acid; iodogorgonic acid; 'agontan', 'apothyrin', 'dityrin', 'flajanina', 'iodoglobin', 'iodogorgon', 'tyrogel').

Diiodo-β-tyrosine *see* Betazine.

'Diiozol' *see* 2,6-Diiodo-1-phenol-4-sulfonic acid.

4,4'-Diisoamyloxythiocarbanilide *see* Tiocarlide.

Diisocyanatotoluene *see* Toluylene diisocyanate.

DIISOPROMINE*** (*N*,*N*-diisopropyl-3,3-
diphenylpropylamine; disopromine;
'agofell', 'bilagol').

N-[2-[(**Diisopropoxyphosphinothioyl**)-
thio]**ethyl**]**benzenesulfonamide** *see*
Bensulide.

DIISOPROPYLAMINE ('disotat').

**DIISOPROPYLAMINE DICHLORO-
ACETATE** (diisopropylamine dichloro-
ethanoate; DIPA; IS-401; 'diedi', 'tensicor')

2'-(**2-Diisopropylaminoethoxy**)**butyrophenone** *see* Ketocaine.

o-(**2-Diisopropylaminoethoxy**)-*α*-**propyl-
benzyl alcohol** *see* Ketocainol.

2-DIISOPROPYLAMINOETHYL
p-**AMINOBENZOATE** ('isocaine').

α-(**2-Diisopropylaminoethyl**)-*α*-**phenyl-2-
pyridineacetamide** *see* Disopyramide.

**4-Diisopropylamino-2-phenyl-2-pyrid-2-
ylbutyramide** *see* Disopyramide.

Diisopropylcarbamothioic acid *S*-(**2,3-
dichloro-2-propenyl**) **ester** *see* Diallate.

Diisopropylcarbamothioic acid *S*-(**2,3,3-
trichloro-2-propenyl**) **ester** *see* Triallate.

Diisopropylfluo(**ro**)**phosph**(**on**)**ate** *see*
Dyflos.

Diisopropyl-methanol-dioxolane *see*
Promoxolane.

Diisopropylmethyl(**diphenylhydroxypropyl**)**ammonium iodide carbamate**
see Isopropamide.

O,*O*-**DIISOPROPYL** *O*-*p*-**NITROPHENYL
PHOSPHATE** ('mioticol', 'propicol').

Diisopropylphosphorodiamidic fluoride
see Mipafox.

Diisopropyl phosphorofluoridate *see*
Dyflos.

Diklorfenidim (tr) *see* Diuron.

'**Dikonirit**' *see* 2,4-Dichlorophenoxy-
acetic acid.

'**Dikotex**' *see* 4-Chloro-2-methylphenoxy-
acetic acid.

'**Dilabron**' *see* Isoetarine.

'**Dilangil**' *see* Mannityl hexanitrate.

'**Dilangio**' *see* Bencyclane.

'**Dilar**' *see* Paramethasone.

'**Dilasmyl**' *see* Choline theophyllinate.

'**Dilatal**' *see* Buphenine.

'**Dilatol**' *see* Buphenine.

'**Dilatropon**' *see* Buphenine.

'**Dilaudid**' *see* Hydromorphone.

'**Dilavase**' *see* Isoxsuprine.

DILAZEP*** (tetrahydro-1H-1,4-diazepine-
1,4(5H)-dipropanol 3,4,5-trimethoxy-
benzoate diester; *N*,*N*'-bis[(3-hydroxy-
propyl)homopiperazine 3,4,5-trimethoxy-
benzoate]; biopropazepan bis(3,4,5-trime-
thoxybenzoate); Asta-C-4898).
See also β-Acetyldigoxin with dilazep.

'**Dilcit**' *see* Inositol nicotinate.

'**Dilexan**' *see* Phloroglucinol with 1,3,5-
trimethoxybenzene.

'**Dillar**' *see* Paramethasone.

DILMEFONE*** (2',4'-dimethoxy-3-pyrid-
4-ylacrylophenone; 4-[2-(2,4-dimethoxy-
benzoyl)vinyl]pyridine).

'**Diloderm**' *see* Dichlorisone acetate.

'**Dilombrin**' *see* Dithiazanine.

'**Dilospan**' *see* Phloroglucinol.

'**Dilosyn**' *see* Methdilazine.

'**Dilovasan**' *see* Isoxsuprine.

DILOXANIDE*** (2,2-dichloro-4'-hydroxy-
N-methylacetanilide; diloxanide hydrochloride; RD-3803; 'entamide').

DILOXANIDE FUROATE (CB-8073;
'furamide').

DILTIAZEM** ((+)-5-(2-dimethylamino-
ethyl)-*cis*-2,3-dihydro-3-hydroxy-2-(*p*-
methoxyphenyl)-1,5-benzothiazepin-4(5H)-
one acetate ester; diltiazem hydrochloride;
CRD-401; 'herbesser').

'**Diluran**' *see* Acetazolamide.

'**Dilvasene**' *see* Oxapropanium iodide.

'**Dilydrin**' *see* Buphenine.

DIMABEFYLLINE*** (7-(*p*-dimethylamino-
benzyl)theophylline; LJ-278).

'**Dimaestad**' *see* Deanol.

**Dimagnesium tetraaluminium hydrox-
ide oxide sulfate hydrate** *see* Almadrate
sulfate.

'**Dimalone**' *see* Dimethyl 5-norbornene-2,3-
dicarboxylate.

DIMANTINE*** (*N*,*N*-dimethyloctadecyl-
amine; dymanthine hydrochloride; GS-
1339; 'thelmesan').

'**Dimapyrin**' *see* Aminophenazone.

DIMAZOLE** (6-(2-diethylaminoethoxy)-2-
dimethylaminobenzothiazole; diamthazole; dimazole dihydrochloride; Ro-2-2453
'asterol', 'atelor', 'atelora').

'**Dimazon**' *see* Diacetazotol.

'**Dimeate**' *see* Thiometon.

Dimebencozamide *see* Cobamamide.

DIMECAMINE*** (3-dimethylamino-2,2,3-
trimethylnorbornane; *N*,*N*,2,3,3-penta-
methyl-2-norbornanamine; methylmecamylamine).

Dimecoline (tr) *see* Dimecolonium iodide.

DIMECOLONIUM IODIDE*** (ester of
2-carboxy-1,1,6-trimethylpiperidinium
iodide with (2-hydroxyethyl)trimethyl-
ammonium iodide; dimethylaminoethyl
ester dimethiodide of 1,6-dimethylpipe-
colic acid; choline iodide dimethylpipecolate methiodide; dimecoline).

'**Dimecron**' *see* Phosphamidon.

DIMECROTIC ACID*** (2,4-dimethoxy-β-
methylcinnamic acid; 3-(2,4-dimethoxy-
phenyl)-3-methylacrylic acid; 3-(2,4-
dimethoxyphenyl)-3-methylpropenoic
acid; 3-(2,4-dimethoxyphenyl)crotonic
acid).

'**Dimedion**' *see* Ethadione.

Dimedrol (tr) *see* Diphenhydramine.

DIMEFADANE*** (*N*,*N*-dimethyl-3-phenyl-
1-indanamine; *N*,*N*-dimethyl-3-phenylin-
dan-1-ylamine; SK&F-1340).

DIMEFILCON A* (2-hydroxyethyl methacrylate polymer with methyl methacrylate
and ethylenebis(oxyethylene) dimethacrylate; 'gelflex').

DIMEFLINE*** (8-dimethylaminomethyl-7-
methoxy-3-methyl-2-phenylbenzo-γ-pyrone;

8-dimethylaminomethyl-7-methoxy-3-methylflavone; dimefline hydrochloride; DW-62; Rec-7-0267; 'remeflin').

DIMEFOX* (tetramethylphosphorodiamidic fluoride; bis(dimethylamido)fluorophosphate; bis(dimethylamino) fluorophosphine oxide; BFP; BFPO; DIFO; DMF; 'hanane', 'pestox XIV', 'terra-sytam').

DIMELAZINE*** (10-(1,3-dimethylpyrrolidin-3-ylmethyl)phenothiazine).

'Dimelor' see Acetohexamide.

DIMEMORFAN** (−)-3,17-dimethylmorphinan; N,3-dimethylmorphinan; AT-17).

'Dimenazone' see Aminophenazone formaldehyde sodium sulfoxylate.

DIMENHYDRINATE*** (2-diphenylmethoxy-N,N-dimethylethylamine compound with 8-chlorotheophylline; 8-chlorotheophyllinate of diphenhydramine; diphenhydramine teoclate; diphenhydramine theoclate; chloranautine).

DIMENHYDRINATE WITH SCOPOLAMINE (G-330; 'gestadramine').

DIMENOXADOL*** (2-dimethylaminoethyl 2-ethoxy-2,2-diphenylacetate; deanol 2-ethoxy-2,2-diphenylacetate; dimenoxadole; esthocine; estocin).

Dimenoxadole* see Dimenoxadol.

DIMEPHEPTANOL*** (6-dimethylamino-4,4-diphenyl-3-heptanol; 5-hydroxy-N,N-dimethyl-4,4-diphenyl-2-heptylamine; 4-hydroxy-N,N,1-trimethyl-3,3-diphenylhexylamine; methadol).

See also Alphamethadol; Betamethadol.

Dimepheptanol acetate see Acetylmethadol.

DIMEPREGNEN*** (3β-hydroxy-6α,16α-dimethylpregn-4-en-20-one; 6α,16α-dimethylpregn-4-en-3β-ol-20-one; St-1411).

Dimepropion* see Metamfepramone.

DIMEPROZAN*** (9-(3-dimethylaminopropylidene)-2-methoxyxanthene; 2-methoxy-N,N-dimethyl-△⁹,ʸ-xanthenepropylamine).

DIMERCAPROL*** (2,3-dimercaptopropanol; British antilewisite; BAL; dicaptol; 1,2-dithioglycol).

Dimercaptopropane sodium sulfonate see Unithiol.

2,3-Dimercaptopropanol see Dimercaprol.

2,3-DIMERCAPTOSUCCINIC ACID (meso-2,3-dimercaptosuccinic acid; DTS; DMS; Ro-1-7977).

2,5-Dimercaptosuccinic acid cyclic thioantimonate (III) S,S-diester see Stibocaptic acid.

Dimerin (tr) see Methyprylon.

'Dimer X' see Meglumine iocarmate.

DIMESONE** (9α-fluoro-11β,21-dihydroxy-16α,17-dimethylpregna-1,4-diene-3,20-dione).

Dimestrol (tr) see Dianisylhexene.

'Di-met' see Disodium methanearsonate.

DIMETACRINE*** (10-(3-dimethylaminopropyl-9,9-dimethylacridan; dimethacrin; 'linostil').

'DIMETACRINE TARTRATE (dimeta-crine bitartrate; SD-709; 'istonil', 'linostil').

DIMETAN* (5,5-dimethyl-1-cyclohexen-1-ol-3-one dimethylcarbamate; 5,5-dimethyl-dihydroresorcinol dimethylcarbamate; 5,5-dimethyl-1-oxocyclohex-2-en-3-yl dimethylcarbamate; G-19258).

Dimetane' see Brompheniramine maleate.

Dimetazine see Mebolazine.

Dimethacrin see Dimetacrine.

DIMETHADIONE*** (5,5-dimethyl-2,4-oxazolidinedione; AC-1198; BAX-1400-Z; DMO; 'eupractone', 'propazone').

Dimethanesulfonoxynonane see Nonamethylene dimesilate.

Dimethanesulfonylmannitol see Mannityl dimesilate.

DIMETHAZAN*** (7-(2-dimethylaminoethyl)theophylline; 1,3-dimethyl-7-(2-dimethylaminoethyl)xanthine).

Dimethenthoate see Phenthoate.

Dimethicone* see Dimeticone.

Dimethindene* see Dimetindene.

DIMETHIODAL SODIUM*** (sodium diiodomethanesulfonate; 'urotrast').

DIMETHIRIMOL* (5-butyl-2-(dimethylamino)-4-hydroxy-6-methylpyrimidine; 5-butyl-2-dimethylamino-6-methyl-4-pyrimidinol; 'milcurb').

Dimethisoquin see Quinisocaine.

DIMETHISTERONE*** (6α,21-dimethylethisterone; 17α-ethynyl-6α,21-dimethyl-androst-4-en-17-ol-3-one; 17α-ethynyl-6α,21-dimethyltestosterone; 17-ethynyl-17β-hydroxy-6α,21-dimethylandrost-4-en-3-one; 17β-hydroxy-6α-methyl-17-(1-propynyl)androst-4-en-3-one; 'secrosteron').

DIMETHISTERONE WITH ETHINYLESTRADIOL ('oracon').

DIMETHOATE* (O,O-dimethyl S-[2-(methylamino)-2-oxoethyl] phosphorodithioate; O,O-dimethyl S-(methylcarbamoylmethyl) phosphorodithioate; 2-[(dimethoxyphosphinothioyl)thio]-N-methylacetamide; HC-8014 bis; fosfamid; phosphamide; 'amidofos', 'cygon', 'fostion MM', 'perfekthion', 'rogor', 'roxion').

DIMETHOCAINE* (3-diethylamino-2,2-dimethylpropyl p-aminobenzoate; 'larocaine').

DIMETHOLIZINE*** (1-(o-methoxyphenyl)-4-(3-methoxypropyl)piperazine; dimetholizine phosphate; HT-1479).

Dimethothiazine* see Dimetotiazine.

DIMETHOXANATE*** (2-dimethylaminoethoxyethyl 10-phenothiazinecarboxylate; dimethoxanate hydrochloride; 'cothera', 'cotrane').

Dimethoxon see Omethoate.

6-(2,6-Dimethoxybenzamido)penicillanic acid see Meticillin.

7-(3,4-Dimethoxybenzoyloxy)-3-ethyl-1-(p-methoxyphenyl)-2-methyl-3-azaheptane see Mebeverine.

4-[2-(2,4-Dimethoxybenzoyl)vinyl]-pyridine see Dilmefone.

3,4-Dimethoxybenzylamine see Veratrylamine.

3,4-DIMETHOXYBENZYLHYDRAZINE
(vetrazin).
**3,3′-(3,3′-Dimethoxy-4,4′-biphenylene)-
bis-(2,5-diphenyl(2H)tetrazolium
chloride** *see* Tetrazolium blue.
**6,7-Dimethoxy-4-(3,4-dimethoxybenzyl-
ideneamino)quinoline** *see* Leniquinsin.
**6,7-Dimethoxy-N-(3-dimethylamino-1,3-
dimethylbutyl)-2,1-benzoxathian-3-
carboxamide 1,1-dioxide** *see* Tisocromide.
**2-(3,6-Dimethoxy-2,4-dimethylbenzyl)-2-
imidazoline** *see* Domazoline.
**2-5-Dimethoxy-α,4-dimethylphenethyl-
amine** *see* 2,5-Dimethoxy-4-methyl-
amphetamine.
Dimethoxy DT *see* Methoxychlor.
**12,13-Dimethoxyibogamine-18-carboxylic
acid methyl ester** *see* Conopharyngine.
**4-(6,7-Dimethoxyisoquinolin-1-ylmethyl)-
pyrocatechol** *see* Papaverine.
Dimethoxymethane *see* Methylal.
**5,6-Dimethoxy-3-[2-[4-(o-methoxyphenyl)-
piperazin-1-yl]ethyl]-2-methylindole**
see Milipertine.
**6,7-Dimethoxy-2-[2-[4-(o-methoxyphenyl)-
piperazin-1-yl]ethyl]-4(3H)-quin-
azolinone** *see* Peraquinsin.
**2,5-DIMETHOXY-4-METHYLAMPHET-
AMINE** (2,5-dimethoxy-α,4-dimethyl-
phenethylamine; 1-(2,5-dimethoxy-4-
methylphenyl)-2-propylamine; 2-amino-1-
(2,5-dimethoxy-4-methylphenyl)propane;
DOM; 'STP').
2,4-Dimethoxy-α-methylbenzhydrol *see*
Fenocinol.
2,4-Dimethoxy-β-methylcinnamic acid
see Dimecrotic acid.
**1-[2-(5,6-Dimethoxy-2-methylindol-3-yl)-
ethyl]-4-(o-methoxyphenyl)piperazine**
see Milipertine.
**1-[2-(5,6-Dimethoxy-2-methylindol-3-yl)-
ethyl]-4-phenylpiperazine** *see* Oxypertine.
**3,4-Dimethoxy-17-methylmorphinan-6β,
14-diol** *see* Drotebanol.
**5,6-Dimethoxy-2-methyl3-[2-(4-phenyl-
piperazin-1-yl)ethyl]indole** *see* Oxypertine.
**1-(2,5-Dimethoxy-4-methylphenyl)-2-
propylamine** *see* Dimethoxy-4-methyl-
amphetamine.
**1-(6,7-Dimethoxy-4(3H)-oxoquinazolin-
2-yl)-4-(o-methoxyphenyl)piperazine** *see*
Peraquinsin.
Dimethoxyphenecillin *see* Meticillin.
3,4-Dimethoxyphenethylamine *see*
Homoveratrylamine.
**2-(3,4-Dimethoxyphenethylimino)-1-
methylpyrrolidine** *see* Mixidine.
**5-[N-(3,4-Dimethoxyphenethyl)methyl-
amino]-2-(3,4-dimethoxyphenyl)-2-iso-
propylvaleronitrile** *see* Verapamil.
2-(3,5-Dimethoxyphenoxy)ethanol *see*
Floverine.
3-(2,4-Dimethoxyphenyl)crotonic acid *see*
Dimecrotic acid.
1-(3,4-Dimethoxyphenyl)-5-ethyl-7,8-

**dimethoxy-4-methyl-5H-2,3-benzo
diazepine** *see* Tofisopam.
**1-(3,4-Dimethoxyphenyl)-4-ethyl-6,7-di-
methoxy-3-methylisoquinoline 2-
imide** *see* Tofisoline.
**2-(3,4-Dimethoxyphenyl)-2-[3-[(N-homo-
veratryl-N-methylamino)propyl]-2-
isopropylacetonitrile** *see* Verapamil.
**3-(2,4-Dimethoxyphenyl)-3-methyl-
acrylic acid** *see* Dimecrotic acid.
**3-(2,4-Dimethoxyphenyl)-3-methyl-
propenoic acid** *see* Dimecrotic acid.
Dimethoxyphenylpenicillin *see* Meticillin.
1-(2,4-Dimethoxyphenyl)-1-phenylethanol
see Fenocinol.
**5,6-Dimethoxy-3-[2-(4-phenylpiperazin-
1-yl)ethyl]indole-2-carboxylic acid
ethyl ester** *see* Alpertine.
**2-[(Dimethoxyphosphinothioyl)thio]-N-
methylacetamide** *see* Dimethoate.
**4-[[(Dimethoxyphosphinothioyl)thio]-
methyl]-2-methoxy-1,3,4-thiadiazol-5-
one** *see* Methidathion.
**2-[[(Dimethoxyphosphinothioyl)thio]-
methyl]phthalimide** *see* Phosmet.
**6-[[(Dimethoxyphosphinothioyl)thio]-
methyl]-1,3,5-triazine-2,4-diamine** *see*
Menazon.
**2-[(Dimethoxyphosphinothioyl)thio]-2-
phenylacetic acid ethyl ester** *see*
Phenthoate.
**[(Dimethoxyphosphinothioyl)thio]-
succinic acid diethyl ester** *see* Malathion.
**3-(Dimethoxyphosphinyloxy)crotonic
acid, esters** *see* Crotoxyphos; Mevinphos.
**3-(Dimethoxyphosphinyloxy)-N,N-di-
methyl-cis-crotonamide** *see* Dicrotophos.
5,6-Dimethoxyphthalaldehydic acid *see*
Opianic acid.
**5,6-Dimethoxyphthalaldehydic acid
isonicotinoylhydrazone** *see* Opiniazide.
Dimethoxyphthalide *see* Meconin.
**(6,7-Dimethoxy-3-phthalidyl)-8-methoxy-
2-methyl-6,7-methylenedioxy-1,2,3,4,
tetrahydroisoquinoline** *see* Noscapine.
**5-(6,7-Dimethoxyphthalidyl)-5,6,7,8-tetra-
hydro-4-methoxy-6-methyl-1,3-di-
oxolo(4,5-g)isoquinoline** *see* Noscapine.
**2′,4′-Dimethoxy-3-pyrid-4-ylacrylo-
phenone** *see* Dilmefone.
**Dimethoxypyrimidylsulfanilamide
isomers** *see* Sulfadimethoxine; Sulfadoxine; Sulfamoprime.
**4-(6,7-Dimethoxyquinazolin-4-yl)pipera-
zine-1-carboxylic acid 2-hydroxy-2-
methylpropyl ester** *see* Hoquizil.
**6,7-Dimethoxy-1-(3,4,5-triethoxyphenyl)-
isoquinoline** *see* Octaverine.
3,5-Dimethoxytoluene *see* Elemicin.
**6,7-Dimethoxy-4-veratrylideneamino-
quinoline** *see* Leniquinsin.
Dimethoxyveratrylisoquinoline *see*
Papaverine.
Dimethpyrindene *see* Dimetindene.
DIMETHRIN* (2,4-dimethylbenzyl chrysanthemate; 2,4-xylylmethyl 2,2-dimethyl-3-

160

(2-methylpropenyl)cyclopropanecarboxyl-
ate; 2,4-dimethylbenzyl 2,2-dimethyl-3-
(2-methyl-1-propenyl)cyclopropane-
carboxylate; ENT-21170).
O,S-**Dimethyl acetylphosphoramidothioate** *see* Acephate.
**9,9-Dimethylacridan-10-carbothioic acid
2-dimethylaminoethyl thioester** *see*
Botiacrine.
2,3-Dimethylacrylic acid *see* Tiglic acid.
2,3-Dimethylacrylic acid tropine ester
see Tropigline.
3,3-Dimethylacrylic acid *see* Senecioic acid.
*N*¹-**(3,3-Dimethylacryloyl)sulfanilamide**
see Sulfadicramide.
3,5-Dimethyl-1-adamantanamine *see*
Memantine.
Dimethylamantadine *see* Memantine.
**Dimethylamido ethoxy phosphoryl
cyanide** *see* Tabun.
**DIMETHYLAMINE 2,4-DICHLORO-
PHENOXYACETATE** ('herbatox D-500').
**DIMETHYLAMINE TRICHLORO-
BENZOATE** (2,3,6-trichlorobenzoic acid
dimethylamine salt; 'benzabor', 'benzac',
'trysben').
**Dimethylaminoacetaldehyde diphenyl-
acetal** *see* Medifoxamine.
6-Dimethylaminoacetylgluconic acid *see*
Pangamic acid.
4-Dimethylaminoantipyrine *see* Aminophenazone.
p-**DIMETHYLAMINOAZOBENZENE**
(*N,N*-dimethyl-*p*-phenylazoaniline; DAB;
butter yellow).
p-**Dimethylaminobenzoic acid 2-ethyl-
hexyl ester** *see* Padimate O.
p-**Dimethylaminobenzoic acid pentyl
ester mixture** *see* Padimate.
**1-(4-DIMETHYLAMINOBENZYLIDENE)-
INDENE** (α-inden-1-ylidene-*N,N*-di-
methyl-*p*-toluidine; DABI; 14M21; NSC-
80087).
7-(*p*-Dimethylaminobenzyl)theophylline
see Dimabefylline.
**3-[[(Dimethylamino)carbonyl]amino]-
phenyl (1,1-dimethylethyl)carbamate**
see Karbutilate.
**1-(Dimethylaminocarbonyl)-5-methyl-
1H-pyrazol-3-yl dimethylcarbamate** *see*
Dimetilan.
3β-Dimethylaminocon-5-ene *see* Conessine.
**5-(4-Dimethylaminocyclohexyl)hydroxy-
methyl-*trans*-2,2′-bithiophene methobromide** *see* Thihexinol methyl bromide.
**3-(Dimethylamino)-2,3-dihydro-2-methyl-
benzopyran** *see* Trebenzomine.
**3-Dimethylamino-1,2-dihydro-7-methyl-
1,2-(propylmalonyl)-1,2,4-benzotriazine**
see Azapropazone.
N-**(3-Dimethylamino-1,3-dimethylbutyl)-
6,7-dimethoxy-2,1-benzoxathian-3-
carboxamide 1,1-dioxide** *see* Tisocromide.
**4-Dimethylamino-3,5-dimethylphenyl
methylcarbamate** *see* Mexacarbate.
**4-(Dimethylamino)-2,3-dimethyl-1-
phenyl-3-pyrazolin-5-one** *see* Amino-

phenazone.
**6-Dimethylamino-2-[2-(2,5-dimethyl-1-
phenyl-3-pyrrolyl)vinyl]-1-methyl-
quinolinium chloride** *see* Pyrvinium
chloride.
**3-Dimethylamino-1,2-dimethylpropyl
p-aminobenzoate** *see* Butamin.
**2-Dimethylamino-5,6-dimethylpyrimidin-
4-yl dimethylcarbamate** *see* Pirimicarb.
**(+)-1-Dimethylamino-1,2-diphenyl-
ethane** *see* *N,N*-Dimethyl-α-phenylphene-
thylamine.
**(−)-1-Dimethylamino-1,2-diphenyl-
ethane** *see* Lefetamine.
**6-Dimethylamino-4,4-diphenyl-3-
heptanol** *see* Dimepheptanol.
**6-Dimethylamino-4,4-diphenyl-3-hepta-
none** *see* Methadone.
**2-Dimethylamino-*N*-(1,3-diphenylpyrazol-
5-yl)propionamide** *see* Difenamizole.
4-Dimethylamino-2,2-diphenylvaleramide
see Dimevamide.
**3-Dimethylamino-1,1-dithien-2-yl-1-
butene** *see* Dimethylthiambutene.
4-Dimethylamino-1,2-dithiolane *see*
Nereistoxin.
2-Dimethylaminoethanethiol *see* Captamine.
2-Dimethylaminoethanol *see* Deanol.
**2-Dimethylaminoethanol salt with 2-(*p*-
biphenylyl)butyric acid** *see* Namoxyrate.
α,α′-**Dimethylaminoethanol-4,4′-biaceto-
phenone** *see* Hemicholinium.
Dimethylaminoethanol methiodide *see*
Choline iodide.
N-**[*p*-(2-Dimethylaminoethoxy)benzyl]-
3,4,5-trimethoxybenzamide** *see* Trimethobenzamide.
**4-(2-Dimethylaminoethoxy)carvacrol
acetate** *see* Moxisylyte.
**5-[2-(Dimethylamino)ethoxy]carvacryl
isopropyl carbonate** *see* Iproxamine.
**2-[α-(2-Dimethylaminoethoxy)-2,6-di-
ethylbenzyl]pyridine** *see* Pytamine.
**11-(2-Dimethylaminoethoxy)-6,11-di-
hydrodibenz(b,e)thiepine** *see* Amethobenzepine.
**4-(2-Dimethylaminoethoxy)-1,2-dihydro-
1-hydroxyiminophthalazine** *see*
Taloximine.
**1-[6-(2-Dimethylaminoethoxy)-4,7-di-
methoxybenzofuran-5-yl]-3-(*p*-methoxy-
phenyl)-2-propen-1-one** *see* Mecinarone.
**6-(2-Dimethylaminoethoxy)-4,7-di-
methoxy-5-[3-(*p*-methoxyphenyl)-1-
oxoprop-2-enyl]benzofuran** *see*
Mecinarone.
**2-(2-Dimethylaminoethoxy)ethyl 10-
phenothiazinecarboxylate** *see* Dimethoxanate.
**2-(2-Dimethylaminoethoxy)ethyl 1-
phenylcyclopentanecarboxylate** *see*
Minepentate.
**4-(2-Dimethylaminoethoxy)-5-isopropyl-
2-methylphenyl acetate** *see* Moxisylyte.
**4-(2-Dimethylaminoethoxy)-5-isopropyl-
2-methylphenyl isopropyl carbonate**

161

see Iproxamine.

trans-1-[*p*-(2-Dimethylaminoethoxy)-
phenyl]-1,2-diphenylbut-1-ene *see*
Tamoxifen.

trans-α-[*p*-(2-Dimethylaminoethoxy)-
phenyl]-α'-ethylstilbene *see* Tamoxifen.

4-(2-Dimethylaminoethoxy)-1(2H)-
phthalazinone oxime *see* Taloximine.

2-Dimethylaminoethyl *p*-acetamido-
benzoate *see* Deanol *p*-acetamidobenzoate.

2-Dimethylaminoethyl 3-amino-4-chloro-
benzoate *see* Clormecaine.

17-[1-(2-Dimethylaminoethyl)amino-
ethyl]androstanol *see* 22,25-Diaza-
cholestanol.

4-(2-Dimethylaminoethylamino)-6-
methoxyquinoline compound with di-
ethylcarbamoylcyclohexenecarboxylic
acid *see* Quinetalate.

2-Dimethylaminoethyl benzilate *see*
Deanol benzilate.

2-Dimethylaminoethyl 1-benzyl-2,3-di-
methylindole-5-carboxylate *see* Indocate.

2-Dimethylaminoethyl 2-(*p*-biphenylyl)-
butyrate *see* Namoxyrate.

2-Dimethylaminoethyl *p*-butylamino-
benzoate *see* Tetracaine.

2-Dimethylaminoethyl 4-butylamino-
salicylate *see* Hydroxytetracaine.

2-Dimethylaminoethyl *p*-chlorophenoxy-
acetate *see* Meclofenoxate.

2-Dimethylaminoethyl cyclohexane-
propionate *see* Cyprodenate.

S-(2-Dimethylaminoethyl) *O,O*-diethyl
phosphorothioate methiodide *see*
Ecothiopate.

5-(2-Dimethylaminoethyl)-*cis*-2,3-dihydro-
3-hydroxy-2-(*p*-methoxyphenyl)-1,5-
benzothiazepin-4(5H)-one acetate *see*
Diltiazem.

10-(2-Dimethylaminoethyl)-5,10-dihydro-
5-methyldibenzo(b,e)(1,4)diazepin-11-
one *see* Dibenzepin.

5-(2-Dimethylaminoethyl)-2,3-dihydro-2-
phenyl-1,5-benzothiazepin-4(5H)-one
see Tiazesim.

2-(Dimethylamino)ethyl 6-(2,6-dimeth-
oxybenzamido)penicillanate *see*
Tameticillin.

S-(2-Dimethylaminoethyl) 9,9-dimethyl-
10-acridancarbothioate *see* Botiacrine.

2-Dimethylaminoethyl 1-(2-dimethyl-
aminoethyl)-2,3-dimethylindole-5-
carboxylate *see* Amindocate.

1-(2-Dimethylaminoethyl)-2,3-dimethyl-
indole-5-carboxylic acid dimethylaminoethyl ester *see* Amindocate.

2-Dimethylaminoethyl 1,6-dimethyl-
pipecolate dimethiodide *see* Dimecolonium iodide.

2-Dimethylaminoethyl *N,N*-diphenyl-
carbamate *see* Dicarfen.

2-Dimethylaminoethyl ethoxydiphenyl-
acetate *see* Dimenoxadol.

2-Dimethylaminoethyl 2-(2-ethylbutoxy)-
2,2-diphenylacetate *see* Denaverine.

1-(2-Dimethylaminoethyl)-9-ethyl-1,3,4,9-

tetrahydro-1-methylthiopyrano(3,4-b)-
indole *see* Tandamine.

2-Dimethylaminoethyl hydrogen *N*-acet-
ylglutamate *see* Deanol aceglumate.

2-Dimethylaminoethyl hydrogen tartrate
see Deanol bitartrate.

1-(2-Dimethylaminoethyl)-3-(1-hydroxy-
iminopropyl)indole *see* Etoprindole.

2-Dimethylaminoethyl 1-hydroxy-α-
phenylcyclopentaneacetate *see* Cyclopentolate.

[(Dimethylaminoethyl)inden-3-ylethyl]-
pyridine *see* Dimetindene.

3-(Dimethylaminoethyl)-4-indolol *see*
Psilocybine.

1-(2-Dimethylaminoethyl)indol-3-yl ethyl
ketone oxime *see* Etoprindole.

α-(2-Dimethylaminoethyl)-α-isopropyl-
1-naphthaleneacetamide *see* Naftypramide.

2-[(2-Dimethylaminoethyl)(*p*-methoxy-
benzyl)amino]pyridine *see* Mepyramine.

2-[(2-Dimethylaminoethyl) (*p*-methoxy-
benzyl)amino]thiazole *see* Zolamine.

5-Dimethylaminoethyl-3-ethyl-2-methylindole
see Medmain.

Dimethylaminoethyl 1-methyl-
pyrrolidine-2-carboxylate dimethiodide *see* Hygronium.

3-[(2-Dimethylaminoethyl)oxyimino]-1,2:
4,5-dibenzocyclohepta-1,4-diene *see*
Noxiptiline.

Dimethylamino-β-ethylphenethyl alcohol
see Trimebutine.

p-(2-Dimethylaminoethyl)phenol *see*
Hordenine.

10-(2-Dimethylaminoethyl)phenothiazine
see Fenethazine.

1-(2-Dimethylaminoethyl)-1-phenylindene
see Indriline.

4-Dimethylamino-2-ethyl-2-phenyl-
valeronitrile *see* Etaminile.

1-(2-Dimethylaminoethyl)-3-propionyl-
indole oxime *see* Etoprindole.

2-Dimethylaminoethyl propynyloxybenzilate *see* Deanol propynyloxybenzilate.

6-(2-Dimethylaminoethyl)pyrido(2,3-b)-
(1,5)benzothiazepin-5(6H)-one *see*
Bepiastine.

Dimethylaminoethyl(pyridylethyl)indene
see Dimetindene.

1-(2-Dimethylaminoethyl)-1,3,4,9-tetra-
hydro-1-methylindeno(2,1-c)pyran *see*
Pirandamine.

2-Dimethylaminoethyl 1,3,4,5-tetrahydro-
thiopyrano(4,3-b)indole-8-carboxylate
see Tipindole.

7-(2-Dimethylaminoethyl)theophylline
see Dimethazan.

N-(2-Dimethylaminoethyl)-*N*-trifluoro-
methylcarbanilic acid ethyl ester *see*
Flubanilate.

1-Dimethylamino-2-hydroxyethyl 2-oxo-
norbornane-3-carboxylate *see* Ethyl-
camphoramine.

5-(4-Dimethylaminoisobutyl)-10,11-

dihydro(5H)dibenzo(a,d)cycloheptene *see* Butriptyline.

Dimethylaminoisopropanol inosine *p*-acetamidobenzoate *see* Methisoprinol.

4-Dimethylamino-2-isopropyl-2-phenyl-valeronitrile *see* Isoaminile.

(Dimethylaminoisopropyl)thiophenyl-pyridylamine *see* Isothipendyl.

2-Dimethylamino-N-[[(methylamino)-carbonyl]oxy]-2-oxoethanimidothioic acid methyl ester *see* Oxamyl.

4-DIMETHYLAMINO-3′-METHYLAZO-BENZENE (*N,N′*-dimethyl-*p*-(*m*-tolylazo)-aniline; 3′-methylDAB; 3′-MeDAB; methyl butter yellow).

10-Dimethylaminomethyldibenzo(b,f)-thiepin *see* Damotepine.

4′-Dimethylaminomethyl-1,11-dihydro-spiro[5H-dibenzo(a,d)cycloheptene-5,2′-(1,3)dioxolane] *see* Ciheptolane.

α-Dimethylaminomethyl-3,4-dihydroxy-benzyl alcohol *see* N-Methylepine-phrine.

4-Dimethylaminomethyl-1,2-dioxolane methiodide *see* Oxapropanium iodide.

4-Dimethylamino-3-methyl-1,2-diphenyl-2-butanol propionate *see* Dextropropoxy-phene; Levopropoxyphene.

3-Dimethylaminomethyl-1,2-diphenyl-3-buten-2-ol propionate *see* Proxibutene; Dexproxibutene.

6-Dimethylamino-5-methyl-4,4-diphenyl-3-hexanone *see* Isomethadone.

3-(Dimethylaminomethyleneamino)-2,4,6-triiodohydrocinnamic acid ethyl ester *see* Ethyl iopodate.

3-(Dimethylaminomethyleneamino)-2,4,6-triiodohydrocinnamic acid sodium salt *see* Sodium iopodate.

1-Dimethylamino-2,3-methylenedioxy-propane methiodide *see* Oxapropanium iodide.

6-(2-Dimethylamino-2-methylethyl)-6,11-dihydro-5H-pyrido(2,3-b)benzo-diazepin-5-one *see* Propizepine.

10-(2-Dimethylamino-1-methylethyl)-phenothiazine *see* Isopromethazine.

1-[2-(Dimethylamino)-1-methylethyl]-2-phenylcyclohexanol acetate ester *see* Nexeridine.

10-(2-Dimethylamino-1-methylethyl)-2-propionylphenothiazine *see* Propioma-zine.

trans-**3-(2-Dimethylaminomethyl-1-hy-droxycyclohexyl)anisole** *see* Tramadol.

3-Dimethylaminomethylindole *see* Gramine.

8-Dimethylaminomethyl-7-methoxy-3-methylflavone *see* Dimefline.

trans-**2-Dimethylaminomethyl-1-(*m*-methoxyphenyl)cyclohexanol** *see* Tramadol.

1-Dimethylaminomethyl-1-methylpropyl benzoate *see* Amylocaine.

3-Dimethylamino-1-methyl-3-oxo-1-propenyl dimethyl phosphate *see* Dicrotophos.

4-Dimethylamino-3-methylphenyl methylcarbamate *see* Aminocarb.

2-Dimethylamino-2-methylpropyl benzilate *see* Difemerine.

5-(3-Dimethylamino-2-methylpropyl)-10,11-dihydrobenz(b,f)azepine *see* Tri-mipramine.

5-(3-Dimethylamino-1-methylpropyl)-10,11-dihydro-5H-dibenzo(a,d)cyclohep-tene *see* Butriptyline.

10-(3-Dimethylamino-2-methylpropyl)-2-ethylphenothiazine *see* Etymemazine.

10-(3-Dimethylamino-2-methylpropyl)-2-methoxyphenothiazine *see* Levome-promazine.

10-(3-Dimethylamino-2-methylpropyl)-2-(methylthio)phenothiazine *see* Methio-meprazine.

10-(3-Dimethylamino-2-methylpropyl)-phenothiazine *see* Alimemazine.

10-(3-Dimethylamino-2-methylpropyl)-phenothiazine-2-carbonitrile *see* Cyamemazine.

5-Dimethylamino-9-methyl-2-propyl-1H-pyrazole(1,2-a)(1,2,4)benzotriazine-1,3(2H)-dione *see* Azapropazone.

10-[3-(Dimethylamino)-2-methylpropyl]-2-trifluoromethylphenothiazine *see* Trifluomeprazine.

O-**[2-(Dimethylamino)-6-methylpyri-midin-4-yl]** *O,O*-diethyl phosphoro-thioate *see* Pyrimitate.

4-Dimethylamino-1,4,4a,5,5a,6,11,12a-octahydro-3,5,10,12,12a-pentahydroxy-6-methyl-1,11-dioxo-2-naphthacene-carboxamide *see* Doxycycline.

4-Dimethylamino-1,4,4a,5,5a,6,11,12a-octahydro-3,5,10,12,12a-pentahydroxy-6-methylene-1,11-dioxo-2-naphthacene-carboxamide *see* Metacycline.

5-[3-(Dimethylamino)-2-oxopropylidene]-10,11-dihydro-5H-dibenzo(a,d)cyclo-heptene *see* Cotriptyline.

Dimethylaminophenazone *see* Amino-phenazone.

2-Dimethylamino-2-phenylbutyl 3,4,5-tri-methoxybenzoate *see* Trimebutine.

2-Dimethylamino-1-phenyl-3-cyclo-hexene-1-carboxylic acid ethyl ester *see* Tilidine.

2-Dimethylamino-5-phenyl-2-oxazolin-4-one *see* Tozalinone.

2-(3-Dimethylamino-1-phenylpropyl-idene)norbornane *see* Heptaverine.

3β-(Dimethylamino)-5α-pregnane-18,20α-diol diacetate ester *see* Stevaladil.

S,S′-**[2-(Dimethylamino)-1,3-propanediyl] carbamothioate** *see* Cartap.

Dimethylamino-2-propanol inosine *p*-acetamidobenzoate *see* Methisoprinol.

5-(2-Dimethylaminopropionamido)-1,3-diphenylpyrazole *see* Difenamizole.

2-Dimethylaminopropiophenone *see* Metamfepramone.

4-(3-Dimethylaminopropoxy)-1,2,2,6,6-pentamethylpiperidine *see* Pemerid.

4-[(3-Dimethylaminopropyl)amino]-7-

iodoquinoline see Iometin.

9-[[3-(Dimethylamino)propyl]amino]-1-nitroacridine see Nitracrine.

10-(2-Dimethylaminopropyl)-1-azaphenothiazine see Isothipendyl.

10-(3-Dimethylaminopropyl)-1-azaphenothiazine see Prothipendyl.

5-(3-Dimethylaminopropyl)-5H-dibenz(b,f)azepine see Depramine.

5-(3-Dimethylaminopropyl)-5,6-dihydro-11H-dibenz(b,e)azepine see Prazepine.

5-(3-Dimethylaminopropyl)-10,11-dihydro-5H-dibenz(b,f)azepine see Imipramine.

5-(3-Dimethylaminopropyl)-5,11-dihydro-10H-dibenz(b,f)azepin-10-one see Ketimipramine.

5-[3-(Dimethylamino)propyl]-5,6-dihydro-11-methylene-11H-dibenzo(b,e)azepine see Enprazepine.

N-[3-(Dimethylamino)propyl]-5,6-dihydromorphanthridine see Prazepine.

10-(3-Dimethylaminopropyl)-9,9-dimethylacridan see Dimetacrine.

10-(2-Dimethylaminopropyl)-2-dimethylsulfamoylphenothiazine see Dimetotiazine.

5-(3-Dimethylaminopropyl)-6,7,8,9,10,11-hexahydrocyclooct(b)indole see Iprindole.

6-(3-Dimethylaminopropylidene)(12H-benzofuro(3,2-c)(1)benzoxepine see Oxetorone.

(Dimethylaminopropylidene)dibenzocycloheptatriene see Cyclobenzaprine.

5-(3-Dimethylaminopropylidene)dibenzocycloheptene see Proheptatriene.

11(6H)-(3-Dimethylaminopropylidene)-dibenz(b,e)oxepine,
cis- see Cidoxepin.
trans- see Doxepine.

5-(3-Dimethylaminopropylidene)-10,11-dihydrodibenzo(a,d)cycloheptene see Amitriptyline.

11-[3-(Dimethylamino)propylidene]-6,11-dihydrodibenzo(b,e)thiepine see Dosulepin.

9-(3-Dimethylaminopropylidene)-9,10-dihydro-10,10-dimethylanthracene see Melitracen.

11-[3-(Dimethylamino)propylidene]-5,6-dihydromorphanthridine see Elantrine.

4-[3-(DIMETHYLAMINO)PROPYL-IDENE]-4,9-DIHYDROTHIENO-(2,3-b)BENZO(e)THIEPINE ('dithiaden').

9-(3-Dimethylaminopropylidene)-2-methoxyxanthene see Dimeprozan.

9-(3-Dimethylaminopropylidene)thioxanthene see Prothixene.

10-(3-Dimethylaminopropyl)-2-methoxyphenothiazine see Methopromazine.

9-(3-Dimethylaminopropyl)-2-methoxythioxanthen-9-ol see Meprotixol.

17β-[(3-Dimethylaminopropyl)methylamino]androst-4-en-3β-ol see Aza-

costerol.

5-(3-Dimethylaminopropyl)phenanthridinone see Fantridone.

10-(2-Dimethylaminopropyl)phenothiazine see Promethazine.

10-(3-Dimethylaminopropyl)phenothiazine see Promazine.

10-(2-Dimethylaminopropyl)phenothiazin-2-yl ethyl ketone see Propiomazine.

10-(2-Dimethylaminopropyl)phenothiazin-3-yl methyl ketone see Aceprometazine.

10-(3-Dimethylaminopropyl)phenothiazin-3-yl methyl ketone see Acepromazine.

1-[10-(2-Dimethylaminopropyl)phenothiazin-2-yl]-1-propanone see Propiomazine.

4′-[4-(3-Dimethylaminopropyl)piperazin-1-yl]acetamide see Piperamide.

10-(2-Dimethylaminopropyl)-2-propionylphenothiazine see Propiomazine.

10-(3-Dimethylaminopropyl)-2-propionylphenothiazine see Propiopromazine.

(+)-3-(3-Dimethylaminopropyl)-1,3,8,8-tetramethyl-3-azabicyclo(3.2.1)octane methyl sulfate methosulfate see Trimethidinium methosulfate.

2′-(3-Dimethylaminopropylthio)cinnamanilide see Cinanserin.

10-(3-Dimethylaminopropyl)-2-trifluoromethylphenothiazine see Triflupromazine.

2-Dimethylaminopyrazine see Ampyzine.

2-[1-[3-[[2-(Dimethylaminosulfonyl)-10H-phenothiazin-10-yl]propyl]-piperidin-4-yl]ethyl] hexadecanoate see Pipotiazine palmitate.

4-Dimethylamino-o-toluenephosphonous acid sodium salt see Sodium 4-dimethylamino-o-toluenephosphonite.

4-Dimethylamino-m-tolyl methylcarbamate see Aminocarb.

4-Dimethylamino-o-tolylphosphinic acid see Toldimfos.

3-Dimethylamino-2,2,3-trimethylnorbornane see Dimecaine.

2-Dimethylamino-3,5,6-trimethylpyrazine see Triampyzine.

3-Dimethylamino-1,1,2-tris(p-methoxyphenyl)-1-propene see Aminoxytriphene.

4-Dimethylamino-3,5-xylyl methylcarbamate see Mexacarbate.

N,N-**DIMETHYLAMPHETAMINE** ('metromin', 'metrotonin').

1,3-DIMETHYLAMYLAMINE (methylhexaneamine; methylhexamine; 'fortane').

1α,17α-DIMETHYLANDROSTAN-17β-OL-3-ONE (dimethylandrostanolone; DMA; 'demalon').

7β,17-Dimethylandrost-4-en-17β-ol-3-one see Calusterone.

'Dimethylane' see Promoxolane.

ar,ar-**Dimethylaniline** see Xylidine.

2-(2,6-Dimethylanilino)-5,6-dihydro-4H-1,3-thiazine see Xylazine.

2-(2,3-Dimethylanilino)nicotonic acid see Nixylic acid.

2-(2,6-Dimethylanilino)nicotinic acid

164

see Metanixin.
Dimethylarsinic acid *see* Cacodylic acid.
ar,ar-**Dimethylbenzamide** *see* Xylamide.
9,10-Dimethyl-1,2-benzanthracene *see*
7,12-Dimethylbenz(a)anthracene.
7,12-DIMETHYLBENZ(a)ANTHRACENE
(9,10-dimethyl-1,2-benzanthracene;
DMBA).
Dimethylbenzene *see* Xylene.
3,3′-Dimethylbenzidine *see* *o*-Tolidine.
5,6-Dimethylbenzimidazole cobamide
coenzyme *see* Cobamamide.
5,6-Dimethylbenzimidazole-5-deoxyade-
nosylcobamide *see* Cobamamide.
α-**(5,6-Dimethylbenzimidazol-2-yl)cob-**
amide methyl *see* Mecobalamin.
5,6-Dimethylbenzimidazolylcyanocob-
amide *see* Cyanocobalamin.
2,2-Dimethyl-1,3-benzodioxol-4-yl
methylcarbamate *see* Bendiocarb.
8,8-Dimethyl-2H,8H-benzo(1,2-b:3,4-b′)-
dipyran-2-one *see* Seselin.
N,N-**Dimethylbenzofuro(3,2-c)(1)benz-**
oxepin-△⁶(¹²ᴴ),γ-**propylamine** *see* Oxetorone.
N¹-**(3,4-Dimethylbenzoyl-sulfanilamide**
see Sulfadimethylbenzoylamide.
*p,*α-**DIMETHYLBENZYL ALCOHOL** (*p*-
tolyl methyl carbinol).
See also Tocamphyl.
2,4-Dimethylbenzyl chrysanthemate
see Dimethrin.
2,4-Dimethylbenzyl 2,2-dimethyl-3-
(2-methyl-1-propenyl)cyclopropane-
carboxylate *see* Dimethrin.
1,1-Dimethylbiguanide *see* Metformin.
1,1′-Dimethyl-4,4′-bipyridinium dichlor-
ide *see* Paraquat.
3,3-Dimethyl-2-butanol *see* Pinacolyl
alcohol.
1-[2-(1,3-Dimethyl-but-2-enylidene)-
hydrazino]phthalazine *see* Budralazine.
3,3-DIMETHYLBUTYL ACETATE (acetylcarbocholine).
3,3-Dimethylbut-2-yl methylphosphoro-
fluoridate *see* Soman.
Dimethylcaramiphen *see* Metcaraphen.
Dimethylcarbamic acid 2-dimethyl-
amino-5,6-dimethylpyrimidin-4-yl
ester *see* Pirimicarb.
Dimethylcarbamic acid ester of 7-
chloro-1,3-dihydro-3-hydroxy-1-
methyl-5-phenyl-2H-1,4-benzodiazepin-
2-one *see* Camazepam.
Dimethylcarbamodithioic acid, salts
see Ferbam; Ziram.
m-**(Dimethylcarbamoylamino)phenyl**
tert-**butylcarbamate** *see* Karbutilate.
5-[(Dimethylcarbamoyl)methoxy]-10,11-
dihydro-5H-dibenzo(a,d)cycloheptene
see Oxitriptyline.
1-Dimethylcarbamoyl-5-methylpyrazol-
3-yl dimethylcarbamate *see* Dimetilan.
2-(Dimethylcarbamoyl)-1-methylvinyl
dimethyl phosphate *see* Dicrotophos.
3-Dimethylcarbamoylpropyl clofibrate
see Clofibride.

Dimethyl carbate *see* Dimethyl 5-norbor-
nene-2,3-dicarboxylate.
2-(Dimethylcarboxamido)-1-methylvinyl
dimethyl phosphate *see* Dicrotophos.
1-(Dimethylcarboxamido)-1-propen-2-yl
dimethyl phosphate *see* Dicrotophos.
*N,*α-**Dimethylcyclohexaneethylamine** *see*
Propylhexedrine.
2,2-Dimethyl-1,3,5-cyclohexanetrione *see*
Filixic acid.
5,5-Dimethyl-1-cyclohexen-1-ol-3-one
dimethylcarbamate *see* Dimetan.
3,3-Dimethylcysteine *see* Penicillamine.
N,N-**Dimethyldibenzo(b,f)thiepin-10-**
methylamine *see* Damotepine.
N,N-**Dimethyldibenzo(b,e)thiepin-**
△¹¹(⁶ᴴ),γ-**propylamine** *see* Dosulepin.
N,N-**Dimethyldibenz(b,e)oxepin-**△¹¹(⁶ᴴ),γ-
propylamine *see* Doxepin.
Dimethyl 1,4-dihydro-2,6-dimethyl-4-(2-
nitrophenyl)pyridine-3,5-dicarboxylate
see Nifedipine.
Dimethyldihydroresorcinol dimethyl-
carbamate *see* Dimetan.
2,3-Dimethyl-4-dimethylamino-1-
phenyl-3-pyrazolin-5-one *see* Aminophenazone.
10,10-Dimethyl-9-(3-dimethylamino-
propylidene)-9,10-dihydroanthracene
see Melitracen.
Dimethyl [1-(dimethylcarboxamido)-1-
propen-2-yl] phosphate *see* Dicrotophos.
1-[3-[(1,3-Dimethyl-2,4-dioxopyrimidin-
6-yl)amino]propyl]-4-(o-methoxy-
phenyl)piperazine *see* Urapidil.
N,N-**Dimethyl-2,2-diphenoxyethylamine**
see Medifoxamine.
N,N-**Dimethyl-2,2-diphenylacetamide** *see*
Diphenamid.
(+)-*N,N*-**Dimethyl-1,2-diphenylethyl-**
amine *see* *N,N*-Dimethyl-α-phenylphen-
ethylamine.
(−)-*N,N*-**Dimethyl-1,2-diphenylethyl-**
amine *see* Lefetamine.
Dimethyl(diphenylhydroxypropyl)ethyl-
ammonium bromide carbamate *see*
Ambutonium bromide.
N,N-**Dimethyl-3,4-diphenyl-2-methyl-3-**
propionoxy-1-butylamine *see* Propoxyphene.
(+)-*threo*-**3,5-Dimethyl-1,6-diphenyl-1-oxa-**
4-azahexane *see* Dextrofemine.
2,9-Dimethyl-4,7-diphenyl-1,10-phenan-
throline sodium disulfonate *see*
Bathocuproine.
1,4-Dimethyl-1,4-diphenyl-2-tetrazene *see*
Simtrazene.
1,1′-Dimethyl-4,4′-dipyridylium di-
chloride *see* Paraquat.
Dimethyldithiocarbamic acid salts *see*
Cupric dimethyldithiocarbamate;
Ferbam; Ziram.
N,N-**Dimethylene oxide bis(pyridinium-**
4-aldoxime) dichloride *see* Obidoxime.
Dimethylenimine *see* Aziridine.
Dimethylergometrine *see* Methysergide.
Dimethylergonovine *see* Methysergide.

165

7α,17-Dimethylestr-4-en-17β-ol-3-one *see* Mibolerone.

16,16-Dimethylestr-4-en-17β-ol-3-one *see* Metogest.

α,α′-Dimethylethanolamino-4,4′-biacetophenone *see* Hemicholinium.

6α,21-Dimethylethisterone *see* Dimethisterone.

α′-[(1,1-Dimethylethyl)aminomethyl]-4-hydroxy-1,3-benzenedimethanol *see* Salbutamol.

N-(1,1-Dimethylethyl)-N′-ethyl-6-methoxy-1,3,5-triazine-2,4-diamine *see* Terbumeton.

N-(1,1-Dimethylethyl)-N′-ethyl-6-(methylthio)-1,3,5-triazine-2,4-diamine *see* Terbutryn.

2-[4-(1,1-Dimethylethyl)phenoxy]cyclohexyl 2-propynyl sulfite *see* Propargite.

2,5-Dimethyl-3-furyl 4-hydroxy-3,5-diiodophenyl ketone *see* Furidarone.

Dimethylhexestrol *see* Methestrol.

1,5-Dimethylhexylamine *see* Octodrine.

N-(1,5-Dimethylhexyl)isopentylamine *see* Octamylamine.

1,1-Dimethylhydrazine (unsymmetrical dimethylhydrazine; UDMH).

N¹-(3,4-Dimethylisoxazol-5-yl)sulfanilamide *see* Sulfafurazole.

N¹-(4,5-Dimethylisoxazol-3-yl)sulfanilamide *see* Sulfatroxole.

Dimethylmeperidine *see* Trimeperidine.

N,N-Dimethylmercaptamine *see* Captamine.

N,N-Dimethyl-N′-[3-[[(methylamino)carbonyl]oxy]phenyl]methanimidamide *see* Formetanate.

O,O-Dimethyl S-[[2-[1-(methylaminocarboxy)ethyl]thio]ethyl] phosphorothioate *see* Vamidothion.

O,O-Dimethyl S-[2-(methylamino)-2-oxoethyl] phosphorodithioate *see* Dimethoate.

O,O-Dimethyl S-[2-(methylamino)-2-oxoethyl] phosphorothioate *see* Omethoate.

2,3-Dimethyl-4-methylamino-1-phenyl-3-pyrazolin-5-one *see* Noramidopyrine.

9,9-Dimethyl-10-(3-methylaminopropyl)-acridan *see* Monometacrine.

10,10-Dimethyl-9-(3-methylaminopropylidene)-9,10-dihydroanthracene *see* Litracen.

3,3-Dimethyl-1-(3-methylaminopropyl)-1-phenylphthalan *see* Talopram.

3,3-Dimethyl-1-(3-methylaminopropyl)-1-phenylthiophthalan *see* Talsupram.

N,N-Dimethyl-2-(α-methylbenzhydryloxy)ethylamine *see* Moxastin.

1,1-Dimethyl-2-(p-methylbenzhydryloxymethyl)piperidinium bromide *see* Pirdonium bromide.

O,O-Dimethyl S-[[2-[1-(methylcarbamoyl)ethyl]thio]ethyl] phosphorothioate *see* Vamidothion.

O,O-Dimethyl S-(methylcarbamoylmethyl) phosphorodithioate *see* Dimethoate.

O,O-Dimethyl S-(methylcarbamoylmethyl) phosphorothioate *see* Omethoate.

Dimethyl (2-methylcarbamoyl-1-methylvinyl) phosphate *see* Monocrotophos.

N,N-Dimethyl-N′-[m-(methylcarbamoyloxy)phenyl]formamidine *see* Formetanate.

Dimethyl (1-methylcarboxamido-1-propen-2-yl) phosphate *see* Monocrotophos.

Dimethyl[2-(N-methyldodecanamido)-ethyl](phenylcarbamoylmethyl)ammonium chloride *see* Dofamium chloride.

4,4-Dimethyl-1-[(3,4-methylenedioxy)-phenyl]-1-penten-3-ol *see* Stiripentol.

O,O-Dimethyl S-[2-[[1-methyl-2-(methylamino)-2-oxoethyl]thio]ethyl] phosphorothioate *see* Vamidothion.

Dimethyl 1-methyl-3-methylamino-3-oxo-1-propenyl phosphate *see* Monocrotophos.

N,N-Dimethyl-2-(o-methyl-α-phenylbenzyloxy)ethylamine *see* Orphenadrine.

1,1-Dimethyl-2-[(p-methyl-α-phenylbenzyloxy)methyl]piperidinium bromide *see* Pirdonium bromide.

2,3-Dimethyl-4-(3-methyl-2-phenylmorpholinomethyl)-1-phenyl-3-pyrazolin-5-one *see* Morazone.

N¹,N¹-Dimethyl-3-(4-methylpiperazin-1-ylcarbonyl)sulfanilamide *see* Delfantrine.

N,N-Dimethyl-9-[3-(4-methylpiperazin-1-yl)propylidene]thioxanthene-2-sulfonamide *see* Tiotixene.

N-[[2,2-Dimethyl-3-(2-methyl-1-propenyl)cyclopropanecarbonyloxy]-methyl] 3,4,5,6-tetrahydrophthalimide *see* Tetramethrin.

2,2-Dimethyl-3-(2-methylpropenyl)cyclopropanecarboxylic acid *see* Chrysanthemic acid.

O,O-Dimethyl O-[2-(methylthio)ethyl] phosphorothioate *see* Demephion-O.

O,O-Dimethyl S-[2-(methylthio)ethyl] phosphorothioate *see* Demephion-S.

3,5-Dimethyl-4-(methylthio)phenyl methylcarbamate *see* Methiocarb.

O,O-Dimethyl O-(p-(methylthio)-m-tolyl) phosphorothioate *see* Fenthion.

3,17-Dimethylmorphinan *see* Dimemorfan.

N,3-Dimethylmorphinan *see* Dimemorfan.

O,O-Dimethyl S-(2-morpholino-2-oxoethyl) phosphorodithioate *see* Morphothion.

O,O-Dimethyl S-(2-morpholin-4-ylacetyl) phosphorodithioate *see* Morphothion.

7α,17-Dimethylnandrolone *see* Mibolerone.

2,3-Dimethyl-4-nicotinamido-1-phenyl-3-pyrazolin-5-one *see* Nifenazone.

1,2-Dimethyl-5-nitroimidazole *see* Dimetridazole.

α,2-Dimethyl-5-nitroimidazole-1-ethanol *see* Secnidazole.

O,O-Dimethyl O-(p-nitrophenyl) phosphorothioate *see* Parathion methyl.

O,S-**Dimethyl** *O*-(*p*-nitrophenyl) **phosphorothioate** *see* Parathion isomethyl.

DIMETHYLNITROSAMINE (nitrosodimethylamine; DMN).

Dimethyl (*p*-**nitro**-*m*-**tolyl**) **phosphate** *see* Fenitrooxon.

O,O-**Dimethyl** *O*-(*p*-nitro-*m*-tolyl) **phosphorothioate** *see* Fenitrothion.

O,O-**DIMETHYL** *S*-(*p*-**NITRO**-*m*-**TOLYL**) **PHOSPHOROTHIOATE** ('isosumithion').

17,17-Dimethyl-18-norandrosta-4,13-dien-11α-ol-3-one *see* Nordinone.

DIMETHYL 5-NORBORNENE-2,3-DICARBOXYLATE (3,6-*endo*-methylene-1,2,3,6-tetrahydrophthalic acid dimethyl ester; dimethyl carbate; RP-50; 'dimalone').

6,6-Dimethyl-2-norpinene *see* Apopinene.

2-[2-(6,6-Dimethylnorpinen-2-yl)ethoxy]-triethylamine *see* Myrtecaine.

7α,17-Dimethyl-19-nortestosterone *see* Mibolerone.

Dimethyloctadecylamine *see* Dimantine.

2-(3,7-Dimethyl-2-octadienyl)hydroquinone *see* Geroquinol.

3,7-Dimethyl-2,6-octadienyl trimethyltetradecatrienoate *see* Gefarnate.

3,5-Dimethyl-*N*-(4,6,6a,7,8,9,10,10a-octahydro-4,7-dimethylindolo(4,3-fg)quinolin-9-yl)pyrazole-1-carboxamide *see* Metoquizine.

1,1-Dimethyl-3-(octahydro-4,7-methano-1H-inden-5-yl)urea *see* Noruron.

4,5-Dimethylol-3-hydroxy-α-picoline *see* Pyridoxine.

Dimethylolurea *see* 1,3-Bis(hydroxymethyl)-urea.

5,5-Dimethyl-2,4-oxazolidinedione *see* Dimethadione.

*N*¹-[(4,5-Dimethyloxazol-2-yl)amidino]-sulfanilamide *see* Sulfaguanole.

*N*¹-(4,5-Dimethyloxazol-2-yl)sulfanilamide *see* Sulfamoxole.

O,O-**Dimethyl** *S*-(4-oxobenzotriazin-3-yl-methyl) **phosphorodithioate** *see* Azinphosmethyl.

5,5-Dimethyl-1-oxocyclohex-2-en-3-yl dimethylcarbamate *see* Dimetan.

3-[2-(3,5-Dimethyl-2-oxocyclohexyl)-2-hydroxyethyl]glutarimide *see* Cycloheximide.

3,7-Dimethyl-1-(5-oxohexyl)xanthine *see* Pentoxifylline.

1,7-DIMETHYL-2-OXO-7-NORBORNANECARBOXALDEHYDE (π-oxocamphor; 8-oxocamphor; 'vitacampher').

4-(4,4-Dimethyl-3-oxopentyl)-1,2-diphenylpyrazolidine-3,5-dione *see* Tribuzone.

6-(2,2-Dimethyl-5-oxo-4-phenylimidazolin-1-yl)penicillanic acid *see* Hetacillin.

3-[[(2,3-Dimethyl-5-oxo-1-phenyl-3-pyrazolin-4-yl)amino]methyl]-4-isopropyl-2-methyl-1-phenyl-3-pyrazolin-5-one *see* Bisfenazone.

[[(2,3-Dimethyl-5-oxo-1-phenyl-3-

pyrazolin-4-yl)methyl]amino]methanesulfonic acid sodium salt *see* Novaminsulfon.

2-(2,2-Dimethyl-1-oxopropyl)-1H-indene-1,3(2H)-dione *see* Pindone.

3,3-Dimethyl-7-oxo-4-thia-1-azabicyclo-(3.2.0)heptane-2-carboxylic acid *see* Penicillanic acid.

Dimethyloxychinizin *see* Phenazone.

N,N-**Dimethyl(3-palmitamidopropyl)-aminoacetic acid** *see* Pendecamaine.

N,α-**Dimethyl-*p*-pentylphenethylamine** *see* Amfepentorex.

α,α-**Dimethylphenethylamine** *see* Phentermine.

N,α-**Dimethylphenethylamine** *see* Methamphetamine.

2,α-Dimethylphenethylamine *see* Ortetamine.

Dimethyl(2-phenoxyethyl)-2-thenyl-ammonium *p*-**chlorobenzenesulfonate** *see* Thenium closilate.

[2-(2,6-Dimethylphenoxy)ethyl]trimethylammonium bromide *see* Xylocholine.

5-(3,5-Dimethylphenoxymethyl)oxazolidin-2-one *see* Metaxalone.

1-(2,6-Dimethylphenoxy)-2-propylamine *see* Mexiletine.

[2-(2,6-Dimethylphenoxy)propyl]trimethylammonium chloride *see* β-Methylxylocholine.

N-(**Dimethylphenyl)anthranilic acid** *see* Mefenamic acid.

N,N-**Dimethyl-*p*-phenylazoaniline** *see* Dimethylaminoazobenzene.

N,N-**Dimethyl-α-phenylbenzeneacet-amide** *see* Diphenamid.

N,N-**Dimethyl-γ-phenylcyclohexane-propylamine** *see* Gamfexine.

Dimethyl [1,2-phenylenebis(iminocarbonothioyl)]bis(carbamate) *see* Thiophanate-methyl.

Dimethyl 4,4′-(*o*-phenylene)bis(3-thioallophanate) *see* Thiophanate-methyl.

1,1-Dimethyl-2-phenylethylamine *see* Phentermine.

N,N-**Dimethyl-3-phenyl-1-indanamine** *see* Dimefadane.

N,N-**Dimethyl-1-phenylindene-1-ethyl-amine** *see* Indriline.

(2,4-Dimethylphenyl)methyl 2,2-dimethyl-3-(2-methyl-1-propenyl)cyclopropanecarboxylate *see* Dimethrin.

3,4-Dimethyl-2-phenylmorpholine *see* Phendimetrazine.

N,N-**Dimethyl-γ-phenyl-△²,γ-norbornane-propylamine** *see* Heptaverine.

6-[(2,2-Dimethyl-4-phenyl-5-oxazolidinyl-idene)amino]-3,3-dimethyl-7-oxa-4-thia-1-azabicyclo(3.2.0)heptane-2-carboxylic acid *see* Hetacillin.

(+)-*N,N*-**DIMETHYL-α-PHENYLPHEN-ETHYLAMINE** ((+)-1-dimethylamino-1,2-diphenylethane; (+)-*N,N*-dimethyl-1,2-diphenylethylamine; (+)-*N,N*-dimethyl-stilbylamine; 'α-spa').

167

(−)-*N*,*N*-**Dimethyl-α-phenylphenethyl-amine** *see* Lefetamine.

1,1-DIMETHYL-4-PHENYLPIPERAZI-NIUM IODIDE (DMPP).

1,3-Dimethyl-4-phenyl-4-propionoxy-azacycloheptane *see* Proheptazine.

1,3-Dimethyl-4-phenyl-4-propionoxy-piperidine *see* Alphaprodine; Betaprodine.

2,3-Dimethyl-1-phenyl-3-pyrazolin-5-one *see* Phenazone.

N,*N*-**Dimethyl-3-phenyl-3-pyrid-2-yl-propylamine** *see* Pheniramine.

1,2-Dimethyl-3-phenyl-3-pyrrolidyl propionate *see* Prodilidine.

Dimethylphenylsuccinimide *see* Mesuximide.

Dimethylphenylthenylethylenediamine *see* Methaphenilene.

N,*N*-**Dimethyl-3-phenyl-3-*p*-tolyl-1-propylamine** *see* Tolpropamine.

1,1-Dimethyl-3-phenylurea *see* Fenuron.

O,*S*-**Dimethyl phosphoramidothioate** *see* Methamidophos.

O,*O*-**Dimethyl phosphorodithioate *S*-ester with 3-(mercaptomethyl)-1,2,3-benzotriazine-4(3H)-one** *see* Azinphos-methyl.

2′,6′-Dimethylphthalanilic acid *see* Ftaxilide.

DIMETHYL PHTHALATE (DMP; methyl phthalate; 'avolin', 'citrola', 'dimp', 'fermine', 'mipax', 'mugia', 'palatinol M', 'sketofax').

O,*O*-**DIMETHYL *S*-PHTHALIMIDO-METHYL PHOSPHORODITHIOATE** ('imidan', 'prolate').

1,6-Dimethylpipecolic acid diethylamino-ethyl ester dimethiodide *see* Dicolinium iodide.

1,6-Dimethylpipecolic acid dimethyl-aminoethyl ester dimethiodide *see* Dimecolonium.

2,5-Dimethylpiperazine *see* Lupetazine.

2,6-Dimethylpiperidine *see* Nanofin.

N-**[4-(2,6-Dimethylpiperid-1-yl)butyl]-2-phenoxy-2-phenylacetamide** *see* Oxir-amide.

1,1-Dimethyl-4-piperidylidenediphenyl-methane methylsulfate *see* Diphemanil metilsulfate.

2,4′-Dimethyl-3-piperid-1-ylpropio-phenone *see* Tolperisone.

6,17-Dimethylpregna-4,6-diene-3,20-dione *see* Medrogestone.

6α,16α-Dimethylpregn-4-en-3β-ol-20-one *see* Demepregnen.

2,2-Dimethylpropane *see* Neopentane.

2,2-Dimethylpropionic acid *see* Pivalic acid.

4-[2-(2,2-Dimethylpropionyl)ethyl]-1,2-diphenyl-3,5-pyrazolidinedione *see* Tribuzone.

2,2′-Dimethyl-2-propylaminopropion-anilide *see* Quatacaine.

1,3-Dimethylpurin-2-one-6-thione *see* 6-Thiotheophylline.

9-(3,5-Dimethylpyrazole-1-carboxamido)-

4-ethyl-7-methyloctahydroindolo-(4,3-fg)quinoline *see* Toquizine.

N,*N*′-**Dimethylpyrazole-3,4-dicarbox-amide** *see* Ethipyrole.

4,6-Dimethyl-3(2H)-pyridazinone *see* Cetohexazine.

N,*N*-**Dimethyl-*N*′-pyrid-2-yl-*N*′-then-2-yl-ethylenediamine** *see* Methapyrilene.

N,*N*-**Dimethyl-*N*′-pyrid-2-yl-*N*′-then-3-yl-ethylenediamine** *see* Thenyldiamine.

5-[*p*-(4,6-Dimethylpyrimidin-2-ylsulfa-moyl)phenylazo]salicylic acid *see* Salazosulfadimidine.

N^1-**(2,6-Dimethylpyrimid-4-yl)sulfanil-amide** *see* Sulfasomidine.

N^1-**(4,6-Dimethylpyrimid-2-yl)sulfanil-amide** *see* Sulfadimidine.

2,5-Dimethyl-1-pyrrolidinepropanol salicylate *see* Pranosal.

1,1-Dimethylpyrrolidinium methosulfate *see* Poldine.

10-(1,3-Dimethylpyrrolidin-3-ylmethyl)-phenothiazine *see* Dimelazine.

Dimethylquinolinyl methyl sulfate urea *see* Quinuronium.

6,6-Dimethyl-L-ribitylbenzimidazole *see* α-Ribazole.

7,8-Dimethyl-10-(1-ribityl)isoalloxazine *see* Riboflavin.

5,6-Dimethyl-1-ribosylbenzimidazole *see* Ribazole.

N,*N*-**Dimethylserotonin** *see* Bufotenine.

Dimethylsiloxane polymer *see* Dimeticone.

N,*N*-**Dimethylspiro[dibenz(b,e)oxepin-11(6H),2′-(1,3)dioxolane]-4′-methyl-amine** *see* Spiroxepin.

(+)-*N*,*N*-**Dimethylstilbylamine** *see* (+)-*N*,*N*-Dimethyl-α-phenylphenethyl-amine.

(−)-*N*,*N*-**Dimethylstilbylamine** *see* Lefet-amine.

2,2-Dimethyl-5-styryloxazolidin-4-one *see* Methastyridone.

Dimethylsulfadiazine *see* Sulfadimidine.

2-(Dimethylsulfamoyl)-10-[3-(1-methyl-piperazin-4-yl)propyl]phenothiazine *see* Thioproperazine.

1-[3-[2-(Dimethylsulfamoyl)pheno-thiazin-10-yl]propyl]-4-(2-hydroxy-ethyl)piperidine *see* Pipotiazine.

3,4-Dimethyl-*N*-sulfanilylbenzamide *see* Sulfadimethylbenzoylamide.

Dimethylsulfapyrimidine *see* Sulfadimidine.

2-[7-[1,1-Dimethyl-3-(4-sulfobutyl)-benz(e)indolin-2-ylidene]-1,3,5-heptatrienyl]-1,1-dimethyl-3-(4-sulfo-butyl)-1H-benz(e)indolium hydroxide *see* Indocyanine green.

DIMETHYLSULFOLANE (2,4-dimethyl-sulfolane; 2,4-dimethyltetrahydrothiophene 1,1-dioxide).

DIMETHYLSULFONAL (bis(ethylsulfonyl)-diethylmethane; 3,3-bis(ethylsulfonyl)-pentane; 'tetronal').

Dimethylsulfonyloxybutane *see* Busulfan.

DIMETHYL SULFOXIDE*** (DMSO; dimexide; methyl sulfoxide; SQ-9453; DM-70; DM-90; 'camesol 90', 'deltan Berna', 'dolicur', 'dromisol', 'hyodur', 'infiltrina', 'phlebolan', 'somnipront', 'syntexan').

7,17-Dimethyltestosterone see Bolasterone.

Dimethyl tetrachloroterephthalate see Chlorthal-dimethyl.

DIMETHYLTHIAMBUTENE* (3-dimethylamino-1,1-dithien-2-yl-but-1-ene; *N*,*N*,1-trimethyl-3,3-dithien-2-ylallylamine; BW-338C48; 'baldon', 'ohton').

2,7-Dimethylthianthrene see Mesulfen.

1-[4-(2,4-Dimethylthiazol-5-yl)butyl]-4-(4-methylthiazol-2-yl)piperazine see Peratizole.

m,*N*-**Dimethylthiocarbanilic acid *O*-indan-5-yl ester** see Tolindate.

m,*N*-**Dimethylthiocarbanilic acid *O*-(1,2,3,4-tetrahydro-1,4-methanonaphth-6-yl) ester** see Tolciclate.

N,*N*-**Dimethylthioxanthene-△⁹,γ-propylamine** see Prothixene.

1,3-Dimethyl-6-thioxanthine see 6-Thiotheophylline.

Dimethyltoluthionine chloride see Tolonium chloride.

N,*N*-**Dimethyl-*p*-(*m*-tolylazo)aniline** see 4-Dimethylamino-3'-methylazobenzene.

5-(3,3-Dimethyl-1-triazeno)imidazole-4-carboxamide see Dacarbazine.

5-(3,3-Dimethyl-1-triazeno)-2-methylimidazole-4-carboxylic acid ethyl ester see Ethyl 5-(3,3-dimethyl-1-triazeno)-2-methylimidazole-4-carboxylate.

5-(3,3-Dimethyl-1-triazeno)-2-phenylimidazole-4-carboxylic acid ethyl ester see Ethyl 5-(3,3-dimethyl-1-triazeno)-2-phenylimidazole-4-carboxylate.

Dimethyl (2,2,2-trichloro-1-hydroxyethyl)phosphonate see Metrifonate.

Dimethyl (2,2,2-trichloro-1-hydroxyethyl)phosphonate butyrate see Butonate.

O,*O*-**Dimethyl *O*-(2,4,5-trichlorophenyl) phosphorothioate** see Fenclofos.

Dimethyl (3,5,6-trichloropyrid-2-yl) phosphate see Fospirate.

O,*O*-**Dimethyl *O*-(3,5,6-trichloropyrid-2-yl) phosphorothioate** see Chlorpyrifos methyl.

2,6-Dimethyl-4-tridecylmorpholine see Tridemorph.

1,1-Dimethyl-3-(*m*-trifluoromethylphenyl)urea see Fluometuron.

1,1-Dimethyl-3-(α,α,α-trifluoro-*m*-tolyl)-urea see Fluometuron.

3,7-Dimethyl-9-(2,6,6-trimethyl-1-cyclohexen-1-yl)nona-2,4,6,8-tetraenal see Retinal.

3,7-Dimethyl-9-(2,6,6-trimethyl-1-cyclohexen-1-yl)nona-2,3,6,8-tetraen-1-oic acid see Tretinoin.

3,7-Dimethyl-9-(2,6,6-trimethyl-1-cyclohexen-1-yl)nona-2,4,6,8-tetraen-1-ol see Retinol.

1,3-Dimethyltrimethylene dimesylate see Dimethyltrimethylene mesilate.

1,3-Dimethyltrimethylene di(methanesulfonate) see Dimethyltrimethylene mesilate.

DIMETHYLTRIMETHYLENE MESILATE (1,3-dimethyltrimethylene di-(methanesulfonate); dimethyltrimethylene dimesylate; 2,4-bis(methanesulfonyloxy)-pentane; CB-2387).

DIMETHYLTUBOCURARINE CHLORIDE* (tubocurarine dimethyl ether; dimethyltubocurarinium chloride; *O*,*O*-dimethyl-(+)-tubocurarine chloride; 'diamethine', 'mecostrin', 'metubine').

N,*N*-**Dimethyltyramine** see Hordenine.

Dimethylurethamide see Meturedepa.

Dimethylurethimine see Meturedepa.

1,3-Dimethylxanthine see Theophylline.

1,7-Dimethylxanthine see Paraxanthine.

3,7-Dimethylxanthine see Theobromine.

2,2-Dimethyl-5-(2,5-xylyloxy)valeric acid see Gemfibrozil.

'Dimethylyn' see Promoxolane.

DIMETICONE* (poly(dimethylsiloxane); dimethylsiloxane polymer; methylpolysiloxane; silidone; dimethicone; polysilane; simethicone; 'aeropax', 'antifoam A', 'asilone', 'barosil', 'bicolon', 'ceolat', 'covicone', 'DC antifoam', 'deselan', 'disflatyl', 'endo-paractol', 'fulguran', 'meteorex', 'minifom', 'mylanta', 'mylicon', 'sicol', 'silane', 'silazulone', 'silicoderm', 'siopel', 'syl', 'vasogen'). *See also* Bisacodyl with dimeticone.

DIMETICONE 350 (dimethicone 350; 'dymasyl').

DIMETICONE WITH ALGELDRATE ('paractol').

DIMETILAN* (1-(dimethylcarbamoyl)-5-methylpyrazol-3-yl dimethylcarbamate; 1-(dimethylaminocarbonyl)-5-methyl-1H-pyrazol-3-yl dimethylcarbamate; OMS-479; 'snip').

'Dimetina' see Phenbenzamine.

DIMETINDENE* (2-[1-[2-(2-dimethyl-aminoethyl)inden-3-yl]ethyl]pyridine; 2-dimethylaminoethyl-3-(1-pyrid-2-ylethyl)-indene; dimethindene; dimethypyrindene; dimetindene hydrogen maleate; Su-6518; 'fenistil', 'fenostil', 'forhistal').

Dimetiotazine* see Dimetotiazine.

DIMETOFRINE* (1-(4-hydroxy-3,5-dimethoxyphenyl)-2-methylaminoethanol; 4-hydroxy-3,5-dimethoxy-α-methylamino-methylbenzyl alcohol; SM-14; 'pressamina').

DIMETOTIAZINE* (10-(2-dimethyl-aminopropyl)-2-dimethylsulfamoylpheno-thiazine; 10-(2-dimethylaminopropyl)-*N*,*N*-dimethylphenothiazine-2-sulfonamide; dimethothiazine; dimetiotazine; fonazine; IL-6302; RP-8599; 'banistyl', 'migristene').

DIMETOTIAZINE MESILATE (dimetotiazine methanesulfonate; fonazine mesylate; 'migristine', 'promaquid').

DIMETRIDAZOLE (1,2-dimethyl-5-nitro-imidazole; RP-8595; 'emtryl', 'entryl').

DIMEVAMIDE* (4-dimethylamino-2,2-

169

diphenylvaleramide).

Dimexide (tr) *see* Dimethyl sulfoxide.

'Dimid' *see* Diphenamid.

DIMIDIUM BROMIDE* (3,8-diamino-5-methyl-6-phenylphenanthridinium bromide; phenanthridinium 1553; 'trypadine').

'Diminal' *see* Vinbarbital.

DIMINAZENE*** (4,4'-(diazoamino)benz-amidine; 1,3-bis(*p*-amidinophenyl)triazene; *p,p'*-diamidino-1,3-diphenyltriazene; di-guanyldiazoaminobenzene; 'berenil').

'Dimite' *see* Chlorfenethol.

'Dimitronal' *see* Cinnarizine.

'Dimocillin' *see* Meticillin.

'Dimorlin' *see* Dextromoramide.

DIMORPHOLAMINE* (*N,N'*-bis(morpho-linocarbonyl)-*N,N'*-dibutylethylenedi-amine; *N,N'*-dibutyl-*N,N'*-dicarboxy-morpholineethylenediamine; Th-1064; 'theraleptique', 'theraptique').

'Dimorphone' *see* Hydromorphone.

'Dimotane' *see* Brompheniramine maleate.

'Dimothyn' *see* Aluminium glycinate.

DIMOXYLINE*** (1-(4-ethoxy-3-methoxy-benzyl)-6,7-dimethoxy-3-methylisoquino-line; dimoxyline phosphate; dioxyline; L-08146; 'paveril').

'Dimp' *see* Dimethyl phthalate.

'Dimplex' *see* Hexachlorophene.

1-(3,3-Diphenylpropyl)hexahydroazepine *see* Hexadiphane.

DIMPYLATE*** (*O,O*-diethyl *O*-(2-iso-propyl-6-methylpyrimidin-4-yl) phos-phorothioate; *O,O*-diethyl *O*-[6-methyl-2-(1-methylethyl)-4-pyrimidinyl] phosphoro-thioate; diazinon; G-24480; 'basudin', 'neocidol', 'nucidol', 'sarolex', 'spectro-cide').

'Dimyril' *see* Isoaminile.

DINEX* (2-cyclohexyl-4,6-dinitrophenyl; dinitro-*o*-cyclohexylphenol; DNOCHP; SN-46; 'pedinex').

DINEX DICYCLOHEXYLAMINE (dinex dicyclohexylamine derivative; dinex bis-(cyclohexanamine) derivative; 'dynone II').

DINEX SODIUM ('anobesina').

Dinezin (tr) *see* Diethazine.

3,6-Dinicotinoylmorphine *see* Nicomor-phine.

'Dinile' *see* Succinonitrile.

'Dinintel' *see* Clobenzorex.

DINIPROFYLLINE*** (7-(2,3-dihydroxy-propyl)theophylline bis(nicotinate ester); diprophylline dinicotinate).

DINIPROFYLLINE WITH PHENO-BARBITAL ('corverum').

DINITOLMIDE** (3,5-dinitro-*o*-toluamide; 2-methyl-3,5-dinitrobenzene; zoalene; 'zoamix').

DINITRAMINE (*N*³,*N*³-diethyl-2,4-dinitro-6-(trifluoromethyl)-*m*-phenylenediamine; *N*⁴,*N*⁴-diethyl-α,α,α-trifluoro-3,5-dinitrotoluene-2,4-diamine; 'cobex').

3,5-Dinitrobenzamide *see* Nitromide.

Dinitrochlorobenzene *see* 1-Chloro-2,4-dinitrobenzene.

DINITRO-*o*-CRESOL (4,6-dinitro-*o*-cresol;

2-methyl-4,6-dinitrophenol; DN; DNOC; 'antinonin', 'dekrysil', 'detal', 'dinitrol', 'dinitrosol', 'ditrosal', 'effusan', 'elgetol', 'elipol', 'K-III', 'K-IV', 'lipan', 'nitrofar', 'prokarbol', 'sinox').

Dinitro-*o*-cyclohexylphenol *see* Dinex.

2,6-Dinitro-*N,N*-dipropyl-α,α,α-trifluoro-*p*-toluidine *see* Trifluralin.

3,5-Dinitro-*N*⁴,*N*⁴-dipropylsulfanilamide *see* Oryzalin.

Dinitrogen monoxide *see* Nitrous oxide.

'Dinitrol' *see* Dinitro-*o*-cresol.

2,6-Dinitro-4-octylphenyl 2-butenoate *see* Dinocap.

2,6-Dinitro-4-octylphenyl crotonate *see* Dinocap.

Dinitropropylacetic acid *see* Dinitrovaleric acid.

3,5-Dinitrosalicylic acid 2-(5-nitrofur-furylidene)hydrazide *see* Nifursol.

'Dinitrosol' *see* Dinitro-*o*-cresol.

3,5-Dinitro-*o*-toluamide *see* Dinitolmide.

DINOBUTON* (2-*sec*-butyl-4,6-dinitro-phenyl isopropyl carbonate; 1-methyl-ethyl [2-(1-methylpropyl)-4,6-dinitro-phenyl] carbonate; dinoseb isopropyl carbonate; 'acrex', 'dessin').

DINOCAP* (2,6-dinitro-4-octylphenyl 2-butenoate with admixture of 2,4-dinitro-6-octylphenyl 2-butenoate; 2,6-dinitro-4-octylphenyl and 2,4-dinitro-6-octylphenyl crotonates; CR-1639; DNOPC; 'arathane', 'crotothane', 'iscothane', 'karathane', mildex').

DINOPROP* (2-isopropyl-3-methyl-4,6-dinitrophenol; 3-methyl-2-(1-methylethyl)-4,6-dinitrophenol; DNOIPP; DNPP; 'motylkopielik').

DINOPROST*** (7-[3α,5α-dihydroxy-2β-(3(*S*)-hydroxy-*trans*-oct-1-enyl)cyclopent-1-yl]*cis*-hept-5-enoic acid; 9α,11α,15-tri-hydroxy-5-*cis*-13-*trans*-prostadienoic acid; prostaglandin F₂α; U-14583).

DINOPROST TROMETAMOL (dinoprost tromethamine; prostaglandin F₂α trometamol; PGF₂αTHAM; U-14583E; 'prostin F2 alpha injectable').

Dinoprost tromethamine* *see* Dinoprost trometamol.

DINOPROSTONE*** (7-[3α-hydroxy-2β-(3(*S*)-hydroxy-*trans*-oct-1-enyl)-5-oxo-cyclopent-1-yl]*cis*-hept-5-enoic acid; 11α,15-dihydroxy-9-oxo-5-*cis*-13-*trans*-prostadienoic acid; prostaglandin E₂; U-12062).

DINOSEB* (2-(1-methylpropyl)-4,6-dinitro-phenol; 2-*sec*-butyl-4,6-dinitrophenol; DNBP; DNIBF; 'dibutox', 'gebutox').

DINOSEB ACETATE ('aretit', 'ivosit').

Dinoseb isopropyl carbonate *see* Dino-buton.

Dinoseb 3-methyl-2-butenoate *see* Bina-pacryl.

Dinoseb senecioate *see* Binapacryl.

DINOSEB TROLAMINE (dinoseb com-pound with 2,2',2''-nitrilotriethanol; DNOSBP; DNSBP; 'premerge').

170

DINSED*** (N,N'-ethylenebis(3-nitroben-zenesulfonamide); N,N'-bis(3-nitroben-zenesulfonyl)ethylenediamine).
'Dinuclan' see Salsalate.
'Dinyl' see Biphenyl.
Diochin (tr) see Dioquin.
'Dioctylal' see Sodium dioctyl sulfosuccinate.
Dioctyl sulfosuccinate calcium see Calcium dioctyl sulfosuccinate.
Dioctyl sulfosuccinate sodium see Sodium dioctyl sulfosuccinate.
'Diocycline' see Diiodohydroxyquin with tetracycline.
'Diocyl' see Dicycloverine.
DIODONE** (3,5-diiodo-4-oxo-1(4H)-pyrid-ineacetic acid diethanolamine salt; iodo-pyracet; RP-3203).
DIODONE MEGLUMINE* (diodone methylglucamine; 'pyelombrine M').
Diodoxyquinoline see Diiodohydroxy-quin.
Diolamine* see Diethanolamine.
'Diolan' see Ethylmorphine.
'Diomax' see Acetazolamide.
'Dionine' see Ethylmorphine.
'Diopal' see Oxyphenisatin and Scopolamine methyl bromide.
DIOQUIN (tr) (2-diethylaminoethyl 2-qui-nuclidinecarboxylate dimethiodide; diochin).
Dioscorea polystacha, steroid saponins see Polisaponin.
'Diothane' see Diperodon.
'Diothoid' see Diperodon.
'Diothyl' see Pyrimitate.
'Diotroxin' see Liotrix.
'Diovac' see Sodium dioctyl sulfosuccinate.
'Diovocyclin' see Estradiol dipropionate.
DIOXACARB* (o-(1,3-dioxolan-2-yl)phenyl methylcarbamate; dioxicarb; dioxocarb; 'elocron', 'famid').
(3,8-Dioxa-4,7-dioxodecamethylene-1,10)-bis(adamant-1-yldimethylammonium iodide) see Diadonium iodide.
DIOXADROL*** (DL-2,2-diphenyl-4-piperid-2-yl-1,3-dioxolane; (±)-2-(2,2-diphenyl-1,3-dioxolan-4-yl)piperidine; oxadrol; CL-639C; 'rydar').
See also Dexoxadrol; Levoxadrol.
3,14-Dioxahexadecamethylene-1,16-bis-[(carbopropoxymethyl)dimethyl-ammonium bromide] see Dioxahexa-dekanium bromide.
DIOXAHEXADEKANIUM BROMIDE* (3,14-dioxahexadecamethylene-1,16-bis-[(carbopropoxymethyl)dimethylammonium bromide]; G-25178; 'prestonal').
DIOXAMATE*** (2-methyl-2-nonyl-1,3-dioxolan-4-ylmethyl carbamate; carbamate of 2-methyl-2-nonyl-1,3-dioxolane-4-methanol; A-2655).
Dioxan see Dioxane.
m-DIOXANE (dihydro-m-dioxin; 1,3-dioxane; m-dioxan).
p-DIOXANE (tetrahydro-p-dioxin; 1,4-dioxane; p-dioxan; diethylene dioxide).
p-Dioxanedithiol bisdiethyl phosphoro-

dithioate see Dioxation.
S,S'-1,4-Dioxane-2,3-diyl-O,O,O',O'-tetra-ethyl phosphorodithioate see Dioxation.
'Dioxanin' see Acetyldigoxin.
1-(2-m-Dioxan-2-ylethyl)-4-(3-pheno-thiazin-10-ylpropyl)piperazine see Oxaprazine.
10-[3-[4-(2-m-Dioxan-2-ylethyl)piperazin-1-yl]propyl]phenothiazine see Oxa-prazine.
10-[3-[4-(2-m-Dioxanylethyl)piperazin-1-yl]propyl]-2-trifluoromethylpheno-thiazine see Oxaflumazine.
3,6-Dioxaoctane-1,8-diol see Triethylene glycol.
DIOXAPHETYL BUTYRATE*** (ethyl α,α-diphenyl-4-morpholinebutyrate; ethyl 4-morpholino-2,2-diphenylbutyrate).
(1,4-Dioxaspiro(4,5)dec-2-ylmethyl)-guanidine see Guanadrel.
Dioxatetradecamethylenebis[(carbo-propoxymethyl)dimethyl ammonium bromide] see Prodeconium.
Dioxathion* see Dioxation.
DIOXATION*** (S,S'-1,4-dioxane-2,3-diyl-O,O,O',O'-tetraethyl phosphorodithioate; S,S'-diester of p-dioxane-2,3-dithiol with O,O-diethylphosphorodithioate; p-dioxane-dithiol bis(diethylphosphorodithioate); S,S',5,5'-p-dioxane-2,3-diyl bis(O,O-diethyl phosphorodithioate); dioxathion; mixture of cis and trans forms of dioxation; Ac-528; 'delnav', 'hercules 528', 'lirofen', 'lirophen', 'navadel').
'Dioxatrine' see Benzetimide.
DIOXETHEDRIN*** (α-(1-ethylamino-ethyl)-3,4-dihydroxybenzyl alcohol; 1-(3,4-dihydroxyphenyl)-2-ethylamino-1-propanol; N-ethylcorbadrine; α-(1-ethyl-aminoethyl)-protocatechuyl alcohol).
Dioxicarb see Dioxacarb.
'Dioxidan' see Dantron with calcium dioctyl sulfosuccinate.
DIOXIDINE (tr) (quinoxaline-2,3-di-methanol 1,4-dioxide).
Dioxidine diacetate see Quinoxidine.
5-(10,10-Dioxido-9-oxothioxanthen-3-yl)-tetrazole see Doxantrazole.
2-[4-[4-(7,9-Dioxo-8-azaspiro(4.5)dec-8-yl)-butyl]piperazin-1-yl]pyrimidine see Buspirone.
4-[4-(7,9-Dioxo-8-azaspiro(4.5)dec-8-yl)-butyl]-1-pyrimidin-2-ylpiperazine see Buspirone.
1,3-Dioxo-1H-benz(de)isoquinoline-2(3H)-acetic acid sodium salt see Alrestatin.
Dioxocarb see Dioxacarb.
1,3-DIOXOLANE (dihydro-1,3-dioxole).
o-(1,3-Dioxolan-2-yl)phenyl methyl-carbamate see Dioxacarb.
3-(1,3-Dioxo-2-methyl-2,8-diazaspiro(4,5)-decan-8-yl)-4'-fluorobutyrophenone see Roxoperone.
'Dioxone' see Diethadione.
N-(2,6-Dioxopiperid-3-yl)phthalimide see Thalidomide.
9,9-Dioxopromethazine see Promethazine

S,S-dioxide.
2,5-Dioxopyrrolidine *see* Succinimide.
4-[(2,5-Dioxopyrrolidin-1-yloxy)car-bonyl]-α,α,4-triphenyl-1-piperidine-butanenitrile *see* Difenoximide.
N,N'-**(1,16-Dioxo-4,7,10,13-tetraoxahexa-decane-1,16-diyl)di(3-amino-2,4,6-triiodobenzoic acid)** *see* Iodoxamic acid.
Dioxyanthranol *see* Dithranol.
DIOXYBENZONE*** (2,2'-dihydroxy-4-methoxybenzophenone; 'spectrasorb UV 24').
Dioxydemeton-S-methyl *see* Demeton-S-methylsulfon.
Dioxyline *see* Dimoxyline.
'Dioxyline' *see* Benzoxiquine.
DIPA *see* Diisopropylamine dichloroacetate.
'Dipar' *see* Phenformin.
'Dipasic' *see* Pasiniazid.
'Dipaxin' *see* Diphenadione.
Dipenine bromide* *see* Diponium bromide.
Diperocaine *see* Diperodon.
DIPERODON*** (dicarbanilate of 3-(1-piperidyl)-1,2-propanediol; diperocaine; 'diothane', 'diothoid').
'Diphacil' *see* Adiphenine.
'Diphacin' *see* Diphenadione.
Diphacinone* *see* Diphenadione.
'Diphantoin' *see* Phenytoin.
Diphasin (tr) *see* 10-(Diethylaminoacetyl)-phenothiazine *and* Promethazine.
Diphazin (tr) *see* 10-(Diethylaminoacetyl)-phenothiazine *and* Promethazine.
'Diphebuzol' *see* Phenylbutazone.
DIPHEMANIL METILSULFATE*** (4-benzhydrylidene-1,1-dimethylpiperidi-nium methylsulfate; 4-diphenylmethylene-1,1-dimethylpiperidinium methylsulfate; *N,N*-dimethyl-4-piperidylidenediphenyl-methane methylsulfate; diphenmethanil; 'demotil', 'diphenatil', 'nivelona', 'pran-tal, 'vagophemanil').
'Diphemin' *see* Deanol benzilate.
'Diphenacin' *see* Diphenadione.
DIPHENADIONE** (2-diphenylacetyl-1,3-indandione; diphacinone; difenatsin; PID; U-1363; 'didandin', 'dipaxin', 'diphacin', 'diphenacin', 'oragulant', 'ratindan 1').
DIPHENAMID* (*N,N*-dimethyl-α-phenyl-benzeneacetamide; *N,N*-dimethyl-2,2-diphenylacetamide; 'dimid', 'dymid', 'enide').
Diphenamizole *see* Difenamizole.
DIPHENAN*** (*p*-benzylphenyl carbamate; α-phenyl-*p*-cresyl carbamate; carphenol; benzylphenylurethan).
Diphenason *see* Dapsone.
'Diphenatil' *see* Diphemanil metilsulfate.
DIPHENAZINE (1,4-bis(3-phenylprop-2-yl)-piperazine; 1,4-bis(α-methylphenethyl)-piperazine; 1,4-bis(phenylisopropyl)-piperazine; diphenazine dihydrochloride; 'quietidine').
Diphencloxazine *see* Difencloxazine.
Diphenetholine *see* Bibenzonium bromide.
N,N'-**Di-*p*-phenethylacetamidine** *see* Phenacaine.

Diphenhexenic acid *see* Xenyhexenic acid.
DIPHENHYDRAMINE*** (2-diphenyl-methoxy-*N,N*-dimethylamine; 2-benz-hydryloxy-*N,N*-dimethylethylamine; benzhydramine; anautine; dimedrol; PM-255; S-51).
Diphenhydramine aminoxide *see* Amoxy-dramine.
DIPHENHYDRAMINE ASCORBATE ('antamin').
DIPHENHYDRAMINE 8-BROMOTHEO-PHYLLINATE (bromanautine).
Diphenhydramine 8-chlorotheophyllinate *see* Dimenhydrinate.
Diphenhydramine *N*-oxide *see* Amoxy-dramine.
Diphenhydramine teoclate *see* Dimen-hydrinate.
DIPHENHYDRAMINE THEOPHYLLIN-ATE (etanautine; 'nautamine').
Diphenidol* *see* Difenidol.
Diphenin (tr) *see* Phenytoin.
Diphenmethanil* *see* Diphemanil metil-sulfate.
DIPHENOXYLATE*** (ethyl ester of 1-(3-cyano-3,3-diphenylpropyl)-4-phenylisoni-pecotic acid; 4-carbethoxy-α,α,4-triphenyl-1-piperidinebutyronitrile; 4-ethoxycarbonyl-α,α,4-triphenyl-1-piperidinebutyronitrile; diphenoxylate hydrochloride; ethyl di-fenoxilate; CB-8049; FH-049-E; R-1132).
DIPHENOXYLATE WITH ATROPINE ('diarsed', 'lomotil', 'reasec', 'retardin').
Di-phenthane-70 *see* Dichlorophen.
Diphenyl (the compound) *see* Biphenyl.
2,2-Diphenylacetic acid esters *see* Adiphen-ine; Anicaine; Aprenal; Mesfenal; Methyladiphenine; Pinolcaine.
Diphenylacetylindandione *see* Diphena-dione.
Diphenylaminechlorarsine *see* Phenars-azine chloride.
Diphenylbutazone *see* Phenylbutazone.
1,3-Diphenyl-2-buten-1-one *see* Dypnone.
2-[*p*-(1,2-Diphenyl-1-butenyl)phenoxy]-*N,N*-dimethylethylamine *see* Tamoxifen.
2,2-DIPHENYLBUTYRIC ACID (diphenyl-ethylacetic acid).
Diphenylcarbamic acid diethylamino-ethyl thioester *see* Fencarbamide.
Diphenylcarbamic acid dimethyl-aminoethyl ester *see* Dicarfen.
DIPHENYLCARBAZONE (phenylazoformic acid phenylhydrazide).
Diphenyl carbinol *see* Benzhydrol.
2,4-Diphenyl-1,3-cyclobutanecarboxylic acid diester with diethyl(3-hydroxy-propyl)methylammonium iodide *see* Truxipicurium iodide.
2,4-Diphenyl-1,3-cyclobutanecarboxylic acid diester with 1-ethyl-1-(3-hydroxy-propyl)piperidinium iodide *see* Truxipicurium iodide.
2,4-Diphenyl-1,3-cyclobutanedicarboxylic acid *see* Truxillic acid.
N,N'-**Diphenyldicarbamate 1,1-dimethyl-**

olcyclopentane *see* Cyclarbamate.
Diphenyl diketone *see* Benzil.
2-(2,2-Diphenyl-1,3-dioxolan-4-yl)piperidine *see* Dioxadrol.
Diphenylene ketone oxide *see* 9-Xanthenone.
Diphenylene oxide *see* Dibenzofuran.
Diphenylenimine *see* Carbazole.
1,2-Diphenylethane *see* Bibenzyl.
1,2-Diphenylethene *see* Stilbene.
Diphenyl ether *see* Phenyl ether.
2-(1,1-Diphenylethoxy)-N,N-dimethylethylamine *see* Moxastin.
[2-(1,2-Diphenylethoxy)ethyl]trimethylammonium bromide *see* Bibenzonium bromide.
Diphenylethylacetic acid *see* 2,2-Diphenylbutyric acid.
1,2-Diphenylethylamine *see* Stilbylamine.
1,2-Diphenylethylene *see* Stilbene.
Diphenylglycolic acid *see* Benzilic acid.
3,4-Diphenylhexamethylenebis(trimethylammonium iodide) *see* Paramyon.
2,2-Diphenyl-4-hexamethyleniminobutyramide *see* Buzepide.
5,5-Diphenylhydantoin *see* Phenytoin.
Diphenylhydracrylic acid acetohydrazide *see* Diphoxazide.
1,2-Diphenylhydrazine *see* Hydrazobenzene.
5,5-Diphenyl-4-imidazolidinone *see* Doxenitoin.
Diphenyl ketone *see* Benzophenone.
2-(Diphenylmethoxy)-N,N-dimethylethylamine *see* Diphenhydramine.
N-(2-Diphenylmethoxyethyl)-N-methylcinnamylamine *see* Cinfenine.
3-Diphenylmethoxy-8-ethylnortropane *see* Etybenzatropine.
1-(2-Diphenylmethoxyethyl)piperidine *see* Perastine.
3-(Diphenylmethoxy)tropane *see* Benzatropine.
2-Diphenylmethylenebutylamine *see* Etifelmine.
3-(Diphenylmethylene)-1,1-diethyl-2-methylpyrrolidinium bromide *see* Prifinium bromide.
4-Diphenylmethylene-1,1-dimethylpiperidinium methylsulfate *see* Diphemanil metilsulfate.
4-Diphenylmethylene-1-[2-[2-(2-hydroxyethoxy)ethoxy]ethyl]piperidine *see* Pipoxizine.
2-[2-[2-(4-Diphenylmethylenepiperid-1-yl)ethoxy]ethoxy]ethanol *see* Pipoxizine.
1-(Diphenylmethyl)-4-[2-(2-hydroxyethoxy)ethyl]piperazine *see* Decloxizine.
1-(Diphenylmethyl)-4-methylpiperazine *see* Cyclizine.
2-[2-[4-(Diphenylmethyl)piperazin-1-yl]ethoxy]ethanol *see* Decloxizine.
1-(Diphenylmethyl)-4-piperonylpiperazine *see* Medibazine.
4,5-Diphenyl-2-oxazolepropionic acid *see* Oxaprozin.
N-(4,5-Diphenyloxazol-2-yl)diethanolamine *see* Ditazole.

2,2'-(4,5-Diphenyloxazol-2-ylimino)-diethanol *see* Ditazole.
Diphenyl oxide *see* Phenyl ether.
4,7-Diphenyl-1,10-phenanthroline *see* Bathophenanthroline.
3,3-Diphenyl-N-(1-phenylethyl)-1-propylamine *see* Fendiline.
3,3-Diphenyl-N-(3-phenylprop-2-yl)-1-propylamine *see* Prenylamine.
1,2-Diphenyl-4-(2-phenylsulfinylethyl)-3,5-pyrazolidinedione *see* Sulfinpyrazone.
2,5-Diphenylpiperazine dipenicillin G *see* Phenyracillin.
α,α-Diphenyl-1-piperidinebutanol *see* Difenidol.
α,α-Diphenyl-2-piperidinemethanol *see* Pipradrol.
α,α-Diphenyl-4-piperidinemethanol *see* Azacyclonol.
α,α-Diphenyl-2-piperidinepropionic acid ethyl ester *see* Pifenate.
2,2-Diphenyl-4-piperidinobutyramide *see* Fenpipramide.
Diphenylpiperidinopropane *see* Fenpiprane.
1,1-Diphenyl-2-piperidino-1-propanol *see* Diphepanol.
1,1-Diphenyl-3-piperidino-1-propanol *see* Pridinol.
1,1-DIPHENYL-3-PIPERID-1-YL-1-BUTANOL (γ-methyl-α,α-diphenyl-1-piperidinepropanol; 'aspaminol').
1,1-Diphenyl-4-piperid-1-yl-1-butanol *see* Difenidol.
2,2-Diphenyl-4-piperid-1-ylbutyramide *see* Fenpipramide.
2,2-Diphenyl-4-piperid-2-yl-1,3-dioxolane *see* Dexoxadrol; Dioxadrol; Levoxadrol.
5,5-Diphenyl-2-(2-piperid-1-ylethyl)-1,3-dioxolan-4-one *see* Pipoxolan.
4,4-Diphenyl-6-piperid-1-yl-3-heptanone *see* Dipipanone.
4,4-Diphenyl-6-piperid-1-yl-3-hexanone *see* Norpipanone.
3,3-Diphenyl-1-piperid-1-ylpropane *see* Fenpiprane.
2,2-Diphenyl-3-piperid-2-ylpropionic acid ethyl ester *see* Pifenate.
1,1-Diphenyl-2-piperid-1-ylpropyl salicylate *see* Diphepanol.
1,2-Diphenyl-4-(2-pivaloylethyl)-3,5-pyrazolidinedione *see* Tribuzone.
1,3-Diphenyl-2-propen-1-one *see* Chalcone.
Diphenylpropionic acid diethylaminoethyl ester *see* Aprofene.
Diphenylpropylacetic acid diethylaminoethyl ester *see* Proadifen.
3-(3,3-Diphenylpropylamino)propyl 3,4,5-trimethoxybenzoate *see* Mepramidil.
N-(3,3-Diphenylpropyl)amphetamine *see* Prenylamine.
1-(3,3-Diphenylpropyl)cyclohexamethylenimine *see* Prozapine.
1-(3,3-Diphenylpropyl)hexamethylenimine *see* Prozapine.
N-(3,3-Diphenylpropyl)-α-methylbenzylamine *see* Fendiline.
N-(3,3-Diphenylpropyl)-α-methylphen-

ethylamine *see* Prenylamine.
N-**(3,3-Diphenylpropyl)-1-phenyl-2-propylamine** *see* Prenylamine.
1,1-Diphenyl-2-propynyl cyclohexanecarbamate *see* Enpromate.
DIPHENYLPYRALINE*** (4-benzhydryloxy-1-methylpiperidine; 4-diphenylmethoxy-1-methylpiperidine; P-253; 'aerogastol', 'diafen', 'hispril', 'histryl', 'hystryl', 'lergoban', 'mepiben').
See also Phenylephrine with diphenylpyraline.
Diphenylpyraline 8-chlorotheophyllinate *see* Piprinhydrinate.
1,2-DIPHENYL-3,5-PYRAZOLIDINEDIONE ('phenopyrazone').
See also Aminophenazone with 1,2-diphenyl-3,5-pyrazolidinedione.
α,α-**Diphenyl-2-pyrid-4-ylcyclopropanemethanol** *see* Cyprolidol.
1,1-Diphenyl-4-pyrrolidin-1-ylbut-2-yn-1-ol *see* Butinoline.
DIPHENYL SULFONE (phenylsulfone; sulfobenzide).
Diphenylthiocarbamic acid *S*-2-diethyl aminoethyl ester *see* Fencarbamide.
Diphenylthiocarbazone *see* Dithizone.
Diphenylthioloacetic acid esters *see* Diprofene; Thiphenamil.
1,3-Diphenylthiourea *see* Thiocarbanilide.
1,3-Diphenyltriazene *see* Diazoaminobenzene.
1,2-Diphenyl-4-(4,4,4-trimethyl-3-oxobutyryl)-3,5-pyrazolidinedione *see* Tribuzone.
1,3-Diphenylurea *see* Carbanilide.
Diphenylvaleric acid diethylaminoethyl ester *see* Proadifen.
Diphenylyl.... *see* Biphenylyl....
DIPHEPANOL* (1,1-diphenyl-2-piperid-1-ylpropyl salicylate; diphenylpiperidinopropanol salicylate; diphepanol hydrochloride; Hö-10682; 'tussilax', 'tussucal', 'tussukal').
DIPHEPANOL WITH (±)-*p*-HYDROXYEPHEDRINE SALICYLATE (J-110-E; 'tussucal forte').
Diphesatine *see* Acetphenolisatin.
Diphesyl (tr) *see* Difezil.
Diphetarsone *see* Difetarsone.
'Diphone' *see* Dapsone.
DIPHOSGENE (trichloromethyl chloroformate; perstoff; superpalite; surpalite).
Diphosphonate *see* Disodium etidronate.
Diphosphopyridine nucleotide *see* Nadide.
DIPHOXAZIDE*** (1-acetyl-2-(3,3-diphenyl-3-hydroxypropionyl)hydrazine; acetylhydrazide of 3,3-diphenylhydracrylic acid).
'Dipidolor' *see* Piritramide.
DIPIN (tr) (1,4-piperazinediylbis[bis(1-aziridinyl)phosphine oxide]; 1,4-bis-(diaziridinylphosphinylidyne)piperazine; 1,4-bis[(*N*,*N*'-bisethylene)diamidophosphoryl]piperazine; tetraethylenamide of piperazine-1,4-diphosphoric acid; *N*,*N*'-diethylenebis(*N*,*N*'-diethylenephosphoric diamide)).

DIPIPANONE*** (4,4-diphenyl-6-piperid-1-yl-3-heptanone; piperidyl amidone; dipipanone hydrochloride; BW-378C48; 'pipadone').
DIPIPANONE WITH CYCLIZINE ('diconal').
2,2',2'',2'''-[(4,8-Dipiperidinopyrimido-(5,4-d)pyrimidine-2,6-diyl)dinitrilo]-tetraethanol *see* Dipyridamole.
Dipiperidyl *see* Bipiperidine.
2β,16β-Dipiperid-1-yl-5α-androstane-3α, 17β-diol 3-acetate dimethobromide *see* Dacuronium bromide.
2β,16β-Dipiperid-1-yl-5α-androstane-3α, 17β-diol diacetate dimethobromide *see* Pancuronium bromide.
'Dipiperon' *see* Pipamperone.
DIPIPROVERINE*** (2-piperid-1-ylethyl α-phenylpiperidineacetate; 2-piperid-1-ylethyl 2-phenyl-2-piperid-1-ylacetate; P-4; 'spasmonol').
DIPLACIN (tr) (4,4'-[*m*-phenylenebis(oxyethylene)]bis[hexahydro-1-hydroxy-7-(hydroxymethyl)(1H)pyrrolizinium chloride]; 1,3-phenylenedioxybis(4-ethyl-1-hydroxy-7-hydroxymethylhexahydro-3H-pyrrolo(1,2-a)pyrrole) dichloride; 1,3-bis-(2-platineciumethoxy)benzene dichloride; diplatineciumethoxybenzene dichloride; diplatsin).
Diplatineciumethoxybenzene dichloride *see* Diplacin.
Diplatsin *see* Diplacin.
'Diplosal' *see* Salsalate.
'Diplosal acetate' *see* Acetylsalicylsalicylic acid.
Dipon* *see* Diponium bromide.
DIPONIUM BROMIDE*** (triethyl(2-hydroxyethyl)ammonium bromide dicyclopentylacetate; (2-dicyclopentyl-acetoxyethyl)triethylammonium bromide; dicyclopentylacetate ester of (2-hydroxyethyl)triethylammonium bromide; dipenine bromide; dipon; DCDE; HL-267; Sa-267; 'unospaston').
DIPOTASSIUM CLORAZEPATE*** ((3-carboxy-7-chloro-2,3-dihydro-2-hydroxy-5-phenyl-1H-1,4-benzodiazepin-2-yloxy)potassium; dipotassium salt of 7-chloro-2,3-dihydro-2,2-dihydroxy-5-phenyl-1H-1,4-benzodiazepine-3-carboxylic acid; clorazepate; potassium clorazepate; AB-35616; Abbott-35616; AH-3232; CB-4306; 'tencilan', 'tranxene', 'tranxilene', 'tranxilium').
'Dipramid' *see* Isopropamide iodide.
Diprazin (tr) *see* Promethazine.
DIPRENORPHINE*** (21-cyclopropyl-6,7,8, 14-tetrahydro-7α-(1-hydroxy-1-methylethyl)-6,14-*endo*-ethenooripavine; *N*-cyclopropylmethyl-7,8-dihydro-7α-(1-hydroxy-1-methylethyl)-*O*⁶-methyl-6,14-*endo*-ethanonormorphine; M-5050; 'revivon').
'Diproderm' *see* Betamethasone dipropionate.
DIPROFENE*** (2-dipropylaminoethyl 2,2-diphenylthioloacetate; diprophen).

174

DIPROGULIC ACID** (2,3:4,6-di-*O*-isopropylidene-α-L-*xylo*-hexulofuranosonic acid).

DIPROLEANDOMYCIN***(oleandomycin 4′,11-dipropionate).

DIPROPAMINE ([*p*-phenylenebis(oxypropylene)]bis(dimethylethylammonium iodide)).

DIPROPETRYN* (6-(ethylthio)-2,4-bis-(isopropylamino)-*s*-triazine; 'cotofor').

Diprophen (tr) *see* Diprofene.

DIPROPHYLLINE*** (7-(2,3-dihydroxypropyl)theophylline; dyphylline; glyphyllinum; glyfillin hyphylline).

DIPROPHYLLINE WITH 7-(2-HYDRO-XYPROPYL)THEOPHYLLINE ('neophylline').

3,5-Dipropionamido-2,3,6-triiodobenzoic acid *see* Diprotrizoic acid.

Dipropylacetamide *see* 2-Propylvaleramide.

Dipropylacetic acid *see* 2-Propylvaleric acid.

4-(Dipropylamino)-3,5-dinitrobenzenesulfonamide *see* Oryzalin.

Dipropylaminoethyl diphenylthioloacetate *see* Diprofene.

5,5-DIPROPYLBARBITURIC ACID (propylbarbital; 'propanal', 'proponal', 'propytal').

Dipropylcarbamothioic acid *S*-ethyl ester *see* Ethyl dipropylcarbamothioate.

Dipropylcarbamothioic acid *S*-propyl ester *see* Vernolate.

Dipropylenediamine *see* Lupetazine.

2,3:4,6-Di-*O*-propylidene-α-L-*xylo*-hexulofuranosonic acid *see* Diprogulic acid.

Dipropyline *see* Alverine.

N,*N*-**Dipropyl-*p*-toluenesulfonamide** *see* Ditolamide.

DIPROQUALONE** (3-(2,3-dihydroxypropyl)-2-methyl-4(3H)-quinazolinone).

'**Diprosone**' *see* Betamethasone dipropionate.

DIPROTRIZOIC ACID (3,5-dipropionamido-2,4,6-triiodobenzoic acid).
See also Sodium diprotrizoate.

DIPROXADOL** (6-chloro-4-(2,3-dihydroxypropyl)-2-methyl-2H-1,4-benzodiazepin-3(4H)-one).

'**Dipsan**' *see* Calcium carbimide.

'**Dipterex**' *see* Metrifonate.

'**Dipterex ER**' *see* Metrifonate plus oxydemeton-methyl.

DIPYRIDAMOLE*** (2,2′,2″,2‴-[(4,8-dipiperidinopyrimido(5,4-d)pyrimidine-2,6-diyl)dinitrilo]tetraethanol; 2,6-bis(diethanolamino)-4,8-dipiperidinopyrimido-(5,4-d)pyrimidine; 2,6-bis[2(2-hydroxyethyl)amino]-4,8-bis(1-piperidyl)pyrimido-(5,4-d)pyrimidine; 2,6-bis[bis(2-hydroxyethyl)amino]-4,8-bis(1-piperidyl)-1,3,5,7-tetraazanaphthalene; RA-8; 'curantyl', 'persantin').

Dipyridyl (the compound) *see* Bipyridine.

α,α-**Di-2-pyridyl-α-[β-di(2-pyridyl)-methylenecyclopenta-1,4-dien-1-yl]-methanol** *see* Pyrinoline.

Di(pyrid-4-ylmethyl)amine *see* Gapicomine.

3-(Dipyrid-2-ylmethylene)-α,α-dipyrid-2-yl-1,4-cyclopentadiene-1-methanol *see* Pyrinoline.

1,2-Dipyrid-3-yl-2-methyl-1-propanone *see* Metyrapone.

'**Di-pyrin**' *see* Aminophenazone.

DIPYRITHIONE*** (2,2′-dithiodipyridine 1,1′-dioxide; OMDS; 'omadine disulfide').

DIPYROCETYL*** (2,3-diacetoxybenzoic acid; diacetylprotocatechuic acid; diacetylpyrocatecholcarboxylic acid; 2,3-dihydroxybenzoic acid diacetate; 'movirene', 'pyrocat').

Dipyrone *see* Novaminsulfon.

Dipyroxime (tr) *see* Trimedoxime.

1,4-Dipyrrolidin-1-yl-2-butyne *see* Tremorine.

DIQUAT* (9,10-dihydro(8a,10a)diazoniaphenanthrene dibromide; 6,7-dihydrodipyrido[1,2-a:2′,1′-c]pyrazinediium dibromide;FB/2; 'acquacide', 'dextrone', 'reglone').

'**Diquel**' *see* Etymemazine.

'**Diquinol**' *see* Ethaverine.

Diquinolylurea bismethosulfate *see* Quinuronium.

'**Diratyl**' *see* Hydroflumethiazide.

Direct red *see* Congo red.

'**Direma**' *see* Hydrochlorothiazide.

Dirhodanethane *see* Dithiocyanoethane.

'**Dirnate**' *see* Carzenide.

'**Disadine**' *see* Povidone iodine.

Disalicylic acid *see* Salsalate.

'**Disalunil**' *see* Hydrochlorothiazide.

'**Disaluril**' *see* Hydrochlorothiazide.

'**Disalyl**' *see* Salsalate.

'**Disamide**' *see* Disulfamide.

'**Discase**' *see* Chymopapain.

'**Disepron**' *see* Spiclomazine.

'**Disflatyl**' *see* Dimeticone.

'**Disipal**' *see* Orphenadrine.

'**Disoderm**' *see* Dichlorisone acetate.

Disodium aurothiomalate *see* Sodium aurothiomalate.

Disodium [(benzylamidino)amidino]-phosphoramidate *see* Benfosformin.

DISODIUM CROMOGLICATE** (disodium 5,5′-(2-hydroxytrimethylenedioxy)bis(4-oxo-4H-1-benzopyran-2-carboxylate); cromoglicic acid disodium salt; disodium cromoglycate; cromolyn sodium; sodium cromoglycate; FPL-670; 'aarane', 'inostral', 'intal', 'rynacrom').

Disodium cromoglycate* *see* Disodium cromoglicate.

Disodium dapsonedisulfonate *see* Dapsonedisulfonic acid disodium salt.

DISODIUM EDETATE (disodium salt of ethylenediaminetetraacetic acid; disodium dihydrogen edetate; sodium edetate; 'decalcinon', 'endrate disodium', 'komplexon II', 'rynacrom', 'sequestrene Na 2', 'titriplex').
See also Sodium calcium edetate; Tetrasodium edetate.

Disodium endothal *see* Endothal sodium.

Disodium 1,2-ethanediylbis(carbamo-

175

dithioate) *see* Nabam.
Disodium ethylenebis(carbamodithioate)
  see Nabam.
DISODIUM ETIDRONATE (EHDP;
  diphosphonate).
  See also Etidronic acid.
DISODIUM HYDROGEN CITRATE (acid
  sodium cirate; 'alkacitron').
DISODIUM METHANEARSONATE
  (disodium methylarsinate; disodium monomethylarsonate; sodium metharsinite;
  'arrhenal', 'arsenyl', 'arsinyl', 'arsynal',
  'cacodyl new', 'crab-E-rad', 'crabgrass
  killer', 'di-met', 'neoarsycodile', 'new
  cacodyle', 'novarscodyle', 'ortho crabgrass
  killer', 'sodar', 'stenosine', 'tonarsin',
  'weedone').
Disodium methylarsinate *see* Disodium
  methanearsonate.
Disodium methylarsonate *see* Disodium
  methanearsonate.
Disodium monomethylarsonate *see*
  Disodium methanearsonate.
**Disodium 4,4′-pyrid-2-ylmethylenedi-
  (phenyl sulfate)** *see* Sodium picosulfate.
'Disomer' *see* Dexbrompheniramine.
'Disonate' *see* Sodium dioctyl sulfosuccinate.
DISOPHENOL (2,6-diiodo-4-nitrophenol;
  'ancylol').
Disopromine * *see* Diisopromine.
DISOPYRAMIDE *** (α-(2-diisopropylami-
  noethyl)-α-phenyl-2-pyridineacetamide;
  4-diisopropylamino-2-phenyl-2-pyrid-2-
  ylbutyramide; disopyramide phosphate;
  SC-7031; 'norpace', 'rhythmodan',
  'rhythmodul', 'ritmodan').
'Disotat' *see* Diisopropylamine.
'Dispamil' *see* Papaverine.
'Disparolene' *see* Chlorpropamide.
'Dispasmol' *see* Phenbenzamine etho-
  bromide.
'Dispermin' *see* Piperazine.
'Dispril' *see* Calcium acetylsalicylate.
'Disprin' *see* Calcium acetylsalicylate.
'Distamine' *see* Penicillamine.
Distamycin A *see* Stallimycin.
'Distaneurine' *see* Clomethiazole edisilate.
DISTIGMINE BROMIDE *** (N,N′-hexa-
  methylenebis[1-methyl-3-(methylcarba-
  moyloxy)pyridinium bromide]; 3-hydroxy-
  1-methylpyridinium bromide hexamethyl-
  enebis(N-methylcarbamate); BC-51;
  'ubretid', 'ulbretid').
'Disto-5' *see* Bithionol sulfoxide.
'Distol-8' *see* Tetrasodium edetate.
'Distolon' *see* Niclofolan.
'Distowet' *see* Hexachloroethane.
'Distrapax' *see* Clomethiazole edisilate.
'Distreptaze' *see* Streptodornase with
  streptokinase.
Distylin *see* Taxifolin.
Disugran * *see* Dicamba-methyl.
DISUL * (2-(2,4-dichlorophenoxy)ethyl
  hydrogen sulfate; dichloresul; 2,4-DES;
  'SES').
DISULFAMIDE ** (5-chloro-2,4-disulfa-
  moyltoluene; 5-chlorotoluene-2,4-

disulfonamide; disulfamide; tolclotide;
  'disamide').
DISULFIRAM *** (bis(diethylthiocarbamyl)
  disulfide; ethyl thiurad; tetraethylthiuram
  disulfide; teturam; TTD; tiuram; thiuram;
  thiuranide; ethyldithiuram).
(Disulfophenylpropyl)sulfathiazole *see*
  Noprylsulfamide.
DISULFORMIN (tr) (1,4,4′-trimethylene-
  bis(4-sulfamoylsulfanilanilide); formalde-
  hyde condensation product of N⁴-sulfanilyl-
  sulfanilamide).
DISULFOTON * (O,O-diethyl S-(2-ethyl-
  thioethyl) phosphorodithioate; dithiodemeton; ethylthiometon; thiodemeton;
  thiometon ethyl; M-74; 'di-syston', 'dithio-
  systox', 'frumin', 'thiosystox').
'Disulone' *see* Dapsone.
Disulphamide * *see* Disulfamide.
Disulph.... *see further* Disulf....
'Disyncran' *see* Methdilazine.
'Di-syston' *see* Disulfoton.
'Disyston-S' *see* Oxydisulfoton.
'Ditaven' *see* Digitoxin.
DITAZOLE *** (2,2′-(4,5-diphenyloxazol-2-
  ylimino)diethanol; N-(4,5-diphenyl-
  oxazol-2-yl)diethanolamine; 2-[bis(2-
  hydroxyethyl)amino]-4,5-diphenyloxazole;
  2,2′-dihydroxy-N-(4,5-diphenyloxazol-2-yl)-
  diethylamine; diethamphenazole; dietam-
  fenazole; S-222).
Ditetrazolium chloride *see* Tetrazolium
  blue.
'Dithane 1740' *see* Nabam.
'Dithane A-40' *see* Nabam.
'Dithane D-14' *see* Nabam.
'Dithane M-22' *see* Maneb.
'Dithane M-45' *see* Mancozeb.
'Dithane manganese' *see* Maneb.
'Dithane S-31' *see* Maneb plus nickel sulfate.
'Dithane-ultra' *see* Mancozeb.
'Dithane Z 78' *see* Zineb.
4,5-Dithia-1-cyclopentene-3-thione *see*
  1,2-Dithiole-3-thione.
'Dithiaden' *see* 4-[3-(Dimethylamino)-
  propylidene]-4,9-dihydrothieno(2,3-b)-
  benzo(e)thiepine.
DITHIANON * (5,10-dihydro-5,10-dioxo-
  naphtho(2,3-b)-1,4-dithiin-2,3-dicarboni-
  trile; 'delan').
DITHIAZANINE IODIDE *** (3-ethyl-2-[5-
  (3-ethyl-2-benzothiazolinylidene)-1,3-
  pentadienyl]benzothiazolium iodide; 3,3′-
  diethylthiadicarbocyanine iodide; L-01748;
  'abminthic', 'anelmid', 'delvex', 'dilombrin', 'omni-passin', 'partel', 'telmid',
  'vercidon').
Dithienyl *see* Bithiophene.
**α-[1-[1-(3,3-Dithien-3-ylallyl)amino]-
  ethyl]benzyl alcohol** *see* Tinofedrine.
**Dithien-2-ylglycolic acid ester with
  6,6,9-trimethyl-9-azabicyclo(3.3.1)-
  nonan-3β-ol** *see* Mazaticol.
**3-(Dithien-2-ylmethylene)-5-methoxy-1,1-
  dimethylpiperidinium bromide** *see*
  Timepidium bromide.
3-(Dithien-2-ylmethylene)-1-methyl-

piperidine see Tipepidine.
Dithio see Sulfotep.
4,4′-Dithiobis(2-aminobutyric acid) see Homocystine.
N,N′-[Dithiobis[2-(2-benzoyloxyethyl)-1-methylvinylene]]bis[N-(4-amino-2-methylpyrimidin-5-ylmethyl)formamide] see Bisbentiamine.
Dithiobisethylamine see Cystamine.
Dithiobis(thionoformic acid) diethyl ester see Dixanthogen.
Dithiocarb see Sodium diethyldithiocarbamate.
DITHIOCYANOETHANE (dirhodanethane; dirodanethane).
Dithiodemeton see Disulfoton.
Dithiodialanine see Cystine.
Dithiodianiline see Diaminodiphenyl disulfide.
3,3′-Dithiodimethylenebis(5-hydroxy-6 methyl-4-pyridinemethanol) see Pyritinol.
2,2′-Dithiodipyridine 1,1′-dioxide see Dipyrithione.
1,2-Dithioglycol see Dimercaprol.
1,3-Dithioisophthalic acid S,S-diethyl ester see Ditophal.
1,3-Dithiolan-2-ylidenephosphoramidic acid diethyl ester see Phosfolan.
5-(1,2-Dithiolan-3-yl)valeric acid see Thioctic acid.
1,2-DITHIOLE-3-THIONE (4,5-dithia-1-cyclopentene-3-thione).
Dithioloisophthalic acid diethyl ester see Ditophal.
1,3-Dithiolo(4,5-b)quinoxaline-2-thione see Thioquinox.
Dithiomethon see Thiometon.
Dithiometon see Thiometon.
Dithion see Sulfotep.
Dithione see Sulfotep.
6,8-Dithiooctanoic acid see Thioctic acid.
Dithiophos (tr) see Sulfotep.
Dithiophosphoric acid see Phosphorodithioic acid.
Dithiopropylthiamine see Prosultiamine.
'Dithio-systox' see Disulfoton.
Dithio-TEPP see Sulfotep.
DITHIZONE (phenylazothionoformic acid 2-phenylhydrazide; diphenylthiocarbazone).
DITHRANOL*** (1,8,9-anthratriol; 1,8-dihydroxyanthranol; 1,8,9-trihydroxyanthracene; anthralin; 'cignaethyl', 'cignolin', 'cigthranol').
DITHRANOL TRIACETATE (1,8,9-triacetoxyanthracene; 'exolan').
DITHYMOL DIIODIDE (bis(thymol iodide); bithymol diiodide; diiododithymol).
Ditilin (tr) see Suxamethonium.
Ditiobisfenol see Probucol.
'Dition' see Coumithoate.
DITOLAMIDE*** (N,N-dipropyl-p-toluenesulfonamide).
DITOPHAL** (S,S-diethyl 1,3-dithioisophthalate; ETIP; ICI-15688; 'etisul').
'Ditox' see Lindane with DDT.

'Ditox L' see Lindane with DDT.
'Ditran' see 1-Ethylpiperid-3-yl phenylcyclopentaneglycolate.
Ditrazin (tr) see Diethylcarbamazine.
'Ditripentat' see Calcium trisodium pentetate.
'Ditrone' see Phenylbutazone 3,4,5-trimethoxybenzoate.
'Ditropan' see Oxybutynin.
'Ditrosal' see Dinitro-o-cresol.
'Dityrin' see Diiodotyrosine.
Diu-60 see Bemetizide.
'Diucardin' see Hydroflumethiazide.
'Diuramide' see Acetazolamide.
'Diuril' see Chlorothiazide.
'Diurilix' see Chlorothiazide.
DIURON* (1-(3,4-dichlorophenyl)-3,3-dimethylurea; DCMU; DMU; dichlorofenidim; diklorfenidim; 'karmex').
'Diurone' see Chlormerodrin.
'Diutazol' see Acetazolamide.
'Divanil' see Cyclovalone.
Divanillylidenecyclohexanone see Cyclovalone.
'Divanon' see Cyclovalone.
'Diveronal' see Quinuronium.
'Dividol' see Viminol p-hydroxybenzoate.
'Divimax' see Spirgetine with paraflutizide.
Diviminol see Viminol.
Divinylbenzene-methacrylic acid polymer see Polacrilin.
Divinylene sulfide see Thiophene.
Divinyl ether see Vinyl ether.
Divinyl oxide see Vinyl ether.
Divinyl sulfone see Vinyl sulfone.
Dixamon bromide see Methantheline.
DIXANTHOGEN*** (O,O-diethyl ester of dithiobis(thionoformic acid); bis(ethylxanthogen); diethyldixanthogen; diethylxanthogen).
'Dixarit' see Clonidine.
'Dixeran' see Melitracen.
2-[2-(Di-2,6-xylylmethoxy)ethoxy]-N,N-dimethylethylamine see Xyloxemine.
DIXYRAZINE (10-[3-[4-(2-(2-hydroxyethoxy)ethyl)piperazin-1-yl]-2-methylpropyl]phenothiazine; UCB-3412; 'esucos').
DJ-1550 see Sulfamethoxine.
DJENKOLIC ACID (3,3′-methylenedithiobis(2-aminopropionic acid); 3,3′-methylenedithiodialanine).
DKB see Dibekacin.
DL-152 see Bietaserpine.
DM see Phenarsazine chloride.
DM-70 (tr) see Dimethyl sulfoxide.
DM-90 (tr) see Dimethyl sulfoxide.
DMBA see 7,12-Dimethylbenz(a)anthracene.
DMC see Chlorfenethol.
DMCT see Demeclocycline.
DMDT see Methoxychlor.
DMF see see Dimefox.
DMI see Desipramine.
DMN see Dimethylnitrosamine.
DMO see Dimethadione.
DMPEA see Homoveratrylamine.
DMPP see Dimethylphenylpiperazinium

iodide.
DMS *see* Dimercaptosuccinic acid.
DMSE *see* Ethylene mesilate.
DMSO *see* Dimethyl sulfoxide.
DMSP *see* Fensulfotion.
DMTT *see* Dazomet.
DMU *see* Diuron.
DNBP *see* Dinoseb.
DNC *see* Dinitro-*o*-cresol.
DNCB *see* 1-Chloro-2,4-dinitrobenzene.
DNIBF *see* Dinoseb.
DNOC * *see* Dinitro-*o*-cresol.
DNOCHP *see* Dinex.
DNOIPP *see* Dinoprop.
DNOPC *see* Dinocap.
DNOSBP *see* Dinoseb trolamine.
DNPP *see* Dinoprop.
DNSBP *see* Dinoseb trolamine.
DO-601 *see* 1-Ethyl-3-(*p*-methoxyphenyl)-1-
propylamine.
'Dobendan' *see* Cetylpyridinium chloride.
'Doberol' *see* Toliprolol.
Dobesilate calcium *see* Calcium dobesilate.
'Dobesin' *see* Amfepramone.
'Dobren' *see* Sulpiride.
'Dobrizon' *see* Methaqualone.
'Doburil' *see* Cyclothiazide.
DOBUTAMINE *** (($\pm$)-4-[2-[3-(*p*-hydroxy-
phenyl)-1-methylpropylamino]ethyl]-
pyrocatechol; ($\pm$)-*N*-[2-(2,3-dihydroxy-
phenyl)ethyl]-4-(*p*-hydroxyphenyl)-2-
butylamine; ($\pm$)-2,3-dihydroxy-*N*-[3-
(*p*-hydroxyphenyl)-1-methylpropyl]-
phenethylamine.
Doc *see* Desoxycortone.
'Doca' *see* Desoxycortone acetate.
'Docabolin' *see* Nandrolone phenpropionate
with desoxycortone phenpropionate.
DOCETRIZOIC ACID * (3-diacetylamino-
2,4,6-triiodobenzoic acid).
See also Propyl docetrizoate.
'Dociton' *see* Propranolol.
'Doclizid-T' *see* Chlorazanil.
Docosanoic acid *see* Behenic acid.
cis-**13-Docosenoic acid** *see* Erucic acid.
trans-**13-Docosenoic acid** *see* Brassidic acid.
'Dodat' *see* DDT.
**Dodecachlorooctahydro-1,3,4-metheno-
1H-cyclobuta(cd)pentalene** *see* Mirex.
**Dodecahydro-2α,11-dimethoxy-3β-(3,4,5-
trimethoxybenzoyloxy)benz(g)indolo-
(2,3-a)quinolizine-1β-carboxylic acid
methyl ester** *see* Reserpine.
**Dodecahydro-2α,11-dimethoxy-3β-(3,4,5-
trimethoxycinnamoyloxy)benz(g)in-
dolo(2,3-a)quinolizine-1β-carboxylic
acid methyl ester** *see* Rescinnamine.
**1α,2β,3α,4,4aα,5,7,8,13,13bβ,14,14aα-Dode-
cahydro-3β-hydroxy-2α,11-dimethoxy-
benz(g)indolo(2,3-a)quinolizine-1β-
carboxylic acid** *see* Reserpic acid.
**1,2,3,4,4a,4b,5,6,7,9,10,10a-Dodecahydro-
2-hydroxy-2,4b-dimethyl-7-oxo-1-
phenanthrenepropionic acid γ-lactone**
see Testolactone.
**Dodecahydro-3-hydroxy-6-(hydroxy-
methyl)-3,3a,6-trimethyl(11H)benz(e)-**

indene-7-acetic acid delta lactone *see*
Oxandrolone.
**Dodecahydro-13-methylbenz(g)indolo-
(2,3a)quinolizine** *see* Mimbane.
Dadecanoic acid *see* Lauric acid.
**[2-(*N*-Dodecanoyl-*N*-methylamino)ethyl]-
dimethyl(phenylcarbamoylmethyl)-
ammonium chloride** *see* Dofamium
chloride.
**1-[*N*-(2-Dodecanoyloxyethyl)carbamoyl-
methyl]pyridinium chloride** *see*
Lapirium chloride.
DODECLONIUM BROMIDE *** ([2-(*p*-
chlorophenoxy)ethyl]dodecyldimethyl-
ammonium bromide).
Dodecylaminoethylaminoethylglycine
see Dodicin.
**Dodecyldimethyl(2-phenoxyethyl)-
ammonium bromide** *see* Domiphen
bromide.
Dodecylguanidine acetate *see* Dodine.
**2-DODECYLISOQUINOLINIUM
BROMIDE** (laurylisoquinolinium bromide;
'isothan Q15').
**1-(2-DODECYLOXYETHYL)PYRROL-
IDINE** (DEP).
**1,1′-(4-Dodecyloxy-*m*-phenylene)diguan-
idine** *see* Lauroguadine.
1-DODECYLPYRIDINIUM BROMIDE
(laurylpyridinium bromide; 'isothan Q4';
'laurosept').
Dodecyl sodium sulfate *see* Sodium
dodecyl sulfate.
Dodecyl sulfate(s) *see* Laurilsulfate(s).
DODECYL SULFOACETATE (lauryl
sulfoacetate; 'lowila').
**DODECYLTRIPHENYLPHOSPHONIUM
BROMIDE** (DTPB; 'mycal', 'myxal').
DODICIN * (2,5,8-triazaeicosane-1-carboxylic
acid; *N*-[2-(2-dodecylamino)ethylamino]-
ethylglycine; 'tego 103S').
DODINE * (dodecylguanidine acetate;
dodecylguanidine monoacetate; citrex;
doguadine; DDGA; 'bilobran', 'cyprex',
'melprex').
DOET *see* 4-Ethyl-2,5-dimethoxyamphet-
amine.
DOFAMIUM CHLORIDE *** (dimethyl[2-
(*N*-methyldodecanamido)ethyl](phenyl-
carbamoylmethyl)ammonium chloride;
[2-(*N*-dodecanoyl-*N*-methylamino)ethyl]-
dimethyl(phenylcarbamoylmethyl)-
ammonium chloride; 'desogen').
'Dogmatyl' *see* Sulpiride.
Doguadine *see* Dodine.
'Doktacillin' *see* Ampicillin.
'Dolicur' *see* Dimethyl sulfoxide.
'Dolipol' *see* Tolbutamide.
'Dolisina' *see* Pethidine.
'Dolitrone' *see* Phenythilone.
'Dolorphen' *see* Dextropropoxyphene.
'Doloxene' *see* Dextropropoxyphene.
DOM *see* 2,5-Dimethoxy-4-methylamphet-
amine.
DOMAZOLINE ** (2-(3,6-dimethoxy-2,4-
dimethylbenzyl)-2-imidazoline; doxa-
zoline).

'Domeboro' *see* Aluminium acetate.
'Dominal' *see* Prothipendyl.
'Dominil' *see* Oxyphencyclimine.
DOMIPHEN BROMIDE*** (dodecyldimethyl(2-phenoxyethyl)ammonium bromide; phenododecinium bromide; PDDB; 'bradosol', 'domittol').
'Domistan' *see* Histapyrrodine.
'Domittol' *see* Domiphen bromide.
DOMOXIN** (1-(1,4-benzodioxan-2-yl-methyl)-1-benzylhydrazine).
DON (L-6-diazo-5-oxonorleucine; L-2-amino-6-diazo-5-ketohexanoic acid; NSC-7365).
Donaxine *see* Gramine.
DOOTC *see* Doxycycline.
DOPA (3-(3,4-dihydroxyphenyl)alanine; dopalanine).
See also Levodopa.
DOPAC *see* Homoprotocatechuic acid.
'Dopaflex' *see* Levodopa.
'Dopal' *see* Levodopa.
Dopalanine *see* Dopa.
'Dopalfher' *see* Levodopa.
DOPAMANTINE** (N-(3,4-dihydroxy-phenethyl)-1-adamantanecarboxamide; N-(1-adamantanecarbonyl)-3,4-dihydroxy-phenethylamine; Sch-15507).
'Dopamet' *see* Methyldopa.
DOPAMINE** (3-hydroxytyramine; 3,4-di-hydroxyphenethylamine; 4-(2-aminoethyl)-pyrocatechol; dopamine hydrochloride; ASL-279; 'dynatra', 'intropin', 'revivan').
DOPAN (tr) (5-[bis(2-chloroethyl)amino]-6-methyluracil; NSC-446297).
'Dopar' *see* Levodopa.
'Dopasol' *see* Levodopa.
'Dopastral' *see* Levodopa.
'Dopegyt' *see* Methyldopa.
'Dopegyt' *see* Methyldopa.
'Dopram' *see* Doxapram.
DORASTINE** (8-chloro-2,3,4,5-tetrahydro-2-methyl-5-[2-(6-methylpyrid-3-yl)ethyl]-1H-pyrido(4,3-b)indole; dorastine dihydrochloride; Ro 5-9110/1).
'Doraxamin' *see* Aluminium glycinate.
'Dorbane' *see* Dantron.
'Dorbanex' *see* Dantron with poloxalkol.
'Dorcalm' *see* Chloralose.
'Doreperol' *see* Cetylpyridinium chloride with hexetidine.
'Dorevane' *see* Propiomazine.
'Dorex' *see* Oxeladin citrate.
'Doriden' *see* Glutethimide.
'Dormiol' *see* Amylene chloral.
'Dormirette' *see* Butethal.
'Dormisan' *see* Cyclopentobarbital.
'Dormodor' *see* Flurazepam.
'Dormogen' *see* Methaqualone.
'Dormuphar' *see* Dichloralphenazone.
'Dormutil' *see* Methaqualone.
Dornase *see* Deoxyribonuclease.
'Dornavac' *see* Pancreatic dornase.
'Dornokinase' *see* Streptodornase with streptokinase.
'Dornwal' *see* Amphenidone.
'Dorsacaine' *see* Ambucaine.
'Dorsedin' *see* Metixine with novamin-

sulfon.
'Dorsiflex' *see* Mephenoxalone.
'Doryl' *see* Carbachol.
'Dosanex' *see* Metoxuron.
'Doseval' *see* Methyprylone.
DOSULEPIN** (11-(3-dimethylamino-propylidene)-6,11-dihydrodibenz(b,e)-thiepine; N,N-dimethyldibenz(b,e)thiepin-△11(6H),γ-propylamine; dothiepin; 'prothiaden').
DOSULEPIN WITH EMBRAMINE ('prothidryl').
DOTEFONIUM BROMIDE*** (1-methyl-1-[2-(N-methyl-α-thien-2-ylmandelamido)-ethyl]pyrrolidinium bromide.).
Dothiepin *see* Dosulepin.
'Dovenix' *see* Nitroxinil.
'Dovine' *see* Prolonium iodide.
Dowco 179 *see* Chlorpyrifos.
Dowco 214 *see* Chlorpyrifos methyl.
'Dowmycin E' *see* Erythromycin stearate.
'Dowpon' *see* Dalapon sodium.
'Dowicide' *see* Phenylphenol.
DOXANTRAZOLE* (3-tetrazol-5-ylthio-xanthen-9-one 10,10-dioxide; 5-(10,10-dioxido-9-oxothioxanthen-3-yl)tetrazole).
DOXAPRAM*** (1-ethyl-4-(2-morpholino-ethyl)-3,3-diphenyl-2-pyrrolidinone; doxapram hydrochloride; AHR-619; 'dopram', 'doxapryl', 'stimulexin').
DOXAPROST** ((1R*,2R*)-2-[(E)-3-hydroxy-3-methyl-1-octenyl]-5-oxocyclo-pentaneheptanoic acid).
'Doxapryl' *see* Doxapram.
Doxazoline *see* Domazoline.
DOXENITOIN** (5,5-diphenyl-4-imidazol-idinone; 2-deoxyphenytoin; LG 1; 'glior').
DOXEPIN** (11(6H)-(3-dimethylamino-propylidene)-6,11-dihydrodibenz(b,e)-oxepine; N,N-dimethyldibenz(b,e)oxepin-*trans*-△11(6H),γ-propylamine; doxepin hydrochloride; MF-10; P-3693A; 'adapin', 'aponal', 'curatin', 'quitaxon', 'sinequan', 'sinquan').
See also Cidoxepin.
'Doxergan' *see* Oxomemazine.
DOXIBETASOL*** (9α-fluoro-11β,17α-dihydroxy-16β-methylpregna-1,4-diene-3,20-dione; doxybetasol).
DOXIBETASOL PROPIONATE (doxibeta-sol 27-propionate; GR2/443).
Doxinate *see* Sodium dioctyl sulfosuccinate.
'Doxium' *see* Calcium dobesilate.
'Doxol' *see* Sodium dioctyl sulfosuccinate.
DOXORUBICIN*** ((1S,3S)-3-glycoloyl-1,2,3,4,6,11-hexahydro-3,5,12-trihydroxy-10-methoxy-6,11-dioxo-1-naphthacenyl 3-amino-2,3,6-trideoxy-α-L-*lyxo*-hexo-pyranoside; 14-hydroxydaunorubicin; adriamycin; NSC-123127; 'adriblastine').
Doxybetasol *see* Doxibetasol.
DOXYCYCLINE*** (6-deoxy-5-hydroxy-tetracycline; 6α-deoxyoxytetracycline; DOOTC; 'doxytrex', 'midoxin', 'vibravenös').
Doxycycline hemiethanolate hydro-

179

chloride *see* Doxycycline hyclate.
DOXYCYCLINE HYCLATE (doxycycline hemiethanolate hydrochloride; GS-3065; 'vibramycin').
DOXYLAMINE*** (2-[α-(2-dimethyl-aminoethoxy)-α-methylbenzyl]pyridine; histadoxylamine).
DOXYLAMINE SUCCINATE* (doxyl-aminium succinate; 'decapryn', 'mere-prine').
'Doxytrex' *see* Doxycycline.
Dp *see* Mazipredone.
2,4-DP *see* Dichlorprop.
DPA *see* Algestone acetofenide *and* Propanil.
DPN *see* Nadide.
Dracylic acid *see* Benzoic acid.
'Dramcillin' *see* Penicillin.
'Drano liquid' *see* 1,1,1-Trichloroethane.
'Dranyl' *see* Hydroflumethiazide.
'Drapolene' *see* Benzalkonium.
'Drat' *see* Chlorophacinone.
'Draza' *see* Methiocarb.
DRAZIDOX** (3-methyl-2-quinoxaline-carboxylic acid hydrazide 1,4-dioxide).
'Drazine' *see* Fenoxypropazine.
'Drenison' *see* Fludroxycortide.
'Drenusil' *see* Polythiazide.
'Drinupal' *see* Proguanil.
'Driol' *see* Osalmid.
'Drocarbil' *see* Arecoline-acetarsol.
DROCINONIDE*** (9-fluoro-11β,16α,17,21-tetrahydroxy-5α-pregnane-3,20-dione cyclic 16,17-acetal with acetone; 9-fluoro-5α-pregnane-11β,16α,17,21-tetrol-3,20-dione cyclic 16,17-acetal with acetone).
DROCLIDINIUM BROMIDE*** (3-hy-droxy-1-methylquinuclidinium bromide α-phenylcyclohexaneglycolate).
'Drocort' *see* Fludroxycortide.
'Droctil' *see* Exiproben sodium.
DROFENINE** (2-diethylaminoethyl α-phenylcyclohexaneacetate; hexahydro-adiphenine; 'cyclospasmol', 'trasentin-6H', 'trasentine-A').
'Drofenite' *see* Tetramisole.
'Drolban' *see* Drostanolone.
'Droleptan' *see* Droperidol.
'Drometil' *see* Azosulfamide.
'Dromisol' *see* Dimethyl sulfoxide.
'Dromoran' *see* Levorphanol.
Dromostalonone* *see* Drostanolone.
DROPEMPINE** (1,2,3,6-tetrahydro-1,2,2,6,6-pentamethylpyridine; dehydro-pempidine).
DROPERIDOL*** (1-[1-[4-(p-fluorophenyl)-4-oxobutyl]-1,2,3,6-tetrahydro-4-pyridyl]-2-benzimidazolinone; 4'-fluoro-4-[4-(2-oxo-benzimidazolin-1-yl)-1,2,3,6-tetrahydro-pyridino]butyrophenone; 1-[1-[3-(p-fluoro-benzoyl)propyl]-1,2,3,6-tetrahydropyrid-4-yl]-2-benzimidazolinone; dehydrobenz-peridol; dehydrobenzoperidol; McN-R-4749; R-4749; 'depridol', 'droleptan', 'inapsine', 'sintodian').
See also Ketamine with droperidol.
DROPERIDOL WITH FENTANYL ('innovan', 'innovar', 'thalamonal').

Dropranolol *see* Idropranolol.
DROPROPIZINE*** (3-(4-phenylpiperazin-1-yl)-1,2-propanediol; 1-(2,3-dihydroxy-propyl)-4-phenylpiperazine; hydro-propizine; idropropizina; UCB-1967; 'catabex', 'katril', 'tussilex').
DROSOPHILIN A (2,3,5,6-tetrachloro-4-hydroxyanisole; 2,3,5,6-tetrachloro-4-methoxyphenol).
DROSTANOLONE*** (4,5α-dihydro-2α-methyltestosterone; 17β-hydroxy-2α-methylandrostan-3-one; 17β-hydroxy-2α-methyl-5α-androstan-3-one; 2α-methyl-androstan-17β-ol-3-one; 2α-methyl-androstanolone; dromostanolone).
DROSTANOLONE PROPIONATE (L-32379; NSC-12198; CS-1507; 'drolban', 'masterid', 'masteril', 'masteron', 'methol-one').
DROTAVERINE*** (1-(3,4-diethoxybenzyl-idene)-6,7-diethoxy-1,2,3,4-tetrahydro-isoquinoline; dihydroethaverine; nos-panum; 'dihydroperparin', 'no-spa').
DROTEBANOL*** (3,4-dimethoxy-17-methylmorphinan-6β,14-diol; 6β,14-dihydroxy-3,4-dimethoxy-17-methyl-morphinan).
'Droxaryl' *see* Bufexamac.
'Droxolan' *see* Desoxycholic acid.
DROXYPROPINE*** (1-[2-(2-hydroxy-ethoxy)ethyl]-4-phenyl-4-propionyl-piperidine; 1-[1-[2-(2-hydroxyethoxy)-ethyl]-4-phenylpiperid-4-yl]-1-propanone).
'Dryptal' *see* Furosemide.
DS-36 *see* Sulfamonomethoxine.
DSDP *see* Amiton.
DSE *see* Nabam.
DSM *see* Mannityl dimesilate.
DSO-16 *see* 4-[(2-Chloroethyl)methyl-amino]-1-(2-oxopyrrolidin-1-yl)but-2-yne.
DS substance *see* Serotonin.
DT-327 *see* Clopamide.
DTIC *see* Dacarbazine.
'DTIC-Dome' *see* Dacarbazine.
DTMC *see* Dicofol.
DTP *see* Prosultiamine.
DTPA *see* Pentetic acid.
DTPB *see* Dodecyltriphenylphosphonium bromide.
DTS *see* Dimercaptosuccinic acid.
Du-21220 *see* Ritodrine.
DU-21445 *see* Tiprenolol.
Du-22550 *see* Caproxamine.
'Dualar' *see* Benzodepa.
DUAZOMYCIN*** (antibiotic from *Str. ambofaciens*; diazomycin A; duazomycin A; NSC-51097).
Duazomycin A *see* Duazomycin.
Duazomycin B *see* Azotomycin.
Duazomycin C *see* Ambomycin.
Duboisine *see* Hyoscyamine.
'Dubronax' *see* Dapsone.
'Ducolax' *see* Bisacodyl.
'Dugro' *see* Ronidazole.
'Dulcin' *see* Phenetylurea.
Dulcite *see* Dulcitol.
DULCITOL (dulcite; dulcose; euonymit;

melampyrin; melampyrit).

10-D-Dulcityl-7,8-dimethylisoalloxazine see Galactoflavin.

'**Dulcolan**' see Bisacodyl.

'**Dulcolax**' see Bisacodyl.

Dulcose see Dulcitol.

'**Dulsivac**' see Sodium dioctyl sulfosuccinate.

'**Dumitone**' see Dapsone.

'**Duodorm**' see Dichloralphenazone.

'**Duogastrone**' see Carbenoxolone sodium.

'**Duoluton**' see Norgestrel with ethynylestradiol.

DUOMETACIN*** (3-(p-anisoyl)-6-methoxy-2-methylindole-1-acetic acid; 3-(p-methoxybenzoyl)-6-methoxy-2-methylindole-1-acetic acid).

'**Duomycin**' see Chlortetracycline.

'**Duo-tran**' see Fentonium bromide with perphenazine.

'**Duperan**' see Clometacin.

'**Duphalac**' see Lactulose.

'**Duphanox**' see Chloral hydrate acetylglycinamide.

'**Duphar**' see Tetradifon.

'**Duphar antisprout**' see Propham.

'**Duphaspasmin**' see Mebeverine.

'**Duphaston**' see Dydrogesterone.

'**Duplexcillin**' see Ampicillin with dicloxacillin.

'**Duponol C**' see Sodium dodecyl sulfate.

'**Durabol**' see Nandrolone cyclohexanecarboxylate.

'**Durabolin**' see Nandrolone phenpropionate.

'**Duraboral**' see Ethylestrenol.

'**Duracaine**' see Procaine.

'**Duraflex**' see Flumetramide.

'**Duranest**' see Etidocaine.

'**Dura-penita**' see Benzathine penicillin.

'**Durasulf**' see Sulfametomidine.

'**Durasuline**' see Protamine zinc insulin.

'**Dura-tab**' see Quinidine gluconate.

'**Durenate**' see Sulfametoxydiazine.

DURENE (1,2,4,5-tetramethylbenzene; durol).

'**Durisan**' see Sulfaperin.

'**Duroliopaque**' see Ethyl iodostearate.

'**Duromine**' see Phentermine resin.

'**Duropenin**' see Benzathine penicillin.

DUROQUINONE (tetramethyl-p-benzoquinone).

'**Durotan**' see Reserpine with xipamide.

'**Dursban**' see Chlorpyrifos.

'**Dusodril**' see Naftidrofuril.

'**Duspatal**' see Mebeverine.

'**Duspatalin**' see Mebeverine.

Dustundan (tr) see under Undecenoic acid.

Dutch liquid see Dichloroethylene.

'**Du-ter**' see Fentin hydroxide.

'**Duvadilan**' see Isoxsuprine.

'**Duvaline**' see 2,6-Pyridinedimethanol bis(methylcarbamate).

'**Duvaron**' see Dydrogesterone.

'**Duxen**' see Diazepam.

DV-714 see Leiopyrrole.

DW-61 see Flavoxate.

DW-62 see Dimefline.

'**Dybar**' see Fenuron.

'**Dybenal**' see Dichlorobenzyl alcohol.

'**Dyclone**' see Dyclonine.

DYCLONINE*** (4'-butoxy-3-piperid-1-yl-propiophenone; dyclonine hydrochloride; 'dyclone').

DYDROGESTERONE*** (9β,10α-pregna-4,6-diene-3,20-dione; 6-dehydro-9β,10α-progesterone; 6-dehydroretroprogesterone; isopregnenone; 'duphaston', 'duvaron', 'gestatron', 'gyno-rest', 'terolut').

DYFLOS* (diisopropyl fluorophosph(on)ate; diisopropyl phosphorofluoridate; DFP; fluostigmine; isofluorophate; diflurophate; 'diflupyl', 'floropryl').

'**Dyfonate**' see Fonofos.

'**Dygratal**' see Dihydrotachysterol.

'**Dykanol**' see Polychlorinated biphenyl mixture.

'**Dylate**' see Clonitrate.

'**Dylox**' see Metrifonate.

Dymanthine* see Dimantine.

'**Dymasyl**' see Dimeticone 350.

'**Dymelor**' see Acetohexamide.

'**Dymid**' see Diphenamid.

'**Dynacaine**' see Pyrrocaine.

'**Dynaltone**' see Aralkonium.

'**Dynamyxin**' see Sulfomyxin.

'**Dynapen**' see Dicloxacillin.

'**Dyneric**' see Clomifene citrate.

'**Dynium**' see Aralkonium.

'**Dynone II**' see Dinex dicyclohexylamine.

'**Dynothel**' see Dextrothyroxine sodium.

'**Dyphonate**' see Fonofos.

Dyphyllin see Diprophylline.

'**Dyphylline**' see Theophylline.

DYPNONE (1,3-diphenyl-2-buten-1-one; β-methylchalcone).

DYPNONE GUANYLHYDRAZONE (WR-5667).

'**Dyren**' see Triamterene.

'**Dyrene**' see Anilazine.

'**Dyrenium**' see Triamterene.

'**Dysedon**' see Oxomemazine.

'**Dysenterol**' see Clioquinol with a macrogol.

'**Dysmalgine**' see Dextrofemine.

'**Dytac**' see Triamterene.

'**Dyta-urese**' see Spironolactone.

'**Dythol**' see Cholesterol.

'**Dytide**' see Benzthiazide with triamterene.

'**Dytransin**' see Ibufenac.

E

E-3 *see* Lachesine.
E-39 *see* Inproquone.
E-106 *see* Furfenorex.
E-106-E *see* Furfenorex cyclamate.
E-111 *see* Propylhexedrine.
E-121-C *see* Reserpine with furosemide.
E-141 *see* Etamsylate.
E-142 *see* Anidoxime.
E-171 *see* Lysine acetylsalicylate.
E-205 *see* Calcium dobesilate.
E-217 *see* Thalidomide.
E-438 *see* Sulfasomizole.
E-600 *see* Paraoxon.
E-605 *see* Parathion.
E-1059 *see* Demeton-O plus demeton-S.
E-3314 *see* Schradan.
E-9002 *see* Naftalofos.
EA-83 *see* Methylheptaminol.
EA-166 *see* Guanoxyfen.
EA-3054 *see* Bioallethrin.
EA-3547 *see* Dibenz(b,f)(1,4)oxazepine.
EACA *see* Aminocaproic acid.
'Eatan' *see* Methaqualone with promazine.
Eazamine *see* Diethazine.
'Ebesal' *see* Allocupreide.
'Ebimar' *see* Poligeenan.
'Ebutol' *see* Ethambutol.
EC-50 *see* Fenitrothion.
'E-carpine' *see* Epinephrine tartrate.
'Ecatox' *see* Parathion.
'Ecatril' *see* Dibenzepin.
Ecboline *see* Ergotoxine.
ECGONINE (3-hydroxy-2-tropanecarboxylic acid; 3-tropanolcarboxylic acid; tropine-2-carboxylic acid).
Echothiopate *see* Ecothiopate.
Echothiophosphate *see* Ecothiopate.
Ecinamine *see* Etifelmine.
'Eclabron' *see* Guaithylline.
'Ecloril' *see* Chlorambucil.
Ecmolin (tr) (antibiotic from fish; ekmolin).
'Ecolid *see* Chlorisondamine.
ECONAZOLE*** (1-[2,4-dichloro-β-(*p*-chlorobenzyloxy)phenethyl]imidazole; 2,4,4'-trichloro-α-imidazol-1-yl-α,α'-ditolyl ether; econazole nitrate; R-14827; 'pevaryl').
Ecostigmine* *see* Ecothiopate iodide.
ECOTHIOPATE IODIDE*** (*S*-(2-dimethylaminoethyl) *O,O*-diethyl phosphorothioate methiodide; diethyl(2-trimethylammoniummethyl) thiophosphate iodide; echothiopate; echothiophosphate; ecostigmine; MI-217; 'phospholine iodide').
'Ecoval 70' *see* Betamethasone valerate.
ECTYLUREA*** (1-(2-ethyl-*cis*-crotonyl)-urea; 'levanil', 'nostyn', 'pacetyn').
'Eczecidin' *see* Clioquinol.
'Edathamil' *see* Edetic acid.
'Edecrin' *see* Etacrynic acid.

'Edemo' *see* Ethyl (2-diethylaminoethyl)-phosphonothioate.
'Edemox' *see* Acetazolamide.
Edetate disodium calcium* *see* Sodium calcium edetate.
Edetate sodium* *see* Tetrasodium edetate.
Edetate trisodium* *see* Trisodium edetate.
EDETIC ACID*** (ethylenediaminetetra-acetic acid; *N,N,N',N'*-tetra(carboxy-methyl)ethylenediamine; ethylenedinitrilo-tetraacetic acid; ethylenebis(iminodiacetic acid); edathamil; EDTA; tetracemine; 'complexic acid', 'komplexic acid', 'verse-nic acid').
See also Disodium edetate; Piperazine calcium edetate; Sodium calcium edetate; Sodium feredetate; Tetrasodium edetate; Trisodium edetate.
EDIFENPHOS* (*O*-ethyl *S,S*-diphenyl phosphorodithioate; 'hinosan').
EDISILATE(S)** (ethane-1,2-disulfonate(s); edisylate(s)).
See also Caramiphen edisilate; Clomethia-zole edisilate.
Edisylate(s)* *see* Edisilate(s).
EDOGESTRONE*** (17-acetoxy-3,3-ethyl-enedioxy-6-methylpregn-5-en-20-one; 3,3-ethylenedioxy-17-hydroxy-6-methylpregn-5-en-20-one acetate; 3,3-ethylenedioxy-6-methylpregn-5-en-20-one-17-ol acetate; 17-hydroxy-6-methylpregn-5-ene-3,20-dione cyclic 3-(ethylene acetal) acetate; Ph-218).
EDPA *see* 2-Ethyl-3,3-diphenylpropen(2)yl-amine.
Edrofuradene *see* Nifurdazil.
EDROPHONIUM CHLORIDE*** (di-methylethyl(*m*-hydroxyphenyl)ammonium chloride; Ro-2-3198; 'tensilon').
EDTA *see* Edetic acid.
EF-185 *see* Framycetin.
'Efferalgan' *see* Paracetamol with ascorbic acid.
'Effilon' *see* Amfepramone.
'Effortil' *see* Etilefrine.
'Effusan' *see* Dinitro-*o*-cresol.
'Efitard' *see* Procaine-penicillin.
EFLOXATE*** (ethyl (4-oxo-2-phenyl-4H-1-benzopyran-7-yloxy)acetate; ethyl 7-flavonoxyacetate; 7-carbethoxymethoxy-flavone; 7-ethoxycarbonylmethoxyflavone; oxyflavyl; 'recordil').
'Efosin' *see* Fenpipramide with fenpiprane.
'Efsiomycin' *see* Fluvomycin.
'Eftolon' *see* Sulfaphenazole.
'Efudix' *see* Fluorouracil.
'Egacen' *see* Hyoscyamine.
'Egalin' *see* Rauwolfia.
'Eggopurin' *see* Calcium mandelate.
'Eglonul' *see* Sulpiride.
'Egmol' *see* Phenolphthalol.

Egyt-13 *see* Benzonatate.
Egyt-201 *see* Bencyclane.
Egyt-739 *see* Guanazodine.
EHDP *see* Disodium etidronate.
EHDP™ *see* Etidronic acid.
Ehrlich 5 *see* Oxophenarsine.
Ehrlich 594 *see* Acetarsol.
Ehrlich 606 *see* Arsphenamine.
Eicosanoic acid *see* Arachidic acid.
5,8,11,14-Eicosatetraenoic acid *see*
    Arachidonic acid.
EICOSA-5,8,11,14-TETRAYNOIC ACID
    (tetraynoic acid).
'Ekaprol' *see* Aminocaproic acid.
'Ekatin' *see* Thiometon.
'Ekatin F' *see* Morphothion.
'Ekatin M' *see* Morphothion.
'Eketebin' *see* Protionamide.
Ekmolin *see* Ecmolin.
'Ekomine' *see* Atropine methonitrate.
'Ektafos' *see* Dicrotophos.
'Ektomin' *see* Chlormebuform.
'Ekvacillin' *see* Cloxacillin.
EL-241 *see* Parinol.
EL-273 *see* Triarimol.
EL-531 *see* Ancymidol.
EL-857 *see* Apramycin.
EL-974 *see* Ticarbodine.
'Eladigal' *see* Lanatoside C.
ELAIDIC ACID (*trans*-9-octadecenoic acid).
'Elamol' *see* Tofenacin.
'Elan' *see* Fenyramidol.
ELANTRINE** (11-(3-dimethylamino-
    propylidene)-5,6-dihydro-5-methyl-
    morphanthridine; EX-10-029).
ELANZEPINE** (3-chloro-11-[3-(dimethyl-
    amino)propylidene]-5,6-dihydromorphan-
    thridine).
'Elarzone' *see* Pipebuzone.
'Elavil' *see* Amitriptyline.
'Elcosal' *see* Aluminium glycinate.
'Elcosine' *see* Sulfasomidine.
ELD-950 *see* Eledoisin.
'Eldopal' *see* Levodopa.
Eldrin *see* Rutoside.
Elecamphane *see* Alantolactone.
Electrocortin *see* Aldosterone.
ELEDOISIN** (5-oxo-L-propyl-L-propyl-L-
    seryl-L-lysyl-L-aspartyl-L-alanyl-L-phenyl-
    alanyl-L-isoleucylglycyl-L-leucyl-L-
    methionamide).
ELEDOISIN SYNTHETIC (ELD-950).
ELEMICIN (3,5-dimethoxytoluene; orcinol
    dimethyl ether).
'Elenium' *see* Chlordiazepoxide.
'Eleocron' *see* Dioxacarb.
'Eleparon' *see* Mucoitin polysulfate.
'Eleudron' *see* Sulfathiazole.
'Elgetol' *see* Dinitro-*o*-cresol.
'Elgetol 30' *see* Dinitro-*o*-cresol.
'Elgetol 313' *see* Dinoseb trolamine.
'Elheparin' *see* Mucoitin polysulfate.
'Elipol' *see* Dinitro-*o*-cresol.
'Elipten' *see* Aminoglutethimide.
'Eliptin' *see* Aminoglutethimide.
'Elisal' *see* Sultiame.
'Elixophylline' *see* Theophylline.

ELLAGIC ACID*** (2,3,7,8-tetrahydroxy-
    (1)benzopyrano(5,4,3-cde)(1)benzopyran-
    5,10-dione; 4,4′,5,5′,6,6′-hexahydroxydi-
    phenic acid dilactone; benzoaric acid;
    'gallogen').
ELLIPTICINE (5,11-dimethyl-6H-pyrido-
    (4,3-b)carbazole; NSC-71795).
'Elobromo' *see* Mitolactol.
'Elocron' *see* Dioxacarb.
'Elorine' *see* Tricyclamol.
'Elozell' *see* Potassium magnesium aspartate.
'Elrodorm' *see* Glutethimide.
'Elsan' *see* Phenthoate.
'Elsix' *see* Hexetidine.
'Elsyl' *see* Metizoline.
'Eltroxin' *see* Levothyroxine sodium.
ELUCAINE** (α-diethylaminomethylbenzyl
    alcohol benzoate ester; *N*,*N*-diethyl-β-
    hydroxyphenethylamine benzoate ester).
'Elvanol' *see* Polyvinyl alcohol.
'Elvaron' *see* Dichlofluanid.
'Elycaine' *see* Butacaine.
'Elyzol' *see* Metronidazole.
'Elzogram' *see* Cefazolin.
'Emanil' *see* Idoxuridine.
'Emanon' *see under* Macrogols.
'Emasols(s)' *see* Polysorbate(s).
'Embadol' *see* Tiomesterone.
'Embanox' *see* Butylated hydroxyanisole.
EMBAY 8440 *see* Praziquantel.
'Embdabol' *see* Tiomesterone.
Embechine (tr) *see* Chlormethine.
Embichin (tr) *see* Chlormethine.
Embichin 7 (tr) *see* Novembichin.
Embikhin (tr) *see* Chlormethine.
EMBONATE(S)** (4,4′-methylenebis(3-
    hydroxynaphthalene-2-carboxylate(s));
    pamoate(s)).
    See also Chloroquine mustard embonate;
    Cycloguanil embonate; Hydroxyzine
    embonate; Noscapine embonate; Pama-
    quine embonate; Pyrantel embonate;
    Pyrvinium embonate.
EMBRAMINE*** (2-(*p*-bromo-α-methyl-α-
    phenylbenzyloxy)-*N*,*N*-dimethylethyl-
    amine; 2-[1-(*p*-bromophenyl)-1-phenyl-
    ethoxy]-*N*,*N*-dimethylethylamine; em-
    bramine hydrochloride; mebromphen-
    hydramine; 'bromadryl', 'embramycin',
    'mebryl').
    See also Dosulepin with embramine.
EMBRAMINE TEOCLATE (embramine
    8-chlorotheophyllinate; embramine theo-
    clate; 'medrin').
'Embramycin' *see* Embramine.
'Embutox' *see* 4-(2,4-Dichlorophenoxy)-
    butyric acid.
EMBUTRAMIDE*** (*N*-[2-ethyl-2-(3-
    methoxyphenyl)butyl]-4-hydroxybutyr-
    amide; *N*-(β,β-diethyl-*m*-methoxy-
    phenethyl)-4-hydroxybutyramide).
EMD-19698 *see* Peratizole.
'Emdabol' *see* Tiomesterone.
'Emedan' *see* Carbutamide.
EMEPRONIUM BROMIDE*** (2-benz-
    hydrylisopropyl)ethyldimethylammonium
    bromide; ethyldimethyl(1-methyl-3,3-

diphenylpropyl)ammonium bromide; 'cetiprin').

Emerald green *see* Brilliant green.

'Emergil' *see* Flupentixol.

'Emete-con' *see* Benzquinamide.

EMETINE (emetine hydrochloride; ipecine; methylcephaeline; NSC-33669).

EMETINE CAMSILATE (emetine camphorsulfonate; emetine camsylate; canforemetina; 'emetoplix').

Emetine camphorsulfonate *see* Emetine camsilate.

'Emeto-Na' *see* Sodium antimonyl tartrate.

'Emetoplix' *see* Emetine camsilate.

'Emex antistaminico' *see* Carbazochrome sodium sulfonate with chlorpheniramine maleate.

'Emivan' *see* Etamivan.

'Emmenin' *see* Estradiol gluconate.

'Emodella' *see* Frangula-emodin.

Emodins *see* Aloe-emodin; Frangula-emodin.

'Emostat' *see* Mepesulfate.

'Emphysin' *see* Quinetalate.

'Empicol' *see* Sodium dodecyl sulfate.

EMPT *see* Fenfluramine.

EMQ *see* Ethoxyquin.

'Emtryl' *see* Dimetridazole.

'Emulax' *see* Sodium dioctyl sulfosuccinate.

EMYLCAMATE**** (1-ethyl-1-methylpropyl carbamate; carbamate of 1-ethyl-1-methyl-1-propanol; carbamate of 2-ethyl-2-butanol; methyl diethyl carbinol urethan; *tert*-hexanol carbamate; carbamate of 3-methyl-3-pentanol; KAB1-925; MK-250; 'nuncital', 'statran', 'striatran').

EN-1010 *see* Pyrrocaine.

EN-1530 *see* Naloxone.

EN-1620A *see* Nalmexone.

EN-1639A *see* Naltrexone.

EN-1661L *see* Bisobrin lactate.

EN-1733A *see* Molindone.

EN-2234-A *see* Nalbuphine.

Enallachrome *see* Esculin.

ENALLYLPROPYMAL* (5-allyl-5-isopropyl-1-methylbarbituric acid).

ENALLYLPROPYMAL SODIUM ('narconumal')

ENANTATE(S)*** (hexane-1-carboxylate(s); heptanoate(s); enanthate(s); oenanthate(s); heptylate(s)).
See also Estradiol enantate; Fluphenazine enantate; Metenolone enantate; Testosterone enantate).

Enanthal *see* Heptyl aldehyde.

Enanthaldehyde *see* Heptyl aldehyde.

ENANTHIC ACID (1-hexanecarboxylic acid; heptanoic acid; heptylic acid; oenanthic acid).
See also Enantate(s).

Enanthol *see* Heptyl aldehyde

'Enavid' *see* Noretynodrel with mestranol.

ENBUCRILATE**** (butyl 2-cyanoacrylate; 'fimomed', 'finomed', 'histoacryl').

'Encephabol' *see* Pyritinol.

ENCLOMIFENE*** (2-[*p*-(2-chloro-*trans*-1,2-diphenylvinyl)phenoxy]triethylamine;

(*E*)-2-[*p*-(2-chloro-1,2-diphenylvinyl)-phenoxy]-triethylamine; (*formerly named*) cisclomifene; cisclomiphene).
See also Clomifene; Zuclomifene.

'Encordin' *see* Peruvoside.

ENCYPRATE**** (ethyl *N*-benzylcyclopropanecarbamate; A-19757; MO-1255).

'Endercin' *see* Etacrynic acid.

'Endiaton' *see* 5,7-Dichloro-8-quinolinol.

Endiemal* *see* Metharbital.

'Endifasept' *see* 2-Phenoxyethanol.

'Endiran' *see* Osalmid.

'Endobil' *see* Iodoxamic acid.

'Endocaine' *see* Pyrrocaine.

'Endogan' *see* Endosulfan.

'Endografin' *see* Adipiodone methylglucamine.

1,4-Endomethylenecyclohexane *see* Norbornane.

1,4-Endomethylene-2-cyclohexene *see* Norbornene.

1,4-Endomethylene-△⁵-cyclohexene-2,3-dicarboxylic acid *see* 5-Norbornene-2,3-dicarboxylic acid.

3,6-Endomethylene-1,2,3,6-tetrahydrophthalic acid *see* 5-Norbornene-2,3-dicarboxylic acid.

'Endomid' *see* Diethyl-5-norbornene-*trans*-2,3-dicarboxamide.

ENDOMYCIN*** (antibiotic from *Streptomyces endus*).
See also Scopafungin.

'Endo-paractol' *see* Dimeticone.

Endophenolphthalein *see* Acetphenolisatin.

'Endosan' *see* Binapacryl.

'Endosprin' *see* Lysine acetylsalicylate.

ENDOSULFAN* (6,7,8,9,10,10-hexachloro-1,5,5a,6,9,9a-hexahydro-6,9-methano-2,4,3-benzodioxathiepin 3-oxide; 5,6-bis-(hydroxymethyl)-1,2,3,4,7,7-hexachloronorbornene sulfite; hexachloronorbornene 5,6-bis(oxymethylene)sulfite; tiodan; 'beosit', 'cyclodan', 'endogan', 'ensawan', 'malix', 'sialan', 'thifor', 'thimul', 'thiodan', 'thionex', 'thyodan', 'thyonex').

'Endothal' *see* Endothal-sodium.

Endothall *see* Endothal-sodium.

ENDOTHAL-SODIUM* (disodium 7-oxa-3,6-*endo*-methylenehexahydrophthalate; disodium *endo-endo*-7-oxabicyclo(2.2.1)-heptane-2,3-dicarboxylate; disodium endothal; endothall; 'endothal').
See also Propham plus endothal-sodium.

ENDOTHION* (*S*-(5-methoxy-4-oxo-4H-pyran-2-ylmethyl) *O,O*-dimethyl phosphorothioate; 'farming S').

'Endoton' *see* Prolonium iodide.

'Endoverine' *see* Papaverine mandelate.

'Endoxan' *see* Cyclophosphamide.

'Endoxana' *see* Cyclophosphamide.

'Endoyodina' *see* Prolonium iodide.

'Endrate' *see* Disodium edetate; Tetrasodium edetate.

ENDRIN* (1,2,3,4,10,10-hexachloro-6,7-epoxy-1,4,4a,5,6,7,8,8a-octahydro-1,4-*endo*-5,8-*endo*-dimethanonaphthalene; 1α,2β, 2aβ,3α,6α,6aβ,7β,7aα-3,4,5,6,9,9-hexa-

chloro-1a,2,2a,3,6,6a,7,7a-octahydro-2,7:
3,6-dimethanonaphth(2,3-6)oxirene; compound 269; nendrin).
ENDRISONE*** (11β-hydroxy-6α-methyl-pregna-1,4-diene-3,20-dione; 6α-methyl-pregna-1,4-dien-11β-ol-3,20-dione; endrysone; 'aldrisone').
Endrysone* *see* Endrisone.
Enduracidin *see* Enramycin.
'Enduron' *see* Methylclothiazide.
'Enduxan' *see* Cyclophosphamide.
'Enelbin' *see* Aluminium sodium silicate.
'Enelone' *see* Pregnenolone acetate.
'Energer' *see* Isocarboxazid.
'Eneril' *see* Paracetamol.
ENESTEBOL*** (4,17β-dihydroxy-17-methylandrosta-1,4-dien-3-one; 17α-methylandrosta-1,4-diene-4,17β-diol-3-one).
ENFLURANE*** (2-chloro-1,1,2-trifluoro-ethyl difluoromethyl ether; methylflur-ether; 'ethrane').
'Enethyl' *see* 2-Methylaminoheptane.
'Enheptin-A' *see* Aminitrozole.
Enhexymal* *see* Hexobarbital.
ENIBOMAL* (5-(2-bromoallyl)-5-isopropyl-1-methyl barbituric acid; narcobarbital; enibomal sodium; 'eunarcon', 'narcodorm', 'narcotal', 'narcovene', 'pronarcon', 'narcovene', 'venopan').
'Enide' *see* Diphenamid.
'Enidran' *see* Osalmid.
'Enidrel' *see* Norethisterone acetate with ethinylestradiol.
Enimal *see* Hexobarbital.
'Enovid' *see* Noretynodrel with mestranol.
ENOXOLONE*** (3β-hydroxy-11-oxoolean-12-en-30-oic acid; glycyrrhetic acid; glycyr-rhetin; glycyrrhetinic acid; 'biogastrone acid', 'bisone').
Enoxolone glycoside *see* Glycyrrhizic acid.
Enoxolone hydrogen succinate *see* Carben-oxolone.
'Enpac' *see* Lactobacillus acidophilus.
Enphenemal* *see* Methylphenobarbital.
ENPIPRAZOLE*** (1-(o-chlorophenyl)-4-[2-(1-methylpyrazol-4-yl)ethyl]piperazine; enpiprazole dihydrochloride; H-3608).
ENPRAZEPINE** (5-(3-dimethylamino-propyl)-5,6-dihydro-11-methylene-11H-di-benz(b,e)azepine).
ENPROMATE*** (1,1-diphenyl-2-propynyl cyclohexanecarbamate).
ENRAMYCIN*** (antibiotic from *Str. fungi-cidicus*; enduracidin).
'Ensawan' *see* Endosulfan.
'Ensidon' *see* Opipramol.
'Ensign' *see* Citicoline.
ENT-7169 *see* Alloxan.
ENT-16275 *see* Bioallethrin.
ENT-21170 *see* Dimethrin.
ENT-24915 *see* Tepa.
ENT-24969 *see* Clofenvinfos.
ENT-25567 *see* Naftalofos.
ENT-26316 *see* Apholate.
ENT-29106 *see* Nimidane.
'Entacyl' *see* Piperazine adipate.
'Entamide' *see* Diloxanide.

'Entefur' *see* Nifuraldezone.
Enteramine *see* Serotonin.
'Enterfram' *see* Framycetin.
'Enturen' *see* Sulfinpyrazone.
'Enterocura' *see* Sulfaguanole.
'Enterokin' *see* Clioquinol.
'Enteromide' *see* Sulfaloxic acid.
'Entero-norm' *see* Albumin tannate.
'Enteroquinol' *see* Clioquinol.
'Entero-septol' *see* Clioquinol.
'Enterotonin' *see* Carbachol.
'Enterovioform' *see* Clioquinol.
'Enterozol' *see* Clioquinol.
'Entex' *see* Fenthion.
'Entizol' *see* Metronidazole.
'Entobex' *see* Phanquinone.
'Entodon' *see* Prolonium iodide.
'Entryl' *see* Dimetridazole.
ENTSUFON (2-[2-[2-[p-(1,1,3,3-tetra-methylbutyl)phenoxy]ethoxy]ethoxy]-ethanesulfonic acid).
ENTSUFON SODIUM* (sodium 2-[2-[2-[p-(1,1,3,3-tetramethylbutyl)phenoxy]-ethoxy]ethoxy]ethanesulfonate).
'Entumine' *see* Clotiapine.
'Envacar' *see* Guanoxan.
ENVIOMYCIN** (stereoisomer of [[15-(3,6-diamino-4-hydroxyhexanamido)-3-(hexa-hydro-2-iminopyrimidin-4-yl)-9,12-bis-(hydroxymethyl)-2,5,8,11,14-pentaoxo-1,4,7,10,13-pentaazacyclohexadec-6-yl-idene]methyl]urea; tuberactinomycin N).
'Enzactin' *see* Triacetin.
'Enzeon' *see* Chymotrypsin.
'Enzopride' *see* Nadide.
'Enzytol' *see* Choline borate.
'Eoden' *see* Heptaminol.
'Eparsulfo' *see* Magnesium methynotrithioglycolate.
EPHEDRINE ((−)-α-(1-methylaminoethyl)-benzyl alcohol; (−)-2-methylamino-1-phenyl-1-propanol; ephedrine hydro-chloride).
See also Pseudoephedrine; Racephedrine.
EPHENAMINE (2-hydroxy-N-methyl-1,2-diphenylethylamine).
L-**EPHENAMINE PENICILLIN** (L-ephen-amine salt of penicillin G; 'compenamine').
Epiandrosterone *see* 5α-Androstan-3β-ol-17-one.
Epichlorhydrine *see* Epichlorohydrin.
EPICHLOROHYDRIN (1-chloro-2,3-epoxy-propane; γ-chloropropylene oxide; chloro-methyloxirane; α-epichlorohydrin; epichlor-hydrine).
Epichlorohydrin dextran reaction products *see* Dextranomer; Polidexide.
Epichlorohydrin polymer with tetra-ethylenepentamine *see* Colestipol.
Epichlorohydrin starch reaction product *see* Amilomer.
EPICILLIN*** (6-(D-2-amino-2-(1,4-cyclo-hexadien-1-yl)acetamido)penicillanic acid; epicillin sodium; dihydroampicillin; SQ-11302; 'dexacillin', 'florispec'; 'spectacillin').
'Epiclase' *see* Phenacemide.
'Epidine' *see* Trimethadione.

'Epido' *see* Phenylmercuric nitrate.
'Epidon' *see* Diacetazotol.
'Epidosin' *see* Valethamate.
'Epidropal' *see* Allopurinol.
EPIESTRIOL*** (estra-1,3,5(10)-triene-3,16β,17β-triol; 16-epiestriol; epioestriol; 'actriol').
Epihydrin alcohol *see* Glycidol.
'Epileptasid' *see* Rattlesnake venom.
'Epilim' *see* Sodium valproate.
EPIMESTROL*** (3-methoxyestra-1,3,5(10)-triene-16α,17α-diol; 16α,17α-dihydroxy-3-methoxyestra-1,3,5(10)-triene; Org.-817).
'Epimide' *see* Phensuximide.
'Epi-monistat' *see* Miconazole.
'Epinal' *see* Epinephryl borate.
Epinefrina *see* Epinephrine.
EPINEPHRINE*** (3,4-dihydroxy-α-methylaminomethylbenzyl alcohol; adrenaline; NSC-62786; epinefrina; epirenamine; levorenin; 'adrenalin').
EPINEPHRYL BORATE ((−)-4-(1-hydroxy-2-methylaminoethyl)-*m*-phenylene cyclic borate; epinephrine 3,4-cyclic borate; adrenaline borate; 'epinal', 'eppy').
'Epinyl' *see* Ethadione.
Epioestriol* *see* Epiestriol.
'Epipol' *see* Dinitro-*o*-cresol.
EPIPROPIDINE*** (1,1′-bis(2,3-epoxy-propyl)-4,4′-bipiperidine; epoxypropidine; L-28002; NSC-56308; 'eponate').
Epirenamine *see* Epinephrine.
EPIRIZOLE** (4-methoxy-2-(5-methoxy-3-methylpyrazol-1-yl)-6-methylpyrimidine; 1-(4-methoxy-6-methylpyrimidin-2-yl)-5-methoxy-3-methylpyrazole; mepirizole; methopyrimazole; DA-398; 'mebron').
'Episcorb' *see* Adrenaline ascorbate.
EPITESTOSTERONE (17α-hydroxyandrost-4-en-3-one; androst-4-en-17α-ol-3-one).
Epithiazide* *see* Epitizide.
2α,3α-Epithio-5α-androstan-17β-ol *see* Epitiostanol.
EPITIOSTANOL** (2α,3α-epithio-5α-androstan-17β-ol; S-10275).
Epitiostanol 1-methoxycyclopentyl ether *see* Mepitiostane.
EPITIZIDE*** (6-chloro-3,4-dihydro-7-sulfamoyl-3-(2,2,2-trifluoroethylthiomethyl)-1,2,4-benzothiadiazine 1,1-dioxide; 6-chloro-3,4-dihydro-3-[(2,2,2-trifluoroethyl)thiomethyl]-2H-1,2,4-benzothiadiazine-7-sulfonamide 1,1-dioxide; epithiazide; 'thiaver').
'Epitone' *see* Ferrous gluconate.
EPN *see* Ethyl *p*-nitrophenyl phenylphosphonothioate.
'Epodyl' *see* Etoglucid.
'Eponate' *see* Epipropidine.
'Epontol' *see* Propanidid.
'Eporal' *see* Dapsone.
4,5-Epoxy-3,14-dihydroxy-N-methyl-6-oxomorphinan *see* Oxymorphone.
6,7-Epoxy-4,5-dihydroxy-2-octenoic acid δ-lactone acetate *see* Asperlin.
21,23-Epoxy-19,24-dinor-17α-chola-1,3,5-(10),7,20,22-hexaene-3,17-diol 3-acetate

see Estrofurate.
2,3-Epoxy-2-ethyl-3-propylpropionic acid *see* Oxanamide.
14,15β-Epoxy-3β-hydroxy-5β-bufa-10,22-dienolide *see* Bufogenin.
4,5-Epoxy-3-hydroxy-5,N-dimethyl-6-oxomorphinan *see* Metopon.
4,5-Epoxy-6-hydroxy-3-methoxy-N-methylmorphinan *see* Dihydrocodeine.
4,5-Epoxy-14-hydroxy-3-methoxy-N-methyl-6-oxomorphinan *see* Oxycodone.
4,5-Epoxy-6-hydroxy-3-methoxymorphin-7-ene *see* Norcodeine.
4,5-Epoxy-3-hydroxy-N-methylmorphinan *see* Desomorphine.
4,5-Epoxy-3-hydroxy-N-methyl-6-oxomorphinan *see* Hydromorphone.
4α,5-Epoxy-17β-hydroxy-3-oxo-5α-androstane-2α-carbonitrile *see* Trilostane.
Epoxymethamine bromide *see* Scopolamine methyl bromide.
4,5-Epoxy-3-methoxy-N-methyl-6-oxomorphinan *see* Hydrocodone.
Epoxypiperazine *see* Epoxypropylpiperazine.
2,3-Epoxy-1-propanol *see* Glycidol.
Epoxypropidine* *see* Epipropidine.
2,3-Epoxypropionic acid *see* Glycidic acid.
6-(1,2-Epoxypropyl)-5-hydroxy-5,6-dihydro-2H-pyran 2-one acetate *see* Asperlin.
1,2-Epoxypropylphosphonic acid *see* Fosfomycin.
EPOXYPROPYLPIPERAZINE (1,4-bis-(2,3-epoxypropyl)piperazine; diepoxypiperazine; epoxypiperazine).
Epoxytropine tropate *see* Scopolamine.
'Eppy' *see* Epinephryl borate.
EPRAZINONE*** (3-[4-(β-ethoxyphenethyl)piperazin-1-yl]-2-methylpropiophenone; 1-(2-ethoxy-2-phenylethyl)-4-(2-methyl-3-oxo-3-phenylpropyl)piperazine; CE-746; 'mucitux').
EPROZINOL*** (4-(β-methoxyphenethyl)-α-phenyl-1-piperazinepropanol; 1-(3-hydroxy-3-phenylpropyl)-4-(β-methoxyphenethyl)piperazine; 'eupneron').
'Epsicapron' *see* Aminocaproic acid.
Epsom salts *see* Magnesium sulfate.
'Eptam' *see* Ethyl dipropylcarbamothioate.
'Eptapur' *see* Buturon.
EPTC* *see* Ethyl dipropylcarbamothioate.
'Equa' *see* Aspartame.
'Equigard' *see* Dichlorvos.
'Equilid' *see* Sulpiride.
EQUILIN (3-hydroxyestra-1,3,5(10),7-tetraen-17-one).
Equine gonadotrophin *see* Serum gonadotrophin.
'Equipax' *see* Procymate.
'Equipertine' *see* Oxypertine.
'Equipoise' *see* Hydroxyzine embonate.
ER-72 *see* Benzydamine with erythromycin.
ER-105 *see* Glyclamide with metformin.
ER-115 *see* Temazepam.
'Eradex' *see* Thioquinox.
'Eraldin' *see* Practolol.

'**Erantin**' *see* Dextropropoxyphene.
'**Erasol**' *see* Chlormethine.
'**Eraverm**' *see* Piperazine adipate.
'**Eraxan**' *see* Magnesium peroxide.
'**Erbaprelina**' *see* Pyrimethamine.
'**Erbocain**' *see* Fomocaine.
ERBON* (2-(2,4,5-trichlorophenoxy)ethyl 2,2-dichloropropionate; dalapon trichlorophenoxyethyl ester; 'baron', 'novon').
'**Ercefuryl**' *see* Nifuroxazide.
'**Ercoquin**' *see* Hydroxychloroquine.
'**Ercoril**' *see* Propantheline.
'**Ercotina**' *see* Propantheline.
Ergadenylic acid *see* Adenosine phosphate.
Ergam (tr) *see* Ergotoxine.
'**Ergenyl**' *see* Sodium valproate.
Ergine *see* Lysergamide.
Ergobasine *see* Ergometrine.
ERGOCALCIFEROL*** (24-methyl-9,10-*seco*-cholesta-5,7,10(19),22-tetraen-3-ol; 9,10-*seco*-ergosta-5,7,10(19),22-tetraen-3-ol; calciferol; irradiated ergosterol; viosterol; vitamin D$_2$).
ERGOCRYPTINE (ergokryptine).
'**Ergoklinine**' *see* Ergometrine.
Ergokryptine *see* Ergocryptine.
ERGOMETRINE*** (*N*-[1-(hydroxymethyl)ethyl]lysergamide; D-lysergic acid 1-hydroxymethylethylamide; hydroxypropyllysergamide; lysergic acid propanolamide; ergobasine; ergonovine; ergotocine; 'ergoklinine', 'ergostetrine').
ERGOMETRINE MALEATE ('basergin', 'cornocentin', 'ermetrine').
ERGOMETRINE TARTRATE ('ergotrate', 'neo-femergen').
Ergonovine* *see* Ergometrine.
9,10-*seco*-Ergosta-5,7,10(19),22-tetraen-3-ol *see* Ergocalciferol.
9,10-*seco*-Ergosta-5,7,22-trien-3β-ol *see* Dihydrotachysterol.
'**Ergostetrine**' *see* Ergometrine.
ERGOTAMINE*** (an alkaloid from ergot).
ERGOTAMINE TARTRATE* ('exmigra', 'femergin', 'gynergen', 'lingraine').
ERGOTAMINE TARTRATE WITH CAFFEINE ('cafergot').
'**Ergoterm TGO**' *see* (Dibenzyltin)bis(isooctylthioglycolate).
Ergothioneine *see* Thioneine.
Ergothionone *see* Thioneine.
Ergotocine *see* Ergometrine.
ERGOTOXINE (mixture of ergocornine, ergocristine and ergocryptine; ergam).
'**Ergotrate**' *see* Ergometrine.
'**Ergotren**' *see* Dihydroergocristine.
'**Eriflogin**' *see* Benzydamine with erythromycin.
Erinit (tr) *see* Pentaerythrityl tetranitrate.
ERIODICTIN (eriodictyol rhamnoside).
ERIODICTYOL (3',4',5,7-tetrahydroxyflavanone).
Eriodictyol glucoside *see* Citrin.
Eriodictyol 3'-methyl ether *see* Homoeriodictyol.
Eriodictyol rhamnoside *see* Eriodictin.
Eriodictyonone *see* Homoeriodictyol.

Erio green B *see* Kiton green.
ERITADENINE (4-(6-aminopurin-9-yl)-2,3-dihydroxybutyric acid; 4-(6-aminopurin-9-yl)-4-deoxy-D-erythronic acid; 4-aden-9-yl-2(*R*),3(*R*)-dihydroxybutyric acid; 9-(3-carboxy-2,3-dihydroxypropyl)adenine; lentysine).
Erithrityl tetranitrate* *see* Erythrityl tetranitrate.
Eritrityl tetranitrate** *see* Erythrityl tetranitrate.
'**Ermetrine**' *see* Ergometrine.
'**Erracalma**' *see* Dextromoramide.
ERUCIC ACID (*cis*-13-docosenoic acid).
'**Ervasin**' *see* Acetylcresotic acid.
'**Erycin**' *see* Erythromycin.
'**Erycinum**' *see* Erythromycin.
Erycorbin *see* Isoascorbic acid.
'**Erypar**' *see* Erythromycin stearate.
'**Erysan**' *see* Chlornaphazine.
Erythorbic acid *see* Isoascorbic acid.
Erythoxylin *see* Cocaine.
Erythrite *see* Erythritol.
ERYTHRITOL (1,2,3,4-butanetetrol; erythrite; erythrol; erythroglucin; *meso*-erythritol; *anti*-erythrite; phlucin; phycitol).
Erythritol anhydride polyethylenimine polymer *see* Polyetadene.
ERYTHRITYL 1,4-DIMESILATE (L-erythritol 1,4-dimethanesulfonate; CB-2562; NSC-39070).
ERYTHRITYL TETRANITRATE (erithrityl tetranitrate; eritrityl tetranitrate; erythryl nitrate; nitroerythrite; nitroerythritol; tetranitrol; 'cardilate', 'cardiwell', 'tetranitrin').
'**Erythrocin**' *see* Erythromycin.
Erythroglucin *see* Erythritol.
Erythrol *see* Erythritol.
ERYTHROMYCIN*** (antibiotic from *Str. erythreus*; 'erycin', 'erycinum', 'erythrocin', 'erythrotil', 'ilotycin', 'lubomycin', 'pantomicina', 'robimycin').
See also Benzydamine with erythromycin.
Erythromycin B *see* Berythromycin.
ERYTHROMYCIN ESTOLATE* (erythromycin propionate ester lauryl sulfate; 'ilosone', 'lauritran', 'PELS').
Erythromycin estolate with tetracycline ('laucetin', 'lautecin').
ERYTHROMYCIN ETHYL SUCCINATE ((2-ethylsuccinyl)erythromycin; 'abboticine', 'erythroped', 'paediathrocin', 'pantomycin', 'pediathrocin').
ERYTHROMYCIN PROPIONATE ('propiocin').
Erythromycin propionate lauryl sulfate *see* Erythromycin estolate.
ERYTHROMYCIN STEARATE ('bristamycin', 'docomycin E', 'erypar', 'gallimycin', 'qidmycin').
ERYTHROMYCIN WITH TETRACYCLINE ('macrocycline').
'**Erythroped**' *see* Erythromycin ethyl succinate.
'**Erythrotil**' *see* Erythromycin.
Erythroxylin *see* Cocaine.

Erythryl nitrate* *see* Erythrityl tetranitrate.
ES-902 *see* Pimefylline nicotinate.
'Esafosfina' *see* Fructose 1,6-diphosphate.
'Esantene' *see* Inositol nicotinate.
Esb-3 *see* Sulfaclozine.
'Esbatal' *see* Betanidine.
'Esberiven' *see* Melilotus extract.
'Escalol 506' *see* Padimate A.
'Escalol 507' *see* Padimate O.
ESCIN (escin sodium; 'concentrin', 'essaven', 'reparil').
   See also Buphenine with escin.
'Escorpal' *see* Fencarbamide.
'Escosyl' *see* Esculin.
ESCULAMINE* (8-[bis(2-hydroxyethyl)-aminomethyl]-6,7-dihydroxy-4-methyl-coumarin).
ESCULETIN (6,7-dihydroxycoumarin; esculetol; aesculetin; 'ultrazeozon', 'zeozon').
Esculetin 6-glucoside *See* Esculin.
Esculetol *see* Esculetin.
ESCULIN (esculetin 6-glucoside; esculoside; aesculin; biocolorin; enallachrome; poly-chrome; 'escosyl').
'Esculol' *see* Padimate.
Esculoside *see* Esculin.
'Esentil' *see* Dicycloverine.
Eseridine *see* Physostigmine *N*-oxide.
Eserine *see* Physostigmine.
'Esfar' *see* Bucloxic acid.
'Esiclene' *see* Formebolone.
'Esidrex' *see* Hydrochlorothiazide.
'Esidrix' *see* Hydrochlorothiazide.
ESILATE(S) ** (ethanesulfonate(s); esylate(s)).
   See also Chloroethyl esilate; Piminodine esilate.
'Esimil' *see* Guanethidine with hydrochloro-thiazide.
'Esiodine' *see* Pronolium iodide.
'Eskacef' *see* Cefradine.
'Eskalith' *see* Lithium carbonate.
'Eskaphen' *see* Thiamine.
'Eskaserp' *see* Reserpine.
'Eskazinyl' *see* Trifluoperazine.
'Esmarin' *see* Trichlormethiazide.
'Esmodil' *see* Meprochol.
'Esoderm' *see* DDT.
'Esoiodine' *see* Prolonium iodide.
'Esopin' *see* Homatropine methyl bromide.
'Esparin' *see* Promazine.
'Espectrin' *see* Co-trimoxazole.
'Esperan' *see* Oxapium iodide.
ESPROQUINE ** (2-[3-(ethylsulfinyl)-propyl]-1,2,3,4-tetrahydroisoquinoline; NC-7197).
'Essavan' *see* Escin.
'Essitol' *see* Aluminium acetate.
'Estax' *see under* Macrogols.
ESTAZOLAM ** (8-chloro-6-phenyl-4H-*s*-triazolo(4,3-a)(1,4)benzodiazepine; D-4OTA).
'Estercol' *see* Mercury oleate.
Esthocin (tr) *see* Dimenoxadol.
'Estil' *see* 2-(4-Allyl-2-methoxyphenoxy)-*N*,*N*-diethylacetamide.

Estocin (tr) *see* Dimenoxadol.
ESTOLATE(S) ** (propionate lauryl sul-fate(s)).
   See also Erythromycin estolate.
'Eston' *see* Aluminium acetate.
'Estonate' *see* DDT.
'Estonmite' *see* Chlorfenson.
'Estonox' *see* Campheclor.
'Estopen' *see* Penethamate hydriodide.
'Estracyt' *see* Estramustine.
ESTRADIOL* (β-estradiol; *cis*-1,3,5(10)-estratriene-3,17β-diol; dihydrofolliculin; dihydromenformon; dihydroxyestrin; oestradiol).
ESTRADIOL BENZOATE* (estradiol 3-benzoate; NSC-9566).
ESTRADIOL BENZOATE WITH TESTOSTERONE ISOBUTYRATE ('folvirin').
Estradiol 3,17-bis[*p*-[bis(2-chloroethyl)-amino]phenyl]acetate *see* Estradiol mustard.
Estradiol 3-[bis(2-chloroethyl)car-bamate] *see* Estramustine.
ESTRADIOL CIPIONATE (estradiol cyclopentanepropionate; estradiol cypio-nate; 'depo-estradiol', 'depofemin').
Estradiol 17-cyclohexen-1-yl ether 3-propionate *see* Orestrate.
Estradiol cyclopentanepropionate *see* Estradiol cipionate.
ESTRADIOL DIPROPIONATE ('agofollin', 'diovocyclin', 'diprovex', 'follicyclin', 'ovocyclin-P', 'progynon-DP').
ESTRADIOL ENANTATE (estradiol 17-heptanoate; estradiol enanthate; SQ-16150).
   See also Algestone acetofenide with estra-diol enantate.
Estradiol enanthate* *see* Estradiol enantate.
ESTRADIOL GLUCONATE ('emmenin').
Estradiol 17-heptanoate *see* Estradiol enantate.
Estradiol 17β-methyl ether 3-propyl ether *see* Promestriene.
ESTRADIOL MUSTARD (estradiol bis[*p*-[bis(2-chloroethyl)amino]phenyl]acetate; chlorphenacyl diester with estradiol; NSC-112259).
Estradiol 17-nicotinate 3-propionate *see* Estrapronicate.
ESTRADIOL PIVALATE (estradiol tri-methylacetate; 'estrotate').
Estradiol polyphosphate *see* Polyestradiol phosphate.
Estradiol 17-trichlorohydroxyethyl ether *see* Cloxestradiol.
Estradiol trimethylacetate *see* Estradiol pivalate.
Estradiol 17-undecanoate *see* Estradiol undecylate.
ESTRADIOL UNDECYLATE* (estradiol 17-undecanoate; SQ-9993; 'delestrec').
ESTRADIOL VALERATE ** (estradiol 17-valerate; NSC-17590; 'delestrogen', 'progynova').
ESTRADIOL VALERATE WITH

188

HYDROXYPROGESTERONE CAPROATE ('gravibindan').
ESTRADIOL VALERATE WITH PROGESTERONE HYDROXY-HEXANOATE (NSC-77622; 'deluteval').
ESTRADIOL VALERATE WITH TESTOSTERONE ENANTATE ('deladumone').
'Estradurin' see Polystradiol phosphate.
ESTRAMUSTINE*** (estradiol 3-[bis-(2-chloroethyl)carbamate]; estramustine phosphate; NSC-89199; 'estracyt').
ESTRANE (19-norandrostane).
ESTRAPRONICATE** (estradiol 17-nicotinate 3-propionate).
Estra-1,3,5(10)-triene-3,17β-diol see Estradiol.
Estra-4,9,11-trien-17β-ol-3-one see Trenbolone.
ESTRAZINOL*** (3-methoxy-8-aza-19-nor-17α-pregna-1,3,5(10)-trien-20-yn-17-ol; DL-trans-3-methoxy-8-aza-19-nor-17α-pregna-1,3,5(10)-trien-20-yn-17-ol; estrazinol hydrobromide; W-4454-A).
Estr-4-ene-3β,17-diol see Bolandiol.
Estr-4-ene-4,17β-diol-3-one 17-cyclopentanepropionate see Oxabolone cipionate.
Estr-4-en-17β-ol-3-one see Nandrolone.
Estr-4-en-17β-ol-3-one adamantane-1-carboxylate see Bolmantalate.
'Estrex' see Delmadinone acetate.
ESTRIOL (1,3,5(10)-estratriene-3β,16α,17β-triol; follicular hormone hydrate; oestriol; theelol; trihydroxyestrin; NSC-12169).
Estriol 3-cyclopentyl ether see Quinestradol.
ESTRIOL SUCCINATE*** (estriol 16,17-bis(hydrogen succinate); estriol dihemisuccinate; 'styptanon', 'synapause').
ESTROFURATE*** (21,23-epoxy-19,24-dinor-17α-chola-1,3,5(10),7,20,22-hexaene-3,17-diol 3-acetate).
Estrogens, conjugated see Conjugated estrogens.
Estrogen sulfate see Conjugated estrogens.
ESTRONE*** (1,3,5(10)-estratrien-3-ol-17-one; 3-hydroxyestra-1,3,5(10)-trien-17-one; oestrone; follicular hormone; folliculin; ketohydroxyestrin; ketohydroxyestratriene; theelin).
ESTRONE ACETATE ('hogival').
'Estrotate' see Estradiol pivalate.
'Estrovis' see Quinestrol.
'Esucos' see Dixyrazine.
Esylate(s)* see Esilate(s).
ET-495 see Piribedil.
ETABENZARONE*** (3-[4-(2-diethylaminoethoxy)benzoyl]-2-ethylbenzofuran; 4-(2-diethylaminoethoxy)phenyl 2-ethylbenzofuran-3-yl ketone; benzarone diethylaminoethyl ether).
'Etacortin' see Fluprednidene acetate.
ETACRYNIC ACID*** (2,3-dichloro-4-(2-ethylacryloyl)phenoxyacetic acid; 2-[2,3-dichloro-4-(2-methylenebutyryl)-phenoxy]acetic acid; ethacrynic acid; MK-595; 'edecrin', 'endercin', 'hydrome-

din', 'uregit' 'uregyt').
See also Sodium etacrynate.
ETAFEDRINE*** (−)-2-(ethylmethylamino)-1-phenylpropan-1-ol; N-ethylephedrine; (−)-α-[1-(ethylmethylamino)-ethyl]benzyl alcohol; etafedrine hydrochloride; 'menethyl', 'netamine', 'nethamine', 'novedrin').
ETAFENONE*** (2'-(2-diethylaminoethoxy)-3-phenylpropiophenone; etafenone hydrochloride; 2-(2-diethylaminoethoxy)phenyl phenethyl ketone; KCA; LG-11457; 'baxacor', 'dialicor').
Etafurazone* see Nifursemizone.
Etambutol see Ethambutol.
Etamid (tr) see Probenecid.
Etamifyllin see Etamiphyllin.
ETAMINILE*** (4-dimethylamino-2-ethyl-2-phenylvaleronitrile).
ETAMIPHYLLIN*** (7-(2-diethylaminoethyl)theophylline; etamifyllin; etamiphylline; R-3588; 'parephylline', 'simesphylline', 'soluphyllin').
Etamiphyllin camphorsulfonate see Etamiphyllin camsilate.
ETAMIPHYLLIN CAMSILATE (etamiphyllin camphorsulfonate; etamiphyllin camsylate; 'millophylline').
ETAMIPHYLLIN DEHYDROCHOLATE ('decofillina').
Etamiphyllin (7-hydroxy-4-methyl-2-oxo-1-benzopyran-6-yloxy)acetate see Metescufylline.
Etamiphylline* see Etamiphyllin.
ETAMIVAN*** (N,N-diethylvanillamide; ethamivan; 'emivan', 'vandid').
ETAMOCYCLINE*** (N,N-[ethylenebis-[(methylimino)methylene]]bistetracycline).
Etampromide see Propetamide.
ETAMSYLATE*** (diethylamine 2,5-dihydroxybenzenesulfonate; diethylammonium 2,5-dihydroxybenzenesulfonate; diethylamine cyclohexadien-1-ol-4-one-1-sulfonate; diethylamine-1,4-dihydroxybenzene-3-sulfonate; ethamsylate; cyclonamine; E-141; MD-141; 'altodor', 'dicinon', 'dicynene', 'dicynone').
'Etamucin' see Hyaluronic acid.
'Etamycin' see Viridofulvin.
Etanautine see Diphenhydramine theophyllinate.
Etaperazine (tr) see Perphenazine.
'Etaphylline' see Acefylline piperazine.
'Etapiam' see Perphenazine.
'Etapirazin' see Perphenazine.
ETAQUALONE** (3-(o-ethylphenyl)-2-methyl-4-(3H)quinazolinone).
ETASULINE*** (6-chloro-2-ethylamino-4-phenyl-4H-3,1-benzothiazine).
'Etazine' see Secmebuton.
(±)-**ETAZOCINE** (5,7-diethyl-2'-hydroxy-2-methyl-6,7-benzomorphan; 6,11-diethyl-1,2,3,4,5,6-hexahydro-3-methyl-2,6-methano-3-benzazocin-8-ol; NIH-7856).
(−)-**ETAZOCINE** (GPA-208).
Etazol (tr) see Sulfaethidole.
ETAZOLATE*** (ethyl 1-ethyl-4-(iso-

propylidene-hydrazino)-1H-pyrazolo-
(3,4-b)pyridine-5-carboxylate; SQ-20009).
ETEBENECID*** (p-diethylsulfamoylben-
zoic acid; p-carboxybenzenesulfondiethyl-
amide; ethebenecid; 'urelim').
Etenzamide* see Ethenzamide.
ETEROBARB*** (5-ethyl-1,3-bis(methoxymethyl)-5-phenylbarbituric acid; EX-12-
095; 'antilon').
ETHACRIDINE*** (6,9-diamino-2-ethoxy-
acridine).
ETHACRIDINE LACTATE (acrinol
lactate; lactacridine; lactoacridine;
'acrinolin', 'acrolactine', 'ethodin',
'metifex', 'rimaon', 'rivanol', 'vucine').
Ethacrynate sodium* see Sodium etacrynate.
Ethacrynic acid* see Etacrynic acid.
ETHADIONE* (5,5-dimethyl-3-ethyl-2,4-
oxazolidinedione; aethadionum; 'didione',
'dimedione', 'epinyl', 'neo-absentol').
Ethal see 1-Hexadecanol.
ETHALLYMAL* (5-allyl-5-ethylbarbituric
acid; aethallymal; 'dormin').
ETHAMBUTOL*** ((+)-2,2'-ethylenedi-
iminodi-1-butanol; (+)-N,N'-bis(1-hydr-
oxymethylpropyl)ethylenediamine; etambutol; (+)-ethambutol hydrochloride;
CL-40881; 'dexambutol', 'ebutol', 'eta-
piam', 'etibi', 'myambutol', 'tibutol').
Ethamicort see Hydrocortamate.
Ethamid (tr) see Probenecid.
Ethaminal see Pentobarbital.
Ethaminol see Monoethanolamine oleate.
Ethamivan* see Etamivan.
ETHAMOXYTRIPHETOL (4-(2-diethyl-
aminoethoxy)-α-hydroxy-4'-methoxy-
α-phenylbibenzyl; 1-[p-(2-diethylamino-
ethoxy)phenyl]-2-(p-methoxyphenyl)-
1-phenylethanol; 2-(p-anisyl)-1-[p-(2-di-
ethylaminoethoxy)phenyl]-1-phenylethanol;
Mer-25).
Ethamsylate* see Etamsylate.
Ethanal see Acetaldehyde.
Ethanedial see Glyoxal.
Ethane diamide see Oxamide.
Ethanedioic acid see Oxalic acid.
1,1-ETHANEDIOL (ethylidene glycol).
1,2-Ethanediol see Ethylene glycol.
ETHANE-1,2-DISULFONIC ACID
(ethylene disulfonate; 'allergosil').
See also Edisilate(s).
1,2-Ethanediylbis(carbamodithioic acid)
salts see Mancozeb; Maneb; Nabam;
Zineb.
1,2-Ethanediylbis(phenylmethyl)
bis[(diethoxyphosphinyl)carbonimido-
dithioate] see Zilantel.
Ethane-1-hydroxy-1,1-diphosphonic acid
see Etidronic acid.
Ethane nitrile see Acetonitrile.
Ethanesulfonic acid, esters and salts
see Esilate(s).
ETHANETHIOL (ethyl mercaptan).
'Ethanion' see Calcium 2-ethylbutyrate.
9,10-ETHANOANTHRACENE (dibenzo-
(b,e)bicyclo(2.2.2)octadiene).
Ethanoic acid see Acetic acid.

ETHANOL (ethyl alcohol).
ETHANOLAMINE (2-aminoethanol;
colamine; olamine).
ETHANOLAMINE ACETYLLEUCINATE
(monoethanolamine salt of DL-N-acetyl-
leucine; RP-7452; 'tanganil').
ETHANOLAMINE IOXITALAMATE
WITH MEGLUMINE IOXITALAMATE
('vasobrix').
ETHANOLAMINE NICOTINATE
(ethanolamine salt of nicotinic acid;
'nicamin').
Ethanolamine nitrate see Itramin.
Ethanolamine oleate see Monoethanol-
amine oleate.
Ethanolamine 2-phenylbutyrate salt see
Cetamifen.
2-Ethanolsulfonic acid see Isethionic acid.
Ethanone see Acetaldehyde.
Ethanoylaminoethanoic acid see Aceturic
acid.
Ethaperazine (tr) see Perphenazine.
'Ethapirazine' see Perphenazine.
'Ethaquin' see Ethaverine.
Ethasulfate sodium* see Sodium etasulfate.
'Ethavan' see Homovanillin.
ETHAVERINE*** (1-(3,4-diethoxybenzyl)-
6,7-diethoxyisoquinoline; ethylpapaverine;
'barbonin', 'diquinol', 'ethaquin',
'papetherine', 'perparine', 'perperin',
'preparin').
Ethazole (tr) see Sulfaethidole.
Ethchlorovynol see Ethchlorvynol.
ETHCHLORVYNOL* (5-chloro-3-ethyl-
pent-4-en-1-yn-3-ol; 1-chloro-3-ethylpent-
4-yn-3-ol; β-chlorovinyl ethynyl carbinol
ethchlorovynol; 'arvynol', 'normoson',
'placididyl', 'serenesil').
Ethebenecid* see Etebenecid.
Ethene see Ethylene.
Ethenone see Ketene.
Ethenyl-p-diethoxydiphenylamidine see
Phenacaine.
ETHENZAMIDE** (o-ethoxybenzamide;
salicylamide ethyl ether; etenzamide;
'ethosalicyl', 'etosalicil', 'meloka',
'trancalgyl').
ETHER (diethyl ether; ethyl ether).
See also Vinycombinum.
Ether hydrochloric see Chloroethane.
Ether muriatic see Chloroethane.
ETHIAZIDE*** (6-chloro-3-ethyl-3,4-
dihydro-2H-1,2,4-benzothiadiazine-7-
sulfonamide-1,1-dioxide; 6-chloro-3-ethyl-
3,4-dihydro-7-sulfamoyl-1,2,4-benzo-
thiadiazine 1,1-dioxide; 'hypertane').
Ethidene chloride see 1,1-Dichloroethane.
ETHIDIUM CHLORIDE** (3,8-diamino-5-
ethyl-6-phenylphenanthridinium chloride;
2,7-diamino-10-ethyl-9-phenylphenan-
thridinium chloride; homidium chloride;
'novidium').
Ethimizole (tr) see Etimizole.
ETHINAMATE*** (1-ethynylcyclohexane-
carboxamide; 1-ethynylcyclohexyl carbamate; 'valamin', 'valmid', 'valmidate').
Ethine see Acetylene.

ETHINYLESTRADIOL*** (17-ethynyl-estradiol; ethinyloestradiol).
See also Chlormadinone acetate with ethinylestradiol; Dimethisterone with ethinylestradiol; Etynodiol diacetate with ethinylestradiol; Levonorgestrel with ethinylestradiol; Medroxyprogesterone acetate with ethinylestradiol; Megestrol acetate with ethinylestradiol; Norethisterone acetate with ethinylestradiol; Norgestrienone with ethinylestradiol.
Ethinylestradiol 3-cyclopentyl ether *see* Quinestrol.
ETHINYLESTRADIOL 3-ISOPROPYL-SULFONATE (ESTER) (J-96; 'deposiston').
Ethinylestradiol 3-methyl ether *see* Mestranol.
ETHINYLESTRADIOL WITH LYN-ESTRENOL ('fisioquens', 'minilyn', 'pregnon 28', 'yermonil').
ETHINYLESTRADIOL WITH QUIN-GESTANOL (S-602-1; 'relovis').
Ethinylestrenol *see* Lynestrenol.
Ethinylnortestosterone *see* Norethisterone.
17α-Ethinyltestosterone *see* Ethisterone.
Ethinyl trichloride *see* Trichlorethylene.
Ethinyltrienolone *see* Norgestrienone.
'Ethiodan' *see* Iofendylate.
ETHIODIZED (^{131}I) **OIL***** (ethyl esters of radioiodinated fatty acids; radioethiodized oil; 'ethiodol-131').
'Ethiodol 131' *see* Ethiodized (^{131}I) oil.
ETHIOLATE* (S-ethyl diethylcarbamothioate; 'prefox').
ETHION (O,O,O',O'-tetraethyl S,S'-methylene diphosphorodithioate; ethyl methylenephosphorodithioate; bis[S-(diethoxyphosphinylthioyl)mercapto]methane; S,S'-methylene-O,O,O',O'-tetraethyl phosphorodithioate; diethion; 'niagara-1240', 'nialate', 'niallate').
ETHIONAMIDE*** (2-ethylisonicotinthioamide; α-ethylisonicotinic thioamide; 2-ethyl-4-thiocarbamoylpyridine; 2-ethyl-pyridine-4-carbothionamide; 2-(ethyl)-thioisonicotinamide; ätina; ethioamide; ethionizine; thianide; Th-1314; 'etionizina', 'iridocin', 'iridozin', 'trecator', 'trescatyl').
ETHIONAMIDE SULFOXIDE (Th-1405).
ETHIONINE (2-amino-4-(ethylthio)butyric acid; NSC-751).
Ethionizine *see* Ethionamide.
'Ethios' *see* Diethyl thiosulfite.
ETHIPYROLE (tr) (N,N'-dimethylpyrazole-3,4-dicarboxamide; pyrazole-3,4-dicarboxylic acid bis(methylamide); etipyrole).
ETHIRIMOL* (5-butyl-2-(ethylamino)-6-methyl-4-pyrimidinol; 5-butyl-2-ethyl-amino-4-hydroxy-6-methylpyrimidine; 'milstem').
Ethiron (tr) *see* 2-Aminoethylisothiuronium bromide.
ETHISTERONE*** (17α-ethynyl-4-an-drosten-17α-ol-3-one; 17-ethynyl-17β-hydroxyandrost-4-en-3-one; anhydrohydr-oxyprogesterone; 17α-ethynyltestosterone; ethinyltestosterone; pregneninolone; pregneninonol; pregnin).
ETHISTERONE ACETATE (ethisterone 17-acetate; SC-8470).
Ethizine *see* Fenethazine.
Ethmozine *see* Moracizine.
ETHOATE-METHYL* (S-(2-ethylamino-2-oxoethyl) O,O-dimethyl phosphorodithio-ate; S-(ethylcarbamoylmethyl) O,O-di-methyl phosphorodithioate; 'fitios').
Ethobrome *see* Bromethol.
'Ethodin' *see* Ethacridine.
Ethofats *see under* Macrogols.
Ethoform* *see* Benzocaine.
ETHOFUMESATE* (2-ethoxy-2,3-dihydro-3,3-dimethylbenzofuran-5-yl methanesul-fonate; 'nortran').
Ethoglucid* *see* Etoglucid.
ETHOHEPTAZINE*** (4-carbethoxy-1-methyl-4-phenylhexamethylenimine; ethyl DL-1-methyl-4-phenylazacyclohept-ane-4-carboxylate; ethyl hexahydro-1-methyl-4-phenyl-4-azepinecarboxylate; Wy-401).
ETHOHEPTAZINE CITRATE ('zactane').
ETHOHEXADIOL* (2-ethyl-1,3-hexanediol; ethohexadiolum; Rutgers-612).
Ethomids *see under* Macrogols.
Ethomorphine *see* Ethylmorphine.
ETHOMOXANE*** (DL-2-butylaminometh-yl-8-ethoxy-1,4-benzodioxan; ethoxybutam-oxane; ethomoxane hydrochloride; 'vortel').
Ethonam* *see* Etonam.
Ethonamidate *see* Etonam nitrate.
'Ethone' *see* Triethyl orthoformate.
ETHOPABATE (methyl 4-acetamido-2-ethoxybenzoate).
ETHOPROP* (O-ethyl S,S-dipropyl phos-phorodithioate; ethoprophos; phosetho-prop; prophos; V-C 9-104; 'mocap').
Ethopropazine* *see* Profenamine.
Ethoprophos *see* Ethoprop.
Ethosalamide* *see* Etosalamide.
'Ethosalicyl' *see* Ethenzamide.
Ethosuccimide *see* Ethosuximide.
ETHOSUXIMIDE*** (2-ethyl-2-methyl-succinimide; 3-ethyl-3-methyl-2,5-pyrro-lidinedione; ethosuccimide; piknolepsin; pyknolepsin; CI-366; H-490; PM-671; 'emeside', 'ethymal', 'mesentol', 'petnidan', 'ronton', 'simatin', 'succinutin', 'suxilep', 'suxinutin', 'zarontin').
ETHOSUXIMIDE WITH MEPACRINE ('acrisuxin').
ETHOTOIN*** (3-ethyl-5-phenylhydantoin; AC-695; 'peganone').
Ethotrimeprazine *see* Etymemazine.
'Ethovan' *see* Homovanillin.
Ethoxarine *see* Oxamarin.
Ethoxazene* Etoxazene.
Ethoxazolamide *see* Ethoxolamide.
ETHOXAZORUTOSIDE*** (morpholinoyl-ethylrutoside; 2-morpholinoethylrutin).
Ethoxide (tr) *see* Etocarlide.
ETHOXOLAMIDE* (1-ethoxy-6-sulfamoyl-

2,1,3-benzothiadiazole; 1-ethoxy-2,1,3-
benzothiadiazole-6-sulfonamide; ethoxazolamide; ethoxyzolamide; 'cardrase',
'cardrax', 'cardraze, 'glaucotensil').

p-**Ethoxyacetanilide** *see* Phenacetin.

4'-**Ethoxyacetanilide** *see* Phenacetin.

Ethoxyacetic acid *p*-menthyl ester *see*
Menglytate.

*N*⁴-(2-**Ethoxyacetyl**)-*N*¹-(5-**methylis-
oxazol-3-yl**)**sulfanilamide** *see* Sulfacecole.

p-**Ethoxyaniline** *see* *p*-Phenetidine.

2-(*p*-**Ethoxyanilino**)-*N*-**propylpropion-
amide** *see* Etapromide.

o-**Ethoxybenzamide** *see* Ethenzamide.

o-**Ethoxybenzoic acid (1-carboxyethyl-
idene)-hydrazide** *see* Ruvazone.

p-**Ethoxybenzoic acid diethylaminoethyl
ester** *see* Parethoxycaine.

Ethoxybutamoxane* *see* Ethomoxane.

p-**Ethoxybutyranilide** *see* *p*-Butyrophen-
etidide.

S-[[[(**Ethoxycarbonyl**)**amino**]**methyl-
carbonyl**]**methyl**] *O,O*-**diethyl
phosphorodithioate** *see* Mecarbam.

S-(α-**Ethoxycarbonylbenzyl**) *O,O*-**dimethyl
phosphorodithioate** *see* Phenthoate.

2-(α-**Ethoxycarbonylbenzyl**)**thiazolidine-
4-carboxylic acid** *see* Leucogen.

18-(4-**Ethoxycarbonyl-3,5-dimethoxy-
benzoyl**)**reserpic acid methyl ester**
see Syrosingopine.

1-[2-[2-(**Ethoxycarbonyl**)-5,6-**dimethoxy-
indol-3-yl**]**ethyl**]-4-**phenylpiperazine**
see Alpertine.

4-**Ethoxycarbonyl-1,3-dimethyl-4-phenyl-
hexamethylenimine** *see* Metethoheptazine.

7-(**Ethoxycarbonylmethoxy**)-3-(2-**diethylaminoethyl**)-4-**methylcoumarin** *see*
Carbocromen.

7-(**Ethoxycarbonylmethoxy**)**flavone** *see*
Efloxate.

2-(**Ethoxycarbonylmethylene**)-3-**methyl-5-
piperid-1-yl-4-thiazolidinone** *see*
Etozolin.

[2-(**Ethoxycarbonyl**)-1-**methylvinyl**]
dimethyl phosphate *see* Mevinphos.

N-**Ethoxycarbonyl-3-morpholinosydnone
imine** *see* Molsidomine.

p-**Ethoxycarbonylphenyl 6-guanidino-
hexanoate** *see* Gabexate.

1-**Ethoxycarbonyl-2-phthalazin-1-yl-
hydrazine** *see* Todralazine.

**Ethoxycarbonylsyringoyl methyl reser-
pate** *see* Syrosingopine.

3-**Ethoxycarbonyl-6,7,8,9-tetrahydro-1,6-
dimethyl-4-oxo-4H-pyrido(1,2-a)-
pyrimidinium methyl sulfate** *see*
Rimazolium metilsulfate.

5-**Ethoxycarbonyl-1-(1,2,3,4-tetrahydro-
naphth-1-yl)imidazole** *see* Etonam.

S-**Ethoxycarbonylthiamine** *see* Cetotiamine.

4-**Ethoxycarbonyl** α,α,4-**triphenyl-1-
piperidinebutyronitrile** *see* Diphenoxylate.

p-**Ethoxychrysoidine** *see* Etoxazene.

Ethoxyd (tr) *see* Etocarlide.

**Ethoxy(2-diethylaminoethylthio)-
phosphine oxide** *see* Ethyl (2-diethyl-
aminoethyl)phosphonothioate.

2-**Ethoxy-2,3-dihydro-3,3-dimethylbenzo-
furan-5-yl methanesulfonate** *see*
Ethofumesate.

6-**Ethoxy-1,2-dihydro-2,2,4-trimethyl-
quinoline** *see* Ethoxyquin.

3-**Ethoxy-1,1-dihydroxy-2-butanone** *see*
Ketoxal.

2-**Ethoxy-2,2-diphenylacetic acid 3-di-
ethylaminopropyl ester** *see* Etpenal.

'**Ethoxydrazone**' *see* Ruvazone.

2-**ETHOXYETHANOL** (ethylene glycol
monoethyl ether; 'cellosolve').

6-(2-**Ethoxyethoxy**)**benzamide** *see* Etosalamide.

2-(2-**ETHOXYETHOXY**)**ETHANOL**
(diethylene glycol monoethyl ether;
'carbitol').

5-[1-[2-(2-**Ethoxyethoxy**)**ethoxy**]**ethyl**]-
1,3-**benzodioxole** *see* Sesamex.

1-[(2-**Ethoxyethoxy**)**ethoxy**]-2-(3,4-
methylenedioxyphenyl)**ethane** *see*
Sesamex.

(1-**Ethoxyethyl**)**glyoxal** *see* 3-Ethoxy-2-oxo-
butyraldehyde.

(1-**Ethoxyethyl**)**glyoxal bisthiosemi-
carbazone** *see* Gloxazone.

2-**Ethoxyethyl *p*-methoxycinnamate** *see*
Cinoxate.

p-**Ethoxy-α-hydroxyacetanilide** *see*
Fenacetinol.

3-**Ethoxy-4-hydroxybenzaldehyde** *see*
Homovanillin.

4-**ETHOXY-3-HYDROXYBENZALDE-
HYDE** (ethylisovanillin).

4'-**Ethoxy-3'-hydroxybutyranilide** *see*
Bucetin.

Ethoxyhydroxyzine *see* Etodroxizine.

**Ethoxylated *tert*-octylphenol formalde-
hydepolymer** *see* Tyloxapol.

1-(4-**Ethoxy-3-methoxybenzyl**)-6,7-**di-
methoxy-3-methylisoquinoline** *see*
Dimoxyline.

**Ethoxymethyl *N*-(2,6-dichloro-*m*-tolyl)-
anthranilate** *see* Terofenamate.

2-**Ethoxy-4'-[(5-methylisoxazol-3-yl)-
sulfamoyl]acetanilide** *see* Sulfacecole.

Ethoxymethyl meclofenamate *see* Terofenamate.

2-**Ethoxy-*N*-methyl-*N*-[2-(methylphenethylamino)ethyl]acetamide** *see* Carbifene.

2-**Ethoxy-*N*-methyl-*N*-[2-(methylphenethylamino)ethyl]-2,2-diphenyl-
acetamide** *see* Etymide.

6-(2-**Ethoxy-1-naphthamido**)**penicillanic
acid** *see* Nafcillin.

2-**Ethoxynaphth-1-yl-penicillin** *see*
Nafcillin.

3-**ETHOXY-2-OXOBUTYRALDEHYDE**
(β-ethoxy-α-ketobutyraldehyde; (1-ethoxy-
ethyl)glyoxal).

3-**Ethoxy-2-oxobutyraldehyde bis-
(thiosemicarbazone)** *see* Gloxazone.

3-[4-(β-**Ethoxyphenethyl**)**piperazin-1-yl**]-

192

2-methylpropiophenone see Eprazinone.
o-**ETHOXYPHENOL** (ethyl 2-hydroxy-phenyl ether; guethol).
2-(*o*-Ethoxyphenoxymethyl)morpholine see Viloxazine.
2-(2-Ethoxyphenoxymethyl)tetrahydro-1,4-oxazine see Viloxazine.
4-(*p*-Ethoxyphenylazo)-*m*-phenylene-diamine see Etoxazene.
N-(*p*-**Ethoxyphenyl)butyramide** see *p*-Butyrophenetidide.
1-(2-Ethoxy-2-phenylethyl)-4-(2-methyl-3-oxo-3-phenylpropyl)piperazine see Eprazinone.
2-[4-(2-Ethoxy-2-phenylethyl)piperazin-1-ylmethyl]propiophenone see Eprazinone.
N-(*p*-**Ethoxyphenyl)glycolamide** see Fenacetinol.
p-(α-**Ethoxy-*p*-phenylphenacylamino)-benzoic acid** see Xenazoic acid.
1-(*p*-Ethoxyphenyl)urea see Phenetylurea.
*N*¹-(6-**Ethoxypyridazin-3-yl) sulfanilamide** see Sulfaethoxypyridazine.
ETHOXYQUIN* (6-ethoxy-1,2-dihydro-2,2,4-trimethylquinoline; polyethoxy-quinoline; EMQ; 'santoquin', 'stop-scald').
8-Ethoxy-5-quinolinesulfonic acid see Actinoquinol.
'Ethoxysclerol' see Polidocanol.
1-Ethoxy-6-sulfamoyl-2,1,3-benzothiadi-azole see Ethoxolamide.
*N*¹-(4-**Ethoxy-1,2,5-thiadiazol-3-yl)-sulfanilamide** see Sulfatrozole.
Ethoxyzolamide see Ethoxolamide.
Ethpenal see Etpenal.
'Ethrane' see Enflurane.
'Ethumine' see Clotiapine.
'Ethussan' see Triethyl orthoformate.
Ethybenztropine* see Etybenzatropine.
Ethychlordiphene see Etofamide.
'Ethycyclin' see Ethinylestradiol.
'Ethydan' see Vinycombinum.
'Ethyl' see Tetraethyllead.
Ethylacetamide see Butyramide.
Ethyl 2-acetamido-3-[*p*-[bis(2-chloro-ethyl)amino]phenyl]propionate see Phenaphan.
2-[2-[3-(*N*-Ethylacetamido)-2,4,6-triiodo-phenoxy]ethoxy]propionic acid see Iolixanic acid.
ETHYL ACETRIZOATE (ethyl ester of 3-acetamido-2,4,6-triiodobenzoic acid; 'bronchiol').
5-(2-Ethylacryloyl)-6-methylbenzofuran-2-carboxylic acid see Furacrinic acid.
'Ethyladrianol' see Etilefrine.
Ethylal see Diethoxymethane.
Ethyl alcohol see Ethanol.
3-Ethylamino-1,2-benzisothiazole see Etisazole.
ETHYL *m*-AMINOBENZOATE (MS-222; 'metacaine').
Ethyl *p*-aminobenzoate see Benzocaine.
Ethyl 2-amino-6-benzyl-4,5,6,7-tetra-hydrothieno(2,3-c)pyridine-3-carboxyl-

ate see Tinoridine.
Ethyl 2-amino-3-(3,4-dihydroxyphenyl)-2-methylpropionate see Methyldopate.
α-(1-**Ethylaminoethyl)-3,4-dihydroxy-benzyl alcohol** see Dioxethedrin.
Ethyl 2-amino-6-[(*p*-fluorobenzyl)-amino]-3-pyridinecarbamate see Flupirtine.
2-Ethylamino-1-hydroxy-1-(3-hydroxy-phenyl)ethane see Etilefrine.
2-Ethylamino-4-isopropylamino-6-methoxy-*s*-triazine see Atraton.
2-Ethylamino-4-isopropylamino-6-(methylthio)-*s*-triazine see Ametryn.
α-**Ethylaminomethyl-3-hydroxybenzyl alcohol** see Etilefrine.
2-(1-Ethylamino-2-oxocyclohexyl)-thiophene see Tiletamine.
S-(2-**Ethylamino-2-oxoethyl) *O*,*O*-di-methyl phosphorodithioate** see Ethoate-methyl.
2-Ethylamino-4-oxo-5-phenyl-2-oxazoline see Fenozolone.
Ethyl 1-(*p*-aminophenethyl)-4-phenyl-isonipecotate see Anileridine.
2-Ethylamino-3-phenylnorbornane see Fenacamfamin.
2-Ethylamino-5-phenyl-2-oxazolin-4-one see Fenozolone.
2-Ethylamino-2-thien-2-ylcyclohexanone see Tiletamine.
2-Ethylamino-1-(3-trifluoromethyl-phenyl)propane see Fenfluramine.
17β-Ethyl-5α-androstane see 5α-Pregnane.
17β-Ethyl-5β-androstane see 5β-Pregnane.
Ethyl 1-(3-anilinopropyl)-4-phenyliso-nipecotate see Piminodine.
Ethylarterenol see Ethylnoradrenaline.
Ethyl 3-benzhydrylcarbazate see Carbenzide.
Ethyl 1-benzhydrylimidazole-5-carboxyl-ate see Etomidate.
Ethyl 2-benzimidazolecarbamate see Lobendazole.
2-Ethylbenzofuran-3-yl 4-hydroxy-3,5-di-iodophenyl ketone see Benziodarone.
2-Ethylbenzofuran-3-yl 4-hydroxyphenyl ketone see Benzarone.
2-(2-Ethylbenzofuran-3-ylmethyl)-2-imidazoline see Coumazoline.
Ethyl *N*-benzoyl-*N*-(3,4-dichlorophenyl)-L-alanine see Benzoylprop-ethyl.
Ethyl *m*-benzoyl-*N*-(trifluoromethylsul-fonyl)carbanilate see Triflumidate.
α-**Ethylbenzyl alcohol** see 1-Phenyl-1-propa-nol.
Ethyl *N*-benzylcyclopropanecarbamate see Encymate.
3-(α-Ethylbenzyl)-4-hydroxycoumarin see Phenprocoumon.
α-**Ethyl-4-biphenylylacetic acid** see Xenbuficin.
α-**Ethyl-4-biphenylylacetic acid com-pound with *trans*-4-phenylcyclohexyl-amine** see Butixirate.
Ethyl bis(1-aziridinyl)phosphinylcarba-mate see Uredepa.

Ethyl 5,6-bis-*O*-(*p*-chlorobenzyl)-
3-*O*-propyl-D-glucofuranoside *see*
Clobenoside.
Ethyl *p*-[2-[*p*-(bis(2-chloroethyl)amino)-
phenyl]acetamido]benzoate *see*
Phenastezin.
Ethyl 2-[*p*-[bis(2-chloroethyl)amino]-
phenylacetamido]-4-(methylthio)-
butyrate *see* Phenamet.
Ethyl 3-[*p*-[bis(2-chloroethyl)amino]-
phenyl]-2-nicotinoylaminopropionate
see Nicosin.
Ethyl 2,2-bis(*p*-chlorophenyl)glycolate
see Chlorobenzilate.
ETHYL BISCOUMACETATE*** (ethyl
ester of 3,3'-carboxymethylenebis(4-hy-
droxycoumarin); Et ester of 2,2-bis(4-hy-
droxy-3-coumarinyl)acetic acid; Et ester
of bis(4-hydroxy-2-oxo-2H-1-benzopyran-
3-yl)acetic acid; aethyldicumarin; ethyldicumarin; BOEA; neodicumarin;
pelentan; G-11765; 'dicumacyl',
'tromexan').
Ethyl 6,7-bis(cyclopropylmethoxy)-
4-hydroxyquinoline-3-carboxylate *see*
Ciproquinate.
Ethyl bis(2,2-dimethylaziridinyl)phos-
phinylcarbamate *see* Meturedepa.
5-Ethyl-1,3-bis(methoxymethyl)-5-
phenylbarbituric acid *see* Eterobarb.
S-Ethyl bis(2-methylpropyl)carbamo-
thioate *see* Butylate.
1-Ethyl-2,6-bis(*p*-pyrrolidin-1-ylstyryl)-
pyridinium iodide *see* Stilbazium iodide.
'Ethyl butex' *see* Ethyl paraben.
2-(2-Ethylbutoxy)-2,2-diphenylacetic acid
2-dimethylaminoethyl ester *see*
Denaverine.
Ethyl 4-butylamino-1-ethyl-1H-pyrazolo-
(3,4-b)pyridine-5-carboxylate *see*
Cartazolate.
ETHYL BUTYLETHYLMALONAMATE
(ethyl ester of 2-but-2-yl-2-ethylmalonamic
acid; 'butesamid').
2-Ethylbutyric acid calcium salt *see*
Calcium 2-ethylbutyrate.
ETHYL CAMPHORAMINE (1-dimethyl-
amino-2-hydroxyethyl 2-oxobornane-3-carb-
oxylate; *N,N*-dimethyl-2-hydroxyethyl-
amine camphocarbonate.
Ethyl carbamate *see* Urethan.
1-(Ethylcarbamoyl)ethyl carbanilate *see*
Carbetamide.
Ethyl 1-(2-carbamoylethyl)-4-phenyl-
isonipecotate *see* Carperidine.
S-(Ethylcarbamoylmethyl) *O,O*-dimethyl
phosphorodithioate *see* Ethoate-methyl.
4-[4-(Ethylcarbonyl)-4-piperid-1-ylpiper-
id-1-yl]-4'-fluorobutyrophenone *see*
Floropipetone.
Ethyl 4-carboxy-α-phenyl-2-thiazolidine-
acetate *see* Leucogen.
ETHYL CARTRIZOATE*** ((3,5-diacet-
amido-2,4,6-triiodobenzoyloxy)acetic acid
ethyl ester; hydroxymethyl 3,5-diacet-
amido-2,4,6-triiodobenzoate ethyl carbonate; ethyl diatrizoate ethyl carbonate).

Ethyl chaulmoograte *see* Chaulmestrol.
Ethyl chloride *see* Chloroethane.
Ethyl *N*-[2-(*p*-chlorobenzyl)prop-2-yl]-
carbamate *see* Cloforex.
Ethyl 4-chloro-α-(4-chlorophenyl)-α-
hydroxybenzeneacetate *see* Chloro-
benzilate.
Ethyl 10-chloro-3-ethoxymethyl-2,3,6,9-
tetrahydro-9-oxo-*p*-dioxino(2,3-g)-
quinoline-8-carboxylate *see* Quincarbate.
Ethyl 2-(*p*-chlorophenoxy)-1-methyl-
propionate *see* Clofibrate.
Ethyl (±)-2-[[α-(*p*-chlorophenyl)-*p*-
tolyl]oxy]-2-methylbutyrate *see*
Beclobrate.
Ethyl cinepazate *see* Cinepazet.
Ethyl clofibrate *see* Clofibrate.
N-Ethylcorbadrine *see* Dioxethedrin.
N-Ethyl-*o*-crotonotoluidide *see* Crotamiton.
Ethyl cyanide *see* Propionitrile.
Ethyl 1-(3-cyano-3,3-diphenylpropyl)-4-
phenylisonipecotate *see* Diphenoxylate.
S-Ethyl cyclohexylethylcarbamido-
thioate *see* Cycloate.
Ethyl 6-decyloxy-7-ethoxy-4-hydroxy-
quinoline-3-carboxylate *see* Decoquinate.
Ethyl (3,5-diacetamido-2,4,6-triiodobenz-
oyloxy)acetate *see* Ethyl cartrizoate.
Ethyl diatrizoate ethyl carbonate *see*
Ethyl cartrizoate.
ETHYL DIBUNATE*** (ethyl 3,6-*ditert*-
butylnaphthalene-1-sulfonate; NDR-304;
'neodyne').
Ethyl 4,4'-dichlorobenzilate *see* Chloro-
benzilate.
Ethyldicumarin *see* Ethyl biscoumacetate.
Ethyl 2-[(diethoxyphosphinothioyl)oxy]-5-
methylpyrazolo(1,5-a)pyrimidine-6-
carboxylate *see* Pyrazophos.
Ethyl [[[(diethoxyphosphinothioyl)-
thio]acetyl]methyl]carbamate *see*
Mecarbam.
Ethyl *N*-(2-diethylaminoethyl)-2-ethyl-
2-phenylmalonate *see* Fenalamide.
Ethyl 3-(2-diethylaminoethyl)-4-methyl-
coumarin-7-yloxyacetate *see* Carbocromen.
O-ETHYL *S*-(2-DIETHYLAMINOETHYL)
PHOSPHONOTHIOATE (ethoxy(2-
diethylamino ethylthio)phosphine oxide;
'edemo').
S-Ethyl diethylcarbamothioate *see*
Ethiolate.
Ethyl difenoxilate *see* Diphenoxylate.
1-Ethyl-3-(10,11-dihydro-5H-dibenzo(a,d)-
cyclohepten-5-ylidene)-2-methyl-
pyrrolidine *see* Piroheptine.
2-Ethyl-9,11-dihydro-8-(hydroxymethyl)-
9-oxoindolizino(1,2-b)quinoline-7-
glycolic acid sodium salt *see* Camptothecin.
1-Ethyl-1,4-dihydro-7-methyl-4-oxo-1,8-
naphthyridine-3-carboxylic acid *see*
Nalidixic acid.
1-Ethyl-4,6-dihydro-3-methyl-8-phenyl-
pyrazolo(4,3-e)(1,4)diazepin-5(1H)-one
see Ripazepam.

1-Ethyl-1,4-dihydro-4-oxo(1,3)dioxolo-(4,5-g)cinnoline-3-carboxylic acid *see* Cinoxacin.

5-Ethyl-5,8-dihydro-5-oxo-1,3-dioxolo-(4,5-g)quinoline-7-carboxylic acid *see* Oxolinic acid.

8-Ethyl-5,8-dihydro-5-oxo-2-piperazin-1-ylpyrido(2,3-d)pyrimidine-6-carboxylic acid *see* Pipemidic acid.

N^1-**(1-Ethyl-1,2-dihydro-2-oxopyrimidin-4-yl)sulfanilamide** *see* Sulfacitine.

8-Ethyl-5,8-dihydro-5-oxo-2-pyrrolidin-1-ylpyrido(2,3-d)pyrimidine-6-carboxylic acid *see* Piromidic acid.

5-Ethyldihydro-5-phenyl-4,6(1H,5H)-pyrimidinedione *see* Primidone.

4-Ethyl-3,4-dihydro-4-phenylthioiso-carbostyril *see* Tisoquone.

Ethyl diiodobrassidate *see* Iodobrassid.

Ethyl diiodostearate *see* Iodetryl.

Ethyl 6,7-diisobutoxy-4-hydroxy-3-quinolinecarboxylate *see* Buquinolate.

4-ETHYL-2,5-DIMETHOXYAMPHET-AMINE (DOET).

Ethyl 5,6-dimethoxy-3-[2-(4-phenyl-piperazin-1-yl)ethyl]indole 2-carboxyl-ate *see* Alpertine.

Ethyl 2-[(dimethoxyphosphinothioyl)-thio]-2-phenylacetate *see* Phenthoate.

4-Ethyl-6,7-dimethoxyquinazoline *see* Quazodine.

Ethyl N-(2-dimethylaminoethyl)-m-trifluoromethylcarbanilate *see* Flubanilate.

Ethyl 2-dimethylamino-2-phenyl-3-cyclo-hexene-1-carboxylate *see* Tilidine.

N-**Ethyl-N,1-dimethyl-3,3-dithien-2-yl-allylamine** *see* Ethylmethylthiambutene.

Ethyl 1,2-dimethyl-5-hydroxyindole-3-carboxylate *see* Mecarbinate.

Ethyldimethyl(1-methyl-3,3-diphenyl-propyl)ammonium bromide *see* Emepronium bromide.

3-Ethyl-5,5-dimethyl-2,4-oxazolidinedione *see* Ethadione.

5-Ethyl-5,5-dimethyl-2,4-oxazolidinedione *see* Paramethadione.

Ethyl dimethylphosphoramidocyanidate *see* Tabun.

($\pm$)-**20-ETHYLDINOPROST** (20-ethyl-PG $F_{2\alpha}$; ICI-74205).

13-Ethyl-18,19-dinor-17α-pregn-4-en-17-ol-3-one *see* Norboletone.

N-**Ethyl-3,3'-diphenyldipropylamine** *see* Alverine.

8-Ethyl-3-diphenylmethoxynortropane *see* Etybenzatropine.

Ethyl α,α-diphenyl-4-morpholinebutyrate *see* Dioxaphetyl butyrate.

O-**Ethyl S,S-diphenyl phosphorodithioate** *see* Edifenphos.

2-ETHYL-3,3-DIPHENYLPROPEN(2)-YLAMINE (3,3-diphenyl-2-ethylpropen-(2)ylamine; EDPA; NA-III; 'gilutensin').

S-**ETHYL DIPROPYLCARBAMOTHIO-ATE** (EPTC; 'eptam').

O-**Ethyl S,S-dipropyl phosphorodithioate** *see* Ethoprop.

Ethyldithiuram *see* Disulfiram.

ETHYLENE (ethene).

Ethylenebis(dithiocarbamic acid) salts *see* Mancozeb; Maneb; Nabam; Zineb.

Ethylenebis(iminodiacetic acid) *see* Edetic acid.

3,3'-Ethylenebis(methylimino)di-1-propanol 3,4,5-trimethoxybenzoate diester *see* Hexobendine.

Ethylenebis[(methylimino)methylene]-bistetracycline *see* Etamocycline.

Ethylenebis(oxyethylene) dimethacrylate polymer with 2-hydroxyethyl methacrylate and methyl methacryl-ate *see* Dimefilcon A.

3,3'-[Ethylenebis(oxyethyleneoxy-ethylenecarbonylimino)]bis(2,4,6-tri-iodobenzoic acid) *see* Iodoxamic acid.

N,N-**Ethylenecarbamic acid** *see* 1-Aziridine-carboxylic acid.

Ethylene chloride *see* 1,2-Dichloroethylene.

Ethylene chlorohydrin *see* 2-Chloroethanol.

ETHYLENEDIAMINE (1,2-diaminoethane; ethanediamine).

Ethylenediaminetetraacetic acid *see* Edetic acid.

N,N'-**Ethylene-1,2-diarsanilic acid** *see* Difetarsone.

cis-**1,3-Ethylenedicarboxylic acid** *see* Maleic acid.

trans-**1,3-Ethylenedicarboxylic acid** *see* Fumaric acid.

Ethylene dichloride *see* 1,2-Dichloroethane.

Ethylene dicyanide *see* Succinonitrile.

2,2'-Ethylenediiminodi-1-butanol *see* Ethambutol.

Ethylene dimesylate *see* Ethylene mesilate.

4,4'-Ethylenedioxybis(N-hexyl-N-methyl-benzylamine) *see* Symetine.

3,3-Ethylenedioxy-17-hydroxy-6-methyl-pregn-5-en-20-one acetate *see* Edogestrone.

3,3-Ethylenedioxy-6-methylpregn-5-en-20-one-17-ol acetate *see* Edogestrone.

Ethylene disulfonate *see* Ethane-1,2-disulfonic acid.

ETHYLENE GLYCOL (1,2-ethanediol; glycol).

Ethylene glycol di(methanesulfonate) *see* Ethylene mesilate.

Ethylene glycol monoethyl ether *see* 2-Ethoxyethanol.

Ethylene glycol monophenyl ether *see* Phenoxyethanol.

Ethylene glycol monosalicylate *see* Glycol salicylate.

Ethylene glycol salicylate *see* Glycol salicylate.

Ethylene glycol terephthalic acid polymer *see* Pegoterate.

Ethylene imine *see* Aziridine.

Ethylene iminoquinone *see* Inproquone.

Ethylene lactic acid *see* Hydracrylic acid.

Ethylene-maleic anhydride polymer *see* Malethamer.

ETHYLENE MESILATE (ethylene glycol

di(methanesulfonate); ethylene dimesylate; 1,2-bis(methylsulfonyloxy)ethane; DMSE).

ETHYLENE OXIDE (oxirane).

1,4-Ethylenepiperidine see Quinuclidine.

Ethylenesulfonic acid polymer sodium salt see Sodium apolate.

Ethylenimine see Aziridine.

N-Ethylephedrine see Etafedrine.

17α-Ethylestrane see 19-Nor-17α-pregnane.

17β-Ethylestrane see 19-Norpregnane.

17α-Ethylestr-4-ene-3,17-diol 3-propionate see Propetandrol.

ETHYLESTRENOL* (17α-ethylestr-4-en-17β-ol; 19-nor-17α-pregn-4-en-17β-ol; 17α-ethyl-17β-hydroxyestr-4-ene; ethylnandrol; ethyloestrenol; 'duraboral', 'maxibolin', 'orabolin', 'orgabolin'). See also Dexamethasone with ethylestrenol.

17α-Ethyl-4-estren-17-ol see Ethylestrenol.

17α-Ethyl-4-estren-17-ol see Bolenol.

17α-Ethyl-4-estren-17-ol-3-one see Norethandrolone.

Ethyl ether see Ether.

Ethylethoxyphosphoryl p-nitrophenolate see Armin.

3-Ethyl-2-[5-(3-ethylbenzothiazolin-2-ylidene)-1,3-pentadienyl]benzothiazolium iodide see Dithiazanine iodide.

5-Ethyl-5-(1-ethylbutyl)barbituric acid see Tetrabarbital.

5-Ethyl-5-(1-ethylbutyl)-2-thiobarbituric acid see Thiotetrabarbital.

Ethyl 1-ethyl-4-(isopropylidenehydrazino)-1H-pyrazolo(3,4-b)pyridine-5-carboxylate see Etazolate.

Ethyl 3-ethyl-4-oxo-5-piperid-1-yl-△²,α-thiazolidine acetate see Piproxolin.

1-Ethyl-2-[3-(1-ethyl-2(1H)-quinolylidene)-propenyl]quinolinium chloride see Quinaldine blue.

α-Ethyl-6-[5-[3-(5-ethyltetrahydro-5-hydroxy-6-methyl-2H-pyran-2-yl)-15-hydroxy-2,10,12-trimethyl-1,6,8-trioxadispiro(4.1.5.3)pentadec-13-en-9-yl]-2-hydroxy-1,3-dimethyl-4-oxo-heptyl]tetrahydro-3,5-dimethyl-2H-pyran-2-acetic acid see Narasin.

6-[7(R)-[5(S)-Ethyl-5-(5(R)-ethyltetrahydro-5-hydroxy-6(S)-methyl-2H-pyran-2(R)-yl)tetrahydro-3(S)-methyl-2(S)-furyl]-4-(S)-hydroxy-3(R),5(S)-dimethyl-6-oxononyl]-2,3-cresotic acid see Lasalocid.

5β-Ethyletioallocholane see 5α-Pregnane.

17β-Ethyletiocholane see 5β-Pregnane.

Ethyl 7-flavonoxyacetate see Efloxate.

Ethyl p-fluorophenyl sulfone see Fluoresone.

Ethyl formate see Triethyl orthoformate.

Ethyl glycol salicylate see Glycol salicylate.

Ethyl green see Brilliant green.

'Ethyl-gusathion' see Azinphosethyl.

'Ethyl guthion' see Azinphos-ethyl.

Ethylhexabital see Cyclobarbital.

S-Ethyl hexahydro-1H-azepine-1-carbothioate see Molinate.

Ethyl hexahydro-1,3-dimethyl-4-phenylazepine-4-carboxylate see Metethheptazine.

m-(3-Ethylhexahydro-1-methyl-1H-azepin-3-yl)phenol see Meptazinol.

2-Ethyl-1,3,4,6,7,11b-hexahydro-10-methyl-2H-benzo(a)quinolizin-2-ol see Tolquinzole.

Ethyl hexahydro-1-methyl-4-phenylazepine-4-carboxylate see Ethoheptazine.

2-Ethyl-1,3-hexanediol see Ethohexadiol.

3-Ethyl-1-hexanol sodium sulfate see Sodium etasulfate.

5-Ethyl-5-hexylbarbituric acid see Hexethal.

N-(2-ETHYLHEXYL)BICYCLO(2.2.1)-HEPT-5-ENE-2,3-DICARBOXIMIDE (2-(2-ethylhexyl)-3a,4,7,7a-tetrahydro-4,7-methano-1H-isoindole-1,3(2H)-dione; N-(2-ethylhexyl)-3,6-endomethylenetetrahydrophthalimide; N-octylbicycloheptenedicarboximide; MGK-264; 'octacide 264', 'VanDyke 264').

2-Ethylhexyl p-dimethylaminobenzoate see Padimate O.

2-Ethylhexyl diphenyl phosphate see Octicizer.

N-(2-Ethylhexyl)-3,6-endomethylenetetrahydrophthalimide see N-(2-Ethylhexyl)bicyclo(2.2.1)hept-5-ene-2,3-dicarboximide.

N-(2-Ethylhexyl)-3-hydroxybutyramide see Butoctamide.

2-Ethylhexyl sodium sulfate see Sodium etasulfate.

2-(2-Ethylhexyl)-3a,4,7,7a-tetrahydro-4,7-methano-1H-isoindole-1,3(2H)-dione see N-(2-Ethylhexyl)bicyclo(2.2.1)hept-5-ene-2,3-dicarboximide.

5-Ethyl-5-hexyl-2-thiobarbituric acid see Thiohexethal.

Ethyl p-hydroxybenzoate see Ethyl paraben.

Ethyl p-hydroxybenzoate 6-guanidino-hexanoate see Gabexate.

2-Ethyl-3-(4-hydroxybenzoyl)benzofuran see Benzarone.

24-Ethyl-3β-hydroxy-5,22-cholestadiene see Stigmasterol.

α-Ethyl-1-hydroxycyclohexaneacetic acid see Cyclobutyrol.

2-Ethyl-3-(4-hydroxy-3,5-diiodobenzoyl)-benzofuran see Benziodarone.

2-Ethyl-3-(4-hydroxy-3,5-diiodobenzoyl)-coumarone see Benziodarone.

Ethyl 5-hydroxy-1,2-dimethylindole 3-carboxylate see Mecarbinate.

13-Ethyl-17-hydroxy-18,19-dinor-17α-pregn-4-en-3-one see Norboletone.

13β-Ethyl-17-hydroxy-18,19-dinor-17α-pregn-4-en-20-yn-3-one see Norgestrel.

(+)-13-Ethyl-17-hydroxy-18,19-dinor-17α-pregn-4-en-20-yn-3-one oxime acetate see Norgestimate.

17α-Ethyl-17β-hydroxyestr-4-ene see Ethylestrenol.

17α-Ethyl-17β-hydroxyestr-5-ene see Bolenol.

17α-Ethyl-17β-hydroxyestr-4-en-3-one see Norethandrolone.

Ethyl 2-hydroxyethyl carbonate ampi-

cillin ester *see* Bacampicillin.
Ethyl(2-hydroxyethyl)dimethylammo-nium chloride benzilate *see* Lachesine.
Ethyl(2-hydroxyethyl)dimethylammo-nium chloride succinate *see* Suxethonium chloride.
Ethyl(2-hydroxyethyl)dimethylammo-nium sulfate dibutylcarbamate *see* Dibutoline.
Ethyl 1-[2-(2-hydroxyethyl)ethyl]-4-phenylisonipecotate *see* Etoxeridine.
1-Ethyl-1-(2-hydroxyethyl)piperidinium bromide benzilate *see* Pipethanate ethobromide.
1-Ethyl-1-(2-hydroxyethyl)pyrrolidinium *p*-toluenesulfonate 3,4,5-trimethoxy-benzoate *see* Troxypyrrolium tosilate.
3-Ethyl-7-hydroxy-1-(*p*-methoxyphenyl)-2-methyl-3-azaheptane 3,4-dimethoxy-benzoate *see* Mebeverine.
1-Ethyl-3-hydroxy-1-methylpiperidinium bromide benzilate *see* Pipenzolate bromide.
2-Ethyl-2-hydroxymethyl-1,3-propanediol trinitrate *see* Propatyl nitrate.
1-[Ethyl(2-hydroxy-2-methylpropyl)-aminoethyl]-4-methylthioxanthen-9-one *see* Becantone.
1-Ethyl-3-hydroxy-1-methylpyrrolidi-nium bromide α-cyclopentylphenyl-acetate *see* Cyclopyrronium.
17α-Ethyl-17-hydroxy-19-norandrost-4-en-3-one *see* Norethandrolone.
β-Ethyl-β-hydroxyphenethyl carbamate *see* Oxyfenamate.
α-Ethyl-1-hydroxy-4-phenylcyclohexane-acetic acid *see* Fencibutirol.
Ethyl(*m*-hydroxyphenyl)dimethyl-ammonium chloride *see* Edrophonium chloride.
Ethyl 1-(2-hydroxy-2-phenylethyl)-4-phenylisonipecotate *see* Oxpheneridine.
3-Ethyl-3-(*m*-hydroxyphenyl)-1-methyl-hexahydroazepine *see* Meptazinol.
3-Ethyl-3-(*m*-hydroxyphenyl)-1-methyl-hexamethylenamine *see* Meptazinol.
Ethyl (*m*-hydroxyphenylmethylpiperidyl) ketone *see* Ketobemidone.
Ethyl 1-(3-hydroxy-3-phenylpropyl)-4-phenylisonipecotate *see* Phenoperidine.
1-Ethyl-1-(3-hydroxypropyl)piperidinium iodide 2,4-diphenyl-1,3-cyclobutanedi-carboxylate *see* Truxipicurium iodide.
3-Ethyl-7-hydroxy-2,8,12,16-tetramethyl-5,13-dioxo-9-(3,4,6-trideoxy-3-dimethyl-amino-β-D-*xylo*-hexapyranosyloxy)-4,17-dioxabicyclo(14.1.0)heptadec-14-ene-10-acetaldehyde *see* Rosamicin.
Ethylideneacetamide *see* Crotonamide.
Ethylidene chloride *see* 1,1-Dichloroethane.
Ethylidene diethyl ether *see* Acetal.
4,4′-Ethylidenedi(2,6-piperazinedione) *see* 1,2-Bis(3,5-dioxopiperazin-1-yl)ethane.
Ethylidene glycol *see* 1,1-Ethanediol.
2-Ethyl-3-(2-imidazolin-2-ylmethyl)-benzofuran *see* Coumazoline.
Ethyl 10-(*p*-iodophenyl)undecanoate *see*

Iofendylate.
Ethyl iodophenylundecylate *see* Iofendylate.
ETHYL IODOSTEARATE (mixture of ethyl esters of 9- and 10-iodostearic acids; 'duroliopaque').
ETHYL IOPODATE (3-(dimethylamino-methyleneamino)-2,4,6-triiodohydro-cinnamic acid ethyl ester; SH-617-L).
5-Ethyl-5-isoamylbarbituric acid *see* Amobarbital.
5-Ethyl-5-isoamyl-2-thiobarbituric acid *see* Thioethamyl.
Ethylisobutrazine *see* Etymemazine.
2-Ethylisonicotinthioamide *see* Ethion-amide.
5-Ethyl-5-isopentylbarbituric acid *see* Amobarbital.
5-Ethyl-5-isopentyl-2-thiobarbituric acid *see* Thioethamyl.
5-Ethyl-5-isopropylbarbituric acid *see* Probarbital.
2-Ethyl-3-isopropylglycidamide *see* Oxanamide.
1-Ethyl-4-(isopropylidenehydrazino)-1H-pyrazolo(3,4-b)pyridine-5-carboxylic acid ethyl ester *see* Etazolate.
Ethylisothiuronium bromide *see* (2-Aminoethyl)isothiuronium bromide.
Ethylisovanillin *see* 4-Ethoxy-3-hydroxy-benzaldehyde.
Ethylkairine *see* 1-Ethyl-1,2,3,4-tetrahydro-8-quinolinol.
N-**ETHYLLYSERGAMIDE** (lysergic acid monoethylamide; LAE-32).
1-Ethyllysergic acid diethylamide *see* Ethyllysergide.
ETHYLLYSERGIDE (1-ethyllysergic acid diethylamide; *N,N*,1-triethyllysergamide; ALD-52).
Ethylmercaptan *see* Ethanethiol.
6-Ethylmercaptopurine *see* Ethylthio-purine.
ETHYLMERCURIC CHLORIDE ('ceresan').
Ethylmercuric chloride with BHC *see* Mercuran.
ETHYLMERCURIC PHOSPHATE (NIUIF-1; 'ruberon').
p-**(Ethylmercurithio)benzenesulfonic acid** *see* Sodium timerfonate.
2-(Ethylmercurithio)benzoxazole-5-carb-oxylic acid *see* Sodium 2-(ethylmercuri-thio)benzoxazole-5-carboxylate.
N-**ETHYLMERCURI-*p*-TOLUENE-SULFONANILIDE** ('ceresan-M').
ETHYL MESILATE (ethyl methane-sulfonate; ethyl mesylate; CB-1528; NSC-26805).
Ethyl methanesulfonate *see* Ethyl mesilate.
Ethyl methimazolate *see* Carbimazole.
β-Ethyl-6-methoxy-α,α-dimethyl-2-naph-thalenepropionic acid *see* Methallenestril.
N-**Ethyl-6-methoxy-*N′*-(1-methylethyl)-1,3,5-triazine-2,4-diamine** *see* Atraton.
N-**[2-Ethyl-2-(3-methoxyphenyl)butyl]-4-hydroxybutyramide** *see* Embutramide.

N-Ethyl-6-methoxy-N'-(1-methylpropyl)-1,3,5-triazine-2,4-diamine *see* Secmebuton.

3-Ethyl-4-(*p*-methoxyphenyl)-2-methyl-3-cyclohexene-1-carboxylic acid *see* Carbestrol.

4-[N-Ethyl-2-(*p*-methoxyphenyl)-1-methylethylamino]butyl 3,4-dimethoxybenzoate *see* Mebeverine.

S-Ethyl 11-methoxy-3,9,11-trimethyl-dodeca-2,4-dienethioate *see* Triprene.

5-Ethyl-5-(2-methylallyl)-2-thiobarbituric acid *see* Methallatal.

3-(Ethylmethylamino)-1,1-dithien-2-yl-but-1-ene *see* Ethylmethylthiambutene.

α-(1-Ethylmethylaminoethyl)benzyl alcohol *see* Etafedrine.

2-Ethyl-2-methylaminoindan-1,3-dione *see* Metindione.

2-(Ethylmethylamino)-1-phenylpropan-1-ol *see* Etafedrine.

Ethyl 3-(α-methylbenzyl)carbazate *see* Carbenzide.

Ethyl 2-(α-methylbenzyl)-1-hydrazine-carboxylate *see* Carbenzide.

Ethyl (+)-1-(α-methylbenzyl)imidazole-5-carboxylate *see* Etomidate.

5-Ethyl-5-(1-methyl-1-butenyl)barbituric acid *see* Vinbarbital.

5-Ethyl-5-(1-methylbutyl)barbituric acid *see* Pentobarbital.

5-Ethyl-5-(3-methylbutyl)barbituric acid *see* Amobarbital.

5-Ethyl-5-(1-methylbutyl)-2-thiobarbituric acid *see* Thiopental.

5-Ethyl-5-(3-methylbutyl)-2-thiobarbituric acid *see* Thioethamyl.

3-Ethyl-2-methyl-5-dimethylaminoindole *see* Medmain.

2-Ethyl-10-(2-methyl-3-dimethylamino-propyl)phenothiazine *see* Etymemazine.

Ethyl methylene phosphorodithioate *see* Ethion.

erythro-4,4'-(1-Ethyl-2-methylethylene)di-(2-fluorophenol) *see* Bifluranol.

N-Ethyl-N'-(1-methylethyl)-6-(methyl-thio)-1,3,5-triazine-2,4-diamine *see* Ametryn.

β-Ethyl-β-methylglutarimide *see* Bemegride.

Ethyl 3-methyl-4-(methylthio)phenyl isopropylphosphoramidate *see* Fenamiphos.

3-Ethyl-2-methyl-5-morpholinomethyl-6,7-dihydroindol-4(5H)-one *see* Molindone.

Ethyl 2-(2-methyl-5-nitroimidazol-1-yl)-ethyl sulfone *see* Tinidazole.

N-(4-Ethyl-7-methyloctahydroindolo-(4,3-fg)quinolin-9-yl)-3,5-dimethyl-pyrazole-1-carboxamide *see* Toquizine.

1-Ethyl-7-methyl-4-oxo-1,8-naphthyridine-3-carboxylic acid *see* Nalidixic acid.

Ethyl 3-methyl-4-oxo-5-piperid-1-ylthia-zolidinylidene-2-acetate *see* Etozolin.

α-Ethyl-*p*-[2-(α-methylphenethylamino)-ethoxy]benzyl alcohol *see* Fenalcomine.

Ethyl 1-methyl-4-phenylazacycloheptane-4-carboxylate *see* Ethoheptazine.

Ethyl-1-methyl-5-phenylbarbituric acid *see* Methylphenobarbital.

Ethyl 6-methyl-2-phenylcinchoninate *see* Neocinchophen.

5-Ethyl-6-methyl-4-phenyl-3-cyclohexane-1-carboxylic acid *see* Fenestrel.

5-Ethyl-1-methyl-5-phenylhydantoin *see* Metetoin.

5-Ethyl-3-methyl-5-phenylhydantoin *see* Mephenytoin.

Ethyl 1-methyl-4-phenylisonipecotate *see* Pethidine.

3-Ethyl-1-methyl-4-phenyl-4-propionoxy-piperidine *see* Alphameprodine; Betameprodine.

3-Ethyl-2-methyl-2-phenylsuccinimide *see* Fenimide.

4-Ethyl-1-(1-methylpiperid-4-yl)-3-phenyl-3-pyrazolin-5-one *see* Piperylone.

5-Ethyl-5-(1-methylpropyl)barbituric acid *see* Secbutabarbital.

1-Ethyl-1-methylpropyl carbamate *see* Emylcamate.

5-Ethyl-5-(1-methylpropyl)-2-thiobarbituric acid *see* Thiobutabarbital.

1-Ethyl-1-methyl-2-propyn-1-ol *see* Methylpentynol.

1-Ethyl-1-methyl-2-propynyl phthalate *see* Ftalofyne.

Ethylmethylsuccinimide *see* Ethosuximide.

2-Ethyl-2-methyltetrahydroisoquino-linium *p*-toluenesulfonate *see* Trethinium tosilate.

ETHYLMETHYLTHIAMBUTENE*** (3-(ethylmethylamino)-1,1-dithien-2-ylbut-1-ene; N-ethyl-N,1-dimethyl-3,3-dithien-2-ylallylamine).

Ethyl 3-methyl-2-thioimidazoline-1-carboxylate *see* Carbimazole.

N-Ethyl-α-methyl-*m*-trifluoromethyl-phenethylamine *see* Fenfluramine.

N-Ethyl-α-methyl-*m*-[(trifluoromethyl)-thio]phenethylamine *see* Tiflorex.

2-Ethyl-3-methylvaleramide *see* Valnoctamide.

1-(2-Ethyl-3-methylvaleryl)urea *see* Capuride.

ETHYLMORPHINE* (morphine ethyl ether; codethyline; ethomorphine; 'diolan', 'dionine', 'tionidel').

Ethyl 4-morpholino-2,2-diphenylbutyrate *see* Dioxaphetyl butyrate.

1-Ethyl-4-(2-morpholinoethyl)-3,3-di-phenyl-2-pyrrolidinone *see* Doxapram.

Ethyl 10-(3-morpholinopropyl)pheno-thiazine-2-carbamate *see* Moracizine.

Ethylnandrol *see* Ethylestrenol.

2-Ethyl-2-naphth-1-ylbutyric acid *see* Nafcaproic acid.

ETHYLNARCEINE HYDROCHLORIDE ('narcyl').

2-[(2-Ethyl-5-nitroimidazol-1-yl)ethyl]-carbamothioic acid *O*-methyl ester *see* Sulnidazole.

Ethyl *p*-nitrophenyl benzenethiophos-

phate *see* Ethyl *p*-nitrophenyl phenyl-phosphonothioate.

Ethyl *p*-nitrophenyl ethylphosphonate *see* Armin.

O-ETHYL O-(*p*-NITROPHENYL) PHENYLPHOSPHONOTHIOATE (ethyl *p*-nitrophenyl benzenethiophosphate; ethyl *p*-nitrophenyl thionobenzene-phosphate; EPN).

Ethyl *p*-nitrophenyl thionobenzene-phosphate *see* Ethyl *p*-nitrophenyl phenyl-phosphonothioate.

1-ETHYL-3-(5-NITROTHIAZOL-2-YL)-UREA (nithiazide).

Ethylnorantitheine (tr) *see* Etimizole.

Ethylnorphenylephrine *see* Etilefrine.

17-Ethyl-19-nortestosterone *see* Norethandrolone.

Ethyloestrenol* *see* Ethylestrenol.

Ethyl orthoformate *see* Triethyl orthoformate.

1-Ethyl-4-oxo(1,3)dioxolo(4,5-g)cinnoline-3-carboxylic acid *see* Cinoxacin.

Ethyl 4-oxo-2-phenyl(4H)-1-benzopyran-7-yloxy)acetate *see* Efloxate.

3-Ethyl-4-oxo-5-piperid-1-yl-△²,ᵅ-thiazo-lidineacetic acid ethyl ester *see* Piproxolin.

Ethylpapaverine *see* Ethaverine.

ETHYL PARABEN (ethyl *p*-hydroxy-benzoate; 'ethyl butex', 'mycocten', 'nipagin A').

5-(1-Ethylpentyl)-3-(trichloromethyl-thio)hydantoin *see* Clodantoin.

ETHYLPHENACEMIDE* (1-(2-phenyl-butyryl)urea; 1-(α-ethyl-α-phenylacetyl)-urea; phenylethylacetylurea; M-551; S-46; 'benuride', 'pheneturide').

Ethyl 1-phenetyl-4-phenylisonipecotate *see* Pheneridine.

Ethylphenylacetamide *see* 2-Phenylbutyr-amide.

Ethylphenylacetic acid *see* 2-Phenylbutyric acid.

1-(α-Ethyl-α-phenylacetyl)urea *see* Ethyl-phenacemide.

N-Ethyl-2-[[(phenylamino)carbonyl]-oxy]propanamide *see* Carbetamide.

5-Ethyl-5-phenylbarbituric acid *see* Phenobarbital.

2-Ethyl-2-phenylbutyric acid diethyl-aminoethoxyethyl ester *see* Oxeladin.

(+)-2-(2-Ethyl-2-phenyl-1,3-dioxolan-4-yl)piperidine *see* Etoxadrol.

Ethyl 1-(1-phenylethyl)imidazole-5-carboxylate *see* Etomidate.

O-Ethyl S-phenyl ethylphosphonodithio-ate *see* Fonofos.

3-Ethyl-5-phenylhydantoin *see* Ethotoin.

Ethyl 4-phenylisonipecotate *see* Nor-pethidine.

Ethyl phenyl ketone *see* Propiophenone.

5-Ethyl-6-phenylmetathiazane-2,4-dione *see* Phenythilone.

3-(o-Ethylphenyl)-2-methyl-4(3H)-quin-azolinone *see* Etaqualone.

N-Ethyl-3-phenyl-2-norbornanamine *see* Fencamfamin.

3-Ethyl-3-phenylpiperazine-2,6-dione *see* Iminophenimide.

(+)-2-Ethyl-2-phenyl-4-piperid-2-yl-1,3-dioxolane *see* Etoxadrol.

Ethyl 4-phenyl-1-(tetrahydrofurfuryloxy-ethyl)isonipecotate *see* Furethidine.

2-Ethyl-2-phenyltetrahydro-1,4-thiazine-3,5-dione *see* Phenythilone.

Ethyl phenylthienylacetate *see* Thiphen.

5-Ethyl-5-phenyl-2-thiobarbituric acid *see* Thiophenobarbital.

Ethylphosphonodithioic acid O-ethyl S-phenyl ester *see* Fonofos.

Ethylphosphonothioic acid O-ethyl O-(2,4,5-trichlorophenyl) ester *see* Tri-chloronat.

Ethyl 3-phthalazin-1-ylcarbazate *see* Todralazine.

Ethyl 2-phthalazin-1-ylhydrazinecarb-oxylate *see* Todralazine.

2-Ethyl-3-(β-piperidino-*p*-phenetidino)-phthalimidine *see* Etomidoline.

1-Ethylpiperid-3-yl benzilate metho-bromide *see* Pipenzolate.

N-Ethyl-3-piperidyl cyclopentyl-mandelate *see* 1-Ethylpiperid-3-yl phenyl-cyclopentaneglycolate.

2-Ethyl-3-[*p*-(2-piperid-1-ylethoxy)-anilino]isoindolin-1-one *see* Etomidoline.

2-Ethyl-3-[*p*-(2-piperid-1-ylethoxy)-anilino]phthalimidine *see* Etomidoline.

1-Ethyl-4-piperidylidene-1,1'-dithienyl-methane *see* Pipendyl methane.

1-ETHYLPIPERID-3-YL PHENYL-CYCLOPENTANEGLYCOLATE (N-ethyl-3-piperidyl cyclopentyl mandelate; JB-329; 'ditran').

N'-Ethylpodophyllohydrazide *see* Mitopodozide.

2-(N-Ethylpropylamino)-2',6'-butyroxyl-idide *see* Etidocaine.

N-[2-(N-Ethylpropylamino)butyryl]-2,6-xylidine *see* Etidocaine.

2-(N-Ethylpropylamino)-2',6'-dimethyl-butyranilide *see* Etidocaine.

2-(Ethylpropylamino)ethyl benzilate *see* Benaprizine.

Ethyl 3-O-propylglucofuranoside 5,6-di-salicylate *see* Salprotoside.

20-Ethylprostaglandin F₂ₐ *see* 20-Ethyl-dinoprost.

Ethyl protal *see* Homovanillin.

Ethylprotocatechuic aldehyde *see* Homo-vanillin.

Ethyl N-[5-(purin-6-ylthio)valeryl]-glycinate *see* Butocin.

N-Ethyl-N-pyrid-4-ylmethyltropamide *see* Tropicamide.

Ethyl pyrophosphate* *see* Tetraethyl pyrophosphate.

Ethyl pyrophosphorothionate *see* Pyrophos.

N-(1-Ethylpyrrolidin-2-ylmethyl)-5-(ethylsulfonyl)-o-anisamide *see* Sultopride.

N-(1-Ethylpyrrolidin-2-ylmethyl)-5-

199

(ethylsulfonyl)-2-methoxybenzamide *see* Sultopride.

N-(1-Ethylpyrrolidin-2-ylmethyl)-2-methoxy-5-sulfamoylbenzamide *see* Sulpiride.

N-(1-Ethylpyrrolidin-2-ylmethyl)-5-sulfamoyl-*o*-anisamide *see* Sulpiride.

O-Ethyl *O*-quinolin-8-yl phenylphosphonothioate *see* Quintiofos.

ETHYL SALICYLATE ('sal-ethyl').

Ethyl salicylate carbonate *see* Carbethyl salicylate.

ETHYLSTIBAMINE* (diethylamine salt of *p*-aminobenzenestibonic acid; stibosamine; Bayer-693; 'neostibosan').

(2-Ethylsuccinyl)erythromycin *see* Erythromycin ethyl succinate.

1-Ethyl-*N*-sulfanilylcytosine *see* Sulfacitine.

S-[2-(Ethylsulfinyl)ethyl] *O,O*-dimethyl phosphorothioate *see* Oxydemetonmethyl.

2-[(3-Ethylsulfinyl)propyl]-1,2,3,4-tetra-hydroisoquinoline *see* Esproquine.

Ethylsulfonal *see* Methylsulfonal.

p-Ethylsulfonylbenzaldehyde thiosemicarbazone *see* Subathizone.

S-[2-(Ethylsulfonyl)ethyl] *O,O*-dimethyl phosphorothioate *see* Demeton-S-methylsulfon.

1-(2-Ethylsulfonylethyl)-2-methyl-5-nitroimidazole *see* Tinidazole.

3-Ethyl-1,6,7,11b-tetrahydro-9,10-dimethoxy-2-(1,2,3,4-tetrahydro-6,7-dimethoxyisoquinolin-1-ylmethyl)-4H-benzo(a)quinolizine *see* Dehydroemetine.

5-[(4-Ethyl-2,3,4,5-tetrahydrofuran-5-on-3-yl)methyl]-1-methylimidazole *see* Pilocarpine.

6-Ethyl-2,3,6,9-tetrahydro-3-methyl-2,6-dioxothiazolo(5,4-f)quinoline-8-carboxylic acid *see* Tioxacin.

2-Ethyl-1,2,3,4-tetrahydro-2-methyliso-quinolinium *p*-toluenesulfonate *see* Trethinium tosilate.

Ethyl 1-(1,2,3,4-tetrahydronaphth-1-yl)-imidazole-5-carboxylate *see* Etonam.

2-[5-Ethyltetrahydro-5-[tetrahydro-3-methyl-5-(tetrahydro-6-hydroxy-6-hydroxymethyl-3,5-dimethylpyran-2-yl)-2-furyl]-2-furyl]-9-hydroxy-β-methoxy-α,γ,2,8-tetramethyl-1,6-dioxaspiro(4.5)decane-7-butyric acid *see* Monensin.

9-Ethyl-1,3,4,9-tetrahydro-*N,N*,1-trimethylthiopyrano(3,4-b)indole-1-ethanamine *see* Tandamine.

*N*¹-(5-ETHYL-1,2,4-THIADIAZOL-3-YL)-SULFANILAMIDE (sulfaethidole isomer; 'isoglobucid').

*N*¹-(5-Ethyl-1,3,4-thiadiazol-2-yl)sulfanilamide *see* Sulfaethidole.

6-(Ethylthio)-2,4-bis(isopropylamino)-*s*-triazine *see* Dipropetryn.

16α-ETHYLTHIO-6-DEHYDRORETRO-PROGESTERONE (16α-(ethylthio)-dydrogesterone; 16α-ethylthio-9β,10α-pregna-4,6-diene-3,20-dione; retro-progestagen; Ro 6-3129).

16α-(Ethylthio)dydrogesterone *see* 16α-Ethylthio-6-dehydroprogesterone.

S-[2-(Ethylthio)ethyl] *O,O*-dimethyl phosphorodithioate *see* Thiometon.

O-[2-(Ethylthio)ethyl] *O,O*-dimethyl phosphorothioate *see* Demeton-O-methyl.

S-[2-(Ethylthio)ethyl] *O,O*-dimethyl phosphorothioate *see* Demeton-S-methyl.

2-Ethylthioisonicotinamide *see* Ethionamide.

2-(Ethylthio)-10-[3-(4-methylpiperazin-1-yl)propyl]phenothiazine *see* Thiethylperazine.

Ethylthiometon *see* Disulfoton.

Ethyl thiurad *see* Disulfiram.

N-Ethyl-*N*-*o*-tolylcrotonamide *see* Crotamiton.

Ethyl 3,5,6-tri-*O*-benzyl-D-glucurofuronoside *see* Tribenoside.

Ethyl trichloramate *see* Carbocloral.

Ethyl (2,2,2-trichloro-1-hydroxyethyl)-carbamate *see* Carbocloral.

O-Ethyl *O*-(2,4,5-trichlorophenyl) ethylphosphonothioate *see* Trichloronat.

N-Ethyl-*m*-trifluoromethylamphetamine *see* Fenfluramine.

N-Ethyl-*m*-[(trifluoromethyl)thio]-amphetamine *see* Tiflorex.

4-[Ethyl-[2,4,6-triiodo-3-(methylamino)-phenyl]amino]-4-oxobutanoic acid *see* Iosumetic acid.

N-Ethyl-2′,4′,6′-triiodo-3′-(methylamino)-succinanilic acid *see* Iosumetic acid.

α-Ethyl-2,4,6-triiodo-3-(2-oxopyrrolidin-1-yl)hydrocinnamic acid *see* Iolidonic acid.

2-Ethyl-3-[2,4,6-triiodo-3-(2-oxopyrrolidin-1-yl)phenyl]propionic acid *see* Iolidonic acid.

1-Ethyl-1-[2-(3,4,5-trimethoxybenzoyloxy)ethyl]pyrrolidinium *p*-toluenesulfonate *see* Troxypyrrolium tosilate.

Ethyl 4-(3,4,5-trimethoxycinnamoyl)-piperazin-1-ylacetate *see* Cinepazet.

α-Ethyltryptamine *see* Etryptamine.

Ethyl urethan *see* Urethan.

Ethyl vanillin* *see* Homovanillin.

ETHYL VINYL ETHER ('vinamar').

'Ethymal' *see* Ethosuximide.

Ethymemazine *see* Etymemazine.

ETHYMIDINE (tr) (2,4-bis(1-aziridinyl)-6-chloropyrimidine; 4-chloro-2,6-diethyleniminopyrimidine; etimidin; A-1).

Ethymisol *see* Ethimizole.

Ethyne *see* Acetylene.

ETHYNERONE* (21-chloro-17-hydroxy-19-nor-17α-pregna-4,9-dien-20-yn-3-one; 21-chloro-19-nor-17α-pregna-4,9-dien-20-yn-17-ol-3-one; 17α-chloroethynyl-19-nor-4,9(10)-androstadien-17β-ol-3-one; etynerone).

ETHYNERONE WITH MESTRANOL (MK-665).

Ethynodiol* *see* Etynodiol.

17-Ethynylandrostane *see* Pregn-20-yne.

17α-Ethynyl-4-androsten-17β-ol-3-one *see*

200

Ethisterone.
α-Ethynylbenzyl alcohol carbamate *see* Carfimate.
1-Ethynylclohexanecarboxamide *see* Ethinamate.
1-Ethynylcyclohexyl carbamate *see* Ethinamate.
1-[3-(1-Ethynylcyclohexyloxy)-2-hydroxypropyl]-4-(*p*-fluorophenyl)piperazine *see* Fluciprazine.
α-[(1-Ethynylcyclohexyloxy)methyl]-4-(*p*-fluorophenyl)-1-piperazineethanol *see* Fluciprazine.
17α-Ethynyl-3β,17β-dihydroxyestr-4-ene *see* Etynodiol.
17α-Ethynyl-3β,17-dihydroxy-11β-methylestr-4-ene *see* Metynodiol.
17α-Ethynyl-6α,21-dimethylandrost-4-en-17-ol-3-one *see* Dimethisterone.
17α-Ethynyl-6α,21-dimethyltestosterone *see* Dimethisterone.
Ethynylestradiol *see* Ethinylestradiol.
17α-Ethynylestra-4,9,11-trien-17-ol-3-one *see* Norgestrienone.
17α-Ethynylestr-4-en-17β-ol *see* Lynestrenol.
17α-Ethynyl-5-estren-17-ol *see* Cingestol.
17α-Ethynyl-5(10)-estren-17-ol *see* Tigestol.
17α-Ethynylestr-5(10)-en-17β-ol-3-one *see* Noretynodrel.
17-Ethynyl-17β-hydroxyandrost-4-en-3-one *see* Ethisterone.
17α-Ethynyl-17-hydroxy-6α,21-dimethylandrost-4-en-3-one *see* Dimethisterone.
17-Ethynyl-17β-hydroxyestr-4-en-3-one *see* Norethisterone.
17α-Ethynyl-17-hydroxy-5(10)-estren-3-one *see* Noretynodrel.
17α-Ethynyl-17-hydroxy-7α-methyl-5(10)-estren-3-one *see* Tibolone.
17-Ethynyl-17β-hydroxy-19-norandrost-4-en-3-one *see* Norethisterone.
17-Ethynyl-11β-methoxyestradiol *see* Moxestrol.
17-Ethynyl-3-methoxy-1,3,5(10)-estratrien-17β-ol *see* Mestranol.
17α-Ethynyl-11β-methylestr-4-ene-3β,17-diol *see* Metynodiol.
17α-Ethynyl-11β-methyl-19-norandrost-4-ene-3β,17-diol *see* Metynodiol.
17α-Ethynyl-19-norandrost-4-ene-3β,17-diol *see* Etynodiol.
17α-Ethynyl-19-nortestosterone *see* Norethisterone.
Ethynyl phenyl carbinol *see* Ethynylbenzyl alcohol.
Ethynyl phenyl carbinol carbamate *see* Carfimate.
17α-Ethynyltestosterone *see* Ethisterone.
ETHYPICONE*** (3,3-diethyl-5-methyl-2,4(1H,3H)-pyridinedione; 3,3-diethyl-1,2,3,4-tetrahydro-5-methyl-2,4-dioxopyridine; dehydromethyprylone).
Ethyrone (tr) *see* (2-Aminoethyl)isothiuronium bromide.
Ethysine (tr) *see* Fenethazine.
Ethyzine (tr) *see* Fenethazine.
Etian *see* 5β-Androstane.

'**Etibi**' *see* Ethambutol.
Eticlordifene *see* Etofamide.
'**Eticol**' *see* Paraoxon.
ETIDOCAINE*** ((±)-2-(*N*-ethylpropylamino)-2′,6′-butyroxylidide; (±)-*N*-[2-(*N*-ethylpropylamino)butyryl]-2,6-xylidine; (±)-2-(*N*-ethylpropylamino)-2′,6′-dimethylbutyranilide; W-19053; 'duranest').
ETIDRONIC ACID*** ((1-hydroxyethylidene)diphosphonic acid; ethane-1-hydroxy-1,1-diphosphonic acid; EHDP™).
See also Disodium etidronate.
ETIFELMINE*** (2-benzhydrylidenebutylamine; 2-diphenylmethylenebutylamine; ecinamine).
ETIFOXINE*** (6-chloro-2-ethylamino-4-methyl-4-phenyl-4H-3,1-benzoxazine; HOE-36801).
ETILEFRINE*** (α-ethylaminomethyl-3-hydroxybenzyl alcohol; α-ethylaminomethyl-*m*-hydroxybenzyl alcohol; 2-ethylamino-1-hydroxy-1-(3-hydroxyphenyl)-ethane; ethylnorphenylephrine; fetanol; phethanol; M-1-36; 'circupon', 'effortil', 'ethyladrianol', 'pressoton', 'trieffortil').
'**Etilon**' *see* Parathion.
Etimidin (tr) *see* Ethymidine.
ETIMIZOLE (tr) (*N*,*N*′-diethylimidazole-4,5-dicarboxamide; imidazole-4,5-dicarboxylic acid bis(ethylamide); ethylnorantitheine; ethimizole; ethymisol; IEM-163).
Etina *see* Ethionamide.
Etioallocholane *see* 5α-Androstane.
Etiocholane *see* 5β-Androstane.
Etiocholanone *see* 5β-Androstan-3α-ol-17-one.
'**Etiol**' *see* Malathion.
'**Etionizina**' *see* Ethinamide.
ETIP *see* Ditophal.
ETIPIRIUM IODIDE*** (1-(2-hydroxyethyl)-1-methylpyrrolidinium iodide benzilate).
Etipyrole *see* Ethipyrole.
Etiron (tr) *see* 2-Aminoethylisothiuronium bromide.
ETIROXATE** (α-methyl-DL-thyroxine ethyl ester; CG-635).
ETISAZOLE*** (3-ethylamino-1,2-benzisothiazole).
Etisine (tr) *see* Fenethazine.
'**Etisul**' *see* Ditophal.
Etizin (tr) *see* Fenethazine.
Etmozine (tr) *see* Moracizine.
ETOCARLIDE*** (4,4′-diethoxythiocarbanilide; ethoxide; ethoxyd; etoxid).
Etoclofene *see* Terofenamate.
ETODOLIC ACID*** (1,8-diethyl-1,3,4,9-tetrahydropyrano(3,4-b)indole-1-acetic acid).
ETODROXIZINE*** (1-(*p*-chlorobenzhydryl)-4-[2-[2-(2-hydroxyethoxy)ethoxy]ethyl]piperazine; 2-[2-[2-[4-(*p*-chloro-α-phenylbenzyl)piperazin-1-yl]ethoxy]ethoxy]ethanol; ethoxyhydroxyzine).

ETODROXIZINE MALEATE (UCB-1414; 'indunox').
See also Methaqualone with etodroxizine maleate.
ETOFAMIDE*** (2,2-dichloro-*N*-(2-ethoxy-ethyl)-*N*-[(*p*-nitrophenoxy)benzyl]acet-amide; ethylchlordiphene; eticlordifene; 'kitnos').
ETOFENAMATE*** (2-(2-hydroxyethoxy)-ethyl *N*-(α,α,α-trifluoro-*m*-tolyl)anthran-ilate; flufenamic acid ester with 2-(2-hydroxyethoxy)ethanol).
ETOFIBRATE** (2-hydroxyethyl nicotinate 2-(*p*-chlorophenoxy)-2-methylpropionate (ester); clofibric acid 2-(nicotinoyloxy)-ethyl ester; nicotinic acid 2-[2-(*p*-chloro-phenoxy)-2-methylpropionoxy]ethyl ester; 'lipo-Merz').
ETOFORMIN** (1-butyl-2-ethylbiguanide; SHE 199).
ETOFURADINE*** (*N*-benzofuran-2-yl-methyl-*N*',*N*'-dimethyl-*N*-pyrid-2-ylethyl-enediamine).
ETOFYLLINE*** (7-(2-hydroxyethyl)-theophylline; 'ascorphylline', 'cordalin', 'oxyphylline', 'phyllocormin-N'.
See also Proscillaridin with etofylline.
ETOFYLLINE NICOTINATE (He-682; 'actemil', 'hesotanol', 'hesotin').
Etofylline pyridoxol salt hydrogen sulfate ester *see* Pyridofylline.
ETOFYLLINE WITH THEOPHYLLINE-EPHEDRINE ('peripherin').
ETOGLUCID*** (1,2:15,16-diepoxy-4,7,10,13-tetraoxahexadecane; triethylene glycol diglycidyl ether; ethoglucid; AY-62013; 'epodyl').
ETOLOREX*** (2-(*p*-chloro-α,α-dimethyl-phenethylamino)ethanol; *p*-chloro-α,α-di-methyl-*N*-(2-hydroxyethyl)phenethyl-amine).
ETOLOXAMINE*** (2-(α-phenyl-*o*-toloxy)-triethylamine; α-[2-(2-diethylaminoethoxy)-phenyl]toluene; 2-(2-diethylaminoethoxy)-diphenylmethane).
ETOMIDATE*** ((+)-ethyl 1-(α-methyl-benzyl)imidazole-5-carboxylate; ethyl 1-benzhydrylimidazole-5-carboxylate; R-7405; R-16659).
Etomide *see* Carbifene.
ETOMIDOLINE** (2-ethyl-3-(β-piperidino-*p*-phenetidino)phthalimidine; 2-ethyl-3-[*p*-(2-piperid-1-ylethoxy)anilino]phthal-imidine; 2-ethyl-3-[*p*-(2-piperid-1-yl-ethoxy)anilino]isoindolin-1-one; amidoline; K-2680).
ETONAM*** (5-ethoxycarbonyl-1-(1,2,3,4-tetrahydronaphth-1-yl)imidazole; ethyl 1-(1,2,3,4-tetrahydronaphth-1-yl)imidazole-5-carboxylate; 1-(1,2,3,4-tetrahydronaphth-1-yl)-5-ethoxycarbonylimidazole; ethonam).
ETONAM NITRATE (ethonam nitrate; ethonamidate; R-10100).
ETONITAZENE*** (1-(2-diethylamino-ethyl)-2-(*p*-ethoxybenzyl)-5-nitrobenz-imidazole).
'Etophylate' *see* Acefylline piperazine.

ETOPOSIDE** (4'-demethylepipodophyllo-toxin 9-(4,6-*O*-ethylidene-β-D-gluco-pyranoside; NSC-141540; VP-16-213).
ETOPRINDOLE** (1-(2-dimethylamino-ethyl)indol-3-yl ethyl ketone oxime; 1-(2-dimethylaminoethyl) 3-propionylindole oxime; 1-(2-dimethylaminoethyl)-3-(1-hydroxyiminopropyl)indole).
Etoquinol *see* Sodium actinoquinol.
ETORPHINE*** (6,7,8,14-tetrahydro-7α-(1-hydroxy-1-methylbutyl)-6,14-*endo*-ethenooripavine; 1,2,3,3a,8,9-hexahydro-5-hydroxy-2α-(1(*R*)-hydroxy-1-methyl-butyl)-3-methoxy-12-methyl-3,9a-etheno-9,9b-iminoethanophenanthro(4,5-bcd)-furan; 7,8-dihydro-7α-(1(*R*)-hydroxy-1-methylbutyl)-*O*⁶-methyl-6,14-*endo*-etheno-morphine; 7α-(1(*R*)-hydroxy-1-methyl-butyl)-6,14-*endo*-ethenotetrahydrooripavine; etorphine hydrochloride; 19-propylnorvi-nol; propylorvinol; M-99).
Etorphine acetate *see* Acetorphine.
ETORPHINE WITH ACEPROMAZINE ('immobilon').
ETORPHINE WITH LEVOMEPROM-AZINE ('immobilon').
ETOSALAMIDE*** (*o*-(2-ethoxyethoxy)-benzamide; salicylamide 2-ethoxyethyl ether; ethosalamide).
'Etosalicil' *see* Ethenzamide.
'Etossidrazone' *see* Ruvazone.
'Etoval' *see* Butethal.
ETOXADROL*** ((+)-2-(2-ethyl-2-phenyl-1,3-dioxolan-4-yl)piperidine; (+)-2-ethyl-2-phenyl-4-piperid-2-yl-1,3-dioxolane; CL-1848C).
ETOXAZENE*** (4-(*p*-ethoxyphenylazo)-*m*-phenylenediamine; 4-(*p*-phenetylazo)-*m*-phenylenediamine; diaminoethoxyazo-benzene; ethoxazene; *p*-ethoxychrysoidine; SQ-2128; 'carmurit', 'crystural', 'serenium').
ETOXERIDINE*** (ethyl ester of 1-[2-(2-hydroxyethoxy)ethyl]-4-phenylisonipecotic acid; carbetidine; UCB-2073).
Etoxid (tr) *see* Etocarlide.
ETOZOLIN*** (ethyl 3-methyl-4-oxo-5-piperid-1-ylthiazolidinylidene-2-acetate; 3-methyl-4-oxo-5-piperidino-Δ²,ᵅ-thia-zolidineacetic acid ethyl ester; 2-carb-ethoxymethylene-3-methyl-5-piperid-1-yl-4-thiazolidinone; 2-(ethoxycarbonyl-methylene)-3-methyl-5-piperid-1-yl-4-thiazolidinone; W-2900A).
ETPENAL (tr) (3-diethylaminopropyl 2-ethoxy-2,2-diphenylacetate; ethpenal).
'Etrafon' *see* Amitriptyline with perphen-azine.
'Etrenol' *see* Hycanthone.
Etrofolan *see* Isoprocarb.
'Etrolene' *see* Fenclofos.
'Etrynit' *see* Propatyl nitrate.
ETRYPTAMINE*** (3-(2-aminobutyl)-indole; α-ethyltryptamine; U-17312-E).
ETRYPTAMINE ACETATE ('monase').
ETTN *see* Propatyl nitrate.
Ettriol nitrate *see* Propatyl nitrate.

'Etumine' *see* Clotiapine.
ETYBENZATROPINE*** (3-diphenyl-
methoxy-8-ethylnortropane; 3-benzhy-
dryloxy-8-ethylnortropane; *N*-ethyl-
nortropane benzhydryl ether; ethybenztropine; methylbenztropine; tropethydryline; UK-738; 'panolid', 'ponalid').
ETYMEMAZINE*** (10-(3-dimethylamino-
2-methylpropyl)-2-ethylphenothiazine;
ethotrimeprazine; ethylisobutrazine;
ethymemazine; RP-6484; 'diquel',
'sergetyl', 'veractil').
Etymide *see* Carbifene.
Etynerone *see* Ethynerone.
ETYNODIOL** (17α-ethynylestr-4-ene-
3β,17β-diol; 17α-ethynyl-19-norandrost-4-
ene-3β,17β-diol; 19-nor-17α-pregn-4-en-
20-yne-3β,17β-diol; 17α-ethynyl-3β,17β-
dihydroxyestr-4-ene; ethynodiol).
ETYNODIOL ACETATE (etynodiol
17-acetate; SC-12222; 'femulen').
ETYNODIOL DIACETATE (etynodiol
3,17-diacetate; CB-8080; SC-11800;
'continuin', 'lutometrodiol').
ETYNODIOL DIACETATE WITH
ETHINYLESTRADIOL ('demulen').
ETYNODIOL DIACETATE WITH
MESTRANOL ('metrulen', 'ovulen',
'planor').
Etyprenaline* *see* Isoetarine.
EU-2200 *see* Inosine.
EU-2826 *see* Benurestat.
EU-4290 *see* Piribedil.
'Eubetin' *see* Chlorpropamide.
'Eubine' *see* Oxycodone.
EUCAINE A (α-eucaine; carbomethoxy-
pentamethyl-4-piperidinol).
EUCAINE B (β-eucaine; benzoate of 2,2,6-
trimethyl-4-piperidinol; benzamine;
'betacaine').
Eucalyptole *see* Cineole.
'Eucast' *see* Nicametate citrate.
EUCATROPINE*** (1,2,2,6-tetramethyl-
piperid-4-yl mandelate; 'euphthalmine').
Euchema spinosum degradation product
see Poligeenan.
'Euchinin' *see* Quinine ethyl carbonate.
'Eucilat' *see* Benfurodil hemisuccinate.
'Euclidan' *see* Nicametate citrate.
'Eucodin' *see* Codeine methyl bromide.
'Eucol' *see* Arginine oxoglurate.
'Eucupine' *see* Euprocin.
'Eudan' *see* Mephebarbital.
'Eudatin' *see* Pargyline.
'Eudemine' *see* Diazoxide.
'Eudyna' *see* Tretinoin.
Euflavine* *see* Acriflavine.
Eugallol *see* Gallacetophenone.
Eugenic acid *see* Eugenol.
EUGENOL (4-allyl-2-methoxyphenol; 4-
allylguaiacol; eugenic acid).
'Euglucin' *see* Chlorpentazide.
'Euglucon' *see* Glibenclamide.
'Euglycin' *see* Metahexamide.
'Eugynon' *see* Norgestrel with ethinyl-
estradiol.
'Eukraton' *see* Bemegride.

'Eumicton' *see* Actazolamide.
'Eumotol' *see* Bumadizone calcium.
'Eumydrine' *see* Atropine methonitrate.
'Eunal' *see* 2-(4-Allyl-2-methoxyphenoxy)-
N,*N*-diethylacetamide.
'Eunarcon' *see* Enibomal.
'Eunasin' *see* Metizoline.
'Eunephran' *see* Butizide.
'Eunoctin' *see* Nitrazepam.
'Eunomin' *see* Chlormadinone acetate with
mestranol.
Euonymit *see* Dulcitol.
'Euparen' *see* Dichlofluanid.
'Eupatal' *see* Alantolactone.
'Eupaverin' *see* Moxaverine.
'Euphagin' *see* Benzocaine.
'Euphoramin' *see* Methamphetamine with
meprobamate.
'Euphthalmine' *see* Eucatropine.
'Euphylline' *see* Aminophylline.
'Eupneron' *see* Epronizol.
'Euporphin' *see* Apomorphine methyl
bromide.
'Eupractone' *see* Dimethadione
'Eupramin' *see* Imipramine.
'Euprax' *see* Albutoin.
EUPROCIN*** (*O*⁶′-isopentylhydro-
cupreine; isoamylhydrocupreine;
'eucupine').
'Euquinine' *see* Quinine ethyl carbonate.
'Eurax' *see* Crotamiton.
'Euraxil' *see* Crotamiton.
'Euresol' *see* Resorcinol acetate.
'Eurinol' *see* Trichlormethiazide.
'Eusaprim' *see* Co-trimoxazole.
EUSARONE (1-allyl-2,4,5-trimethoxy-
benzene).
'Eusidon' *see* Opipramol.
Eusintomicine *see* Chloramphenicol stearate.
'Eustidil' *see* Haloxon.
Eusynthomycin *see* Chloramphenicol
stearate.
'Euthroid' *see* Liotrix.
'Eutizon' *see* Isoniazid.
'Eutonyl' *see* Pargyline.
'Eutrophyl' *see* α-Tocopherylquinone.
'Euvernil' *see* Sulfacarbamide.
'Euvitol' *see* Fencamfamin.
'Evadyne' *see* Butriptyline.
EVANS BLUE** (tetrasodium salt of 4,4′-
bis[7-(8-amino-1-hydroxy-5,7-disulfo-
naphth-2-ylazo)]-3,3′-bitolyl; azovan blue;
diazo bleu; T-1824).
'Evaspirine' *see* Fenyramidol.
'Eventin' *see* Propylhexedrine.
'Evramicina' *see* Troleandomycin.
'Evramycin' *see* Troleandomycin.
'Evronal' *see* Secobarbital.
EX-12-095 *see* Eterobarb.
EX-4355 *see* Desipramine.
EX-4810 *see* Ambuside.
EX-4883 *see* Rolicyprine.
EX-10029 *see* Elantrine.
EX-10781 *see* Benazoline.
'Exacyl' *see* Tranexamic acid.
'Ex-adipos' *see* Phentermine.
'Exalgin' *see* Methylacetanilide.

'**Exangit**' *see* Benzonatate.
EXAPROLOL*** (1-(*o*-cyclohexylphenoxy)-3-isopropylamino-2-propanol).
'**Exelmin**' *see* Piperazine citrate.
EXIPROBEN*** (*o*-(3-hexyloxy-2-hydroxy-propoxy)benzoic acid; 1-(2-carboxy-phenoxy)-3-hexyloxy-2-propanol; X-40).
EXIPROBEN SODIUM (sodium *o*-(3-hexyloxy-2-hydroxypropoxy)benzoate; 'droctil').
'**Exluto**' *see* Lynestrenol.
'**Exluton**' *see* Lynestrenol.
'**Exmigra**' *see* Ergotamine tartrate.
'**Exna**' *see* Benzthiazide.
'**Exofene**' *see* Hexachlorophene.
'**Exolan**' *see* Dithranol triacetate.
'**Exomycol**' *see* Phenylmercuric borate.

'**Exopon**' *see* Cyclexanone.
'**Exosterol**' *see* Dexametasone pivalate with phenylmercuric borate.
'**Exotherm termul**' *see* Chlorothalonil.
EXP-105-1 *see* Amantadine.
EXP-126 *see* Rimantadine.
EXP-338 *see* Midaflur.
EXP-999 *see* Metopimazine.
'**Expandex**' *see* Dextran.
'**Exponcit**' *see* Norpseudoephedrine.
'**Extencillin**' *see* Benzathine penicillin.
'**Exton reagent**' *see* Sulfosalicylic acid.
Extraline (tr) Methylaniline.
'**Extramycin**' *see* Sisomicin.
'**Extranase**' *see* Bromelains.
Extrinsic factor *see* Cyanocobalamin.

F

F-1 *see* 5-Nitro-2-furfuryl methyl ether.
F-2 *see* Zearalenone.
F-8 *see* 5-Nitro-2-furaldehyde thiosemicar-bazone.
F-19 *see* Amikhellin.
F-26 *see* Nidroxyzone.
F-28 *see* Nitrofurylideneaminoguanidine sulfate.
F-30 *see* Nitrofurantoin.
F-35 *see* Furazidin.
F-60 *see* Furazolidone.
F-70 *see* Oxitefonium bromide.
F-74 *see* Nitrofurylideneisoniazid.
F-75 *see* Prazocillin.
F-151 *see* Methafurylene.
F-309 *see* Suramin.
F-368 *see* Dantrolene.
F-440 *see* Dantrolene sodium.
F-461 *see* Carboxin dioxide.
F-710 *see* Plasmocide.
F-831 *see* Carboxin oxide.
F-883 *see* (Diethylaminomethyl)-1,4-benzo-dioxan.
F-933 *see* Piperoxan.
F-1052 *see* Butamoxane.
F-1162 *see* Sulfanilamide.
F-1358 *see* Dapsone.
F-1399 *see* Acedapsone.
F-1500 *see* Succinyldapsone.
F-1983 *see* Pyrovalerone.
F-2249 *see* Oxapropanium.
F-2559 *see* Gallamine triethiodide.
F-6066 *see* Cyclofenil.
'**Fabahistin**' *see* Mebhydrolin napadisilate.
'**Fabantol**' *see* Propanidid.
'**FAC**' *see* Prothoate.
FAD *see* Flavine-adenine dinucleotide.
'**Falepsin**' *see* Phenobarbital-norpseudo-ephedrine.

'**Falicaine**' *see* Propipocaine.
'**Falicor**' *see* Prenylamine lactate.
'**Falignost**' *see* Iomeglamic acid.
'**Falmonox**' *see* Teclozan.
'**Falone**' *see* 2,4-DEP.
'**Famid**' *see* Dioxacarb.
FAMOTINE*** (1-(*p*-chlorophenoxy-methyl)-3,4-dihydroisoquinoline; UK-2054).
FAMPHUR* (*O*-[*p*-(dimethylamino)sul-fonyl]phenyl *O*,*O*-dimethyl phosphoro-thioate; 'warbex').
FAMPROFAZONE*** (4-isopropyl-2-methyl-3-[*N*-methyl-*N*-(α-methylphenethyl)-aminomethyl]-1-phenyl-3-pyrazolin-5-one; *N*-(4-isopropyl-2-methyl-5-oxo-1-phenyl-3-pyrazolin-3-ylmethyl)-*N*-methylamphet-amine).
FAMPROFAZONE WITH PROPYPHEN-AZONE ('gevodin').
'**Fanasil**' *see* Sulfadoxine.
'**Fanerom**' *see* Bromofenoxim.
Fankinon *see* Phanquinone.
'**Fansidar**' *see* Sulfadoxine with pyrimeth-amine.
Fanthridone* *see* Fantridone.
'**Fantorin**' *see* Stibophen.
FANTRIDONE*** (5-(-3-dimethylamino-propyl)-6-(5H)phenanthridinone; fan-thridone; AGN-616).
'**Fanzil**' *see* Sulfadoxine.
FAOP *see* Pralidoxime phenacyl chloride.
'**Farlutal**' *see* Medroxyprogesterone.
'**Farmiglucina**' *see* Paromomycin.
'**Farming S**' *see* Endothion.
'**Farmiserina**' *see* Cycloserine.
'**Farmocaine**' *see* Diethylaminoethyl *p*-butylaminobenzoate.
'**Farmotal**' *see* Thiopental.

FARNESOL (3,7,11-trimethyl-2,6,10-dodecatrien-1-ol).

FARNOQUINONE (3-difarnesyl-2-methyl-1,4-naphthoquinone; 2-methyl-3-*all-trans*-tetraprenyl-1,4-naphthoquinone; menaquinone-4; pharnoquinone; vitamin K_2).

Fasciolin (tr) *see* Hexachloroethane.

'Fasciophene' *see* Hexachlorophene.

'Fasigyn' *see* Tinidazole.

Fast green *see* Malachite green.

Fast green J *see* Brilliant green.

'Fat Ponceau R' *see* Scarlet red.

'Faustan' *see* Diazepam.

FAZADINIUM BROMIDE*** (1,1'-azobis(3-methyl-2-phenyl-1H-imidazo-(1,2-a)pyridin-4-ium bromide); AH-8165-D; phenazidinium).

FB/2 *see* Diquat.

FBA-140 *see* Propanidid.

FBA-1464 *see* Guanacline.

FBA-1500 *see* Mefruside.

FBA-4503 *see* Propiram.

FB b-4231 *see* Glisoxepide.

FB b-5097 *see* Clotrimazole.

FB b-6366 *see* L-Asparaginase.

FC-1 *see* Clobenztropine.

'F-cortef' *see* Fludrocortisone acetate.

'Fe-3-specific' *see* Bis(2-hydroxyethyl)glycine.

FEBARBAMATE*** (1-(3-butoxy-2-hydroxypropyl)-5-ethyl-5-phenylbarbituric acid carbamate ester; 1-(3-butoxy-2-hydroxypropyl)phenobarbital carbamate; Go-560; 'getryl', 'G-TRIL', 'solium').

'Febramine' *see* Cetoxime.

FEBRIFUGINE (tr) (3-[3-(3-hydroxypiperid-2-yl)acetonyl]-4(3H)-quinazolinone).

'Febrimin' *see* Phenicarbazide.

'Febrinina' *see* Aminophenazone.

FEBUPROL*** (1-butoxy-3-phenoxy-2-propanol; H-33).

'Febutol' *see* Fenyramidol oxyphenbutazone salt.

FEBUVERINE*** (1,4-bis(2-phenylbutyryloxyethyl)piperazine; 2-phenylbutyrate diester of 1,4-bis(2-hydroxyethyl)piperazine; 1,4-piperazinediethanol di(2-phenylbutyrate) ester; phebutazine).

'Febuzine isopirin' *see* 4-Isopropylaminophenazone with phenylbutazone.

'Fecatest' *see* o-Tolidine.

FECLOBUZONE*** (4-butyl-4-hydroxymethyl-1,2-diphenyl-3,5-pyrazolidinedione ester of *p*-chlorobenzoic acid).

FEDRILATE*** (1-methyl-3-morpholinopropyl tetrahydro-4-phenyl-2H-pyran-4-carboxylate; fenhydropyxilate; 'tussefane').

'Feguanide' *see* Phenformin.

'Felagol' *see* Cholic acid.

'Felicur' *see* 1-Phenyl-1-propanol.

FELIPYRINE*** (1-phenyl-3-piperid-1-yl-2-pyrrolidinone).

'Felkreon' *see* Ox bile.

'Felogen' *see* 6-(1-Hydroxyethyl)norbornene acid succinate.

'Felotrast' *see* Phenobutiodil.

Fel tauri *see* Ox bile.

'Felviten' *see* Anethole trithione.

FELYPRESSIN*** (2-phenylalanine-8-lysine vasopressin; PLV-2; 'octapressin').

'Femergin' *see* Ergotamine tartrate.

'Femigen' *see* Chlormadinone acetate with mestranol.

'Feminor sequential' *see* Noretynodrel with mestranol.

'Femulen' *see* Etynodiol diacetate.

Fen..... *see also* Phen.....

FENABUTENE*** (*p*-(1-methylpropenyl)-phenyl acetate; *p*-(2-buten-2-yl)phenyl acetate; CB-309; 'isotyl AO12').

FENACETINOL** (*p*-glycolophenetidide; *N*-glycoloyl-*p*-phenetidine; *N*-(*p*-ethoxyphenyl)glycolamide; *p*-ethoxy-α-hydroxyacetanilide; α-hydroxyphenacetin).

FENACLON** (3-chloro-*N*-phenethylpropionamide; *N*-(3-chloropropionyl)-phenethylamine; fenacon; fenakon; phenacon).

Fenacon *see* Fenaclon.

FENADIAZOLE*** (*o*-(1,3,4-oxadiazol-2-yl)-phenol; 2-(*o*-hydroxyphenyl)-1,3,4-oxadiazole; JL-512; 'hyphazol').

Fenafan (tr) *see* Phenaphan.

FENAFTIC ACID*** (1-(diethylcarbamoyl)-1,2,3,4,5,6,7,8-octahydro-6,6-dimethyl-8-oxo-3-phenyl-2-naphthoic acid).

Fenakon (tr) *see* Fenaclon.

FENALAMIDE*** (ethyl *N*-(2-diethylaminoethyl)-2-ethyl-2-phenylmalonamate; phenylethylmalonic acid monoethyl ester diethylaminoethylamide; Sch-5706; 'spasmamide').

FENALCOMINE*** (α-ethyl-*p*-[2-(α-methylphenethylamino)ethoxy]benzyl alcohol; *N*-[2-[*p*-(1-hydroxypropyl)phenoxy]ethyl]-α-methylphenethylamine; fenalcomine hydrochloride; 'cordoxene').

Fenamet (tr) *see* Phenamet.

FENAMIFURIL*** (tetrahydrofurfuryl (2-carbamoylphenoxy)acetate).

Fenamin (tr) *see* Amphetamine.

FENAMIPHOS* (ethyl 3-methyl-4-(methylthio)phenyl isopropylphosphoramidate; 'nemacur P').

FENAMISAL*** (phenyl 4-aminosalicylate; phenyl-PAS; *p*-aminosalol; FR-7; 'pheny-pas-tebamin', 'tebamin', 'tebanyl').

'Fenamizol' *see* Amiphenazole.

FENAMOLE** (5-amino-1-phenyl-1H-tetrazole; AL-0559; P-463).

FENAPERONE*** (4-[3-(*p*-fluorobenzoyl)-propyl]-1-piperazinecarboxylic acid cyclohexyl ester; cyclohexyl 4-[3-(*p*-fluorobenzoyl)propyl]-1-piperazinecarboxylate; 4-[(4-cyclohexyloxycarbonyl)piperazin-1-yl]-4'-fluorobutyrophenone).

'Fenarol' *see* Hydroxyzine.

Fenasal (tr) *see* Niclosamide.

Fenasprate *see* Benorilate.

Fenastezin (tr) *see* Phenastezin.

Fenatin (tr) *see* Phenatin.

FENAZAFLOR* (phenyl 5,6-dichloro-2-(trifluoromethyl)-1H-benzimidazole-1-

carboxylate; fenoflurazole; NC-5016; 'lovozal').

FENBENDAZOLE*** (methyl 5-(phenylthio)-2-benzimidazolecarbamate; 'panacur').

FENBENICILLIN*** (6-(α-phenoxyphenylacetamido)penicillanic acid; α-phenoxybenzylpenicillin; phenbenicillin).

FENBENICILLIN POTASSIUM ('penspek').

'Fen-bridal' *see* Promethazine.

FENBUFEN* (3-(4-biphenylylcarbonyl)-propionic acid; γ-oxo(1,1'-biphenyl)-4-butanoic acid; CL-82204).

Fenbutazona *see* Phenylbutazone.

FENBUTRAZATE*** (2-(3-methyl-2-phenylmorpholino)ethyl 2-phenylbutyrate; phenbutrazate).

FENCAMFAMIN*** (N-ethyl-3-phenyl-2-norbornanamine; N-ethyl-3-phenylnorcamphanamine; fencamfamin hydrochloride; H-610; 'euvitol').

FENCARBAMIDE*** (2-diethylaminoethyl N,N-diphenylthiolocarbamate; S-(2-diethylaminoethyl) diphenylthiocarbamate; diphenylcarbamate ester of diethylaminoethanethiol; phencarbamide; Bayer-1355; Wh-3363; 'escorpal').

Fenchlorfos *see* Fenclofos.

Fenchlorophos* *see* Fenclofos.

Fenchlorphos* *see* Fenclofos.

FENCIBUTIROL** (α-ethyl-1-hydroxy-4-phenylcyclohexaneacetic acid).

FENCLEXONIUM METILSULFATE*** (1-(3-cyclohexen-1-yl-3-phenylpropyl)-1-methylpiperidinium methylsulfate; Hoe-019).

FENCLOFENAC** (o-(2,4-dichlorophenoxy)-phenylacetic acid; RX-67408).

FENCLOFOS*** (O,O-dimethyl O-(2,4,5-trichlorophenyl) phosphorothioate; fenchlorfos; fenchlorophos; fenchlorphos; phenchlorphos; Dau ET-14; Dau ET-57; ronnel; 'dermafos', 'etrolene', 'korlan', 'nankor', 'rovan', 'trolen', 'trolene', 'viozen', 'viozene').

FENCLONINE*** (DL-3-(p-chlorophenyl)-alanine; CP-10188).

FENCLORAC*** (chloro(3-chloro-4-cyclohexylphenyl)acetic acid).

FENCLOZIC ACID*** (2-(p-chlorophenyl)-thiazol-4-ylacetic acid; ICI-54450; 'myalex').

FENDILINE** (N-(3,3-diphenylpropyl)-α-methylbenzylamine; N-benzhydryl-1'-phenyldiethylamine; N-(2-benzhydrylethyl)-1-phenylethylamine; 3,3-diphenyl-N-(1-phenylethyl)-1-propylamine; N-(α-methylbenzyl)-3,3-diphenyl-1-propylamine; fendiline hydrochloride; 'sensit').

FENDIZOATE(S)** (2-[(2'-hydroxybiphenyl-4-yl)carbonyl]benzoate(s)).

FENDOSAL** (5-(4,5-dihydro-2-phenyl-3H-benz(e)indol-3-yl)salicylic acid; 3-(3-carboxy-4-hydroxyphenyl)-4,5-dihydro-2-phenyl-3H-benz(e)indole).

FENERITROL*** (pentaerythritol tetrakis-(2-phenylbutyrate)).

'Fenesina' *see* Butetamate.

Fenesterin (tr) *see* Phenesterin.

FENESTREL** (5-ethyl-6-methyl-4-phenyl-3-cyclohexene-1-carboxylic acid).

FENETHAZINE*** (10-(2-dimethylaminoethyl)phenothiazine; aethyzine; ethizine; etizin; ethysine; etisine; fenethiazine; phenethazine; phenetizin; RP-3015; SC-1627).

Fenethiazine *see* Fenethazine.

Fenethylazocine *see* Phenazocine.

Fenethylline* *see* Fenetylline.

FENETRADIL** (1-(isobutoxymethyl)-2-(4-methylpiperazin-1-yl)ethyl 2-phenylbutyrate; 1-[2-hydroxy-3-(isobutylmethoxy)propyl]-4-methylpiperazine 2-phenylbutyrate ester).

FENETYLLINE*** (7-[2-(α-methylphenethylamino)ethyl]theophylline; amfetyline; amphetyline; fenethylline hydrochloride; R-720-11; 'captagon').

FENFLURAMINE*** (2-ethylamino-1-(3-trifluoromethylphenyl)propane; N-ethyl-α-methyl-m-trifluoromethylphenethylamine; N-ethyl-m-trifluoromethylamphetamine; fenfluramine hydrochloride; phenfluoramine; AHR-965; EMPT; S-768; 'minifage', 'ponderal', 'ponderax').

FENHARMANE*** (1-benzyl-2,3,4,9-tetrahydro-1H-pyrido(3,4-b)indole; fenoharman).

'Fenhydren' *see* Phenindione.

Fenhydropyxylate *see* Fedrilate.

Fenidim (tr) *see* Fenuron.

'Fenidina' *see* Phenacetin.

'Fenidrone' *see* Oxycinchophen.

'Fenilin' *see* Phenindione.

'Fenilor' *see* Broxyquinoline with broxaldine.

FENIMIDE** (3-ethyl-2-methyl-2-phenylsuccinimide; CI-419; PM-1807).

'Fenina' *see* Phenacetin.

FENIODIUM CHLORIDE*** (bis(2,4-dichlorophenyl)iodonium chloride; chlodofen).

Feniodol *see* Pheniodol.

FENIPENTOL*** (α-butylbenzyl alcohol; 1-phenyl-1-pentanol; PC-1).

FENIPENTOL CAMPHORATE (phenylpentyl camphorate; phenylamyl camphorate; 'flubilar').

FENISOREX** ((±)-cis-7-fluoro-1-phenyl-3-isochromanmethylamine; (±)-cis-3-(aminomethyl)-7-fluoro-1-phenylisochroman).

'Fenistil' *see* Dimetindene.

FENITRON (tr) (3-hexamethylenimino-3'-nitropropiophenone; β-hexamethylenimino-m-nitropropiophenone; 2-(azacycloheptyl) ethyl m-nitrophenyl ketone; 3-hexahydroazepin-1-yl-3'-nitropropiophenone; phenitron).

FENITROOXON (dimethyl (p-nitro-m-tolyl) phosphate; 'sumioxon').

FENITROTHION* (O,O-dimethyl O-(p-nitro-m-tolyl) phosphorothioate; methylnitrophos; metathion; Bay-41831; Bayer

206

41831; EC-50; HC-8057; OMS-43; 'accothion', 'folithion', 'metathion', 'owadofos', 'sumithion').

Fenizin (tr) *see* Phenelzine.

Fenizon *see* Fenson.

Fenmedifam *see* Phenmedipham.

FENMETOZOLE** (2-(3,4-dichlorophenoxymethyl)-2-imidazoline; fenmetozole hydrochloride; DH-524).

FENMETRAMIDE*** (5-methyl-6-phenyl-3-morpholinone; McN-1075).

FENOCINOL** (2,4-dimethoxy-α-methyl-benzhydrol; 2,4-dimethoxy-α-methyl-α-phenylbenzyl alcohol; 1-(2,4-dimethoxyphenyl)-1-phenylethanol; 'pancreabil').

FENOFIBRATE** (isopropyl 2-[*p*-(*p*-chlorobenzoyl)phenoxy]-2-methyl-propionate).

FENOFIBRIC ACID*** (2-[*p*-(*p*-chloro-phenoxy)phenoxy]propionic acid).

Fenoflurazole *see* Fenazaflor.

Fenoharman *see* Fenharmane.

Fenolactina *see* Lactylphenetidin.

Fenolovo (tr) *see* Fentin hydroxide.

Fenoperidine *see* Phenoperidine.

Fenophosphon *see* Trichloronat.

Fenoprain *see* Propafenone.

FENOPROFEN ((±)-2-(3-phenoxyphenyl)-propionic acid; (±)-*m*-phenoxyhydratropic acid; 'feprona', 'nalfon').

FENOPROFEN CALCIUM ('fenopron').

'Fenopron' *see* Fenoprofen calcium.

FENOPROP* (2-(2,4,5-trichlorophenoxy)-propionic acid; 245-TP; silvex).

FENOPROP ESTER MIXTURE ('kuron').

FENOPROP POTASSIUM ('kurosal').

'Fenostil' *see* Dimetindene.

FENOTEROL*** (3,5-dihydroxy-α-(*p*-hydroxy-α-methylphenethylaminomethyl)-benzyl alcohol; 1-(3,5-dihydroxyphenyl)-1-hydroxy-2-[(*p*-hydroxyphenyl)isopropyl-amino]ethane; 3,5-dihydroxy-α-[[2-(*p*-hydroxyphenyl)-1-methylethyl]amino-methyl]benzyl alcohol; *N*-[2-(3,5-di-hydroxyphenyl)-2-hydroxyethyl]-*p*-hydroxyamphetamine; fenoterol hydro-bromide; hydroxyphenylorciprenaline; β',3',4,5'-tetrahydroxy-α-methyldiphen-ethylamine; Th-1165*a*; 'berotec', 'partusi-sten').

FENOVERINE*** (10-[(4-piperonylpiper-azin-1-yl)acetyl]phenothiazine; 1-(pheno-thiazin-10-ylmethylcarbonyl)-4-piperonyl-piperazine; phenothiazin-10-yl 4-piper-onylpiperazin-1-ylmethyl ketone).

'Fenoverm' *see* Phenothiazine.

'Fenoxazol' *see* Pemoline.

FENOXAZOLINE*** (2-(2-isopropylphen-oxymethyl)-2-imidazoline).

Fenoxazoline prednisolone compound *see* Prednazoline.

FENOXEDIL*** (2-(*p*-butoxyphenoxy)-*N*-(2,5-diethoxyphenyl)-*N*-(2-diethylamino-ethyl)acetamide; *N*-[2-(*p*-butoxyphenoxy)-acetyl]-*N*-(2,5-diethoxyphenyl)-*N'*,*N'*-diethylethylenediamine; 'suplexedil').

'Fenoxypen' *see* Penicillin V.

FENOXYPROPAZINE*** (1-(1-methyl-2-phenoxyethyl)hydrazine; phenoxy-propazine; HP-1275).

FENOXYPROPAZINE HYDROGEN MALEATE ('drazine').

FENOZOLONE*** (2-ethylamino-5-phenyl-2-oxazolin-4-one; LD-3394; 'ordinator').

FENPENTADIOL*** (2-(*p*-chlorophenyl)-4-methyl-2,4-pentanediol; Rd-292; 'tredum').

FENPERATE*** (2-piperid-1-ylethyl α-benzyl-α-hydroxyhydrocinnamate acetate (ester); 2-piperid-1-ylethyl α-ace-toxy-α-benzylhydrocinnamate).

FENPIPALONE** (5-[2-(3,6-dihydro-4-phenyl-1(2H)-pyridyl)ethyl]-3-methyl-2-oxazolidinone; 3,6-dihydro-1(2H)-[2-(3-methyl-2-oxooxazolidin-5-yl)ethyl]-4-phenylpyridine; AHR-1680).

FENPIPRAMIDE*** (2,2-diphenyl-4-piper-idinobutyramide; 2,2-diphenyl-2-(2-piperid-1-ylethyl)acetamide; 2,2-di-phenyl-4-piperid-1-ylbutyramide; α,α-di-phenyl-1-piperidinebutyramide; fenpi-pramide hydrochloride; Hö-9980; R-14; U-229; 'resantin').

FENPIPRAMIDE WITH FENPIPRANE ('efosin').

FENPIPRANE*** (1-(3,3-diphenylpropyl)-piperidine; 3,3-diphenyl-1-piperid-1-yl-propane; diphenylpiperidinopropane; fenpiprane hydrochloride; Hö-10116).
See also Fenpipramide with fenpiprane.

FENPIVERINIUM BROMIDE*** (1-(3-carbamoyl-3,3-diphenylpropyl)-1-methyl-piperidinium bromide).

'Feprona' *see* Fenoprofen.

FENPROPOREX*** (DL-3-(α-methyl-phenethylamino)propionitrile; *N*-(2-cyano-ethyl)amphetamine).

FENQUIZONE** (7-chloro-1,2,3,4-tetra-hydro-4-oxo-2-phenyl-6-quinazolinesulfon-amide; 7-chloro-1,2,3,4-tetrahydro-4-oxo-2-phenyl-6-sulfamoylquinazoline).

FENSON* (4-chlorophenyl benzenesulfonate; *p*-chlorophenyl besilate; CPBS; PCBS; PCI; PCPBS; fenizon; 'murvesco', 'nitri-cide').

FENSPIRIDE*** (8-phenethyl-1-oxa-3,8-di-azaspiro(4.5)decan-2-one; JP-428; decaspiride; 'espiran', 'pneumorel', 'viarespan').

FENSULFOTHION* (*O*,*O*-diethyl *O*-(4-methylsulfinylphenyl) phosphorothioate; DMSP; Bayer 25141; 'dasanil', 'terracur P').

'Fentanest' *see* Fentanyl.

FENTANYL*** (1-phenethyl-4-*N*-propionyl-anilinopiperidine; *N*-(1-phenethylpiperid-4-yl)propionanilide; phentanyl; R-4263; 'fentanest').

FENTANYL CITRATE (fentanyl dihydr-ogen citrate; McN-JR-4263-49; 'leptanal', 'sublimaze').
See also Droperidol with fentanyl.

'Fentazin' *see* Perphenazine.

FENTHION* (*O*,*O*-dimethyl *O*-[4-(methyl-

thio)-*m*-tolyl] phosphorothioate; Bayer
29493; Bayer S-1752; 'bayten', 'baytex',
'entex', 'lebaycid', 'mercaptophos',
'queleton', 'tiguvon').
FENTIAZAC*** (4-(*p*-chlorophenyl)-2-
phenyl-5-thiazoleacetic acid; BR-700;
'norvedan').
FENTICLOR*** (bis(5-chloro-2-hydroxy-
phenyl) sulfide; 5,5'-dichloro-2,2'-di-
hydroxydiphenyl sulfide; 2,2'-thiobis-
(4-chlorophenol); D-25; HL-1050; OMS-2;
S-7; 'novex', 'ovitrol').
FENTICLOR WITH TRIAMCINOLONE
('fentiderm').
'Fentiderm' *see* Fenticlor with triamcinolone.
FENTIN* (triphenyltin).
FENTIN ACETATE* (acetoxytriphenylstannane; 'brestan', 'brestan 66').
FENTIN CHLORIDE* (chlorotriphenylstannane; TPTC).
FENTIN HYDROXIDE* (hydroxytriphenylstannane; fenolovo; triphenylhydroxytin;
triphenyltin hydroxide; TPTH; 'du-ter').
FENTONIUM BROMIDE*** (3α-hydroxy-
8-(*p*-phenylphenacyl)-1αH,5αH-tropanium
bromide (−)-tropate; hyoscyamine (4'-
phenylphenacyl) bromide; Z-326; 'ketoscilium', 'ulcesium').
**FENTONIUM BROMIDE WITH PER-
PHENAZINE** (FZ-484; 'duo-tran').
'Fentrinol' *see* Amidefrine mesilate.
FENURON* (1,1-dimethyl-3-phenylurea;
fenidim; 'dybar').
FENURON TRICHLOROACETATE
(fenuron-TCA; 'urab').
FENYRAMIDOL*** (α-(2-pyridylamino-
methyl)benzyl alcohol; 2-(β-hydroxyphenethylamino)pyridine; β-hydroxy-*N*-pyrid-
2-ylphenethylamine; phenyramidol;
fenyramidol hydrochloride; IN-511;
MJ-505; 'analexin', 'bonapar', 'elan',
'evaspirine', 'vilexin').
**FENYRAMIDOL OXYPHENBUTAZONE
SALT** (CG-21; 'febutol').
FENYRIPOL*** (α-(2-pyrimidinylamino-
methyl)benzyl alcohol; 2-(β-hydroxyphenethylamino)pyrimidine; β-hydroxy-
N-pyrimidin-2-ylphenethylamine;
IN-836).
FEPENTOLIC ACID** (α-butyl-α-hydroxy-
4,3-cresotic acid; 4-hydroxy-3-(1-hydroxy-
pentyl)benzoic acid; α-butyl-5-carboxy-
2-hydroxybenzyl alcohol).
FEPRACET (tr) (*N*-(*p*-aminophenylacetyl)-
amphetamine; amphetamine *p*-amino-
phenylacetate; *p*-amino-*N*-(1-methyl-2-
phenylethyl)phenylacetamide; *p*-amino-
phenylacetic acid phenylisopropylamide;
phepracet; IEM-366).
FEPRAZONE** (4-(3-methyl-2-butenyl)-
1,2-diphenyl-3,5-pyrazolidinedione; 4-
prenyl-1,2-diphenyl-3,5-pyrazolidinedione;
phenylprenazone; prenazone; DA-2370;
'zepelin').
FEPROMIDE*** (3,4,5-trimethoxy-*N*-
(1-phenoxymethyl-2-pyrrolidin-1-ylethyl)-

benzamide).
FERBAM* (*S,S,S*''-tris(dimethylcarbamo-
dithioato)iron; ferric dimethyldithio-
carbamate; ferric dimethylcarbamodithio-
ate; 'ferberk', 'fermate', 'ferradow',
'fuklasin ultra', 'karbam black').
'Ferberk' *see* Ferbam.
Ferbitol (tr) *see* Iron sorbitex.
'Fergon' *see* Ferrous gluconate.
'Ferlucon' *see* Ferrous gluconate.
'Fermate' *see* Ferbam.
'Fermine' *see* Dimethyl phthalate.
'Fernasan' *see* Thiram.
'Ferradow' *see* Ferbam.
Ferric.... *See also* Iron....
Ferric chloride-phenazone compound *see*
Ferripyrine.
FERRIC (^{59}Fe) CITRATE INJECTION***
(sterile solution containing radioactive
iron, sodium citrate and sodium chloride).
Ferric cyanoferrate *see* Prussian blue.
Ferric dimethylcarbamodithioate *see*
Ferbam.
Ferric dimethyldithiocarbamate *see*
Ferbam.
Ferric ferrocyanide *see* Prussian blue.
FERRIC FRUCTOSE*** (fructose-iron
complex compound with potassium (2:1)).
Ferriclate calcium sodium* *see* Calcium
sodium ferriclate.
FERRICYANIDES (cyanoferrates (III)).
'Ferridextran' *see* Iron dextran.
'Ferrigen' *see* Dextriferron.
Ferriheme chloride *see* Hemin.
Ferriheme hydroxide *see* Hematin.
Ferriporphyrin chloride *see* Hemin.
Ferriporphyrin hydroxide *see* Hematin.
FERRIPYRINE (compound of phenazone
with ferric chloride; ferropyrine).
Ferritetraceminnatrium* *see* Sodium
feredetate.
Ferrocene *see* Dicyclopentadienyliron.
'Ferrochel' *see* Ferrocholinate.
FERROCHOLINATE*** (chelate of ferric
hydroxide with choline dihydrogen citrate;
'ferrochel', 'ferrolip').
FERROCYANIDES (cyanoferrates (II)).
FERROGLYCINE-SULFATE COMPLEX*
(iron-glycine complex; 'ferronord',
'orferon', 'plesmet').
Ferroheme *see* Heme.
'Ferrolip' *see* Ferrocholinate.
'Ferronascin' *see* Sodium dipantoylferrate.
'Ferronat' *see* Ferrous gluconate.
'Ferronicum' *see* Ferrous gluconate.
'Ferronord' *see* Ferroglycine-sulfate complex.
FERROPOLIMALER*** (maleic acid
polymer with methylvinyl ether iron
(ferrous) salt; 'tetucur').
Ferroporphyrin *see* Heme.
Ferropyrine *see* Ferripyrine.
FERROTRENINE*** (bis(*N*-ethylidene-
threoninato) hydrogen diaquoferrate (II)).
Ferrous.... *See also* Iron....
FERROUS FUMARATE ('fersamal',
'ferumat', 'fumafer').
FERROUS GLUCONATE ('epitone',

'fergon', 'ferlucon', 'ferronat', 'ferronicum', 'glistron', 'gluco-ferrum', 'iromin', 'ironate', 'irox', 'nionate').

Ferrous sodium pantoate *see* Sodium dipantoylferrate.

'Fersamal' *see* Ferrous fumarate.

'Fertodur' *see* Cyclofenil.

FERULIC ACID (4-hydroxy-3-methoxy-cinnamic acid).

o-**FERULIC ACID** (2-hydroxy-3-methoxy-cinnamic acid).

'Ferumat' *see* Ferrous fumarate.

'Fesovite' *see* Ferrous sulfate.

Fetanol (tr) *see* Etilefrene.

FETOXILATE*** (2-phenoxyethyl 1-(3-cyano-3,3-diphenylpropyl)-4-phenyl-isonipecotate; 2-phenoxyethyl 1-(3-cyano-3,3-diphenylpropyl)-4-phenylpiperidine-4-carboxylate; fetoxylate hydrochloride; 2-phenoxyethyl difenoxilate; McN-JR-13558-11; R-13558).

Fetoxylate* *see* Fetoxilate.

FEXICAINE*** (2-(*p*-butoxyphenoxy)-*N*-(*o*-methoxyphenyl)-*N*-(2-pyrrolidin-1-ylethyl)-acetamide; *N*-[2-(*p*-butoxyphenoxy)acetyl]-*N*-(2-pyrrolidin-1-ylethyl)-*o*-anisidine; *N*-[2-(*p*-butoxyphenoxy)acetyl]-*o*-methoxy-*N*-(2-pyrrolidin-1-ylethyl)aniline; 1-[2[[[2-(*p*-butoxyphenoxy)acetyl]-*o*-methoxy-phenyl]amino]ethyl]pyrrolidine).

'Feximac' *see* Bufexamac.

FEZATIONE*** (3-(*p*-methylbenzylidene-amino)-4-phenyl-4-thiazoline-2-thione).

FG-5111 *see* Melperone.

FGA *see* Flugestone acetate.

FH-049-E *see* Diphenoxylate.

FI-5631 *see* Methopromazine.

FI-5853 *see* Paromomycin.

FI-6337 *see* Metergoline.

FI-6642 *see* Metiazinic acid.

FI-6654 *see* Caroxazone.

FI-6714 *see* Nicergoline.

FI-6927 *see* Pipotiazine palmitate.

'Fibocil' *see* Aprindine.

'Fiboran' *see* Aprindine.

FIBRACILLIN** (D-6-[2-[2-(*p*-chloro-phenoxy)-2-methylpropionamido]-2-phenylacetamido]penicillanic acid).

'Fibrase' *see* Pentosan polysulfate.

FIBRINOGEN (human fibrinogen; 'fibrogen', 'parenogen').

FIBRINOLYSIN (HUMAN)** ('actase', 'thrombolysin').
See also Brinase; Plasmin.

'Fibrogen' *see* Fibrinogen.

'Ficam' *see* Bendiocarb.

'Ficoid' *see* Fluocortolone caproate.

FIGLU *see* Formiminoglutamic acid.

'Filair' *see* Terbutaline.

Filicic acid *see* Filixic acid.

Filicin *see* Filixic acid.

Filicinic acid *see* Filixic acid.

FILIPIN** (4,6,8,10,12,14,16,27-octahydroxy-3-(1-hydroxyhexyl)-17,28-dimethyloxa-cyclooctacosa-17,19,21,23,25-pentaen-2-one; 3,5,7,9,11,13,15,26,27-nonahydroxy-2-(1-hydroxyhexyl)-16-methyl-16,18,20,22,

24-octacosapentaenoic acid 1,27-lactone; NSC-3364).

FILIXIC ACID (2,2-dimethyl-1,3,5-cyclo-hexanetrione; 3,5-dihydroxy-6,6-dimethyl-2,4-cyclohexadien-1-one; filicic acid; filicin; filicinic acid).

'Filmaron' *see* Male fern.

'Filmoderm' *see* Trichloroacetic acid.

'Filon' *see* Phenmetrazine teoclate.

'Filoral' *see* Choline theophyllinate.

'Fimomed' *see* Enbucrilate.

'Finalin' *see* Benactyzine methobromide.

'Finimal' *see* Paracetamol.

'Finomed' *see* Enbucrilate.

'Finovakil' *see* Fluoroacetic acid.

'Fintozid' *see* Pasiniazid.

FIPEXIDE*** (1-(*p*-chlorophenoxyacetyl)-4-piperonylpiperazine; 'vigilor').

'Fisiogamma' *see* Oxybate sodium.

'Fisioquens' *see* Ethinylestradiol with lynestrenol.

'Fisohex' *see* Sodium octylphenoxyethyl ether sulfate.

'Fissancort' *see* Dexamethasone.

Fitios *see* Ethoate-methyl.

'Fixanol' *see* Cetylpyridinium.

FK-880 *see* Sulpiride.

FK-1320 *see* Glipizide.

FL-1039 *see* Pivmecillinam.

FL-1060 *see* Mecillinam.

'Flabellin' *see* Meticillin.

'Flac' *see* Fluoroacetic acid.

'Flagicidin' *see* Anisomycin.

'Flagyl' *see* Metronidazole.

'Flajanina' *see* Diiodotyrosine.

'Flamanil' *see* Pifoxime.

FLAMENOL** (5-methoxyresorcinol).

'Flammazin' *see* Sulfadiazine silver.

'Flanthin' *see* Calcium levulinate.

FLAVAMINE** (6-diethylaminomethyl-3-methylflavone; flavamine hydrochloride; Rec-7-0052).

FLAVAN (3,4-dihydro-2-phenyl-2H-1-benzopyran; 2-phenylchroman).

3,3′,4,4′,5,7-Flavanhexol *see* Leucocianidol.

FLAVANONE (2,3-dihydro-2-phenyl(4H)-1-benzopyran-4-one; 2-phenyl-4-chroman-one; dihydroflavone).

3,3′,4′,5,7-Flavanpentol *see* Catechol.

Flavin *see* Quercetin.

FLAVIN-ADENINE DINUCLEOTIDE (riboflavin 5′-adenosine diphosphate; isoalloxazine-adenine dinucleotide; FAD).

FLAVIN MONONUCLEOTIDE (ribo-flavin 5′-phosphate sodium salt; 'AMM', 'coflavinase', 'cytoflav', 'hyryl').

FLAVODIC ACID*** ([[(4-oxo-2-phenyl-4H-1-benzopyran-5,7-diyl)dioxy]diacetic acid; 5,7-bis(carboxymethoxy)flavone).

FLAVODIC ACID SODIUM SALT ('pericel').

'Flavomycin' *see* Bambermycin.

FLAVONE (2-phenylchromone; 2-phenyl-(4H)-1-benzopyran-4-one).

7-Flavonoxyacetic acid ethyl ester *see* Efloxate.

'Flavoquine' *see* Amodiaquine.

'Flavoteben' see Hydroxybenzylideneisoniazid.
FLAVOTINE (6-chloro-9-(1-sorbityl)iso-
alloxazine).
FLAVOVIOLET (3-hydroxy-6,7-dimethyl-
2-(ribit-1-yloxy)quinoxaline).
FLAVOXATE*** (2-piperid-1-ylethyl
3-methyl-4-oxo-2-phenyl-4H-1-benzo-
pyran-8-carboxylate; piperidinoethyl
methylflavonecarboxylate; AK-123;
DW-61; Rec 7-0040; 'urispas').
'Flavugal' see Cyclovalone.
'Flaxedil' see Gallamine triethiodide.
FLAZALONE** (p-fluorophenyl 4-(p-fluoro-
phenyl)-4-hydroxy-1-methylpiperid-3-yl
ketone; 3-(p-fluorobenzoyl)-4-(p-fluoro-
phenyl)-4-hydroxy-1-methylpiperidine;
flumefenine; R-760).
'Fleboside' see Carbazochrome with trox-
erutin.
'Flectar' see Butixirate.
FLETAZEPAM** (7-chloro-5-(o-fluoro-
phenyl)-2,3-dihydro-1-(2,2,2-trifluoro-
ethyl)-1H-1,4-benzodiazepine; Sch-15698).
'Flexartal' see Carisoprodol.
'Flexin' see Zoxazolamine.
'Flit' see Chlordane-kerosene mixture.
FLOCTAFENINE*** (2,3-dihydroxypropyl
N-(8-trifluoromethylquinolin-4-yl)anthr-
anilate; RU-15750; 'idarac').
'Flonatril' see Clorexolone.
FLOPROPIONE*** (2',4',6'-trihydroxy-
propiophenone; phloropropiophenone;
THPP; RP-13907; 'labroda', 'labrodax',
'supanate').
FLORANTYRONE*** (4-(fluoranthren-8-
yl)-4-ketobutyric acid; γ-oxo-8-fluoranthr-
enebutyric acid; SC-1674; 'zanchol').
FLOREDIL*** (4-[2-(3,5-diethoxyphenoxy)-
ethyl]morpholine; 1,3-diethoxy-5-(2-
morpholinoethoxy)benzene).
FLORENAL (tr) (9-oxofluoren-2-ylglyoxal
bisulfite compound; fluorenal).
Floretione see Fluoresone.
Florimycin (tr) see Viomycin.
'Florinef' see Fludrocortisone acetate.
'Florisil' see Magnesium trisilicate.
'Florispec' see Epicillin.
'Florocid' see Sodium fluoride.
Floropipamide see Pipamperone.
FLOROPIPETONE** (4-[4-(ethylcarbonyl)-
4-piperid-1-ylpiperid-1-yl]-4'-fluoro-
butyrophenone; R-4082).
'Floropryl' see Dyflos.
FLOVERINE** (2-(3,5-dimethoxyphenoxy)-
ethanol; 5-(2-hydroxyethyl)-1,3-di-
methoxybenzene).
FLOXACILLIN* see Flucloxacillin.
FLOXACRINE** (7-chloro-3,4-dihydro-
10-hydroxy-3-(α,α,α-trifluoro-p-tolyl)-
1,9(2H)-acridandione).
'Floxapen' see Flucloxacillin.
FLOXURIDINE*** (5-fluoro-2'-deoxy-
uridine; fluorodeoxyuridine; FUDR;
NSC-27640).
FLUACIZINE*** (10-(3-diethylaminopropio-
nyl)-2-(trifluoromethyl)phenothiazine;

2-diethylaminoethyl 2-(trifluoromethyl)-
phenothiazin-10-yl ketone; fluoracizine;
ftoracizine).
FLUALAMIDE*** (2-allyloxy-N-(2-diethyl-
aminoethyl)-α,α,α-trifluoro-p-toluamide;
2-allyloxy-N-(2-diethylaminoethyl)-4-tri-
fluoromethylbenzamide; CE-305).
FLUANISONE*** (4'-fluoro-4-[4-(o-methoxyphenyl)piperazin-1-yl]butyrophenone;
1-[3-(p-fluorobenzoyl)propyl]-4-(o-
methoxyphenyl)piperazine; fluanisone
dihydrochloride; MD-2028; R-2028;
'anti-pica', 'haloanisone', 'metorin',
'sedalande', 'solusediv').
'Fluanxol' see Flupentixol.
FLUAZACORT* (21-acetoxy-9-fluoro-11β-
hydroxy-2'-methyl-5'βH-pregna-1,4-dieno-
(17,16-d)oxazole-3,20-dione; 9-fluoro-
11β,21-dihydroxy-2'-methyl-5'βH-pregna-
1,4-dieno(17,16-d)oxazole-3,20-dione
21-acetate; L-6400; fluazacortenol; 'azacortid').
Fluazacortenol see Fluazacort.
FLUBANILATE*** (ethyl N-(2-dimethyl-
aminoethyl)-m-trifluoromethylcarbanilate-
HCl; flubanilate hydrochloride).
FLUBENDAZOLE** (methyl 5-(p-fluorobenzoyl)-2-benzylimidazolecarbamate).
Flubenisolone see Betamethasone.
FLUBEPRIDE** (N-[[1-(p-fluorobenzyl)-
pyrrolidin-2-yl]methyl]-5-sulfamoyl-o-
anisamide; 1-(p-fluorobenzyl)-2-[(2-
methoxy-5-sulfamoylbenzamido)methyl]-
pyrrolidine).
'Flubiral' see Fenipentol camphorate.
FLUCARBRIL*** (1-methyl-2-oxo-6-tri-
fluoromethylquinoline).
FLUCETOREX** (α-[[α-methyl-m-(trifluoromethyl)phenethyl]carbamoyl]-p-acet-
anisidide; N-[(p-acetamidophenoxymethyl)-
carbonyl]-α-methyl-m-trifluoromethyl-
phenethylamine; p-[[(α-methyl-m-trifluoro-
methylphenethyl)carbamoyl]methoxy]-
acetanilide).
FLUCIPRAZINE** (α-[(1-ethynylcyclo-
hexyloxy)methyl]-4-(p-fluorophenyl)-1-
piperazineethanol; 1-[3-(1-ethynylcyclo-
hexyloxy)-2-hydroxypropyl]-4-(p-fluoro-
phenylpiperazine)).
FLUCLOROLONE* (9α,11β-dichloro-6α-
fluoro-16α,17α,21-trihydroxypregna-1,4-
diene-3,20-dione; 9α,11β-dichloro-6α-
fluoropregna-1,4-diene-16α,17α, 21-triol-
3,20-dione).
FLUCLOROLONE ACETONIDE***
(fluclorolone cyclic 16,17-acetal with acetone; 9α,11β-dichloro-6α-fluoro-21-hydroxy-
16α,17α-isopropylidenedioxypregna-1,4-
diene-3,20-dione; RS-2252).
FLUCLOXACILLIN*** (6-[3-(2-chloro-6-
fluorophenyl)-5-methyl-4-isoxazolecarb-
oxamido]penicillanic acid; 3-(2-chloro-
6-fluorophenyl)-5-methyl isoxazol-4-yl-
penicillin; floxacillin; BRL-2039; 'floxapen', 'staphylex').
See also Ampicillin with flucloxacillin.
'Flucort' see Flumetasone.

210

FLUCRILATE*** (2,2,2-trifluoro-1-methyl-ethyl 2-cyanoacrylate).
FLUCYTOSINE*** (5-fluorocytosine; Ro-2-9915; 'alcobon', 'ancobon', 'ancotil').
FLUCYTOSINE ARABINOSIDE (5-fluorocytosine arabinoside; 1β-D-arabinofuranosyl-5-fluorocytosine; ara-F).
FLUCYTOSINE DEOXYRIBOSIDE (5-fluoro-2′-deoxycytidine).
FLUDAZONIUM CHLORIDE*** (1-[2,4-dichloro-β-[(2,4-dichlorobenzyl)oxy]-phenethyl]-3-(p-fluorophenacyl)imidazolium chloride).
'Fluderma' see Formocortal.
'Fludex' see Indapamide.
'Fludilat' see Bencyclane furoate.
FLUDOREX** (β-methoxy-N-methyl-m-trifluoromethylphenethylamine; WIN-11464).
'Fludrocortisate' see Fludrocortisone acetate.
FLUDROCORTISONE*** (9α-fluoro-11β,17α,21-trihydroxypregn-4-ene-3,20-dione; 9α-fluoro-pregn-4-ene-11β,17α,21-triol-3,20-dione; 9α-fluorohydrocortisone; 9α-fluorocortisol; fluohydrisone; fluohydrocortisone; fluorhydrocortisone; fluorocortisone).
FLUDROCORTISONE ACETATE* (fludrocortisone 21-acetate; STC-1400; 'alflorone', 'astinon', 'astonin', 'F-cortef', 'florinef', 'fludrocortisate', 'fludrocortone', 'fludrone', 'scherofluron').
'Fludrocortone' see Fludrocortisone acetate.
'Fludrone' see Fludrocortisone acetate.
FLUDROXYCORTIDE*** (6α-fluoro-16α,17-dihydroxycorticosterone cyclic 16,17-acetal with acetone; fluorodihydroxycorticosterone acetonide; 6α-fluoro-11β,16α,17,21-tetrahydroxypregn-4-ene-3,20-dione cyclic 16,17-acetal with acetone; 6α-fluoro-16α,17α-isopropylidenedioxypregn-4-ene-11β,21-diol-3,20-dione; 6α-fluoro-16α,17α-isopropylidenedioxyhydrocortisone; 6α-fluoro-16α-hydroxyhydrocortisone 16,17-acetonide; fluorandrenolone; flurandrenolone; flurandrenolide; L-33379; 'cordran', 'drenison', 'drocort', 'haelan', 'sermaka').
Fluenethyl see Fluenetil.
FLUENETIL* (2-fluoroethyl(1,1′-biphenyl)-4-acetate; 2-fluoroethylbiphenylylacetate; 2-fluoroethyl xenylacetate; fluenethyl; 'lambrol').
FLUFENAMIC ACID*** (N-(α,α,α-trifluoro-m-tolyl)anthranilic acid; 2-carboxy-3′-trifluoromethyldiphenylamine; CI-440; INF-1837; 'arlef').
See also Aluminium flufenamate.
Flufenamic acid glycolamide ester see Colfenamate.
Flufenazine* see Fluphenazine.
FLUFENISAL*** (4-acetoxy-4′-fluorobiphenyl-3-carboxylic acid; 4′-fluoro-4-hydroxy-3-biphenylcarboxylic acid acetate).
FLUGESTONE*** (9α-fluoropregn-4-ene-11β,17-diol-3,20-dione; 9α-fluoro-11β,17-dihydroxypregn-4-ene-3,20-dione; 9α-fluoro-11β,17α-dihydroxyprogesterone;

fluorogestone; flurogestone).
FLUGESTONE ACETATE (flugestone 17-acetate; flurogestone acetate; FGA; SC-9880; 'cronolone', 'syncro-mate').
'Fluidemin' see Bromindione.
'Fluidex' see Dextran 40.
'Fluimucil' see Acetylcysteine.
FLUINDAROL*** (2-(α,α,α-trifluoro-p-tolyl)-indan-1,3-dione).
'Fluitran' see Trichlormethiazide.
'Flukanide' see Rafoxanide.
'Flumamine' see Metformin.
'Flumazine' see Fluphenazine.
FLUMEDROXONE*** (17-hydroxy-6α-trifluoromethylprogesterone; 6α-trifluoromethylpregn-4-ene-17-ol-3,20-dione).
FLUMEDROXONE ACETATE (Wg-537; 'demigran').
Flumefenine see Flazalone.
FLUMEQUINE** (9-fluoro-6,7-dihydro-5-methyl-1-oxo-1H,5H-benzo(ij)quinolizine-2-carboxylic acid).
FLUMETASONE*** (6α,9α-difluoro-16α-methylpregna-1,4-diene-11β,17α,21-triol-3,20-dione; 6α,9α-difluoro-16α-methylprednisolone; 6α,9-difluoro-11β,17,21-trihydroxy-16α-methylpregna-1,4-diene-3,20-dione; flumethasone; RS-2177; U-10974; 'cortexilar', 'flucort').
FLUMETASONE PIVALATE (flumetasone 21-pivalate; 'locacorten', 'locorten', 'losalen').
FLUMETASONE PIVALATE WITH SALICYLIC ACID AND COAL TAR ('psocorten').
FLUMETHIAZIDE*** (6-trifluoromethyl-2H-1,2,4-benzothiadiazine-7-sulfonamide 1,1-dioxide; 7-sulfamoyl-6-trifluoromethyl-1,2,4-benzothiadiazine 1,1-dioxide; trifluoromethylthiazide; 'ademil').
FLUMETRAMIDE*** (6-(α,α,α-trifluoro-p-tolyl)-3-morpholinone; McN-1546; 'duraflex').
'Flumidin' see Moroxydine.
FLUMINOREX*** (2-amino-5-(α,α,α-trifluoro-p-tolyl)-2-oxazoline; McN-1231).
FLUMIZOLE*** (4,5-bis(p-methoxyphenyl)-2-trifluoromethylimidazole; 4,5-bis(p-anisyl)-2-trifluoromethylimidazole; CP-22665).
Flumoperon see Trifluperidol.
FLUNAMINE** (2-[bis(p-fluorophenyl)-methoxy]ethylamine; 2-(4,4′-difluorobenzhydryloxy)ethylamine).
FLUNARIZINE*** (1-[bis(p-fluorophenyl)-methyl]-4-cinnamylpiperazine; 1-cinnamyl-4-(p,p′-difluorobenzhydryl)piperazine).
FLUNIDAZOLE*** (2-(p-fluorophenyl)-5-nitroimidazole-1-ethanol; 2-(p-fluoro-phenyl)-1-(2-hydroxyethyl)-5-nitroimidazole; MK-915).
FLUNISOLIDE*** (6α-fluoropregna-1,4-diene-11β,16α,17,21-tetrol-3,20-dione cyclic 16,17-acetal with acetone; 6α-fluoro-11β,16α,17,21-tetrahydroxypregna-1,4-diene-3,20-dione acetonide).
FLUNISOLIDE ACETATE* (flunisolide

211

21-acetate; RS-1320).

FLUNITRAZEPAM*** (5-(*o*-fluorophenyl)-
1,3-dihydro-1-methyl-7-nitro-2H-1,4-benzo-
diazepin-2-one; Ro 5-4200; 'rohypnol',
'rophynal').

FLUNIXIN** (2-[(2-methyl-3-trifluoro-
methylphenyl)amino]-3-pyridinecarboxylic
acid; 2-(2-methyl-3-trifluoromethylanilino)-
nicotinic acid; 2-($\alpha^3,\alpha^3,\alpha^3$-trifluoro-2,3-
xylidino)nicotinic acid; Sch-14714).

FLUNIXIN MEGLUMINE (flunixin
methylglucamine).

'Fluobate' *see* Betamethasone benzoate.

FLUOCINOLONE (6α,9-difluoro-11β,16α,
17,21-tetrahydroxypregna-1,4-diene-
3,20-dione).

FLUOCINOLONE ACETONIDE*** (6α,9-
difluoro-11β,16α,17,21-tetrahydroxy-
pregna-1,4-diene-3,20-dione acetonide;
6α,9α-difluoropregna-1,4-diene-11β,16α,
17,21-tetrol-3,20-dione cyclic 16,17-acetal
with acetone; 6α,9α-difluoro-16α,17α-
isopropylidenedioxy-1,4-pregnadiene-
11β,21-diol-3,20-dione; 6α,9α-difluoro-16α-
hydroxyprednisolone 16,17-acetonide;
RS-1401-AT; 'dermalar', 'jellin', 'monoderm', 'sinalar', 'synalar', 'synandone').

Fluocinolone acetonide 21-acetate *see*
Fluocinonide.

FLUOCINONIDE*** (fluocinolone acetonide
21-acetate; RS-410 FAPG; 'lidex', 'metosine', 'metosyn', 'topsym', 'topsyne').

FLUOCORTIN** (6α-fluoro-11β-hydroxy-
16α-methyl-3,20-dioxopregna-1,4-dien-21-
oic acid).

FLUOCORTIN BUTYL* (butyl 6α-fluoro-
11β-hydroxy-16α-methyl-3,20-dioxo-
pregna-1,4-dien-21-oate; fluocortin butyl
ester; SH K-203).

FLUOCORTOLONE*** (6α-fluoro-16α-
methyl-1-dehydrocorticosterone; 6α-fluoro-
11β,21-dihydroxy-16α-methylpregna-1,4-
diene-3,20-dione; 6α-fluoro-16α-methyl-
pregna-1,4-diene-11β,21-diol-3,20-dione;
SH-742).

FLUOCORTOLONE CAPROATE (fluocortolone 21-hexanoate; SH-770; 'ficoid',
'ultralan').

**FLUOCORTOLONE OCTANOATE
WITH FLUOCORTOLONE PIVALATE**
('ultracur').

FLUOCORTOLONE PIVALATE (fluocortolone trimethylacetate).

Fluocortolone trimethylacetate *see*
Fluocortolone pivalate.

Fluohydrisone *see* Fludrocortisone.

Fluohydrocortisone *see* Fludrocortisone.

FLUOMETURON* (1,1-dimethyl-3-
(*m*-trifluoromethylphenyl)urea; 1,1-di-
methyl-3-(α,α,α-trifluoro-*m*-tolyl)urea;
'cotoran').

'Fluon' *see* Politef.

Fluophosphonic acid *see* Fluorophosphoric
acid.

Fluophosphoric acid *see* Fluorophosphoric
acid.

Fluopromazine* *see* Triflupromazine.

Fluoracizine *see* Fluacizine.

Fluorafur *see* Ftorafur.

'Fluorakil' *see* Fluoroacetic acid.

Fluorandrenolone *see* Fludroxycortide.

FLUORANIL (2,3,5,6-tetrafluoro-*p*-benzo-
quinone).

4-(Fluoranthren-8-yl)-4-ketobutyric acid
see Florantyrone.

FLUORBENSIDE* (1-[(*p*-chlorobenzyl)-
thio]-4-fluorobenzene; 1-chloro-4-[[(4-
fluorophenyl)thio]methyl]benzene; 4-
chloro-α-[(*p*-fluorophenyl)thio]toluene;
'fluoroparacide', 'fluorosulphacide').

Fluordopan (tr) *see* Ftordopan.

Fluorenal *see* Florenal.

FLUORENE (2,2'-methylenebiphenyl; di-
phenylenemethane).

FLUOREN-2-YLACETAMIDE (*N*-fluoren-
2-ylacetamide; 2-acetamidofluorene).

**FLUORENYLACETOHYDROXAMIC
ACID** (*N*-fluoren-2-yl-*N*-hydroxyacet-
amide; *N*-hydroxy-2-acetylaminofluorene).

***N*-Fluoren-2-yl-*N*-hydroxyacetamide** *see*
Fluorenylacetohydroxamic acid.

α-Fluoren-9-ylidene-*p*-toluamidine *see*
Renytoline.

2-Fluoren-2-ylpropionic acid *see*
Cicloprofen.

FLUORESCEIN (9-(*o*-carboxyphenyl)-
6-hydroxy-3-isoxanthenone; 3',6'-di-
hydroxyfluoran; resorcinolphthalein). †

FLUORESCEIN DISODIUM SALT
(obiturin; uranin).

FLUORESCIN (reduced fluorescein;
resorcinolphthalin).

FLUORESONE** (ethyl *p*-fluorophenyl
sulfone; floretione; 'bripadon', 'caducid').

'Fluorformylon' *see* Formocortal.

Fluorhydrocortisone *see* Fludrocortisone.

FLUOROACETAMIDE (2-fluoroacetamide;
'fussol').

Fluormetolon* *see* Fluorometholone.

FLUOROACETIC ACID (2-fluoroacetic
acid (or its salts); 'finovakil', 'flac',
'fluorakil', 'fluoron', 'fluron', 'furatol',
'megatox', 'tritox', 'vitax F-15').

***N*-(2-FLUOROACETYL)-*N*-METHYL-
1-NAPHTHYLAMINE** (2-fluoro-*N*-
methyl-*N*-naphth-1-ylacetamide; *N*-
methyl-*N*-naphth-1-ylfluoroacetamide;
MNFA; 'nissol').

**5-(*p*-Fluorobenzoyl)-2-benzimidazole-
carbamic acid methyl ester** *see*
Flubendazole.

**3-(*p*-Fluorobenzoyl)-4-(*p*-fluorophenyl)-4-
hydroxy-1-methylpiperidine** *see*
Flazalone.

**1'-[3-(*p*-Fluorobenzoyl)propyl]-1,4'-
bipiperidine-4'-carboxamide** *see*
Pipamperone.

**8-[3-(*p*-Fluorobenzoyl)propyl]-1-(*p*-
fluorophenyl)-1,3,8-triazaspiro(4.5)-
decan-4-one** *see* Fluspiperone.

**2-[3-(*p*-Fluorobenzoyl)propyl]hexa-
hydropyrrolo(1,2-a)pyrazine** *see*
Azabuperone.

1-[3-(*p*-Fluorobenzoyl)propyl]-4-(*o*-

methoxyphenyl)piperazine *see*
Fluanisone.
8-[3-(*p*-Fluorobenzoyl)propyl]-2-methyl-
2,8-diazaspiro(4.5)decane-1,3-dione *see*
Roxoperone.
1-[3-(*p*-Fluorobenzoyl)propyl]-4-methyl-
piperidine *see* Melperone.
8-[3-(*p*-Fluorobenzoyl)propyl]-1-oxo-4-
phenyl-2,4,8-triazaspiro(4.5)decane *see*
Spiperone.
8-[3-(*p*-Fluorobenzoyl)propyl]-1-phenyl-
1,3,8-triazaspiro(4.5)decan-4-one *see*
Spiperone.
4-[3-(*p*-Fluorobenzoyl)propyl]-1-piper-
azinecarboxylic acid cyclohexyl ester
see Fenaperone.
1-[3-(*p*-Fluorobenzoyl)propyl]piperidine
see Primaperone.
1-[1-[3-(*p*-Fluorobenzoyl)propyl]piperid-
4-yl]-2-benzimidazolinone *see* Benperidol.
1-[3-(*p*-Fluorobenzoyl)propyl]-4-piperid-
1-ylisonipecotamide *see* Pipamperone.
1′-[3-(*p*-Fluorobenzoyl)propyl]-4′-pro-
pionyl-1,4′-bipiperidine *see* Propyperone.
1-[3-(*p*-Fluorobenzoyl)propyl]-4-pyrid-
2-ylpiperazine *see* Azaperone.
1-[3-(*p*-Fluorobenzoyl)propyl]-4-(pyrro-
lidin-1-ylcarbonyl)-4-*m*-tolylpiperidine
see Meperidide.
1-[1-[3-(*p*-Fluorobenzoyl)propyl]-1,2,3,6-
tetrahydropyrid-4-yl]-2-benzimidazol-
inone *see* Droperidol.
1-[3-(*p*-Fluorobenzoyl)propyl]-4-(*p*-tolyl)-
4-piperidinol *see* Moperone.
1-[3-(*p*-Fluorobenzoyl)propyl]-4-(*m*-tri-
fluoromethylphenyl)-4-piperidinol *see*
Trifluperidol.
1-(*p*-Fluorobenzyl)-2-[(2-methoxy-5-
sulfamoylbenzamido)methyl]pyrrol-
idine *see* Flubepride.
N-[[1-(*p*-Fluorobenzyl)pyrrolidin-2-
yl]methyl]-5-sulfamoyl-*o*-anisamide
see Flubepride.
2-(2-Fluoro-4-biphenyl)propionic acid *see*
Flurbiprofen.
2-(3′-Fluoro-4-biphenylyl)propionic acid
see Fluprofen.
4′-Fluoro-4-(4-carbamoyl-4-piperid-1-yl-
piperidino)butyrophenone *see* Pipamperone.
Fluorocortisol *see* Fludrocortisone.
Fluorocortisone *see* Fludrocortisone.
5-Fluorocytosine *see* Flucytosine.
5-Fluoro-2′-deoxycytidine *see* Fluocytosine
deoxyriboside.
5-Fluoro-2′-deoxyuridine *see* Floxuridine.
FLUORODIFEN* (2-nitro-1-(*p*-nitro-
phenoxy)-4-(trifluoromethyl)benzene;
α,α,α-trifluoro-3-nitro-4-(*p*-nitrophenoxy)-
toluene; 'preforan').
9-Fluoro-6,7-dihydro-5-methyl-1-oxo-
1H,5H-benzo(ij)quinolizine-2-carboxylic
acid *see* Flumequine.
6α-Fluoro-16α,17-dihydroxycorticosterone
acetonide *see* Fludroxycortide.
9α-Fluoro-11β,21-dihydroxy-16α,17-di-
methylpregna-1,4-diene-3,20-dione *see*
Dimesone.
9α-Fluoro-11β,21-dihydroxy-16α,17α-iso-
propylidenedioxypregna-1,4-diene-
3,20-dione *see* Triamcinolone acetonide.
9-Fluoro-11β,17α-dihydroxy-17-lactoyl-
androst-1,4-dien-3-one *see* Fluperolone.
9α-Fluoro-11β,17β-dihydroxy-17α-methyl-
androst-4-en-3-one *see* Fluoxymesterone.
9α-Fluoro-11β,17α-dihydroxy-6α-methyl-
pregna-1,4-diene-3,20-dione *see* Fluorometholone.
9α-Fluoro-11β,17α-dihydroxy-16β-methyl-
pregna-1,4-diene-3,20-dione *see* Doxibetasol.
9-Fluoro-11β,21-dihydroxy-16α-methyl-
pregna-1,4-diene-3,20-dione *see* Desoximetasone.
9-Fluoro-11β,21-dihydroxy-2′-methyl-
5′βH-pregna-1,4-dieno(17,16-d)oxazole-
3,20-dione 21-acetate *see* Fluazacort.
9-Fluoro-11β,17-dihydroxypregn-4-ene-
3,20-dione *see* Flugestone.
9α-Fluoro-11β,17α-dihydroxyprogesterone
see Flugestone.
Fluorodopan *see* Ftordopan.
2-Fluoroethyl (1,1′-biphenyl)-4-acetate
see Fluenetil.
2-Fluoroethyl biphenylylacetate *see*
Fluenetil.
FLUOROETHYL DIMESILATE (2-fluoro-
ethyl di(methanesulfonate); fluoroethyl
dimesylate; CB-1522; NSC-52142).
2-Fluoroethyl di(methanesulfonate) *see*
Fluoroethyl dimesilate.
2-Fluoroethyl xenylacetate *see* Fluenetil.
'Fluorofen' *see* Triflupromazine.
4′-Fluoro-4-[4-(*p*-fluorobenzoyl)piperid-1-
yl]butyrophenone *see* Lenperone.
FLUOROFORM (trifluoromethane;
'genetron-23').
Fluoroformylon *see* Formocortal.
5-Fluoro-1-(2-furanidyl)uracil *see* Ftorafur.
Fluorogestone* *see* Flugestone.
4′-Fluoro-4-(hexahydropyrrolo(1,2-a)-
pyrazin-2(1H)yl)-butyrophenone *see*
Azabuperone.
4′-Fluoro-4-hydroxy-3-biphenylcarboxylic
acid acetate *see* Flufenisal.
6-Fluoro-9-[3-[4-(2-hydroxyethyl)-
piperazin-1-yl]propyl]-2-(trifluoromethyl)thioxanthene *see* Teflutixol.
6-Fluoro-9-[3-[4-(2-hydroxyethyl)piperid-
1-yl]propylidene]-2-(trifluoromethyl)-
thioxanthene *see* Piflutixol.
6α-Fluoro-16α-hydroxyhydrocortisone
acetonide *see* Fludroxycortide.
6α-Fluoro-11β-hydroxy-16α-methyl-3,20-
dioxopregna-1,4-dien-21-oic acid *see*
Fluocortin.
6α-Fluoro-11β-hydroxy-16α-methyl-3,20-
dioxopregna-1,4-dien-21-oic acid butyl
ester *see* Fluocortin butyl.
9α-Fluoro-11β-hydroxy-17α-methyl-
testosterone *see* Fluoxymesterone.
4′-Fluoro-4-(4-hydroxypiperid-1-yl)-
butyrophenone isopropylcarbamate
see Carperone.

213

9α-Fluoro-16α-hydroxyprednisolone *see*
Triamcinolone.
4'-Fluoro-4-(4-hydroxy-4-*p*-tolylpiperid-1-yl)butyrophenone *see* Moperone.
4'-Fluoro-4-[4-hydroxy-4-(*m*-trifluoromethylphenyl)piperid-1-yl]butyrophenone *see* Trifluperidol.
4'-Fluoro-4-[4-hydroxy-4-(α,α,α-trifluoro-*m*-tolyl)piperid-1-yl]butyrophenone *see*
Trifluperidol.
5-Fluoro-*N*-(2-imidazolin-2-yl)-*o*-toluidine
see Flutonidine.
6α-Fluoro-16,17α-isopropylidenedioxy-pregn-4-ene-11β,21-diol-3,20-dione *see*
Fludroxycortide.
9-Fluoro-17-lactoylandrosta-1,4-diene-11β,17α-diol-3-one *see* Fluperolone.
'Fluoromar' *see* Fluroxene.
FLUOROMETHOLONE*** (9α-fluoro-6α-methyl-1,4-pregnadiene-11β,17α-diol-3,20-dione; 9α-fluoro-11β,17α-dihydroxy-6α-methylpregna-1,4-diene-3,20-dione; 21-desoxy-9α-fluoro-6α-methylprednisolone; fluormetolon; 'delmeson', 'oxylone').
FLUOROMETHOLONE ACETATE
(fluorometholone 17-acetate; NSC-47438; U-17323).
N-**(5-Fluoro-2-methoxy-α-methylbenzyl)-2-[*p*-[(5-isobutylpyrimidin-2-yl)-sulfamoyl]phenyl]acetamide** *see*
Gliflumide.
4'-Fluoro-4-[4-(*o*-methoxyphenyl)piper-azin-1-yl]butyrophenone *see* Fluanisone.
2-Fluoro-α-methylbiphenyl-4-acetic acid
see Flurbiprofen.
6α-Fluoro-16α-methyl-1,2-dehydrocorti-costerone *see* Fluocortolone.
9α-Fluoro-16α-methyl-17-deoxypredni-solone *see* Desoximetasone.
9α-Fluoro-6α-methyl-21-desoxypredni-solone *see* Fluorometholone.
α-FLUOROMETHYL-3,4-DIHYDROXY-BENZYL ALCOHOL (fluorarterenol).
4'-Fluoro-3-(2-methyl-1,3-dioxo-2,8-diazaspiro(4.5)dec-8-yl)butyrophenone
see Roxoperone.
9-Fluoro-16-methyleneprednisolone *see*
Fluprednidene.
9-Fluoro-16-methylenepregna-1,4-diene-11β,17,21-triol-2,20-dione *see* Flupred-nidene.
9α-Fluoro-2-methylhydrocortisone *see*
Methylfludrocortisone.
5-Fluoro-2-methyl-1-[*p*-(methylsulfinyl)-benzylidene]indene-3-acetic acid *see*
Sulindac.
2-Fluoro-*N*-methyl-*N*-naphth-1-yl-acetamide *see* *N*-(2-Fluoroacetyl)-*N*-methyl-1-naphthylamine.
4'-Fluoro-4-(4-methylpiperid-1-yl)butyro-phenone *see* Melperone.
6α-Fluoro-16α-methylprednisolone *see*
Paramethasone.
9α-Fluoro-16α-methylprednisolone *see*
Dexamethasone.
9α-Fluoro-16β-methylprednisolone *see*
Betamethasone.

9α-Fluoro-21-methylprednisolone *see*
Fluperolone.
6α-Fluoro-16α-methylpregna-1,4-diene-11β,21-diol-3,20-dione *see* Fluocortolone.
9-Fluoro-16α-methylpregna-1,4-diene-11β,21-diol-3,20-dione *see* Desoximetasone.
9α-Fluoro-6α-methylpregna-1,4-diene-11β,17α-diol-3,20-dione *see* Fluorome-tholone.
6α-Fluoro-16α-methylpregna-1,4-diene-11β,17α,21-triol-3,20-dione *see* Para-methasone.
9α-Fluoro-16α-methylpregna-1,4-diene-11β,17α,21-triol-3,20-dione *see* Dexa-methasone.
9α-Fluoro-16β-methylpregna-1,4-diene-11β,17α,21-triol-3,20-dione *see* Beta-methasone.
9α-Fluoro-21-methylpregna-1,4-diene-11β,17α,21-triol-3,20-dione *see* Fluper-olone.
Fluoromethyl 2,2,2-(trifluoro-1-trifluoro-methyl)ethyl ether *see* Sevoflurane.
'Fluoron' *see* Fluoroacetic acid.
4'-Fluoro-4-(octahydro-4-hydroxy-1(2H)-quinolyl)butyrophenone carbanilate
see Cicarperone.
4'-Fluoro-4-[4-(2-oxobenzimidazolin-1-yl)-piperid-1-yl]butyrophenone *see*
Benperidol.
4'-Fluoro-4-[4-(2-oxobenzimidazolin-1-yl)-1,2,3,6-tetrahydropyrid-1-yl]butyro-phenone *see* Droperidol.
'Fluoroparacide' *see* Fluorbenside.
'Fluorophene' *see* Flusalan.
8-[3-(*p*-Fluorophenoxy)propyl]-1-phenyl-1,3,8-triazaspiro(4.5)decan-4-one *see*
Spiramide.
4-(*p*-Fluorophenyl)-3,6-dihydro-1(2H)-[[2-[1-(2-hydroxyethyl)-5-methyl-pyrazol-4-yl]carbonyl]ethyl]pyridine
see Flupranone.
5-(*o*-Fluorophenyl)-1,3-dihydro-1-methyl-7-nitro-2H-1,4-benzodiazepin-2-one *see*
Flunitrazepam.
4-(*p*-Fluorophenyl)-3,6-dihydropyrid-1(2H)-yl 1-(2-hydroxyethyl)-5-methyl-pyrazol-4-yl ketone *see* Flupranone.
3-[4-(*p*-Fluorophenyl)-3,6-dihydro-1(2H)-pyridyl]-1-[1-(2-hydroxyethyl)-5-methylpyrazol-4-yl]-1-propanone *see*
Flupranone.
4-[3-[4-(*p*-Fluorophenyl)-3,6-dihydropyrid-1(2H)yl]propionyl]-1-(2-hydroxyethyl)-5-methylpyrazole *see* Flupranone.
4-(*o*-Fluorophenyl)-6,8-dihydro-1,2,8-tri-methylpyrazolo(3,4-e)(1,4)diazepin-7(1H)-one *see* Zolazepam.
***p*-Fluorophenyl 4-(*p*-fluorophenyl)-4-hydroxy-1-methylpiperid-3-yl ketone**
see Flazalone.
2-(*p*-Fluorophenyl)-1-(2-hydroxyethyl)-5-nitroimidazole *see* Flunidazole.
7-Fluoro-1-phenylisochroman-3-yl-methylamine *see* Fenisorex.
α-(*p*-Fluorophenyl)-4-(*o*-methoxyphenyl)-1-piperazinebutanol *see* Anisopirol.

2-(*p*-Fluorophenyl)-5-nitroimidazole-1-ethanol *see* Flunidazole.

1-[1-[4-(*p*-Fluorophenyl)-4-oxobutyl]-1,2,3,6-tetrahydropyrid-4-yl]-2-benzimidazolinone *see* Droperidol.

4′-Fluoro-4-(4-phenylpiperazin-1-yl)-butyrophenone *see* Butyropipazone.

N-[3-[4-(*p*-Fluorophenyl)piperazin-1-yl]-1-methylpropyl]nicotinamide *see* Niaprazine.

2′-(*p*-Fluorophenyl)-2′H-17α-pregna-2,4-dien-20-yno(3,2-c)pyrazol-17-ol *see* Nivacortol.

4′-Fluoro-4-piperid-1-ylbutyrophenone *see* Primaperone.

4′-Fluoro-4-(4-piperid-1-yl-4-propionyl-piperid-1-yl)butyrophenone *see* Propyperone.

'Fluoroplex' *see* Fluorouracil.

6α-Fluoroprednisolone *see* Fluprednisolone.

9α-Fluoropregna-1,4-diene-11β,16α,17α,21-tetrol-3,20-dione *see* Triamcinolone.

6α-Fluoropregna-1,4-diene-11β,16α,17,21-tetrol-3,20-dione acetonide *see* Flunisolide.

6α-Fluoropregna-1,4-diene-11β,17α,21-triol-3,20-dione *see* Fluprednisolone.

9-Fluoropregna-1,4-diene-11β,16α,17-triol-3,20-dione *see* Descinolone.

9-Fluoro-5α-pregnane-11β,16α,17,21-tetrol-3,20-dione cyclic 16,17-acetal with acetone *see* Drocinonide.

9-Fluoropregn-4-ene-11β,17-diol-3,20-dione *see* Flugestone.

6α-Fluoropregn-4-ene-11β,16α,17α,21-tetrol-3,20-dione acetonide *see* Fludroxycortide.

4′-Fluoro-4-(4-pyrid-2-ylpiperazin-1-yl)-butyrophenone *see* Azaperone.

5-FLUORO-4-PYRIMIDINOL ('fluoxydin').

4′-Fluoro-4-(4-pyrrolidinamido-4-*m*-tolylpiperid-1-yl)butyrophenone *see* Meperidide.

Fluorosalan* *see* Flusalan.

4′-Fluoro-4-[spiro(5-oxo-3-phenylimidazolidin-4,4′-piperidin)-1′-yl]butyrophenone *see* Spiperone.

'Fluorosulphacide' *see* Fluorbenside.

5-Fluoro-1-(tetrahydro-2-furyl)uracil *see* Ftorafur.

9-Fluoro-11β,16α,17,21-tetrahydroxypregna-1,4-diene-3,20-dione *see* Triamcinolone.

9-Fluoro-11β,16α,17,21-tetrahydroxy-5α-pregnane-3,20-dione cyclic 16,17-acetal with acetone *see* Drocinonide.

6α-Fluoro-11β,16,17,21-tetrahydroxypregn-4-ene-3,20-dione cyclic 16,17-acetal with acetone *see* Fludroxycortide.

2-(5-Fluoro-*o*-toluidino)-2-imidazoline *see* Flutonidine.

1-[3-[6-Fluoro-2-(trifluoromethyl)thioxanthen-9-ylidene]propyl]-4-piperidineethanol *see* Piflutixol.

4-[3-[6-Fluoro-2-(trifluoromethyl)thioxanthen-9-yl]propyl]-1-piperazineethanol *see* Teflutixol.

9-Fluoro-11β,17,21-trihydroxy-16-methylenepregna-1,4-diene-3,20-dione *see* Fluprednidene.

6α-Fluoro-11β,15,21-trihydroxy-16α-methylpregna-1,4-diene-3,20-dione *see* Paramethasone.

9α-Fluoro-11β,17,21-trihydroxy-16β-methylpregna-1,4-diene-3,20-dione *see* Betamethasone.

6α-Fluoro-11β,17,21-trihydroxypregna-1,4-diene-3,20 dione *see* Fluprednisolone.

FLUOROURACIL*** (5-fluorouracil; 5-FU; fluracil; NSC-19893; Ro-2-9757; 'efudix', 'fluoroplex', 'fluril').

Fluoroxene *see* Fluroxene.

2-(3′-Fluoroxenyl)propionic acid *see* Fluprofen.

'Fluosterone' *see* Fluoxymesterone.

Fluostigmine* *see* Dyflos.

'Fluotestin' *see* Fluoxymesterone.

'Fluothane' *see* Halothane.

FLUOXETINE** ((±)-*N*-methyl-3-phenyl-3-[(α,α,α-trifluoro-*p*-tolyl)oxy]propylamine; (±)-α,α,α-trifluoro-*p*-[3-(methylamino)1-phenylpropoxy]toluene; *N*-methyl-3-phenyl-3-[*p*-(trifluoromethyl)phenoxy]propylamine; L-110140).

'Fluoxydin' *see* 5-Fluoro-4-pyrimidinol.

FLUOXYMESTERONE*** (9α-fluoro-17α-methyl-4-androstene-11β,17β-diol-3-one; 9α-fluoro-11β,17β-dihydroxy-17α-methylandrost-4-en-3-one; 9α-fluoro-11β-hydroxy-17α-methyltestosterone; NSC-12165; 'fluosterone', 'fluostestin', 'halotestin', 'oratestryl', 'ultandren').

Fluoxyprednisolone *see* Triamcinolone.

Flupenthixol *see* Flupentixol.

FLUPENTIXOL*** (9-[3-[4-(2-hydroxyethyl)piperazin-1-yl]propylidene]-2-(trifluoromethyl)thioxanthene; flupenthixol; 'emergil', 'fluanxol').

FLUPENTIXOL DECANOATE ('depixol').

FLUPENTIXOL WITH MELITRACEN ('deanxit').

FLUPERAMIDE*** (4-(4-chloro-α,α,α-trifluoro-*m*-tolyl)-4-hydroxy-*N*,*N*-dimethyl-α,α-diphenyl-1-piperidinebutyramide; 4-(4-chloro-3-trifluoromethylphenyl)-4-hydroxy-piperid-1-yl)-*N*,*N*-dimethyl-2,2-diphenylbutyramide; R-18910).

FLUPEROLONE*** (9α-fluoro-21-methylprednisolone; 9α-fluoro-21-methylpregna-1,4-diene-11β,17,21-triol-3,20-dione; 9-fluoro-11β,17α-dihydroxy-17-lactoylandrosta-1,4-dien-3-one).

FLUPEROLONE ACETATE (fluperolone 17-acetate; P-1742; 'alacortril', 'methral').

FLUPHENAZINE*** (10-[3-[4-(2-hydroxyethyl)piperazin-1-yl]propyl]-2-trifluoromethylphenothiazine; flufenazine; 4-[3-(2-trifluoromethylphenothiazin-10-yl)propyl]-1-piperazineethanol; fluphenazine dihydrochloride; 'anatensol', 'antasol', 'lyogen', 'lyorodin', 'moditen', 'omca', 'pacinol', 'permitil', 'prolixin', 'sevinal', 'sevinol', 'siqualone', 'siquoline', 'tensofin', 'trancin', 'vespazin').

FLUPHENAZINE DECANOATE ('dapotum D', 'lyogen', 'modecate').

FLUPHENAZINE ENANTATE (fluphenazine heptanoate; fluphenazine enanthate; 'dapotum').

Fluphenazine heptanoate see Fluphenazine enantate.

FLUPHENAZINE WITH NORTRIPTYLINE ('motipress', 'motival').

FLUPIMAZINE** (2-[[1-[3-[2-(trifluoromethyl)phenothiazin-10-yl]propyl]piperid-4-yl]oxy]ethanol; 10-[3-[4-(2-hydroxyethoxy)piperid-1-yl]propyl]-2-(trifluoromethyl)phenothiazine; 4-(2-hydroxyethoxy)-1-[3-[2-(trifluoromethyl)phenothiazin-10-yl]propyl]piperidine).

FLUPIRTINE** (ethyl 2-amino-6-[(p-fluorobenzyl)amino]-3-pyridinecarbamate).

FLUPRANONE*** (3-[4-(p-fluorophenyl)-3,6-dihydro-1(2H)-pyridyl]-1-[1-(2-hydroxyethyl)-5-methylpyrazol-4-yl]-1-propanone; 4-[3-[4-(p-fluorophenyl)-3,6-dihydropyrid-1(2H)-yl]propionyl]-1-(2-hydroxyethyl)-5-methylpyrazole; 4-(p-fluorophenyl)-3,6-dihydro-1(2H)-[[2-[1-(2-hydroxyethyl)-5-methylpyrazol-4-yl]carbonyl]ethyl]pyridine; 4-(p-fluorophenyl)-3,6-dihydropyrid-1(2H)-yl 1-(2-hydroxyethyl)-5-methylpyrazol-4-yl ketone).

FLUPREDNIDENE** (9-fluoro-11β,17,21-trihydroxy-16-methylenepregna-1,4-diene-3,20-dione; 9-fluoro-16-methylenepregna-1,4-diene-11β,17,21-triol-3,20-dione; 9-fluoro-16-methyleneprednisolone; fluprednylidene; fluprednilidene).

FLUPREDNIDENE ACETATE (fluprednidene 21-acetate; StC-1106; 'corticoderm', 'decoderm', 'etacortin').

Fluprednilidene see Fluprednidene.

FLUPREDNISOLONE*** (6α-fluoroprednisolone; 6α-fluoropregna-1,4-diene-3,20-dione-11β,17α,21-triol; 6α-fluoro-11β,17α, 21-trihydroxypregna-1,4-diene-3,20-dione; U-7800).

FLUPREDNISOLONE ACETATE ('alphadrol').

Fluprednylidene see Fluprednidene.

FLUPROFEN*** (2-(3'-fluoro-4-biphenylyl)-propionic acid; 2-(3'-fluoroxenyl)propionic acid; RD-17435).

FLUPROSTENOL*** ((±)-Z-[(1R*,2R*, 3R*,5S*)-3,5-dihydroxy-2-[(E)-(3R*)-3-hydroxy-4-[(α,α,α-trifluoro-m-tolyl)oxy]-1-butenyl]cyclopentyl]-5-heptenoic acid).

Fluracil* see Fluorouracil.

Flurandrenolide* see Fludroxycortide.

Flurandrenolone* see Fludroxycortide.

FLURANTEL*** (2,6-dihydroxy-3-nitro-3',5'-bis(trifluoromethyl)benzanilide diacetate (ester)).

FLURAZEPAM*** (7-chloro-1-(2-diethylaminoethyl)-5-(o-fluorophenyl)-1,3-dihydro-2H-1,4-benzodiazepin-2-one; ID-480; Ro 5-6901; 'dalmadorm', 'dalmane', 'dormodor').

FLURBIPROFEN*** (2-(2-fluoro-4-biphenylyl)propionic acid; 2-fluoro-α-methylbiphenyl-4-acetic acid; BTS-18322).

Flurecol see Flurenol.

FLURENOL* (9-hydroxy-9H-fluorene-9-carboxylic acid; flurecol).

FLURENOL-BUTYL (butyl 9-hydroxy-9H-fluorene-9-carboxylate; 'aniten').

'Fluril' see Fluorouracil.

'Fluron' see Fluoroacetic acid.

Flurogestone see Flugestone.

Flurothyl* see Flurotyl.

FLUROTYL** (bis(2,2,2-trifluoroethyl) ether; hexafluorodiethyl ether; HFE; fluorothyl; SK&F-6539; 'indokolon').

Flurotyl isomer see Hexafluoroisopropyl methyl ether.

FLUROXENE** (2,2,2-trifluoroethylvinyl ether; fluoroxene; 'fluoromar').

FLUSALAN*** (3,5-dibromo-α,α,α-trifluoro-m-salicylotoluidide; 3,5-dibromo-3'-trifluoromethylsalicylanilide; fluorosalan; 'fluorophene').

FLUSPIPERONE** (8-[3-(p-fluorobenzoyl)-propyl]-1-(p-fluorophenyl)-1,3,8-triazaspiro(4.5)decan-4-one).

FLUSPIRILENE*** (8-[4,4-bis(p-fluorophenyl)butyl]-1-phenyl-1,3,8-triazaspiro-(4.5)decan-4-one; spirodiflamine; R-6218; 'imap', 'redeptin').

FLUTAMIDE*** (α,α,α-trifluoro-2-methyl-4'-nitro-m-propionotoluamide; 4'-nitro-3'-(trifluoromethyl)isobutyranilide; 2-methyl-4'-nitro-3'-(trifluoromethyl)propionanilide; Sch-13521).

FLUTAZOLAM*** (10-chloro-11b-(o-fluorophenyl)-2,3,7,11b-tetrahydro-7-(2-hydroxyethyl)oxazolo(3,2-d)(1,4)benzodiazepin-6(5H)-one).

FLUTIAZIN*** (8-trifluoromethylphenothiazine-1-carboxylic acid; SK&F-22908).

FLUTIZENOL*** (4-[3-(6-trifluoromethyl-4H-thieno(2,3-b)(1,4)benzothiazin-4-yl)propyl]-1-piperazineethanol; 4-[3-[4-(2-hydroxyethyl)piperazin-1-yl]propyl]-6-(trifluoromethyl)-4H-thieno(2,3-b)(1,4)-benzothiazine).

FLUTONIDINE** (2-(5-fluoro-o-toluidino)-2-imidazoline; 5-fluoro-N-(2-imidazolin-2-yl)-o-toluidine).

'Flutra' see Trichlormethiazide.

FLUVOMYCIN (polypeptide antibiotic from Bac. subtilis; 'efsiomycin', 'riomycin', 'vivicil').

FLUVOXAMINE** (5-methoxy-4'-(trifluoromethyl)valerophenone (E)-O-(2-aminoethyl)oxime).

'Fobex' see Benactyzine.

'Focusan' see Tolnaftate.

Folacin see Folic acid.

'Folbex' see Chlorobenzilate.

'Folcid' see Captafol.

216

FOLESCUTOL*** (6,7-dihydroxy-4-(morpholinomethyl)coumarin; 4-morpholinomethylesculetin; LD-2988; 'covalan').

'Folex' see Tributyl phosphorotrithioite.

FOLIC ACID*** (pteroylglutamic acid; N-[p-[(2-amino-4-hydroxy-6-pteridyl-methyl)amino]benzoyl]-L-(+)-glutamic acid; folacin; vitamin B$_c$; vitamin M; *Lactobacillus casei* factor; PGA; NSC-3073).

'Folidol E' see Parathion.

'Folidol M' see Parathion-methyl.

'Folimat' see Omethoate.

FOLINIC ACID (N^5-formyltetrahydrofolic acid).
See also Calcium folinate.

'Foliosan' see Chlorophyll.

'Folithion' see Fenitrothion.

Follicle stimulating hormone, human see Human menopausal gonadotrophin.

Follicular hormone see Estrone.

Folliculin see Estrone.

Folliculin hydrate see Estriol.

'Follinett' see Norgestrel with ethinyl-estradiol.

'Follistrel' see Levonorgestrel.

Follotropin see Human menopausal gonadotrophin.

'Folosan' see Tecnazene.

FOLPET* (N-(trichloromethylthio)phthalimide; 2-(trichloromethylthio)-1H-iso-indole-1,3(2H)-dione; 'ortho-phaltan', 'phaltan').

'Folvirin' see Estradiol benzoate with testosterone isobutyrate.

FOMINOBEN*** (3'-chloro-α-[methyl-(morpholinocarbonylmethyl)amino]-o-benzotoluidide; N-[2-[(6-benzamido-2-chlorobenzyl)methylamino]acetyl]-morpholine; clobenmetamide; PB-89; 'noleptan').
See also Bromhexine with fominoben.

FOMOCAINE** (4-[3-(4-phenoxymethyl-phenyl)propyl]morpholine; 4-(3-morpho linopropyl)benzyl phenyl ether; P-652; 'erbocain', 'panacaine').

Fonazine* see Dimetotiazine.

'Fonderma' see Pyrithione sodium.

'Fonlipol' see Tiadenol.

FONOPHOS* (O-ethyl S-phenyl ethyl-phosphonodithioate; 'dyfonate', 'dyphonate').

'Fontamide' see Sulfathiourea.

'Fontilix' see Meticrane.

'Fonurit' see Acetazolamide.

Food blue 3 see Sulfan blue.

Food red 1 see Ponceau SX.

FOPIRTOLINE*** (4-[2-(6-chloropyrid-2-ylthio)ethyl]morpholine; 2-chloro-6-(2-morpholinoethylthio)pyridine).

'Foralamin' see Methafurylene.

'Forane' see Isoflurane.

'Forapin' see Bee venom.

'Fordonal' see Thiazolinobutazone.

'Forenol' see Niflumic acid.

'Forhistal' see Dimetindene.

'Forit' see Oxypertine.

Formal see Methylal.

FORMALDEHYDE (formalin; formol; methanal; methyl aldehyde; oxomethane; oxymethylene; methylene oxide).

Formaldehydeacetamide see Formicin.

Formaldehydeaniline see Formaniline.

Formalin see Formaldehyde.

FORMAMIDE (methenamide).

FORMAMIDE OXIME (isouretin; isuretin).

FORMAMIDINE (methanimidamide).

Formamine see Methenamine.

'Formamint' see Paraformaldehyde.

Formamol see Methenamine anhydromethyl-enecitrate.

FORMANILIDE (N-phenylformamide).

FORMANILINE (formaldehydeaniline).

'Formanol' see Methenamine anhydro-methylenecitrate.

FORMEBOLONE** (11α,17β-dihydroxy-17-methyl-3-oxoandrosta-1,4-diene-2-carbox-aldehyde; 2-formyl-11α,17β-dihydroxy-17α-methylandrosta-1,4-dien-3-one; 2-formyl-17α-methylandrosta-1,4-diene-11α,17β-diol-3-one; formyldienolone; 'esiclene').

FORMETANATE* (N,N-dimethyl-N'-[3-(methylcarbamoyloxy)phenyl]forma-midine; N,N-dimethyl-N'-[3-[[(methyl-amino)carbonyl]oxy]phenyl]methanimid-amide; 'carzol', 'dicarzol').
See also Chlorphenamidine with formetanate.

FORMETOREX*** (N-(α-methylphenethyl)-formamide; N-formyl-α-methylphenethyl-amine).

FORMIC ACID (aminic acid).

FORMICIN (formaldehydeacetamide; methylalacetamide).

'Formiloxine' see Gitoformate.

FORMIMINOGLUTAMIC ACID (N-formimidoylglutamic acid; FIGLU).

Formin see Methenamine.

FORMINITRAZOLE*** (2-formamido-5-nitrothiazole; BW-291C51; 'aroxine').

'Forminitrol' see Paraformaldehyde.

'Formitrol' see Paraformaldehyde.

FORMOCORTAL*** (21-acetoxy-3-(2-chloroethoxy)-9α-fluoro-6-formyl-11β-hydroxy-16α,17α-isopropylidenedioxy-pregna-3,5-dien-20-one; 3-(2-chloro-ethoxy)-9α-fluoro-6-formyl-11β,21-di-hydroxy-16α,17α-isopropylidenedioxy-pregna-3,5-dien-20-one 21-acetate; 3-(2-chloroethoxy)-9α-fluoro-11β,16α,17α,21-tetrahydroxy-20-oxo-3,5-pregnadiene-6-carboxaldehyde cyclic 16,17-acetal with acetone 21-acetate; 3-(2-chloroethoxy)-9α-fluoro-6-formyl-3,5-pregnadiene-11β,16α,17α,21-tetrol-20-one 16α,17α-acetonide 21-acetate; fluoroformylon; 'deflamene', 'fluderma', 'fluorformylon').

Formoguanamine see 2,4-Diamino s-triazine.

Formol see Formaldehyde solution.

FORMONETIN (7-hydroxy-4'-methoxyiso-flavone; formononetin; ononein).

Formononetin see Formonetin.

FORMOTHION* (S-(N-formyl-N-methyl-carbamoylmethyl) O,O-dimethyl phos-phorodithioate; S-(2-formylmethylamino)-2-oxoethyl O,O-dimethyl phosphorodithioate; isoformothion; 'anfix', 'anthio', 'antio').

FORMYCIN A (7-amino-3-(β-D-ribofuranosyl)pyrazolo(4,3-d)pyrimidine).

FORMYCIN B (7-hydroxy-3-(β-D-ribofuranosyl)pyrazolo(4,3-d)pyrimidine; larusin).

4'-Formylacetanilide thiosemicarbazone see Thiacetazone.

16-Formylacetylgitoxin see Acetylgitaloxin.

o-**Formylbenzoic acid** see Phthalaldehydic acid.

p-**Formylbenzoic acid** see Benzaldehyde-4-carboxylic acid.

Formyldienolone see Formebolone.

2-Formyl-11α,17β-dihydroxy-17α-methylandrosta-1,4-dien-3-one see Formebolone.

Formylformic acid see Glyoxylic acid.

16-Formylgitoxigenin see Gitaloxigenin.

16-Formylgitoxin see Gitaloxin.

4-Formyl-3-hydroxy-5-hydroxymethyl-2-methylpyridine see Pyridoxal.

FORMYLMELPHALAN (N-formylmelphalan; L-3-[p-[bis(2-chloroethyl)amino]-phenyl]-N-formylalanine; N-formyl-L-sarcolysin; CB-3208; NSC-37024).

Formylmerphalan see Formylsarcolysin.

S-(**2-Formylmethylamino)-2-oxoethyl O,O-dimethyl phosphorodithioate** see Formothion.

2-Formyl-17α-methylandrosta-1,4-diene-11α,17β-diol-3-one see Formebolone.

S-(**N-Formyl-N-methylcarbamoylmethyl) O,O-dimethyl phosphorodithioate** see Formothion.

7-(Formylmethyl)-4,10-dihydroxy-5-methoxy-9,16-dimethyl-2-oxooxacyclohexadeca-11,13-dien-6-yl 3,6-dideoxy-4-O-(2,6-dideoxy-3-C-methyl-α-L-ribo-hexopyranosyl)-3-dimethylamino-β-D-glucopyranoside 4,4''-dipropionate see Midecamycin.

10-(Formylmethyl)-7,13-dihydroxy-8-methoxy-3,12-dimethyl-5-oxo-4,17-dioxabicyclo(14.1.0)heptadec-14-en-9-yl 3,6-dideoxy-4-O-(2,6-dideoxy-3-C-methyl-α-L-ribo-hexopyranosyl)-3-dimethylamino-β-D-glucopyranoside 4'',7'-dipropionate (ester) see Maridomycin.

N-Formyl-α-methylphenethylamine see Formetorex.

2-Formyl-1-methylpyridinium iodide oxime see Pralidoxime.

o-**Formylphenoxyacetic acid isonicotinoylhydrazone** see Aconiazide.

18-Formyl-4-pregnen-11β,21-diol-3,20-dione see Aldosterone.

2-Formylpyridine see Picolinaldehyde.

FORMYLSARCOLYSIN (DL-3-[p-[bis-(2-chloroethyl)amino]phenyl]-N-formylalanine; N-formylmerphalan; MP-506; NSC-39274).
See also Formylmelphalan.

Formyl terchloride see Chloroform.

N⁵-Formyltetrahydrofolic acid see Folinic acid.

5-Formyl-2-thiophenecarbonitrile thio-

semicarbazone see Citenazone.

5-Formyl-4,6,8-trihydroxy-1-(methoxycarbonyl)phenazine see Lomofungin.

'Forstan' see Chinomethionat.

'Fortal' see Pentazocine.

'Fortalgesic' see Pentazocine.

'Fortasept' see Lauralkonium.

'Fortecortin' see Dexamethasone.

'Forthane' see Dimethylamylamine.

'Fortivenat' see Chymotrypsin with trypsin.

'Fortombrine' see Sodium acetrizoate.

'Fortombrine M' see Meglumine acetrizoate.

'Fortral' see Pentazocine.

'Fortralin' see Pentazocine.

'Fortrol' see Cyanazine.

Fosarbin see Pyrophos.

FOSAZEPAM*** ((7-chloro-1,3-dihydro-2-oxo-5-phenyl-2H-1,4-benzodiazepin-1-ylmethyl)dimethylphosphine oxide; 7-chloro-1-[(dimethylphosphinyl)methyl]-1,3-dihydro-5-phenyl-2H-1,4-benzodiazepin-2-one; HR-930).

'Foschlor' see Metrifonate.

FOSCOLIC ACID*** (2,2'-phosphinicodilactic acid).

Fosfakol see Paraoxon.

Fosfamid (tr) see Dimethoate.

'Fosferno' see Parathion.

FOSFESTROL*** (trans-α,α'-diethyl-4,4'-stilbenediol bis(dihydrogen phosphate); stilbestrol diphosphate; diethylstilbestrol phosphate; NSC-10481; ST-52; 'cytonal', 'honvan', 'khonvan', 'phosphoestrol', 'stilphostrol').

FOSFOMYCIN** ((−)(1R,2S)-1,2-epoxypropylphosphonic acid; phosphonomycin).

FOSFONET SODIUM** (phosphonoacetic acid disodium salt monohydrate).

'Fosfothion' see Malathion.

'Fosgran' see Metrifonate.

'Fosgren' see Metrifonate.

FOSPIRATE*** (dimethyl (3,5,6-trichloropyrid-2-yl) phosphate; 'torelle').

'Fossyol' see Metronidazole.

'Fostion' see Prothoate.

'Fostion MM' see Dimethoate.

'Fouadin' see Stibophen.

'Fovane' see Benzthiazide.

'Foxalin' see Digitoxin.

Fox green see Indocyanine green.

'Foy' see Gabexate mesilate.

FPL-670 see Disodium cromoglicate.

FR-7 see Fenamisal.

FR-33 see Roxoperone.

'Fragivix' see Benzarone.

FRAMYCETIN* (neomycin B; streptothricin B-II; EF-185; 'actilin', 'enterfram', 'framygen', 'soframycin').

Framycin (tr) see Neomycin.

'Framygen' see Framycetin.

'Francaine' see Procaine teoclate.

FRANGULA-EMODIN (1,3,8-trihydroxy-6-methylanthraquinone; frangulahaemodin; rheum; 'emodella').

FRANGULIN (frangula-emodin rhamnoside; franguloside; avorin; rhamnoxanthin).

Franguloside see Frangulin.

218

'Fraustan' see Diazepam.
'Frekentine' see Amfepramone.
'Frenactyl' see Benperidol.
'Frenemo' see Calcium polygalacturonate.
'Frenodosa' see Amyl nitrite.
'Frenolon' see Metofenazate.
'Frenolyse' see Tranexamic acid.
'Frenquel' see Azacyclonol.
FRENTIZOLE** (1-(6-methoxy-2-benzo-
  thiazolyl)-3-phenylurea; 6-methoxy-2-
  [(phenylcarbamyl)amino]benzothiazole).
'Freon 12' see Dichlorodifluoromethane.
'Freon 112' see Tetrachlorodifluoroethane.
'Freon 114' see Cryofluorane.
'Freon C-138' see Octafluorocyclobutane.
'Frescon' see Trifenmorph.
Frey inhibitor see Aprotinin.
'Frideron' see Zeranol.
'Frigen 12' see Dichlorodifluoromethane.
'Frigen 112' see Tetrachlorodifluoroethane.
'Frigen 113' see 1,1,2-Trichloro-1,2,2-tri-
  fluoroethane.
'Frigen 114' see Cryofluorane.
'Frigiderm' see Cryofluorane.
'Fringanor' see Phendimetrazine embonate.
'Fructergyl' see Ascorbic acid with disodium
  fructose 1,6-diphosphate.
Fructofuranose tetranicotinate see
  Nicofuranose.
β-D-Fructofuranoside fructohydrolase see
  Invertase.
FRUCTOSE (D-fructose; fruit sugar;
  laevulose; levulose).
FRUCTOSE 1,6-DIPHOSPHATE (Harden-
  Young ester; 'esafosfina').
  See also Calcium fructose 1,6-diphosphate.
Fructose-iron complex see Ferric fructose.
Fructose nicotinate see Nicofuranose.
FRUCTOSE 6-PHOSPHATE (hexose mono-
  phosphate; Neuberg ester).
Fructose tetranicotinate see Nicofuranose.
'Frugalan' see Furfenorex.
Fruit sugar see Fructose.
'Frumin' see Disulfoton.
Frusemide* see Furosemide.
'Frutone CPA' see Cloprop.
FT-81 see Bendroflumethiazide.
FT-207 see Ftorafur.
Ftalicetimida see Phthalylsulfacetamide.
Ftalofos (tr) see Phosmet.
FTALOFYNE*** (3-methyl-1-pentyn-3-yl
  acid phthalate; 1-ethyl-1-methyl-2-propynyl
  phthalate; methylpentynol phthalate;
  phthalofyne; 'whipicide').
FTAXILIDE*** (2',6'-dimethylphthalanilic
  acid; N-(2,6-xylyl)phthalamic acid).
F₃TDR see Trifluorothymidine.
FTIVAZIDE*** (4-hydroxy-3-methoxybenz-
  aldehyde isonicotinoylhydrazone;
  N'-vanillideneisoniazid; vanillin isonicotinoylhydrazone; isonicotinic acid vanillylidene-
  hydrazide; phthivazid; 'vanizide',
  'vanzide').
Ftoracizine (tr) see Fluacizine.
FTORAFUR (tr) (5-fluoro-1-(tetrahydro-2-
  furyl)uracil; 5-fluoro-1-(2-furanidyl)uracil;
  fluorafur; FT-207).

FTORDOPAN (tr) (5-[(2-chloroethyl)(2-
  fluoroethyl)amino]-6-methyluracil;
  fluordopan; fluorodopan).
FTORMETAZINE*** (10-[3-(4-methyl-
  piperazin-1-yl)propionyl]-2-trifluoro-
  methylphenothiazine; 2-(4-methylpiper-
  azin-1-yl)ethyl 2-trifluoromethylpheno-
  thiazin-10-yl ketone).
Ftoroplast (tr) see Politef.
Ftorotan (tr) see Halothane.
FTORPROPAZINE*** (10-[3-[4-(2-hy-
  droxyethyl)piperazin-1-yl]propionyl]-2-
  trifluoromethylphenothiazine; 2-[4-(2-
  hydroxyethyl)piperazin-1-yl]ethyl 2-tri-
  fluoromethylphenothiazin-10-yl ketone).
'Fuadin' see Stibophen.
FUBERIDAZOLE* (2-furan-2-yl-1H-
  benzimidazole; 'voronit').
FUBROGONIUM IODIDE*** (diethyl-
  (3-hydroxybutyl)methylammonium iodide
  5-bromo-2-furoate; [3-(5-bromo-2-furoyl-
  oxy)butyl]diethylmethylammonium iodide;
  fubromegan).
Fubromegan (tr) see Fubrogonium iodide.
FUCHSINE (mixture of hydrochlorides of
  pararosaniline and rosaniline; magenta;
  rosein; aniline red; 'solferino').
FUCHSINE SULFONATE (acid fuchsine;
  mixture of NH₄ or Na salts of fuchsine di-
  and trisulfonic acids).
FUCHSONE (4-benzhydrylidene-2,5-cyclo-
  hexadien-1-one).
'Fucidin' see Fusidic acid.
'Fuclasin' see Ziram.
FUDR see Floxuridine.
'Fugacillin' see Carbenicillin.
'Fugillin' see Fumagillin.
'Fugin' see under Polyoxyalkylene compounds.
'Fugipaverin' see Alverine.
'Fugoa' see Norpseudoephedrine.
'Fuklasin' see Ziram.
'Fuklasin ultra' see Ferbam.
'Fulcin' see Griseofulvin.
'Fulguran' see Dimeticone.
Fulmicoton' see Pyroxylin.
'Fulvicin' see Griseofulvin.
'Fumafer' see Ferrous fumarate.
FUMAGILLIN*** (antibiotic from Aspergillus
  fumigatus; NSC-9168; 'amebacilin',
  'amebacillin', 'fugillin', 'fumidil').
FUMAGILLIN DICYCLOHEXYLAMINE
  SALT (NSC-58368).
FUMARIA OFFICINALIS EXTRACT
  (AN-1320; 'oddibil').
FUMARIC ACID (trans-butenedioic acid;
  trans-1,2-ethylenedicarboxylic acid;
  allomaleic acid; boletic acid).
  See also Ferrous fumarate.
Fumarin see Coumafuryl.
Fumarine see Protopine.
'Fumasol' see Coumafuryl sodium.
'Fumidil' see Fumagillin.
FUMIGATIN (6-hydroxy-5-methoxy-p-
  toluquinone; 3-hydroxy-4-methoxy-2,5-
  toluquinone).
'Fumigrain' see Acrylonitrile.
'Fumite TCNB' see Tecnazene.

219

'Fundal' *see* Chlorphenamidine.
'Fundal forte' *see* Chlorphenamidine plus formetanate.
'Fungi-ban' *see* Bis(tributyltin)oxide.
Fungicidin *see* Nystatin.
'Fungifral' *see* Hedaquinium.
FUNGIMYCIN* (perimycin; NC-1968; WX-2412).
'Fungiplex' *see* Sulbentine.
'Fungitin' *see* Amphotericin B.
'Fungizone' *see* Amphotericin B.
FUNTUMIDINE (3α-aminoallopregnan-2-ol; 3α-amino-5α-pregnan-2-ol).
Furacilin *see* Nitrofural.
'Furacin' *see* Nitrofural.
FURACRINIC ACID*** (6-methyl-5-(2-methylenebutyryl)-2-benzofurancarboxylic acid; 5-(2-ethylacryloyl)-6-methylbenzo-furan-2-carboxylic acid; GP-48674).
FURACRYLIN (tr) (1-(5-nitrofurylacryl-ideneamino)-1,3,4-triazole).
'Furadan' *see* Carbofuran.
'Furadantin' *see* Nitrofurantoin.
'Furadantoin' *see* Nitrofurantoin.
Furadoine *see* Nitrofurantoin.
Furadonin (tr) *see* Nitrofurantoin.
'Furadroxyl' *see* Nidroxyzone.
Furaguanidine (tr) *see* Nitrofurfurylidene-aminoguanidine sulfate.
FURALAZINE** (3-amino-6-(5-nitro-furfurylidenemethyl)-1,2,4-triazine; 3-amino-6-(5-nitrofurylethenyl)-1,2,4-triazine; 3-amino-6-[2-(5-nitro-2-furyl)-vinyl]-*as*-triazine; furatrizine; nifuralazin; nitrofuralazin).
2-FURALDEHYDE (furfural; furfuraldehyde; pyromucic aldehyde).
Furaloxon (tr) *see* Nidroxyzone.
FURALTADONE*** (DL-5-morpholino-methyl-3-(5-nitrofurfurylideneamino)-2-oxazolidinone; 5-morpholinomethyl-furazolidone; furmethonol; 'altafur'). *See also* Levofuraltadone.
'Furamazone' *see* Nifuraldezone.
Furamicid (tr) *see* 5-Nitro-2-furfuryl methyl ether.
'Furamide' *see* Diloxanide furoate.
Furamon (tr) *see* Furtrethonium.
FURAN (furfuran).
'Furanace' *see* Nifurpirinol.
2-Furancarboxylic acid *see* Furoic acid.
Furaniozid (tr) *see* 5-Nitro-1-furfurylidene-isoniazid.
2-Furanmethanol *see* Furfuryl alcohol.
6,7-Furanochromone *see* (5H)-Furo(3,2-g)-(1)benzopyran-5-one.
FURANOMYCIN (α-amino-2,5-dihydro-5-methyl-2-furanacetic acid; (2,5-dihydro-5-methyl-2-furan)glycine).
'Furantoin' *see* Nitrofurantoin.
2-Furan-2-yl-1H-benzimidazole *see* Fuberidazole.
3-(1-Furan-2-yl-3-oxobutyl)-4-hydroxy-2H-1-benzopyran-2-one *see* Coumafuryl.
'Furaspore' *see* 5-Nitro-2-furfuryl methyl ether.
'Furatin' *see* Nitrofurantoin.

'Furatol' *see* Fluoroacetic acid.
Furatrizine *see* Furalazine.
Furaxone (tr) *see* Furazolidone.
FURAZABOL** (17β-hydroxy-17α-methyl-5α-androstano(2,3-c)furazan; 17-methyl-5α-androstano(2,3-c)furazan-17β-ol; andro-furazanol).
FURAZIDIN (tr) (1-[3-(5-nitro-2-furyl)-allylideneamino]hydantoin).
Furazole* *see* Furazolium.
FURAZOLIDONE*** (3-(5-nitro-2-furfuryl-ideneamino)-2-oxazolidinone; furaxone; nifurazolidone; F-60; 'furoxone', 'nifuli-done', 'trichofuron', 'tricofuron').
FURAZOLIUM CHLORIDE*** (6,7-di-hydro-3-(5-nitro-2-furyl)-5H-imidazo-(2,1-b)thiazolium chloride; furazole; NF-963; 'novofur').
FURAZOLIUM TARTRATE* (NF-1425).
Furazosin* *see* Prazosin.
'Furbenal' *see* 5-Nitro-2-furyl methyl ether.
FURBUCILLIN** (6-((R)-2-hydroxy-4-methylvaleramido)penicillanic acid 2-furoate ester; 6-((R)-2-furoyloxy-4-methylvaleramidopenicillanic acid).
'Furedeme' *see* Furterene.
Furenapyridazine *see* Nifurprazine.
Furenazine *see* Nifurprazine.
FURETHIDINE*** (ethyl ester of 1-(tetra-hydrofurfuryloxyethyl)-4-phenylisonipecotic acid; ethyl 1-(tetrahydrofurfuryloxyethyl)-4-phenylpiperidine-4-carboxylate).
FURFENOREX*** ((+)-N-methyl-N-(α-methylphenethyl)furfurylamine; (+)-N-furfuryl-N-methylamphetamine; (+)-N-furfurylmethamphetamine; (+)-N-methyl-N-(1-methylprop-2-yl)-2-furfurylamine; E-106; 'frugalan').
FURFENOREX CYCLAMATE (furfenorex cyclohexylsulfamate; E-106-E; SD-27115).
Furfural *see* 2-Furaldehyde.
Furfuraldehyde *see* 2-Furaldehyde.
Furfuran *see* Furan.
Furfurol(e) *see* 2-Furaldehyde.
FURFURYL ALCOHOL (2-furanmethanol; 2-(hydroxymethyl)furan).
2-FURFURYLAMINOPURINE (kinetin).
N-Furfuryl-N,α-dimethylphenethylamine *see* Furfenorex.
N-Furfuryl-N',N'-dimethyl-N-pyrid-2-ylethylenediamine *see* Methafurylene.
N'-[1-(2-Furfuryl)ethylidene]isoniazed *see* Menazone.
N-Furfuryl-N-methylamphetamine *see* Furfenorex.
2-Furfuryl methyl ketone isonicotinoyl-hydrazone *see* Menazone.
FURFURYLTRIMETHYLAMMONIUM BENZENESULFONATE (benzamon).
Furfuryltrimethylammonium iodide *see* Furtrethonium iodide.
FURIDARONE*** (2,5-dimethyl-3-furyl 4-hydroxy-3,5-diiodophenyl ketone; 3,5-diiodo-4-hydroxyphenyl 2,5-dimethyl-3-furyl ketone; 3-(4-hydroxy-3,5-diiodo-benzoyl)-2,5-dimethylfuran; furodiarone; DB-136).

'Furidin' see Thiofuradene.
Furmarin see Coumafuryl.
Furmethonol see Furaltadone.
FURMETHOXADONE*** (5-methyl-3-(5-nitro-2-furfurylideneamino)-2-oxazolidinone; 5-methylfurazolidone).
5H-FURO(3,2-g)(1)BENZOPYRAN-5-ONE (6,7-furanochromone; furo-2′,3′,6,7-chromone).
7H-Furo(3,2-g)(1)benzopyran-7-one see Psoralen.
FUROBUFEN** (2-[(2-carboxyethyl)-carbonyl]dibenzofuran; 2-carboxyethyl dibenzofuran-2-yl ketone; γ-oxo-2-dibenzo-furanbutyric acid; AY-21367).
Furodiarone see Furidarone.
2-FUROIC ACID (2-furancarboxylic acid; furoic acid; pyromucic acid; brenzschleim-säure).
See also Diloxanide furoate; Furostilbestrol; Guaiacyl furoate.
FUROMAZINE*** (3-[1-[3-(2-chloro-phenothiazin-10-yl)propyl]-4-hydroxy-piperid-4-yl]dihydro-1(3H)-furanone; 2-chloro-10-[3-[4-(dihydro-2(3H)-oxo-furan-3-yl)-4-hydroxypiperid-1-yl]propyl]-phenothiazine; 1-[3-(2-chlorophenothiazin-10-yl)propyl]-4-(dihydro-2(3H)-oxofuran-3-yl)-4-hydroxypiperidine).
FUROSEMIDE*** (4-chloro-N-furfuryl-5-sulfamoylanthranilic acid; 4-chloro-N-(2-furylmethyl)-5-sulfamoylanthranilic acid; frusemide; fursemide; LB-502; 'dryptal', 'impugan', 'lasix', 'nicorol').
See also Reserpine with furosemide.
FUROSTILBESTROL*** (diethylstilbestrol di(2-furoate); stilbestrol furoate; stil-bestrol 2-furancarboxylate; trans-3,4-bis-[4-(2-furoyloxy)phenyl]hex-3-ene).
'Furoxone' see Furazolidone.
6-((R)-2-Furoyloxy-4-methylvaleramido)-penicillanic acid see Furbucillin.
FURSALAN** (3,5-dibromo-N-tetrahydro-furfurysalicylamide).
Fursemide see Furosemide.
FURSULTIAMINE*** (N-(4-amino-2-methylpyrimidin-5-ylmethyl)-N-[4-hy-droxy-1-methyl-2-(tetrahydrofurfuryl-dithio)-1-butenyl]formamide; thiamine tetrahydrofurfuryl disulfide; TTFD; 'judolor').
FURTERENE*** (2,4,7-triamino-6-(2-furyl)-pteridine; 6-(2-furyl)-2,4,7-triamino-pteridine; 'furedeme').
FURTRETHONIUM IODIDE*** (furfuryl-trimethylammonium iodide; furamon).
FURYLFURAMIDE (2-(2-furyl)-3-(5-nitro-2-furyl)acrylamide; 2-(2-furyl)-2-(5-nitro-2-furfurylidene)acetamide; AF-2).
7-[2-(2-Furyl)glyoxylamido]-3-(hydroxy-methyl)-2-cephem-2-carboxylic acid mono-(O-methyloxime) carbamate see Cefuroxime.
2-(2-Furyl)-2-(5-nitro-2-furfurylidene)-acetamide see Furylfuramide.
2-(2-Furyl)-3-(5-nitro-2-furyl)acrylamide see Furylfuramide.
6-(2-Furyl)-2,4,7-triaminopteridine see Furterene.
FUSAFUNGINE*** (antibiotic from a fusarium of Lateritium Wr. section; 'lo-cabiotal').
'Fusarex' see Tecnazene.
FUSARIC ACID (5-butylpicolinic acid; 5-butylpyridine-2-carboxylic acid).
Fusaric acid amide see Bupicomide.
FUSIDIC ACID*** (3α,11α,16β-trihydroxy-29-nor-8α,9β,13α,14β-dammara-17(20),24-dien-21-oic acid 16-acetate; cis-3α,11α,16β-trihydroxy-4α,8,14-trimethyl-18-nor-5α,8α,9β,13α,14β-cholesta-17(20),24-dien-21-oic acid 16-acetate; SQ-16603; ZN-6; 'caviject', 'fucidine').
See also Sodium fusidate.
Fusidium coccineceum, antibiotic, see Fusidic acid.
'Fussol' see Fluoroacetamide.
FW-152 see Hydroxy-DDD.
FX-501 see Xenytropium bromide.
'Fyracyl' see Magnesium acetylsalicylate.
Fytic acid** see Phytic acid.
FZ-484 see Fentonium bromide with perphenazine.

G

G-4 see Dichlorophen.
G-11 see Hexachlorophene.
G-330 see Dimenhydrinate with scopolamine.
G-469 see Nicothiazone.
G-491 see Tiabendazole.
G-605 see Sulfoniazid.
G-610 see Trichlorophen.
G-867 see Sulfadimethylbenzoylamide.
G-2747 see Caramiphen.

G-3012 see Metcaraphen.
G-5668 see Prethcamide.
G-7225 see Mecloralurea.
G-11765 see Ethyl biscoumacetate.
G-12114 see Chloropyramine.
G-13289 see Sulfaproxyline.
G-13871 see Phenylbutazone.
G-19258 see Dimetan.
G-22150 see Imipramine.

G-22355 see Imipramine.
G-23350 see Acenocoumarol.
G-23611 see 1-Isopropyl-3-methylpyrazol-5-yl dimethylcarbanilate.
G-23922 see Chlorobenzilate.
G-24480 see Dimpylate.
G-24483 see Diethyl 3-methylpyrazol-5-yl phosphate.
G-25178 see Dioxahexadekanium.
G-25766 see Clorindione.
G-25804 see Chlorazine.
G-27202 see Oxyphenbutazone.
G-28315 see Sulfinpyrazone.
G-30027 see Atrazine.
G-30320 see Clofazimine.
G-31150 see Calcium methyl polygalacturonate sulfonate.
G-32883 see Carbamazepine.
G-33040 see Opipramol.
G-33182 see Clortalidone.
G-34586 see Clomipramine.
G-35020 see Desipramine.
G-35359 see Ketipramine.
GABA see 4-Aminobutyric acid.
'Gabbromycin' see Paromomycin.
'Gabbroral' see Paromomycin.
GABEXATE** (ethyl p-hydroxybenzoate 6-guanidinohexanoate; p-ethoxycarbonyl-phenyl 6-guanidinohexanoate).
GABEXATE MESILATE (gabexate methanesulfonate; 'foy').
GABOB see 4-Amino-3-hydroxybutyric acid.
'Gadexyl' see Pipradrol.
'Gadusan' see Cupric morrhuate.
'Gaiacyl' see Calcium guaiacolsulfonate.
'Gaiamar' see Guaifenesin.
Galactin see Luteotrophin.
GALACTOFLAVIN (10-D-dulcityl-7,8-dimethylisoalloxazine; NSC-3099).
4-O-β-D-Galactopyranosyl-D-fructose see Lactulose.
GALACTOSAMINE (chondrosamine).
Galactosidogluconic acid see Lactobionic acid.
GALANGIN (3,5,7-trihydroxyflavone).
GALANTAMINE*** (1,2,3,4,6,7,7a,11c-octahydro-9-methoxy-2-methylbenzofuro-(4,3,2-e,f,g)(2)benzazocin-2-ol; galanthamine; nivaline).
Galanthamine see Galantamine.
GALASCORBIN (tr) (potassium ascorbate flavonoid complex; vitamin C plus vitamin P).
'Galatone' see Isoniazid glucuronolactone.
'Galatur' see Iprindole.
'Galecron' see Chlorphenamidine.
'Galidor' see Bencyclane furoate.
Gallabis see Bismuth gallate.
GALLACETOPHENONE (2',3',4'-tri-hydroxyacetophenone; 4-acetylpyrogallol; pyrogallol monoacetate; alizarin yellow C; eugallol).
GALLAMINE TRIETHIODIDE** (1,2,3-tris(2-diethylaminoethoxy)benzene triethiodide; pyrogallol trisdiethylaminoethyl ether triethiodide; bencurine iodide; [v-phenenyltris(oxyethylene)]tris(triethyl-

ammonium iodide); benzcurine iodide; gallammonium iodide; pyrolaxon; sinocurarine; F-2559; RP-3697).
Gallammonium iodide* see Gallamine triethiodide.
GALLIC ACID (3,4,5-trihydroxybenzoic acid).
See also Methyl gallate.
Gallic acid glucosides see Tannins.
'Gallicin' see Methyl gallate.
'Gallimycin' see Erythromycin stearate.
GALLIUM (⁶⁷Ga) CITRATE*** (radio-gallium citrate (1:1)).
Gallodeoxycholic acid see Chenodeoxy-cholic acid.
'Gallogen' see Ellagic acid.
Gallotannic acid see Tannins.
GALOSEMIDE*** (N-[[4-(α,α,α-trifluoro-m-toluidino)pyrid-3-yl]sulfonyl]propion-amide; 3-(propionamidosulfonyl)-4-[(m-trifluoromethyl)anilino]pyridine).
'Gamaquil' see Phenprobamate.
Gamatran see Alverine.
'Gamefar' see Pamaquin.
Gametocidum see Pamaquin.
GAMFEXINE*** (N,N-dimethyl-γ-phenyl-cyclohexanepropylamine; 3-cyclohexyl-N,N-dimethyl-3-phenyl-1-propylamine; WIN-1344).
'Gamibetol' see 4-Amino-3-hydroxybutyric acid.
'Gamiso' see Lindane.
'Gamma 666' see Lindane.
Gammabenzene hexachloride see Lindane.
'Gammacorten' see Dexamethasone.
Gamma-OH see Oxybate sodium.
'Gammexane' see Lindane.
GAMOLENIC ACID*** (cis,cis,cis-octadeca-6,9,12-trienoic acid; Z,Z,Z-octadeca-6,9,12-trienoic acid).
'Gamonil' see Lofepramine.
'Gamophen' see Hexachlorophene.
GANGLEFENE*** (3-diethylamino-1,2-di-methylpropyl ester of p-isobutoxybenzoic acid; ganglerone).
Ganglerone (tr) see Ganglefene.
'Ganibetal' see 4-Amino-3-hydroxybutyric acid.
'Ganlion' see Azamethonium.
'Gantanol' see Sulfamethoxazole.
'Gantrisin' see Sulfafurazole.
'Gantrosan' see Sulfafurazole.
GAPICOMINE** (4,4'-(iminodimethylene)-dipyridine; di(pyrid-4-ylmethyl)amine; 4-(pyrid-4-ylmethylaminomethyl)pyridine).
'Garamycin' see Gentamicin.
Garantose see Saccharin.
'Gardenal' see Phenobarbital.
'Gardol' see Sodium lauroylsarcosinate.
'Gardona' see Stirofos.
'Gargilon' see Dequalinium.
Garlic see Allium sativum.
'Garoin' see Phenytoin with phenobarbital.
'Garrathion' see Carbofenotion.
'Gastomag' see Magnesium trisilicate.
'Gastracid-test' see Phenazopyridine.
'Gastramine' see Betazole.

'Gastrazid' see Phenazopyridine.
Gastrin-like pentapeptide see Pentagastrin.
Gastrin-like tetrapeptide see Tetragastrin.
'Gastripon' see Xenytropium.
'Gastrixone' see Trantelinium bromide.
'Gastrodiagnost' see Pentagastrin.
'Gastrografin' see Meglumine diatrizoate.
'Gastronilo' see Zolimdine.
'Gastropin' see Xenytropium.
'Gastrotest' see Phenazopyridine.
'Gastrovit' see Magnesium hydroxide.
'Gatalone' see Gluconiazone.
'Gatnon' see Benzthiazuron.
Gaultheria oil see Methyl salicylate.
GB see Sarin.
GB-94 see Mianserin.
GC-4072 see Clofenvinfos.
'Geabol' see Metandienone.
'Gebutox' see Dinoseb.
'Gecolate' see Guaifenesin.
GEFARNATE*** (trans-3,7-dimethyl-2,6-
octadienyl 5,9,13-trimethyltetradeca-4,8,12-
trienoate; geranyl farnesylacetate;
'gefarnil', 'gefarnyl').
'Gefarnil' see Gefarnate.
'Gefarnyl' see Gefarnate.
Geksan (tr) see Lindane.
'Gelafusal' see Gelatin solution.
GELATIN BROMOTANNATE (bromtan-
nigel; 'bromocoll').
GELATIN SOLUTION ('gelafusal',
'gelifundin').
See also Polygeline.
GELATIN SPONGE ('marbagelan').
'Gelflex' see Dimefilcon A.
'Gelifundin' see Gelatin solution.
'Geloverm' see Hexylresorcinol.
'Gelstaph' see Cloxacillin.
'Gelvatol' see Polyvinyl alcohol.
GEMAZOCINE*** (3-cyclopropylmethyl-
6-ethyl-1,2,3,4,5,6-hexahydro-11,11-di-
methyl-2,6-methano-3-benzazocin-8-ol;
R-15497).
GEMCADIOL** (2,2,9,9-tetramethyl-1,10-
decanediol).
Gemfa (tr) see Hempa.
GEMFIBROZIL** (2,2-dimethyl-5-(2,5-
xylyloxy)valeric acid; 2,2-dimethyl-5-(2,5-
dimethylphenoxy)valeric acid).
Gemodex (tr) see Dextran(s).
'Gemodez' see Povidone.
'Gemonil' see Metharbital.
'Genabil' see Menbutone.
'Genabilene' see Menbutone.
'Genabol' see Norboletone.
'Genacort' see Hydrocortisone.
Genatropine see Atropine N-oxide.
'Genebile' see Menbutone.
'Geneserine' see Physostigmine N-oxide.
'Genetron 23' see Fluoroform.
'Genetron 113' see Trichlorotrifluoroethane.
'Genetron 152A' see 1,1-Difluoroethane.
'Genicide' see 9-Xanthenone.
'Geniphene' see Campheclor.
GENISTEIN (4',5,7-trihydroxyisoflavone;
prunetol).
Genistein 4-methyl ether see Biochanin A.

'Genite' see Dichlorophenyl besilate.
GENKWANIN (4',5'-dihydroxy-7-methoxy-
flavone; puddmetin).
'Genomorphine' see Morphine N-oxide.
'Genoscopolamine' see Scopolamine
N-oxide.
'Genostrychnine' see Strychnine N-oxide.
'Genovul' see Cloxestradiol acetate.
'Genoxal' see Cyclophosphamide.
'Gentallin' see Gentamicin.
'Gentalyn' see Gentamicin.
GENTAMICIN** (O-2,6-diamino-2,3,4,6-
tetradeoxy-α-D-erythro-hexopyranosyl-
(1→4)-O-[3-deoxy-4-C-methyl-3-(methyl-
amino)-β-L-arabinopyranosyl-(1→6)]-2-
deoxy-D-streptamine; gentamycin; gento-
mycin; gentamicin sulfate; 'cidomycin',
'garamycin', 'gentallin', 'gentalyn',
'genticin', 'geomycin', 'refobacin', 'sul-
mycin').
'Gentamidon' see Aminophenazone
gentisate.
Gentamycin see Gentamicin.
Gentian violet see Crystal violet.
'Genticin' see Gentamicin.
GENTISIC ACID*** (2,5-dihydroxybenzoic
acid; 5-hydroxysalicylic acid).
See also Sodium gentisate.
'Gentisod' see Sodium gentisate.
Gentomycin see Gentamicin.
'Gentran' see Dextran 70.
'Gentron 12' see Dichlorodifluoromethane.
'Geomycin' see Gentamicin.
Geranyl farnesylacetate see Gefarnate.
2-Geranylhydroquinone see Geroquinol.
6-Geranyl-7-hydroxycoumarin see
Ostruthin.
'Germa-medica see Hexachlorophene.
'Germanin' see Suramin.
'Germidine' see Cetylpyridinium.
'Germinol' see Benzalkonium.
'Germitol' see Benzalkonium.
'Gernebcin' see Tobramycin.
'Gerodyl' see Pipradrol.
Gerontine see Spermine.
GEROQUINOL*** (2-geranylhydroquinone;
2-(3,7-dimethyl-2,6-octadienyl)hydro-
quinone).
'Gerovital H3' see Procaine.
'Gesabel' see Ipazine.
'Gesagard' see Prometryn.
'Gesamil' see Propazine.
'Gesapax' see Ametryn.
'Gesapon' see DDT.
'Gesaprim' see Atrazine.
'Gesarex' see DDT.
'Gesaran 25' see Methoprotryn.
'Gesaran 207' see Methoprotryn plus
simazine.
'Gesaran 211' see Methoprotyn plus
simazine.
'Gesaran 2079' see Methoprotryn plus
simazine.
Gesarol see DDT.
'Gesatop' see Simazine.
GESTACLONE*** (17β-acetyl-6-chloro-1β,
1a,2β,8β,9α,10,11,12,13,14α,15,16β,16a,17-

223

tetradecahydro-10β,13β-dimethyl-3H-di-
cyclopropa(1,2:16,17)cyclopenta(a)phen-
anthren-3-one).
GESTADIENOL*** (17-hydroxy-19-nor-
pregna-4,6-diene-3,20-dione).
GESTADIENOL ACETATE(Ba-31458).
'Gestadramine' *see* Dimenhydrinate with
scopolamine.
'Gestafortin' *see* Chlormadinone.
'Gestamestrol' *see* Chlormadinone acetate
with mestranol.
'Gestamin' *see* Atraton.
'Gestanin' *see* Allylestrenol.
'Gestanol' *see* Allylestrenol.
'Gestapuran' *see* Medroxyprogesterone
acetate.
'Gestatron' *see* Dydrogesterone.
'Gestogan' *see* Chlormadinone acetate.
GESTONORONE (17-hydroxy-19-norpregn-
4-ene-3,20-dione; 19-norpregn-4-en-17-ol-
3,20-dione; 17α-hydroxy-19-norproge-
sterone; 17β-ethyl-17α-hydroxyestr-4-ene
3,20-dione; gestronol).
GESTONORONE CAPROATE*** (gest-
onorone hexanoate; gestronol hexanoate;
SH-582; 'depostat').
Gestonorone hexanoate *see* Gestonorone
caproate.
'Gestranol' *see* Chlormadinone acetate with
mestranol.
Gestronol* *see* Gestonorone.
'Getryl' *see* Febarbamate.
'Gevelina' *see* Properidine.
'Gevilon' *see* Sodium hexacyclonate.
'Gevodin' *see* Famprofazone with propy-
phenazone.
GEWO-339 *see* Pasiniazid.
'Gexane' *see* Lindane.
GHBA *see* 4-Hydroxybutyric acid.
GHRH *see* Somatomedin.
'Gichtex' *see* Allopurinol.
Gigantic acid *see* Penicillin F.
'Gilurtymal' *see* Ajmaline.
'Gilutensin' *see* 2-Ethyl-3,3-diphenylpropen-
(2)ylamine.
'Gimid' *see* Glutethimide.
'Gina' *see* Propatyl nitrate.
'Ginapect' *see* Propatyl nitrate.
'Ginebatin' *see* Bacitracin.
'Ginetris' *see* Cloponone with myralact.
'Gingicaine' *see* Tetracaine.
'Gingivit' *see* Dichlorophen.
GINK (tr) *see* Isoniazid.
GINKGO BILOBA EXTRACT ('ginkor',
'tebonin').
'Ginkor' *see* Ginkgo biloba extract.
GINSENG (Panax; Panax ginseng; Panax
quinquefolium root; hiyaku).
**GINSENG EXTRACT WITH TROME-
TAMOL** ('panabolide').
GIRACTIDE*** (1-glycine-18-L-arginin-
amide-α¹⁻¹⁸-corticotrophin; renactide).
'Girostan' *see* Thiotepa.
'Gitalide' *see* Gitalin.
'Gitaligin' *see* Gitalin.
GITALIN AMORPHOUS** ('gitalide',
'gitaligin', 'verodigen').

GITALIN CRYSTALLINE (Ψ-digitonin;
pseudigitonin).
GITALOXIGENIN (16-formylgitoxigenin).
Gitaloxigenin monodigitoxoside *see*
Lanadoxin.
Gitaloxigenin tridigitoxoside *see* Gitaloxin.
GITALOXIN (16-formylgitoxin; gitaloxigenin tridigitoxoside).
GITOFORMATE*** (gitoxin 3',3'',3''',4''',
16-pentaformate; 3β-[(2,6-dideoxy-β-D-*ribo*-
hexopyranosyl)-(1→4)-*O*-2,6-dideoxy-β-D-
ribo-hexopyranosyl(→4)-2,6-dideoxy-β-D-
ribo-hexopyranosyl)oxy]-14,16β-dihydroxy-
5β-card-20(22)-enolide 3',3'',3''',4''',16-
pentaformate; pentaformylgitoxin; AC-
2770; 'formiloxine').
GITOXIGENIN (△²⁰,²²-3,14,16,21-tetra-
hydronorcholenic acid lactone; aglycone of
gitoxin).
GITOXIN (gitoxigenin glycoside; anhydrogitalin; bigitalin; Ψ-digitoxin; pseudodigitoxin).
Gitoxin pentaformate *see* Gitoformate.
'Gix' *see* 1,1,1-Trichloro-2,2-bis(*p*-fluoro-
phenyl)ethane.
GL-7 *see* Glycol salicylate.
'Glacialin' *see* Boroglyceride.
GLADIOLIC ACID (4-methoxy-5-methyl-
o-phthalaldehyde-3-carboxylic acid).
GLAFENINE*** (2,3-dihydroxypropyl *N*-
(7-chloro-4-quinolyl)anthranilate;
glaphenine; R-1707; 'glifanan').
Glaphenine* *see* Glafenine.
'Glarubin' *see* Glaucarubin.
Glauber salt *see* Sodium sulfate.
'Glaucadrin' *see* Aceclidine with epinephrine.
GLAUCARUBIN (MK-53; 'glarubin',
'glaumeba').
'Glaucomide' *see* Acetazolamide.
Glaucostat *see* Aceclidine.
'Glaucotensil' *see* Ethoxolamide.
'Glaumarin' *see* Carbachol.
'Glaumeba' *see* Glaucarubin.
'Glaurin' *see* Diethylene glycol monolaurate.
'Glaxoridin' *see* Cefaloridine.
GLAZIOVINE** ((±)-glaziovine; PM-297).
GLIAMILIDE*** (*endo*-1-[[4-[2-(2-methoxy-
nicotinamido)ethyl]piperid-1-yl]sulfonyl]-
3-(5-norbornen-2-ylmethyl)urea).
'Glianimon' *see* Benperidol.
GLIBENCLAMIDE*** (1-[*p*-[2-(5-chloro-
2-methoxybenzamido)ethyl]benzenesulf-
onyl]-3-cyclohexylurea; 1-[*p*-[2-(5-chloro-
o-anisamido)ethyl]phenylsulfonyl]-3-cyclo-
hexylurea; glybenclamide; glybenzcyclamide; glyburide; HB-419; U-26452;
'daonil', 'diabeta', 'euglucon', 'glidiabet',
'hemi-daonil', 'maninil', 'miglucan').
**GLIBENCLAMIDE WITH PHENFOR-
MIN** ('bi-euglucon').
'Glibenese' *see* Glipizide.
GLIBORNURIDE*** (1-(2-*endo*-hydroxy-
3-*endo*-bornyl)-3-(*p*-toluenesulfonyl)urea;
Ro 6-4563; 'gluborid', 'glutril').
GLIBUTIMINE** (*N*-[*p*-[[3-(3-cyclohexen-
1-yl)-2-iminoimidazolidin-1-yl]sulfonyl]-

phenethyl]butyramide; 1-[[*p*-(2-butyr-amidoethyl)phenyl]sulfonyl]-3-(3-cyclo-hexen-1-yl)-2-iminoimidazoline; *N*-butyryl-*p*-[[(3-cyclohexen-1-yl)-2-imino-imidazolidin-1-yl]sulfonyl]phenethyl-amine; glybutamide; 'glucidol').

GLICARAMIDE** (1-cyclohexyl-3-[[*p*-[2-[1-ethyl-4-(isopentyloxy)-3-methyl-1H-pyrazolo(3,4-b)pyridine-5-carboxamido]-ethyl]phenyl]sulfonyl]urea).

GLICLAZIDE*** (1-(3-azabicyclo(3.3.0)-oct-3-yl)-3-(*p*-toluenesulfonyl) urea; Se-1702; 'diamicron').

'Glicotron' *see* Tolbutamide.

GLIDANILE** (5'-chloro-2-[*p*-[(5-isobutyl-pyrimidin-2-yl)sulfamoyl]phenyl]-*o*-acet-anisidide).

GLIDAZAMIDE*** (1-(hexahydro-1H-azepin-1-yl)-3-(indan-5-ylsulfonyl)urea).

'Glidiabet' *see* Glibenclamide.

Glidiazine* *see* Glymidine.

'Glifanan' *see* Glafenine.

GLIFLUMIDE*** ((−)-(*S*)-*N*-(5-fluoro-2-methoxy-α-methylbenzyl)-2-[*p*-[(5-isobutylpyrimidin-2-yl)sulfamoyl]phenyl]-acetamide; (−)-(*S*)-4-[*N*-(5-isobutylpyrimi-din-2-yl)sulfamoyl]phenylacetic acid 1-(5-fluoro-2-methoxyphenyl)ethylamide; Z-28200).

'Glimid' *see* Glutethimide.

'Glior' *see* Doxenitoin.

'Glipasol' *see* Glybuthiazole.

GLIPENTIDE** (1-[*p*-[2-(*o*-anisamido)-ethyl]benzenesulfonyl]-3-cyclopentylurea; 1-cyclopentyl-3-[[*p*-[2-(*o*-anisamido)ethyl]-phenyl]sulfonyl]urea; 1-cyclopentyl-3-[*p*-[2-(*o*-methoxybenzamido)ethyl]benzene-sulfonyl]urea; glypentide; UR-661).

GLIPIZIDE** (*N*-[2-[4-[[[(cyclohexyl-amino)carbonyl]amino]sulfonyl]phenyl]-ethyl]-5-methylpyrazine-2-carboxamide; 1-cyclohexyl-3-[[*p*-[2-(5-methylpyrazine-2-carboxamido)ethyl]phenyl]sulfonyl]urea; 1-cyclohexyl-3-[*p*-[2-(5-methylpyrazine-2-carboxamido)ethyl]benzenesulfonyl]-urea; glydiazinamide; FK-1320; CP-28720; K-4024; 'glibenese', 'minidiab', 'minodiab').

'Gliptide' *see* Sulglicotide.

GLIQUIDONE*** (1-cyclohexyl-3-[*p*-[2-(3,4-dihydro-7-methoxy-4,4-dimethyl-1,3-dioxo-2(1H)-isoquinolyl)ethyl]benzene-sulfonyl]urea; ARDF-26; 'glurenon').

'Glirona' *see* Ferrous gluconate.

GLISOXEPIDE*** (1-(hexahydro-1H-azepin-1-yl)-3-[[*p*-[2-(5-methyl-3-isoxazole-carboxamido)ethyl]phenyl]sulfonyl]urea; 3-[4-(hexahydroazepin-1-ylureidosulfonyl)-phenethylcarbamoyl]-5-methylisoxazole; 4-[4-[3-(5-methylisoxazole-3-carboxamido)-ethyl]benzenesulfonyl]-1,1-hexamethylene-semicarbazide; BS-4231; FB b-4231; RP-22410; 'pro-diaban').

'Glissitol' *see* Ox bile.

'Glistelone' *see* Prednisolone steaglate.

'Glistron' *see* Ferrous gluconate.

'Glitisol' *see* Thiamphenicol.

'Globacillin' *see* Azidocillin.

'Globenicol' *see* Chloramphenicol.

'Globucid' *see* Sulfaethidole.

Globulariacitrin *see* Rutoside.

'Glofil' *see* Sodium iotalamate.

GLOMERULOTROPHIN (1,2,3,4-tetra-hydro-6-methoxy-1-methyl-9H-pyrido-(3,4-b)indole; 1,2,3,4-tetrahydro-6-meth-oxy-1-methyl-β-carboline).

Glonoin *see* Glyceryl trinitrate.

GLOXAZONE*** (3-ethoxy-2-oxobutyral-dehyde bis(thiosemicarbazone); (1-ethoxy-ethyl)glyoxal bis(thiosemicarbazone); kethoxal bis(thiosemicarbazone); BW-356C61; NSC-82116; 'contrapar', 'KTS').

GLIPS *see* Sulglicotide.

'Gluborid' *see* Glibornuride.

GLUCAGON** (hyperglycaemic-glycogeno-lytic factor of pancreas; glukagon; HG factor; HGF).

'Glucal' *see* Calcium gluconate.

Glucaldrate *see* Potassium glucaldrate; Sodium glucaldrate.

GLUCALOX*** (polymerized complex of glycerol and aluminium hydroxide; glycalox; 'manalox AG').

GLUCAMETACIN*** (2-[2-[1-(*p*-chloro-benzoyl)-5-methoxy-2-methylindol-3-yl]-acetamido]-2-deoxy-D-glucose; indometa-cin amide deoxyglucose derivative).

GLUCAMINE (1-amino-1-deoxy-D-glucitol; glycamine).

'Glucantime' *see* Meglumine antimonate.

D-**Glucaric acid** *see* Saccharic acid.

'Glucaron' *see* Aceglatone.

Glucaspaldrate *see* Sodium glucaspaldrate.

GLUCEPTATE(S)** (glucoheptonate(s)).

'Glucidol' *see* Glibutimine.

'Glucidoral' *see* Carbutamide.

'Glucifrene' *see* Carbutamide with phen-formin.

'Glucinan' *see* Metformin *p*-chlorophenoxy-acetate.

'Glucirenan' *see* Metformin *p*-chlorophen-oxyacetate.

Glucitol *see* Sorbitol.

D-**Glucitol hexanicotinate** *see* Sorbinicate.

'Glucobasin' *see* Adenosine triphosphate.

'Glucobiogen' *see* Calcium gluconate.

Glucochloral *see* Chloralose.

Glucochloralose *see* Chloralose.

Glucodiazine *see* Glymidine.

'Glucodigin' *see* Digitoxin.

'Gluco-ferrum' *see* Ferrous gluconate.

'Glucofos' *see* Calcium fructose 1,6-di-phosphate.

Glucofuranoic acid lactone *see* Glucuro-lactone.

Glucofuranoside *see* Tribenoside.

Glucoheptonate(s) *see* Gluceptate(s).

Glucohexitol *see* Sorbitol.

'Glucomycin' *see* Streptomycin sulfate glucurolactone.

(D-**Gluconato**)(**lactobionato**)**calcium monohydrate** *see* Calcium glubionate.

GLUCONIAZONE (isoniazid glucurono-lactone; glyconiazide; isoniazid *N*²-D-

225

glucuronolactone; 'gatalone', 'INGH, 'INHG, 'gluronazid', 'mycobactyl', 'neoniazide').

GLUCONIC ACID (D-gluconic acid; dextronic acid; glyconic acid; glycogenic acid; maltonic acid; pentahydroxycaproic acid; pentahydroxyhexanoic acid).
See also Calcium gluconate; Ferrous gluconate; Magnesium gluconate; Potassium gluconate; Sodium antimonylgluconate; Sodium stibogluconate.

Glucophage *see* Metformin.

'Glucopostin' *see* Phenformin.

Glucoproscillaridin A *see* Scillaren A.

α-D-Glucopyranosyl-β-D-fructofuranoside *see* Sucrose.

3β-(β-D-Glucopyranosyloxy)-14,23-dihydroxy-24-nor-5β,14β-chol-20(22)-en-21-oic acid γ-lactone *see* Actodigin.

D-Glucosaccharic acid *see* Saccharic acid.

1,4-Glucosaccharolactone *see* Saccharic acid 1,4-lactone.

Glucosaccharonic acid *see* Isoascorbic acid.

GLUCOSAMINE** (2-amino-2-deoxy-D-glucose; 2-amino-2-deoxy-β-D-glucopyranose; chitosamine; glucosamine hydrochloride; NSC-758).

Glucosaminedesoxystreptamine ribosediaminohexose *see* Paromomycin.

GLUCOSE (α-D-glucopyranose; D-glucose; corn sugar; dextrose; glycose; grape sugar; saccharum amylaceum; starch sugar; Traubenzucker).

GLUCOSE 1-PHOSPHATE (Cori ester).

GLUCOSE 6-PHOSPHATE (Robinson ester).

'Glucosulfa' *see* Metformin with tolbutamide.

GLUCOSULFAMIDE** (glucose sodium bisulfite compound of N^1-hydroxymethylsulfanilamide; glucose sodium bisulfite compound of sulfanilamidomethanol; p-aminobenzenesulfonoxymethylamide N-D-glucose sodium sulfite; glycosulfamide; 'ladogal').

GLUCOSULFONE** (N,N'-di(glucose sodium sulfonate) of 4,4'-diaminodiphenyl sulfone; p,p'-sulfonyldianiline N,N'-di-(D-glucose sodium bisulfite compound); dapsone di(glucose sodium sulfonate); P-501; SN-166).

1-D-Glucos-2-yl-3-methyl-3-nitrosourea *see* Streptozocin.

'Glucoxy' *see* Glucurolactone.

GLUCUROLACTONE** (γ-lactone of D-glucofuranuronic acid; glucuronolactone; 'glucoxy', 'glucurone').

'Glucurone' *see* Glucurolactone.

GLUCURONIC ACID (D-glucofuranuronic acid; 'guronsan').

Glucuronolactone *see* Glucurolactone.

'Gludiase' *see* Glybuzole.

'Gluferate' *see* Ferrous gluconate.

Gluk..... *see* Gluc....

'Glumorin' *see* Kallidinogenase.

'Gluquinate' *see* Quinidine gluconate.

'Glurenon' *see* Gliquidone.

'Gluronazid' *see* Gluconiazone.

'Gluside' *see* Saccharin.

'Glutadenyl' *see* Adenosine phosphate.

GLUTAMIC ACID** (2-aminopentanedioic acid; 2-aminoglutaric acid; glutaminic acid; glutamic acid hydrochloride).

Glutamic acid lactam *see* Pyroglutamic acid.

Glutamic acid monoamide *see* Glutamine.

Glutamic acid salts *see* Ammonium glutamate; Arginine glutamate; Calcium glutamate; Sodium glutamate.

GLUTAMINE (2-aminoglutaramic acid; glutamic acid monoamide; DL-glutamine; NSC-97925).

L-Glutamine *see* Levoglutamide.

Glutaminic acid *see* Glutamic acid.

Glutamyltaurine *see* Glutaurine.

GLUTARAL** (glutaraldehyde; pentanedial; 'alhydex, 'cidex).

Glutaraldehyde *see* Glutaral.

GLUTARAMIC ACID (4-carbamoylbutyric acid; glutaric acid monoamide).

GLUTARANILIC ACID (4-(phenylcarbamoyl)butyric acid; N-phenylglutaramic acid).

GLUTARIC ACID (pentanedioic acid).

Glutaric acid monoamide *see* Glutaramic acid.

GLUTARIMIDE (2,6-piperidinedione).

GLUTATHIONE (L-glutamyl-L-cysteinylglycine; GSH; 'tathion').

GLUTATHIONE SODIUM SALT ('triptide').

GLUTAURINE** (N-(2-sulfoethyl)-L-glutamine; glutamyltaurine).

'Glutavene' *see* Sodium glutamate.

GLUTETHIMIDE** (α-ethyl-α-phenylglutarimide; 2-ethyl-2-phenylglutarimide; 3-ethyl-3-phenyl-2,6-piperidinedione; 'doriden', 'elrodorm', 'gimid, 'glimid', 'noxiron', 'noxyron', 'ondasil', 'redimyl', 'sarodormin').

Glutimic acid *see* Pyroglutamic acid.

Glutiminic acid *see* Pyroglutamic acid.

'Glutril' *see* Glibornuride.

Glybenclamide *see* Glibenclamide.

Glybenzcyclamide *see* Glibenclamide.

'Glyboral' *see* Boroglyceride.

Glyburide* *see* Glibenclamide.

Glybutamide* *see* Glibutimine.

GLYBUTHIAZOL** (N^1-(5-tert-butyl-1,3,4-thiadiazol-2-yl)sulfanilamide; 5-tert-butyl-2-sulfanilamido-1,3,4-thiadiazole; glybuthiazole; sulfatertiobutylthiadiazole; RP-2259; Th-1395; 'glipasol').

GLYBUZOLE** (N-(5-tert-butyl-1,3,4-thiadiazol-2-yl)benzenesulfonamide; 5-tert-butyl-2-benzenesulfonyl-1,3,4-thiadiazole; desaglybuzole; AN-1324; RP-7891; 'gludiase', 'theraplix').

Glycalox* *see* Glucalox.

'Glycamide' *see* 4,5-Imidazoledicarboxamide.

'Glycamine-AM' *see* Aluminium magnesium glycinate.

Glycarbylamide *see* 4,5-Imidazoledicarboxamide.

226

GLYCARSAMIDE (*N*-glycoloylarsanilic acid; 'astryl').
See also Tryparsamide.
GLYCERALDEHYDE (2,3-dihydroxypropionaldehyde; 2,3-dihydroxypropanal; NSC-67934).
Glycérides oléiques polyoxyéthylènes *see* Peglicol 5 oleate.
Glycerin *see* Glycerol.
GLYCEROL*** (1,2,3-propanetriol; glycerin).
Glycerol α-monobromohydrin *see* Bromohydrin.
Glycerol α-monochlorohydrin *see* Chlorohydrin.
Glycerol α-monoiodohydrin *see* Iodohydrin.
Glycerosalicylic acid *see* Glyceryl glycerosalicylate.
Glyceryl diacetate *see* Diacetin.
Glyceryl guaiacolate *see* Guaifenesin.
Glyceryl iodopropylidene ether *see* (2-Iodopropylidenedioxy)propanol.
GLYCERYL SALICYLATE (glyceryl monosalicylate; 'glycosal', 'saliceral').
Glyceryl triacetate *see* Triacetin.
Glyceryl trilinoleate *see* Trilinolein.
GLYCERYL TRINITRATE (nitroglycerin; nitroglycerol; trinitrin; trinitroglycerin; trinitroglycerol; glonoin).
Glycide *see* Glycidol.
GLYCIDIC ACID (2,3-epoxypropionic acid).
See also Oxanamide.
GLYCIDOL (2,3-epoxy-1-propanol; epihydrin alcohol; glycide).
GLYCINAMIDE (α-aminoacetamide).
GLYCINE (aminoacetic acid; glycocoll; sucre de gelatine).
1-Glycine-18-L-argininamide-α$^{1-18}$-corticotrophin *see* Giractide.
Glycine-*p*-phenetidine *see* Phenocoll.
GLYCLOPYRAMIDE*** (1-(*p*-chlorobenzenesulfonyl)-3-pyrrolidin-1-ylurea).
GLYCOBIARSOL** (bismuth glycolylarsanilate; bismuthoxy salt of *N*-glycolylarsanilic acid; WIN-1011).
See also Chloroquine diphosphate with glycobiarsol.
GLYCOCHOLIC ACID (cholylglycine; glycinecholic acid conjugate).
Glycocoll *see* Glycine.
GLYCOCYAMIDINE (2-imino-4-imidazolidinone).
GLYCOCYAMINE (*N*-amidinoglycine; guanidoacetic acid).
Glycodiazine *see* Glymidine.
GLYCOGEN (animal starch; hepatin).
Glycogenic acid *see* Gluconic acid.
Glycol *see* Ethylene glycol.
GLYCOLALDEHYDE (hydroxyacetaldehyde).
Glycolamide ester with flufenamic acid *see* Colfenamate.
Glycol chlorohydrin *see* 2-Chloroethanol.
Glycoleucine *see* Norleucine.
GLYCOLIC ACID (2-hydroxyacetic acid; glycollic acid).
Glycolic acid 8-ester with octahydro-5,8-dihydroxy-4,6,9,10-tetramethyl-6-vinyl-3a,9-propano-3aH-cyclopentacycloocten-1(4H)-one *see* Pleuromulin.
Glycolic acid indometacin(ester) derivative *see* Acemetacin.
Glycolic acid polyester with lactic acid *see* Polyglactin.
Glycolic acid polymer *see* Polyglycolic acid.
Glycollic acid *see* Glycolic acid.
***p*-Glycolophenetidide** *see* Fenacetinol.
***N*-Glycoloylarsanilic acid** *see* Glycarsamide.
(1*S*,3*S*)-3-Glycoloyl-1,2,3,4,6,11-hexahydro-3,5,12-trihydroxy-10-methoxy-6,11-dioxo-1-naphthacenyl-3-amino-2,3,6-trideoxy-α-L-*lyxo*-hexopyranoside *see* Doxorubicin.
***N*-Glycoloyl-*p*-phenetidine** *see* Fenacetinol.
GLYCOL SALICYLATE (2-hydroxyethyl salicylate; monoglycol salicylate; ethyl glycol salicylate; ethylene glycol salicylate; ethylene glycol monosalicylate; GL-7; 'glysal', 'rheumacyl', 'spirosal').
***N*-Glycolylarsanilic acid** *see* Glycarsamide.
Glycolyltheophylline sodium *see* Sodium theophyllin-7-ylacetate.
Glycolylurea *see* Hydantoin.
Glyconiazide *see* Gluconiazone.
Glyconic acid *see* Gluconic acid.
Glycopyrrolate* *see* Glycopyrronium.
GLYCOPYRRONIUM BROMIDE*** (1,1-dimethyl-3-hydroxypyrrolidinium bromide α-cyclopentylmandelate; glycopyrrolate; AHR-504; 'nodapton', 'robinul', 'tarodyl', 'tarodyn').
'Glycosal' *see* Glyceryl salicylate.
Glycose *see* Glucose.
Glycosulfamide *see* Glucosulfamide.
'Glycotron' *see* Tolbutamide.
GLYCYCLAMIDE*** (1-cyclohexyl-3-(*p*-toluenesulfonyl)urea; cyclamide; tolhexamide; K-836; 'agliral', 'diaboral').
GLYCYCLAMIDE WITH METFORMIN (ER-105).
4-Glycylamidobenzenearsonic acid sodium salt *see* Tryparsamide.
Glycyrrhetic acid *see* Enoxolone.
Glycyrrhetin *see* Enoxolone.
Glycyrrhetinic acid *see* Enoxolone.
Glycyrrhiza *see* Liquorice.
GLYCYRRHIZIC ACID (enoxolone glycoside; glycyrrhetic acid glycoside; glycyrrhetic acid diglucuronate; glycyrrhizin; glycyrrhizinic acid).
Glycyrrhizin *see* Glycyrrhizic acid.
Glycyrrhizinic acid *see* Glycyrrhizic acid.
Glydiazinamide *see* Glipizide.
Glyfillin *see* Diprophylline.
GLYHEXAMIDE*** (1-cyclohexyl-3-indan-5-ylsulfonylurea; SQ-15860; 'serbose', 'subose').
Glyhexylamide* *see* Metahexamide.
Glykresin *see* Mephenesin.

'Glymaxil' see Sodium glucaldrate.

GLYMIDINE SODIUM** (sodium derivative of 2-benzenesulfonamido-5-(2-methoxyethoxy)pyrimidine; *N*-[5-(2-methoxyethoxy)pyrimidin-2-yl]benzenesulfonamidosodium; glucodiazine; glycodiazine; glidiazine; sodium glymidine; SH-717; 'gondafin', 'gondafon', 'lycanol', 'redul').

'Glyo 6' see Piridoxilate.

GLYOCTAMIDE*** (1-cyclooctyl-3-*p*-toluenesulfonylurea).

GLYODIN* (2-heptadecyl-4,5-dihydro-1H-imidazole monoacetate; 'glyoxide').

GLYOXAL (biformyl; diformyl; dihydroxyacetaldehyde; ethanedial; oxalaldehyde).

Glyoxalic acid see Glyoxylic acid.

Glyoxalidine see Imidazolidine.

Glyoxaline see Imidazole.

Glyoxaline-5-alanine see Histidine.

trans-**3-Glyoxylamidoacrylamide oxime** see Zedalan.

'Glyoxide' see Glyodin.

Glyoxyldiureide see Allantoin.

GLYOXYLIC ACID (ketoacetic acid; oxoacetic acid; formylformic acid; glyoxalic acid).

GLYPARAMIDE* (1-*p*-chlorobenzenesulfonyl-3-*p*-dimethylaminophenylurea; P-1306).

'Glyped' see Triacetin.

Glypentide see Glipentide.

Glyphenarsine see Tryparsamide.

Glyphyllin see Diprophylline.

GLYPINAMIDE*** (1-*p*-chlorobenzenesulfonyl-3-hexahydro-1H-azepin-1-ylurea; azepinamide; U-12504).

GLYPROTHIAZOL*** (N^1-(5-isopropyl-1,3,4-thiadiazol-2-yl)sulfanilamide; 5-isopropyl-2-sulfanilamido-1,3,4-thiadiazole; glyprothiazole; sulfaisopropylthiadiazole; RP-2254; VK-57; 'IPTD', 'PASIT').

Glyptide sulfate see Sulglicotide.

'Glysal' see Glycol salicylate.

GLYSOBUZOLE*** (*N*-(5-isobutyl-1,3,4-thiadiazol-2-yl)-*p*-methoxybenzenesulfonamide; 5-isobutyl-2-(*p*-methoxybenzenesulfonamido)-1,3,4-thiadiazole; isobuzole; 'stabinol').

'Glyvenol' see Tribenoside.

GMP see Guanylic acid.

GNOSCOPINE (α-gnoscopine; DL-narcotine; DL-noscapine).
See also Noscapine.

Go-560 see Febarbamate.

Gö-919 see Piprozolin.

Gö-1261 see Tilidine.

Gö-1733 see Suloxifen oxalate.

Gö-3026A see Ciclafrine.

'Goalgan' see Calcium alginate.

Goa powder see Chrysarobin.

GOBAB see 3-Amino-4-hydroxybutyric acid.

Goetsch's vitamin see Vitamin T.

GOHBA see 4-Hydroxybutyric acid.

GOITRIN (5-vinyl-2-oxazolidinethione).

'Golaval' see Cloponone.

GOLD (^{198}Au) **COLLOIDAL**** (colloidal radiogold; radiogold solution; radioaurum (^{198}Au); 'aurcoloid-198').

Gold sodium allylthioureidobenzoate see Sodium auroallylthioureidobenzoate.

Gold sodium thiomalate see Sodium aurothiomalate.

Gold sodium thiosulfate see Sodium aurotiosulfate.

Gold thioglucose see Aurothioglucose.

Gold tribromide see Gold bromide.

'Gomaxine' see Cetrimonium.

GONADORELIN*** (luteinizing hormone releasing factor (pig); 5-oxo-L-prolyl-L-histidyl-L-tryptophyl-L-seryl-L-tyrosylglycyl-L-leucyl-L-arginyl-L-prolylglycinamide; L-pyroglutamyl-L-histidyl-L-tryptophyl-L-seryl-L-tyrosylglycyl-L-leucyl-L-arginyl-L-prolylglycinamide; LH-RH; HOE-471; 'relefact LH-RH').

Gonadotrophins see Chorionic gonadotrophin; Follitropin; Human pituitary gonadotrophin; Serum gonadotrophin.

'Gondafin' see Glymidine.

'Gondafon' see Glymidine.

'Gonosan' see Kavain.

'Gontochin' see Chloroquine.

'Gophicide' see Bis(*p*-chlorophenyl) *N*-acetimidoylphosphoramidothioate.

GOSSYPETIN (3,3',4',5,7,8-hexahydroxyflavone).

GOSSYPOL (1,1',6,6',7,7'-hexahydroxy-5,5'-diisopropyl)3,3'-dimethyl-(2,2'-binaphthalene)-8,8'-dicarboxaldehyde).

'Goutin' see Sodium anhydromethylenecitrate.

GP-121 see Phencyclidine.

GP-41299 see Damotepine.

GP-41353 see Triclosan.

GP-45840 see Diclofenac sodium.

GP-48674 see Furacrinic acid.

GPA-2087 see (−)-Etazocine.

GPT see Glutamic-pyruvic transaminase.

GR2/234 see Alfaxalone.

GR2/443 see Doxibetasol propionate.

GR2/541 see Betamethasone acibutate.

GR2/925 see Clobetasol propionate.

GR2/1214 see Clobetasone butyrate.

GR2/1574 see Alfadolone.

GR-62 see Isoxsuprine.

'Gracidin' see Phenmetrazine.

'Gramaxin' see Cefazolin.

GRAMICIDIN*** (cyclo(L-valyl-L-ornithyl-L-leucyl-D-phenylalanyl-L-prolyl-L-valyl-L-ornithyl-L-leucyl-D-phenylalanyl-L-prolyl)).

GRAMICIDIN S*** (antibiotic from *Bac. brevis*; 'gramoderm', 'gromidin').

GRAMINE (3-dimethylaminomethylindole; donaxine).

'Gramoderm' see Gramicidin.

'Gramoxone' see Paraquat.

Granatan see Granatanine.

GRANATANINE (9-azabicyclo(3.3.1)-nonane; granatan).

Granatol see Granatoline.

GRANATOLINE (9-azabicyclo(3.3.1)nonan-3-ol; granatol).

Grape sugar see Glucose.

'Gratibain' see Ouabain.
Gratus strophanthin see Ouabain.
'Gravibinan' see Estradiol valerate with hydroxyprogesterone caproate.
'Gravistat' see Levonorgestrel with ethinylestradiol.
'Gravosan' see Clomifene citrate.
Green of bitter almonds see Malachite green.
'Grenolon' see Perphenazine.
'Gricin' see Griseofulvin.
'Grifulvin' see Griseofulvin.
'Grillocin' see Zinc ricinoleate.
'Grisactin' see Griseofulvin.
GRISEIN (antibiotic from Streptomyces griseus, identical with Albomycin (q.v)).
GRIS-2'-ENE-3,4'-DIONE (coumaran-3-one-2-spiro-1'-(cyclohex-2'-en-4'-one)).
GRISEOFULVIN*** (7-chloro-4,6,2'-trimethoxy-6'-methylgris-2'-ene-3,4'-dione; 7-chloro-2',4,6-trimethoxy-6'-methylspiro-(benzofuran-2-(3H),1'-(2)-cyclohexene)-3,4'-dione; 7-chloro-4,6-dimethoxycoumaran-3-one-2-spiro-1'-(2'-methoxy-6'-methylcyclohex-2'-en-4'-one); curling factor; NSC-34533; 'fulcin', 'fulvicin', 'gricin', 'grifulvin', 'grisactin', 'grisovin', 'lamoryl', 'likudin').
'Grisovin' see Griseofulvin.
'Gromidin' see Gramicidin.
GROWTH HORMONE (somatotrophic hormone; somatotrophin; SF; ST; STH). See also Human growth hormone.
Growth hormone release inhibiting factor see Somatostatin.
Growth hormone releasing hormone see Somatomedin.
GS-95 see Thiethylperazine.
GS-1339 see Dimantine.
GS-2147 see Sancycline.
GS-2876 see Metacycline.
GS-2989 see Meclocycline.
GS-3065 see Doxycycline.
GS-6244 see Carbadox.
GS-6742 see Sulfomyxin.
GS-7443 see Mequidox.
GSH see Glutathione.
'GT 41' see Busulfan.
'GT 75' see Cyclopentolate.
GTP see Guanosine triphosphate.
'G-TRIL' see Febarbamate.
GUABENXAN*** ((1,4-benzodioxan-6-ylmethyl)guanidine; 6-(guanidinomethyl)-1,4-benzodioxan).
'Guacamphol' see Guaiacyl camphorate.
'Guacetin' see Guaiacetin.
GUAIACETIN (Na pyrocatechol monoacetate; Na phenone acetate; 'guacetin').
GUAIACOL (o-methoxyphenol; pyrocatechol methyl ether; o-hydroxyanisole; 'anastil').
Guaiacol glyceryl ether see Guaifenesin.
Guaiacolsulfonic acid calcium salt see Calcium guaiacolsulfonate.
GUAIACTAMINE*** (2-(o-methoxyphenoxy)triethylamine).
Guaiacyl potassium sulfate see Sulfogaiacol.

'Guaiamar' see Guaifenesin.
GUAIAPATE*** (1-[2-[2-(2-(o-methoxyphenoxy)ethoxy)ethoxy]ethyl]piperidine).
GUAIAZULENE (S-guaiazulene; 1,4-dimethyl-7-isopropylazulene; AZ-8; 'azulon').
Guaicuran see Guaifenesin.
GUAIFENESIN*** (3-(o-methoxyphenoxy)-1,2-propanediol; glyceryl guaiacolate; guaiacol glyceryl ether; guaicuran; guaiphenesin; XL-90; 'gaiamar', 'gecolate', 'guaiamar', 'guajacuran', 'guayanesin', 'miorelax', 'My 301', 'myocaine', 'myoscaine', 'oresol', 'oreson', 'reorganin', 'resil', 'respenyl', 'resyl', 'robitussin', 'tolseron'). See also Noscapine with guaifenesin.
Guaifenesin carbamate see Methocarbamol.
Guaifenesin theophylline derivative see Guaifylline.
GUAIFYLLINE** (3-(o-methoxyphenoxy)-1,2-propanediol compound with theophylline; guaiphenesin theophylline derivative; guaithylline; 'eclabron').
Guaiphenesin* see Guaifenesin.
Guaithylline* see Guaifylline.
'Guajacuran' see Guaifenesin.
GUAMECYCLINE** (N-[4-(amidinoamidino)piperazin-1-ylmethyl]tetracycline; N-(4-diguanidopiperazin-1-ylmethyl)-tetracycline; N-(4-guanidinoformimidoyl-piperazin-1-ylmethyl)tetracycline; 'guanamycin', 'xantocyclina').
GUANABENZ*** (1-(2,6-dichlorobenzyl-ideneamino)guanidine; DCBAG; BR-750).
GUANABENZ ACETATE (Wy-8678).
GUANACLINE** (1-(2-guanidinoethyl)-1,2,3,6-tetrahydro-4-picoline; [2-(4-methyl-3,6-dihydro(2H)pyrid-1-yl)ethyl]-guanidine; 1-[2-(3,6-dihydro-4-methyl-1-(2H)-pyridyl)ethyl]guanidine; 1-(2-guanidinoethyl)-1,2,3,6-tetrahydro-4-methyl-pyridine; cyclazenin; cyclozanin; guanacline sulfate; FBA-1464; 'leron').
GUANACLINE WITH METHYLDOPA ('tadip').
GUANADREL*** ((1,4-dioxaspiro(4.5)dec-2-ylmethyl)guanidine; guanadrel sulfate; CL-1388R; U-28288D).
Guanamprazine see Amiloride.
'Guanamycin' see Guamecycline.
'Guanatol' see Proguanil.
GUANAZODINE*** (1-(octahydroazocin-2-ylmethyl)guanidine; 2-(guanidylmethyl)-octahydroazocine; guanidinomethylaza-cyclooctane; 2-(guanidylmethyl)hepta-methylenimine; 1-(2-heptamethylenimino-methyl)guanidine; Egyt-739; 'sanegyt').
GUANAZOLE (3,5-diamino-1,2,4-triazole; NSC-1895).
'Guanazolo' see 8-Azaguanine.
GUANCIDINE** (1-cyano-3-tert-pentyl-guanidine; 1-cyano-3-(1,1-dimethylpropyl)-guanidine; guancydine; CL-2422).
GUANCLOFINE** ([2-(2,6-dichloro-anilino)ethyl]guanidine; 2,6-dichloro-N-(2-guanidinoethyl)aniline).
Guancydine* see Guancidine.

'**Guaneran**' see Tiamiprine.

GUANETHIDINE*** (1-[2-(1-azacyclooctyl)-ethyl]guanidine; 1-[2-(hexahydro-1(2H)-azocinyl)ethyl]guanidine; 1-(2-guanidino-ethyl)azacyclooctane; 1-(2-guanidino-ethyl)azocine; 1-(2-guanidinoethyl)hepta-methylenimine; [1-(2-perhydroazocin-1-yl)-ethyl]guanidine; 1-[2-(octahydro-1-azo-cinyl)ethyl]guanidine; 1-[2-(hexahydro-1(2H)-azocinyl)ethyl]guanidine; guanizol; isobarin; octadine; octatensin; oktadin; 'sanotensin').

Guanethidine hydrogen sulfate see Guan-ethidine monosulfate.

GUANETHIDINE MONOSULFATE* (guanethidine hydrogen sulfate; 'esimil').

GUANETHIDINE SULFATE* (C-5864-Su; Su-5864; 'ismelin').

GUANETHIDINE WITH HYDRO-CHLOROTHIAZIDE ('esimil').

GUANICAINE (1,3-bis(*p*-methoxyphenyl)-2-phenetylguanidine; 1,3-dianisyl-2-phenetyl-guanidine; 2-(*p*-ethoxyphenyl)-1,3-bis(*p*-methoxyphenyl) guanidine; di-*p*-anisyl monophenetylguanidine; guanicaine hydro-chloride; phenodianisyl; 'acoin').

GUANIDINE (aminoformamidine; carb-amidine; iminourea; uramine).

4-Guanidinobutyramide see Tiformin.

N-**(2-Guanidinoethyl)aza-6-spiro(2.5)-octane** see Spirgetine.

1-(2-Guanidinoethyl)-1,2,3,6-tetrahydro-4-picoline see Guanacline.

N-**(Guanidinoformimidoyl)morpholine** see Moroxydine.

N-**(4-Guanidinoformimidoylpiperazin-1-ylmethyl)tetracycline** see Guamecy-cline.

6-Guanidinohexanoic acid *p*-**(ethoxy-carbonyl)phenyl ester** see Gabexate.

Guanidinomethylazacyclooctane see Guanazodine.

2-(Guanidinomethyl)-1,4-benzodioxan see Guanoxan.

6-(Guanidinomethyl)-1,4-benzodioxan see Guabenxan.

Guanidoacetic acid see Glycocyamine.

Guanidotaurine see Taurocyamine.

2-(Guanidylmethyl)heptamethylenimine see Guanazodine.

2-(Guanidylmethyl)octahydroazocine see Guanazodine.

GUANINE (2-amino-6-hydroxypurine; 2-aminohypoxanthine).

GUANINE ARABINOSIDE (9β-D-arabino-furanosylguanine; ara-G).

Guanine phosphate see Guanylic acid.

GUANINE PROPIONATE (2-(α-propion-amido)-6-hydroxypurine).

Guanine riboside see Guanosine.

Guanisochin* see Guanisoquine.

Guanisoquin* see Guanisoquine.

GUANISOQUINE*** (7-bromo-3,4-dihydro-2(1H)-isoquinoline carboxamidine; guanisoquin sulfate; guanisochin; P-3896).

Guanizol see Guanethidine.

GUANOCLOR*** (1-[2-(2,6-dichloro-phenoxy)ethylamino]guanidine; 1-[2-(2,6-dichlorophenoxy)ethyl]-2-guanylhydrazine; guanoclor sulfate; P-1029; 'vatensol').

GUANOCTINE*** (1-(1,1,3,3-tetramethyl-butyl)guanidine; *tert*-octylguanidine; guanoctine hydrochloride; A-7283; BP-1184).

'**Guanofuracin**' see Nitrofurfurylideneamino guanidine sulfate.

GUANOSINE (guanine riboside; 2-amino-6-hydroxypurine riboside; vernine).

Guanosine monophosphate see Guanylic acid.

Guanosine phosphate see Guanylic acid.

GUANOSINE TRIPHOSPHATE (GTP).

GUANOXABENZ** (1-[(2,6-dichlorobenzyl-idene)amino]-3-hydroxyguanidine; 2-[(2,6-dichlorophenyl)methylene]-*N*-hydroxycarboximidamide).

GUANOXAN*** (1-(1,4-benzodioxan-2-yl-methyl)guanidine; 2-guanidinomethyl-1,4-benzodioxan; guanoxan sulfate; P-1003; 'envacar').

GUANOXYFEN*** (1-(3-phenoxypropyl)-guanidine; guanoxyfen sulfate; CI-515; EA-166).

Guanylhydrazine see Aminoguanidine.

GUANYLIC ACID (guanosine monophos-phate; guanosine phosphate; GMP).

N-**Guanyl-*N*-methylglycine** see Creatine.

GUANYLTHIOUREA (gutimine).

Guaranine see Caffeine.

'**Guarin**' see Caffeine.

'**Guayanesin**' see Guaifenesin.

'**Gubernal**' see Alprenolol.

Guethol see Ethoxyphenol.

'**Gumbix**' see *p*-Aminomethylbenzoic acid.

'**Guronsan**' see Glucuronic acid.

'**Gusathion**' see Azinphos-ethyl plus azinphos-methyl.

'**Gusathion A**' see Azinphos-ethyl.

'**Gusathion M**' see Azinphos-methyl.

'**Gusathion MS**' see Azinphos-methyl plus demeton-S-methylsulfon.

'**Guthion**' see Azinphos-methyl.

Gutimine (tr) see Guanylthiourea.

'**Gutron**' see Midodrine.

'**Guttalax**' see Sodium picosulfate.

GUVACINE (1,2,5,6-tetrahydronicotinic acid).

GUVACOLINE (methyl 1,2,5,6-tetrahydro-nicotinate).

'**Gyn**' see Magnesium gluconate.

'**Gynergen**' see Ergotamine tartrate.

'**Gynesin**' see Trigonelline.

'**Gyno-daktarin**' see Miconazole.

'**Gynodal**' see Diethylaminoethyl butyl-aminosalicylate.

'**Gyno-monistat**' see Miconazole.

'**Gynophase**' see Norethisterone acetate with ethinylestradiol.

'**Gyno-rest**' see Dydrogesterone.

'**Gyno-sterosan**' see Chlorquinaldol.

'**Gynovlar**' see Norethisterone acetate with ethinylestradiol.

H

H *see* Mustard gas.
H₃ *see* Procaine.
H-9/88 *see* Metirosine.
H-22/54 *see* 2-(3,4-Dihydroxyphenyl)-valeramide.
H-33 *see* Febuprol.
H-44/68 *see* Metirosine methyl ester.
H-56/28 *see* Alprenolol.
H-93/26 *see* Metoprolol.
H-115 *see* Chlormidazole.
H-365 *see* Paroxypropione.
H-490 *see* Ethosuximide.
H-610 *see* Fencamfamin.
H-853 *see* Cafedrine with theodrenaline.
H-990 *see* Oxymetazoline.
H-3452 *see* Cyclofenil.
H-3608 *see* Enpiprazole.
H-4007 *see* Mepiprazole.
H-4170 *see* Topiprazole.
Ha-242 *see* (Methoxypropylaminomethyl)-1,4-benzodioxan.
HACHIMYCIN** (antibiotic from *Str. hachijoensis*; 'cambimycin', 'trichomycin', 'trichonat', 'trichosept').
'Haelan' *see* Fludroxycortide.
Haem.... *see also* Hem.....
'Haemaccel' *see* Polygeline.
Haffkynine *see* Mepacrine.
'Haflutan' *see* Clofenamide.
'Halan' *see* Halothane.
'Halane' *see* Sodium troclosene.
HALAZEPAM** (7-chloro-1,3-dihydro-5-phenyl-1-(2,2,2-trifluoroethyl)-2H-1,4-benzodiazepin-2-one; Sch-12041).
HALAZONE* (*p*-(*N,N*-dichlorosulfamoyl)-benzoic acid).
HALAZONE SODIUM (sodium *p*-(*N,N*-dichlorosulfamoyl)benzoate; 'pantocide', 'pantosept').
HALCINONIDE** (21-chloro-9-fluoro-11β,16α,17-trihydroxypregn-4-ene-3,20-dione cyclic 16,17-acetal with acetone; 21-chloro-9-fluoropregn-4-ene-11β,16α,17-triol-3,20-dione cyclic 16,17-acetal with acetone; 21-chloro-9α-fluoro-11β-hydroxy-16α,17α-isopropylidenedioxypregn-4-ene-3,20-dione; SQ-18566).
'Haldol' *see* Haloperidol.
'Haldrate' *see* Paramethasone.
'Haldrone' *see* Paramethasone.
'Halenol' *see* Dichlorophen.
HALETAZOLE** (5-chloro-2-[*p*-(2-diethylaminoethoxy)phenyl]benzothiazole; halethazole; 'episol').
Halethazole* *see* Haletazole.
'Halidor' *see* Bencyclane furoate.
'Halinone' *see* Bromindione.
'Haloanisone' *see* Fluanisone.
HALOCARBAN** (4,4'-dichloro-3-(trifluoromethyl)carbanilide cloflucarban; 'irgasan CF3').

HALOCORTOLONE** (9-chloro-6α,11β-difluoro-21-hydroxy-16α-methylpregna-1,4-diene-3,20-dione; 9-chloro-6α,11β-difluoro-16α-methylpregna-1,4-dien-21-ol-3,20-dione).
HALOFENATE** (2-(*p*-chlorophenyl)-2-(α,α,α-trifluoro-*m*-toloxy)acetic acid ester with *N*-(2-hydroxyethyl)acetamide; 2-acetamidoethyl (*p*-chlorophenyl)(3-trifluoromethylphenoxy)acetate; MK-185; 'livipas').
HALOFUGINONE** ((±)-*trans*-7-bromo-6-chloro-[3-(3-hydroxypiperid-2-yl)-acetonyl]-4(3H)-quinazolinone; 7-bromo-6-chlorofebrifugine).
'Halon' *see* Dichlorodifluoromethane.
HALONAMINE** (2-[[*p*-chloro-α-(*p*-fluorophenyl)benzyl]oxy]ethylamine; 2-(4-chloro-4'-fluorobenzhydryloxy)ethylamine).
HALOPENIUM CHLORIDE** ((*p*-bromobenzyl)[3-(4-chloro-2-isopropyl-5-methylphenoxy)propyl]dimethylammonium chloride).
HALOPERIDIDE (4-(*m*-chlorophenyl)-1-[3-(*p*-fluorophenyl)propyl]-4-(pyrrolidin-1-ylcarbonyl)piperidine; 4-[(4-*m*-chlorophenyl)(4-pyrrolidinamido)piperidino]-4'-fluorobutyrophenone.
HALOPERIDIDE OXALATE (R-3201).
HALOPERIDOL** (4-[4-(*p*-chlorophenyl)-4-hydroxypiperidino]-4'-fluorobutyrophenone; 4-(*p*-chlorophenyl)-1-[3-(*p*-fluorobenzoyl)propyl]-4-piperidinol; McN-JR-1625; R-1625; 'haldol', 'serenace', 'serenase').
See also Buzepide metiodide with haloperidol.
HALOPROGESTERONE** (17α-bromo-6α-fluoro-4-pregnene-3,20-dione; 17α-bromo-6α-fluoroprogesterone; 'prohalone').
HALOPROGIN** (3-iodo-2-propynyl 2,4,5-trichlorophenyl ether; 2,4,5-trichlorophenyl γ-iodopropargyl ether; 2,4,5-trichloro-1-(3-iodo-2-propyn-1-yloxy)benzene; 2,4,5-trichloro-1-(3-iodo-2-propyn-1-yloxy)-benzene; M-1028(Meiji); 'halotex', 'mycanden').
HALOPROPANE (3-bromo-1,1,2,2-tetrafluoropropane).
Halopyramine* *see* Chlorpyramine.
'Halotestin' *see* Fluoxymesterone.
'Halotex' *see* Haloprogin.
HALOTHANE** (2-bromo-2-chloro-1,1,1-trifluoroethane; ftorotan; 'fluothane', 'halan').
HALOXON** (bis(2-chloroethyl)(3-chloro-4-methylcoumarin-7-yl) phosphate; 3-chloro-7-hydroxy-4-methylcoumarin bis(2-chloroethyl)phosphate; 'eustidil').
HALQUINOLS* (mixture of 5-chloro-,

7-chloro- and 5,7-dichloro-8-quinolinols in proportions resulting from chlorination of 8-quinolinol; chlorquinol; CHQ; SQ-16401; 'quinolor', 'quixalin', 'silital', 'tarquinor'). *See also* Chlorquinaldol with halquinols; Triamcinolone with halquinols.

HAMA *see* Aluminium magnesium glycinate.

HAMYCIN** (antibiotic from *Str. pimprina*; 'primamycin').

'**Hanane**' *see* Dimefox.

'**Hansolar**' *see* Acedapsone.

'**Hapamine**' *see* Histamine azoprotein.

Harden-Young ester *see* Fructose 1,6-diphosphate.

HARMALINE (4,9-dihydro-7-methoxy-1-methyl(3H)pyrido(3,4-b)indole).

HARMAN (1-methyl(9H)pyrido(3,4-b)-indole).

HARMINE (7-methoxyharman; banisterine; leucoharmine; telepathine; yageine).

'**Harmogen**' *see* Piperazine estrone sulfate.

'**Harmonyl**' *see* Deserpidine.

'**Harnosal**' *see* Sulfaethidole with sulfamethizole.

'**Harvatrate**' *see* Atropine methonitrate.

'**Harzol**' *see* β-Sitosterol.

Hashimycin *see* Hachimycin.

'**Hasivin**' *see* Oxymetazoline.

'**Hazol**' *see* Oxymetazoline.

HB-113 *see* Chlorpentazide.

HB-419 *see* Glibenclamide.

HBF-386 *see* Cactinomycin.

HBT *see* Tioxolone.

HC-3 *see* Hemicholinium.

HC-606 *see* Hexcarbacholine bromide.

HC-1528 *see* Decoquinate.

HC-8014bis *see* Dimethoate.

HC-8056 *see* Parathion methyl.

HC-8057 *see* Fenitrothion.

HC-8059 *see* Malathion.

HC-8061 *see* Parathion isomethyl.

HCC *see* 25-Hydroxycolecalciferol.

HCG *see* Chorionic gonadotrophin.

HCS-3260 *see* Chlordane.

'**H-dulapine**' *see* Clofedanol noscapine succinate.

HE-111 *see* Dexamethasone isonicotinate.

He-682 *see* Etofylline nicotinate.

'**Hebaral**' *see* Hexethal.

'**Hebucol**' *see* Cyclobutyrol.

'**Heclox**' *see* Cloxacillin with hetacillin.

HECYLAMINE (2-cyclohexyl-*N*-hexylethylamine; (2-hexylaminoethyl)cyclohexane).

HEDAQUINIUM CHLORIDE*** (2,2'-hexadecamethylenebis(isoquinolinium chloride); BIQ-16; 'fungifral', 'teoquil').

'**Hedex**' *see* Paracetamol.

HEDONOL (2-pentyl carbamate; methyl propyl carbinol carbamate).

HEFILCON A* (poly(2-hydroxyethyl 2-methyl-2-propenoate); poly(2-hydroxyethyl methacrylate); 'Brucker lens').

'**Helbucol**' *see* Cyclobutyrol sodium.

'**Helcosol**' *see* Bismuth gallate.

Helenin *see* Alantolactone.

'**Helfergin**' *see* Meclofenoxate.

'**Helfo-dopa**' *see* Levodopa.

HELIOMYCIN*** (antibiotic from *Actinomyces flavochromogenes* var. *heliomycini*).

'**Heliophan**' *see* Homosalate.

'**Helmex**' *see* Pyrantel embonate.

'**Helmezine**' *see* Piperazine citrate.

'**Helmicid**' *see* Piperazine.

'**Helminal**' *see* Kainic acid.

'**Helminthex**' *see* Piperazine citrate.

'**Helmitol**' *see* Methenamine anhydromethylenecitrate.

'**Helmodym-88**' *see* Levulinic acid rare earth salts.

'**Helmox**' *see* Cyacetacide.

HEMATIN (ferriheme hydroxide; ferriporphyrin hydroxide; hydroxyhemin; 'phenodin').

Hematin-protein *see* Cytochrome c.

Hematin reduction product *see* Heme.

HEMATOPORPHYRIN (2,4-bis(1-hydroxyethyl)-1,3,5,8-tetramethylporphine-6,7-dipropionic acid; 'photodyn', 'porfyron'). *See also* Mercury hematoporphyrin.

HEME (ferroheme; ferroporphyrin; haem; protoheme; reduced hematin; ferrous complex of 1,3,5,8-tetramethyl-2,4-divinyl-porphine-6,7-dipropionic acid).

'**Hemeran**' *see* Calcium methyl polygalacturonate sulfonate complex(es).

HEMICHOLINIUM No. 3 (4',4'''-biacetophenone-2,2''-bis[dimethyl(2-hydroxyethyl)ammonium bromide]; α,α'-dimethylethanolamino-4,4'-biacetophenone; HC-3).

'**Hemi-daonil**' *see* Glibenclamide.

Hemiglobin *see* Methemoglobin.

3,4,5-Hemimellitinol *N*-methylcarbamate ester *see* 3,4,5-Trimethylphenyl methylcarbamate.

HEMIN (chlorohemin; ferriheme chloride; ferriporphyrin chloride; Teichmann's crystals; ferrichloride of 2,4-divinyl-1,3,5,8-tetramethylporphine-6,7-dipropionic acid).

'**Hemineurine**' *see* Clomethiazole edisilate.

'**Heminevrine**' *see* Clomethiazole edisilate.

Hemitiamine (tr) *see* Clomethiazole edisilate.

'**Hemiton**' *see* Clonidine.

'**Hemocaprol**' *see* Aminocaproic acid.

HEMOCOAGULASE ('reptilase').

'**Hemodyn I**' *see* Povidone.

'**Hemo-pak**' *see* Oxidized cellulose.

'**Hemostat**' *see* Mepesulfate.

'**Hemostop**' *see* Naftazone.

'**Hemostypt**' *see* Snake venom(s).

'**Hemotabs**' *see* Cetaceum.

HEMPA (hexamethylphosphoric triamide; hexamethylphosphamide; hexamethylphosphoramide; gemfa; HMPA; HMPT; 'hexametapol').

Hendecanoic acid *see* Undecanoic acid.

Hendecenoic acid *see* Undecenoic acid.

HEOD *see* Dieldrin.

'**Hepa-Merz**' *see* Ornithine aspartate.

'**Hepaldine**' *see* Timonacic.

'**Heparcholine**' *see* Choline.

'**Heparegene**' *see* Timonacic.

HEPARIN** (heparin sodium; 'contusol',

'pularin', 'thromboliquin', 'thrombophob', 'thrombo-vetren', 'trombo-vetren', 'vetren'). *See also* Batroxobin with heparin; Magnesium heparinate.

β-HEPARIN (chondroitinsulfuric acid B; 'beparin').

HEPARIN CALCIUM ('caliparin').

'Heparin-degranol' *see* Mannomustine heparinate.

HEPARIN POTASSIUM ('clarin', 'lipohepin', 'liquaemin', 'liquemin', 'panhepin').

Heparin sodium *see* Heparin.

'Heparlipon' *see* Thioctic acid.

'Heparoid' *see* Mepesulfate.

'Hepartest' *see* Sulfobromphthalein.

'Hep-A-stat' *see* Nitarsone.

'Hepasulfol' *see* Anethole trithione.

Hepatin *see* Glycogen.

'Hepatotestbrom' *see* Sulfobromphthalein.

'Hepbisul' *see* Heptyl aldehyde bisulfite compound.

'Hepoid' *see* Sodium polyanhydromannuronic acid sulfate.

'Heporal' *see* Anethole trithione.

HEPRONICATE*** (2-hexyl-2-hydroxymethyl-1,3-propanediol trinicotinate).

'Hepsan' *see* Acetylmethionine choline salt.

HEPTABARB*** (5-cyclohept-1-enyl-5-ethylbarbituric acid; heptabarbital; heptabarbitone; heptamal; 'medapan', 'medomin').

Heptabarbital* *see* Heptabarb.

Heptabarbitone* *see* Heptabarb.

HEPTACHLOR* (1,4,5,6,7,8,8-heptachloro-3a,4,7,7c-tetrahydro-4,7-methanoindene).

Heptachlorotetrahydromethanoindene *see* Heptachlor.

2-Heptadecyl-4,5-dihydro-1H-imidazole acetate *see* Glyodin.

Heptadrine *see* Tuaminoheptane.

Heptaldehyde *see* Heptyl aldehyde.

Heptamal* *see* Heptabarb.

HEPTAMETHYLENIMINE (azacyclooctane; octahydroazocine; perhydroazocine).

1-(2-Heptamethyleniminomethyl)guanidine *see* Guanazodine.

'Heptamine' *see* Octodrine *and* Tuaminoheptane.

HEPTAMINOL*** (6-amino-2-methyl-2-heptanol; heptaminol hydrochloride; 6-hydroxy-6-methyl-2-heptylamine; RP-2831).
See also Deanol pyroglutamate with heptaminol.

Heptaminol acefyllinate *see* Heptaminol theophyllineacetate.

HEPTAMINOL THEOPHYLLINE-ACETATE (heptaminol acefyllinate; heptaminol theophylline ethanoate; TEH; MD-6260; 'cariamyl', 'theo-heptylon').
See also Cinnarizine with heptaminol theophyllineacetate.

Heptaminol theophylline ethanoate *see* Heptaminol theophyllineacetate.

'Heptanal' *see* Methadone.

1-Heptanecarboxylic acid *see* Octanoic acid.

1,7-Heptanedicarboxylic acid *see* Azelaic acid.

Heptanedioic acid *see* Pimelic acid.

Heptanoic acid *see* Enanthic acid.

4-HEPTANONE (butyrone; dipropyl ketone).

HEPTAVERINE*** (2-(3-dimethylamino-1-phenylpropylidene)norbornane; N,N-dimethyl-γ-phenyl-$\Delta^{2,\gamma}$-norbornanepropylamine).

'Heptedrine' *see* Tuaminoheptane.

Heptobarbital *see* Mephebarbital.

HEPTOLAMIDE*** (1-cycloheptyl-3-(p-toluenesulfonyl)urea).

HEPTYL ALDEHYDE (enanthaldehyde; enanthal; heptaldehyde; heptanal; oenanthal).

HEPTYL ALDEHYDE BISULFITE COMPOUND ('hepbisul').

2-Heptylamine *see* Tuaminoheptane.

Heptylic acid *see* Enanthic acid.

Heptylpenicillin *see* Penicillin K.

HEPZIDINE*** (4-(10,11-dihydro-5H-dibenzo(a,d)cyclohepten-5-yloxy)-1-methylpiperidine; BS-7051).

'Heraclene' *see* Cobamamide.

'Heraldium' *see* Mecloralurea.

'Herban' *see* Noruron.

'Herbatox-D-500' *see* Dimethylamine dichlorophenoxyacetate.

'Herbesser' *see* Diltiazem.

HERBIPOLIN (2-amino-6-7,7-dimethylhydroxypurine).

'Hercules-528' *see* p-Dioxane-2,3-diyl ethyl phosphorodithioate.

'Herkol' *see* Dichlorvos.

Heroin *see* Diamorphine.

'Herplex' *see* Idoxuridine.

'Heruclin' *see* Histidine.

'Herulcin' *see* Histidine.

'Hesotanol' *see* Etofylline nicotinate.

'Hesotin' *see* Etofylline nicotinate.

'Hespan' *see* Hetastarch.

'Hespander' *see* Hetastarch.

HESPERETIN (trihydroxy-4'-methoxy-3',5,7-flavanone; hesperitin).

HESPERIDIN (hesperetin 7-rhamnoglucoside).

HESPERIDIN METHYL CHALCONE ('acti-5', 'pev-gram').

Hesperitin *see* Hesperetin.

'Hetabiotic' *see* Hetacillin.

HETACILLIN** (6-(2,2-dimethyl-5-oxo-4-phenyl-1-imidazolidinyl)penicillanic acid; phenazacillin; hetacillin potassium; penicinate; BL-P-804; BRL-804; 'hetabiotic', 'penplenum', 'versapen').
See also Cloxacillin with hetacillin; Dicloxacillin with hetacillin.

HETAFLUR*** (hexadecylamine hydrofluoride; SK&F-2208).

HETASTARCH* (2-hydroxyethyl starch; 'hespan', 'hespander').

Heteroauxin *see* 3-Indoleacetic acid.

HETERONIUM BROMIDE*** (3-hydroxy-1,1-dimethylpyrrolidinium bromide α-phenyl-2-thiopheneglycolate; L-31814; 'hetrum bromide').

'Hetol' see Sodium cinnamate.

'Hetolin' see Tris(p-chlorophenyl)propionic acid 4-methylpiperazide.

HETP see Hexaethyl tetraphosphate.

'Hetrazan' see Diethylcarbamazine.

'Hetrum' see Heteronium.

'Hexabalm' see Hexachlorophene.

Hexabendine see Hexobendine.

'Hexabolan' see Trenbolone cyclohexyl-methylcarbonate.

HEXACAMPHAMINE[*] (methenamine (+)-camphorate; 'amphotropin', 'arocan', 'zymarocan').

Hexacarbacholine see Hexcarbacholine.

'Hexachloran' see Lindane.

Hexachlorane (tr) see Lindane.

HEXACHLOROBENZENE (perchloro-benzene; Julin's carbon chloride; 'anti-carie', 'bunt-cure', 'bunt-no-more').

1,2,3,4,7,7-Hexachloro-5,6-bis(chloro-methyl)bicyclo(2.2.1)hept-2-ene see Chlorbicyclen.

1,4,5,6,7,7-Hexachloro-5,6-bis(chloro-methyl)norbornene see Chlorbicyclen.

Hexachlorocyclohexane see Lindane.

HEXACHLOROETHANE (fasciolin; carbon hexachloride; perchloroethane; 'alvothane', 'distowet').

6,7,8,9,10,10-Hexachloro-1,5,5a,6,9,9a-hexahydro-6,9-methano-2,4,3-benzo-dioxathiepin 3-oxide see Endosulfan.

Hexachloronorbornene 5,6-bis(oxy-methylene) sulfite see Endosulfan.

3,4,5,6,9,9-Hexachloro-1a,2,2a,3,6,6a,7,7a-octahydro-2,7:3,6-dimethanonaphth-(2,3-b)oxirene see Dieldrin and Endrin.

Hexachlorophane[*] see Hexachlorophene.

HEXACHLOROPHENE[***] (2,2'-methyl-enebis(3,4,6-trichlorophenol); hexachloro-dihydroxydiphenylmethane; hexachloro-phane; AT-7; G-11; 'almederm', 'cidal', 'curaglymol', 'dial', 'dimiplex', 'exofene', 'fasciophene', 'gamophen', 'germa-medica', 'hexabalm', 'hex-o-san', 'pHisohex', 'surgi-cen', 'surofene', 'tod'l', 'trisophene').

HEXACHLOROPHENE WITH PHENYL-MERCURIC BORATE ('remanex').

HEXACHLOROPHENE PHOSPHATE (hexachlorophene monophosphate; Ph-1503).

Hexachloro-p-xylene see 1,4-Bis(trichloro-methyl)benzene.

Hexacitramine see Methenamine anhydro-methylenecitrate.

'Hexacol' see Alloclamide.

HEXACYCLINE (tetracycline addition product with sodium hexametaphosphate; tetracycline phosphate complex; 'bristaci-clina A', 'sumycin', 'tetrex', 'tevacycl-ine').

HEXACYCLINE WITH AMPHOTERI-CIN B ('amphocycline').

Hexacyclonate see Sodium hexacyclonate.

HEXACYCLONIC ACID (1-(hydroxy-methyl)cyclohexaneacetic acid; 4-hydroxy-3,3-pentamethylenebutyric acid; β,β-penta-methylene-γ-hydroxybutyric acid).
See also Sodium hexacyclonate.

HEXACYPRONE[***] (1-benzyl-2-oxocyclo-hexanepropionic acid).

Hexadecadrol see Dexamethasone.

2,2'-Hexadecamethylenebis(isoquino-linium chloride) see Hedaquinium chloride.

Hexadecanoic acid see Palmitic acid.

1-HEXADECANOL (cetyl alcohol; cetanol; ethal).

HEXADECYLAMINE (cetylamine).

Hexadecylamine hydrofluoride see Hetaflur.

α-Hexadecylcitric acid see Agaricic acid.

Hexadecyl(hydroxycyclohexyl)dimethyl-ammonium bromide see Cethexonium.

Hexadecyltrimethylammonium bromide see Cetrimonium.

HEXADECYLTRIMETHYLAMMONIUM PENTACHLOROPHENATE (cetyl-trimethylammonium pentachlorophenate; TCAP).

2,4-Hexadienoic acid see Sorbic acid.

HEXADILINE[***] (2-(2,2-dicyclohexylvinyl)-piperidine).

HEXADIMETHRINE BROMIDE[***] (N,N,N',N'-tetramethyl-1,6-hexanedi-amine polymer with 1,3-dibromopropane; polymer of N,N,N',N'-tetramethyl-N-tri-methylenehexamethylenediammonium dibromide; N,N,N',N'-tetramethyl-hexamethylenediamine trimethylene bromide polymer; 'polybrene').

HEXADIPHANE[*] (1-(3,3-diphenylpropyl)-hexahydroazepine; 1,1-diphenyl-3-hexa-methyleniminopropane).

HEXADIPHANE WITH MOPERONE ('sedalium').

Hexadiphensulfonium[*] see Hexasonium.

HEXADISTIGMINE (hexamethylene-1,6-bis[[m-(N-methylcarbamoyloxy)phenyl]-trimethylammonium bromide]; BC-40).

'Hexadrol' see Dexamethasone.

HEXAETHYL TETRAPHOSPHATE (HETP; hexastigmine; 'bladan', 'blodon').

Hexafluorenium[*] see Hexafluronium.

Hexafluorodiethyl ether see Flurotyl.

HEXAFLUOROISOPROPYL METHYL ETHER (flurotyl isomer; 'isoindokolon').

HEXAFLURONIUM BROMIDE[***] (hexamethylenebis(fluoren-9-yldimethyl-ammonium bromide); hexafluorenium; IN-117; 'mylaxen').

HEXAHOMOSERINE (2-amino-6-hydroxy-hexanoic acid; α-amino-ε-hydroxycaproic acid; 6-hydroxynorleucine).

Hexahydroadiphenine see Drofenine.

Hexahydroaminoethanophenanthrene see Morphinan.

Hexahydroazepine see Hexamethylenimine.

Hexahydro-1H-azepine-1-carbothioic acid S-ethyl ester see Molinate.

4-Hexahydroazepin-1-yl-2,2-diphenyl-butyramide methiodide see Buzepide

234

metiodide.

2-(Hexahydro-1H-azepin-1-yl)ethyl α-cyclohexyl-3-thiopheneacetate *see* Cetiedil.

1-(2-Hexahydroazepin-1-ylethyl)-2-oxo-cyclohexanecarboxylic acid benzyl ester *see* Amicibone.

1-(Hexahydro-1H-azepin-1-yl)-3-(indan-5-ylsulfonyl)urea *see* Glidazamide.

6-[[(Hexahydro-1H-azepin-1-yl)-methylene]amino]penicillanic acid *see* Mecillinam.

6-[(Hexahydroazepin-1-ylmethylene)-amino]penicillanic acid pivaloyloxy-methyl ester *see* Pivmecillinam.

1-(Hexahydro-1H-azepin-1-yl)-3-[[p-[2-(5-methyl-3-isoxazolecarboxamido)ethyl]-phenyl]sulfonyl]urea *see* Glisoxepide.

3-Hexahydroazepin-1-yl-3'-nitro-propiophenone *see* Fenitron.

1-(Hexahydro-1H-azepin-1-yl)-3-(p-tolu-enesulfonyl)urea *see* Tolazamide.

3-[4-(Hexahydroazepin-1-ylureidosul-fonyl)phenethylcarbamoyl]-5-methyl-isoxazole *see* Glisoxepide.

1-[(2-Hexahydro-1(2H)-azocinyl)ethyl]-guanidine *see* Guanethidine.

1,2,3,4,5,6-Hexahydro-2,3'-bipyridine *see* Anabasine.

Hexahydrodesoxyephedrine *see* Propyl-hexedrine.

HEXAHYDRO-1H-1,4-DIAZEPINE
(1,4-diazacycloheptane; homopiperazine).

Hexahydro-3,6-dimethyl-γ-carboline *see* Dicarbine.

Hexahydro-3α,7α-dimethyl-4,7-epoxyiso-benzofuran-1,3-dione *see* Cantharidin.

1,2,3,4,5,6-Hexahydro-6,11-dimethyl-3-(3-methyl-2-butenyl)-2,6-methano-3-benzazocin-8-ol *see* Pentazocine.

8,9,10,11,11a,12-Hexahydro-8,10-dimethyl-7aH-naphtho(1',2':5,6)pyrano(3,2-c)-pyridin-7a-ol *see* Naranol.

1,2,3,4,5,6-Hexahydro-6,11-dimethyl-3-phenethyl-2,6-methano-3-benzazocin-8-ol *see* Phenazocine.

Hexahydro-1,3-dimethyl-4-phenylazepine-4-carboxylic acid ethyl ester *see* Metethoheptazine.

Hexahydro-1,2-dimethyl-4-phenylazepine-4-carboxylic acid methyl ester *see* Metheptazine.

Hexahydro-1,3-dimethyl-4-phenylazepin-4-ol propionate ester *see* Proheptazine.

2,3,4,4a,5,9b-Hexahydro-2,8-dimethyl-1H-pyrido(4,3-b)indole *see* Dicarbine.

Hexahydro-α,α-diphenylpyrrolo(1,2-a)-pyrazine-2(1H)-butyramide *see* Pirolazamide.

1,2,3,4,5,6-Hexahydro-8-hydroxy-6,11-dimethyl-3-(3-methyl-2-butenyl)-2,6-methano-3-benzazocine *see* Pentazocine.

8,9,14,15,24,25-Hexahydro-14-hydroxy-4,12-dimethyl-3-(1-methylethyl)-3H-21,18-nitrilo-1H,22H-pyrrolo(2,1-c)-(1,8,4,19)dioxadiazacyclotetracosine-1,7,16,22(4H,17H)-tetrone *see* Virginia-

mycin M_1.

1,2,3,4,5,6-Hexahydro-8-hydroxy-6,11-di-methyl-3-phenethyl-2,6-methanobenz-azocine *see* Phenazocine.

5-[3-[Hexahydro-1-(2-hydroxyethyl)-1H-1,4-diazepin-4-yl]propyl]-5H-dibenzo-(b,f)azepine *see* Homopipramol.

10-[3-[Hexahydro-1-(2-hydroxyethyl)-1H-1,4-diazepin-4-yl]propyl]-2-(trifluoro-methyl)phenothiazine *see* Homofenazine.

8,9,14,15,24,25-Hexahydro-14-hydroxy-3-isopropyl-4,12-dimethyl-3H-21,18-nitrilo-1H,22H-pyrrolo(2,1-c)(1,8,4,19)-dioxadiazacyclotetracosine-1,7,16,22-(4H,17H)-tetrone *see* Virginiamycin M_1.

2,3,5,6,7,7aα-Hexahydro-7β-hydroxy-1H-pyrrolizine-1β-methanol *see* Platynecine.

1,2,3,4,5,6-Hexahydro-8-hydroxy-3,6,11-tri-methyl-2,6-methanobenzazocine *see* Metazocine.

1,3,4,6,7,11b-Hexahydro-3-isobutyl-9,10-dimethoxy-2H-benzo(a)quinolizin-2-one *see* Tetrabenazine.

1-(3a,4,5,6,7,7a-Hexahydro-4,7-methano-indan-5-yl)-3,3-dimethylurea *see* Noruron.

(+)-cis-1,3,4,9,10,10a-Hexahydro-6-meth-oxy-11-methyl-2H-10,4a-iminoethano-phenanthrene *see* Dextromethorphan.

5,6,7,7a,8,9-Hexahydro-3-methoxy-10-methyl-4aH-8,9c-iminoethanophenan-thro(4,5-bcd)furan-5-ol *see* Dihydroco-deine.

1,2,3,4,10,14b-Hexahydro-2-methyldi-benzo(c,f)pyrazino(1,2-a)azepine *see* Mianserin.

(+)-cis-1,3,4,9,10,10a-Hexahydro-11-methyl-2H-10,4a-iminoethanophenan-thren-6-ol *see* Dextrorphan.

2-(Hexahydro-1-methylindolin-3-yl)ethyl benzilate *see* Metindizate.

4,6,6a,7,8,9-Hexahydro-7-methylindolo-(4,3-fg)quinoline-9-carboxylic acid diethylamide *see* Lysergide.

Hexahydro-1-methyl-4-phenylazepine-carboxylic acid ethyl ester *see* Ethohept-azine.

1,3,6,7,8,9-Hexahydro-5-phenyl-2H-(1)-benzothieno(2,3-e)-1,4-diazepin-2-one *see* Bentazepam.

Hexahydropicolinic acid *see* Pipecolic acid.

Hexahydropyrazine *see* Piperazine.

1,3,4,6,7,11b-Hexahydro-2H-pyrazino-(2,1-a)isoquinoline *see* Azaquinzole.

Hexahydropyridine *see* Piperidine.

2-(Hexahydropyrrolo(1,2-a)pyrazin-2(1H)-yl)ethyl 2-trifluoromethylpheno-thiazin-10-yl ketone *see* Azaftozine.

10-(3-(Hexahydropyrrolo(1,2-a)pyrazin-2-(1H)-yl)propionyl)-2-trifluoromethyl-phenothiazine *see* Azaftozine.

Hexahydro-2(1H)-[2-[(2-trifluoromethyl-phenothiazin-10-yl)carbonyl]ethyl]-pyrrolo(1,2-a)pyrazine *see* Azaftozine.

Hexahydro-4-[3-(2-trifluoromethylpheno-thiazin-10-yl)propyl]-(1H)1,4-diazepine-

235

1-ethanol see Homofenazine.
Hexahydroxycyclohexane see Inositol.
1,1',6,6',7,7'-Hexahydroxy-5,5'-diiso-propyl-3,3'-dimethyl(2,2'-dinaphthal-ene)-8,8'-dicarboxaldehyde see Gossypol.
1β,3β,5,11α,14,19-Hexahydroxy-5β-card-20(22)-enolide 3-L-rhamnoside see Ouabain.
4,5,7,4',5',7'-Hexahydroxy-2,2'-dimethyl-naphthodianthone see Hypericin.
Hexahydroxydiphenic acid dilactone see Ellagic acid.
5,6,9,17,19,21-Hexahydroxy-23-methoxy-2,4,12,16,18,20,22-heptamethyl-2,7-(epoxypentadeca(1,11,13)trienimino)-naphtho(2,1-b)furan-1,11(2H)-dione 21-acetate see Rifamycin.
Hexakis(1-aziridinyl) phosphonitrilate see Apholate.
Hexakis(hydroxymethyl)melamine see Hexamethylolmelamine.
Hexakis(1-methyl-2-phenylpropyl)-distannoxane see Neostanox.
Hexaklor see BHC.
'Hexal' see Methenamine sulfosalicylate.
'Hexalet' see Methenamine sulfosalicylate.
'Hexalgon' see Norpipanone.
'Hexaloid' see Methenamine.
'Hexamandelate' see Methenamine mande-late.
'Hexametapol' see Hempa.
Hexamethonium benzenesulfonate see Hexamethonium besilate.
HEXAMETHONIUM BESILATE (hexa-methonium benzenesulfonate; hexonium B).
HEXAMETHONIUM BROMIDE*** (hexa-methylene-1,6-bis(trimethylammonium bromide); hexonium; C-6; P-4420).
Hexamethylenamine see Methenamine.
Hexamethylene see Cyclohexane.
Hexamethylenebis[(2-carbamoyloxy-ethyl)dimethylammonium bromide] see Hexcarbacholine bromide.
1,1'-Hexamethylenebis[5-(p-chlorophen-yl)biguanide] see Chlorhexidine.
Hexamethylene-1,6-bis[dimethyl-[1-methyl-3-(2,2,6-trimethylcyclohexyl)-propyl]ammonium chloride] see Tri-clobisonium.
1,1'-Hexamethylenebis[5-(2-ethylhexyl)-biguanide] see Alexidine.
Hexamethylenebis(fluoren-9-yldimethyl-ammonium bromide) see Hexafluronium bromide.
α,α'-[Hexamethylenebis(iminomethyl-ene)]bis(3,4-dihydroxybenzyl alcohol) see Hexoprenaline.
Hexamethylene-1,6-bis[[m-(N-methyl-carbamoyloxy)phenyl]trimethyl-ammonium bromide] see Hexadistig-mine.
Hexamethylene-1,6-bis[1-methyl-3-(methylcarbamoyloxy)pyridinium bromide] see Distigmine.
N,N'-Hexamethylenebis(noradrenaline) see Hexoprenaline.
Hexamethylene-1,6-bis(trimethylam-

monium bromide) see Hexamethonium.
4,4'-Hexamethylenedioxydibenzamidine see Hexamidine.
6-[N,N-(1,6-Hexamethylene)formami-dino]penicillanic acid see Mecillinam.
Hexamethylenetetramine see Methenamine.
1,1-Hexamethylene-4-(p-toluenesulfonyl)-semicarbazide see Tolazamide.
HEXAMETHYLENIMINE (hexahydro-azepine; azacycloheptane; perhydro-azepine).
4-(N-Hexamethylenimino)-2,2-diphenyl-butyramide methiodide see Buzepide metiodide.
2-Hexamethyleniminoethyl α-cyclohexa-ne-3-thiopheneacetate see Cetiedil.
2-Hexamethyleniminoethyl α-thien-2-ylcyclohexaneacetate see Cetiedil.
3-Hexamethylenimino-3'-nitropropio-phenone see Fenitron.
HEXAMETHYLMELAMINE (NSC-13875).
HEXAMETHYLOLMELAMINE (2,4,6-tris-[di(hydroxymethyl)amino]-3-triazine; hexakis(hydroxymethyl)melamine; (s-tri-azine-2,4,6-triyltrinitrilo)hexamethanol; trimethylolmelamine; Cilag-61; 'cealysin').
Hexamethylpararosaniline hydrochloride see Crystal violet.
Hexamethylphosphamide see Hempa.
Hexamethylphosphoramide see Hempa.
Hexamethylphosphoric triamide see Hempa.
HEXAMETHYLTEPA (tris(2,2-dimethyl-aziridin-1-yl)phosphine oxide; tepa-132).
Hexamethyltetracosahexaene see Squalene.
Hexamethyl violet see Crystal violet.
Hexamic acid see Cyclamic acid.
Hexamidin (tr) see Primidone.
HEXAMIDINE*** (4,4'-hexamethylene-dioxydibenzamidine; 'hexomilone').
Hexamidine diisethionate see Hexamidine isetionate.
HEXAMIDINE ISETIONATE (hexamidine di(ethanol-2-sulfonate); hexamidine diisethionate; RP-2535; 'hexomedine', 'ophtamedine').
See also Benzydamine with hexamidine isetionate.
Hexamine* see Methenamine.
Hexanaphthene see Cyclohexane.
1-Hexanecarboxylic acid see Enanthic acid.
1,6-Hexanedioic acid see Suberic acid.
'Hexanicit' see Inositol nicotinate.
'Hexanicotol' see Inositol nicotinate.
'Hexanitrin' see Mannityl hexanitrate.
'Hexanitrol' see Mannityl hexanitrate.
HEXANOIC ACID (1-pentanecarboxylic acid; caproic acid; butylacetic acid).
tert-Hexanol carbamate see Emylcamate.
HEXANOPHENONE (caprophenone; pentyl phenyl ketone).
HEXAPHOSPHAMIDE (tr) (N-cyclohexyl-N',N''-diethylenephosphorotioic triamide; bis(1-aziridinyl)(cyclohexylamino)phos-phine sulfide).
'Hexapneumine' see Biclotymol.

HEXAPRADOL* (α-(1-aminohexyl)benzhydrol).
HEXAPROFEN (2-(4-cyclohexylphenyl)propionic acid; p-cyclohexylhydratropic acid; BTS-13622).
HEXAPROPYMATE* (1-(2-propynyl)-cyclohexanol carbamate; propargylcyclohexanol carbamate; propynylcyclohexyl carbamate; L-2103; 'merinax', 'modirax').
Hexasone* see Hexasonium.
HEXASONIUM IODIDE* ((2-hydroxyethyl)dimethylsulfonium iodide α-phenylcyclohexaneacetate; [2-(cyclohexylphenylacetoxyethyl)]dimethylsulfonium iodide; hexadiphensulfonium iodide; hexasone; 'thiospasmin').
Hexastigmine see Hexaethyl tetraphosphate.
'Hexatrione' see Triamcinolone hexacetonide.
'Hexaverm' see Lindane.
'Hexayodina' see Prolonium iodide.
HEXCARBACHOLINE BROMIDE* (choline bromide hexamethylenedicarbamate; hexamethylenebis[(2-carbamoyloxyethyl)dimethylammonium bromide]; carbolonium bromide; hexacarbacholine bromide; HC-606; 'imbretil').
'Hexchloran' see Lindane.
HEXEDINE* (2,6-bis(2-ethylhexyl)hexahydro-7a-methyl-1H-imidazo (1,5-c)-imidazole; W-4701; 'sterisol').
Hexemal see Cyclobarbital.
Hexenal (tr) see Hexobarbital.
3-Hexenoic acid see Hydrosorbic acid.
δ-Hexenolactone see Parasorbic acid.
Hexenolide see Parasorbic acid.
HEXESTROL* (4,4'-(1,2-diethylethylene)-diphenol; α,α'-diethyl-4,4'-dihydroxybibenzyl; 3,4-bis(p-hydroxyphenyl)hexane; hexoestrol; synestrol; dihydrodiethylstilbestrol; dihydrostilbestrol; NSC-9894).
HEXETHAL* (5-ethyl-5-hexylbarbituric acid; hexethal sodium; 'hebaral', 'ortal').
HEXETIDINE* (5-amino-1,3-bis(2-ethylhexyl)hexahydro-5-methylpyrimidine; 'elsix', 'hexetril', 'hexoral', 'oraldene', 'sterisil', 'triocil').
See also Cetylpyridinium chloride with hexetidine.
'Hexetril' see Hexetidine.
Hexicide see Lindane.
HEXOBARBITAL* (5-cyclohexen-1-yl-1,5-dimethylbarbituric acid; ciclobarbital; enhexymal; enimal; hexenal; hexobarbitone; hexobarbitural; methexenyl; methylhexabital; methylhexobarbital; methylcyclobarbital; hexobarbital sodium).
HEXOBENDINE* (3,3'-[ethylenebis-(methylimino)]di-1-propanol 3,4,5-trimethoxybenzoate diester; N,N'-bis[3-(3,4,5-trimethoxybenzoyloxy)propyl]-N,N'-dimethylethylenediamine; hexabendine; hexobendine dihydrochloride; ST-7090; 'andramine', 'reoxyl', 'ustimon').
HEXOCYCLIUM METILSULFATE* (1-(2-cyclohexyl-2-hydroxy-2-phenylethyl)-4,4-dimethylpiperazinium methylsulfate;

4-(β-cyclohexyl-β-hydroxyphenethyl)-1,1-dimethylpiperazinium methylsulfate; 'tral').
Hexoestrol* see Hexestrol.
'Hexo-imotryl' see Benzydamine with hexamidine isetionate.
Hexol see Inositol.
'Hexomedine' see Hexamidine isetionate.
'Hexomilone' see Hexamidine.
Hexonate (tr) see Hexamethonium nicotinate.
'Hexone' see Hexamethonium bromide.
Hexonium (tr) see Hexamethonium bromide.
Hexonium B (tr) Hexamethonium besilate.
'Hexopal' see Inositol nicotinate.
HEXOPRENALINE* (α,α'-[hexamethylenebis(iminomethylene)]bis(3,4-dihydroxybenzyl alcohol); N,N'-hexamethylenebis-(noradrenaline); N,N'-bis[2-(3,4-dihydroxyphenyl)-2-hydroxyethyl]hexamethylenediamine; hexoprenaline hydrochloride; ST-1512; 'ipradol').
HEXOPYRRONIUM BROMIDE* (3-hydroxy-1,1-dimethylpyrrolidinium bromide α-phenylcyclohexaneglycolate; AHR-483).
'Hexoral' see Hexetidine.
'Hex-o-san' see Hexachlorophene.
'Hexyclan' see Lindane.
'Hexydal' see Methenamine mandelate.
'Hexydaline' see Methenamine mandelate.
2-Hexylaminoethylcyclohexane see Hecylamine.
HEXYLCAINE* (benzoate of 1-cyclohexylamino-2-propanol; D-109; 'cyclaine').
1-Hexyl-3,7-dimethylxanthine see Pentifylline.
2-Hexyl-2-hydroxymethyl-1,3-propanediol trinicotinate see Hepronicate.
1-Hexyl-4-(N-isobutylbenzimidoyl)-piperazine see Bucainide.
Hexyl methyl carbinol see 2-Octanol.
1-Hexyl-4-[N-(2-methylpropyl)benzimidoyl]piperazine see Bucainide.
p-HEXYLOXYHYDROCINNAMIC ACID (3-(p-hexyloxyphenyl)propionic acid).
See also Nandrolone p-hexyloxyhydrocinnamate; Testosterone p-hexyloxyhydrocinnamate.
2-(3-Hexyloxy-2-hydroxypropoxy)benzoic acid see Exiproben.
9-(p-Hexyloxyphenyl)-10-methylacridinium chloride see Phenacridan.
3-(p-Hexyloxyphenyl)propionic acid see p-Hexyloxyhydrocinnamic acid.
HEXYLRESORCINOL* (4-hexylresorcinol; 6-hexylresorcinol; 1,3-dihydroxy-4-hexylbenzene; dihydroxyphenylhexane; 4-hexylbenzene-1,3-diol; ST-37; 'caprokol', 'crystoids', 'geloverm', 'prensol', 'prentif', 'sucrets').
Hexylresorcinol 9-aminoacridinium salt see Acrisorcin.
3-Hexyl-7,8,9,10-tetrahydro-6,6,9-trimethyl-6H-dibenzo(b,d)pyran-1-ol see Pyrahexyl.
1-Hexyltheobromine see Pentifylline.
Hexyphenidyl* see Trihexyphenidyl.
Heyden-611 see Stibophen potassium.

HF-1854 see Clozapine.
HF-1927 see Dibenzepin.
HF-2159 see Clotiapine.
HF-2333 see Perlapine.
HFE see Flurothyl.
4-HFU (tr) see p-Chlorophenoxyacetic acid.
HCG see Chorionic gonadotrophin.
HGF see Glucagon.
HH-50 see Vanillylnonamide.
HH-197 see Butamirate.
HHDN see Aldrin.
HHG see Human pituitary gonadotrophin.
HI-56 see Ampicillin with dicloxacillin.
5-HIAA see 5-Hydroxy-3-indoleacetic acid.
HIBENZATE(S) ** (2-(4-hydroxybenzoyl)-
  benzoate(s); 4-hydroxybenzophenone-2-
  carboxylate(s)).
  See also Tipepidine hibenzate.
'Hibicon' see Beclamide.
'Hibiscrub' see Chlorhexidine digluconate.
'Hibitane' see Chlorhexidine.
'Hiconcil' see Amoxicillin.
'Hidacian' see Cyacetacide.
'Hidrea' see Hydroxycarbamide.
'Hidrix' see Hydroxycarbamide.
'Hidrofugal' see Aluminium oxychloride.
'Hi-enterol' see Clioquinol.
'Hi-glucon' see Calcium glucoheptonate.
'Hilomid' see Dibromsalan with tribrom-
  salan.
HINDERIN (3-[4-(3,5-ditert-butyl-4-hydroxy-
  phenoxy)-3,5-diiodophenyl]propionic acid;
  4-(3,5-ditert-butyl-4-hydroxyphenoxy)-3,5-
  diiodohydrocinnamic acid).
Hinokitiol see β-Thujaplicin.
'Hinosan' see Edifenphos.
Hiochic acid see Mevalonic acid.
'Hippocras' see Magnesium orotate.
'Hippodine' see Sodium iodohippurate.
'Hippramine' see Methenamine hippurate.
'Hippuran' see Sodium iodohippurate.
HIPPURIC ACID (N-benzoylglycine).
Hippuric acid hexamine complex see
  Methenamine hippurate.
Hippuric acid methenamine complex see
  Methenamine hippurate.
'Hiprex' see Methenamine hippurate.
Hisfen (tr) see Hisphen.
Hisindamone (tr) see Chlorisondamine.
HISPHEN (tr) (methyl 2-[p-[bis(2-chloro-
  ethyl)amino]phenylacetamido]-3-imidazol-
  4-ylpropionate; N-[p-[bis(2-chloroethyl)-
  amino]phenylacetyl]-L-histidine methyl
  ester; methyl-N-[p-[bis(2-chloroethyl)-
  amino]phenylacetyl]-L-histidinate; hisfen;
  MD-2).
'Hispril' see Diphenylpyraline.
'Histabromazine' see Bromazine.
'Histabutazine' see Buclizine.
Histadoxylamine see Doxylamine.
HISTAGLOBIN (tr) (histamine-γ-globulin
  complex ; 'biobasal AG').
'Histalog' see Betazole.
'Histamethine' see Meclozine.
Histametizine* see Meclozine.
Histaminase see Diamine oxidase.
HISTAMINE (4-(2-aminoethyl)imidazole;

4-imidazoleethylamine).
HISTAMINE AZOPROTEIN COMPLEX
  ('hapamine', 'lertigon').
Histamine-γ-globulin complex see Histaglobin.
Histapyridamine see Pheniramine.
HISTAPYRRODINE** (N-phenyl-N-(2-
  pyrrolid-1-ylethyl)benzylamine; 1-(2-N-
  benzylanilinoethyl)pyrrolidine; 'domistan',
  'luvistin').
Histazylamine see Thonzylamine.
HISTIDINE (L-2-amino-3-(4-imidazole)-
  propionic acid; glyoxaline-5-alanine;
  histidine hydrochloride; 'heruclin', 'herul-
  cin', 'laristin', 'larostidin', 'stellidin',
  'ulcostidine').
'Histoacryl' see Enbucrilate.
'Histol' see Chlorphenoxamine.
'Histostat' see Nitarsone.
'Histryl' see Diphenylpyraline.
'Hitreman' see Dibromsalan with tribrom-
  salan.
Hiyaku see Ginseng.
HL-267 see Diponium bromide.
HL-523 see Tiformin.
HL-1050 see Fenticlor.
HL-7746 see Chlorpromazine.
HLS-831 see Tolbutamide.
HM-11 see Pheniprazine.
HM-51 see Dihydroergotoxine with thiorid-
  azine.
HMD see Oxymetholone.
HMG see Human menopausal gonadotrophin.
HMPA see Hempa.
HMPT see Hempa.
HMS see Medrysone.
HN2 see Chlormethine.
HN3 see Trichlormethine.
Hö-..... see also HOE-.....
Hö-1/93 see Tretamine.
Hö-2374 see Tetranitrocarbazole.
Hö-9980 see Fenpipramide.
Hö-10116 see Feniprane.
Hö-10446 see Hydroxypethidine.
Hö-10582 see Normethadone.
Hö-10600 see Phenadoxone.
Hö-10682 see Diphepanol.
Hö-10720 see Ketobemidone.
Hö-10820 see Methadone.
Hö-11513 see Pheniramine.
Hö-16842 see Bitoscanate.
HOE-..... see also Hö-.....
HOE-019 see Fenclexonium metilsulfate.
HOE-045 see Carticaine.
HOE-105 see Citenazone.
HOE-440 see Tiamenidine.
HOE-471 see Gonadorelin.
HOE-757 see Toprilidine.
HOE-16842 see Bitoscanate.
HOE-36801 see Etifoxine.
HOE-36984 see Nomifensine maleate.
HOE-40045 see Carticaine.
'Hog' see Phencyclidine.
'Hogival' see Estrone acetate.
Holarrhena antidysenterica bark see
  Kurchi.
'Holfidal' see Tetranitrocarbazole.

'**Hollicide**' *see* Bis(tributyltin) oxide.
'**Holocaine**' *see* Phenacaine.
'**Homactid**' *see* Tosactide.
'**Homapin**' *see* Homatropine methyl bromide.
HOMARINE (picolinic acid methylbetaine).
HOMARYLAMINE*** (4-(2-methyl-aminoethyl)-1,2-methylenedioxybenzene; *N*-methyl-3,4-methylenedioxyphenethyl-amine; *N*-methylhomopiperonylamine; homarylamine hydrochloride; MK-7).
'**Homatromide**' *see* Homatropine methyl bromide.
HOMATROPINE (tropine mandelate; mandelyl tropeine).
HOMATROPINE METHYL BROMIDE*** (8-methyltropinium bromide mandelate; 'arkitropin', 'camatropin', 'esopin', 'homapin', 'homatromide', 'malcotran', 'mesopin', 'methatropin', 'novatrin', 'novatropine', 'sethyl').
HOMATROPINE METHYL NITRATE ('atoxatrin').
Homatropine phenacyl chloride *see* Phenactropinium.
Homidium chloride *see* Ethidium chloride.
HOMOANSERINE (*N*-(4-aminobutyryl)-1-methylhistidine).
Homoarterenol *see* Corbadrine.
HOMOCARNOSINE (*N*-(4-aminobutyryl)-histidine).
HOMOCHLORCYCLIZINE*** (1-(*p*-chloro-α-phenylbenzyl)hexahydro-4-methyl-1H-1,4-diazepine; 1-(*p*-chloro-diphenylmethyl)-4-methyl-1,4-diazacyclo-heptane; 1-(*p*-chlorobenzhydryl)-4-methylhomopiperazine; 'homoclomin').
HOMOCHOLINE ((3-hydroxypropyl)-trimethylammonium ion).
'**Homoclomin**' *see* Homochlorcyclizine.
HOMOCOCAINE (ecgonine 3-benzoate 2-ethyl ester; cocaethylin).
Homocodeine *see* Pholcodine.
HOMOCYSTEINE (2-amino-4-mercapto-butyric acid).
HOMOCYSTINE (4,4'-dithiobis(2-amino-butyric acid)).
HOMOERIODICTYOL (3'-methoxy-4',5,7-trihydroxyflavanone; eriodictyol 3'-methyl ether; eriodictyonone).
HOMOFENAZINE*** (hexahydro-4-[3-(2-trifluoromethylphenothiazin-10-yl)propyl]-1H-1,4-diazepine-1-ethanol; 10-[3-[hexa-hydro-1-(2-hydroxyethyl)-1H-1,4-diazepin-4-yl]propyl]-2-(trifluoromethyl)phenothia-zine; 10-[3-[4-(2-hydroxyethyl)-1,4-diaza-cyclohept-1-yl]propyl]-2-trifluoromethyl-phenothiazine; 1-(2-hydroxyethyl)-4-[3-(2-trifluoromethyl)phenothiazin-10-ylpropyl]-homopiperazine; homofenazine hydro-chloride; 'pasaden').
HOMOGENTISIC ACID (2-(2,5-dihydroxy-phenyl)acetic acid; 2,5-dihydroxy-α-toluic acid; alcapton; alcaptonic acid).
Homomenthyl salicylate *see* Homosalate.
Homomyrtenyloxytriethylamine *see* Myrtecaine.

Homopantothenic acid *see* Hopantenic acid.
Homophenothiazine *see* 10,11-Dihydrodi-benzo(b,f)(1,4)thiazepine.
Homopiperazine *see* Hexahydro-1,4-diazepine.
Homopiperazine-1,4-dipropanol *see* Biopropazepan.
HOMOPIPRAMOL*** (4-[3-(5H-dibenz-(b,f)azepin-5-yl)propyl]hexahydro-1H-1,4-diazepine-1-ethanol; 4-[3-(5H-dibenz-(b,f)azepin-5-yl)propyl]-1-(2-hydroxyethyl)-homopiperazine; 5-[3-[hexahydro-1-(2-hydroxyethyl)-1H-1,4-diazepin-4-yl]-propyl]-5H-dibenz(b,f)azepine).
Homoproline *see* Pipecolic acid.
HOMOPROTOCATECHUIC ACID (3,4-dihydroxyphenylacetic acid; DOPAC).
Homopyrimidazole *see* 4H-Pyrido(1,2-a)-pyrimidine.
HOMOSALATE*** (3,3,5-trimethyl-cyclohexyl salicylate; homomenthyl salicyl-ate; 'heliophan').
p-**Homosalicylic acid** *see* 2,5-Cresotic acid.
HOMOSERINE (2-amino-4-hydroxybutyric acid).
Homosulfamide *see* Mafenide.
Homosulfamine *see* Mafenide.
Homosulfanilamide *see* Mafenide.
HOMOTHIAMINE (3-(4-amino-2-ethyl-5-pyrimidylmethyl)-5-(2-hydroxyethyl)-4-methylthiazolium chloride).
HOMOVANILLIC ACID (2-(4-hydroxy-3-methoxyphenyl)acetic acid).
HOMOVANILLIDENEISONIAZID (*N*'-homovanillideneisoniazid; 3-ethoxy-4-hydroxybenzaldehyde isonicotinoyl-hydrazone; homovanillin isonicotinoyl-hydrazone; isonicotinic acid homovanillid-enehydrazide; 'bourbonal-IHN').
HOMOVANILLIN (3-ethoxy-4-hydroxy-benzaldehyde; O-desmethyl-O-ethyl-vanillin; ethylprotocatechuic aldehyde; ethylprotal; ethylvanillin; 'bourbonal', 'ethavan', 'ethovan', 'vanillal').
Homovanillin isonicotinoylhydrazone *see* Homovanillideneisoniazid.
HOMOVERATRYLAMINE (3,4-dimeth-oxyphenethylamine; DMPEA).
HOMPRENORPHINE*** (*N*-cyclopropyl-methyl-7α-(1-(R)-hydroxy-1-methylpropyl)-6,14-*endo*-ethenotetrahydronorthebaine; 22-cyclopropyl-7α-((R)-1-hydroxy-1-methyl-propyl)-6,14-*endo*-ethenotetrahydro-thebaine; R&S 5205-M).
'**Honvan**' *see* Fosfestrol.
HOPA *see* Hopantenic acid.
HOPANTENIC ACID*** (D-(+)-4-(2,4-di-hydroxy-3,3-dimethylbutyramido)butyric acid; homopantothenic acid; HOPA).
HOQUIZIL*** (2-hydroxy-2-methylpropyl 4-(6,7-dimethoxyquinazolin-4-yl)piper-azine-1-carboxylate; hoquizil hydrochloride; CP-14185-1).
HORDENINE (*p*-(2-dimethylaminoethyl)-phenol; *p*-hydroxyl-*N*,*N*-dimethylphen-ethylamine; *N*,*N*-dimethyltyramine; anhaline).

'Horizon' see Amitriptyline.
'Hormoformin' see Prasterone.
'Hormofort' see Hydroxyprogesterone caproate.
'Hormoslyr' see Chlorinated phenoxyacetic acid mixture.
Horse chestnut see Aesculus hippocastanum.
'Hostacaine' see Butanilicaine.
'Hostaginan' see Prenylamine lactate.
'Hostathion' see Phentriazophos.
HP-170 see Calcium benzamidosalicylate.
HP-213 see Salinazid.
HP-1275 see Fenoxypropazine.
HPC see Oxycinchophen.
HPEK see Tetroquinone.
HP-FSH see Human pituitary gonadotrophin.
HPG see Human pituitary gonadotrophin.
HPP see Allopurinol.
HR-376 see Clobazam.
HR-930 see Fosazepam.
HR-4723 see Clobazam.
HS see Mustard gas.
HS-592 see Clemastine.
Hsp-2916 see Pramiverine.
HT-11 see Cloperastine.
HT-1479 see Dimetholizine.
5-HT see Serotonin.
5-HTP see 5-Hydroxytryptophan.
'Hubersona' see Dexamethasone sodium m-sulfobenzoate.
Hudorex see Hydrochlorothiazide.
'Humachtid' see Tosactide.
Human chorionic gonadotrophin see Chorionic gonadotrophin.
Human α^{1-28} corticotrophin see Tosactide.
HUMAN GROWTH HORMONE ('crescormon').
See also Growth hormone.
HUMAN MENOPAUSAL GONADO-TROPHIN (follicle stimulating hormone, human; follotropin (human); menotrophin; menotropin; menotropins; HMG; 'humegon', 'pergonal', 'pregova').
HUMAN PITUITARY GONADO-TROPHIN (HHG; HPG; HP-FSH).
'Humatin' see Paromomycin.
'Humegon' see Human menopausal gonadotrophin.
'Humorsol' see Demecarium bromide.
'Humycin' see Paromomycin.
'Hungazin' see Atrazine.
HY-185 see Carbocloral.
HYALURONIC ACID ('etamucin').
HYALURONIDASE(S)*** (mesomucinase; diffusing factor; spreading factor; hyaluronate glycanohydrolase; lidase; lydasa).
'Hyamate' see Buramate.
'Hyamine 10X' see Methylbenzethonium.
'Hyamine 1622' see Benzethonium.
'Hyamine 3528' see Octriphenate.
'Hybamate' see Buramate.
HYCANTHONE*** (1-(2-diethylamino-ethylamino)-4-(hydroxymethyl)thioxanthen-9-one; hydroxylucanthone; lucanthone metabolite; 'etrenol').
'Hycodan' see Hydrocodone.
HYDANTOIN (2,4-(3H,5H)imidazolidine-

dione; glycolylurea).
Hydantoinal see Phenytoin.
'Hydeltrasol' see Prednisolone phosphate.
'Hydergin' see Dihydroergotoxine.
HYDNOCARPIC ACID (11-(2-cyclopenten-1-yl)undecanoic acid).
Hydnocarpylacetic acid see Chaulmoogric acid.
HYDRABAMINE PENICILLIN (N,N'-bis-(dehydroabietyl)ethylenediamine-di-penicillin G; 'compocillin').
HYDRACARBAZINE*** (6-hydrazino-3-pyridazinecarboxamide; TH-1325).
Hydracetin see Acetylphenylhydrazine.
'Hydracoll' see Algeldrate.
HYDRACRYLIC ACID (3-hydroxypropionic acid; ethylene lactic acid).
Hydracrylic acid β-lactone see β-Propiolactone.
'Hydral' see Chloral hydrate.
HYDRALAZINE*** (1-hydrazinophthalazine; apressin; hydrallazine; hydralazine hydrochloride or sulfate; Ba-5968; C-5968; 'apresoline', 'depressan', 'plethorit-C').
Hydrallazine* see Hydralazine.
Hydramitrazine see Meladrazine.
'Hydraphen' see Hydrargaphen.
HYDRARGAPHEN*** (phenylmercuric 3,3'-methylenebis(2-naphthalenesulfonate); phenylmercuric salt of dinaphthylmethane-disulfonic acid; 'conotrane', 'hydraphen', 'instrumer', 'penotrane').
HYDRATROPIC ACID (2-phenylpropionic acid; α-methyl-α-phenylacetic acid; Th-4082).
Hydrazinecarboxylic acid see Carbazic acid.
α-Hydrazino-3,4-dihydroxy-α-methyl-hydrocinnamic acid see Carbidopa.
2-Hydrazino-3-(3,4-dihydroxyphenyl)-2-methylpropionic acid see Carbidopa.
Hydrazinomethyldopa see Carbidopa.
α-Hydrazino-α-methyldopa see Carbidopa.
2-Hydrazinooctane see Octamoxin.
Hydrazinophthalazine see Hydralazine.
6-Hydrazino-3-pyridinecarboxamide see Hydracarbazine.
1-Hydrazino-4-pyrid-4-ylmethyl-phthalazine see Picodralazine.
HYDRAZOBENZENE (1,2-diphenylhydrazine).
'Hydrea' see Hydroxycarbamide.
'Hydrenox' see Hydroflumethiazide.
'Hydril' see Hydrochlorothiazide.
'Hydrion' see Ambuside.
Hydroaminacridine see Tacrine.
Hydroaminacrine see Tacrine.
HYDROBENTIZIDE*** (3-benzylthio-methyl-6-chloro-3,4-dihydro-7-sulfamoyl-1,2,4-benzothiadiazine 1,1-dioxide; di-hydrobenzthiazide; hydrobenzthiazide).
Hydrobenzthiazide see Hydrobentizide.
Hydroberberine see Tetrahydroberberine.
Hydrobutamine see Butidrine.
Hydrochloric ether see Chloroethane.
HYDROCHLOROTHIAZIDE*** (6-chloro-3,4-dihydro-7-sulfamoyl-1,2,4-benzothiadiazine 1,1-dioxide; dihydrochlorothiazide;

hypothiazide; chlorosulthiadil; 'dichlo-
tride', 'diclotride', 'direma', 'disalunil',
'disaluril', 'esidrex', 'esidrix', 'hidril',
'hudorex', 'hydro-diuril', 'hydro-saluric',
'hydro-tonuron', 'nefrix', 'niagar', 'oretic',
'thiuretic').
See also Amiloride with hydrochlorothiazide;
Bietaserpine with hydrochlorothiazide;
Guanethidine with hydrochlorothiazide;
Methyldopa with hydrochlorothiazide.
HYDROCINNAMIC ACID (3-phenyl-
propionic acid; benzylacetic acid).
Hydrocodeine see Dihydrocodeine.
'Hydrocodin' see Dihydrocodeine.
HYDROCODONE*** (4,5-epoxy-3-methoxy-
N-methyl-6-oxomorphinan; dihydroco-
deinone; hydrocon).
HYDROCODONE BITARTRATE
(hydrocodone acid tartrate; 'bekadid',
'bi-cotussin', 'biocodone', 'codinovo',
'codone', 'cofacodide', 'dico', 'dicodid',
'hycodan', 'mercodinone', 'stocodon',
'synkonin').
Hydrocodone O-carboxymethyloxime see
Codoxime.
Hydrocodone enol acetate see Thebacon.
Hydrocon see Hydrocodone.
HYDROCORTAMATE*** (hydrocortisone
21-(2-diethylaminoacetate); hydrocorta-
mate hydrochloride; ethamicort; 'mag-
nacort').
HYDROCORTISONE*** (4-pregnene-
11β,17α,21-triol-3,20-dione; 11β,17α,21-
trihydroxypregn-4-ene-3,20-dione; 17-
hydroxycorticosterone; cortisol; compound
F; NSC-10483).
HYDROCORTISONE 21-ACETATE
(NSC-741; 'cortiphate', 'hydrocortisate').
**HYDROCORTISONE WITH OXY-
TETRACYCLINE** ('terra-cortril').
Hydrocortisone-21-*tert*-butylacetate see
Hydrocortisone tebutate.
HYDROCORTISONE BUTYRATE
(hydrocortisone 17-butyrate; 'locoid').
Hydrocortisone diethylaminoacetate see
Hydrocortamate.
Hydrocortisone hemisuccinate see Hydro-
cortisone sodium succinate.
**HYDROCORTISONE 21-SODIUM
PHOSPHATE** ('actocortin').
**HYDROCORTISONE 21-SODIUM
SUCCINATE** (hydrocortisone hemi-
succinate; 'buccalsone', 'corlan', 'ef-
cortelan soluble', 'solu-cortef').
HYDROCORTISONE TEBUTATE
(hydrocortisone-21-*tert*-butylacetate;
'hydrocortone-TBA').
'Hydrocortone-TBA' see Hydrocortisone
tebutate.
'Hydro-diuril' see Hydrochlorothiazide.
HYDROFLUMETHIAZIDE*** (3,4-di-
hydro-7-sulfamoyl-6-trifluoromethyl-1,2,4-
benzothiadiazine 1,1-dioxide; dihydroflumethiazide; metflorylthiadiazine; trifluoromethylhydrothiazide; 'ademol',
'bristab', 'di-ademil', 'diratyl', 'diucardin',
'dranyl', 'hydrenox', 'leodrine', 'naclex',

'plurine', 'rodiuran', 'rontyl', 'saluron',
'sisuril', 'vergonil').
**HYDROFLUMETHIAZIDE WITH
SPIRONOLACTONE** ('aldactide').
**Hydrogen bis(N-ethylidenethreoninato)
diaquoferrate (II)** see Ferrotrenine.
HYDROGEN PEROXIDE (hydrogen
dioxide; NSC-19892).
HYDROGEN PEROXIDE SOLUTIONS
('albone', 'perhydrol', 'pyrozone', 'super-
oxol').
**HYDROGEN PEROXIDE UREA
DERIVATIVE** ('hydroperit', 'hyperol',
'lapurol', 'ortizon', 'percarbamid', 'perhydrit').
**α-Hydro-ω-hydroxypoly(oxyethylene)-
poly(oxypropylene)poly(oxyethylene)
block copolymer** see Poloxamer.
HYDROMADINONE*** (6α-chloro-17-
hydroxyprogesterone).
'Hydromedin' see Etacrynic acid.
'Hydromerfene' see Phenylmercuric borate.
HYDROMORPHINOL** (14-hydroxy-7,8-
dihydromorphine).
HYDROMORPHONE*** (7,8-dihydro-
morphinone; 4,5-epoxy-3-hydroxy-N-
methyl-6-oxomorphinan; hydromorphone
hydrochloride; laudaconum; morficon;
morphicon; 'biomorphyl', 'cofalaudid',
'dilaudid', 'dimorphone', 'hymorphan',
'novolaudon', 'semcox').
'Hydromox' see Quinethazone.
'Hydronol' see Isosorbide.
'Hydroperit' see Hydrogen peroxide urea
derivative.
Hydropropizine see Dropropizine.
HYDROQUINONE (p-dihydroxybenzene;
hydroquinol; quinol; 'achromin', 'tec-
quinol').
**HYDROQUINONE β-D-GLUCOPYRAN-
OSIDE** (arbutin; ursin; 'uvasol').
'Hydro-saluric' see Hydrochlorothiazide.
'Hydrosarpan' see Raubasine.
'Hydrosarpan 711' see Raubasine with
pipratecol.
HYDROSORBIC ACID (3-hexenoic acid).
'Hydrosulfosol' see Calsulfhydryl.
HYDROTALCITE*** (aluminium
magnesium hydroxide carbonate hydrate).
Hydrothroxin see Merethoxylline.
'Hydro-tonuron' see Hydrochlorothiazide.
HYDROTRICHLOROTHIAZIDE
(6-chloro-3-dichloromethyl-3,4-dihydro-
7-sulfamoyl-1,2,4-benzothiadiazine
1,1-dioxide).
HYDROXINDASATE*** (5-acetoxy-
1-(p-methoxybenzyl)-2-methyltryptamine;
5-acetoxy-3-(2-aminoethyl)-1-(p-methoxybenzyl)-2-methylindole; 3-(2-aminoethyl)-
1-(p-methoxybenzyl)-2-methylindol-5-ol
acetate ester; hydroxindasol acetate).
HYDROXINDASOL*** (5-hydroxy-
1-(p-methoxybenzyl)-2-methyltryptamine;
(2-aminoethyl)-5-hydroxy-3-1-(p-methoxybenzyl)-2-methylindole; 3-(2-aminoethyl)-
1-(p-methoxybenzyl)-2-methylindol-5-ol).
Hydroxindasol acetate see Hydroxindasate.

241

'Hydroxobase' see Hydroxocobalamin.
HYDROXOCOBALAMIN*** (α-(5,6-di-
methylbenzimidazolyl)hydroxocobamide;
hydroxycobalamin; OH-cobalamin;
vitamin B₁₂ₐ; 'hydroxobase').
Hydroxyacetaldehyde see Glycolaldehyde.
N-Hydroxyacetamide see Acetohydroxamic
acid.
2-(N-Hydroxyacetamido)fluorene see
Fluorenylacetohydroxamic acid.
3'-Hydroxyacetanilide see Metacetamol.
4'-Hydroxyacetanilide see Paracetamol.
4'-Hydroxyacetanilide salicylate see
Acetaminosalol.
2-Hydroxyacetic acid see Glycolic acid.
HYDROXYACETONE (1-hydroxy-2-pro-
panone; acetol; acetyl carbinol).
Hydroxyacetone salicylate see Salicyl
acetol.
2-HYDROXYACETOPHENONE (benzoyl
carbinol).
N-Hydroxy-2-acetylaminofluorene see
Fluorenylacetohydroxamic acid.
β-Hydroxyalanine see Serine.
Hydroxy aluminium magnesium aminoacetate see Aluminium magnesium glycinate.
HYDROXYAMPHETAMINE***
(p-(2-aminopropyl)phenol; p-hydroxy-
amphetamine; p-hydroxy-α-methyl-
phenethylamine; α-methyltyramine; norpholedrine; oxamphetamine; 'paradrine',
'paredrine', 'paredrinex', 'pulsoton').
17β-Hydroxyandrosta-1,4-dien-3-one see
Boldenone.
3α-Hydroxy-5β-androstan-17-one see
5β-Androstan-3α-ol-17-one.
17β-Hydroxy-5α-androstan-3-one see
Androstanolone.
3β-Hydroxyandrost-5-en-17-one see
Prasterone.
17α-Hydroxyandrost-4-en-3-one see
Epitestosterone.
17β-Hydroxyandrost-4-en-3-one see
Testosterone.
p-Hydroxyanisole see Mequinol.
9-Hydroxyanthracene see 9-Anthrol.
9-HYDROXY-1(10)-ARISTOLEN-2-ONE
('debilon').
4-HYDROXY-m-ARSANILIC ACID
(3-amino-4-hydroxybenzenearsonic acid).
5-Hydroxybarbituric acid see Dialuric acid.
o-Hydroxybenzaldehyde see Salicylaldehyde.
p-Hydroxybenzaldehyde isonicotinoylhydrazone see p-Hydroxybenzylidene-
isoniazid.
o-Hydroxybenzamide see Salicylamide.
o-Hydroxybenzoic acid see Salicylic acid.
p-Hydroxybenzoic acid esters see Parabens.
p-Hydroxybenzoic acid ethyl ester
6-guanidinohexanoate see Gabexate.
p-Hydroxybenzoic acid 5-nitrofurfuryl-
idenehydrazide see Nitrofuroxazide.
4'-Hydroxybenzophenone-2-carboxy-
late(s) see Hibenzate(s).
4-Hydroxy-1,3-benzoxathiol-2-one see
Tioxolone.

2-(4-Hydroxybenzoyl)benzoic acid,
esters and salts see Hibenzate(s).
o-Hydroxybenzyl alcohol see Saligenin.
N'-(p-HYDROXYBENZYLIDENE)ISONI-
AZID (p-hydroxybenzaldehyde isonicotinoylhydrazone; isonicotinic acid (p-hydroxybenzylidene)hydrazide; 'flavoteben').
p-Hydroxybenzylpenicillin see Penicillin X.
cis-1-Hydroxy(bicyclohexyl)-2-carboxylic
acid 2-(diethylamino)-1-methylethyl
ester see Rociverine.
2-Hydroxybiphenyl see Phenylphenol.
2-[(2'-Hydroxybiphenyl-4-yl)carbonyl]-
benzoic acid, esters and salts see
Fendizoate(s).
1-(2-endo-Hydroxy-3-endo-bornyl)-3-(p-
toluenesulfonyl)urea see Glibornuride.
Hydroxybutanedioic acid see Malic acid.
2-Hydroxy-3-butanone see Acetoin.
1-(3-Hydroxybutyl)-4-[6-(6-methoxy-
quinolin-8-ylamino)hexyl]piperazine
see Moxipraquine.
8-[6-[4-(3-Hydroxybutyl)piperazin-1-yl]-
hexylamino]-6-methoxyquinoline see
Moxipraquine.
8-[6-[1-(3-Hydroxybutyl)piperazin-4-yl]-
hexylamino]-6-methoxyquinoline see
Moxipraquine.
4-HYDROXYBUTYRIC ACID (GHBA;
GOHBA).
4-Hydroxybutyric acid acetate see
Aceburic acid.
4-Hydroxybutyric acid sodium salt see
Oxybate sodium.
3-Hydroxy-p-butyrophenetidide see
Bucetin.
N-(4-Hydroxybutyryl)-2-ethyl-2-
(3-methoxyphenyl)-1-butylamine see
Embutramide.
HYDROXYCARBAMIDE*** (hydroxyurea; NSC-32065; SQ-1089; 'hidrea',
'hidrix', 'hydrea', 'litalair').
HYDROXYCHLOROQUINE*** (7-chloro-
4-[4-[ethyl-(2-hydroxyethyl)amino]-
1-methylbutylamino]quinoline; 4-(7-
chloroquinolin-4-ylamino)-N-ethyl-N-
(2-hydroxyethyl)-4-methyl-1-butylamine;
oxychloroquine; oxichlorochin; SN-8137;
'ercoquin', 'plaquenil').
3-Hydroxycholanic acid see Lithocholic
acid.
25-Hydroxycholecalciferol see 25-Hydroxy-
colecalciferol.
24-Hydroxycholesterol see Cholestenediol.
6-Hydroxycinchonine see Cupreine.
3-Hydroxycinchophen see Oxycinchophen.
cis-o-HYDROXYCINNAMIC ACID
(coumarinic acid).
trans-o-HYDROXYCINNAMIC ACID
(o-coumaric acid).
p-HYDROXYCINNAMIC ACID (p-coumaric acid).
Hydroxycobalamine see Hydroxocobalamin.
Hydroxycodeine see Neopine.
25-HYDROXYCOLECALCIFEROL
(25-hydroxycholecalciferol; HCC; vitamin
D₄).

242

7-Hydroxycoumarin *see* Umbelliferone.
3-Hydroxy-*cis*-crotonic acid dimethyl
phosphate methyl ester *see* Mevinphos.
4-Hydroxy-2,5-cyclohexadienone *see*
Quinol.
α-HYDROXYCYCLOHEXANEBUTYRIC
ACID (4-cyclohexyl-2-hydroxybutyric
acid; 'lipotrin').
2-Hydroxy-1,1,3,3-cyclohexanetetra-
methanol tetranicotinate *see* Nicomol.
HYDROXYCYCLOHEXIMIDE (3-[2-
hydroxy-2-(5-hydroxy-3,5-dimethyl-2-oxo-
cyclohexyl)-ethyl]glutarimide; NSC-39147;
U-9361; 'resactin A', 'streptovitacin A').
2-(1-Hydroxycyclohexyl)butyric acid *see*
Cyclobutyrol.
14-Hydroxydaunorubicin *see* Doxorubicin.
HYDROXY-DDD (2,2-dichloro-1,1-bis-
(*p*-chlorophenyl)ethanol; 4,4′-dichloro-
α-dichloromethylbenzhydrol; FW-152).
Hydroxy-DDT *see* Dicofol.
N-(3-Hydroxydecanoyl)serine *see*
Serratamic acid.
12-Hydroxydigitoxin *see* Digoxin.
14-Hydroxydihydrocodeinone *see* Oxycodone.
14-Hydroxy-7,8-dihydromorphine *see*
Hydromorphinol.
Hydroxydihydromorphinone* *see* Oxymorphone.
14-Hydroxydihydro-6β-thebainol 4-methyl
ether *see* Oxymethanol.
3-Hydroxy-4,5-di(hydroxymethyl)-2-
methylpyridine *see* Pyridoxine.
4-Hydroxy-3,5-diiodobenzonitrile *see*
Ioxynil.
3-(4-Hydroxy-3,5-diiodobenzoyl)-2,5-di-
methylfuran *see* Furidarone.
2-(4-HYDROXY-3,5-DIIODOBENZYL)-
CYCLOHEXANECARBOXYLIC ACID
('monophen').
4-Hydroxy-3,5-diiodo-α-[1-(1-methyl-
3-phenylpropylamino)ethyl]benzyl
alcohol *see* Bufeniode.
[3-(4-Hydroxy-3,5-diiodophenoxy)-3,5-di-
iodophenyl]alanine *see* Dextrothyroxine;
Levothyroxine; Thyroxine.
4-Hydroxy-3,5-diiodophenylalanine *see*
Diiodotyrosine.
3-(4-Hydroxy-3,5-diiodophenyl)-β-alanine
see Betasin.
4-Hydroxy-3,5-diiodophenyl 2,5-dimethyl-
3-furyl ketone *see* Furidarone.
(4-Hydroxy-3,5-diiodophenyl)-2-phenyl-
propionic acid *see* Pheniodol.
4-Hydroxy-6,7-diisobutoxyquinoline-
3-carboxylic acid ethyl ester *see*
Buquinolate.
4-Hydroxy-6,7-diisopropoxy-3-quinoline-
carboxylic acid methyl ester *see*
Proquinolate.
4-Hydroxy-3,5-dimethoxybenzoic acid
see Syringic acid.
4-Hydroxy-3,5-dimethoxy-α-methyl-
aminomethylbenzyl alcohol *see* Dimetofrine.
1-(4-Hydroxy-3,5-dimethoxyphenyl)-

2-methylaminoethanol *see* Dimetofrine.
2-Hydroxy-1-dimethylaminoethyl 2-oxo-
bornane-3-carboxylate *see* Ethyl
camphoramine.
17β-Hydroxy-2α,17-dimethyl-5α-andro-
stan-3-one azine *see* Mebolazine.
17β-Hydroxy-7α,17-dimethylandrost-
4-en-3-one *see* Bolasterone.
17β-Hydroxy-7β,17-dimethylandrost-
4-en-3-one *see* Calusterone.
4-Hydroxy-*N*,*N*-dimethylbutyramide
ester of clofibric acid *see* Clofibride.
3-Hydroxy-*N*,*N*-dimethyl-*cis*-croton-
amide dimethyl phosphate *see* Dicrotophos.
5-Hydroxy-*N*,*N*-dimethyl-4,4-diphenyl-
2-heptylamine *see* Dimepheptanol.
3-Hydroxy-6,*N*-dimethyl-4,5-epoxy-
morphin-6-ene *see* Methyldesorphine.
17β-Hydroxy-7α,17-dimethylestr-4-en-
3-one *see* Mibolerone.
17β-Hydroxy-16,16-dimethylestr-4-en-
3-one *see* Metogest.
2-Hydroxy-*N*,*N*-dimethylethylamine
camphocarbonate *see* Ethyl camphoramine.
(−)-5-(1-Hydroxy-1,5-dimethylhex-4-en-
1-yl)-2-methyl-1-cyclohexene *see*
Levomenol.
5-Hydroxy-1,2-dimethylindole-3-carb-
oxylic acid ethyl ester *see* Mecarbinate.
2′-Hydroxy-5,9-dimethyl-2-(3-methyl-
2-butenyl)-6,7-benzomorphan *see*
Pentazocine.
2-Hydroxy-*N*,*N*-dimethyl-*N*-(1-methyl-
ethyl)-3-(1-naphthalenyloxy)-1-
propanaminium chloride *see* Pranolium
chloride.
11α-Hydroxy-17,17-dimethyl-18-nor-
androsta-4,13-dien-3-one *see* Nordinone.
5-(3-Hydroxy-4,4-dimethyl-1-pentenyl)-
1,3-benzodioxole *see* Stiripentol.
p-Hydroxy-*N*,*N*-dimethylphenethylamine
see Hordenine.
2′-Hydroxy-5,9-dimethyl-2-phenethyl-
6,7-benzomorphan *see* Phenazocine.
3-Hydroxy-1,1-dimethylpiperidinium
bromide benzilate *see* Mepenzolate
bromide.
4-Hydroxy-1,1-dimethylpiperidinium
bromide benzilate *see* Parapenzolate
bromide.
4-Hydroxy-1,1-dimethylpiperidinium
methylsulfate 3-methyl-2-phenyl-
valerate ester *see* Pentapiperium metilsulfate.
3β-Hydroxy-6α,16α-dimethyl-4-pregnen-
20-one *see* Demepregnen.
1-Hydroxy-4,6-dimethylpyridin-2(1H)-one
see Metipirox.
3-Hydroxy-1,1-dimethylpyrrolidinium
bromide benzilate *see* Benzopyrronium
bromide.
erythro-3-Hydroxy-1,1-dimethylpyrro-
lidinium bromide α-cyclopentylmandelate *see* Ritropirronium bromide.
3-Hydroxy-1,1-dimethylpyrrolidinium

bromide α-phenylcyclohexaneglycolate *see* Hexopyrronium bromide.

3-Hydroxy-1,1-dimethylpyrrolidinium bromide α-phenylcyclopentaneglycolate *see* Glycopyrronium bromide.

3-Hydroxy-1,1-dimethylpyrrolidinium bromide α-phenyl-2-thiopheneglycolate *see* Heteronium bromide.

3-Hydroxy-6,7-dimethyl-2-(1-ribityloxy)-quinoxaline *see* Flavoviolet.

4-Hydroxy-*N*,*N*-dimethyltryptamine *see* Psilocin.

5-Hydroxy-*N*,*N*-dimethyltryptamine *see* Bufotenine.

HYDROXYDIONE SODIUM SUCCIN-ATE*** (21-hydroxy-5β-pregnane-3,20-dione 21-(sodium hemisuccinate); sodium 21-(3-carboxypropionyloxy)pregnane-3,20-dione; pregnocin; 'presuren', 'viadril').

7-Hydroxy-5,9-dioxatridecane *see* Dibuprol.

2-[[(3-Hydroxy-11,29-dioxoolean-12-en-29-yl)oxy]methyl]-1,1-dimethylpyrrolidinium methylsulfate *see* Roxolonium metilsulfate.

trans-[4-(Hydroxydi-2-thienylmethyl)-cyclohexyl]trimethylammonium bromide *see* Thihexinol methylbromide.

6-HYDROXYDOPA (2,4,5-trihydroxy-phenylalanine).

6-HYDROXYDOPAMINE (2,4,5-tri-hydroxyphenethylamine).

p-HYDROXYEPHEDRINE (*p*-hydroxy-α-(1-methylaminoethyl)benzyl alcohol; 1-(*p*-hydroxyphenyl)-2-methylamino-1-propanol; 'methylsympathol', 'suprifen'). *See also* Diphepanol with *p*-hydroxy-ephedrine salicylate.

3-Hydroxyestra-1,3,5(10),7-tetraen-17-one *see* Equilin.

3-Hydroxyestra-1,3,5(10)-trien-17-one *see* Estrone.

17β-Hydroxyestra-4,9,11-trien-3-one *see* Trenbolone.

17β-Hydroxyestr-4-en-3-one *see* Nandrolone.

17β-Hydroxyestr-4-en-3-one 1-adamantanecarboxylate *see* Bolmantalate.

2-Hydroxyethanesulfonic acid *see* Isethionic acid.

2-Hydroxyethanethiol *see* 2-Mercaptoethanol.

8a-Hydroxy-6,10-ethano-5-azoniaspiro-(4,5)decane chloride benzilate *see* Trospium chloride.

1-[2-(2-Hydroxyethoxy)ethyl]-4-phenyl-isonipecotic acid ethyl ester *see* Etoxeridine.

1-[2-(2-Hydroxyethoxy)ethyl]-4-phenyl-4-propionylpiperidine *see* Droxypropine.

10-[3-[4-(2-(2-Hydroxyethoxy)ethyl)-piperazin-1-yl]-2-methylpropyl]-phenothiazine *see* Dixyrazine.

2-(2-Hydroxyethoxy)ethyl *N*-(α,α,α-tri-fluoro-*m*-tolyl)anthranilate *see* Etofenamate.

4-(2-Hydroxyethoxy)-3-methoxycinnamic acid *see* Cinametic acid.

10-[3-[4-(2-Hydroxyethoxy)piperid-1-yl]-propyl]-2-(trifluoromethyl)pheno-thiazine *see* Flupimazine.

4-(2-Hydroxyethoxy)-1-[3-[2-(trifluoro-methyl)phenothiazin-10-yl]propyl]-piperidine *see* Flupimazene.

N-(2-Hydroxyethyl)acetamide 2-(*p*-chlorophenyl)-2-(α,α,α-trifluoro-*m*-toloxy)acetate ester *see* Halofenate.

1-(2-Hydroxyethyl)aziridine *see* Aziridine-ethanol.

2-Hydroxyethyl benzylcarbamate *see* Buramate.

1-[(2-Hydroxyethyl)carbamoylmethyl]-pyridinium chloride laurate *see* Lapirium chloride.

N-(2-Hydroxyethyl)cinnamamide *see* Idrocilamide.

10-[2-[4-(2-Hydroxyethyl)-1,4-diazacyclo-hept-1-yl]propyl]-2-trifluoromethyl-phenothiazine *see* Homofenazine.

(4-(2-Hydroxyethyl)diethylenediamino-methyl]tetracycline *see* Pipacycline.

(2-Hydroxyethyl)diisopropylmethyl-ammonium bromide xanthene-9-carb-oxylate *see* Propantheline bromide.

5-(2-Hydroxyethyl)-1,3-dimethoxy-benzene *see* Floverine.

(2-Hydroxyethyl)dimethyl-[1-(10-pheno-thiazinylmethyl)ethyl]ammonium chloride *see* Promethazine hydroxyethyl chloride.

(2-Hydroxyethyl)dimethylsulfonium chloride succinylbis ester *see* Succinyl-disulfocholine.

(2-Hydroxyethyl)dimethylsulfonium iodode α-phenylcyclohexaneacetate *see* Hexasonium iodide.

(2-Hydroxyethyl)dimethylsulfonium iodide α-phenylcyclohexaneglycolate *see* Oxysonium iodide.

2-(1-Hydroxyethyl)-β-(hydroxymethyl)-3-methyl-5-benzofuranacrylic acid γ-lactone *see* Benfurodil.

(1-Hydroxyethylidene)diphosphonic acid *see* Etidronic acid.

2,2'-(2-Hydroxyethylimino)bis-[*N*-(α,α-di-methylphenethyl)-*N*-methylacetamide] *see* Oxetacaine.

3-(2-Hydroxyethyl)indole *see* Tryptophol.

2-Hydroxyethyl methacrylate polymers *see* Dimefilcon A; Hefilcon A; Vifilcon A.

2-Hydroxyethyl methacrylate polymer with methyl methacrylate and ethyl-enebis(oxyethylene) dimethacrylate *see* Dimefilcon A.

8-[(2-Hydroxyethyl)methylamino]-caffeine *see* Cafaminol.

7-[3-[(2-Hydroxyethyl)methylamino]-2-hydroxypropyl]theophylline nico-tinate *see* Xantinol nicotinate.

1-(2-Hydroxyethyl)-1-methylguanidine dihydrogen phosphate ester *see* Creatinolfosfate.

1-(2-Hydroxyethyl)-2-methyl-5-nitro-imidazole *see* Metronidazole.

244

1-(2-Hydroxyethyl)-1-methylpyrrolidi-
nium iodide benzilate *see* Etipirium
iodide.

N-(2-Hydroxyethyl)-3-methyl-2-quinox-
alinecarboxamide 1,4-dioxide *see*
Olaquindox.

2-Hydroxyethyl 3-methylquinoxaline-
2-carboxylate 2,4-dioxide *see* Temodox.

N-(2-Hydroxyethyl)nicotinamide ester
with clofibric acid *see* Picafibrate.

2-Hydroxyethyl nicotinate 2-(*p*-chloro-
phenoxy)-2-methylpropionate ester
see Etofibrate.

1-(2-Hydroxyethyl)-3-(5-nitrofurfuryl-
ideneamino)-2-imidazolinone *see*
Nifurdazil.

N-(2-Hydroxyethyl)-α-(5-nitro-2-furyl)-
nitrone *see* Nifuratrone.

6-(1-HYDROXYETHYL)NORBORNENE
(6-(1-hydroxyethyl)bicyclo(2.2.1)hept-
2-ene; hydroxyethylnorcamphene).

6-(1-HYDROXYETHYL)NORBORNENE
ACID SUCCINATE ('felogen').

2,2′-[[3-(2-Hydroxyethyl)octadecylamino-
propyl]imino]diethanol dihydrofluoride *see* Olaflur.

N-(2-Hydroxyethyl)palmitamide *see*
Palmidrol.

N-(2-HYDROXYETHYL)PHENMETRA-
ZINE 2-PHENYLBUTYRATE (*N*-(2-
hydroxyethyl)-3-methyl-2-phenylmorpho-
line 2-phenylbutyrate; R-381).
See also Phenmetrazine teoclate with *N*-(2-
hydroxyethyl)phenmetrazine 2-phenyl-
butyrate.

N-[[4-(2-Hydroxyethyl)piperazin-1-yl]-
carboxymethyl]tetracycline *see*
Apicycline.

2-[4-(2-Hydroxyethyl)piperazin-1-yl]-
ethyl 2-trifluoromethylphenothiazin-10-
yl ketone *see* Ftorpropazine.

N-[4-(2-Hydroxyethyl)piperazin-1-yl-
methyl]tetracycline *see* Pipacycline.

10-[3-[4-(2-Hydroxyethyl)piperazin-1-yl]-
propionyl]-2-trifluoromethylpheno-
thiazine *see* Ftorpropazine.

3-[4-(2-Hydroxyethyl)piperazin-1-yl]-
propyl DL-4-benzamido-*N*,*N*-dipropyl-
glutaramate 1-(*p*-chlorobenzoyl)-5-
methoxy-2-methylindole-3-acetate
see Proglumetacin.

5-[3-[3-(2-Hydroxyethyl)piperazin-1-yl]-
propyl]dibenz(b,f)azepine *see* Opipramol.

9-[3-[4-(2-Hydroxyethyl)piperazin-1-yl]-
propylidene]-2-trifluoromethylthio-
xanthene *see* Flupentixol.

10-[3-[4-(2-Hydroxyethyl)piperazin-1-yl]-
propyl]phenothiazin-2-yl methyl
ketone *see* Acetophenazine.

10-[3-[4-(2-Hydroxyethyl)piperazin-1-yl]-
propyl]-2-propionylphenothiazine *see*
Carfenazine.

10-[3-[4-(2-Hydroxyethyl)piperazin-1-yl]-
propyl]-2-trifluoromethylphenothi-
azine *see* Flufenazine.

4-[3-[4-(2-Hydroxyethyl)piperazin-1-yl]-

propyl]-6-trifluoromethyl-4H-thieno-
(2,3-b)(1,4)benzothiazine *see* Flutizenol.

10-[4-[3-(2-Hydroxyethyl)piperid-1-yl]-
propyl]-*N*,*N*-dimethylphenothiazine
2-sulfonamide *see* Pipotiazine.

10-[3-[4-(2-Hydroxyethyl)piperid-1-yl]-
propyl]phenothiazin-2-yl methyl
ketone *see* Piperacetazine.

N-Hydroxyethylpromethazine *see* Promethazine hydroxyethyl chloride.

1-(2-Hydroxyethyl)-4-[3-(pyrido(3,2-b)-
(1,4)benzothiazin-10-yl)propyl]piper-
azine *see* Oxypendyl.

7-*O*-(2-Hydroxyethyl)rutoside *see* Monoxerutin.

2-Hydroxyethyl salicylate *see* Glycol
salicylate.

2-Hydroxyethyl starch *see* Hetastarch.

2-Hydroxyethyl *p*-sulfamoylcarbanilate
see Sulocarbilate.

4-(2-Hydroxyethyl)-α-tetracyclinyl-
1-piperazineacetic acid *see* Apicycline.

7-(2-Hydroxyethyl)theophylline *see*
Etofylline.

1-(2-Hydroxyethyl)-4-[3-(2-trifluoro-
methyl)phenothiazin-10-ylpropyl]-
homopiperazine *see* Homofenazine.

(2-Hydroxyethyl)trimethylammonium
hydroxide *see* Choline.

(2-Hydroxyethyl)trimethylammonium
iodide benzilate *see* Metocinium iodide.

9-Hydroxy-9H-fluorene-9-carboxylic acid
see Flurenol.

3-HydroxyGABA *see* 4-Amino-3-hydroxy-
butyric acid.

Hydroxyhemin *see* Hematin.

5-Hydroxy-2-hexenoic acid lactone *see*
Parasorbic acid.

p-Hydroxyhydrocinnamic acid *see*
Phloretic acid.

7-[2-Hydroxy-3-[(2-hydroxyethyl)methyl-
amino]propyl]theophylline compound
with 2-(*p*-chlorophenoxy)-2-methyl-
propionic acid *see* Xantifibrate.

7-[2-Hydroxy-3-[(2-hydroxyethyl)methyl-
amino]propyl]theophylline compound
with nicotinic acid *see* Xantinol nicotinate.

N-[2-Hydroxy-2-(4-hydroxy-3-hydroxy-
methylphenyl)ethyl]-4-methoxy-α-
methylphenethylamine *see* Salmefamol.

2′-Hydroxy-5′-(1-hydroxy-2-isopropyl-
aminoethyl)methanesulfonanilide *see*
Soterenol.

o-(6-Hydroxy-5-hydroxymercuri-2,7-di-
iodo-3-oxo(3H)xanthen-9-yl)benzene-
sulfonic acid sodium salt *see* Meralein
sodium.

o-[[2-Hydroxy-3-(hydroxymercuri)-
propyl]carbamoyl]phenoxyacetic acid
see Mercuderamide.

2′-Hydroxy-5′-[1-hydroxy-2-(*p*-methoxy-
phenethylamino)propyl]methanesul-
fonanilide *see* Mesuprine.

17β-Hydroxy-2-hydroxymethylene-17-
methyl-5α-androstan-3-one *see* Oxymetholone.

4-Hydroxy-3-hydroxymethyl-α-(4-methoxy-α-methylphenethylamino-methyl)benzyl alcohol see Salmefamol.
3-Hydroxy-5-hydroxymethyl-2-methyl-isonicotinaldehyde see Pyridoxal.
3-Hydroxy-5-hydroxymethyl-2-methyl-isonicotinic acid see Pyridoxic acid.
2-[(5-HYDROXY-4-HYDROXYMETHYL-6-METHYLPYRID-3-YL)METHOXY]-GLYCOLIC ACID (5-hydroxy-6-methyl-3,4-pyridinedimethanol 3-ether with glycolic acid; pyridoxine 3-ether with glycolic acid).
See also Piridoxilate.
2-[(5-Hydroxy-4-hydroxymethyl-6-methylpyrid-3-yl)methoxy]glycolic acid compound with [4,5-bis(hydroxy-methyl)-2-methylpyrid-3-yloxy]-glycolic acid see Piridoxilate.
7-[3-Hydroxy-2-[(3R)-(3-hydroxy-3-methyl-1-octenyl)]-5-oxocyclopentyl]-5-heptenoic acid see Arbaprostil.
1-(4-Hydroxy-3-hydroxymethylphenyl)-2-(4-methoxy-α-methylphenethyl-amino)ethanol see Salmefamol.
5-Hydroxy-2-hydroxymethyl-4-pyrone see Kojic acid.
N-[2-Hydroxy-2-[4-hydroxy-5-(methyl-sulfonamido)phenyl]-1-methylethyl]-p-methoxyphenethylamine see Mesuprine.
7-[3α-Hydroxy-2β-[3(S)-hydroxy-trans-oct-1-enyl]-5-oxo-cyclopent-1-yl]-cis-hept-5-enoic acid see Dinoprostone.
4-Hydroxy-3-(1-hydroxypentyl)benzoic acid see Fepentolic acid.
p-Hydroxy-α-[1-(p-hydroxyphenethyl-amino)ethyl]benzyl alcohol see Ritodrine.
Hydroxyimine see Aziridineethanol.
4-[[p-[1-(Hydroxyimino)ethyl]phenoxy]-acetyl]morpholine see Mofoxime.
1-[[p-[1-(Hydroxyimino)ethyl]phenoxy]-acetyl]piperidine see Pifoxime.
4-(Hydroxyiminomethyl)-1-methyl-pyridinium iodide see Pralidoxime iodide.
1-(2-Hydroxyindan-2-yl)propylamine see Indanorex.
3-Hydroxyindole see Indoxyl.
5-HYDROXYINDOLEACETIC ACID (5-hydroxyindol-3-ylacetic acid; 5-HIAA).
5-Hydroxyindol-3-ylacetic acid see 5-Hydr-oxyindoleacetic acid.
4-Hydroxy-3-iodo-5-nitrobenzonitrile see Nitroxinil.
4-(4-Hydroxy-3-iodophenoxy)-3,5-diiodo-benzoic acid acetate see Acetiromate.
4-(4-Hydroxy-3-iodophenoxy)-3,5-di-iodohydrocinnamic acid see Thyropropic acid.
2-[4-(4-Hydroxy-3-iodophenoxy)-3,5-di-iodophenyl]acetic acid see Triac.
3-[4-(4-Hydroxy-3-iodophenoxy)-3,5-di-iodophenyl]alanine see Detrothyronine; Liothyronine; Rathyronine.
3-[4-(4-Hydroxy-3-iodophenoxy)-3,5-diiodophenyl]propionic acid see Thyro-

propic acid.
8-Hydroxy-7-iodoquinolin-5-sulfonic acid see 7-Iodo-8-quinolinol-5-sulfonic acid.
1-[2-Hydroxy-3-(isobutylmethoxy)-propyl]-4-methylpiperazine 2-phenyl-butyrate see Fenetradil.
8-Hydroxyisocoumarin-4-yl hydroxy-methyl ketone see Oosponol.
4-(2-Hydroxy-3-isopentyloxypropyl)-morpholine 3,4,5-trimethoxybenzoate see Amoproxan.
4'-(1-Hydroxy-2-isopropylaminoethyl)-methanesulfonanilide see Sotalol.
5-(1-Hydroxy-2-isopropylaminoethyl)-8-quinolinol see Quinprenaline.
p-Hydroxy-α-(isopropylaminomethyl)-benzyl alcohol see Deterenol.
4-Hydroxy-α-isopropylaminomethyl-3-methanesulfonamidobenzyl alcohol see Soterenol.
4-Hydroxy-α-isopropylaminomethyl-3-methoxybenzyl alcohol see Metipren-aline.
8-Hydroxy-α-isopropylaminomethyl-5-quinolinemethanol see Quinprenaline.
4'-(2-Hydroxy-3-isopropylaminoprop-oxy)acetanilide see Practolol.
4-(2-Hydroxy-3-isopropylaminopropoxy)-indole see Pindolol.
1-(2-Hydroxy-3-isopropylaminopropoxy)-naphthalene see Propranolol.
p-(2-Hydroxy-3-isopropylaminopropoxy)-phenylacetamide see Atenolol.
2-(2-Hydroxy-3-isopropylaminopropoxy)-thiazole see Tazolol.
4-(2-Hydroxy-3-isopropylaminopropoxy)-2,3,6-trimethylphenyl acetate see Trime-pranol.
2-Hydroxy-3-isopropylaminopropyl 2,6,2',6'-tetramethylbenzhydryl ether see Xipranolol.
1-Hydroxy-2-isopropyl-5-methylbenzene see Thymol.
2-(4-Hydroxy-2-isopropyl-5-methyl-phenoxy)-N,N-dimethylethylamine acetate ester see Moxisylyte.
N-[2-(4-Hydroxy-2-isopropyl-5-methyl-phenoxy)ethyl]dimethylamine acetate ester see Moxisylyte.
β-Hydroxy-p-(isopropylthio)-α-methyl-N-octylphenethylamine see Suloctidil.
1-Hydroxy-1-[p-(isopropylthio)phenyl]-N-octyl-2-propylamine see Suloctidil.
3α-Hydroxy-8-isopropyl-1αH,5αH-tropa-nium bromide (±)-tropate see Ipratropium bromide.
Hydroxyisosparteine see Retamine.
3-Hydroxy-7-ketocholanic acid see Ketolithocholic acid.
HYDROXYLAMINE (oxammonium).
Hydroxylucanthone see Hycanthone.
17-Hydroxy-7-mercapto-3-oxo-17α-pregn-4-ene-21-carboxylic acid γ-lactone 7-acetate see Spironolactone.
Hydroxymercurichlorophenol see 2-Chloro-4-(hydroxymercuri)phenol.
4-Hydroxymercuri-2,7-diiodoresorcinol-

246

sulfonphthalein *see* Meralein sodium.

1-(3-Hydroxymercuri-2-methoxypropyl)-biuret *see* Merbiurelidin.

o-[*N*-(**3-Hydroxymercuri-2-methoxy-propyl)carbamoyl]phenoxyacetic acid sodium salt** *see* Mersalyl.

3-[*N*-(3-Hydroxymercuri-2-methoxy-propyl)carbamoyl]-1,2,2-trimethyl-cyclopentanecarboxylic acid theophylline derivative *see* Mercurophylline.

8-[3-(Hydroxymercuri)-2-methoxy-propyl]coumarin-3-carboxylic acid sodium salt with theophylline *see* Mercumatilin sodium.

1-(3-Hydroxymercuri-2-methoxypropyl)-3-succinylurea theophylline derivative *see* Meralluride.

3-Hydroxymercuri-4-nitro-*o*-cresol *see* Nitromersol.

1-Hydroxymercuri-2-propanol *see* Merisoprol.

2'-Hydroxy-4'-methoxyacetophenone *see* Peonol.

4-Hydroxy-3-methoxybenzaldehyde *see* Vanillin.

4-Hydroxy-3-methoxybenzaldehyde isonicotinoylhydrazone *see* Ftivazide.

4-Hydroxy-3-methoxybenzoic acid *see* Vanillic acid.

2-Hydroxy-4-methoxybenzophenone *see* Oxybenzone.

β-**Hydroxy-*N*-[2-(*m*-methoxybenzoyl)-ethyl]amphetamine** *see* Oxyfedrine.

2-Hydroxy-3-methoxycinnamic acid *see* *o*-Ferulic acid.

4-Hydroxy-3-methoxycinnamic acid *see* Ferulic acid.

7-Hydroxy-6-methoxycoumarin *see* Scopoletin.

4-Hydroxy-3-methoxymandelic acid *see* Vanilmandelic acid.

4-Hydroxy-3-methoxy-*α*-methylamino-methylbenzyl alcohol *see* Metanephrine.

2-Hydroxy-4-methoxy-4'-methylbenzo-phenone *see* Mexenone.

6-Hydroxy-5-methoxy-2-methyl-*p*-benzo-quinone *see* Fumigatin.

11-Hydroxy-10-methoxy-1,2-methylene-dioxyaporphine *see* Bulbocapnine.

11-Hydroxy-10-methoxy-6-methyl-1,2-methylenedioxy-4H-dibenzo(de,g)-quinoline *see* Bulbocapnine.

6-(4-Hydroxy-6-methoxy-7-methyl-3-oxo-phthalan-5-yl)-4-methyl-4-hexenoic acid *see* Mycophenolic acid.

4-Hydroxy-*α*-[(*p*-methoxy-*α*-methyl-phenethylamino)methyl]-*m*-xylene-*α*,*α*'-diol *see* Salmefamol.

4-Hydroxy-*α*-[1-(*p*-methoxyphenethyl-amino)ethyl]-5-(methylsulfonamido)-benzyl alcohol *see* Mesuprine.

4-Hydroxy-3-methoxyphenylacetic acid *see* Homovanillic acid.

4-(4-Hydroxy-3-methoxyphenyl)-2-butanone *see* Zingerone.

6-Hydroxy-7-methoxy-4-phenylcoumarin *see* Dalbergin.

1-(4-Hydroxy-3-methoxyphenyl)-1,2-ethanediol *see* 4-Hydroxy-*α*-hydroxy-methyl-3-methoxybenzyl alcohol.

2-(4-Hydroxy-3-methoxyphenyl)ethyl methyl ketone *see* Zingerone.

4-Hydroxy-3-methoxyphenylglycolic acid *see* Vanilmandelic acid.

1-(2-Hydroxy-3-methoxy-3-phenyl-propyl)-4-(2-methoxy-2-phenylethyl)-piperazine *see* Zipeprol.

3-Hydroxy-7-methoxy-7-(2-thien-2-ylacet-amido)-2-cephem-2-carboxylic acid *see* Cefoxitin.

6-Hydroxy-5-methoxy-*p*-toluquinone *see* Fumigatin.

p-**Hydroxy-*α*-(1-methylaminoethyl)benzyl alcohol** *see* *p*-Hydroxyephedrine.

3'-(1-Hydroxy-2-methylaminoethyl)-methanesulfonanilide methanesulfon-ate *see* Amidefrine mesilate.

Hydroxymethyl 6-D(−)-(*α*-aminophenyl-acetamido)penicillinate pivalate *see* Pivampicillin.

20-Hydroxy-3*β*-methylamino-5-preg-nene-18-carboxylic acid lactone *see* Paravallarine.

4'-(1-Hydroxy-2-methylaminopropyl)-methanesulfonanilide *see* Metalol.

17*β*-Hydroxy-17-methylandrosta-1,4-dien-3-one *see* Metandienone.

17*β*-Hydroxy-17*α*-methyl-5*α*-androstano-(2,3-c)furazan *see* Furazabol.

17*β*-HYDROXY-17*α*-METHYL-5*α*-ANDROSTANO(3,2-c)ISOXAZOLE (androisoxazole).

17*β*-Hydroxy-1*α*-methyl-5*α*-androstan-3-one *see* Mesterolone.

17*β*-Hydroxy-2*α*-methylandrostan-3-one *see* Drostanolone.

17*β*-Hydroxy-2*α*-methyl-5*α*-androstan-3-one azine *see* Bolazine.

17*β*-Hydroxy-17*α*-methylandrostano-(3,2-c)pyrazole *see* Stanozolol.

17*β*-Hydroxy-2-methyl-5*α*-androst-1-en-3-one *see* Stenbolone.

2-Hydroxy-3-methylbenzamide *see* Cresotamide.

2-Hydroxy-3-methylbenzoic acid *see* Hydroxytoluic acid.

2-Hydroxy-5-methylbenzoic acid *see* 2,5-Cresotic acid.

14-Hydroxy-*N*-(3-methyl-2-butenyl)-7,8-dihydronormorphinone *see* Nal-mexone.

2-Hydroxy-3-(3-methyl-2-butenyl)-1,4-naphthoquinone *see* Lapachol.

7*α*-(1-Hydroxy-1-methylbutyl)tetra-hydro-6,14-*endo*-ethenooripavine *see* Etorphine.

7*α*-(1-Hydroxy-1-methylbutyl)tetra-hydro-6,14-*endo*-ethenooripavine 3-acetate *see* Acetorphine.

N-[**2-Hydroxy-1-(methylcarbamoyl)-ethyl]-2,4,6-triiodo-5-(2-methoxyacet-amido)isophthalamidic acid** *see* Ioseric acid.

4'-[[(Hydroxymethyl)carbamoyl]-

247

sulfamoyl]phthalanilic acid *see*
Sulfaloxic acid.

2-(3-Hydroxy-3-methyl-5-carboxypentyl)-
3,5,6-trimethyl-*p*-benzoquinone lactone
see Tocopheronic acid.

3-Hydroxymethyl-2-cephem-2-carboxylic
acid acetate *see* Cephalosporanic acid.

Hydroxymethylchrysazin *see* Aloe-emodin.

7-Hydroxy-4-methylcoumarin *see*
Hymecromone.

(6-Hydroxy-4-methylcoumarin-7-yloxy)-
acetic acid, esters and salts *see*
Cromacate(s).

3-Hydroxy-*N*-methyl-*cis*-crotonamide
dimethyl phosphate *see* Monocrotophos.

1-(Hydroxymethyl)cyclohexaneacetic
acid *see* Hexacyclonic acid.

β-Hydroxy-*β*-methylcyclohexane-
propionic acid *see* Cyclobutoic acid.

5-Hydroxymethylcytosine *see* Desmethylbacimethrin.

2-Hydroxymethyl-2,3-dimethylpentyl
carbamate isopropylcarbamate *see*
Nisobamate.

2-Hydroxymethyl-2,3-dimethylpentyl
dicarbamate *see* Mebutamate.

2-Hydroxymethyl-1,1-dimethylpiperid-
inium methyl sulfate benzilate *see*
Bevonium metilsulfate.

2-Hydroxymethyl-1,1-dimethylpyrrolid-
inium bromide *α*-phenylcyclohexane-
glycolate *sdee* Oxypyrronium bromide.

2-Hydroxymethyl-1,1-dimethylpyrrolid-
inium methylsulfate benzilate *see*
Poldine metilsulfate.

2-(Hydroxymethyl)-1,1-dimethylpyrrolid-
inium methylsulfate 3*β*-hydroxy-11-
oxoolean-12-en-30-oate *see* Roxolonium
metilsulfate.

2-Hydroxy-*N*-methyl-1,2-diphenyl-
methylamine *see* Ephenamine.

2-Hydroxy-2-(3,4-methylenedioxyphenyl)-
acetamidine *see* Olmidine.

2-Hydroxymethylene-17*α*-methylan-
drostan-17-ol-3-one *see* Oxymetholone.

17*α*-HYDROXY-16-METHYLENE-
PREGNA-4,6-DIENE-3,20-DIONE
(16-methylene-4,6-pregnadien-17*α*-ol-3,20-
dione; 6-dehydro-17*α*-hydroxy-16-methyl-
eneprogesterone).

17*α*-HYDROXY-16-METHYLENE-
PREGNA-4,6-DIENE-3,20-DIONE
ACETATE (17*α*-acetoxy-6-dehydro-16-
methyleneprogesterone; 'superlutin').

17*α*-HYDROXY-16-METHYLENE-
PREGNA-4,6-DIENE-3,20-DIONE
ACETATE WITH MESTRANOL
('antigest').

5-Hydroxy-6-methylenetetracycline *see*
Metacycline.

3-Hydroxy-17*α*-methylestra-1,3,5(10)-
trien-17-one *see* Almestrone.

17*β*-Hydroxy-7*α*-methylestr-4-en-3-one
see Trestolone.

N-[1-(Hydroxymethyl)ethyl]lysergamide
see Ergometrine.

D-(+)-2-(1-Hydroxy-1-methylethyl)-1-

methylpiperidine diphenylacetate
(ester) *see* Pinolcaine.

Hydroxymethylgramicidin *see* Methocidin.

6-Hydroxy-6-methyl-2-heptylamine *see*
Heptaminol.

3-Hydroxy-1-methyl-5,6-indolinedione *see*
Adrenochrome.

3-Hydroxy-1-methyl-5,6-indolinedione
semicarbazone *see* Carbazochrome.

7-Hydroxymethyl-4-methoxybenzopyran-
5-one *see* Khellol.

8*β*-Hydroxymethyl-10-methoxy-1,6-di-
methylergoline 5-bromonicotinate *see*
Nicergoline.

2-Hydroxymethyl-5-methoxy-6,7-furano-
chromone *see* Khellol.

7-Hydroxymethyl-4-methoxy-5H-furo-
(3,2-g)(1)benzopyran-5-one glucoside
see Khelloside.

3-[[[1-(Hydroxymethyl)-2-(methylamino)-2-oxoethyl]amino]carbonyl]-
2,4,6-triiodo-5-[(methoxyacetyl)amino]-
benzoic acid *see* Ioseric acid.

17-Hydroxy-6-methyl-16-methylene-
pregna-4,6-diene-3,20-dione *see* Melengestrol.

4-Hydroxy-2-methyl-*N*-(5-methylisoxazol-
3-yl)-2H-1,2-benzothiazine-3-carbox-
amide 1,1-dioxide *see* Isoxicam.

4-Hydroxy-2-methyl-2-nonyl-
1,3-dioxolane carbamate *see* Dioxamate.

2-Hydroxymethyl-2-methyl-1-pentanol
butylcarbamate carbamate *see*
Tybamate.

2-(Hydroxymethyl)-2-methyl-1-pentanol
cyclopropanecarbamate carbamate
see Lorbamate.

2-Hydroxymethyl-2-methyl-1-pentanol
p-tolylborate *see* Tolboxane.

2-Hydroxymethyl-2-methylpentyl butylcarbamate carbamate *see* Tybamate.

2-Hydroxymethyl-1-methylpyrrolidine
benzilate *see* Poldine.

2-Hydroxymethyl-3-methylquinoxaline
1,4-dioxide *see* Mequidox.

1-Hydroxymethyl-3-methyl-2-thiourea
see Noxytiolin.

3-Hydroxy-*N*-methylmorphinan *see*
Dextrorphan; Levorphanol; Racemorphan.

2-Hydroxy-3-methyl-1,4-naphthoquinone
see Phthiocol.

5-Hydroxy-2-methyl-1,4-naphthoquinone
see Plumbagin.

3-(Hydroxymethyl)-1-[3-(5-nitro-2-furyl)-
allylideneamino]hydantoin *see* Nifurmazole.

2-(Hydroxymethyl)-6-[2-(5-nitro-2-furyl)-
vinyl]pyridine *see* Nifurpirinol.

17*β*-Hydroxy-17*α*-methyl-19-norandrosta-
4,9,11-trien-3-one *see* Methyltrienolone.

17*β*-Hydroxy-17-methyl-B-norandrost-
4-en-3-one *see* Benorterone.

17-Hydroxy-11*β*-methyl-19-norpregn-4-
ene-3,20-dione acetate *see* Norgestomet.

17-Hydroxy-7*α*-methyl-19-nor-17*α*-pregn-
5(10)-en-20-yn-3-one *see* Tibolone.

2-[(E)-3-Hydroxy-3-methyl-1-octenyl]-

5-oxocyclopentaneheptanoic acid *see* Doxaprost.

2-(3-Hydroxy-3-methyloctyl)-5-oxocyclopentaneheptanoic acid *see* Deprostil.

17β-Hydroxy-17-methyl-2-oxa-5α-androstan-3-one *see* Oxandrolone.

15-Hydroxy-15-methyl-9-oxoprostan-1-oic acid *see* Deprostil.

4-Hydroxy-3-methyl-2-(2,4-pentadienyl)-2-cyclopenten-1-one *see* Pyrethrolone.

4-Hydroxy-4-methyl-2-pentanone *see* Diacetone alcohol.

p-Hydroxy-α-methylphenethylamine *see* Hydroxyamphetamine.

7-[2-(2-Hydroxy-1-methylphenethyl-amino)ethyl]theophylline *see* Cafedrine.

3-(β-Hydroxy-α-methylphenethylamino)-3′-methoxypropiophenone *see* Oxyfedrine.

1-(3-Hydroxy-5-methyl-4-phenylhexyl)-1-methylpiperidinium bromide *see* Piperphenamine.

p-Hydroxy-α-[1-(1-methyl-3-phenyl-propylamino)ethyl]benzyl alcohol *see* Buphenine.

5-[1-Hydroxy-2-(1-methyl-3-phenyl-propylamino)ethyl]salicylamide *see* Labetalol.

11β-Hydroxy-6α-methylpregna-1,4-diene-3,20-dione *see* Endrisone.

17-Hydroxy-6-methylpregna-4,6-diene-3,20-dione *see* Megestrol.

11β-Hydroxy-6α-methylpregn-4-ene-3,20-dione *see* Medrysone.

17α-Hydroxy-6α-methylpregn-4-ene-3,20-dione *see* Medroxyprogesterone.

17-Hydroxy-6-methylpregn-5-ene-3,20-dione cyclic 3-(ethylene acetal) acetate *see* Edogestrone.

11β-Hydroxy-6α-methylprogesterone *see* Medrysone.

17α-Hydroxy-6α-methylprogesterone *see* Medroxyprogesterone.

2-Hydroxy-2-methylpropyl 4-(4-amino-6,7,8-trimethoxyquinazolin-2-yl)-piperazine-1-carboxylate *see* Trimazosin.

2-Hydroxy-2-methylpropyl 4-(6,7-di-methoxyquinazolin-4-yl)piperazine-1-carboxylate *see* Hoquizil.

N-(1-Hydroxymethylpropyl)lysergamide *see* Methylergometrine.

N-(1-Hydroxymethylpropyl)-1-methyl-lysergamide *see* Methysergide.

17β-Hydroxy-6α-methyl-17-(1-propynyl)-androst-4-en-3-one *see* Dimethisterone.

3-Hydroxy-2-methyl-4,5-pyridinedi-methanol *see* Pyridoxine.

5-Hydroxy-6-methyl-3,4-pyridinedi-methanol *see* Pyridoxine.

5-Hydroxy-6-methyl-3,4-pyridinedi-methanol 3-ether with glycolic acid *see* 2-[(5-Hydroxy-4-hydroxymethyl-6-methyl-pyrid-3-yl)methoxy]glycolic acid.

3-Hydroxy-1-methylpyridinium bromide dimethylcarbamate *see* Pyridostigmine.

3-Hydroxy-1-methylpyridinium bromide hexamethylenebis(*N*-methyl-

carbamate) *see* Distigmine.

4-Hydroxy-2-methyl-*N*-pyrid-2-yl-2H-1,2-benzothiazine-3-carboxamide 1,1-dioxide *see* Piroxicam.

3-Hydroxymethyl-7-[2-(4-pyridylthio)-acetamido]-2-cephem-2-carboxylic acid acetate *see* Cefapirin.

3-Hydroxy-1-methylquinuclidinium bromide benzilate *see* Clidinium.

3-Hydroxy-1-methylquinuclidinium bromide α-phenylcyclohexaneglycolate *see* Droclidinium bromide.

14-Hydroxy-3-(4-*O*-methyl-α-L-rhamno-pyranosyloxy)-14β-bufa-4,20,22-tri-enolide *see* Rambufaside.

*N*¹-Hydroxymethylsulfanilamide glucose sodium bisulfite compound *see* Glucosulfamide.

4-Hydroxy-2-methyl-*N*-thiazol-2-yl-2H-1,2-benzothiazine-3-carboxamide 1,1-dioxide *see* Sudoxicam.

5-Hydroxymethyl-3-*m*-tolyloxazolidin-2-one *see* Toloxatone.

5-Hydroxy-6-methyluracil *see* Pentoxyl.

2-[4-(Hydroxymethylureidosulfonyl)-phenylcarbamoyl]benzoic acid *see* Sulfaloxic acid.

6-((*R*)-2-Hydroxy-4-methylvaleramido)-penicillanic acid 2-furoate *see* Furbucillin.

3-Hydroxymorphinan *see* Norlevorphanol.

7-Hydroxy-4-morpholinomethylcoumarin *see* Oxazorone.

2′-Hydroxy-3-morpholinopropiophenone *see* Romifenone.

Hydroxymycin *see* Paromomycin.

N-Hydroxynaphthalamide diethyl phosphate *see* Naftalofos.

6-Hydroxy-1-naphthalenepropionic acid *see* Allenolic acid.

3-HYDROXY-2-NAPHTHOIC ACID ('bona').

3-Hydroxy-2-naphthoic acid (3-acetyl-5-chloro-2-hydroxybenzyl)dimethyl(2-phenoxyethyl)ammonium salt *see* Difezil.

3-Hydroxy-2-naphthoic acid benzyl-dimethyl(2-phenoxyethyl)ammonium salt *see* Bephenium hydroxynaphthoate.

5-Hydroxy-1,4-naphthoquinone *see* Juglone.

2-(2-Hydroxynaphth-1-yl)cyclohexanone *see* Naphthonone.

N-Hydroxynaphthylimide diethyl phosphate *see* Naftalofos.

3-Hydroxy-4-naphth-1-yloxybutyr-amidoxime *see* Nadoxolol.

(2-Hydroxy-3-naphth-1-yloxypropyl)iso-propyldimethylammonium chloride *see* Pranolium chloride.

2-Hydroxy-2′,6′-nicotinoxylidide *see* Isonixin.

4-Hydroxy-3-nitrobenzenearsonic acid *see* Roxarsone.

p-Hydroxy-*N*²-(5-nitro-2-furfurylidene)-benzohydrazide *see* Nifuroxazide.

8-Hydroxy-4-nitroquinoline *see* Nitroxoline.

17β-Hydroxy-19-norandrosta-4,9,11-trien-

3-one *see* Trienolone.
m-**Hydroxynorephedrine** *see* Metaraminol.
6-Hydroxynorleucine *see* Hexahomoserine.
17-Hydroxy-19-norpregna-4,6-diene-3,20-dione *see* Gestadienol.
17-Hydroxy-19-nor-17α-pregna-4,9,11-trien-20-yn-3-one *see* Norgestrienone.
20β-Hydroxy-19-norpregn-4-en-3-one *see* Oxogestone.
17-Hydroxy-19-nor-17α-pregn-5(10)-en-20-yn-3-one *see* Noretynodrel.
17α-Hydroxy-19-norprogesterone *see* Gestonorone.
12-Hydroxy-9-octadecenoic acid *see* Ricinoleic acid.
2-Hydroxy-4-octyloxybenzophenone *see* Octabenzone.
3-(17β-Hydroxy-3-oxoandrosta-4,6-dien-17-yl)propionic acid *see* Canrenoic acid.
17-(2-Hydroxyethyl)-4-androstene-3,11-dione *see* Dehydrocorticosterone.
3-Hydroxy-11-oxoolean-12-en-30-oic acid *see* Enoxolone.
3β-Hydroxy-11-oxoolean-12-en-30-oic acid hydrogen *cis*-1,2-cyclohexanedicarboxylate *see* Cicloxolone.
4-Hydroxy-3-(3-oxo-1-phenylbutyl)-2H-1-benzopyran-2-one *see* Warfarin.
17β-Hydroxy-3-oxo-17α-pregna-4,6-diene-21-carboxylic acid *see* Canrenoic acid.
17-Hydroxy-3-oxo-17α-pregn-4-ene-7,21-dicarboxylic acid 7-methyl ester 21-potassium salt *see* Mexrenoate potassium.
15α-Hydroxy-9-oxo-10,13-*trans*-prostadienoic acid *see* Prostaglandin A₁.
15-Hydroxy-9-oxo-5-*cis*-8(12),13-*trans*-prostatrienoic acid *see* Prostaglandin B₂.
3-Hydroxy-4-oxo-1(4H)-pyridinealanine *see* Minosine.
6-(10-Hydroxy-6-oxo-*trans*-1-undecenyl)-β-resorcyclic acid lactone *see* Zearalenone.
4-Hydroxy-2,4-pentadienoic acid γ-lactone *see* Protoanemonin.
4-Hydroxy-3,3-pentamethylenebutyric acid *see* Hexacyclonic acid.
Hydroxypentenoic acid lactones *see* Angelica lactones.
HYDROXYPETHIDINE*** (ethyl 4-(*m*-hydroxyphenyl)-1-methylisonipecotate; bemidone; Hö-10446; WIN-771; 'biphenal', 'demidone').
α-Hydroxyphenacetin *see* Fenacetinol.
3-Hydroxy-*N*-phenacylmorphinan *see* Levophenacylmorphan.
Hydroxyphenamate* *see* Oxyfenamate.
4-Hydroxyphenethylamine *see* Tyramine.
2-(*p*-Hydroxyphenethylamino)-1-(*p*-hydroxyphenyl)propan-1-ol *see* Ritodrine.
2-(β-Hydroxyphenethylamino)pyridine *see* Fenyramidol.
2-(β-Hydroxyphenethylamino)pyrimidine *see* Fenyripol.
β-Hydroxyphenethyl carbamate *see* Styramate.
α-(*p*-Hydroxyphenethyl)-4,7-dimethoxy-

6-(2-piperid-1-ylethoxy)-5-benzofuranmethanol *see* Piprofurol.
2-(β-Hydroxyphenethyl)-1-methyl-6-phenacylpiperidine *see* Lobeline.
2-[6-(β-Hydroxyphenethyl)-1-methyl-piperid-2-yl]acetophenone *see* Lobeline.
7-Hydroxyphenothiazin-3-one *see* Thionol.
β-(4-Hydroxyphenoxy)phenethylamine *see* Thyronamine.
2-[4-(4-Hydroxyphenoxy)phenyl]acetic acid *see* Thyroacetic acid.
3-[4-(4-Hydroxyphenoxy)phenyl]alanine *see* Thyronine.
3-[4-(4-Hydroxyphenoxy)phenyl]propionic acid *see* Thyropropionic acid.
5-(*m*-Hydroxyphenoxy)-1H-tetrazole *see* Melizame.
α-Hydroxyphenylacetic acid *see* Mandelic acid.
p-Hydroxyphenylbutazone *see* Oxyphenbutazone.
4-(*o*-Hydroxyphenyl)-3-buten-2-one *see* Salicylidene acetone.
2-Hydroxy-2-phenylbutyl carbamate *see* Oxyfenamate.
3-Hydroxy-2-phenylcinchoninic acid *see* Oxycinchophen.
cis-**2-Hydroxy-2-phenylcyclohexane-carboxylic acid** *see* Cicloxilic acid.
6-[4-(*p*-Hydroxyphenyl)-2,2-dimethyl-5-oxoimidazolidin-1-yl]penicillanic acid *see* Oxetacillin.
3-(*m*-Hydroxyphenyl)-2,3-dimethyl-1-phenacylpiperidine *see* Myfadol.
2-[3-(*m*-Hydroxyphenyl)-2,3-dimethyl-piperid-1-yl]acetophenone *see* Myfadol.
2-(*m*-Hydroxyphenyl)ethanolamine *see* Norphenylephrine.
2-(*p*-Hydroxyphenyl)ethanolamine *see* Octopamine.
N-(*p*-**Hydroxyphenyl)ethanolamine** *see* 2-(*p*-Hydroxyanilino)ethanol.
2-(*p*-Hydroxyphenyl)ethylamine *see* Tyramine.
2-(2-Hydroxy-2-phenylethylamino)-pyridine *see* Fenyramidol.
2-(2-Hydroxy-2-phenylethylamino)-pyrimidine *see* Fenyripol.
2-Hydroxy-2-phenylethyl carbamate *see* Styramate.
3-Hydroxy-*N*-(2-phenylethyl)morphinan *see* Phenomorphan.
1-(*p*-Hydroxyphenyl)-2-isopropylamino-ethanol *see* Deterenol.
3-(1-Hydroxy-1-phenylisopropylamino)-3′-methoxypropiophenone *see* Oxyfedrine.
1-(*p*-Hydroxyphenyl)-2-methylamino-1-propanol *see* *p*-Hydroxyephedrine.
1-(*p*-Hydroxyphenyl)-2-(1-methyl-2-phenoxyethylamino)-1-propanol *see* Isoxsuprine.
1-(*p*-Hydroxyphenyl)-2-(1-methyl-3-phenylpropylamino)-1-propanol *see* Buphenine.
1-[4-(*m*-Hydroxyphenyl)-1-methylpiperid-4-yl]-1-propanone *see* Ketobemidone.

4-(*m*-Hydroxyphenyl)-1-methyl-4-propion-
ylpiperidine *see* Ketobemidone.
4-[2-[3-(*p*-Hydroxyphenyl)-1-methyl-
propylamino]ethyl]pyrocatechol *see*
Dobutamine.
3-(*m*-Hydroxyphenyl)-1-methyl-3-propyl-
pyrrolidine *see* Profadol.
o-Hydroxyphenyl-2-morpholinoethyl
ketone *see* Romifenone.
Hydroxyphenylorciprenaline *see* Fenoterol.
2-(*o*-Hydroxyphenyl)-1,3,4-oxadiazole *see*
Fenadiazole.
3α-Hydroxy-8-(*p*-phenylphenacyl)-
1αH,5αH-tropanium bromide (−)-
tropate *see* Fentonium bromide.
2-Hydroxy-2-phenylpropionamide *see*
Atrolactamide.
2-Hydroxy-2-phenylpropionic acid *see*
Atrolactic acid.
3-Hydroxy-2-phenylpropionic acid *see*
Tropic acid.
4-Hydroxy-3-(1-phenyl-2-propion-
ylethyl)coumarin sodium salt *see*
Nafarin.
4-Hydroxy-3-(1-phenylpropyl)coumarin
see Phenprocoumon.
1-(3-Hydroxy-3-phenylpropyl)-4-(β-
methoxyphenethyl)piperazine *see*
Eprozinol.
1-(3-Hydroxy-3-phenylpropyl)-4-phenyl-
isonipecotic acid ethyl ester *see*
Phenoperidine.
N-(*p*-Hydroxyphenyl)salicylamide *see*
Osalmid.
4-(3-Hydroxy-3-phenyl-3-thien-2-yl-
propyl)-4-methylmorpholinium iodide
see Tiemonium iodide.
2-[(*N*-(*m*-Hydroxyphenyl)-*p*-toluidino)-
methyl]-2-imidazoline *see* Phentolamine.
(*m*-Hydroxyphenyl)trimethylammonium
bromide decamethylenebis(methylcarbamate) *see* Demecarium bromide.
(*m*-Hydroxyphenyl)trimethylammonium
methosulfate methylcarbamate *see*
Neostigmine.
3-Hydroxyphthalide ampicillin ester *see*
Talampicillin.
N-(3-Hydroxypicolinylcarbonyl)-L-
threonyl-D-α-aminobutyryl-L-prolyl-
N-methyl-L-phenylalanyl-4-oxo-L-
pipecolyl-L-2-phenylglycine β-lactone
see Virginiamycin S.
3-(3-Hydroxypiperid-2-ylacetonyl)-
4(3H)-quinazolinone *see* Febrifugine.
3-(1-Hydroxy-2-piperid-1-ylethyl)-5-
phenylisoxazole *see* Perisoxal.
10-[3-(4-Hydroxypiperid-1-yl)-2-methyl-
propyl]-2-methoxyphenothiazine *see*
Perimetazine.
10-[2-(4-Hydroxypiperid-1-yl)propyl]-
phenothiazine-1-carbonitrile *see*
Periciazine.
α-Hydroxypiperonylformamidine *see*
Olmidine.
Hydroxypolyethoxydodecane *see*
Polidocanol.
16α-Hydroxyprednisolone 16,17-acetonide

see Desonide.
17β-Hydroxy-17α-pregna-4,6-diene-3-one-
21-carboxylic acid *see* Canrenoic acid.
3α-Hydroxy-5α-pregnane-11,20-dione *see*
Alfaxalone.
3α-Hydroxy-5β-pregnane-11,20-dione *see*
Renanolone.
3β-Hydroxy-pregn-5-en-20-one *see* Pregnenolone.
HYDROXYPROCAINE*** (2-diethylamino-
ethyl 4-aminosalicylate; pascain; 'hydroxy-
novocaine', 'oxycaine', 'oxyprocaine').
HYDROXYPROCAINE-PENICILLIN
('citocillin').
HYDROXYPROGESTERONE*** (17α-
hydroxypregn-4-ene-3,20-dione; 17α-
hydroxyprogesterone).
17α-Hydroxyprogesterone *see* Hydroxyprogesterone.
21-Hydroxyprogesterone *see* Desoxycortone.
HYDROXYPROGESTERONE ACE-
TATE*** ('prodox').
HYDROXYPROGESTERONE CAPRO-
ATE*** (hydroxyprogesterone hexanoate;
'delalutin', 'hormofort', 'neolutin',
'primolut-depot', 'proluton-depot').
See also Estradiol valerate with hydroxyprogesterone caproate.
1-Hydroxy-2-propanone *see* Hydroxyacetone.
6-Hydroxy-2-(α-propionamido)purine *see*
Guanine propionate.
4'-Hydroxypropionanilide *see* Parapropamol.
3-Hydroxypropionic acid *see* Hydracrylic
acid.
2-HYDROXYPROPIOPHENONE (lactophenone).
4'-Hydroxypropiophenone *see* Paroxypropione.
p-Hydroxypropiophenone *see* Paroxypropione.
2'-(2-Hydroxy-3-propylaminopropoxy)-3-
phenylpropiophenone *see* Propafenone.
2-Hydroxypropyl 14-deoxyvincaminate
see Vinpoline.
1-(2-Hydroxypropyl)-2-methyl-5-nitro-
imidazole *see* Secnidazole.
1-(3-Hydroxypropyl)-2-methyl-4-nitro-
imidazole *see* Ternidazole.
N-[2-[*p*-(1-Hydroxypropyl)phenoxy]-
ethyl]-α-methylphenethylamine *see*
Fenalcomine.
3-Hydroxypropyl phosphate *see* Propylene
glycol 1-phosphate.
N-(3-Hydroxypropyl)picoline *p*-cyclo-
hexyloxybenzoate *see* Cyclomethycaine.
5-(2-Hydroxypropyl)-5-(2-propenyl)-
2,4,6(1H,3H,5H)-pyrimidinetrione *see*
Proxibarbal.
1-(2-Hydroxypropyl)theobromine *see*
Protheobromine.
(2-Hydroxypropyl)trimethylammonium
ion *see* β-Methylcholine.
(3-Hydroxypropyl)trimethylammonium
ion *see* Homocholine.
6-Hydroxypurine *see* Hypoxanthine.

4-Hydroxypyrazole-3-carboxamide 5-riboside see Pirazofurin.

4-Hydroxypyrazolopyrimidine see Allopurinol.

HYDROXYPYRIDINE TARTRATE*** (3-pyridinol tartaric ester; 3-hydroxypyridine tartrate).

1-HYDROXYPYRIDO(3,2-a)PHENOXAZIN-5-ONE-3-CARBOXYLIC ACID ('catalin').

5-(α-Hydroxy-α-pyrid-2-ylbenzyl)-7-(α-pyrid-2-ylbenzylidene)norborn-5-ene-2,3-dicarboxamide see Norbormide.

N-[(**3-Hydroxypyrid-2-yl)carbonyl**]-L-threonyl-D-α-aminobutyryl-L-prolyl-*N*-methyl-L-phenylalanyl-4-oxo-L-pipecolyl-L-2-phenylglycine β-lactone see Virginiamycin S.

β-Hydroxy-*N*-pyrid-2-ylphenethylamine see Fenyramidol.

β-Hydroxy-*N*-pyrimid-2-ylphenethylamine see Fenyripol.

4-Hydroxyquinaldic acid see Kynurenic acid.

8-Hydroxyquinoline see 8-Quinolinol.

14β-Hydroxy-3β-(rhamnoglucosyloxy)-bufa-4,20,22-trienolide see Scillaren A.

14-Hydroxy-3β-rhamnosyloxybufa-4,20,22-trienolide see Proscillaridin.

4-Hydroxy-5-β-D-ribofuranosyl-1H-pyrazole-3-carboxamide see Pirazofurin.

7-Hydroxy-3-(β-D-ribofuranosyl)pyrazolo-(4,3-d)pyrimidine see Formycin B.

4′-Hydroxysalicylanilide see Osalmid.

5-Hydroxysalicylic acid see Gentisic acid.

3α-Hydroxyspiro(1αH,5αH-nortropane-8,1′-pyrrolidinium)chloride benzilate see Trospium chloride.

HYDROXYSTENOZOLE*** (17β-hydroxy-17α-methyl-4-androsteno(3,2-c)pyrazole).

HYDROXYSTILBAMIDINE*** (1-(4-amidino-2-hydroxyphenyl)-2-(4-amidinophenyl)ethylene; 2-hydroxy-4,4′-stilbenedicarboxamidine).

Hydroxysuccinic acid see Malic acid.

4-Hydroxy-3-(4-sulfonaphth-1-ylazo)-naphthionic acid see Carmoisine.

HYDROXYTETRACAINE*** (2-dimethylaminoethyl 4-butylaminosalicylate; deanol 4-butylaminosalicylate; 'rhenocaine', 'salicaine').

2-HYDROXYTETRACOSANOIC ACID (cerebronic acid).

Hydroxytetracycline see Oxytetracycline.

4-Hydroxy-3-(1,2,3,4-tetrahydronaphth-1-yl)coumarin see Coumatetralyl.

4′-HYDROXY-5,6,7,8-TETRAMETHOXY-FLAVONE (4′-demethyltangeretin).

o-[**2-Hydroxy-3-(2,2,5,5-tetramethyl-pyrrolidin-1-yl)propoxy]toluene** see Lotucaine.

N-[**3-(2-Hydroxy-2-thien-2-ylethyl)-4-thiazolin-2-ylidene]acetamide** see Antazonite.

p-[**2-[[2-Hydroxy-3-(*o*-toloxy)propyl]-amino]ethoxy]benzamide** see Tolamolol.

1-[2-Hydroxy-3-(*o*-toloxy)propyl]-2,2,5,5-

tetramethylpyrrolidine see Lotucaine.

HYDROXYTOLUIC ACID*** (2-hydroxy-*m*-toluic acid; 2-hydroxy-3-methylbenzoic acid; 2,3-cresotic acid; *o*-cresotinic acid; 3-methylsalicylic acid; hydroxytoluinic acid).

2-Hydroxy-*m*-toluic acid see Hydroxytoluic acid.

6-Hydroxy-*m*-toluic acid see 2,5-Cresotic acid.

α-Hydroxy-α-toluic acid see Mandelic acid.

Hydroxytoluinic acid see Hydroxytoluic acid.

Hydroxytricarballylic acids see Citric acid; Isocitric acid.

3-Hydroxy-17β-(2,2,2-trichloro-1-hydroxyethoxy)estra-1,3,5(10)-triene see Cloxestradiol.

2-Hydroxytriethylamine ribonucleate see Ribaminol.

17-Hydroxy-6α-trifluoromethylprogesterone see Flumedroxone.

Hydroxytrimethonium see Prolonium.

6-Hydroxy-β,2,7-trimethyl-5-benzofuranacrylic acid δ-lactone see Trioxysalen.

2′-Hydroxy-2,5,9-trimethyl-6,7-benzomorphan see Metazocine.

4-Hydroxy-*N*,*N*,1-trimethyl-3,3-diphenylhexylamine see Dimepheptanol.

3-Hydroxy-3,7,11-trimethyldodecanoic acid see Trethocanic acid.

2-Hydroxytrimethylene-1,3-bis(trimethylammonium iodide) see Prolonium.

5,5′-(2-Hydroxytrimethylenedioxy)bis-(4-oxo-4H-1-benzopyran-2-carboxylic acid) see Cromoglicic acid.

8-Hydroxy-3,6,11-trimethyl-2,6-methanohexahydro-3-benzazocine see Metazocine.

Hydroxytriphenylstannane see Fentin hydroxide.

5-Hydroxytryptamine see Serotonin.

5-HYDROXYTRYPTOPHAN (5-HTP; Ro 0783/B).

5-Hydroxytyramine see Dopamine.

4-Hydroxy-5,6-undecadiene-8,10-diynoic acid γ-lactone see Memotin.

Hydroxyurea* see Hydroxycarbamide.

γ-Hydroxyvinylacrylic acid γ-lactone see Protoanemonin.

17β-Hydroxy-17α-vinylestr-4-en-3-one see Norvinisterone.

17β-Hydroxy-17α-vinyl-5(10)-estren-3-one see Norgesterone.

17β-Hydroxy-17α-vinyl-19-norandrost-4-en-3-one see Norvinisterone.

4-Hydroxy-3-(3,5-xylyl)coumarin see Xylocoumarol.

17α-Hydroxyyohimban-16α-carboxylic acid see Yohimbic acid.

HYDROXYZINE*** (2-[2-[4-(*p*-chloro-α-phenylbenzyl)-1-piperazinyl]ethoxy]-ethanol; 1-(*p*-chlorobenzhydryl)-4-[2-(2-hydroxyethoxy)ethyl]piperazine; hydroxyzine dihydrochloride; UCB-4492; 'arcanax', 'atarax', 'fenarol', 'kombistrat', 'masmoran', 'parenteral', 'tran-Q',

252

'visatril', 'vistaril').

HYDROXYZINE EMBONATE (hydroxyzine 4,4'-methylenebis(3-hydroxynaphthalene-4-carboxylate); hydroxyzine pamoate; 'equipoise', 'masmoran', 'paxistil').

HYDROXYZINE EMBONATE WITH CALCIUM 2-ETHYLBUTYRATE ('sedocalene').

Hydroxyzine pamoate *see* Hydroxyzine embonate.

HYDURILIC ACID (5,5'-bibarbituric acid).

'**Hyflavin**' *see* Methylolriboflavin.

HYGRONIUM (tr) (1-methylpyrrolidine-2-carboxylic acid dimethylaminoethyl ester dimethiodide).

'**Hygroton**' *see* Chlortalidone.

HYMECROMONE*** (7-hydroxy-4-methylcoumarin; 4-methylumbelliferone; 'cantabilin').

'**Hyminal**' *see* Methaqualone.

'**Hymorphan**' *see* Hydromorphone.

HYOCHOLIC ACID (3α,6α,7α-trihydroxycholanic acid).

HYODEOXYCHOLIC ACID (3α,6α-dihydroxycholanic acid).

'**Hyodur**' *see* Dimethyl sulfoxide.

'**Hyosan**' *see* Dichlorophen.

HYOSCINE (DL-atroscine).
See also Scopolamine.

HYOSCYAMINE (tropine L-tropate; duboisine; daturine; hyoscyamine sulfate; 'egacen', 'levsin').

D-**Hyoscyamine** *see* Atropine.

L-**Hyoscyamine** *see* Hyoscyamine.

Hyoscyamine (4'-phenylphenacyl) bromide *see* Fentonium bromide.

'**Hypaque**' *see* Sodium diatrizoate.

'**Hypaque 50**' *see* Sodium diatrizoate.

'**Hypaque 60**' *see* Meglumine diatrizoate.

'**Hypaque 76**' *see* Meglumine diatrizoate with sodium diatrizoate.

'**Hypaque 90**' *see* Meglumine diatrizoate with sodium diatrizoate.

HYPERICIN (4,5,7,4',5',7'-hexahydroxy-2,2'-dimethylnaphthodianthone; hypericium red; 'cyclosan', 'cyclo-werrol').

HYPEROSIDE (quercetin 3-galactoside).

'**Hyperpax**' *see* Methyldopa.

'**Hyperstat**' *see* Diazoxide.

'**Hypertane**' *see* Ethiazide.

Hypertensin *see* Angiotensin.

Hypertensin-Ciba *see* Angiotensinamide.

'**Hypertonal**' *see* Diazoxide.

'**Hyphilline**' *see* Diprophylline.

'**Hypnal**' *see* Chloralphenazone.

'**Hypnazol**' *see* Fenadiazole.

'**Hypnodil**' *see* Metomidate.

Hypnone *see* Acetophenone.

'**Hypnorex**' *see* Lithium carbonate.

'**Hypnotal**' *see* Diethyloxyacetylurea.

'**Hypnotrol**' *see* Secobarbital.

Hypo *see* Sodium thiosulfate.

HYPOGLYCIN A (L-2-amino-3-(2-methylenecyclopropyl)propionic acid; α-amino-2-methylenecyclopropanepropionic acid).

HYPOGLYCIN B (L-glutamyl dipeptide with hypoglycin A).

'**Hypoglycone**' *see* Tolbutamide.

Hyponitrous acid anhydride *see* Nitrous oxide.

α-**Hypophamine** *see* Oxytocin.

β-**Hypophamine** *see* Vasopressin.

'**Hyposan**' *see* Sodium hypochlorite.

'**Hypostamine**' *see* Tritoqualine.

'**Hyposterol**' *see* 2-Phenylbutyramide.

Hyposulfite *see* Sodium thiosulfate.

'**Hyposulphene**' *see* Sodium thiosulfate.

HYPOTAURINE (2-aminoethanesulfinic acid).

Hypothiazide (tr) *see* Hydrochlorothiazide.

'**Hypotrol**' *see* Secobarbital.

'**Hypovase**' *see* Prazosin.

HYPOXANTHINE (6-hydroxypurine; 6(1H)-purinone; sarcine; sarkin).

Hypoxanthine riboside *see* Inosine.

HYPROMELLOSE*** (a partial mixed methyl and hydroxypropyl ether of cellulose).

'**Hyptor**' *see* Methaqualone.

'**Hyryl**' *see* Flavin mononucleotide.

'**Hystryl**' *see* Diphenylpyraline.

'**Hytacherol**' *see* Dihydrotachysterol.

'**Hytakerol**' *see* Dihydrotachysterol.

'**Hyton**' *see* Pemoline.

'**Hytrast**' *see* Iopydol with iopydone.

'**Hyvar**' *see* Isocil.

'**Hyvar X**' *see* Bromacil.

I

IA-307 *see* Sulfadiasulfone.

IAA *see* 3-Indoleacetic acid.

'**Iatropur**' *see* Triamterene.

Ibenzmethyzin* *see* Procarbazine.

'**Ibition**' *see* Thiobarbital.

IBOGAINE (alkaloid from *Tabernanthe iboga*; ibogine; 'bogadin-TM').

IBOTENIC ACID (α-amino-3-hydroxy-5-isoxazoleacetic acid).

IBROTAMIDE*** (2-bromo-N-ethyl-N-isopropylacetamide; 'neodorm', 'vagoprol').

IBUFENAC*** (p-isobutylphenylacetic acid; RD-11654; 'dytransin').

IBUPROFEN*** (2-(p-isobutylphenyl)-

253

propionic acid; *p*-isobutylhydratropic acid;
B-80; IP-82; U-181573; UCB-79171;
'brufen', 'motrin').

IBUPROXAM** (*p*-isobutylhydratropo-
hydroxamic acid; 2-(*p*-isobutylphenyl)-
propionohydroxamic acid).

IBUTEROL** (5-(2-*tert*-butylamino-1-
hydroxyethyl)-*m*-phenylene diisobutyrate;
isobutyric acid diester with 5-(2-*tert*-
butylamino-1-hydroxyethyl)resorcinol).

IBUVERINE*** (isobutyl α-phenylcyclohexaneglycolate).

ICG *see* Indocyanine green.

Ichthammol *see* Ammonium sulfobituminate.

Ichthammonium *see* Ammonium sulfobituminate.

Ichthium *see* Ammonium sulfobituminate.

Ichthosulfol *see* Ammonium sulfobituminate.

ICI-350 *see* Aminochlorthenoxazine.

ICI-15688 *see* Ditophal.

ICI-24223 *see* Isobutyltritylamine.

ICI-28257 *see* Clofibrate.

ICI-32525 *see* Sulfamonomethoxine.

ICI-33828 *see* Metallibure.

ICI-45520 *see* Propranolol.

ICI-45763 *see* Toliprolol.

ICI-46474 *see* Tamoxifen.

ICI-47319 *see* Dexpropranolol.

ICI-48213 *see* Cyclofenil.

ICI-50123 *see* Pentagastrin.

ICI-50172 *see* Practolol.

ICI-51426 *see* Cyheptamide.

ICI-54450 *see* Fenclozic acid.

ICI-55052 *see* Nequinate.

ICI-55695 *see* Methyl clofenapate.

ICI-58834 *see* Viloxazine.

ICI-59118 *see* Razoxane.

ICI-66082 *see* Atenolol.

ICI-74205 *see* 20-Ethyldinoprost.

ICI-74917 *see* Bufrolin sodium.

ICN-542 *see* Ribaminol.

ICN-1229 *see* Ribavirin.

'Icobudon' *see* Allopyrine.

ICRF-159 *see* Razoxane.

'Icteryl' *see* Menbutone.

ID-480 *see* Flurazepam.

ID-530 *see* Nimetazepam.

'Idarac' *see* Floctafenine.

IDC *see* Iododeoxycytidine.

'Ideaxan' *see* Piracetam.

'Idemin' *see* Meprobamate with benactyzine.

'Idexur' *see* Idoxuridine.

'Idogenabil' *see* Menbutone.

IDOXURIDINE*** (2'-deoxy-5-iodouridine;
1-(2-deoxy-β-D-ribofuranosyl)-5-iodouracil;
iduridine; IDU; IUDR; NSC-39661;
SK&F-14287; allergan 211; 'dendrid',
'emanil', 'herplex', 'idexur', 'iduviran',
'kerecid', 'stoxil', 'synmiol', 'virunguent').

IDP *see* Inosine diphosphate.

'Idril' *see* 8-Quinolinol potassium sulfate.

Idrobutamina *see* Butidrine.

IDROCILAMIDE** (*N*-(2-hydroxyethyl)-
cinnamamide; LCB-29; 'brolitene').

'Idroestril' *see* Diethylstilbestrol disulfate.

'Idro P-3' *see* Oxamarin.

IDROPRANOLOL** (1-(5,6-dihydronaphth-

1-yloxy)-3-isopropylamino-2-propanol; 5,6-
dihydro-1-(2-hydroxy-3-isopropylamino-
propoxy)naphthalene; dihydropropranolol;
dropranolol).

Idropropizina *see* Dropizine.

IDU *see* Idoxuridine.

'Idulian' *see* Azatadine maleate.

Iduridine *see* Idoxuridine.

'Iduviran' *see* Idoxuridine.

IEM-163 (tr) *see* Etimizole.

IEM-366 (tr) *see* Fepracet.

IFENPRODIL*** (4-benzyl-α-(*p*-hydroxy-
phenyl)-β-methyl-1-piperidineethanol;
4-benzyl-1-[3-hydroxy-3-(*p*-hydroxy-
phenyl)prop-2-yl]piperidine; α-[1-(4-ben-
zylpiperid-1-yl)ethyl]-*p*-hydroxybenzyl
alcohol; 2-(4-benzylpiperid-1-yl)-1-(*p*-
hydroxyphenyl)-1-propanol; 'vadilex').

IFK (tr) *see* Propham.

IFOSFAMIDE*** (3-(2-chloroethyl)-2-(2-
chloroethylamino)tetrahydro-2H-1,3,2-
oxaphosphorine 2-oxide; 3-(2-chloroethyl)-
2-(2-chloroethylamino)-1-oxa-3-aza-2-
phosphocyclohexane 2-oxide; 3-(2-chloro-
ethyl)-2-(2-chloroethylamino)-2H-1,3,2-
oxazaphosphorinane 2-oxide; isofosfamide;
isophosphamide; Asta-4942; NSC-109724;
Z-4942; 'iso-endoxan').

'Igepal' *see* Nonoxinol.

Ignotine *see* Carnosine.

'Igran' *see* Terbutryn.

'Igroton' *see* Chlortalidone.

I-K-1 *see* Metofoline.

'Ikapharm' *see* Phenmetrazine.

IL-5902 *see* Spiramycin.

IL-6001 *see* Trimipramine.

IL-6302 *see* Dimetotiazine.

IL-17803A *see* Acebutolol.

IL-19552 *see* Pipotiazine palmitate.

'Ildamen' *see* Oxyfedrine.

'Iletin' *see* Insulin zinc suspension.

'Iliadin' *see* Oxymetazoline.

'Ilidar' *see* Azapetine.

'Ilopan' *see* Dexpanthenol.

'Ilosone' *see* Erythromycin estolate.

'Ilotycin' *see* Erythromycin.

'Ilozoft' *see* Sodium dioctyl sulfosuccinate.

ILUDIN M (antibiotic from *Clitocybe
illudens*; NSC-400978).

ILUDIN S (NSC-400979).

'Ilvin' *see* Brompheniramine.

IMA *see* Isopropylmethoxamine.

IMAFEN** (2,3,5,6-tetrahydro-5-phenyl-
1H-imidazo(1,2-a)imidazole).

'Imagon' *see* Chloroquine diphosphate.

'Imagotan' *see* Sulforidazine.

'Imakol' *see* Oxomemazine.

'Imap' *see* Fluspirilene.

'Imbretil' *see* Hexcarbacholine bromide.

Imequin *see* Tetramethylquinuclidine
methiodide.

'Imesonal' *see* Secobarbital.

'Imferdex' *see* Iron dextran.

'Imferon' *see* Iron dextran.

IMICLOPAZINE*** (1-[2-[4-(3-(2-chloro-
phenothiazin-10-yl)propyl)piperazin-1-yl]-
ethyl]-3-methyl-2-imidazolidinone; 2-

chloro-10-[3-[4-(2-(3-methyl-2-oxoimida-zolidin-1-yl)ethyl)piperazin-1-yl]propyl]-phenothiazine; chlorimpiphenine; imiclo-pazine dihydrochloride; Astra-4241; 'ponsital').
'Imidaline' *see* Phentolamine mesilate.
Imidamin *see* Antazoline.
'Imidan' *see* Dimethyl phthalimidomethyl phosphorodithioate.
IMIDAZOLE (1,3-diazole; glyoxaline; iminazole; miazole).
Imidazoleacrylic acid *see* Urocanic acid.
Imidazoleacryloylcholine *see* Murexine.
4,5-IMIDAZOLEDICARBOXAMIDE (glycarbylamide; 'glycamide').
Imidazole-4,5-dicarboxylic acid bis-(ethylamide) *see* Etimizole.
4,5-Imidazoledicarboxylic acid diethyldi-amide *see* Etimizole.
2-IMIDAZOLEETHYLAMINE (2-(2-aminoethyl)imidazole; 2-isohistamine).
4-Imidazoleethylamine *see* Histamine.
IMIDAZOLIDINE (tetrahydroimidazole tetrahydroglyoxaline).
2,4-Imidazolidinedione *see* Hydantoin.
Imidazolidinetrione *see* Parabanic acid.
2-IMIDAZOLINE (4,5-dihydroimidazole).
3-(2-Imidazolin-2-ylmethyl)-2-methyl-benzo(b)thiophene *see* Metizoline.
Imidazolinylureidoaluminium compounds *see* Alcloxa; Aldioxa.
1-(4-Imidazol-4(5)-ylbutyl)-3-methyl-thiourea *see* Burimamide.
Imidazolylthioguanine *see* Tiamiprine.
7-Imidazo(4,5-d)pyrimidine *see* Purine.
IMIDECYL IODINE* (complex of 2-alkyl-(C_7H_{15} to $C_{17}H_{35}$)-1-carboxymethyl-1-(2-hydroxyethyl)-2-imidazolinium chloride with 3,6,9,12,15,18,21,24,27,30,33,36,39-tridexaoxapentaconan-1-ol and iodine; 'amfodyne', 'amphodyne').
IMIDOCARB*** (3,3'-bis(2-imidazolin-2-yl)-carbanilide; 1,3-bis[m-(2-imidazolin-2-yl)-phenyl]urea; 3,3'-diimidazolin-2-ylcarb-anilide; 'imizol').
IMIDOLINE** (1-(m-chlorophenyl)-3-(2-dimethylaminoethyl)-2-imidazolidinone; imidoline hydrochloride; CL-48156).
Iminazole *see* Imidazole.
Iminobibenzyl *see* Dihydrodibenzazepine.
Iminodibenzyl *see* Dihydrodibenzazepine.
2,2'-Iminodiethanol *see* Diethanolamine.
4,4'-(Iminodimethylene)dipyridine *see* Gapicomine.
3,3'-Iminodi-1-propanol dimesilate *see* Improsulfan.
(1-Iminoethyl)phosphoramidothioic acid O,O-bis(p-chlorophenyl) ester *see* Phosacetim.
2-Imino-1-methyl-4-imidazolinone *see* Creatinine.
2-Imino-3-methyl-1-phenyl-4-imidazolidi-none *see* Azolimine.
IMINOPHENIMIDE*** (3-ethyl-3-phenyl-piperazine-2,6-dione).
2-Imino-5-phenyl-4-oxazolidinone *see* Pemoline.

Iminopromazine *see* Aminopromazine.
Iminostilbene *see* Dibenzazepine.
IMIPRAMINE*** (5-(3-dimethylamino-propyl)-10,11-dihydro-5H-dibenzo(b,f)-azepine; 1(3-dimethylaminopropyl)-4,5-dihydro-2,3,6,7-dibenzazepine; 2,2'-(3-dimethylaminopropylimino)bibenzyl; imipramine hydrochloride; imizine; meli-pramine; G-22150; G-22355; 'antidepin', 'berkomin', 'deprinol', 'eupramin', 'irmin', 'meliprimin', 'promiben', 'pryleugan', 'psychoforine', 'surplix', 'tofranil').
IMIPRAMINE OXIDE (imipramine N-oxide; 'imiprex').
'Imiprex' *see* Imipramine oxide.
Imizine (tr) *see* Imipramine.
'Imizol' *see* Imidocarb.
'Immenoctal' *see* Secobarbital.
'Immenox' *see* Secobarbital.
'Immobilon' *see* Etorphine with aceproma-zine *and* Etorphine with levomepromazine.
'Imodium' *see* Loperamide.
IMOLAMINE*** (4-(2-diethylaminoethyl)-5-imino-3-phenyl-△²-1,2,4-oxadiazoline; imolamine hydrochloride; LA-1211; 'angolon', 'irrigor').
'Imotryl' *see* Benzydamine.
IMP *see* Inosinic acid.
'Imperacin' *see* Oxytetracycline.
Imperatorin *see* Pentosalen.
'Impletol' *see* Procaine-caffeine complex.
IMPROSULFAN** (3,3'-iminodi-1-propanol dimethanesulfonate (ester); 3,3'-iminodi-1-propanol dimesilate; NSC-102627).
'Impruvol' *see* Butylated hydroxytoluene.
'Impugan' *see* Furosemide.
'Imugan' *see* Chloraniformethan.
'Imuran' *see* Azathioprine.
'Imurel' *see* Azathioprine.
IN-29-5931 *see* Triclofenol piperazine.
IN-73 *see* Isoniazid.
IN-117 *see* Hexafluronium.
IN-379 *see* Pimetine.
IN-391 *see* Methindethyrium.
IN-461 *see* Benzindopyrine.
IN-511 *see* Fenyramidol.
IN-836 *see* Fenyripol.
IN-1060 *see* Cyprolidol.
'Inactin' *see* Thiobutabarbital.
'Inaktin' *see* Thiobutabarbital.
'Inamycin' *see* Novobiocin.
'Inappetyl' *see* Benzphetamine.
'Inapsine' *see* Droperidol.
'Incidal' *see* Mebhydrolin napadisilate.
In:Cn *see* Poly I:C.
'Indalitan' *see* Clorindione.
Indalone *see* Butopyronoxyl.
INDAN (2,3-dihydroindene).
INDANOREX** (2-(1-aminopropyl)-2-indanol; 1-(2-hydroxyindan-2-yl)-propylamine).
Indanylcarbenicillin *see* Carindacillin.
6-[2-(Indan-5-ylcarbonyl)-2-phenylaceta-mido]penicillanic acid *see* Carindacillin.
Indan-5-yl N-(2-carboxy-3,3-dimethyl-7-oxo-4-thia-1-azabicyclo(3.2.0)hept-6-yl)-

2-phenylmalonamate *see* Carindacillin.
N-**Indan-2-yl-*N*-(3-dimethylaminopropyl)**
aniline *see* Aprindine.
O-**Indan-5-yl** *m*,*N*-**dimethylthiocarbani-**
late *see* Tolindate.
[3-([*N*-**Indan-2-yl**)-*N*-**phenylamino**]-
propyl]diethylamine *see* Aprindine.
INDAPAMIDE*** (4-chloro-*N*-(2-methyl-
indolin-1-yl)-3-sulfamoylbenzamide;
2-chloro-5-[(2-methylindolin-1-yl)carbam-
oyl]benzenesulfonamide; 'fludex').
α-**Inden-1-ylidene-*N*,*N*-dimethyl-*p*-tolui-**
dine *see* 1-(4-Dimethylaminobenzylidene)-
indene.
'**Inderal**' *see* Propranolol.
Indican *see* Indoxylsulfuric acid.
Indicarmin *see* Indigo carmine.
Indigo blue *see* Indigotin.
INDIGO CARMINE (indigotin-5,5-disulf-
onic acid disodium salt; carminum
coeruleum; indicarmin; soluble indigo
blue).
INDIGOTIN (2,2'-bipseudoindoxyl; diindogen; indigo blue).
Indigotin-5,5'-disulfonate *see* Indigo
carmine.
'**Indoarginine**' *see* Indometacin arginine
salt.
INDOCATE** (2-dimethylaminoethyl
1-benzyl-2,3-dimethylindole-5-carboxylate;
deanol ester of 1-benzyl-2,3-dimethyl-
indole-5-carboxylic acid).
'**Indocid**' *see* Indometacin.
'**Indocin**' *see* Indometacin.
INDOCYANINE GREEN* (2-[7-[1,1-di-
methyl-3-(4-sulfobutyl)benz(e)indolin-2-
ylidene]-1,3,5-heptatrienyl]-1,1-dimethyl-
3-(4-sulfobutyl)-1H-benz(e)indolium
hydroxide internal salt sodium salt; Fox
green; tricarbocyanine II; ICG; 'cardio-
green', 'ujoviridin', 'wofaverdin').
'**Indocybin**' *see* Psilocybine.
'**Indokolon**' *see* Flurotyl.
INDOLE (1-benzazole; 2,3-benzopyrrole;
ketole).
3-**INDOLEACETIC ACID** (heteroauxin;
IAA).
2,3-**Indoledione** *see* Isatin.
Indole-3-ethanol *see* Tryptophol.
3-**Indoleethylamine** *see* Tryptamine.
2-**Indolinone** *see* Oxindole.
INDOLMYCIN (tr) (5-(1-indol-3-ylethyl)-
2-methylaminooxazolin-4-one; antibiotic
PA-155).
2(3H)-**Indolone** *see* Oxindole.
5-(1-**Indol-3-ylethyl)-2-methylaminooxa-**
zolin-4-one *see* Indolmycin.
N-[1-(2-**Indol-3-ylethyl)piperid-4-yl]-**
benzamide *see* Indoramin.
Indol-4-yloxy-3-isopropylamino-2-propa-
nol *see* Pindolol.
'**Indomee**' *see* Indometacin.
INDOMETACIN*** (1-(*p*-chlorobenzoyl)-5-
methoxy-2-methyl-3-indoleacetic acid;
indomethacin; 'amuno', 'confortid',
'indocid', 'indocin', 'indomee', 'metindol').
See also Dexamethasone with indometacin;

Meglumine indometacinate.
Indometacin amide deoxyglucose deri-
vative *see* Glucametacin.
INDOMETACIN ARGININE SALT (PIR-
353; 'combiflex', 'indoarginine').
Indometacin ester with glycolic acid *see*
Acemetacin.
Indometacin ester with 3-[4-(2-hydroxy-
ethyl)piperazin-1-yl]propyl DL-**4-benz-**
amido-*N*,*N*-dipropylglutaramate *see*
Proglumetacin.
INDOMETACIN WITH ZOLIMIDINE
('solitacin').
Indomethacin* *see* Indometacin.
Indopan (tr) *see* 2-Methyltryptamine.
INDOPINE*** (3-[2-(1-phenethylpiperid-4-
yl)ethyl]indole).
INDOPROFEN*** (*p*-(1-oxoisoindolin-2-
yl)hydratropic acid; 2-[*p*-(1-oxoiso-indo-
lin-2-yl)phenyl]propionic acid; 2-[*p*-(1-
carboxyethyl)phenyl]isoindol-1-one; 2-[*p*-
(1-carboxyethyl)phenyl]phthalimidine;
K-4277).
INDORAMIN*** (3-[2-(4-benzamidopiperid-
1-yl)ethyl]indole; 4-benzamido-1-(2-indol-
3-ylethyl)piperidine; *N*-[1-(2-indol-3-yl-
ethyl)piperid-4-yl]benzamide; Wy-21901).
'**Indorm**' *see* Propiomazine.
INDOXOLE** (2,3-bis(*p*-methoxyphenyl)-
indole; U-22020).
INDOXYL (3-hydroxyindole; indol-3-ol).
INDOXYL β-D-**GLUCOSIDE** (indican;
plant indican).
3-**INDOXYLSULFURIC ACID** (indican;
urinary indican).
INDRILENE*** (*N*,*N*-dimethyl-1-phenyl-
indene-1-ethylamine; 1-(2-dimethyl-
aminoethyl)-1-phenylindene).
'**Indunox**' *see* Etodroxizine.
'**Indusil T**' *see* Cobamamide.
'**Inerteen**' *see* Polychlorinated biphenyl
mixture.
'**Inezin**' *see* Benzyl ethyl phenylphosphono-
thioate.
INF *see* Menazone.
INF-1837 *see* Flufenamic acid.
INF-3355 *see* Mefenamic acid.
'**Infecundin**' *see* Noretynodrel with
mestranol.
'**Inferno**' *see* Amiton.
'**Infiltrina**' *see* Dimethyl sulfoxide.
'**Inflacine**' *see* Dexamethasone with indo-
metacin.
'**Inflaryl**' *see* Niflumic acid.
Inflatine *see* Lobeline.
'**Infukoll M-40**' *see* Dextran 40.
'**Infundin**' *see* Oxytocin.
Ingalan (tr) *see* Methoxyflurane.
'**INGH**' *see* Gluconiazone.
INH *see* Isoniazid.
Inhalan (tr) *see* Methoxyflurane.
'**INHA-PAS**' *see* Pasiniazid.
'**INHG**' *see* Gluconiazone.
'**Inhibostamin**' *see* Tritoqualine.
'**Inhiston**' *see* Pheniramine.
'**INHM**' *see* Isoniazid mesilate.
'**INHS**' *see* Salinazid.

INICARONE*** (2-isopropylbenzofuran-3-yl pyrid-4-yl ketone; 3-isonicotinoyl-2-isopropylbenzofuran).
'Inimur' *see* Nifuratel.
'Innovan' *see* Droperidol with fentanyl.
'Innovar' *see* Droperidol with fentanyl.
INO-502 *see* Cetiedil.
'Inofal' *see* Sulforidazine.
'Inolin' *see* Tretoquinol.
'Inophylline' *see* Aminophylline.
INOSINE (hypoxanthine riboside; oxiamin; Eu-2200; 'atorel').
'Inosine' *see* Phytic acid.
Inosine dimethylamino-2-propanol *p*-**acetamidobenzoate** *see* Methisoprinol.
Inosine monophosphate *see* Inosinic acid.
INOSINE TRIPHOSPHATE (inosine triphosphoric acid; ITP).
INOSINIC ACID (inosinephosphoric acid; inosine 5'-phosphate; IMP).
'Inosiplex' *see* Methisoprinol.
Inosite *see* Inositol.
Inositocalcium *see* Calcium magnesium phytate.
INOSITOL (*meso*-inositol; *meso*-1,2,3,4,5,6-hexahydroxycyclohexane; *myo*-inositol; cyclohexanehexol; cyclohexitol; mesoinosite; bios-I; mouse antialopecia factor; rat antispectacled eye factor; betitol; dambose; hexol; inosite; *i*-inositol; *m*-inositol; meat sugar; nucite; phaseomannitol; scyllite; 'mesitol').
Inositol hexanicotinate *see* Inositol nicotinate.
INOSITOL HEXANITRATE ('mesonitrol', 'nitrositol', 'tolanate').
Inositolhexaphosphoric acid *see* Phytic acid.
Inositol niacinate* *see* Inositol nicotinate.
INOSITOL NICOTINATE*** (*meso*-inositol hexanicotinate; inositol niacinate; cyclohexanehexol hexanicotinate; WIN-9154; 'dilcit', 'esantene', 'hexanicit', 'hexanicotol', 'hexopal', 'linodil', 'mesonex', 'palohex').
See also Bamethan with inositol nicotinate.
'Inostral' *see* Disodium cromoglicate.
INPC *see* Propham.
INPEA *see* Nifenalol.
INPROQUONE*** (2,5-bis(1-aziridinyl)-3,6-dipropoxy-1,4-benzoquinone; 2,5-bis-ethylenimino-3,6-dipropoxy-*p*-benzoquinone; ethylene iminoquinone; E-39; NSC-17261; RP-6870; 'cytostaticum', 'zytostatika').
'INSH' *see* Isoniazid.
'Insidon' *see* Opipramol.
'Insoral' *see* Phenformin.
'Instrumer' *see* Hydrargaphen.
Insulin *see below* and Biphasic insulin injection; Dalanated insulin; Isophane insulin; Neutral insulin.
'Insulin actrapid' *see* Neutral insulin injection.
INSULIN ZINC SUSPENSION*** (lente insulin; 'insulin lente', 'lente iletin').
  amorphous ('insulin semilente').

crystalline ('insulin ultralente').
'Intal' *see* Disodium cromoglicate.
'Integrin' *see* Oxypertine.
'Intenkordin' *see* Carbocromen.
'Intensain' *see* Carbocromen.
'Intercordin' *see* Carbocromen.
INTERFERON*** (protein formed by interaction of animal cells with virus).
INTERMEDIN** (chromatophore-expanding hormone; melanophore-stimulating hormone; MSH; melanotropin(s); A-732179).
'Intestopan' *see* Broxyquinoline with broxaldine.
'Intex' *see* Medroxyprogesterone acetate with ethinylestradiol.
'Intrabilix' *see* Adipiodone meglumine.
'Intracaine' *see* Parethoxycaine.
'Intracillin' *see* Penicillin.
'Intradex' *see* Dextran.
'Intraion' *see* Potassium magnesium aspartate.
'Intranarcon' *see* Thialbarbital.
'Intrathion' *see* Thiometon.
'Intration' *see* Thiometon.
'Intraval' *see* Thiopental.
'Intraxium' *see* Penimocycline.
INTRAZOLE** (1-(*p*-chlorobenzoyl)-3-(1H-tetrazol-5-ylmethyl)indole; BL-R743).
INTRIPTYLINE*** (4-(5H-dibenzo(a,d)-cyclohepten-5-ylidene)-*N*,*N*-dimethyl-2-butynylamine).
'Intropin' *see* Dopamine.
'Inubuse' *see* Naringenin.
Inula camphor *see* Alantolactone.
INULIN (alantin; alant starch; dahlin; 'synanthrin').
'Invenol' *see* Carbutamide.
'Inversine' *see* Mecamylamine.
'Inzellon' *see* Potassium magnesium aspartate.
'Inzolen' *see* Potassium magnesium aspartate.
IOBENZAMIC ACID*** (*N*-(3-amino-2,4,6-triiodobenzoyl)-*N*-phenyl-β-alanine; 3-[(3-amino-2,4,6-triiodobenzoyl)phenylamino]-propionic acid; *N*-(3-amino-2,4,6-triiodobenzoyl)-*N*-(2-carboxyethyl)aniline; ST-5066; 'osbil', 'razebil', 'tracebyl').
IOBUTOIC ACID*** (4-[2,4,6-triiodo-3-(morpholinocarbonyl)phenoxy]butyric acid).
IOCARMIC ACID*** (5,5'-(adipoyldiimino)-bis(2,4,6-triiodo-*N*-methylisophthalamic acid); bis[3-carboxy-2,4,6-triiodo-5-(*N*-methylcarboxamido)anilide] of adipic acid).
See also Meglumine iocarmate.
IOCETAMIC ACID** (*N*-acetyl-*N*-(3-amino-2,4,6-triiodophenyl)-2-methyl-β-alanine; *N*-acetyl-*N*-(2-carboxypropyl)-2,4,6-tri-iodo-*m*-phenylenediamine; 3-[*N*-(3-amino-2,4,6-triiodophenyl)acetamido]-2-methyl-propionic acid; 'cholebrine', 'colebrina').
IODAMIDE*** (3-acetamido-5-acetamido-methyl-2,4,6-triiodobenzoic acid; α,5-diacetamido-2,4-6-triiodo-*m*-toluic acid; jodamide; 'radiomiro', 'rayomiro', 'trimiro', 'urombrine', 'uromiro').

IODANIL (2,3,5,6-tetraiodo-*p*-benzoquinone).
Iodeosin *see* Tetraiodofluorescein.
IODETRYL* (ethyl 9,10-diiodooctadeca-noate; ethyl diiodostearate).
IODINATED GLYCEROL* (2-(1-iodo-ethyl)-1,3-dioxolane-4-methanol; iodinated dimers of glycerol; 'organidin').
IODINATED (^{125}I) **HUMAN SERUM ALBUMIN** (radioiodinated (^{125}I) h.s.e).
IODINATED (^{131}I) **HUMAN SERUM ALBUMIN** (radioiodinated (^{131}I) h.s.e.).
Iodinated (^{131}I) **macroaggregated human albumin** *see* Macrosalb (^{131}I).
IODINATED POPPYSEED OIL (di-, tetra- and hexaiodinated addition products of triolein and trilinolein; iodized oil; oleum iodatum; oleum iodisatum; iodolipol).
Iodipamide* *see* Adipiodone.
'Iodisan' *see* Prolonium iodide.
Iodized oil* *see* Iodinated poppyseed oil.
IODOACETYLSALICYLIC ACID ('aspriodine').
See also Methyl iodoacetylsalicylate.
Iodoalphionic acid *see* Pheniodol.
Iodoantipyrine *see* Iodophenazone.
ω-(*p*-Iodobenzyl)-2-(2-oxopyrrolidin-1-yl) ethamer *see* Tolpovidone.
IODOBRASSID* (ethyl ester of 9,10-diiodo-brassidic acid).
Iodochlorhydroxyquin* *see* Clioquinol.
Iodochlorhydroxyquinoline *see* Clioquinol.
5-IODO-2-DEOXYCYTIDINE (IDC).
Iododeoxyuridine *see* Idoxuridine.
Iododiazoate *see* Sodium diatrizoate.
'Iodoenterol' *see* Clioquinol.
2-(1-Iodoethyl)-1,3-dioxolane-4-methanol *see* Iodinated glycerol.
IODOFENPHOS (*O*-(2,5-dichloro-4-iodo-phenyl) *O,O*-dimethyl phosphorothioate; jodphenphos; 'nuvacron N', 'nuvanol M').
IODOFORM (triiodomethane).
'Iodoglobin' *see* Diiodotyrosine.
Iodogorgoic acid *see* Diiodotyrosine.
'Iodogorgon' *see* Diiodotyrosine.
Iodogorgonic acid *see* Diiodotyrosine.
o-**Iodohippuric acid sodium salt** *see* Sodium iodohippurate.
IODOHYDRIN (3-iodo-1,2-propanediol; 3-iodopropylene glycol; α-iodohydrin; glycerol α-monoiodohydrin).
Iodolipol (tr) *see* Iodinated poppyseed oil.
'Iodolysin' *see* Thiosinamine ethyl iodide.
Iodomethamate *see* Iodoxyl.
Iodomethanesulfonic acid sodium salt *see* Methiodal.
N¹-(4-Iodo-3-methylisoxazol-3-yl)sulfanil-amide *se* Sulfiodizole.
'Iodopact' *see* Sodium acetrizoate.
Iodopanoic acid* *see* Iopanoic acid.
'Iodopaque' *see* Sodium acetrizoate.
IODOPHENAZONE (iodinated phenazone; iodoantipyrine; iodopyrine).
Iodophenylundecanoic acid ethyl ester *see* Iofendylate.
IODOPHTHALEIN SODIUM* (disodium salt of tetraiodophenolphthalein; iodognost; tetraiodophthalein-Na; tetraiodum; tetro-thalein-Na).
3-Iodo-1,2-propanediol *see* Iodohydrin.
(2-IODOPROPYLIDENEDIOXY)-PROPANOL (glyceryl iodopropylidene ether; 'mucantil').
1-(3-Iodo-2-propyn-1-yloxy)-2,4,5-tri-chlorobenzene *see* Haloprogin.
3-Iodo-2-propynol 2,4,5-trichlorophenyl ether *see* Haloprogin.
Iodopyracet *see* Diodone.
IODOPYRIDONE* (sodium 3,5-diiodo-4-oxo-1(4H)-pyridineacetate; 'iopax', 'pyelosil', 'uroselectan').
Iodopyrine *see* Iodophenazone.
Iodoquinine sulfate *see* Quinine iodosulfate.
Iodoquinoline *see* Chiniofon.
7-IODO-8-QUINOLINOL-5-SULFONIC ACID (8-hydroxy-7-iodoquinoline-5-sulfonic acid).
7-Iodo-8-quinolinol-5-sulfonic acid chloroquine salt *see* Cloquinate.
Iodostearic acid ethyl ester(s) *see* Ethyl iodostearate.
3-Iodosulfamethoxole *see* Sulfiodizole.
Iodotetroxide *see* Meglumine iodoxamate.
IODOTHIOURACIL* (5-iodo-2-thio-uracil; iothiouracil).
IODOTHIOURACIL SODIUM ('itrumil').
Iodothymol *see* Dithymol diiodide.
IODOXAMIC ACID* (3,3'-[ethylenebis-(oxyethyleneoxyethylenecarbonylimino)]-bis(2,4,6-triiodobenzoic acid); 4,7,10,13-tetraoxahexadecane-1,16-dioylbis(3-carboxy-2,4,6-triiodoanilide); N,N'-(1,16-dioxo-4,7,10,13-tetraoxahexadecane-1,16-diyl)di(3-amino-2,4,6-triiodobenzoic acid); BC-17; 'endobil').
See also Meglumine iodoxamate.
Iodoxine *see* Diiodohydroxyquin.
IODOXYL* (disodium 3,5-diiodo-N-methyl-4-pyridone-2,6-dicarboxylate; disodium salt of 3,5-diiodo-1-methylchemidamic acid; iodomethamate sodium; D-40; 'neo-iopax', 'pyelectan', 'ultraren', 'uridognost', 'uropac', 'uroselectan-B', 'urumbrin').
'Iodozol' *see* 2,6-Diiodo-1-phenol-4-sulfonic acid.
IOFENDYLATE* (ethyl 10-(*p*-iodophenyl)-undecanoate; iophendylate; neurotrast; 'ethiodan', 'jodsal', 'myodil', 'mulsopaque', 'neirotrast', 'pantopaque').
IOGLICIC ACID* (5-acetamido-2,4,6-tri-iodo-N-[(methylcarbamoyl)methyl]iso-phthalamidic acid; 3-(acetylamino)-2,4,6-triiodo-5-[[[[(methylamino)carbonyl]-methyl]amino]carbonyl]benzoic acid).
Ioglycamate meglumine* *see* Ioglycamide.
IOGLYCAMIC ACID* (3,3'-[oxybis-(methylenecarbonylimino)]bis(2,4,6-triiodo-benzoic acid); N,N'-diglycoloyldi(3-carboxy-2,4,6-triiodoaniline); diglycolic acid bis(3-carboxy-2,4,6-triiodoanilide); 3,3'-(diglycoloyldiimino)bis(2,4,6-triiodo-benzoic acid); BE-419).
See also Ioglycamide; Sodium ioglycamate.
IOGLYCAMIDE** (methylglucamine salt of ioglycamic acid; ioglycamate meglumine;

meglumine ioglycamate; 'biligram').
**IOGLYCAMIDE WITH SODIUM
IOGLYCAMATE** ('bilivistan').
IOLIDONIC ACID*** (α-ethyl-2,4,6-triiodo-
3-(2-oxopyrrolidin-1-yl)hydrocinnamic
acid; 2-ethyl-3-[2,4,6-triiodo-3-(2-oxo-
pyrrolidin-1-yl)phenyl]propionic acid;
2-[2,4,6-triiodo-3-(2-oxopyrrolidin-1-yl)-
benzyl]butyric acid; 1-[3-(2-carboxybutyl)-
2,4,6-triiodophenyl]pyrrolidin-2-one).
IOLIXANIC ACID*** (2-[2-[3-(N-ethylacet-
amido)-2,4,6-triiodophenoxy]ethoxy]-
propionic acid; 3-[2-(1-carboxyethoxy)-
ethoxy]-N-ethyl-2,4,6-triiodoacetanilide).
IOMEGLAMIC ACID*** (3'-amino-2',4',6'-
triiodo-N-methylglutaranilic acid; N-(3-
amino-2,4,6-triiodophenyl)-N-methyl-
glutaramic acid; 4-[N-(3-amino-2,4,6-tri-
iodophenyl)-N-methylcarbamoyl]butyric
acid; RG270; 'falignost').
IOMETIN (4-[(3-dimethylaminopropyl)-
amino]-7-iodoquinoline).
IOMETIN (¹²⁵I)** (iometin labeled with
radioactive iodine (¹²⁵I)).
IOMETIN (¹³¹I)** (iometin labeled with
radioactive iodine (¹³¹I)).
'Ionamine' see Phentermine resin.
'Ionol' see Butylated hydroxytoluene.
'Ionosteril' see Mannitol.
IOPANOIC ACID*** (2-(3-amino-2,4,6-tri-
iodobenzyl)butyric acid; 3-amino-α-ethyl-
2,4,6-triiodohydrocinnamic acid; 3-(3-
amino-2,4,6-triiodophenyl)-2-ethylpropionic
acid; iodopanoic acid; 'bilijodon',
'choladine', 'cistobil', 'jopagnost',
'panjopaque', 'telepaque', 'teletrast').
'Iopax' see Iodopyridone.
Iophendylate* see Iofendylate.
Iophenoic acid*** see Iophenoxic acid.
IOPHENOXIC ACID* (2-(3-hydroxy-2,3,6-
triiodobenzyl)butyric acid; α-ethyl-3-
hydroxy-2,4,6-triiodohydrocinnamic acid;
iophenoic acid; triiodoethanoic acid;
'teridax', 'trilombrine').
IOPODIC ACID (3-(dimethylaminomethyleneamino)-2,4,6-triiodobenzoic acid).
See also Ethyl iopodate; Sodium iopodate.
IOPRONIC ACID*** (2-[2-(3-acetamido-
2,4,6-triiodophenoxy)ethoxymethyl]-
butyric acid).
IOPYDOL** (1-(2,3-dihydroxypropyl)-3,5-
diiodo-4(1H)-pyridone).
IOPYDOL WITH IOPYDONE ('hytrast').
IOPYDONE** (3,5-diiodo-4(1H)-pyridone).
IOSEFAMIC ACID*** (5,5'-(sebacoyldi-
imino)bis(2,4,6-triiodo-N-methyliso-
phthalamic acid); MP-271).
IOSERIC ACID*** (N-[2-hydroxy-2-
(methylcarbamoyl)ethyl]-2,4,6-triiodo-
5-(2-methoxyacetamido)isophthalamidic
acid; 3-[[[1-(hydroxymethyl)-2-(methylamino)-2-oxoethyl]amino]carbonyl]-
2,4,6-triiodo-5-[(methoxyacetyl)amino]-
benzoic acid).
IOSUMETIC ACID*** (N-ethyl-2',4',6'-tri-
iodo-3'-(methylamino)succinanilic acid;
4-[ethyl-[2,4,6-triiodo-3-(methylamino)-

phenyl]amino]-4-oxobutanoic acid).
IOTALAMIC ACID*** (5-acetamido-
2,4,6-triiodo-N-methylisophthalamic acid;
iothalamic acid; 5-acetylamino-2,4,6-tri-
iodoisophthalamic acid 3-methalamide;
jodtalmin; methalamic acid).
See also Meglumine iotalamate; Sodium
iotalamate.
Iothalamic acid* see Iotalamic acid.
Iothiouracil see Iodothiouracil.
IOTRANIC ACID*** (3,3'-[oxybis(ethylene-
oxyethylenecarbonylimino)]bis(2,4,6-tri-
iodobenzoic acid)).
IOTRIZOIC ACID*** (2,4,6-triiodo-3-[2-[2-
[2-[2-(methoxy)ethoxy]ethoxy]ethoxy]-
acetamido]benzoic acid).
IOTROXIC ACID*** (3,3'-[oxybis(ethyl-
eneoxymethylenecarbonylimino)]bis(2,4,6-
triiodobenzoic acid)).
IOXITALAMIC ACID*** (5-acetamido-N-
(2-hydroxyethyl)-2,4,6-triiodoisophthalamic
acid; 'vasombrix').
See also Ethanolamine ioxitalamate with
meglumine ioxitalamate.
IOXOTRIZOIC ACID*** (3-acetamido-5-
glycolamido-2,4,6-triiodobenzoic acid).
IOXYNIL* (4-hydroxy-3,5-diiodobenzo-
nitrile; 'actril', 'certrol', 'toxynil').
IOXYNIL OCTANOATE ('totril').
**IOXYNIL PLUS (2,4-DICHLORO-
PHENOXY)ACETIC ACID** ('actril D').
IOZOMIC ACID*** (3,3'-[tetramethylenebis-
[oxy(2-hydroxytrimethylene) (acetylim-
ino)]]bis[2,4,6-triiodo-5-(N-methylacet-
amido)benzoic acid]).
IP-82 see Ibuprofen.
IPA see Riboprine.
IPAS see Isopropylideneazastreptonigrin.
IPAZINE* (6-chloro-2-diethylamino-4-iso-
propylamino-s-triazine; 6-chloro-N,N-di-
ethyl-N'-(1-methylethyl)-1,3,5-triazine-
2,4-diamine; 'gesabel').
IPC see Propham.
Ipecine see Emetine.
IPM see Isoprocarb.
IPMC see Propoxur.
'Ipoglicone' see Tolbutamide.
'Ipradol' see Hexoprenaline.
IPRAGRATINE** (9-isopropylgranatoline
(±)-tropate (ester)).
'Ipral' see Probarbital.
IPRATROPIUM BROMIDE*** ((8r)-3α-
hydroxy-8-isopropyl-1αH,5αH-tropanium
bromide (±)-tropate; 8-isopropyl-3-(±)-
tropoyloxy-1αH,5αH-tropanium bromide;
N-isopropylatropinium bromide; Sch-1000;
'atrovent').
Iprazide (tr) see Iproniazid.
'Iprenol' see Isoprenaline.
IPRIFLAVONE** (7-isopropoxyisoflavone;
7-isopropoxy-3-phenylchromone).
IPRINDOLE*** (5-(3-dimethylamino-
propyl)-6,7,8,9,10,11-hexahydro-5H-cyclo-
oct(b)-indole; iprindole hydrochloride;
pramindole; Wy-3263; 'galatur', 'prondol',
'tertran').
IPROCLOZIDE*** (p-chlorophenoxyacetic

259

acid 2-isopropylhydrazide; 1-(*p*-chloro-phenoxyacetyl)-2-isopropylhydrazine; 'sinderesin').

Ipronal (tr) *see* Proxibarbal.

IPRONIAZID*** (2-isopropylhydrazide of isonicotinic acid; *N'*-isopropylisoniazid; iprazide; 'ipronin', 'marsalid').

IPRONIDAZOLE*** (2-isopropyl-1-methyl-5-nitroimidazole; Ro 7-1554; 'ipropan').

'Ipronin' *see* Iproniazid.

'Ipropan' *see* Ipronidazole.

Iproveratril *see* Verapamil.

IPROXAMINE** (5-[2-(dimethylamino)-ethoxy]carvacryl isopropyl carbonate; 4-[2-(dimethylamino)ethoxy]-5-isopropyl-2-methylphenyl isopropyl carbonate).

'Ipsilon' *see* Aminocaproic acid.

'IPTD' *see* Glyprothiazole.

IQUINDAMINE** (1-[[2-(diethylamino)-ethyl]amino]-3,4-dihydroisoquinoline).

'Irenat' *see* Potassium perchlorate.

'Irgafen' *see* Sulfadimethylbenzoylamide.

'Irgalon' *see* Tetrasodium edetate.

'Irgamide' *see* Sulfadicramide.

'Irgapyrin' *see* Aminophenazone with phenylbutazone.

'Irgasan CF3' *see* Cloflucarban.

'Irgasan DP-30' *see* Triclosan.

'Iricoline' *see* Carbachol.

'Iridocin' *see* Ethionamide.

'Iridozin' *see* Ethionamide.

'Iridus' *see* Naftidrofuryl.

'Irium' *see* Sodium dodecyl sulfate.

'Irmin' *see* Imipramine.

'Iromin' *see* Carbasalate calcium; Ferrous gluconate.

Iron.... *See also* Ferr....

'Ironate' *see* Ferrous gluconate.

Iron choline citrate *see* Ferrocholinate.

IRON DEXTRAN INJECTION* (iron-dextran complex; 'ferridextran', 'imferon', 'imferdex').

Iron-dextrin complex *see* Dextriferron.

Iron-fructose complex *see* Ferric fructose.

Iron-glycine complex *see* Ferroglycine-sulfate complex.

Iron salt of maleic acid polymer with methyl vinyl ether *see* Ferropolimaler.

IRON-SERINE COMPLEX ('aktiferrin').

Iron sodium edetate *see* Sodium feredetate.

IRON SORBITEX* (iron sorbitol; iron sorbitol-citric acid complex; Astra-1572; 'ferbitol', 'jectofer').

Iron-sucrose-polymer complex *see* Polyferose.

'Irox' *see* Ferrous gluconate.

'Irrigor' *see* Imolamine.

IS-121 *see* Naftidrofuryl oxalate.

IS-362 *see* Suxethonium.

IS-370 *see* Suxamethonium.

IS-401 *see* Diisopropylamine dichloroacetate.

IS-499 *see* Poldine.

Isadrin (tr) *see* Isoprenaline.

Isaphenin (tr) *see* Acetphenolisatin.

Isatidine *see* Retrorsine *N*-oxide.

ISATIN (2,3-indoledione; 2,3-indolinedione).

ISATROPIC ACID (1,2,3,4-tetrahydro-1-phenyl-1,4-naphthalenedicarboxylic acid).

Isatropylditropeine *see* Belladonnin.

'Iscothane' *see* Dinocap.

'I-sedrin' *see* Ephedrine.

ISETHIONIC ACID (ethanol-2-sulfonic acid; 2-hydroxyethanesulfonic acid). *See also* Isetionate(s).

ISETIONATE(S)** (2-hydroxyethane-sulfonate(s); isethionate(s)). *See also* Amicarbalide isethionate; Dibrompropamidine isetionate; Hexamidine isetionate; Pentamidine isetionate; Propamidine isetionate; Stilbamidine isetionate.

'Iskedyl' *see* Raubasine with dihydroergocristine mesilate.

'Ismelin' *see* Guanethidine.

'Ismicetina' *see* Chloramphenicol.

'Ismipur' *see* Mercaptopurine.

'Isoadanon' *see* Isomethadone.

Isoadrenaline *see* Corbadrine.

ISOALLOXAZINE (benzo(g)pteridine-2,4-(3H,10H)-dione; pyrimido(4,5-b)quinox-aline-2,4(3H,10H)-dione).

Isoalloxazine-adenine dinucleotide *see* Flavin-adenine dinucleotide.

Isoamidone *see* Isomethadone.

ISOAMINILE*** (4-dimethylamino-2-iso-propyl-2-phenylvaleronitrile; (β-dimethyl-aminopropyl)-α-isopropylphenylaceto-nitrile).

ISOAMINILE CITRATE ('dimyril', 'peracon').

2-Isoamylamino-6-methylheptane *see* Octamylamine.

N-Isoamylcadaverine *see* Isoverine.

Isoamyl N-(2-diethylaminoethyl)-2-phenylglycinate *see* Camylofin.

N-Isoamyl-1,5-dimethyl-1-hexylamine *see* Octamylamine.

Isoamylenoxypsoralen *see* Pentosalen.

Isoamylhydrocupreine *see* Euprocin.

Isoamyl nitrite *see* Amyl nitrite.

1-(2-Isoamyloxy-2-phenylethyl)pyrrol-idine *see* Amixetrine.

N-[3-Isoamyloxy-2-(3,4,5-trimethoxy-benzoyloxy)propyl]morpholine *see* Amoproxan.

'Isoamytal' *see* Pentobarbital.

Isoandrosterone *see* 5α-Androstan-3β-ol-17-one.

5-Isoandrosterone *see* 5β-Androstan-3α-ol-17-one.

ISOASCORBIC ACID (D-erythro-3-keto-hexonic acid lactone; D-erythro-3-oxo-hexonic acid lactone; D-araboascorbic acid; erycorbin; erythorbic acid; gluco-saccharonic acid; isovitamin C; saccharo-sonic acid; 'mercate-5', 'neo-cebicure'). *See also* Sodium isoascorbate.

Isobarin (tr) *see* Guanethidine.

ISOBENZAN* (1,3,4,5,6,7,8,8-octachloro-3a,4,7,7a-tetrahydro-4,7-methanophthalan; 1,3,4,5,6,7,8,8-octachloro-1,3,3a,4,7,7a-hexahydro-4,7-methanoisobenzofuran; SD-4402; 'telodrin').

1-Isobenzofuranone *see* Phthalide.

Isobornylamine *see* 2-Bornanamine.

6-Isobornyl-3,4-xylenol *see* Xibornol.
ISOBROMANIL (3,4,5,6-tetrabromo-*o*-benzoquinone).
p-**Isobutoxybenzoic acid diethylamino-dimethylpropyl ester** *see* Ganglefene.
1-(Isobutoxymethyl)-2-(4-methylpiperazin-1-yl)ethyl 2-phenylbutyrate *see* Fenetradil.
Isobutyl alcohol *see* 2-Methyl-1-propanol.
Isobutyl *p*-aminobenzoate *see* Isobutylcaine.
4-Isobutylamino-2,3-dimethyl-1-phenyl-5-pyrazolin-3-one methanesulfonate *see* Dibupyrone.
2-Isobutylaminoethyl *p*-aminobenzoate *see* Butethamine.
ISOBUTYLCAINE (isobutyl *p*-aminobenzoate; 'benzamelid', 'cyclocaine', 'cycloform', 'cyclogesin', 'isocaine').
Isobutyl 2-cyanoacrylate *see* Bucrilate.
Isobutyl 4-(6,7-dimethoxyquinazolin-4-yl)-1-piperazinecarboxylate *see* Piquizil.
p-**Isobutylhydratropic acid** *see* Ibuprofen.
p-**Isobutylhydratropohydroxamic acid** *see* Ibuproxam.
Isobutylhydrochlorothiazide *see* Butizide.
Isobutylphenazone methanesulfonate *see* Dibupyrone.
p-**Isobutylphenylacetic acid** *see* Ibufenac.
2-(*p*-Isobutylphenyl)butyric acid *see* Butibufen.
Isobutyl α-phenylcyclohexaneglycolate *see* Ibuverine.
2-(*p*-Isobutylphenyl)propionic acid *see* Ibuprofen.
2-(*p*-Isobutylphenyl)propionohydroxamic acid *see* Ibuproxam.
(−)-(*S*)-4-[*N*-(5-Isobutylpyrimidin-2-yl)-sulfamoyl]phenylacetic acid 1-(5-fluoro-2-methoxyphenyl)ethylamide *see* Gliflumide.
N-**(5-Isobutyl-1,3,4-thiadiazol-2-yl)-*p*-methoxy benzenesulfonamide** *see* Glysobuzole.
N-**Isobutyl(triphenylmethyl)amine** *see* Isobutyltritylamine.
ISOBUTYLTRITYLAMINE (*N*-isobutyl-(triphenylmethyl)amine; ICI-24223; 'molucid').
ISOBUTYRIC ACID (2-methylpropionic acid).
Isobutyric acid diester with 5-(2-*tert*-butylamino-1-hydroxyethyl)resorcinol *see* Ibuterol.
Isobuzole * *see* Glysobuzole.
Isocaine *see* Pseudococaine.
Isocaramidine *see* Debrisoquin.
ISOCARBOXAZID*** (5-methylisoxazole-3-carboxylic acid 2-benzylhydrazide; 1-benzyl-2-(6-methylisoxazol-3-ylcarbonyl)-hydrazine; 3-(*N*-benzylhydrazinocarbonyl)-5-methylisoxazole; BMIH; Ro-5-0831; U-10387; 'energer', 'marplan', 'marplon').
ISOCHLORANIL (3,4,5,6-tetrachloro-*o*-benzoquinone).
ISOCHROMAN (3,4-dihydro-2,1H-benzo-pyran).

ISOCIL * (5-bromo-3-isopropyl-6-methyl-uracil; 5-bromo-6-methyl-3-(1-methyl-ethyl)-2,4(1H,3H)-pyrimidinedione; iso-procil; 'hyvar').
'Isocillin' *see* Penicillin V.
ISOCITRIC ACID (1-hydroxy-1,2,3-propanetricarboxylic acid; α-hydroxytri-carballylic acid).
ISOCONAZOLE** (1-[2,4-dichloro-β-(2,6-dichlorobenzyloxy)phenethyl]imidazole; 1-[2-(2,4-dichlorophenyl)-2-[(2,6-dichloro-phenyl)methoxy]ethyl]-1H-imidazole; iso-conazole nitrate; R-15454).
'Iso-cornox' *see* Mecoprop.
1-Isocoumaranone *see* Phthalide.
ISOCROTONIC ACID (*cis*-2-butenoic acid).
'Isocurine' *see* 1,4-Bis(2-diethylaminoethyl)-piperazine.
Isodemeton *see* Demeton-S.
Isodemeton methyl *see* Demeton-S-methyl.
'Isodine' *see* Povidone-iodine.
ISODRIN * (1,2,3,4,10,10-hexachloro-1,4,4a,5,8,8a-hexahydro-1,4:5,8-dimethanonaph-thalene *endo-endo* form; OMS-198).
Isodrin * *see* Pholedrine.
'Iso-endoxan' *see* Ifosfamide.
Isoephedrine *see* Pseudoephedrine.
ISOETARINE*** (3,4-dihydroxy-α-(1-iso-propylaminopropyl)benzyl alcohol; α-ethyl-*N*-isopropylnoradrenaline; 1-(3,4-dihydr-oxyphenyl)-2-isopropylamino-1-butanol; etyprenaline; isoetharine; WIN-3046; 'asthmalitan', 'dilabron', 'neoisuprel', 'numotac').
Isoethadione *see* Paramethadione.
Isoetharine * *see* Isoetarine.
'Isoflav' *see* Proflavine.
ISOFLAVONE (3-phenylchromone).
ISOFLUORANIL (2,3,5,6-tetrafluoro-*o*-benzoquinone).
Isofluorophate * *see* Dyflos.
ISOFLURANE*** (1-chloro-2,2,2-trifluoro-ethyl difluoromethyl ether; 'forane').
Isoformothion *see* Formothion.
Isofosfamide *see* Ifosfamide.
'I-so-gel' *see* Ispagula.
'Isoglaucon' *see* Clonidine.
'Isoglobucid' *see* *N*¹-(5-Ethyl-1,2,4-thia-diazol-3-yl)sulfanilamide.
ISOGLUTAMINE (4-aminoglutaramic acid).
Isogranatanamine *see* 3-Azabicyclo(3.3.1)-nonane.
ISOGUANOSINE (6-amino-2-hydroxy-purine D-riboside).
Isohesperidin *see* Aurantiin.
2-Isohistamine *see* 2-Imidazoleethylamine.
ISOIDIDE (1,4:3,6-dianhydroiditol).
Isoidide isomers *see* Isomannide; Iso-sorbide.
'Isoindokolon' *see* Hexafluoroisopropyl methyl ether.
1,3-Isoindoledione *see* Phthalimide.
ISOINDOLINE (1,3-dihydro-2-benzazole; 1,3-dihydroisoindole).
1,3-Isoindolinedione *see* Phthalimide.

261

Isoindolin-1-one see Phthalimidine.
'Isoket' see Isosorbide dinitrate.
'Isolan' see 1-Isopropyl-3-methylpyrazol-5-yl dimethylcarbanilate.
ISOLEUCINE (2-amino-3-methylvaleric acid; 2-amino-3-ethyl-3-methylpropionic acid).
ISOMANNIDE (1,4:3,6-dianhydromannitol).
Isomannide isomers see Isoidide; Isosorbide.
ISOMETAMIDIUM CHLORIDE*** (8-[3-(*m*-amidinophenyl)-2-triazeno]-3-amino-5-ethyl-6-phenylphenanthridinium chloride; anthridonium chloride; antridonium chloride; M&B-4180A; 'samorin').
ISOMETHADONE*** (6-dimethylamino-5-methyl-4,4-diphenyl-3-hexanone; isoamidone; isomethadone hydrochloride; WIN-1783; 'isoadanon', 'liden').
ISOMETHEPTENE*** (6-methyl-2-methylaminohept-5-ene; *N*-1,5-trimethyl-4-hexenylamine; *N*-methylisooctenylamine; methylaminoisooctane; 'octanil', 'octin', 'octon').
Isomethyl parathion see Parathion isomethyl.
'Isomyl nitrite' see Amyl nitrite.
ISONIAZID** (isonicotinic acid hydrazide; 4-pyridinecarboxylic acid hydrazide; isonicotinoylhydrazine; INH; tubazid; AB-41; GINK; IN-73; RP-5015).
ISONIAZID COBALT COMPLEX ('isonicco').
Isoniazid glucuronolactone see Gluconiazone.
ISONIAZID METHANESULFONATE (sodium salt of isoniazid *N*-methanesulfonic acid; INHM; 'neotizide', 'pyridizin').
'Isonicco' see Isoniazid cobalt complex.
ISONICOTINALDEHYDE (4-pyridyl aldehyde; γ-pyridyl aldehyde).
ISONICOTINIC ACID (4-pyridinecarboxylic acid; γ-picolinic acid).
Isonicotinic acid hydrazide see Isoniazid. See also Aconiazide; Crotoniazide; Ftivazide; Homovanillideneisoniazid; Hydroxybenzylideneisoniazid; Iproniazid; Larusan; Menazone; Metazide; Methaniazide; Nialamide; 5-Nitro-2-furylideneisoniazid; Opiniazide; Phenylisopropylisoniazid; Salinazid; Streptoniazid; Sulfoniazid; Verazide.
Isonicotinic thioamide see Isonicotinthioamide.
6-[2-[2-(Isonicotinimidoylamino)-acetamido]-2-phenylacetamido]-penicillanic acid see Pirbenicillin.
3-Isonicotinoyl-2-isopropylbenzofuran see Inicarone.
ISONICOTINTHIOAMIDE (isonicotinic thioamide; thioisonicotinic acid amide; Th-3624).
Isonipecaine see Pethidine.
ISONIPECOTAMIDE (4-piperidinecarboxamide).
ISONIPECOTIC ACID (4-piperidinecarboxylic acid).

ISONITROSOACETONE (acetone monoxime; monoisonitroso acetone; MINA).
ISONIXIN** (2-hydroxy-2',6'-nicotinoxylidide; 2-hydroxynicotinic acid 2,6-dimethylanilide).
ISONORURON* (1,1-dimethyl-3-(octahydro-4,7-methano-1H-inden-1-yl)urea mixture with ...... inden-2-yl isomer). See also Brompyrazon plus isonoruron; Buturon plus isonoruron.
'Isonox' see Methaqualone with etodroxizine maleate.
ISO-OMPA (*N*,*N*',*N*'',*N*'''-tetraisopropylpyrophosphoramide; tetraisopropylphosphorodiamidic anhydride; tetraisopropylpyrophosphorotetramide).
Isooxazole see Isoxazole.
'Isopaque' see Sodium metrizoate.
'Isopaque 440' see Sodium metrizoate with calcium and magnesium metrizoates.
'Isopaque cerebral' see Meglumine metrizoate with calcium metrizoate.
'Isopaque coronary' see Meglumine metrizoate with calcium and sodium metrizoates.
'Iso-par' see Coparaffinate.
'IsoPC' see Propham.
ISOPELLETIERINE (2-acetonylpiperidine; 1-piperid-2-yl-2-propanone).
Isopenicillin N see (−)-Adicillin.
8-ISOPENTENYL-7-METHOXYCOUMARIN ('osthol').
ISOPENTYLAMINE (3-methylbutylamine).
2-Isopentylaminomethyl-1,4-benzodioxan see Pentamoxane.
N-Isopentyl-1,5-dimethylhexylamine see Octamylamine.
Isopentyl hydrocupreine see Euprocin.
α-Isopentyloxymethyl-4-morpholineethanol 3,4,5-trimethoxybenzoate see Amoproxan.
1-(β-Isopentyloxyphenethyl)pyrrolidine see Amixetrine.
Isopentyl 2-phenyl-2-[(2-pyrrolidin-1-ylethyl)amino]acetate see Camiverine.
Isopestox (tr) see Mipafox.
ISOPHANE INSULIN* (NPH insulin; protamine insulin; 'NPH-iletin'). See also Protamine zinc insulin.
Isophenylephrine see Metaraminol.
Isophosphamide see Ifosfamide.
ISOPHTHALAMIC ACID (*m*-carbamoylbenzoic acid; isophthalic acid monoamide).
ISOPHTHALIC ACID (*m*-benzenedicarboxylic acid).
Isophthalic acid monoamide see Isophthalamic acid.
ISOPREDNIDENE** (11β,17α,21-trihydroxy-16-methylenepregna-4,6-diene-3,20-dione; 16-methylenepregna-4,6-diene-11β,17α,21-triol-3,20-dione).
Isopregnenone see Dydrogesterone.
ISOPRENALINE*** (3,4-dihydroxy-α-(isopropylaminomethyl)benzyl alcohol; α-(isopropylaminomethyl)protocatechuyl alcohol; *N*-isopropylnoradrenaline; isopropydrine; isoproterenol; levoisoprenaline; isadrin;

isoprenaline bitartrate, chloride or sulfate; isopropylarterenol; A-21; WIN-5162).

'Isoprinosine' see Methisoprinol.

ISOPROCARB* (o-isopropylphenyl methylcarbamate; 2-(1-methylethyl)phenyl methylcarbamate; IPM; MIPC; OMS-32; 'carbamat', 'etrofolan', 'mipicin').

Isoprocil see Isocil.

Isopromedol (tr) see Isotrimeperidine.

ISOPROPALIN* (4-isopropyl-2,6-dinitro-*N,N*-dipropylaniline; 4-(1-methylethyl)-2,6-dinitro-*N,N*-dipropylbenzenamine; 'paarlan').

ISOPROPAMIDE IODIDE*** ((3-carbamoyl-3,3-diphenylpropyl)diisopropylmethylammonium iodide; methiodide of 4-diisopropylamino-2,2-diphenylbutyramide; isopropon; R-55; R-79; 'darbid', 'dipramide', 'priamide', 'tyrimide').

ISOPROPAMIDE METHOSULFATE (R-192).

Isopropenyl nitrile see Methacrylonitrile.

Isoprophenamine see Clorprenaline.

ISOPROPICILLIN*** (6-(2-methyl-2-phenoxypropionamido)penicillanic acid; (1-methyl-1-phenoxyethyl)penicillin).

Isopropon* see Isopropamide.

Isopropoxamine see Isopropylmethoxamine.

N[1]-**(4-Isopropoxybenzoyl)sulfanilamide** see Sulfaproxyline.

7-Isopropoxyisoflavone see Ipriflavone.

7-Isopropoxy-9-oxoxanthene-2-carboxylic acid see Xanoxic acid.

7-Isopropoxy-3-phenylchromone see Ipriflavone.

o-**Isopropoxyphenyl methylcarbamate** see Propoxur.

Isopropydrine* see Isoprenaline.

Isopropyl alcohol see 2-Propanol.

Isopropylamine see 2-Propylamine.

3-Isopropylamino-1-(di-2,6-xylylmethoxy)-2-propanol see Xipranolol.

α-**(1-Isopropylaminoethyl)-2,5-dimethoxybenzyl alcohol** see Isopropylmethoxamine.

1-Isopropylamino-3-[*p*-(2-methoxyethyl)-phenoxy]-2-propanol see Metoprolol.

2-Isopropylamino-4-(3-methoxypropyl-amino)-6-(methylthio)-*s*-triazine see Methoprotryn.

α-**Isopropylaminomethyl-2-naphthalenemethanol** see Pronetalol.

α-**Isopropylaminomethyl-*p*-nitrobenzyl alcohol** see Nifenalol.

1-Isopropylamino-3-(3-methylphenoxy)-2-propanol see Toliprolol.

1-Isopropylamino-3-[*o*-(methylthio)-phenoxy]-2-propanol see Tiprenolol.

α-**Isopropylaminomethylvanillyl alcohol** see Metiprenaline.

1-Isopropylamino-3-(1-naphthyloxy)-2-propanol see Propranolol.

8-(5-Isopropylaminopentylamino)-6-methoxyquinoline see Pentaquine.

4-ISOPROPYLAMINOPHENAZONE (2,3-dimethyl-4-isopropylamino-1-phenyl-3-pyrazolin-5-one; 'isopyrin').

4-ISOPROPYLAMINOPHENAZONE WITH PHENYLBUTAZONE ('febuzine isopirin', 'tomanol').

3-Isopropylamino-1-(2,6,2′,6′-tetramethyl-benzhydryloxy)-2-propanol see Xipranolol.

(±)-**1-Isopropylamino-3-thiazol-2-yloxy-2-propanol** see Tazolol.

1-Isopropylamino-3-(*m*-toloxy)-2-propanol see Toliprolol.

N-**Isopropylatropinium bromide** see Ipratropium bromide.

p-**Isopropylbenzaldehyde thiosemicarbazone** see Cutizone.

2-Isopropylbenzofuran-3-yl pyrid-4-yl ketone see Inicarone.

p-**ISOPROPYLBENZOIC ACID** (cumic acid).
See also Isopropylcaine.

3-Isopropyl-1H-2,1,3-benzothiadiazin-4(3H)-one 2,2-dioxide see Bentazon.

Isopropyl 2,2-bis(*p*-bromophenyl)glycolate see Bromopropylate.

Isopropyl 2,2-bis(*p*-chlorophenyl)-glycolate see Chloropropylate.

ISOPROPYLCAINE (2-diethylaminoethyl ester of *p*-isopropylbenzoic acid).

Isopropylcarbamic acid ester with 4′-fluoro-4-(4-hydroxypiperid-1-yl)but-yrophenone see Carperone.

3-[[(Isopropylcarbamoyl)amino]sulfon-yl]-4-(*m*-toluidino)pyridine see Torasemide.

1-(4-Isopropylcarbamoylbenzyl)-2-methylhydrazine see Procarbazine.

1-(Isopropylcarbamoylmethyl)-4-(3,4,5-trimethoxycinnamoyl)piperazine see Cinpropazide.

Isopropyl carbanilate see Propham.

S-**(Isopropylcarboxymethyl)cysteine** see Isovalthine.

Isopropyl 2-[*p*-(*p*-chlorobenzoyl)phen-oxy]-2-methylpropionate see Fenofibrate.

Isopropyl *m*-chlorocarbanilate see Chlorpropham.

3-Isopropyl-2,4,6-cycloheptatrien-2-ol-1-one see α-Thujaplicin.

4-Isopropyl-2,4,6-cycloheptatrien-2-ol-1-one see β-Thujaplicin.

α-**Isopropylcyclohexanemethanol** see Cimepanol.

Isopropyl 4,4′-dibromobenzilate see Bromopropylate.

Isopropyl 4,4′-dichlorobenzilate see Chloropropylate.

5-Isopropyl-4-(2-dimethylaminoethoxy)-2-methylphenyl acetate see Moxisylyte.

α-**Isopropyl-α-(2-dimethylaminoethyl)-1-naphthaleneacetamide** see Naftypramide.

2-Isopropyl-4-dimethylamino-2-phenyl-valeronitrile see Isoaminile.

7-Isopropyl-1,4-dimethylazulene see Guaiazulene.

5-Isopropyl-3,8-dimethyl-1-azulenesul-fonic acid sodium salt see Sodium

263

gualenate.

4-Isopropyl-2,3-dimethyl-1-phenyl-3-pyrazolin-4-one see Propyphenazone.

4-Isopropyl-2,6-dinitro-*N*,*N*-dipropylaniline see Isopropalin.

N-**Isopropyl-4,4-diphenylcyclohexylamine** see Pramiverine.

1-Isopropyl-4,4-diphenylpiperidine see Propidine.

9-Isopropylgranatoline ($\pm$)**-tropate** see Ipragratine.

2-Isopropyl-2-[3-(*N*-homoveratryl-*N*-methylamino)propyl]-2-(3,4-dimethoxyphenyl)acetonitrile see Verapamil.

ISOPROPYLIDENEAZASTREPTO-NIGRIN (5-amino-4-(2-hydroxy-3,4-dimethoxyphenyl)-6-(5-hydroxy-4-methoxy-2,2-dimethyl-2H-imidazo(4,5-h)-quinolin-8-yl)-3-methylpicolinic acid; IPAS; NSC-62709).

16α,17α-Isopropylidenedioxypregn-4-ene-3,20-dione see Algestone acetonide.

4,4′-Isopropylidenedithiobis(2,6-*tert*-butylphenol) see Probucol.

2-Isopropylindol-3-yl pyrid-3-yl ketone see Nictindole.

Isopropylmeprobamate see Carisoprodol.

ISOPROPYLMETHOXAMINE (α-(1-isopropylaminoethyl)-2,5-dimethoxybenzyl alcohol; 2,5-dimethoxy-α-(1-isopropylaminoethyl)benzyl alcohol; *N*-isopropylmethoxamine; isopropoxamine; IMA; BW-61-43).

5-Isopropyl-4-methoxyfurobenzopyran-7-one see Peucedanin.

Isopropyl 11-methoxy-3,7,11-trimethyl-2,4-dodecadienoate see Methoprene.

2-Isopropyl-5-methylbenzoquinone see Thymoquinone.

2-Isopropyl-5-methylcyclohexanol see Menthol.

3-Isopropyl-1-methylcyclopentanecarboxylic acid see Fencholic acid.

2-Isopropyl-3-methyl-4,6-dinitrophenol see Dinoprop.

ISOPROPYL METHYL ETHER ('isopryl').

N-**Isopropyl-α-(2-methylhydrazino)-*p*-toluamide** see Procarbazine.

2-Isopropyl-5-methylhydroquinone see Thymohydroquinone.

4-Isopropyl-2-methyl-3-[*N*-methyl-*N*-(α-methylphenethyl)aminomethyl]-1-phenyl-3-pyrazolin-5-one see Famprofazone.

2-Isopropyl-1-methyl-5-nitroimidazole see Ipronidazole.

N-**(4-Isopropyl-2-methyl-5-oxo-1-phenyl-3-pyrazolin-3-ylmethyl)-*N*-methylamphetamine** see Famprofazone.

2-Isopropyl-5-methylphenol see Thymol.

2-[(2-Isopropyl-5-methylphenoxy)methyl]-2-imidazoline see Tymazoline.

3-Isopropyl-5-methylphenyl methylcarbamate see Promecarb.

1-Isopropyl-7-methyl-4-phenylquinazolin-2(1H)-one see Proquazone.

Isopropyl methylphosphonofluoridate see Sarin.

1-ISOPROPYL-3-METHYLPYRAZOL-5-YL DIMETHYLCARBAMATE (G-23611; 'isolan', 'primin').

4-[(Isopropyl)(nicotinamidomethyl)-amino]-2,3-dimethyl-1-phenyl-3-pyrazolin-5-one see Niprofazone.

4-[(Isopropyl)(nicotinamidomethyl)-amino]phenazone see Niprofazone.

N-**Isopropyl-*p*-nitrophenylethanolamine** see Nifenalol.

4-Isopropylphenazone see Propyphenazone.

o-**Isopropylphenyl methylcarbamate** see Isoprocarb.

Isopropylphosphoramidic acid ethyl 3-methyl-4-(methylthio)phenyl ester see Fenamiphos.

10-[(4-Isopropylpiperazin-1-yl)carbonyl]-phenothiazine see Sopitazine.

4-Isopropylpiperazin-1-yl phenothiazin-10-yl ketone see Sopitazine.

'Isopropyl-systral' see Mecloxamine.

N^1-**(5-Isopropyl-1,3,4-thiadiazol-2-yl)-sulfanilamide** see Glyprothiazole.

Isopropyl 2-thiazol-4-yl-5-benzimidazole-carbamate see Cambendazole.

p-**(Isopropylthio)-α-(1-octamylamino-ethyl)benzyl alcohol** see Suloctidil.

1-[*p*-(Isopropylthio)phenyl]-2-octamyl-amino-1-propanol see Suloctidil.

1-Isopropyl-3-[(4-*m*-toluidinopyrid-3-yl)-sulfonyl]urea see Torasemide.

4-Isopropyl-2-(α,α,α-trifluoro-*m*-tolyl)-morpholine see Oxaflozane.

N-**Isopropyl-4-(3,4,5-trimethoxy-cinnamoyl)-1-piperazineacetamide** see Cinpropazide.

Isopropyltropolone(s) see Thujaplicin(s).

8-Isopropyl-3-($\pm$)-tropoyloxy-1αH,5αH-tropanium bromide see Ipratropium bromide.

Isoprotan (tr) see Carisoprodol.

Isoproterenol* see Isoprenaline.

Isoprothane see Carisoprodol.

'Isopryl' see Isopropyl methyl ether.

'Isoptin' see Verapamil.

'Isopyrin' see Isoniazid; Isopropylamino-phenazone.

ISOQUERCITRIN (quercetin 3-glucoside).

ISOQUINOLINE (2-benzazine; leucoline).

'Isordil' see Isosorbide dinitrate.

ISORHAMNETIN (3,4′,5,7-tetrahydroxy-3′-methoxyflavone).

ISORIBOFLAVIN (6,7-dimethyl-10-(1-D-ribityl)isoalloxazine; NSC-3100).

ISOSERINE (3-amino-2-hydroxypropionic acid; 3-aminolactic acid).

ISOSORBIDE (1,4:3,6-dianhydrosorbitol; 1,4:3,6-dianhydro-D-glucitol; AT-101; 'hydronol').

ISOSORBIDE DINITRATE*** (1,4:3,6-dianhydrosorbitol 2,5-dinitrate; sorbide nitrate; 'carvasin', 'cedocard', 'conovliss', 'isoket', 'isordil', 'maycor', 'rigedal', 'risordan', 'sorbangil', 'sorbidilat', 'sorbi-trate', 'vascardin', 'vasorbate').

See also Proscillaridin with isosorbide dinitrate.

Isosorbide isomers *see* Isoidide; Isomannide.

'Isosumithion' *see* O,O-Dimethyl S-(p-nitro-m-tolyl) phosphorothioate.

Isosystox *see* Demeton-S.

'Isoteben' *see* Benzylideneisoniazid.

'Isotense' *see* Syrosingopine.

'Isotensen' *see* Methindethyrium.

'Isothan' *see* Dodecylpyridinium bromide; Dodecylisoquinolinium bromide.

Isothazine *see* Prophenamine.

Isothiazine *see* Prophenamine.

Isothiocyanic acid allyl ester *see* Allyl isothiocyanate.

Isothiourea *see* Pseudothiourea.

ISOTHIPENDYL*** (10-(2-dimethylaminopropyl)-10H-pyrido(3,2-b) (1,4)benzothiazine; 10-(2-dimethylaminopropyl)-1-azaphenothiazine; 10-(2-dimethylaminopropyl)-9-thia-1,10-diazaanthracene; dimethylaminoisopropylthiophenylpyridylamine; thipendyl; thypendyl; isothipendyl hydrochloride; D-201; 'andantol', 'nilergex', 'theruhistin').

'Isoton 12' *see* Dichlorodifluoromethane.

ISOTRIMEPERIDINE (4-phenyl-4-propionoxy-1,2,5-trimethylpiperidine; isopromedol).

'Isotyl AO12' *see* Fenabutene.

Isourea *see* Pseudourea.

Isouretin *see* Formamide oxime.

ISOVALERIC ACID (3-methylbutyric acid).

N-Isovaleryl-p-phenetidine *see* Valeridin.

Isovaleryl-L-valyl-L-valyl-4-amino-3-hydroxy-6-methylheptanoyl-L-alanyl-4-amino-3-hydroxy-6-methylheptanoic acid *see* Pepstatin.

ISOVALTHINE (S-(1-carboxy-2-methylpropyl)cysteine; S-(1-isopropylcarboxymethyl)cysteine).

ISOVERINE (tr) (N-isoamylcadaverine).

Isovitamin C *see* Isoascorbic acid.

Isoxacillin *see* Oxacillin.

ISOXICAM** (4-hydroxy-2-methyl-N-(5-methylisoxazol-3-yl)-2H-1,2-benzothiazine-3-carboxamide 1,1-dioxide).

ISOXSUPRINE*** (p-hydroxy-N-(1-methyl-2-phenoxyethyl)norephedrine; 1-(p-hydroxyphenyl)-2-(1-methyl-2-phenoxyethylamino)-1-propanol; p-hydroxy-N-(2-phenoxyisopropyl)norephedrine; p-hydroxy-α-[1-(3-phenoxy-2-propylamino)-ethyl]benzyl alcohol; isoxsuprine hydrochloride; Caa-40; GR-62; 'defencin', 'dilavase', 'dilovasan', 'duvadilan', 'fenam', 'phenoxyisopropylnorsuprifen', 'vasodilan', 'vasodilian', 'vasosuprine', 'vasotran').

'Isoxyl' *see* Tiocarlide.

'Ispaghul' *see* Ispagula.

ISPAGULA* (mucilage of *Plantago ovata* seeds; *Plantago ovata* coating; psyllium hydrophilic mucilloid; 'arcolax', 'betajel', 'ispaghul', 'i-so-gel', 'konsyl', 'L.A.', 'metamucil', 'mucilose', 'vi-siblin').

'Istin' *see* Dantron.

'Istizin' *see* Dantron.

'Istonil' *see* Dimetacrine tartrate.

'Isuretin' *see* Formamide oxime.

ITACONIC ACID (methylenesuccinic acid).

Italchine *see* Mepacrine.

ITG *see* Tiamiprine.

'Itinerol' *see* Meclozine.

Itobarbital *see* Butalbital.

ITP *see* Inosine triphosphate.

ITRAMIN (2-aminoethyl nitrate; 2-aminoethanol nitrate ester; ethanolamine nitrate; 2-nitratoethylamine).

ITRAMIN TOSILATE*** (2-aminoethyl-nitrate p-toluenesulfonate; 'nilatil').

'Itrumil' *see* Iodothiouracil.

'Ituran' *see* Nitrofurantoin.

IUDR *see* Idoxuridine.

Iuglone (tr) *see* Juglone.

'Ivalon' *see* Polyvinyl alcohol.

'Ivepirine' *see* Acetylsalicylic acid.

'Iversal' *see* Ambazone.

'Ivosit' *see* Dinoseb acetate.

J

J-51 *see* Diathymosulfone silver.

J-66 *see* Norethisterone acetate with ethinylestradiol.

J-96 *see* Ethinylestradiol 3-isopropylsulfonate.

J-110-E *see* Diphepanol with p-hydroxyephedrine salicylate.

'Jacuta' *see* Lindane.

'Jacutin' *see* Lindane.

'Jadit' *see* Buclosamide with salicylic acid.

'Jatroneural' *see* Trifluoperazine.

'Jatropur' *see* Triamterene.

JAV-852 *see* Benfosformin.

Javel water *see* Sodium hypochlorite.

JB-251 *see* Protokylol.

JB-305 *see* Piperidolate.

JB-323 *see* Pipenzolate.

JB-329 *see* 1-Ethylpiperid-3-yl phenylcyclopentaneglycolate.

JB-340 *see* Mepenzolate.

JB-516 *see* Pheniprazine.

JB-821 *see* Phenylisopropylisoniazid.

JB-835 *see* Phenylisobutylhydrazine.

JB-840 *see* Oxyclipine.
JB-8181 *see* Desipramine.
JD-177 *see* Aminocaproic acid.
JDL-37 *see* Niflumic acid.
JDL-38 *see* Troflocin.
'Jectofer' *see* Iron sorbitex.
'Jefron' *see* Polyferose.
'Jellin' *see* Fluocinolone acetonide.
'Jenotone' *see* Aminopromazine.
'Jestryl' *see* Carbachol.
'Jetrium' *see* Dextromoramide.
JL-512 *see* Fenediazole.
JL-998 *see* Dicycloverine.
JL-1078 *see* Dihexyverine.
'Jodozoat' *see* Meglumine acetrizoate.
Jodphenphos* *see* Iodofenphos.

Jodtalamin* *see* Iotalamic acid.
'Jomezol' *see* Thiamazole methiodide.
'Jonctum' *see* Oxaceprol.
'Jonit' *see* Bitoscanate.
'Jopagnost' *see* Iopanoic acid.
JOSAMYCIN*** (macrolide antibiotic from *Str. narbonensis* var. *josamceticus* var. *nova*).
JP-428 *see* Fenspiride.
JR-7904 *see* Lidoflazine.
'Jubalon' *see* Carbifene.
'Judolor' *see* Fursultiamine.
JUGLONE (5-hydroxy-1,4-naphthoquinone; iuglone; nucin).
Julin's carbon chloride *see* Hexachlorobenzene.

K

K-III *see* Dinitro-*o*-cresol.
K-IV *see* Dinitro-*o*-cresol.
K-17 *see* Thalidomide.
K80-KBOT *see* Tramazoline with oxytetracycline.
K-206 (tr) *see* Tipindole methiodide.
K-315 *see* Tramadol.
K-386 *see* Glycyclamide.
K-1875 *see* Bis(*p*-chlorophenoxy)methane.
K-1900 *see* Nimorazole.
K-2680 *see* Etomidoline.
K-3712 *see* Morclofone.
K-3717 *see* Aluminium histidinate with magnesium hydroxide.
K-4024 *see* Glipizide.
K-4049 *see* Glipizide.
K-4277 *see* Indoprofen.
'Kabikinase' *see* Streptokinase.
Kabl-925 *see* Emylcamate.
KAEMPFEROL (3,4',5,7-tetrahydroxyflavone).
Kaempferol 3-galactoside *see* Trifolin.
'Kafocin' *see* Cefaloglycin.
KAINIC ACID*** (2-carboxy-4-isopropenyl-3-pyrrolidineacetic acid; *xylo*-kainic acid; α-kainic acid; digenic acid; 'digenin', 'helminal').
KALAFUNGIN** (antibiotic from *Str. tanashiensis* strain *kala*; kalamycin; U-19718).
Kalamycin *see* Kalafungin.
'Kalex' *see* Tetrasodium edetate.
'Kalipin' *see* Calcium alginate.
Kallidin I *see* Lysylbradykinin.
Kallidin II *see* Bradykinin.
KALLIDINOGENASE*** (callicrein; 'angioxyl', 'depropanex', 'glumorin', 'kallikrein', 'padreatin', 'padutin', 'tardokrein').
'Kallikrein' *see* Kallidinogenase.
'Kalmerid' *see* Potassium mercuric iodide.

'Kalmettum-somniferum' *see* Chloralose.
'Kalmin' *see* Phlorizin.
'Kalsetal' *see* Calcium acetylsalicylate.
'Kalypnon' *see* Barotal.
'Kalzan' *see* Calcium gluconate.
Kamfochlor *see* Campheclor.
Kampfstoff *see* Mustard gas.
'Kamycin' *see* Kanamycin.
'Kamynex' *see* Kanamycin.
'Kanabristol' *see* Kanamycin.
'Kanacillin' *see* Kanamycin with penicillin.
'Kanacine' *see* Kanamycin.
KANAMYCIN*** (4,6-diamino-2-hydroxy-1,3-cyclohexene 3,6'-diamino-3,6'-dideoxy-di-α-D-glucoside; kanamycin sulfate; 'cantrex', 'kamycin', 'kamynex', 'kanabristol', 'kanacine', 'kanamytrex', 'kannasyn', 'kantrex', 'kappaxan', 'ophthalmokalixan', 'otokalixan', 'resistomycin').
KANAMYCIN WITH PENICILLIN ('kanacillin').
Kanamycin B *see* Bekanamycin.
'Kanamytrex' *see* Kanamycin.
KANENDOMYCIN (2'-amino-2'-deoxykanamycin).
'Kanechlor' *see* Polychlorinated biphenyl mixture.
'Kanesten' *see* Clotrimazole.
'Kannasyn' *see* Kanamycin.
'Kantrex' *see* Kanamycin.
'Kaon' *see* Potassium gluconate.
'Kappaxan' *see* Kanamycin.
'Kaprolsin' *see* Aminocaproic acid.
'Kaprylex' *see* Sodium octanoate.
'Karathane' *see* Dinocap.
'Karbam black' *see* Ferbam.
'Karbam white' *see* Ziram.
Karbation (tr) *see* Metam-sodium.
'Karbatox' *see* Carbaril.
'Karbinone' *see* Naftazone.

Karbofos (tr) see Malathion.
'Karbosep' see Carbaril.
KARBUTILATE* (3-[[(dimethylamino)-carbonyl]amino]phenyl (1,1-dimethyl-ethyl)carbamate; m-(dimethylcarbamoyl-amino)phenyl tert-butylcarbamate; 1-[m-(tert-butylcarbamoyloxy)phenyl]-3,3-dimethylurea; 'tandex').
'Kardylan' see Nicofuranose.
'Karion' see Pimeclone and Sorbitol.
'Karmex' see Diuron.
'Karsil' see 3,4-Dichloro-2-methylvaler-anilide.
KAT-256 see Clobutinol.
'Katapyrin' see Aminometradine.
Kathine see Norpseudoephedrine.
'Katin' see Sodium menadiol-3-sulfonate.
Katine see Norpseudoephedrine.
'Katonil' see Chlormerodrin.
'Katovit' see Prolintane.
'Katril' see Dropropizine.
'Kavaform' see Kavain plus magnesium orotate.
Kavahin see Methysticin.
KAVAIN (DL-5,6-dihydro-4-methoxy-6-styryl-2-pyrone; kava pyrone; kawain; 'gonosan').
KAVAIN PLUS MAGNESIUM OROTATE ('kavaform').
Kava pyrone see Kavain.
Kavatin see Methysticin.
Kawain see Kavain.
'Kaylene' see Aluminium silicate.
KB-77 see Tramazoline.
KB-95 see Benzpiperylone.
KB-227 see Tramazoline.
KCA see Etafenone.
KE see Cortisone.
KEBUZONE* (4-(2-acetylethyl)-1,2-di-phenyl-3,5-pyrazolidinedione; 4-(3-oxo-butyl)-1,2-diphenyl-3,5-pyrazolidinedione; ketophenylbutazone; 'ketazone').
'Kefglycin' see Cefaloglycin.
'Keflex' see Cefalexin.
'Keflin' see Cefalotin.
'Keflodin' see Cefaloridine.
'Keflordin' see Cefaloridine.
'Keforal' see Cefalexin.
'Kefspor' see Cefaloridine.
'Kefzol' see Cefazolin.
'Keithon' see Clofenetamine.
'Kelacid' see Alginic acid.
'Kelatin' see Penicillamine.
'Kelene' see Chloroethane.
'Kelfizine' see Sulfalene.
'Kelgin' see Sodium alginate.
'Kelin' see Chloroethane.
Kellofylline see Visnafylline.
'Kelox' see Tetroquinone.
'Keltan' see Dicofol.
'Kelthane' see Dicofol.
'Kemadrin' see Procyclidine.
'Kemate' see Anilazine.
'Kemithal' see Thialbarbital.
'Kenacort' see Triamcinolone.
'Kenalog' see Triamcinolone acetonide.
'Kepone' see Chlordecone.

'Keracaine' see Proxymetacaine.
KERACYANIN* (3-[6-O-(6-deoxy-α-L-mannopyranosyl)-β-D-glucopyranosyloxy]-3',4',5,7-tetrahydroxyflavylium chloride).
'Kerb' see Propyzamide.
'Kerecid' see Idoxuridine.
'Ketaject' see Ketamine.
'Ketalar' see Ketamine.
KETAMINE* (2-(o-chlorophenyl)-2-methylaminocyclohexanone; ketamine hydrochloride; CI-581; CL-369; 'ketalar', 'ketaject').
KETAMINE WITH DROPERIDOL ('ketanest').
'Ketanest' see Ketamine with droperidol.
KETAZOCINE* ((2R*,6R*,11S*)-3-(cyclo-propylmethyl)-3,4,5,6-tetrahydro-8-hydr-oxy-6,11-dimethyl-2,6-methano-3-benzazo-cin-1(2H)-one).
KETAZOLAM* (11-chloro-8,12b-dihydro-2,8-dimethyl-12b-phenyl-4H(1,3)-oxazino(3,2-d)(1,4)benzodiazepine-4,6-(6H)-dione; U-28774).
'Ketazone' see Kebuzone.
KETENE (carbomethene; ethenone).
'Kethamed' see Pemoline.
Kethoxal* see Ketoxal.
Kethoxal bis(thiosemicarbazone)see Gloxazone.
KETIMIPRAMINE* (5-(3-dimethyl-aminopropyl)-5,11-dihydro-10H-dibenz-(b,f)azepine-10-one; ketipramine; ketoimipramine).
KETIMIPRAMINE FUMARATE (keti-pramine fumarate; G-35259).
Ketipramine* see Ketimipramine.
Keto.... See also Oxo....
Ketoacetic acid see Glyoxylic acid.
KETOBEMIDONE* (4-(m-hydroxy-phenyl)-1-methyl-4-propionylpiperidine; ethyl 4-[4-(m-hydroxyphenyl)-N-methyl-piperidyl]ketone; 1-[4-(m-hydroxyphenyl)-1-methylpiperid-4-yl]-1-propanone; cétobemidone; A-21; C-5511; C-7115; Hö-10720; WIN-1539; 'cliradon', 'cymidon').
KETOCAINE* (2'-(2-diisopropylamino-ethoxy)butyrophenone; N-[2-(o-propionyl-phenoxy)ethyl]diisopropylamine; Rec-7-0518).
KETOCAINOL* (o-(2-diisopropyl-aminoethoxy)-α-propylbenzyl alcohol).
3-Ketocaproic acid see 3-Oxohexanoic acid.
2-Ketoglutaric acid see 2-Oxoglutaric acid.
3-Ketohexanoic acid see 3-Oxohexanoic acid.
3-Ketohexonic acid lactone see Isoascorbic acid.
Ketohydroxyestratriene see Estrone.
Ketoimipramine see Ketimipramine.
α-Ketoisocaproic acid see 4-Methyl-2-oxovaleric acid.
Ketole see Indole.
7-KETOLITHOCHOLIC ACID (3α-hydroxy-7-ketocholanic acid).
Ketomalonic acid see Mesoxalic acid.
KETOMYCIN ((R)-3-cyclohexenylglyoxylic acid).

Ketophenylbutazone see Kebuzone.
KETOPROFEN*** (2-(3-benzoylphenyl)-propionic acid; *m*-benzoylhydratropic acid; 3-(1-carboxyethyl)benzophenone; RP-19583; 'orudis', 'profenid').
11-Ketoprogesterone see Pregnenetrione.
1-Ketopropionaldehyde see Methylglyoxal.
2-Ketopropionic acid see Pyruvic acid.
'Ketoscilium' see Fentonium bromide.
'Ketostix' see Sodium nitroprusside.
Ketosuccinic acid see Oxalacetic acid.
KETOTIFEN** (4,9-dihydro-4-(1-methyl-piperid-4-ylidene)-10H-benzo(4,5)cyclo-hepta(1,2-b)thiophen-10-one).
4-Ketovaleric acid see Levulinic acid.
KETOXAL*** (3-ethoxy-1,1-dihydroxy-2-butanone; kethoxal).
'Ketrax' see Levamisole.
'Keuten' see Sodium dibunate.
KHELLIN*** (4,9-dimethoxy-7-methyl-4-oxo-1,8-dioxabenz(f)indene; 4,9-dimethoxy-7-methyl-5H-furo(3,2-g)(1)benzopyran-5-one; 5,8-dimethoxy-2-methyl-6,7-furano-chromone; ammicardin; visammin).
Khellinin see Khelloside.
KHELLOL (7-hydroxymethyl-4-methoxy-5H-furo(3,2-g)(1)benzopyran-5-one; 2-hydroxymethyl-5-methoxy-6,7-furano-chromone).
Khellol glucoside see Khelloside.
KHELLOSIDE*** (2-hydroxymethyl-5-methoxy-6,7-furanochromone glucoside; 7-hydroxymethyl-4-methoxy-5H-furo(3,2-g)(1)benzopyran-5-one glucoside; khellinin; khellol glucoside).
'Khonvan' see Fosfestrol.
'Kidrolase' see Asparaginase.
'Kikuthrin' see Prothrin.
'Killavon' see Benzalkonium.
Killifolin see Quillifolin.
'Kilval' see Vamidothion.
'Kinalysin' see Streptokinase.
Kindekamin see Quindecamine.
Kinetin see Furfurylaminopurine.
'Kinevac' see Sincalide.
Kinic acid see Quinic acid.
KINO* (Pterocarpus marsupium).
KINOPRENE* (*E,E*-2-propynyl 3,7,11-trimethyldodeca-2,4-dienoate; 'altodel').
Kinozol (tr) see 8-Quinolinol.
'Kiron' see Sulfametoxydiazine.
'Kitamycin' see Kitasamycin.
KITASAMYCIN*** (antibiotic from *Str. kitasatoensis*; leucomycin; 'kitamycin', 'syneptine').
'Kitazin P' see Benzyl diisopropyl phosphorothioate.
'Kitnos' see Etofamide.
KITON GREEN (erio green B; lissamine green V).
KL-255 see Bupranolol.
'Klinomycin' see Minocycline.
'Klinium' see Lidoflazine.
'Klion' see Metronidazole.
'Kloben' see Neburon.

Klofibrat* see Clofibrate.
Kloretazin see Chlormethine.
'Klorex' see Clorexolone.
Klorfenidim (tr) see Monuron.
Klor-IFK (tr) see Chlorpropham.
Klorinat (tr) see Barban.
Klorofos (tr) see Metrifonate.
Kloroksifenidim (tr) see Chloroxuron.
Klorpromazine see Chlorpromazine.
'Klot' see Tolonium.
'Klyx' see Sodium dioctyl sulfosuccinate.
KM-65 see Benzonatate.
K-MV see Pheneticillin.
Kö-339 see 3,4-Dihydroxy-3-methyl-4-phenyl-1-butyne.
Kö-592 see Toliprolol.
Kö-1173 see Mexiletine.
Kö-1366 see Bunitrolol.
'Koglucoid' see Alseroxylon.
KOJIC ACID (5-hydroxy-2-hydroxymethyl-4-pyrone).
'Kolantyl' see Dicycloverine.
'Kollidon' see Povidone.
'Kolton' see Piprinhydrinate.
'Koluphthisin' see Viomycin.
'Kombetin' see Strophanthin.
'Kombistrat' see Hydroxyzine.
'Komplexic acid' see Edetic acid.
'Komplexon' see Trisodium edetate.
'Komplexon IV' see 1,2-Diaminocyclo-hexanetetraacetic acid.
'Konsyl' see Ispagula.
Korelborin (tr) see Veratrum viride.
Korkonium (tr) see Dicholine suberate.
'Korlan' see Fenclofos.
'Krasnitin' see L-Asparaginase.
'Krecalvin' see Dichlorvos with calcium 2,2-dichlorovinyl methyl phosphate.
'Kresatin' see *m*-Cresyl acetate.
'Kresival' see Calcium cresolsulfonate.
'Kronitex' see Tricresyl phosphate.
'Kryogenin' see Phenicarbazide.
'Krysid' see Antu.
KSW-786 see Clofenciclan.
KTS see Gloxazone.
'Kumatoks' see Warfarin.
'Kumatox' see Warfarin.
'Kumoran' see Dicoumarol.
KURCHI* (Holarrhena antidysenterica bark; Conessi bark; Telicherry bark).
KURCHI BISMUTH IODIDE* (total kurchi alkaloids with Bi iodide).
'Kuron' see Fenoprop ester mixture.
'Kurosal' see Fenoprop potassium.
Kutizon (tr) see Cutizone.
KW-110 see Aceglutamide aluminium hydroxide complex.
KWD-2019 see Terbutaline.
'Kwells' see Scopolamine hydrobromide.
KXM see Proglumide.
'Kynex' see Sulfamethoxypyridazine.
KYNURENIC ACID (4-hydroxyquinaldic acid).
KYNURENINE (β-anthranoylalanine).
Kynurine see 4-Quinolinol.

L

L-01516 *see* Promethazine.
L-01748 *see* Dithiazanine.
L-08146 *see* Dimoxyline.
L-2 *see* Butoctamide hemisuccinate.
L-11-6 (tr) *see* Phorate.
L-30 *see* Sulfasomidine.
L-67 *see* Prilocaine.
L-84 *see* Diethylcarbamazine.
L-554 *see* Tritoqualine.
L-566 *see* Dibemethine.
L-1418 *see* Sultopride.
L-1573 *see* Mercaptamine.
L-1591 *see* Cystamine.
L-1633 *see* Sodium dibunate.
L-1718 *see* Osalmid.
L-2013 *see* Hexapropymate.
L-2197 *see* Benzarone.
L-2214 *see* Benzbromarone.
L-2329 *see* Benziodarone.
L-3428 *see* Amiodarone.
L-5418 *see* Diftalon.
L-6257 *see* Oxetorone fumarate.
L-6842 *see* Bitoscanate.
L-7810 *see* Cicarperone.
L-8027 *see* Nictindole.
L-8109 *see* Tianafac.
L-14045 *see* Tricyclamol.
L-16298 *see* Dextropropoxyphene.
L-16726 *see* Symetine.
L-20025 *see* Chlorprenaline.
L-20522 *see* DCI.
L-21679 *see* Maletamer.
L-25398 *see* Methohexital.
L-26383 *see* Tifencillin.
L-28002 *see* Epipropidine.
L-29060-LE *see* Vinblastine.
L-29275 *see* Capreomycin.
L-29866 *see* Levopropoxyphene.
L-30109 *see* Noracymethadol.
L-30639 *see* Polyetadene.
L-31814 *see* Heteronium.
L-32379 *see* Drostalone.
L-32645 *see* Vinleurosine.
L-33355 *see* Mestranol.
L-33379 *see* Fludroxycortide.
L-33876 *see* Antelmycin.
L-35483 *see* Cyclothiazide.
L-36781 *see* Vinrosidine.
L-37231 *see* Vincristine.
L-38000 *see* Clometerone.
L-38389 *see* Levopropicillin.
L-38489 *see* Nortriptyline.
L-39435 *see* Cefaloglycin.
L-40602 *see* Cefaloridine.
L-42339 *see* Acronine.
L-42406 *see* Metoquizine.
L-44106 *see* Toquizine.
L-46083 *see* Cefazolin.
L-47599 *see* Pirazofurin.
L-47663 *see* Tobramycin.
L-60284 *see* Ciclofenazine.

L-64000 *see* Fluazacort.
L-66873 *see* Cefalexin.
L-67314 *see* Monensin.
L-110140 *see* Fluoxetine.
'L.A.' *see* Ispagula
LA-012 *see* Quatacaine.
LA-1 *see* Nitrazepam.
LA-6 *see* Clonazepam.
LA-111 *see* Diazepam.
La-271 *see* Bisoxatin.
La-271a *see* Bisoxatin diacetate.
La-391 *see* Sodium picosulfate.
LA-956 *see* Pemoline.
LA-1211 *see* Imolamine.
LA-1221 *see* Butalamine.
'LA-6023' *see* Metformin.
LA-6024 *see* Metformin.
Labarraque's solution *see* Sodium hypo-
chlorite.
'Labazene' *see* Valproic acid.
'Labazil' *see* Salacetamide.
LABETALOL** (5-[1-hydroxy-2-(1-methyl-
3-phenylpropylamino)ethyl]salicylamide;
3-carboxamido-4-hydroxy-α-[(1-methyl-
3-phenylpropylamino)methyl]benzyl
alcohol; AH-5158A; Sch-15719W).
'Laboran' *see* Diethylhexadecylmethyl-
ammonium methosulfate.
'Labotropine' *see* Deanol benzilate.
'Labrafil M-1944CS' *see* Peglicol 5 oleate.
'Labroda' *see* Flopropione.
'Labrodax' *see* Flopropione.
Laburnine *see* Cytisine.
LAC-43 *see* Bupivacaine.
'Lacarnol' *see* Adenosine.
'Lacfer' *see* Lactobacillus acidophilus.
LACHESINE ((2-benzilyloxyethyl)dimethyl-
ethylammonium chloride; ethyl(2-hydr-
oxyethyl)dimethylammonium chloride
benzilate; E-3).
Lactacridine *see* Ethacridine lactate.
LACTIC ACID (2-hydroxypropionic acid).
Lactic acid polyester with glycolic acid
see Polyglactin.
Lactic acid 3,3,5-trimethylcyclohexyl
ester *see* Ciclactate.
Lactoacridine *see* Ethacridine lactate.
LACTOBACILLUS ACIDOPHILUS
CULTURES ('enpac', 'lacfer', 'lactophil',
'viacil').
Lactobacillus bulgaricus factor *see*
Pantetheine.
Lactobacillus casei factor *see* Folic acid.
Lactobacillus casei fermentation factor
see Pteropterin.
LACTOBIONIC ACID (4-(β-D-galactosido)-
D-gluconic acid).
See also Calcium lactobionate.
Lactoflavin *see* Riboflavin.
'Lactol' *see* 2-Naphthyl lactate.
Lactonaphthol *see* 2-Naphthyl lactate.

Lactophenin *see* Lactylphenetidin.
Lactophenone *see* 2-Hydroxypropiophenone.
'Lactophenymer' *see* Phenylmercuric lactate.
'Lactophil' *see* Lactobacillus acidophilus.
LACTULOSE* (4-*O*-β-D-galactopyranosyl-D-fructose; 'bifiteral', 'duphalac', 'laevilac', 'laevolac').
LACTYLPHENETIDIN* (*N*-lactyl-*p*-phenetidine; *N*-(*p*-ethoxyphenyl)lactamide; fenolactine; lactophenin).
'Lacumin' *see* Pecazine.
'Ladogal' *see* Glucosulfamide.
LAE-32 *see* Ethyllysergamide.
'Laevilac' *see* Lactulose.
Laevo.... *see also* Levo....
'Laevolac' *see* Lactulose.
'Laevostrophan' *see* Strophanthin.
'Lakarnol' *see* Adenosine.
'Lambrol' *see* Flunenetil.
'Lammacorten' *see* Dexamethasone.
'Lamoryl' *see* Griseofulvin.
'Lampit' *see* Nifurtimox.
'Lamprene' *see* Clofazimine.
'Lamuran' *see* Raubasine.
'Lanadigin' *see* Acetyldigoxin.
LANADOXIN (gitaloxigenin monodigitoxoside).
'Lanatilin' *see* Acetyldigoxin.
LANATOSIDE A ('adigal', 'aglunat').
LANATOSIDE C* (3β,12,14-trihydroxy-5β-card-20(22)-enolide 3-(acetylglucosyl)-tridigitoxoside; digoxigenin 3-acetyl-glucosyltridigitoxoside; 'cedilanid oral', 'cedisanol', 'ceglunat', 'celadigal', 'eladigal', 'lanimerck').
LANATOSIDES (mixture of lanatosides A, B & C; 'cardiolanata', 'cordilan', 'digil-anid', 'digimed', 'diglanex', 'lanostabil', 'pandigal', 'panlanat', 'tridigal').
'Landrax' *see* Cytochrome c.
'Landrin' *see* Trimethylphenyl methyl-carbamate.
'Landrina' *see* Xantinol nicotinate.
'Landromil' *see* Ticlatone.
'Lanesta' *see* Clorindanol.
'Lanettes' *see* Clorindanol with laureth 9.
'Lanicor' *see* Digoxin.
'Lanimerck' *see* Lanatoside C.
'Lanitop' *see* Medigoxin.
'Lannate' *see* Methomyl.
'Lanostabil' *see* Lanatosides.
'Lanoxalin' *see* Bisoxatin diacetate.
'Lanoxin' *see* Digoxin.
LANTHIONINE (3,3'-thiodialanine; bis(2-amino-2-carboxyethyl) sulfide).
'Lanvis' *see* Tioguanine.
Laokon *see* Oxycodone.
LAPACHOL (2-hydroxy-3-(3-methyl-2-butenyl)-1,4-naphthoquinone).
LAPIRIUM CHLORIDE* 1-[(2-hydroxy-ethyl)carbamoylmethyl]pyridinium chloride laurate (ester); 1-[*N*-(2-dodecano-yloxyethyl)carbamoylmethyl]pyridinium chloride; 1-[*N*-(2-lauroyloxyethyl)carb-amoylmethyl]pyridinium chloride; lapyrium chloride; 'emcol E-607').
'Lapudrine' *see* Chlorproguanil.

'Lapurol' *see* Hydrogen peroxide urea derivative.
Lapyrium chloride* *see* Lapirium chloride.
'Larex' *see* Polynoxylin.
'Largactil' *see* Chlorpromazine.
'Largon' *see* Propiomazine.
'Largophren' *see* Prothipendyl.
Laricic acid *see* Agaric acid.
'Laristin' *see* Histidine.
'Larocaine' *see* Dimethocaine.
'Larocin' *see* Amoxicillin.
'Larodon' *see* Propyphenazone.
'Larodopa' *see* Levodopa.
'Larostidin' *see* Histidine.
'Larotid' *see* Amoxicillin.
'Laroxyl' *see* Amitriptyline.
LARUSAN (tr) (*N*'-(1-methyl-2-furfuryl-ideneethylidene)isoniazid; 2-isonicotinoyl-hydrazone of 1-furfurylideneacetone; iso-nicotinic acid [1-methyl-1-(2-furfuryl-idene)ethylidene]hydrazide).
Larusin *see* Formycin B.
LAS-11871 *see* Thiazolinobutazone.
LASALOCID ** (6-[7(*R*)-[5(*S*)-ethyl-5-(5(*R*)-ethyltetrahydro-5-hydroxy-6(*S*)-methyl-2H-pyran-2(*R*)-yl)tetrahydro-3(*S*)-methyl-2(*S*)-furyl]-4(*S*)-hydroxy-3(*R*),5(*S*)-dimethyl-6-oxononyl]-2,3-cresotic acid; Ro 2-2985; 'avatec').
'Lasix' *see* Furosemide.
'Lasso' *see* Alachlor.
'Lastanox' *see* Bis(tributyltin) iodide.
'Latépyrine' *see* Aminophenazone ethyl salicylate.
Lateritium Wr., antibiotic, *see* Fusafungine.
Lathyrus factor *see* Aminopropionitrile.
'Laucetin' *see* Erythromycin estolate with tetracycline.
Laudacon *see* Hydromorphone.
'Laudamonium' *see* Benzalkonium.
Laudanum *see* Opium alkaloids.
LAUDEXIUM METILSULFATE*
(2,2'-decamethylenebis(1,2,3,4-tetrahydro-6,7-dimethoxy-2-methyl-1-veratryliso-quinolinium methylsulfate); decamethyl-ene-1,10-bis[1-(3,4-dimethoxybenzyl)-1,2,3,4-tetrahydro-6,7-dimethoxy-2-methyl-isoquinolinium methosulfate]; curarexium methylsulfate; curarexine methylsulfate; laudexium methylsulfate; compound 20; 'laudolissin').
'Laudolissin' *see* Laudexium metilsulfate.
Laughing gas *see* Nitrous oxide.
LAURALKONIUM CHLORIDE* (benzyl-[2-(*p*-dodecoylphenoxy)ethyl]dimethyl-ammonium chloride; laurophenonium chloride; 'fortasept', 'pyrgasol').
LAURETH 9* (mixture of polyoxyethylene lauryl esters having a statistical average of 9 ethylene oxide groups per molecule).
LAURIC ACID (dodecanoic acid).
LAURILSULFATE(S) ** (dodecyl sulfate(s); lauryl sulfate(s)).
'Lauritran' *see* Erythromycin estolate.
'Laurodin' *see* Laurolinium acetate.
LAUROGUADINE* (1,1'-dodecyloxy-*m*-phenylene)diguanidine; 1,3-diguanyl-4-

lauryloxybenzene).

LAUROLINIUM ACETATE*** (4-amino-1-dodecylquinaldinium acetate; 'laurodin').

LAUROMACROGOL 400*** (mixture of monolauryl ethers of polyoxyethylene glycols having a statistical average of 8 ethylene oxide groups per molecule; 'brij'). *See also* Laureth.

'Lauron' *see* Aurothioglycanide.

Laurophenonium *see* Lauralkonium.

'Laurosept' *see* Dodecylpyridinium bromide.

1-[N-(2-Lauroyloxyethyl)carbamoylmethyl]pyridinium chloride *see* Lapirium chloride.

'Laurycuivre' *see* Cuprammonium dodecyl sulfonate.

Laurylpyridinium *see* Dodecylpyridinium.

Laurylisoquinolinium *see* Dodecylisoquinolinium.

Lauryl sodium sulfate *see* Sodium dodecyl sulfate.

Lauryl sulfate(s) *see* Laurilsulfate(s).

Lauryl sulfoacetate *see* Dodecyl sulfoacetate.

'Lautecin' *see* Erythromycin estolate with tetracycline.

Lauth's violet *see* Thionine.

'Lavasyl' *see* Phenobarbital-ethylenediamine.

'Laxanthrene' *see* Dantron.

'Laxatin' *see* Phenisatin.

'Laxbene' *see* Bisacodyl with dimeticone.

'Laxoberal' *see* Sodium picosulfate.

'Laxoberon' *see* Sodium picosulfate.

LB-46 *see* Pindolol.

LB-125 *see* Cyprodenate maleate.

LB-502 *see* Furosemide.

LBF *see* Pantetheine.

LC-44 *see* Flupentixol.

LCB-29 *see* Idrocilamide.

LD-2480 *see* Piprocurarium iodide.

LD-2988 *see* Folescutol.

LD-3394 *see* Fenozolone.

LD-3598 *see* Spirgetine.

LD-3612 *see* Paraflutizide.

LD-3695 *see* Cyclazodone.

LD-4610 *see* Oxazidone.

LE-29060 *see* Vinblastine.

Lead tetraethyl *see* Tetraethyllead.

'Lealgin' *see* Phenoperidine.

'Leandin' *see* Cyacetacide.

'Lebaycid' *see* Fenthion.

Lecithin *see* Phosphatidylcholine.

'Ledacrin' *see* Nitracrine.

'Ledclair' *see* Sodium calcium edetate.

'Ledercort' *see* Triamcinolone.

'Lederkyn' *see* Sulfamethoxypyridazine.

'Ledermix' *see* Demeclocycline with triamcinolone.

'Ledermycin' *see* Demeclocycline.

'Lederspan' *see* Triamcinolone hexacetonide.

'Ledertepa' *see* Thiotepa.

'Ledertrexate' *see* Methotrexate.

'Ledopa' *see* Levodopa.

'Ledosten' *see* Diethadione.

LEFETAMINE** ((−)-N,N-dimethyl-1,2-diphenylethylamine; (−)-N,N-dimethyl-α-phenylphenethylamine; (−)-N,N-di-methyl-1,2-diphenylethylamine; (−)-1-dimethylamino-1,2-diphenylethane; (−)-N,N-dimethylstilbylamine; 'spa').

'Legalon' *see* Silymarin sodium.

'Legumex extra' *see* Benazolin.

'Legurame' *see* Carbetamide.

LEIOPYRROLE*** (1-[o-(2-diethylaminoethoxy)phenyl]-2-methyl-5-phenylpyrrole; DV-714).

'Leiormone' *see* Vasopressin.

'Lekamin' *see* Trichlormethine.

LENACIL* (3-cyclohexyl-6,7-dihydro-1H-cyclopentapyrimidine-2,4(3H,5H)-dione; 'venzar').

'Lenetran' *see* Mephenoxalone.

'Lenicet' *see* Aluminium acetate.

'Lenigallol' *see* Acetpyrogall.

'Lenigesal' *see* Dextropropoxyphene theobromin-1-ylacetate.

LENIQUINSIN*** (6,7-dimethoxy-4-veratrylideneaminoquinoline; 4-(3,4-dimethoxybenzylideneamino) 6,7-dimethoxyquinoline; U-1085).

'Lenopect' *see* Pipazetate.

LENPERONE*** (4'-fluoro-4-[4-(p-fluorobenzoyl)piperid-1-yl]butyrophenone; lenperone hydrochloride; AHR-2277).

'Lente iletin' *see* Insulin zinc suspension.

Lente insulin *see* Insulin zinc suspension.

'Lentin' *see* Carbachol.

'Lentizol' *see* Amitriptyline.

'Lentostamin' *see* Chlorpheniramine maleate.

Lentysine *see* Eritadenine.

Leo-114 *see* Polyestradiol phosphate.

Leo-640 *see* Lofepramine.

'Leocentyl' *see* Bendroflumethiazide.

'Leocillin' *see* Penethamate hydriodide.

'Leodrine' *see* Hydroflumethiazide.

'Leofungin' *see* Pecilocin.

'Leopental' *see* Thiopental.

Lepargylic acid *see* Azelaic acid.

'Lepitoin' *see* Phenytoin.

'Lepivane' *see* Profenamine.

'Leponex' *see* Clozapine.

'Lepsiral' *see* Primidone.

LEPTACLINE*** (1-cyclohexylmethylpiperidine; piperid-1-ylmethylcyclohexane; piperidinomethylcyclohexane; leptacline hydrochloride; PMC; SD-210-32).

LEPTACLINE CAMSILATE (leptacline DL-camphorsulfonate; leptacline camsylate; SD-210-37).

'Leptanal' *see* Fentanyl citrate.

Leptazol *see* Pentetrazole.

'Lepticur' *see* Tropatepine.

'Leptidrol' *see* Pipradrol.

'Lepton' *see* Leptophos.

LEPTOPHOS* (O-(4-bromo-2,5-dichlorophenyl) O-methyl phenylphosphonothioate; OMS-1438; 'abar', 'lepton', 'phosvel').

'Leptryl' *see* Perimetazine.

'Lergigan' *see* Promethazine.

'Lergine' *see* Tricyclamol.

'Lergitin' *see* Phenbenzamine.

'Lergoban' *see* Diphenylpyraline.

'Lergopenin' *see* Clemizole-penicillin.

LERGOTRILE*** (2-chloro-6-methyl-ergoline-8β-acetonitrile; 2-chloro-8β-(cyanomethyl)-6-methylergoline).
'Leritin' see Anileridine.
'Leron' see Guanacline.
'Lertigon' see Histamine azoprotein complex.
'Lescopine' see Scopolamine methyl bromide.
'Lete' see Promazine.
'Lethidrone' see Nalorphine.
LETIMIDE*** (3-(2-diethylaminoethyl)-2H-1,3-benzoxazine-2,4(3H)-dione).
'Letter' see Levothyroxine sodium.
'Letusin' see Levopropoxyphene napsilate.
Leucenine see Leucenol.
LEUCENOL (DL-2-amino-3-(3-hydroxy-4-oxopyrid-1-yl)propionic acid; α-amino-(3-hydroxy-4-pyridinone)propionic acid; leucenine).
(−)Leucenol see Mimosine.
LEUCINE (2-amino-4-methylvaleric acid; α-aminoisocaproic acid).
LEUCINOCAINE*** (2-diethylamino-4-methylpentyl p-aminobenzoate; N,N-diethylleucinol ester of p-aminobenzoic acid; 'stadacaine').
LEUCINOCAINE MESILATE (leucinocaine methanesulfonate; leucinocaine mesylate; 'panthesin').
See also Dihydroergotoxine with leucinocaine mesilate.
LEUCINOL (2-amino-4-methyl-1-pentanol).
'Leuco-4' see Adenine.
Leucoalizarin see Anthrarobin.
LEUCOCIANIDOL** (3,3',4,4',5,7-flavanhexol; leucocyanidol; 'resivit').
'Leucocristine' see Vincristine.
Leucocyanidol see Leucocianidol.
'Leucofen' see Chlorphentermine.
LEUCOGEN (tr) (4-carboxy-α-phenyl-2-thiazolidineacetic acid ethyl ester; 2-(α-carbethoxybenzyl)thiazolidine-4-carboxylic acid; 2-(α-ethoxycarbonylbenzyl)thiazolidine-4-carboxylic acid).
Leucoharmine see Harmine.
Leucoline see Isoquinoline.
Leucomycin see Kitasamycin.
'Leucomycin N' see Azidamfenicol.
'Leucovorin' see Calcium folinate.
'Leukeran' see Chlorambucil.
'Leukerin' see Mercaptopurine.
'Leukomycin' see Chloramphenicol.
'Leupurin' see Mercaptopurine.
Leurocristine see Vincristine.
Leurosine see Vinleurosine.
LEVACETYLMETHADOL** ((−)-3-acetoxy-6-dimethylamino-4,4-diphenyl-heptane).
See also Acetylmethadol.
'Levadenyl' see Adenosine triphosphate.
LEVALLORPHAN*** ((−)-N-allyl-3-hydroxymorphinan).
See also Pethidine with levallorphan.
LEVALLORPHAN ACETATE (Ro-1-7929).
LEVALLORPHAN TARTRATE (Ro-1-7700; 'lorfan').
LEVAMFETAMINE*** ((−)-amphetamine;

(−)-α-methylphenethylamine; levamphetamine).
LEVAMFETAMINE ALGINATE ('levonor').
LEVAMFETAMINE SUCCINATE* ('cydril').
See also Amphetamine; Dexamphetamine.
LEVAMISOLE*** ((−)-2,3,5,6-tetrahydro-6-phenylimidazo(2,1-b)thiazole; (−)-tetramisole; R-12456; 'ketrax', 'nilverm GL').
See also Dexamisole; Tetramisole.
Levamphetamine* see Levamfetamine.
'Levanil' see Ectylurea.
'Levanxol' see Temazepam.
Levarterenol** see Noradrenaline.
'Levicor' see Metaraminol.
Levisoprenaline*** see Isoprenaline.
'Levium' see Diazepam.
'Levius' see Acetylsalicylic acid.
Levo-BC-2627 see Butorphanol.
Levocarbinoxamine* see Rotoxamine.
LEVODOPA*** ((−)-3-(3,4-dihydroxy-phenyl)-L-alanine; (−)-dopa; 'berkdopa', 'brocadopa', 'dopaflex', 'dopal', 'dopal-fher', 'dopar', 'dopasol', 'dopastral', 'eldopal', 'helfo-dopa', 'larodopa', 'ledopa', 'levopa', 'rigakin', 'rigitrem', 'sobiodopa', 'speciadopa', 'veldopa').
LEVODOPA WITH BENSERAZIDE (Ro 8-0576; 'madopar').
LEVODOPA WITH CARBIDOPA ('nacom', 'sinemet').
'Levo-dromoran' see Levorphanol.
LEVOFURALTADONE*** ((−)-5-morpholinomethyl-3-(5-nitrofurfurylideneamino)-2-oxazolidinone; levofuraltadone hydrochloride; NF-602; NF-902).
See also Furaltadone.
LEVOGLUTAMIDE** (L-glutamine; levoglutamine).
Levoglutamine* see Levoglutamide.
LEVOMENOL*** ((−)-6-methyl-2-(4-methyl-3-cyclohexen-1-yl)-5-hepten-2-ol; (−)-5-(1-hydroxy-1,5-dimethylhex-4-en-1-yl)-2-methyl-1-cyclohexene; (−)-α-bisabolol).
Levomepate* see Atromepine.
LEVOMEPROMAZINE*** ((−)-10-(3-dimethylamino-2-methylpropyl)-2-methoxyphenothiazine; levopromazine; mepromazine; methotrimeprazine; methoxypromazine; Bayer-1213; CL-39743; CL-36467; RP-7044; SK&F-5116; 'sinogan', 'tisercin').
LEVOMEPROMAZINE MALEATE (levomepromazine hydrogen maleate; 'levoprome', 'minozinan', 'neozine', 'neuractil', 'neurocil', 'nozinan', 'tiserci-netta', 'veractil').
See also Etorphine with levomepromazine.
LEVOMETHORPHAN*** ((−)-3-methoxy-N-methylmorphinan; levomethorpan hydrobromide; Ro-1-5470/6; R-1-7788).
LEVOMETIOMEPRAZINE*** ((−)-10-(3-dimethylamino-2-methylpropyl)-2-(methyl-thio)phenothiazine).
See also Methiomeprazine.

LEVOMORAMIDE*** ((−)-4-(2-methyl-4-
oxo-3,3-diphenyl-4-pyrrolidin-1-ylbutyl)-
morpholine; (−)-1-(3-methyl-4-morpho-
lino-2,2-diphenylbutyryl)pyrrolidine;
levomoramide bitartrate).
See also Dextromoramide; Racemoramide.
Levomycetin (tr) *see* Chloramphenicol.
LEVOMYCIN (tr) (antibiotic from an
unidentified Streptomyces).
'Levonor' *see* Levamfetamine alginate.
Levonordefrin *see* (−)-Corbadrine.
LEVONORGESTREL** (D-(−)-13-ethyl-
17-hydroxy-18,19-dinor-17α-pregn-4-en-
20-yn-3-one; (*formerly named*) dexnorgestrel;
'follistrel', 'microluton', 'mikro-30',
'mivroval'). *See also* Norgestrel.
**LEVONORGESTREL WITH ETHINYL-
ESTRADIOL** (SH-71144; SH-71155;
'gravistat', 'microgynon', 'neogynon',
'ovran', 'ovranette', 'sequilar', 'stediril-d').
'Levopa' *see* Levodopa.
Levophacetoperane* Phacetoperan.
LEVOPHENACYLMORPHAN*** ((−)-3-
hydroxy-*N*-phenacylmorphinan).
Levopromazine* *see* Levomepromazine.
'Levoprome' *see* Levomepromazine.
LEVOPROPICILLIN*** ((−)-6-(α-
phenoxybutyramido)penicillanic acid; 1-
phenoxypropylpenicillin; levopropylcillin;
levopropylcillin potassium; BRL-284;
L-38389; P-248; 'delprosyn').
See also Propicillin.
LEVOPROPOXYPHENE*** (α-(−)-4-
dimethylamino-3-methyl-1,2-diphenyl-
2-butanol propionate ester; α-(−)-*N,N*,2-
trimethyl-3,4-diphenyl-3-propionoxy-1-
butylamine).
See also Dextropropoxyphene.
LEVOPROPOXYPHENE DIBUDINATE
(levopropoxyphene 2,6-di-*tert*-butylnaph-
thalenedisulfonate; 'probunafon', 'sotorni').
LEVOPROPOXYPHENE NAPSILATE*
(levopropoxyphene 2-naphthalenesulfonate
hydrate; levopropoxyphene napsylate;
L-29866; 'letusin', 'novrad').
Levopropylcillin *see* Levopropicillin.
Levorenin *see* Epinephrine.
LEVORIN** (polyene antibiotic from
Actinomyces levoris).
Levorphan *see* Levorphanol.
LEVORPHANOL*** ((−)-3-hydroxy-*N*-
methylmorphinan; levorphan).
LEVORPHANOL TARTRATE ('dromo-
ran', 'levo-dromoran').
'Levothyl' *see* Methadone.
LEVOTHYROXINE SODIUM*** (L-3,5,
3',5'-tetraiodothyronine sodium; L-[3-(4-
hydroxy-3,5-diiodophenoxy)-3,5-diiodo-
phenyl]alanine sodium salt; sodium
levothyroxine; 'eltroxin', 'letter', 'levoxin',
'proloid', 'synthroid').
See also Liotrix.
LEVOXADROL*** ((−)-2,2-diphenyl-4-
piperid-2-yl-1,3-dioxolane; (−)-2-(2,2-
diphenyl-1,3-dioxolan-4-yl)piperidine;
(−)-dioxadrol; levoxadrol hydrochloride;
CL-912-C; 'levoxan').

'Levoxan' *see* Levoxadrol.
'Levoxin' *see* Levothyroxine sodium.
'Levsin' *see* Hyoscyamine.
'Levucalcin' *see* Calcium levulinate.
Levulic acid *see* Levulinic acid.
LEVULINIC ACID (3-acetylpropionic acid;
4-ketovaleric acid; laevulic acid; levulic
acid).
See also Calcium levulinate.
**LEVULINIC ACID PHENYLHYDR-
AZONE** ('antithermin').
LEVULINIC ACID RARE-EARTH SALTS
(neodymium and praesodymium levulin-
ates; 'helodym 88').
Levulose *see* Fructose.
LEWISITE (dichloro(2-chlorovinyl)arsine).
'Lexatin' *see* Bromazepam.
'Lexinol-cal' *see* Phosphatidylcholine.
'Lexotan' *see* Bromazepam.
'Ley cornox' *see* Benazolin.
LF-77 *see* Pifoxime.
LG-1 *see* Doxenitoin.
LG-206 *see* Prothipendyl.
LG-278 *see* Xenazoic acid.
LG-11457 *see* Etafenone.
LH-150 *see* Phenylbutazone 3,4,5-trimethoxy-
benzoate.
LH-RH *see* Gonadorelin.
LIBECILLIDE*** (2-[[(5-carboxy-5-
formamidopentyl)carbamoyl](2-phenyl-
acetamido)methyl]-5,5-dimethyl-4-
thiazolidinecarboxylic acid; lisocillide).
'Libratar' *see* Chlorbenoxamine.
'Librax' *see* Chlordiazepoxide with clidinium.
'Libraxin' *see* Clidinium bromide.
'Librium' *see* Chlordiazepoxide.
'Licaran' *see* Phenetamine.
'Licosin' *see* Camylofin.
'Lidanar' *see* Mesoridazine.
'Lidanil' *see* Mesoridazine.
Lidase (tr) *see* Hyaluronidase.
'Liden' *see* Isomethadone.
'Lidepran' *see* Phacetoperan.
'Lidex' *see* Fluocinonide.
LIDIMYCIN** (antibiotic from *Str. lydicus*;
lydimycin).
LIDOCAINE*** (2-diethylamino-2',6'-acet-
oxylidide; (*N'*-(2,6-dimethylphenyl)-*N,N*-
diethylglycinamide; α-diethylamino-2,6-
dimethylacetanilide; lignocaine; xylcaine;
DDA; lidocaine hydrochloride; LL-30).
LIDOCAINE ETHOBROMIDE (QX-314).
LIDOFLAZINE*** (4-[4,4-bis(*p*-fluoro-
phenyl)butyl]piperazin-1-yl-2',6'-acetoxy-
lidide; *N*-[4-[4,4-bis(*p*-fluorophenyl)butyl]-
piperazin-1-ylacetyl]-2,6-xylidine; McN-
JR-7904; R-7904; 'clinium', 'corflazine',
'klinium').
Lidol (tr) *see* Pethidine.
'Lifene' *see* Phensuximide.
LIFIBRATE** (1-methylpiperid-4-yl
glyoxalate 2-[bis(*p*-chlorophenyl)acetal];
1-methylpiperid-4-yl bis(4-chlorophenoxy)-
acetate; SaH-42-348; 'melipan').
Lignocaine* *see* Lidocaine.
Lignoceric acid *see* Tetracosanoic acid.
'Likudin' *see* Griseofulvin.

273

'**Limbatril**' *see* Amitriptyline with chlordiazepoxide.
'**Limbitrol**' *see* Amitriptyline with chlordiazepoxide.
'**Limclair**' *see* Trisodium edetate.
'**Lincocin**' *see* Lincomycin.
LINCOMYCIN*** (methyl 6,8-dideoxy-6-(1-methyl-*trans*-4-propyl-L-2-pyrrolidine-carboxamido)-1-thio-D-erythro-α-D-galactooctopyranoside; U-10149A; 'albiotic', 'cillimycin', 'lincocin', 'mycivin').
'**Linctussal**' *see* Sodium dibunate.
LINDANE* (γ-1,2,3,4,5,6-hexachlorocyclohexane; γ-BHC; benzenehexachlor; benzhexachlor; gamma-benzenehexachloride; geksan; hexachlorane; hexicide; 'aparasin', 'aphthiria', 'ben-hex', 'chloresene', 'dagicide', 'devoran', 'gamiso', 'gamma 666', 'gammexane', 'gexane', 'hexachloran', 'hexaverm', 'hexchloran', 'hexyclan', 'jacuta', 'jacutin', 'lorexane', 'neo-scabicidol', 'nourycid', 'streunex', 'tri-6', 'trisix', 'vermexane').
LINDANE WITH DDT (BHC with DDT; 'ditox L', 'omyl', 'trix', 'zoralin').
Lindane with ethylmercuric chloride *see* Mercuran.
'**Lindol**' *see* Tricresyl phosphate.
'**Linfolysin**' *see* Chlorambucil.
'**Lingraine**' *see* Ergotamine tartrate.
Link's compound 63 *see* Cyclocoumarol.
'**Linodil**' *see* Inositol nicotinate.
N-**Linoleamido-*p*-methyl-α-phenylphenethylamine** *see* Moctamide.
LINOLEIC ACID (*cis*,*cis*-9,12-octadecadienoic acid; linolic acid).
See also Trilinolein.
LINOLENIC ACID (9,12,15-octadecatrienoic acid).
Linolexamide *see* Clinolamide.
Linolic acid *see* Linoleic acid.
'**Linostil**' *see* Dimetacrine tartrate.
'**Lintex**' *see* Niclosamide.
LINURON* (1-(3,4-dichlorophenyl)-3-methoxy-3-methylurea; methoxydiuron; 'afalon', 'lorox').
'**Linyl**' *see* Phentermine resin.
'**Lio-metacen**' *see* Meglumine indometacinate.
'**Lioresal**' *see* Baclofen.
'**Liosol**' *see* Xenbucin.
LIOTHYRONINE*** (L-[3-(4-hydroxy-3-iodophenoxy)-3,5-diiodophenyl]alanine; L-3,5,3'-triiodothyronine; T-3; 'triomet', 'trionine').
LIOTHYRONINE SODIUM (sodium liothyronine; 'cynomel', 'cytomel', 'tertroxin', 'thybon', 'triothyrone').
See also Liotrix.
LIOTRIX* (mixture of levothyroxine sodium and liothyronine sodium; 'diotroxin', 'euthroid', 'thyrolar').
'**Lioxone**' *see* 3-Pyridineacetic acid.
'**Lipan**' *see* Dinitro-*o*-cresol.
Lipancreatin *see* Pancrelipase.
'**Lipavlon**' *see* Clofibrate.
'**Lipect**' *see* Pholcodine.

'**Lipenan**' *see* Clofibride.
'**Liphadione**' *see* Chlorophacinone.
'**Lipogantrisin**' *see* Acetylsulfafurazole.
'**Lipo-hepin**' *see* Heparin.
α-**Lipoic acid** *see* Thioctic acid.
'**Lipo-Merz**' *see* Etofibrate.
α-**Liponic acid** *see* Thioctic acid.
'**Lipotam**' *see* Trometamol thioctate.
'**Lipotril**' *see* Choline.
'**Lipotrin**' *see* α-Hydroxycyclohexanebutyric acid.
'**Liprodene**' *see* Pentorex tartrate.
'**Liquaemin**' *see* Heparin.
'**Liquamar**' *see* Phenprocoumon.
'**Liquemin**' *see* Heparin.
'**Liquoid**' *see* Sodium polyanetholesulfonate.
LIQUORICE EXTRACT OR JUICE (succus liquiritiae; 'réglisse', 'sucsan').
See also Deglycyrrhizinized liquorice; Glycyrrhizin; Nitrofurantoin with liquorice.
'**Liranol**' *see* Promazine.
'**Liro antisprout**' *see* Propham.
'**Lirofeen**' *see* *p*-Dioxation.
'**Liromidon**' *see* Phosphamidon.
'**Lironox**' *see* Butyl dichlorophenoxyacetate.
'**Lirophen**' *see* *p*-Dioxation.
'**Liro-trithion**' *see* Carbofenotion.
'**Lisdonil**' *see* Meladrazine.
'**Liserdol**' *see* Metergoline.
'**Lisergan**' *see* Acepromazine.
'**Liskantin**' *see* Primidone.
Lisocillide *see* Libecillide.
'**Lispamol**' *see* Aminopromazine.
'**Lispasmol**' *see* Aminopromazine.
Lissamine green V *see* Kiton green.
'**Lissapol(s)**' *see* Polyoxyalkylene compounds.
'**Lissolamine**' *see* Cetrimonium.
'**Listenon**' *see* Suxamethonium.
'**Listica**' *see* Oxyfenamate.
'**Listrocol**' *see* Cynarine.
LISURIDE*** (3-(9,10-didehydro-6-methyl ergolin-8α-yl)-1,1-diethylurea; 3,3-diethyl-1-(D-6-methylisoergolen-8-yl)urea; 9-(3,3-diethylureido)-4,6,6a,7,8,9-hexahydro-7-methylindolo(4,3-f,g)quinoline; lysuride; mesorgydine).
LISURIDE HYDROGEN MALEATE ('lysenil', 'lysenyl').
'**Litalir**' *see* Hydroxycarbamide.
'**Litec**' *see* Pizotifen maleate.
'**Lithane**' *see* Lithium carbonate.
Lithic acid *see* Uric acid.
'**Lithiofor**' *see* Lithium sulfate.
'**Lithionit**' *see* Lithium sulfate.
LITHIUM ACETATE ('quilonum').
LITHIUM CARBONATE (CP-15467-61; 'candamide', 'carbolith', 'eskalith', 'hypnorex', 'lithane', 'lithonate', 'lito', 'litoduron', 'neurolepsin', 'phasal', 'priadel', 'teralithe').
LITHIUM SALICYLATE WITH PROCAINE ('lithocaine').
LITHIUM SULFATE ('lithiofor', 'lithionit').
'**Lithocaine**' *see* Lithium salicylate with procaine.
LITHOCHOLIC ACID (3α-hydroxycholanic acid).

'**Lithonate**' *see* Lithium carbonate.
'**Lito**' *see* Lithium carbonate.
'**Litoduron**' *see* Lithium carbonate.
LITRACEN** (9,10-dihydro-10,10-dimethyl-9-(3-methylaminopropylidene)-anthracene).
LIVIDOMYCIN*** (lividomycin A; *O*-2-amino-2,3-dideoxy-α-D-*ribo*-hexopyranosyl-(1→4)-*O*-[*O*-α-D-mannopyranosyl-(1→4)-*O*-2,6-diamino-2,6-dideoxy-β-L-idopyranosyl-(1→3)-β-D-ribofuranosyl-(1→5)]-2-deoxy-D-streptamine).
Lividomycin A *see* Lividomycin.
'**Livipas**' *see* Halofenate.
'**Lixophen**' *see* Phenobarbital.
LJ-30 *see* Lidocaine.
LJ-278 *see* Dimabefylline.
LL-172 *see* Phloroglucinol with 1,3,5-trimethoxybenzene.
LL-705W *see* Neutramycin.
LL-1418 *see* Olmidine.
LL-1530 *see* Nadoxolol.
LL-1558 *see* Tiadenol.
LL-1656 *see* Buflomedil.
LLD factor *see* Cyanocobalamin.
LM-203A *see* Biperiden.
LM-208 *see* Quinupramine.
LM-2717 *see* Clobazam.
'**LMD**' *see* Dextran 40.
'**Lobamine**' *see* Methionine.
LOBELINE** (2-(β-hydroxyphenethyl)-1-methyl-6-phenacylpiperidine; 2-[6-(β-hydroxyphenethyl)-1-methylpiperid-2-yl]-acetophenone; inflatine; lobeline hydrochloride or sulfate; 'lobeton', 'nikoban', 'no-kotin', 'unilobin').
LOBENDAZOLE*** (ethyl 2-benzimidazole-carbamate; SK&F-24529).
'**Lobeton**' *see* Lobeline.
'**Locabiotal**' *see* Fusafungine.
'**Locacorten**' *see* Flumethasone pivalate.
'**Locastine**' *see* Amoxecaine.
'**Locoid**' *see* Hydrocortisone butyrate.
'**Locorten**' *see* Flumethasone pivalate.
LOFENAL (tr) (2-[*p*-[bis(2-chloroethyl)-amino]phenylacetamido]-3-phenylpropionic acid; *N*-[*p*-[bis(2-chloroethyl)-amino]phenylacetyl]-DL-phenylalanine; lophenal).
LOFENDAZAM* (8-chloro-4,5-dihydro-1-phenyl-3H-1,5-benzodiazepin-2-one).
LOFEPRAMINE*** (4'-chloro-2-[[3-(10,11-dihydro-5H-dibenz(b,f)azepin-5-yl)propyl]-methylamino]acetophenone; *N*-(*p*-chlorobenzoylmethyl)-3-(10,11-dihydro-5H-dibenz(b,f)azepin-5-yl)-*N*-methylpropylamine; 5-[3-[(*p*-chlorobenzoyl methyl)methylamino]propyl]-10,11-dihydro-5H-dibenz(b,f)azepine; 5-[3-[*N*-(*p*-chlorophenacyl)methylamino]propyl]-10,11-dihydro-5H-dibenz(b,f)azepine; chopramine; Leo-640; lopramine; 'gamonil').
LOFEXIDINE*** (2-[1-(2,6-dichlorophenoxy)ethyl]-2-imidazoline).
LOMETRALINE*** (8-chloro-1,2,3,4-tetrahydro-5-methoxy-*N*,*N*-dimethyl-1-naphthylamine; lometraline hydrochloride;

CP-14368-1).
'**Lomidine**' *see* Pentamidine isetionate.
'**Lomodex**' *see* Dextran 40.
LOMOFUNGIN (antibiotic from *Str. lomodensis*; 5-formyl-4,6,8-trihydroxy-1-(methoxycarbonyl)phenazine; lomondomycin).
Lomondomycin *see* Lomofungin.
'**Lomotil**' *see* Diphenoxylate with atropine.
LOMUSTINE*** (1-(2-chloroethyl)-3-cyclohexyl-1-nitrosourea; CCNU; NSC-79037).
'**Lonacol**' *see* Zineb.
LONAZOLAC** (3-(*p*-chlorophenyl)-1-phenylpyrazole-4-acetic acid).
'**Longacid**' *see* Butacid.
'**Longacilina**' *see* Benzathine penicillin.
'**Longacor**' *see* Quinidine arabogalactan sulfate.
'**Longamex**' *see* Noscapine.
'**Longanoct**' *see* Butethal.
'**Longestrol**' *see* Broparestrol.
'**Longicid**' *see* Benzathine penicillin.
'**Longifene**' *see* Buclizine.
'**Longoperidol**' *see* Penfluridol.
'**Longum**' *see* Sulfalene.
'**Lontanyl**' *see* Testosterone cyclohexane-carboxylate.
LOPERAMIDE*** (4-(*p*-chlorophenyl)-4-hydroxy-*N*,*N*-dimethyl-α,α-diphenyl-1-piperidinebutyramide; 4-[4-(*p*-chlorophenyl)-4-hydroxypiperidino]-*N*,*N*-dimethyl-2,2-diphenylbutyramide; loperamide hydrochloride; R-18553; 'imodium').
Lophenal (tr) *see* Lofenal.
'**Lopion**' *see* Sodium auroallylthioureidobenzoate.
Lopramine *see* Lofepramine.
Lopremone* *see* Protirelin.
'**Lopresor**' *see* Metoprolol.
'**Lora**' *see* Chloralodol.
LORAJMINE** (ajmaline chloroacetate; 17-chloroacetylajmaline; 'viaductor').
'**Lorakon**' *see* Benzalkonium.
LORAZEPAM*** (7-chloro-5-(*o*-chlorophenyl)-1,3-dihydro-3-hydroxy-2H-1,4-benzodiazepin-2-one; Wy-4036; 'ativan', 'lorenin', 'tavor', 'temesta').
LORBAMATE*** (2-(hydroxymethyl)-2-methylpentyl cyclopropanecarbamate carbamate (ester)).
'**Lorenin**' *see* Lorazepam.
'**Lorexane**' *see* Lindane.
'**Lorfan**' *see* Levallorphan.
'**Loridine**' *see* Cefaloridine.
'**Lorinal**' *see* Chloral hydrate.
'**Lormin**' *see* Chlormadinone.
'**Lorol**' *see* Sodium dodecyl sulfate.
'**Lorox**' *see* Linuron.
'**Lorusil**' *see* Aminopromazine.
'**Losalen**' *see* Flumetasone pivalate.
Lost *see* Mustard gas.
'**Lostinil**' *see* Cyclophosphamide.
'**Lotagen**' *see* Methylenedi(*m*-cresolsulfonic acid) polymer.
'**Lotone**' *see* Spermine.

LOTUCAINE*** (2,2,5,5-tetramethyl-α-(*o*-toloxymethyl)-1-pyrrolidineethanol; 1-[2-hydroxy-3-(*o*-toloxy)propyl]-2,2,5,5-tetramethylpyrrolidine; *o*-[2-hydroxy-3-(2,2,5,5-tetramethylpyrrolidin-1-yl)propoxy]toluene).

'**Lotusate**' *see* Talbutal.

'**Lovozal**' *see* Fenazaflor.

'**Lowila**' *see* Dodecyl sulfoacetate.

Low molecular weight dextran *see* Dextran 40.

LOXAPINE*** (2-chloro-11-(4-methylpiperazin-1-yl)dibenz(b,f)(1,4)oxazepine; oxilapine; CL-62362; S-805; SUM-3170). †

LOXAPINE SUCCINATE (CL-72563).

LP-1 (tr) *see* Chromocarb.

LRCL-3794 *see* Benoxaprofen.

LS-121 *see* Naftidrofuryl oxalate.

LS-701 *see* Benzydamine phenylbutazone-5-enolate.

LSD 25 *see* Lysergide.

LT-1 *see* Suxamethonium.

Lu-3-010 *see* Talopram.

Lu-5-003 *see* Talsupram.

Lü-274 *see* Cyclomethone.

'**Lubergal**' *see* 5-Allyl-5-phenylbarbituric acid.

'**Lubomycine**' *see* Erythromycin.

'**Lucaine**' *see* Piridocaine.

'**Lucamid**' *see* Ethenzamide.

LUCANTHONE*** (1-(2-diethylaminoethylamino)-4-methylthioxanthen-9-one; lucanthone hydrochloride; BW-57-233; BW-79T61; MS-752; NSC-14574; 'miracil D', 'miracol', 'nilodin', 'tixantone').

'**Lucel**' *see* Chlorquinox.

'**Lucidil**' *see* Benactyzine.

'**Lucidryl**' *see* Meclofenoxate.

LUCIMYCIN** (antibiotic from *Str. lucensis*).

'**Lucofen**' *see* Chlorphentermine.

'**Lucopenin**' *see* Meticillin.

'**Lucosil**' *see* Sulfamethizole.

'**Ludicril**' *see* Meclofenoxate.

'**Ludilat**' *see* Bencyclane.

'**Ludiomil**' *see* Maprotiline.

'**Ludobal**' *see* Quinuronium.

Lü-H-6 *see* Obidoxime.

'**Ludozan**' *see* Aluminium sodium silicate.

'**Lumbrical**' *see* Piperazine.

'**Lumetrodiol**' *see* Etynodiol diacetate.

LUMIFLAVIN (7,8,10-trimethylisoalloxazine).

'**Luminal**' *see* Phenobarbital.

'**Lumirelax**' *see* Methocarbamol.

LUPETAZINE (2,5-dimethylpiperazine; dipropylenediamine).

2,6-Lupetidine *see* Nanofin.

Lupinidine *see* Sparteine.

'**Lutazol**' *see* Salazosulfamide.

Luteinizing hormone releasing factor (pig) *see* Gonadorelin.

Luteinizing hormone releasing factor (synthetic) *see* Gonadorelin.

Luteohormone *see* Progesterone.

LUTEOLIN (3′,4′,5,7-tetrahydroxyflavone).

'**Luteran**' *see* Chlormadinone acetate.

'**Lutionex**' *see* Demegestone.

'**Lutometrodiol**' *see* Etynodiol diacetate.

'**Lutrexin**' *see* Lututrin.

LUTUTRIN* (uterus-relaxing factor from corpus luteum; 'lutrexin').

'**Luvatren**' *see* Moperone.

'**Luvistin**' *see* Histapyrrodine.

'**Luxan**' *see* Thiometon.

LX-100-129 *see* Clozapine.

Lyapolate *see* Sodium apolate.

'**Lycanol**' *see* Glymidine.

'**Lycedan**' *see* Adenosine phosphate.

Lycine *see* Betaine.

Lydasa (tr) *see* Hyaluronidase.

Lydimycin* *see* Lidimycin.

LYMECYCLINE*** (N^2-((+)-5-amino-5-carboxypentylaminomethyl)tetracycline; tetracycline-L-methylene-lysine; 'tetralysal').

'**Lymphochin**' *see* Aniline mustard.

'**Lymphoquine**' *see* Aniline mustard.

'**Lympholysin**' *see* Chlorambucil.

'**Lyndiol**' *see* Lynestrenol with mestranol.

LYNESTRENOL** (19-nor-17α-pregn-4-en-20-yn-1-ol; 17α-ethinylestr-4-en-17β-ol; ethinyloestrenol; lynoestrenol; 'exluto', 'exluton', 'orgametil', 'orgametril').
See also Ethinylestradiol with lynestrenol.

LYNESTRENOL WITH MESTRANOL ('lyndiol', 'noracycline', 'ovanon', 'ovariostat', 'restovar', 'sistometril').

Lynoestrenol* *see* Lynestrenol.

'**Lyochym**' *see* Chymotrypsin.

'**Lyogen**' *see* Fluphenazine; Fluphenazine decanoate.

'**Lyopect**' *see* Nicocodine.

'**Lyorodin**' *see* Fluphenazine.

'**Lyorthol**' *see* *o*-Phenylphenol.

'**Lyovac diuril**' *see* Chlorothiazide sodium.

'**Lyovac sodium edecrin**' *see* Sodium etacrynate.

LYPRESSIN*** (8-lysinevasopressin; 'diapid', 'syntopressin').

LYPRESSIN TANNATE ('pitressin').

'**Lyseen**' *see* Pridinol mesilate.

'**Lysenil**' *see* Lisuride.

'**Lysenyl**' *see* Lisuride.

LYSERGAMIDE (lysergic acid amide; ergine).

LYSERGIC ACID (7-methyl-4,6,6a,7,8,9-hexahydroindolo(4,3-f,g)quinoline-9-carboxylic acid).

Lysergic acid amide *see* Lysergamide.

Lysergic acid butanolamide *see* Methylergometrine.

Lysergic acid diethylamide *see* Lysergide.

Lysergic acid ethylamide *see* Ethyllysergamide.

Lysergic acid propanolamide *see* Ergometrine.

LYSERGIDE*** (4,6,6a,7,8,9-hexahydro-7-methylindolo(4,3-f,g)quinoline-9-carboxylic acid diethylamide; *N*,*N*-diethyllysergamide; lysergic acid diethylamide; LSD; LSD 25; 'delysid').

LYSIDINE (4,5-dihydro-2-methylimidazole; methylglyoxalidine; 2-methyl-2-imidazoline; ethyleneethenyldiamine).

Lysin *see* Plasmin.
LYSINE (2,6-diaminohexanoic acid; α,ε-diaminocaproic acid).
LYSINE ACETYLSALICYLATE (lysine soluble aspirin; E-171; 'aspegic', 'endosprin').
Lysine soluble aspirin *see* Lysine acetylsalicylate.
8-Lysinevasopressin *see* Lypressin.
'Lysobex' *see* Bibenzonium.
'Lysodren' *see* Mitotane.
'Lysoform' *see* Formaldehyde.
'Lysothiazole' *see* Sulfathiazole-aluminium.

Lysozyme with metronidazole *see* Metronidazole with lysozyme.
'Lyspafen' *see* Pentapiperide.
Lysuride* *see* Lisuride.
LYSYLBRADYKININ (kallidin I).
'Lyteca' *see* Paracetamol.
10-(L-Lyxityl)-7,8-dimethylisoalloxazine *see* Lyxoflavin.
LYXOFLAVIN (6,7-dimethyl-9-(1'-L-lyxityl)isoalloxazine).
LZ-544 *see* Tris(*p*-chlorophenyl)propionic acid 4-methylpiperazide.

M

M-1-36 *see* Etilefrine.
M6/42 *see* Ruvazone.
14-M-21 *see* 1-(4-Dimethylaminobenzylidene)-indene.
M40 (tr) *see* Chlordane.
M-74 (tr) *see* Disulfoton.
M-81 (tr) *see* Thiometon.
M-82 (tr) *see* Demephion-S.
M-99 *see* Etorphine.
M-115 *see* Suxethonium.
M-141 *see* Spectinomycin.
M-144 *see* Atrolactamide.
M-183 *see* Acetorphine.
M-285 *see* Cyprenorphine.
M-410 (tr) *see* Chlordane.
M-551 *see* Ethylphenacemide.
M-640 *see* Sulfathiazole-aluminium.
M-1028(Meiji) *see* Haloprogin.
M-4000 *see* Dichlorophenarsine.
M-4888 *see* Proguanil.
M-5050 *see* Diprenorphine.
M-5512 *see* Antazoline.
M-5943 *see* Chlorproguanil.
M-7555 *see* Quinapyramine.
M-9500 *see* Tretamine.
M-33536 *see* Dicycloverine.
M-2H *see* Butoctamide hemisuccinate.
MA-1277 *see* Zolertine.
MA-1291 *see* Quipazine.
MA-1337 *see* Cloperidone.
'Maalox' *see* Aluminium magnesium hydroxide.
'Mablin' *see* Busulfan.
'Mace' *see* Chloroacetophenone.
'Machete' *see* Butoclor.
Macleyine *see* Protopine.
Maclicine *see* Dicloxacillin.
'Macmirror' *see* Nifuratel.
'Macocyn' *see* Oxytetracycline.
Macrisalb (^{131}I) *see* Macrosalb (^{131}I).
Macroaggregated iodinated (^{131}I)**human albumin** *see* Macrosalb (^{131}I).
'Macrocycline' *see* Erythromycin with tetracycline.
'Macrodantin' *see* Nitrofurantoin.
'Macrodex' *see* Dextran 70.
MACROGOL(S)* (polyethylene glycol(s); PEG; 'carbowax', 'nycoline', 'solbase').
Macrogol cetyl ether *see* Cetomacrogol.
MACROGOL DI(POLYOXYETHYLENE) FATTY ACID AMIDES (ethomids).
Macrogol dodecyl ether *see* Lauromacrogol.
MACROGOL ESTER(S)*** (macrogol monoacid esters of fatty acids; ethofats; 'emanon' 'estax', 'neugen', 'nonex', 'polygol', 'postonal', 'sta-soft').
See also Macrogol laurate; Macrogol oleate; Macrogol stearate.
MACROGOL ETHERS ('sorbolen', 'tergitols', 'texofors', 'tritons').
See also Cetomacrogol; Lauromacrogol; Polysorbate(s); Ricinomacrogol; Tyloxapol.
Macrogol hexadecyl ether *see* Cetomacrogol.
MACROGOL LAURATE 600* (polyethylene glycol 600 monolaurate).
Macrogol lauryl ether *see* Lauromacrogol.
MACROGOL OLEATE 600* (polyethylene glycol 600 monooleate).
MACROGOL STEARATE(S) ('cithrol', 'myrj', 'polymal').
MACROGOL STEARATE 8 (polyoxyethylene 8 stearate; polyoxyl 8 stearate; 'myrj 45').
MACROGOL STEARATE 40 (polyethylene glycol 40 monostearate; polyoxyethylene 40 stearate; polyoxyl 40 stearate; 'myrj 52').
MACROGOL STEARATE 600* (polyethylene glycol 600 monostearate).
MACROGOL STEARATE 1000* (polyethylene gycol 1000 monostearate).
Macrogol (tetramethylbutyl)phenyl ether *see* Octylphenoxy polyethoxyethanol.
MACROSALB (^{131}I)** (macroaggregated

iodinated (^{131}I) human albumin; (*formerly named*) macrisalb (^{131}I)).
MACROSALB (^{99m}**Tc**)*** (technetium (^{99m}Tc) labeled macroaggregated human serum albumin).
'Macrose' *see* Dextran.
MACROZAMIN (methylazoxymethanol primeveroside).
'Madar' *see* Demethyldiazepam.
'Madecassol' *see* Asiaticoside.
'Madomicetina' *see* Chloramphenicol.
'Madopar' *see* Levodopa with benserazide.
'Madribon' *see* Sulfadimethoxine.
'Madroxin' *see* Sulfadimethoxine.
MAFENIDE** (*p*-aminomethylbenzene-sulfonamide; α-amino-*p*-toluenesulfonamide; bensulfamide; 4-homosulfanilamide; *p*-sulfamoylbenzylamine; homosulfamide; homosulfamine; maphenide; sulfabenz-amine; mafenide hydrochloride).
MAFENIDE ACETATE ('napaltan').
Mafenide sulfathiourea salt *see* Sulfatol-amide.
MAGALDRATE (tetrakis(hydroxymagne-sium) decahydroxydialuminate dihydrate; AY-5710; 'monalium hydrate', 'riopan').
'Magaspirin' *see* Magnesium acetylsali-cylate.
'Magcyl' *see* Poloxalkol.
Magenta *see* Fuchsine.
'Magisal' *see* Magnesium acetylsalicylate.
'Maglactis' *see* Magnesium hydroxide.
'Magmasil' *see* Magnesium trisilicate.
'Magmilor' *see* Nifuratel.
'Magna-cort' *see* Hydrocortamate.
'Magnamycin' *see* Carbomycin.
'Magnapen' *see* Ampicillin with flucloxa-cillin.
'Magnepurin' *see* Magnesium mandelate.
Magnesia *see* Magnesium carbonate.
MAGNESIUM ACETYLSALICYLATE ('apyron', 'canocyl', 'fyracyl', 'magaspirin', 'magisal', 'magnespirin', 'magsyn', 'noca-vetyl', 'novacyl').
Magnesium aluminium glycinate *see* Aluminium magnesium glycinate.
Magnesium aluminosilicate *see* Simal-drate.
MAGNESIUM ASPARTATE (Wy-2838).
MAGNESIUM ASPARTATE WITH POTASSIUM ASPARTATE ('cardilan', 'tromcardin').
See also Potassium magnesium aspartate.
MAGNESIUM CARBONATE (Mg sub-carbonate; magnesia; light Mg carbonate).
MAGNESIUM CLOFIBRATE (bis[2-(*p*-chlorophenoxy)-2-methylpropionato]-magnesium; UR-112; 'clomag').
See also Clofibric acid.
Magnesium dioxide *see* Magnesium peroxide.
MAGNESIUM GLUCONATE ('almora', 'gyn', 'menesia', 'relaxin').
MAGNESIUM GLUTAMATE HYDRO-BROMIDE ('psicosoma', 'psychoverlan').
MAGNESIUM HEPARINATE ('cuthe-parin').

MAGNESIUM HYDROXIDE ('alkavit', 'gastrovit', 'maglactis', 'polysan').
See also Aluminium histidinate with magnesium hydroxide.
MAGNESIUM MANDELATE ('magne-purin').
Magnesium mesosilicate *see* Magnesium trisilicate.
Magnesium 3-(4-methoxy-1-naphthoyl)-propionate *see* Menbutone magnesium.
MAGNESIUM METHYNOTRITHIO-GLYCOLATE ('eparsulfo').
MAGNESIUM OROTATE ('hippocras').
See also Kavain plus magnesium orotate.
Magnesium pemoline *see* Pemoline with magnesium hydroxide.
'Magnesium perhydrol' *see* Magnesium peroxide.
MAGNESIUM PEROXIDE (magnesium dioxide; 'eraxan', 'magnesium perhydrol', 'magnesium superoxol', 'sanoma').
MAGNESIUM SALICYLATE WITH SODIUM SALICYLATE ('magsalyl', 'salimagol').
Magnesium sodium chlorophyllin *see* Sodium magnesium chlorophyllin.
Magnesium subcarbonate *see* Magnesium carbonate.
MAGNESIUM SULFATE (Epsom salts; sel anglais; sel de Seidlitz).
Magnesium sulfate choline salicylate compound *see* Salcolex.
'Magnesium superoxol' *see* Magnesium peroxide.
MAGNESIUM TRISILICATE (Mg meso-silicate; 'adsorbon', 'florisil', 'gastomag', 'magmasil', 'magsorbent', 'novabsorb', 'salisil', 'trinesium', 'trisillac', 'trisomin').
'Magnespirin' *see* Magnesium acetylsali-cylate.
'Magnipen' *see* Metampicillin.
'Magsalyl' *see* Magnesium salicylate with sodium salicylate.
'Magsyn' *see* Magnesium acetylsalicylate.
MAHP *see* Methioprim.
'Maidex' *see* Dexamethasone.
'Majeptil' *see* Thioproperazine mesilate.
MALACHITE GREEN (acid oxalate, chloride or sulfate of anhydrobis(2-di-methylaminophenyl)phenylmethanol; benzyl green; fast green; China green; Victoria green; green of bitter almonds).
Malachite green G *see* Brilliant green.
'Maladone' *see* Allomethadione.
'Malafos' *see* Malathion.
'Malakin' *see* Salicylidene-*p*-phenetidine.
MALAOXON (*S*-(1,2-dicarbethoxyethyl *O,O*-dimethyl) phosphorothioate).
'Malaston' *see* Malathion.
MALATHION* (*S*-(1,2-dicarbethoxyethyl) *O,O*-dimethyl phosphorodithioate; diethyl [(dimethoxyphosphinothioyl)thio]-butanedioate; diethyl [(dimethoxyphosph-inothioyl)thio]succinate; carbophos; maldison; HC-8063; OMS-1; TM-4049; 'etiol', 'fosfothion', 'karbofos', 'malafos', 'malaston', 'malathon', 'mercaptothion',

278

'prioderm', 'sadofos', 'sumitox').
MALATHION PLUS PARATHION
('malatox').
'Malathon' *see* Malathion.
'Malatox' *see* Malathion plus parathion.
'Malazol' *see* Allomethadione.
'Malcotran' *see* Homatropine methyl
bromide.
Maldison* *see* Malathion.
MALEAMIC ACID (maleic acid mono-
amide).
MALEANILIC ACID (*N*-phenylmaleamic
acid).
MALE FERN EXTRACTS (aspidinolfilicin;
filicin; 'filmaron').
See also Filixic acid.
MALEIC ACID (*cis*-butenedioic acid; toxilic
acid).
**Maleic acid polymer with methylvinyl
ether, iron salt** *see* Ferropolimaler.
Maleic anhydride ethylene polymer *see*
Maletamer.
MALETAMER** (maleic anhydride
ethylene polymer; malethamer; L-21679-
CH).
Malethamer* *see* Maletamer.
MALEURIC ACID (*N*-carbamoylmaleamic
acid; *N*-carbamoyl monoamide of maleic
acid; maleylurea).
MALEYLSULFATHIAZOLE** (*p*-(2-thia-
zolylsulfamyl)maleanilic acid; 'carbothia-
zole').
Maleylurea *see* Maleuric acid.
'Maliasin' *see* Barbexaclone.
MALIC ACID (hydroxybutanedioic acid;
hydroxysuccinic acid).
See also Arginine malate.
'Malidone' *see* Allomethadione.
'Malix' *see* Endosulfan.
'Mallophene' *see* Phenazopyridine.
'Mallorol' *see* Thioridazine.
'Malloryl' *see* Thioridazine.
'Malocide' *see* Pyrimethamine.
MALONAMIC ACID (malonic acid mono-
amide).
MALONAMIDE (malonic acid diamide;
malondiamide).
Malondiamide *see* Malonamide.
MALONIC ACID (propanedioic acid;
methanedicarboxylic acid).
Malonic acid diamide *see* Malonamide.
Malonic acid monoamide *see* Malonamic
acid.
Malonic acid mononitrile *see* Cyanato-
acetic acid.
Malononitrile *see* Cyanatoacetic acid.
MALONURIC ACID (*N*-carbamoylmalon-
amic acid).
N,*N*'-**MALONYLBIS(PROCAINAMIDE)**
('nobamide').
N,*N*'-**MALONYLBIS(PROCAINE)**
('novdimal').
Malonylurea *see* Barbituric acid.
'Maloran' *see* Chlorbromuron.
Maltonic acid *see* Gluconic acid.
'Maltrate' *see* Mannityl hexanitrate.
'Malysol' *see* Bemegride.

MAM *see* Cycasin.
'Manalox AG' *see* Glucalox.
'Manalox AS' *see* Sucralox.
MANCOZEB* (mixture of maneb and zineb;
'dithane-ultra', 'manzate 200').
'Mandamine' *see* Methenamine mandelate.
'Mandecal' *see* Calcium mandelate.
**7-D-Mandelamido-3-[[(1-methyl-1H-
tetrazol-5-yl)thio]methyl]-2-cephem-
2-carboxylic acid** *see* Cefamandole.
'Mandelamine' *see* Methenamine mandelate.
MANDELIC ACID (2-phenylglycolic acid;
α-hydroxyphenylacetic acid; α-hydroxy-
α-toluic acid; amygdalic acid; paraman-
delic acid; racemic acid).
See also Ammonium mandelate; Calcium
mandelate; Isoamyl mandelate; Magnesium
mandelate; Sodium mandelate.
'Mandelix' *see* Sodium mandelate.
Mandelonitrile gentiobioside *see* Amygdalin.
Mandelyl tropeine *see* Homatropine.
'Mandicid' *see* Ammonium mandelate.
'Mandrax' *see* Methaqualone with diphen-
hydramine.
'Manduryl' *see* Ammonium mandelate.
MANEB* ([[1,2-ethanediylbis(carbamo-
dithioato)](2)]manganese; manganous
N,*N*'-ethylenebis(dithiocarbamate);
manganous *N*,*N*'-ethylenebis(carbamodi-
thioate); MEB; MnEDB; 'dithane
manganese', 'dithane M22', 'manzate').
MANEB PLUS NICKEL(II) SULFATE
('dithane S31').
Maneb with zineb *see* Mancozeb.
'Manexin' *see* Mannityl hexanitrate.
**Manganous ethylenebis(carbamodithio-
ate)** *see* Maneb.
Manganous ethylenebis(dithiocarbamate)
see Maneb.
'Manicole' *see* Mannityl hexanitrate.
'Maninil' *see* Glibenclamide.
'Manipal' *see* Dihydrotachysterol.
'Manite' *see* Mannityl hexanitrate.
'Mannex' *see* Mannityl hexanitrate.
Mannite *see* Mannitol.
MANNITOL (mannite; 'ionosteril', 'osmitrol',
'osmofundin').
D-Mannitol 1,6-di(methanesulfonate) *see*
Mannityl dimesilate.
Mannitol hexanitrate** *see* Mannityl
hexanitrate.
'Mannitol myleran' *see* Mannityl dimesilate.
Mannitol nitrogen mustard *see* Manno-
mustine.
D-Mannitol 1,2,5,6-tetramethanesulfonate
see Mannosulfan.
'Mannitrate' *see* Mannityl hexanitrate.
MANNITYL DIMESILATE (D-mannitol
1,6-di(methanesulfonate); 1,6-bis(methylsulfonyl)mannitol; dimethanesulfonylmannitol; mannityl dimesylate; DSM; CB-
2511; NSC-37538; 'mannitol myleran').
MANNITYL HEXANITRATE* (mannitol
hexanitrate; hexanitromannitol; nitromannite; nitromannitol; 'dilangil', 'hexanitrin', 'hexanitrol', 'maltrate', 'manexin',

'manicole', 'manite', 'manitrin', 'mannex', 'mannitrate', 'maxitate', 'medemanol', 'nitrangin', 'nitranitol', 'nitroman').

Mannityl tetramesilate *see* Mannosulfan.

MANNOMUSTINE*** (1,6-bis(2-chloroethylamino)-1,6-dideoxy-D-mannitol; mannitol nitrogen mustard; mannomustine dihydrochloride; BCM; NSC-9698; 'degranol').

MANNOMUSTINE HEPARINATE ('heparin-degranol', 'zitofenton').

MANNOSULFAN*** (D-mannitol 1,2,5,6-tetramethanesulfonate; tetrakis(methylsulfonyl)mannitol; tetramesylmannitol; mannityl tetramesilate; R-52; 'zitostop', 'zytostop').

Mannuronic acid polymers *see* Alginic acid; Sodium polyanhydromannuronic acid sulfate.

'Manoxol' *see* Sodium dioctyl sulfosuccinate.

'Mansonil' *see* Niclosamide piperazine salt.

'Mantadan' *see* Amantadine.

'Mantadix' *see* Amantadine.

Mantheline *see* Methantheline.

'Mantomide' *see* Chlorbetamide.

'Mantropina' *see* Methenamine mandelate.

'Manucol' *see* Sodium alginate.

'Manuronate' *see* Sodium polyanhydromannuronic acid sulfate.

'Manvene' *see* Mytatrienediol.

'Manzate' *see* Maneb.

'Manzate 200' *see* Mancozeb.

MAO *see* Monoamine oxidase.

'Maolate' *see* Chlorphenesin carbamate.

'MAO-rem' *see* Phenelzine.

MAP *see* Medroxyprogesterone acetate.

MAP (tr) *see* Adenosine phosphate.

Maphenide* *see* Mafenide.

'Mapiprin' *see* Piperazine adipate.

MAPO *see* Metepa.

Mappine *see* Bufotenine.

MAPROTILINE*** (N-methyl-9,10-ethanoanthracene-9(10H)-propylamine; 1-(3-methylaminopropyl)dibenzo(b,e)bicyclo-(2.2.2)octadiene; benzylamine; Ba-34276; C-34276-Ba; 'ludiomil').

'Maratan' *see* Bisoxatin diacetate.

'Marbadal' *see* Sulfatolamide.

'Marbagelan' *see* Gelatin sponge.

'Marboran' *see* Metisazone.

'Marcain' *see* Bupivacaine.

'Marcoumar' *see* Phenprocoumon.

'Marcumar' *see* Phenprocoumon.

Maretin' *see* Naftalofos.

'Marevan' *see* Warfarin.

'Margeryl' *see* Tenylidone.

MARIDOMYCIN*** (10-(formylmethyl)-7,13-dihydroxy-8-methoxy-3,12-dimethyl-5-oxo-4,17-dioxabicyclo(14.1.0)heptadec-14-en-9-yl 3,6-dideoxy-4-O-(2,6-dideoxy-C-methyl-α-L-*ribo*-hexopyranosyl)-3-dimethylamino-β-D-glucopyranoside 4'',7'-dipropionate (ester)).

Marihuana *see* Cannabis.

'Marlate' *see* Methoxychlor.

'Marplan' *see* Isocarboxazid.

'Marplan bromide' *see* Clidinium bromide.

'Marplon' *see* Isocarboxazid.

'Marsalid' *see* Iproniazid.

'Marsin' *see* Phenmetrazine.

'Marvosan' *see* Paraformaldehyde.

'Maryosan' *see* Paraformaldehyde.

'Masmoran' *see* Hydrozyzine embonate.

'Masterid' *see* Drostanolone propionate.

'Masteril' *see* Drostanolone propionate.

'Masteron' *see* Drostanolone.

'Matacil' *see* Aminocarb.

'Matadan' *see* Amantadine.

Matecite *see* Pinitol.

Matezite *see* Pinitol.

'Matromycin' *see* Oleandomycin.

'Matulane' *see* Procarbazine.

'Maxibolin' *see* Ethylestrenol.

'Maxicaine' *see* Parethoxycaine.

'Maxifen' *see* Pivampicillin.

'Maxilase' *see* α-Amylase.

'Maxipen' *see* Pheneticillin.

'Maxisporin' *see* Cefradine.

'Maxitate' *see* Mannityl hexanitrate.

'Maxolon' *see* Metoclopramide.

'Maycor' *see* Isosorbide dinitrate.

'Mayeptil' *see* Thioproperazine mesilate.

MAZATICOL*** (6,6,9-trimethyl-9-azabicyclo(3.3.1)non-3β-yl dithien-2-ylglycolate; 6,6,9-trimethylgranatoline dithienylglycolate; mazaticol hydrochloride; PG-501).

MAZIDOX* (azidophosphonic bisdimethylamide; tetramethylphosphorodiamidic azide).

MAZINDOL*** (5-(p-chlorophenyl)-2,5-dihydro-3H-imidazo(2,1-a)isoindol-5-ol; AN-448; SAH-42-548; 'sanorex', 'teronac').

MAZIPREDONE*** (11β,17-dihydroxy-21-(4-methylpiperazin-1-yl)pregna-1,4-diene-3,20-dione; 21-deoxy-21-(4-methylpiperazin-1-yl)prednisolone; 21-(4-methylpiperazin-1-yl)deprodone; mazipredone hydrochloride; dp; 'depersolone').

MBA *see* Chlormethine.

MBAO *see* Chlormethine N-oxide.

M &B-125 *see* Benzylsulfamide.

M &B-693 *see* Sulfapyridine.

M &B-744 *see* Stilbamidine isetionate.

M &B-760 *see* Sulfathiazole.

M &B-782 *see* Propamidine isetionate.

M &B-800 *see* Pentamidine isetionate.

M &B-1948-A *see* Amphotalide.

M &B-2050-A *see* Pentolonium tartrate.

M &B-2207 *see* Suxamethonium.

M &B-2210 *see* Suxethonium.

M &B-4180A *see* Isometamidium chloride.

M &B-4486 *see* Pempidine.

M &B-8430 *see* Clorexolone.

M &B-9302 *see* Clorgiline.

M &B-15497 *see* Decoquinate.

M &B-17803A *see* Acebutolol.

MBBA *see* Bromebric acid.

MBLA *see* Melinamide.

MBR-4164-8 *see* Diflumidone.

MBR-4223 *see* Triflumidate.

2-M-4-C *see* 4-Chloro-2-methylphenoxyacetic acid.

MC-4703 *see* Triflupromazine.

4-(MCB) *see* 4-(4-Chloro-2-methylphenoxy)-butyric acid.
MCE *see* Metergoline.
McN-485 *see* Zoxazolamine.
McN-742 *see* Aminorex.
McN-1025 *see* Norbormide.
McN-1075 *see* Fenmetramide.
McN-1107 *see* Clominorex.
McN-1231 *see* Fluminorex.
McN-1564 *see* Flumetramide.
McN-1589 *see* Mixidine.
McN-A-343 *see* [4-(*m*-Chlorophenylcarbamoyloxy)-2-butynyl]trimethylammonium chloride.
McN-JR-1625 *see* Haloperidol.
McN-JR-2498 *see* Trifluperidol.
McN-JR-4263-49 *see* Fentanyl citrate.
McN-JR-4584 *see* Benperidol.
McN-JR-4749 *see* Droperidol.
McN-JR-4929 *see* Benzetimide.
McN-JR-7242-11 *see* Difluanazine.
McN-JR-7904 *see* Lidoflazine.
McN-JR-8299 *see* Tetramisole.
McN-JR-13558-11 *see* Fetoxilate.
McN-R-73-Z *see* Rotoxamine.
McN-R-1162-22 *see* Potassium glucaldrate.
McN-X-94 *see* Capuride.
McN-X-181 *see* Valnoctamide.
MCP *see* (4-Chloro-2-methylphenoxy)acetic acid.
MCPA *see* 2-(4-Chloro-2-methylphenoxy)-acetic acid.
MCPB* *see* 4-(4-Chloro-2-methylphenoxy)-butyric acid.
2,4-MCPB *see* 4-(4-Chloro-2-methylphenoxy)-butyric acid.
4-(MCPB) *see* 4-(4-Chloro-2-methylphenoxy)-butyric acid.
MCPP *see* Mecoprop.
2-MCPP *see* Mecoprop.
MD-2 *see* Hisphen.
MD-154 *see* Etamsylate.
MD-205 *see* Calcium dobesilate.
MD-516 *see* Cinnarizine.
MD-1035 *see* Cinnarizine with heptaminol theophyllineacetate.
MD-2028 *see* Fluanisone.
MD-6134 *see* Warfarin-deanol.
MD-6260 *see* Heptaminol theophyllineacetate.
MD-6753 *see* Cinepazet.
MD-67350 *see* Cinepazide maleate.
MDA *see* 3,4-Methylenedioxyamphetamine.
MDi-193 *see* Cyclothiazide.
Me-3625 *see* Niclofolan.
MEA *see* Mercaptamine.
Meat sugar *see* Inositol.
MEB *see* Maneb.
'Mebacid' *see* Sulfamerazine.
'Mebadin' *see* Dehydroemetine.
Meballymal* *see* Secobarbital.
MEBANAZINE*** (1-(α-methylbenzyl)-hydrazine; 1-(1-phenylethyl)hydrazine; 'actamol', 'actomol', 'astomol').
'Mebaral' *see* Methylphenobarbital.
MEBENDAZOLE*** (methyl 5-benzoyl-2-benzimidazolecarbamate; R-17635; 'vermox').

MEBENOSIDE*** (methyl 3,5,6-tri-*O*-benzyl-D-glucofuranoside).
MEBEVERINE** (7-(3,4-dimethoxybenzoyloxy)-3-ethyl-1-(*p*-methoxyphenyl)-2-methyl-3-azaheptane; 4-[ethyl-(*p*-methoxy-α-methylphenethyl)amino]butyl 3,4-dimethoxybenzoate; 4-[ethyl-(*p*-methoxy-α-methylphenethyl)amino]butyl veratrate; mebeverine hydrochloride; CSAG-144; 'colofac', 'duphaspasmin', 'duspatal', 'duspatalin').
MEBEZONIUM IODIDE*** (4,4'-methylenebis(cyclohexyltrimethylammonium iodide); (methylenedi-1,4-cyclohexylene)-bis(trimethylammonium iodide)).
MEBHYDROLIN*** (5-benzyl-1,2,3,4-tetrahydro-2-methyl-2H-pyrid(4,3-b)indole; 9-benzyl-3-methyl-γ-carboline; diazoline).
MEBHYDROLIN NAPADISILATE (mebhydrolin 1,5-naphthalenedisulfonate; mebhydrolin napadisylate; 'fabahistin', 'incidal', 'omeril').
Mebhydrolin napadisylate* *see* Mebhydrolin napadisilate.
'Mebichloramine' *see* Chlormethine.
'Mebinol' *see* Clefamide.
MEBIQUINE** (dihydroxy(6-methyl-8-quinolinolato)bismuth; 6-methyl-8-quinolinol compound with bismuth hydroxide).
MEBOLAZINE*** (17β-hydroxy-2α,17-dimethyl-5α-androstan-3-one azine; dimetazine; 'roxilon').
Mebromphenhydramine *see* Embramine.
'Mebron' *see* Epirizole.
'Mebryl' *see* Embramine.
Mebubarbital *see* Pentobarbital.
Mebumal* *see* Pentobarbital.
MEBUTAMATE*** (2-*sec*-butyl-2-methyl-1,3-propanediol dicarbamate; 2,2-di(carbamoyloxymethyl)-3-methylpentane; W-583; 'capla', 'preminex').
MEBUTIZIDE*** (6-chloro-3-(1,2-dimethylbutyl)-3,4-dihydro-2H-1,2,4-benzothiadiazine-7-sulfonamide-1,1-dioxide; 'neoniagar').
'Mecadox' *see* Carbadox.
Mecamine (tr) *see* Mecamylamine.
MECAMYLAMINE*** (*N*,2,3,3-tetramethylnorbornamine; 3-methylaminoisobornane; 2,2,3-trimethyl-3-(methylamino)-norbornane; 3-methylaminoisocamphane; camphanamine; mecamine; mecamylamine hydrochloride; 'inversine', 'mekamine', 'mevasine', 'revertina', 'revertine', 'suversin', 'versamine').
MECARBAM* (ethyl [[[(diethoxyphosphinothioyl)thio]acetyl]methyl]carbamate; *S*-[[[(ethoxycarbonyl)amino]methylcarbonyl]methyl] *O*,*O*-diethyl phosphorodithioate; 'afos', 'murfotox', 'murtox', 'pestan').
MECARBINATE*** (ethyl 5-hydroxy-1,2-dimethylindole-3-carboxylate).
MeCCNU *see* Semustine.
'Mechloral' *see* Chloralodol.
Mechlorethamine *see* Chlormethine.
'Mechothane' *see* Bethanechol.

281

MECILLINAM*** ((2S,5R,6R)-6-[[(hexa-hydro-1H-azepin-1-yl)methylene]amino]-penicillanic acid; 6-[N,N-(1,6-hexamethyl-ene)formamidino]penicillanic acid; (2S,5R,6R)-6-(perhydroazepin-1-ylmethyl-eneamino)penicillanic acid; amidino-penicillin HX; F1-1060).

Mecillinam hydroxymethyl ester pivalate see Pivmecillinam.

MECINARONE** (1-[6-(2-dimethylamino-ethoxy)-4,7-dimethoxybenzofuran-5-yl]-3-(p-methoxyphenyl)-2-propen-1-one; 6-(2-dimethylaminoethoxy)-4,7-dimethoxy-5-[3-(p-methoxyphenyl)-1-oxoprop-2-enyl]-benzofuran).

Meclastine see Clemastine.

Meclizine* see Meclozine.

MECLOCYCLINE*** (7-chloro-4-(dimethyl-amino)-1,4,4a,5,5a,6,11,12a-octahydro-3,5,10,12,17-pentahydroxy-6-methylene-1,11-dioxonaphthacene-2-carboxamide; 7-chloro-6-demethyl-6-methylenetetra-cycline; GS-2989; chlormethylenecycline; 'meclosorb').

MECLOFENAMIC ACID*** (N-(2,6-di-chloro-m-tolyl)anthranilic acid; 2-carboxy-2',6'-dichloro-3'-methyldiphenylamine; N-(2-carboxyphenyl)-2,6-dichloro-m-toluidine; Cl.-583).

Meclofenamic acid ethoxymethyl ester see Terofenamate.

MECLOFENOXATE*** (2-dimethylamino-ethyl p-chlorophenoxyacetate; deanol p-chlorophenoxyacetate; centrophenoxine; clofenoxine; ANP-235; 'cerutil', 'helfergin', 'lucidril', 'lucidryl', 'ludicril').

MECLOFENOXATE METHIODIDE (dimethylaminoethyl p-chlorophenoxy-acetate methiodide; p-chlorophenoxyacetyl-choline iodide).

Mecloprodine see Clemastine.

MECLOQUALONE*** (3-(o-chlorophenyl)-2-methyl-4(3H)-quinazolinone; W-4744).

MECLORALUREA** (1-methyl-3-(2,2,2-trichloro-1-hydroxyethyl)urea; G-7225; 'heraldium').

'Meclosorb' see Meclocycline.

MECLOXAMINE*** (2-[α(p-chlorophenyl)-α-methyl-α-phenylmethoxy]propyldimethyl-amine; 2-(p-chloro-α-methylbenzhydryl-oxy)-N,N-dimethylpropylamine; 2-(p-chloro-α-methyl-α-phenylbenzyloxy)-N,N-dimethylpropylamine; methylchlorphenox-amine; 'isopropyl-systral').

MECLOZINE** (1-(p-chloro-α-phenyl-benzyl)-4-(m-methylbenzyl)piperazine; 1-(p-chlorobenzhydryl)-4-(m-methyl-benzyl)piperazine; meclizine; parachlor-amine; meclozine dihydrochloride; 1-[α-(p-chlorophenyl)benzyl]-4-(3-methyl-benzyl)piperazine; 1-[(4-chlorophenyl)-phenylmethyl]-4-(3-methylphenyl)-piperazine; histametizine; UCB-5062; 'ancolan', 'bonamine', 'bonine', 'calmonal', 'histamethine', 'itinerol', 'navicalm', 'neoistafene', 'postafene', 'sea-legs', 'supri-mal').

MECOBALAMIN** (α-(5,6-dimethylbenz-imidazol-2-yl)cobamide methyl; cobin-amide Co-methyl derivative hydroxide, di-hydrogen phosphate (ester), inner salt, 3'-ester with 5,6-dimethyl-1-α-D-ribo-furanosyl benzimidazole).

MECONIC ACID (3-hydroxy-4-oxo-1(4H)-pyran-2,6-dicarboxylic acid).
See also Morphine noscapine meconate.

MECONIN (6,7-dimethoxyphthalide).

m-MECONIN (5,6-dimethoxyphthalide; meconic acid lactone; opianyl).

Meconium see Opium.

'Mecopar' see Mecoprop.

'Mecopex' see Mecoprop.

MECOPROP* ((±)-2-(4-chloro-2-methyl-phenoxy)propionic acid; CMPP; MCPP; 2-MCPP; 'iso-cornox', 'mecopar', 'mecopex').

'Mecoral' see Chloralodol.

'Mecortolone' see Prednisolone trimethyl-octanoate.

'Mecostrin' see Dimethyltubocurarine.

'Mecothane' see Bethanechol.

MECRILATE*** (methyl 2-cyanoacrylate).

MECYSTEINE*** (methyl 2-amino-3-mer-captopropionate; cysteine methyl ester; methylcysteine; mecysteine hydrochloride; 'acdrile').

3'-MeDAB see 4-Dimethylamino-3'-methyl-azobenzene.

'Medapan' see Heptabarb.

MEDAZEPAM*** (7-chloro-2,3-dihydro-1-methyl-5-phenyl-1H-1,4-benzodiazepine; medazepam hydrochloride; Ro-5-4556; 'anxitol', 'nobrium', 'rudotel').
See also Metoclopramide with medazepam.

MEDAZOMIDE*** (1,4,5,6-tetrahydro-1-methylpyridazin-6-one-3-carboxamide; 1,4,5,6-tetrahydro-1-methyl-6-oxo-3-pyrid-azinecarboxamide; medazonamide).

Medazonamide* see Medazomide.

'Medemanol' see Mannityl hexanitrate.

'Medemycin' see Midecamycin.

'Mederel' see Amoproxan.

Medfalan see Medphalan.

MEDIBAZINE** (1-benzhydryl-4-piperonyl-piperazine; 1-(diphenylmethyl)-4-(3,4-methylenedioxyphenyl)piperazine; S-4105; 'valibran').

'Mediben' see Dicamba.

MEDIFOXAMINE*** (dimethylaminoacet-aldehyde diphenyl acetal; N,N-dimethyl-2,2-diphenoxyethylamine; 'gerdaxyl').

MEDIGOXIN** (3β-[O-(2,6-dideoxy-4-O-methyl-D-ribo-hexopyranosyl)-(1→4)-O-(2,6-dideoxy-D-ribo-hexopyranosyl)-(1→4)-(2,6-dideoxy-D-ribo-hexopyranosyl)oxy]-12β,14-dihydroxy-5β,14β-card-20(22)-enolide; 3β,12β,14β-trihydroxy-5β-card-20(22)-enolide 3-(4'''-O-methyl)tridigitoxo-side; 4'''-O-methyldigoxin; β-methyl-digoxin; 'lanitop').

'Medinal' see Barbital.

'Medipectol' see Bibenzonium bromide.

Meditrene see Chiniofon.

MEDMAIN (5-(dimethyl-amino)-(3-ethyl-2-

methyl-indole; methylethyldimethylamino-indole).

'Medobis' see Bismuth 2-allyl-4-pentenoate.

'Medopaque' see Sodium iodohippurate.

MEDPHALAN (D-p-[bis(2-chloroethyl)-amino]phenylalanine; D-phenylalanine mustard; D-sarcolysin; medfalan; CB-3206; NSC-35051).
See also Melphalan; Sarcolysin.

'Medrifar' see Medrysone.

'Medrin' see Embramine teoclate.

'Medrocort' see Medrysone.

MEDROGESTONE*** (6,17-dimethyl-pregna-4,6-diene-3,20-dione; metrogestone; AY-62022; 'colprone', 'prothil').

'Medrol' see Methylprednisolone.

'Medrone' see Methylprednisolone.

MEDROXYPROGESTERONE*** (17α-hydroxy-6α-methylpregn-4-ene-3,20-dione; 6α-methylpregn-4-en-17α-ol-3,20-dione; 17α-hydroxy-6α-methylprogesterone; methylpregnone).

MEDROXYPROGESTERONE ACETATE* (17α-acetoxy-6α-methylprogesterone; 17α-hydroxy-6α-methylpregn-4-ene-3,20-dione acetate; depoprogesterone; MAP; NSC-26386; 'clinovir', 'depo-clinovir', 'depo-prodasone', 'depo-provera', 'farlutal', 'gestaputan', 'oragest', 'perlutex', 'provera').

MEDROXYPROGESTERONE ACETATE WITH ETHINYLESTRADIOL ('intex', 'nogest', 'provest', 'verafen').

MEDRYLAMINE*** (2-(p-methoxy-α-phenylbenzyloxy)-N,N-dimethylethylamine; 2-(p-methoxybenzhydryloxy)-N,N-dimethyl-ethylamine; p-methoxydiphenhydramine; 2-dimethylaminoethyl p-methoxybenz-hydryl ether; BS-556).

MEDRYSONE** (11β-hydroxy-6α-methyl-pregn-4-ene-3,20-dione; 11β-hydroxy-6α-methylprogesterone; 6α-methylpregn-4-en-11β-ol-3,20-dione; HMS; U-8471; 'medrifar', 'medrocort').

MEFECLORAZINE*** (1-(o-chlorophenyl)-4-(3,4-dimethoxyphenethyl)piperazine; mephechlorazine; DCF).

MEFENAMIC ACID** (N-(2,3-xylyl)-anthranilic acid; N-(2,3-dimethylphenyl)-anthranilic acid; CL-473; INF-3355; 'parkemed', 'ponstan', 'ponstel', 'ponstyl', 'pontal').

MEFENOREX** (N-(3-chloropropyl)-amphetamine; N-(3-chloropropyl)-α-methylphenethylamine; mefenorex hydro-chloride; Ro-4-5282; 'anexate', 'pondinil', 'rondimen').

MEFESERPINE*** (p-methoxyphenoxy-acetic acid ester of methyl reserpate; methoxyphenoserpine).

'Mefexadyne' see Mefexamide.

MEFEXAMIDE*** (N-(2-diethylamino-ethyl)-2-(p-methoxyphenoxy)acetamide; ANP-297; NP-297; 'mefexadyne', 'per-neuron', 'timodyne').

MEFLOQUINE*** (DL-erythro-α-piperid-2-yl-2,8-bis(trifluoromethyl)-4-quinoline-methanol).

MEFRUSIDE*** (4-chloro-N1-methyl-N1-(tetrahydro-2-methylfuryl)-m-benzenedi-sulfonamide; 2-[[N-(4-chloro-3-sulfamoyl-benzenesulfonyl)-N-methylamino]-methyl]-2-methyltetrahydrofuran; B-1500; FBA-1500; 'baycaron').
See also Methyldopa with mefruside.

'Megace' see Megestrol acetate.

'Megachlor' see Clomocycline.

'Megacillin' see Clemizole penicillin.

MEGALLATE(S)** (3,4,5-trimethoxy-benzoate(s)).

'Megatox' see Fluoroacetic acid.

Megestranol (tr) see Megestrol acetate with mestranol.

MEGESTROL** (6-methylpregna-4,6-diene-17α-ol-3,20-dione; 17α-hydroxy-6-methylpregna-4,6-diene-3,20-dione).

MEGESTROL ACETATE* (BDH-1296; SC-10363; 'megace', 'niagestin').

MEGESTROL ACETATE WITH ETHINYLESTRADIOL ('novoquens', 'oraconal', 'planovin', 'serial', 'tri-ervo-num', 'volidan', 'volplan').

MEGESTROL ACETATE WITH MESTRANOL (megestranol; 'delpreg-nen').

'Megimide' see Bemegride.

MEGLITINIDE** (p-[2-(5-chloro-o-anis-amido)ethyl]benzoic acid; p-[2-(5-chloro-2-methylbenzamido)ethyl]benzoic acid; N-(p-carboxyphenethyl)-5-chloro-2-methylbenzamide).

MEGLUCYCLINE*** (2-deoxy-2-(tetra-cyclinylmethylamino)-β-D-glucopyranose; 2-deoxy-2-methylaminoglucose compound with tetracycline).

MEGLUMINE*** (N-methylglucamine; 1-deoxy-1-methylamino-D-glucitol).
See also below and Adipiodone meglumine; Flunixin meglumine; Nitroxinil meglu-mine; Papaveroline meglumine; Theo-phylline meglumine.

MEGLUMINE ACETRIZOATE (acetrizoic acid methylglucamine salt; 'angiombrine', 'fortoshade M', 'fortombrine M', 'jodozoat R', 'plexombrine', 'vasurix').

Meglumine amidotrizoate see Meglumine diatrizoate.

MEGLUMINE ANTIMONATE (N-methyl-glucamine antimonate; RP-2168; 'glu-cantime', 'protostib').

MEGLUMINE DIATRIZOATE (diatrizoic acid methylglucamine salt; meglumine amidotrizoate; SH-20932; 'angiografin', 'cardiografin', 'gastrografin', 'hypaque 60', 'reno 60', 'renografin', 'urografin', 'uro-vist').

MEGLUMINE DIATRIZOATE WITH ADIPIODONE MEGLUMINE ('sino-grafin').

MEGLUMINE DIATRIZOATE WITH SODIUM DIATRIZOATE ('cystografin', 'hypaque 76', 'hypaque 90', 'reno 76', 'renografin', 'renovist', 'urografin 76', 'uropolin', 'urovison', 'verografin', 'viso-trast').

283

MEGLUMINE IOCARMATE (DB-2041; 'dimer X').
See also Iocarmic acid.
MEGLUMINE IODOXAMATE (iodoxamic acid meglumine salt; iodotetroxide; B-10610).
Meglumine ioglycamate *see* Ioglycamide.
MEGLUMINE IOTALAMATE (iotalamic acid methylglucamine salt; meglumine iothalamate; 'conray 30', 'conray 60', 'contrix 28').
MEGLUMINE IOTALAMATE WITH SODIUM IOTALAMATE ('conray 70', 'conray FL', 'vascoray').
MEGLUMINE IOXITALAMATE ('telebrix 300').
Meglumine ioxitalamate with ethanol-amine ioxitalamate *see* Ethanolamine ioxitalamate with meglumine ioxitalamate.
MEGLUMINE IOXITALAMATE WITH SODIUM IOXITALAMATE ('telebrix 38', 'vasobrix 32').
MEGLUMINE METRIZOATE WITH CALCIUM METRIZOATE ('isopaque cerebral', 'ronpacon cerebral').
MEGLUMINE METRIZOATE WITH CALCIUM & SODIUM METRI-ZOATES ('isopaque coronary').
MEGLUMINE METRIZOATE WITH SODIUM, CALCIUM & MAGNESIUM METRIZOATES ('ronpacon').
MEGLUMINE SALICYLATE* (PFA-186).
'Meguan' *see* Metformin.
'Mekamine' *see* Mecamylamine.
'Meladinin' *see* Methoxsalen.
MELADRAZINE*** (2,4-bis(diethylamino)-6-hydrazino-*s*-triazine; hydramitrazine; C-13155).
MELADRAZINE TARTRATE (meladra-zine (+)-tartrate; 'lisdonil').
MELAMINE (2,4,6-triamino-*s*-triazine; azamin; cyanurotriamide).
Melaminsulfone *see* Sulfamidopyrine.
Melampyrin *see* Dulcitol.
Melampyrit *see* Dulcitol.
'Melanex' *see* Metahexamide.
Melanophore-stimulating hormone *see* Intermedin.
Melanotropin(s) *see* Intermedin.
'Melantoin' *see* Methylphenytoin.
Melarsenoxide-BAL *see* Melarsoprol.
MELARSONYL POTASSIUM*** (dipotas-sium salt of 2-[4-(4,6-diamino-*s*-triazin-2-ylamino)phenyl]-1,3,2-dithiaarsolane-4,5-dicarboxylic acid; mel W; 'trimelarsan').
MELARSOPROL*** (2-[*p*-(4,6-diamino-*s*-triazin-2-ylamino)phenyl]-1,3,2-dithiaar-solane-4-methanol; 2-[*p*-(4,6-diamino-*s*-triazin-4-ylamino)phenyl]-4-hydroxymethyl-1,3-dithia-2-arsenolidine; dimercaprol deriv. of *p*-[(4,6-diamino-*s*-triazin-2-yl)-amino]benzenearsonous acid; melarsen-oxide-BAL; mel B; RP-3854; 'arsobal').
MELATONIN (*N*-acetyl-5-methoxytrypt-amine; *N*-acetyl-*O*-methylserotonin; *N*-acetylserotonin methyl ether; *N*-[2-(5-methoxyindol-3-yl)ethyl]acetamide; NSC-

56423).
Mel B *see* Melarsoprol.
'Meldian' *see* Chlorpropamide.
MELENGESTROL*** (6-methyl-16-methyl-enepregna-4,6-diene-17α-ol-3,20-dione; 17-hydroxy-6-methyl-16-methylenepregna-4,6-diene-3,20-dione).
MELENGESTROL ACETATE* (BDH-1921; NSC-70968).
MELETIMIDE*** (DL-2-[1-(*p*-methyl-benzyl)-4-piperidyl]-2-phenylglutarimide; R-5183).
Meletin *see* Quercetin.
Melfalan *see* Melphalan.
MELILOTUS OFFICINALIS EXTRACT ('esberiven', 'venalot').
See also Coumarin.
Melin *see* Rutoside.
MELINAMIDE*** (*N*-(α-methylbenzyl)-linoleamide; MBLA; AC-223).
'Melipan' *see* Lifibrate.
Melipramine *see* Imipramine.
'Meliprimin' *see* Imipramine.
'Melitase' *see* Chlorpropamide.
'Melitoxin' *see* Dicoumarol.
Melittin *see* Bee venom.
MELITRACEN*** (9-(3-dimethylamino-propylidene)-9,10-dihydro-10,10-dimethyl-anthracene; *N,N*,10,10-tetramethyl-Δ$^{9(10H),γ}$ anthracenepropylamine; melitracen hydro-chloride; N-7001; U-24973A; 'dixeran', 'trausabun').
See also Flupentixol with melitracen.
MELIZAME*** (*m*-(1H-tetrazol-5-yloxy)-phenol; 5-(*m*-hydroxyphenoxy)-1H-tetra-zole).
'Mellaril' *see* Thioridazine.
'Mellerette' *see* Thioridazine.
'Melleril' *see* Thioridazine.
Mellictine *see* Methylisaconitine.
'Meloka' *see* Ethenzamide.
'Melonex' *see* Metahexamide.
'Meloxine' *see* Methoxsalen.
MELPERONE** (4'-fluoro-4-(4-methyl-piperid-1-yl)butyrophenone; 1-[3-(*p*-fluorobenzoyl)propyl]-4-methylpiperidine; methylperone; metylperone; FG-6111; 'buronil', 'eunerpan').
MELPHALAN*** (L-[*p*-bis(2-chloroethyl-amino)phenyl]alanine; melfalan; L-phenyl-alanine mustard; PAM; L-sarcolysin; CB-3025; NSC-8806; 'alkeran').
See also Medphalan; Sarcolysin.
'Melprex' *see* Dodine.
'Melsedin' *see* Methaqualone.
'Meltrol' *see* Phenformin.
'Melubrin' *see* Sulfamidopyrine.
'Melufin' *see* Dibupyrone.
Mel W *see* Melarsonyl potassium.
MEMANTINE** (3,5-dimethyl-1-adamantan-amine; dimethylamantadine).
MEMOTINE** (3,4-dihydro-1-(*p*-methoxy-phenoxymethyl)isoquinoline; memotine hydrochloride; UK-2371).
'Menacor' *see* Cloridarol hemisuccinate.
MENADIOL*** (2-methyl-1,4-naphthalene-diol).

Menadiol diacetate see Acetomenaphthone.
Menadiol diphosphate see Menadiol sodium phosphate.
Menadiol disulfate see Menadiol sodium sulfate.
MENADIOL POTASSIUM SULFATE (dipotassium salt of 2-methyl-1,4-naphthalenediol bis(hydrogen sulfate); dipotassium menadiol 1,4-disulfate).
MENADIOL SODIUM PHOSPHATE (tetrasodium salt of 2-methyl-1,4-naphthalenediol bis(hydrogen phosphate); tetrasodium menadiol 1,4-diphosphate; naftidon).
MENADIOL SODIUM SULFATE*** (disodium salt of 2-methyl-1,4-naphthalenediol bis(hydrogen sulfate); disodium menadiol 1,4-disulfate).
Menadiol 3-sulfonic acid sodium salt see Sodium menadiolsulfonate.
MENADIONE*** (2-methyl-1,4-naphthoquinone; menaquinone; menaphthone; vitamin K$_3$).
Menadione carboxymethoxime see Menadoxime.
MENADIONE SODIUM BISULFITE*** (sodium salt of 1,2,3,4-tetrahydro-2-methyl-1,4-dioxo-2-naphthalenesulfonic acid; 2-methyl-1,4-naphthoquinone bisulfite compound; vikasol).
MENADOXIME (menadione 4-oxime carboxymethyl ether NH$_4$ salt; menadione carboxymethoxime ammonium salt).
Menaphthone see Menadione.
Menaquinone see Menadione.
Menaquinone-4 see Farnoquinone.
MENATETRENONE*** (2-methyl-3-(3,7,11,15-tetramethylhexadecatetraenyl)-1,4-naphthoquinone).
MENAZON* (S-(4,6-diamino-s-triazin-2-ylmethyl) O,O-dimethyl phosphorodithioate; 6-[[(dimethoxyphosphinothioyl)thio]-methyl]-1,3,5-triazine-2,4-diamine; 'azidithion', 'saphi-col', 'saphizon', 'sayfos').
MENAZONE (2-furfuryl methyl ketone isonicotinoylhydrazone; isonicotinic acid 1-(2-furfurylethylidene)hydrazide; N'-[1-(2-furfuryl)ethylidene]isoniazid; INF; 'clitizina').
MENBUTONE*** (3-(4-methoxy-1-naphthoyl)propionic acid; SC-1749; 'genabil', 'genabiline', 'genebile', 'icteryl', 'idogenabil').
MENBUTONE MAGNESIUM (magnesium 3-(4-methoxy-1-naphthoyl)propionate; 'agolene').
'Menesia' see Magnesium gluconate.
'Menest' see Conjugated estrogens.
MENGLYTATE*** (p-menth-3-yl ethoxyacetate; menthyl ethylglycolate; 'col-menthol', 'coryfin').
Menichlopholan see Niclofolan.
'Menine' see Methionine.
MENITRAZEPAM*** (5-(1-cyclohexen-1-yl)-1,3-dihydro-1-methyl-7-nitro-2H-1,4-benzodiazepin-2-one).
'Menocil' see Aminorex fumarate.

MENOCTONE*** (2-(8-cyclohexyloctyl)-3-hydroxy-1,4-naphthoquinone: WIN-11530).
'Menolysin' see Yohimbine.
Menotrophin see Human menopausal gonadotrophin.
Menotropin* see Human menopausal gonadotrophin.
Menotropins* see Human menopausal gonadotrophin.
'Menstridyl' see Chlormadinone acetate.
p-Mentha-3,6-diene-2,5-dione see Thymoquinone.
p-Menthan-3-ol see Menthol.
p-MENTHAN-3-ONE (menthone).
(+)-p-Menthene-8,9-diol see Uroterpenol.
2-p-Menthene 1,4-peroxide see Ascaridole.
MENTHOL (2-isopropyl-5-methylcyclohexanol; hexahydrothymol; p-methan-3-ol; peppermint camphor).
Menthone see p-Menthan-3-one.
Menthyl ethoxyacetate see Menglytate.
Menthyl ethylglycolate see Menglytate.
'Meobal' see 3,4-Xylyl methylcarbamate.
'Meonine' see Methionine.
MEPACRINE*** (6-chloro-9-(4-diethylamino-1-methylbutylamino)-2-methoxyacridine; acriquine; akrichin; antimalarina; haffkinine; italchine; mepacrine dihydrochloride; SN-390; 'quinacrine' (trademark in some countries, nonproprietary name in others)).
See also Ethosuximide with mepacrine.
Meparfynol see Methylpentynol.
MEPARTRICIN** (partricin methyl ester; methyl partricin; SPA-S-160).
Mepasin see Pecazine.
Mepazine see Pecazine.
'Mepedyl' see Piprinhydrinate.
MEPENZOLATE BROMIDE*** (1-methyl-3-piperidyl benzilate methobromide; benzilate methobromide of 1-methyl-3-piperidinol; 3-hydroxy-1,1-dimethylpiperidinium bromide benzilate; JB-340; 'cantil').
MEPERIDIDE (1-[3-(p-fluorobenzoyl)-propyl]-4-(pyrrolidin-1-ylcarbonyl)-4-(m-tolyl)piperidine; 4'-fluoro-4-[4-(pyrrolidin-amido)]-4-(m-tolyl)butyrophenone; methylperidide; R-2963).
Meperidine* see Pethidine.
MEPESULFATE (polysulfonated methoxylated polygalacturonic acid; polysulfonated pectin; Ro-2-3053; 'emostat', 'haemostat', 'stypturon', 'treburon').
'Mephanac' see (4-Chloro-2-methylphenoxy)-acetic acid.
MEPHEBARBITAL* (5-methyl-5-phenylbarbituric acid; heptobarbital; 'eudan', 'rutonal').
Mephechlorazine see Mefeclorazine.
'Mephenamine' see Orphenadrine.
MEPHENESIN*** (3-(o-toloxy)-1,2-propanediol; 3-(o-methylphenoxy)-1,2-propanediol; methylphenoxypropanediol; o-cresyl glyceryl ether; o-tolylglycerol; cresoxydiol; glykresin; BDH-312; Byk-M-1; RP-3602).

285

Mephenetoin see Mephenytoin.
Mephenhydramine see Moxastine.
MEPHENOXALONE*** (5-(o-methoxy-phenoxymethyl)-2-oxazolidinone; methoxy-done; AHR-233; OM-518; 'dorsiflex', 'lenetran', 'riself', 'tranpoise', 'trepidone', 'xerene').
MEPHENTERMINE*** (N,α,α-trimethyl-phenethylamine; N-methyl-ω-phenyl tert-butylamine; mephetedrine; 'mephine', 'vialin', 'wyamin').
MEPHENYTOIN*** (5-ethyl-3-methyl-5-phenylhydantoin; methoin; methyl-phenetoin; mephenetoin; phenantoin; tri-antoin).
Mephetedrine see Mephentermine.
'Mephine' see Mephentermine.
Mephobarbital see Methylphenobarbital.
MEPHOSFOLAN* (diethyl (4-methyl-1,3-dithiolan-2-ylidene)phosphoramidate; methocarbolane; 'cytrolane').
'Mepiben' see Diphenylpyraline.
Mepicycline see Pipacycline.
'Mepilon' see Pipacycline.
Mepiperphenidol see Piperphenamine.
MEPIPRAZOLE*** (1-(m-chlorophenyl)-4-[2-(5-methylpyrazol-3-yl)ethyl]piperazine; mepiprazole dihydrochloride; H-4007).
Mepirizole see Epirizole.
MEPIROXOL *** (3-pyridinemethanol 1-oxide).
'Mepiserpate' see Metoserpate.
MEPITIOSTANE** (cyclopentanone 2α,3α-epithio-5α-androstan-17β-yl methyl acetal; epitiostanol 1-methoxycyclopentyl ether; S-10364).
MEPIVACAINE*** (DL-1,2',6'-trimethyl-pipecolanilide; DL-1-methyl-2',6'-pipecol-oxylidide; N-methylpipecolic acid 2,6-di-methylanilide; N-methylpipecolic acid 2,6-xylidide; 1-methyl-2-(2,6-xylylcarb-amoyl)piperidine; mepivacaine hydro-chloride; 'betapar', 'carbocaine', 'scandi-caine').
See also Dexivacaine.
MEPRAMIDIL*** (3,4,5-trimethoxybenzoic acid 3-(3,3-diphenylpropyl amino)propyl ester).
'Meprane' see Methestrol dipropionate.
MEPREDNISONE*** (17,21-dihydroxy-16β-methylpregna-1,4-diene-3,11,20-trione; 16β-methylpregna-1,4-diene-17α,21-diol-3,11,20-trione; 16β-methylprednisone; 'betalone').
MEPROBAMATE*** (2-methyl-2-propyl-1,3-propanediol dicarbamate; meprotan; procalmadiol).
See also Aceprometazine with meprobamate.
MEPROBAMATE WITH BENACTYZINE ('deprol', 'idemin').
MEPROBAMATE WITH OXYPHEN-CYCLIMINE ('daritran').
See also Methamphetamine with meprob-amate.
MEPROCHOL* ((2-methoxy-2-propenyl)-trimethylammonium bromide; (2-methoxy-allyl)trimethylammonium bromide;

'esmidil', 'parastimal').
Mepromazine see Levomepromazine.
'Mepronizine' see Aceprometazine. with meprobamate.
MEPROPHENIDOL* (3-(o-methoxy-p-propionylphenoxy)-1,2-propanediol; MPD; DA-1128).
Meprotan (tr) see Meprobamate.
Meprothixol* see Meprotixol.
MEPROTIXOL*** (9-(3-dimethylamino-propyl)-2-methoxythioxanthen-9-ol; N-7020; meprothixol).
MEPRYLCAINE*** (2-methyl-2-propyl-aminopropyl benzoate; 'oracaine').
MEPTAZINOL** (3-ethyl-3-(m-hydroxy-phenyl)-1-methylhexahydroazepine; 3-ethyl-3-(m-hydroxyphenyl)-1-methyl-hexamethylenimine; m-(3-ethylhexahydro-1-methyl-1H-azepin-3-yl)phenol; mept-azinol hydrochloride; Wy-22811).
MEPYRAMINE****(N-(p-methoxybenzyl)-N',N-dimethyl-N-pyrid-2-ylethylenedi-amine; 2-[(2-dimethylaminoethyl)(p-methoxybenzyl)amino]pyridine; mepyr-amide; pyranisamine; pyrilamine; PM-273).
MEPYRAMINE MALEATE (RP-2786).
MEQUIDOX*** (3-methyl-2-quinoxaline-methanol 1,4-dioxide; 2-hydroxymethyl-3-methylquinoxaline 1,4-dioxide; GS-7443).
MEQUINOL*** (4-methoxyphenol; p-hydroxyanisole; hydroquinone monomethyl ether).
Mequinolate* see Proquinolate.
MEQUITAZINE** (10-(quinuclidin-3-yl-methyl)phenothiazine; 3-(phenothiazin-10-ylmethyl)quinuclidine).
Mer-17 see Azacyclonol.
Mer-25 see Ethamoxytriphetol.
Mer-29 see Triparanol.
Meractinomycin see Dactinomycin.
MERALEIN SODIUM*** (o-[6-hydroxy-5-(hydroxymercuri)-2,7-diiodo-3-oxo-3H-xanthen-9-yl]benzenesulfonic acid sodium salt; 'mercurex', 'merodicein').
MERALLURIDE*** (N-[[3-(hydroxy-mercuri)-2-methoxypropyl]carbamoyl]-succinamic acid or its sodium salt with theophylline; theophylline deriv. of 1-(2-methoxy-3-hydroxymercuripropyl)-3-succinylurea).
'Merapid' see Polyoxymethylene glycol.
'Meratonic' see Pipradrol.
'Meratran' see Pipradrol.
'Merbak' see Acetomeroctol.
MERBAPHEN (2-chloro-6-(hydroxy-mercuri)phenoxyacetic acid barbital derivative sodium salt; 'novasurol').
'Merbentul' see Chlorotrianisene.
'Merbentyl' see Dicycloverine.
MERBIURELIDIN (1-[3-(hydroxymercuri)-2-methoxypropyl]biuret; 'meterox').
MERBROMIN*** (disodium salt of 2,7-di-bromo-4-(hydroxymercuri)fluorescein; mercurochrome; mercurescein sodium; bromochromium; rhodochromium).
'Mercaleukin' see Mercaptopurine.
Mercamine (tr) see Mercaptamine.

'**Mercaprol**' *see* Dimercaprol.
MERCAPTAMINE*** (2-aminoethanethiol;
decarboxycysteine; 2-mercaptoethylamine;
cysteamine; cysteinamine; mercamine;
thioethanolamine; L-1573).
MERCAPTAMINE-*N*-ACETIC ACID
(2-(2-mercaptoethylamino)acetic acid;
N-carboxymethyl 2-mercaptoethylamine;
N-carboxymethylmercaptamine; cyste-
amine-*N*-acetic acid).
Mercaptamine *S*-phosphate *see* Cystafos.
2-Mercaptoacetanilide *S*-gold derivative
see Aurothioglycanide.
2-Mercaptoacetic acid *see* Thioglycolic
acid.
β-**Mercaptoalanine** *see* Cysteine.
Mercaptoarsenol *see* Arsthinol.
Mercaptodimethur *see* Methiocarb.
**2-Mercaptoethanesulfonic acid sodium
salt** *see* Mesna.
2-MERCAPTOETHANOL (2-hydroxy-
ethanethiol; monothioglycol).
2-Mercaptoethylamine *see* Mercaptamine.
N-**(2-Mercaptoethyl)dimethylamine** *see*
Captamine.
**(2-Mercaptoethyl)trimethylammonium
hydroxide** *see* Thiocholine.
MERCAPTOMERIN*** (disodium salt of
N-[3-(carboxymethylthiomercuri)-
2-methoxypropyl]camphoramic acid).
2-Mercapto-1-methylimidazole *see*
Thiamazole.
Mercaptophas *see* Demeton-O plus
demeton-S.
'**Mercaptophos**' *see* Fenthion.
Mercaptophossystox *see* Demeton-O.
**7-Mercapto-17α-pregn-4-en-17-ol-3-one-
21-carboxylic acid γ-lactone acetate** *see*
Spironolactone.
**1-(3-Mercaptopropionic acid)-8-D-argi-
nine vasopressin** *see* Desmopressin.
**1-(3-Mercaptopropionic acid)-2-iso-
leucine vasopressin** *see* 1-Deamino-2-iso-
leucine vasopressin.
1-(3-Mercaptopropionic acid)oxytocin
see Demoxytocin.
N-**(2-Mercaptopropionyl)glycine** *see*
Tiopronin.
MERCAPTOPURINE*** (6-mercapto-
purine; 6-purinethiol; 6-MP; NSC-755;
'ismipur', 'leukerin', 'leupurin', 'mercaleukin', 'mycaptine', 'puri-nethol').
MERCAPTOPURINE ARABINOSIDE
(9-*β*-D-arabinofuranosyl(9H)purine-6-thiol).
MERCAPTOPURINE RIBONUCLEOSIDE
(6-MP-R; NSC-4911; thioinosine).
4-Mercaptopyrazolo(3,4-d)pyrimidine
see Tisopurine.
Mercaptosuccinic acid *see* Thiomalic acid.
**Mercaptosuccinic acid *S*-gold derivative
disodium salt** *see* Sodium aurothiomalate.
2-Mercaptothiazoline *see* 4-Thiazoline-2-
thione.
'**Mercaptothion**' *see* Malathion.
3-Mercaptovaline *see* Penicillamine.
'**Mercarbolide**' *see* Mercocresols.

'**Mercardox**' *see* Chlormerodrin.
'**Mercate**' *see* Isoascorbic acid; Sodium
ascorbate.
Mercazolyl (tr) *see* Thiamazole.
'**Mercloran**' *see* Chlormerodrin.
MERCOCRESOLS* (*o*-(chloromercuri)-
phenol with *sec*-amyltricresol; 'mercarb-
olide', 'mercresin').
'**Mercoral**' *see* Chlormerodrin.
'**Mercreol**' *see* Mercury oleate.
'**Mercresin**' *see* Mercocresols.
'**Mercryl**' *see* Mercurobutol.
MERCUDERAMIDE*** (*o*-[[2-hydroxy-3-
(hydroxymercuri)propyl]carbamoyl]-
phenoxyacetic acid; *o*-carboxyphenoxy-
acetic acid hydroxymercuripropanolamide;
'neptal', 'unephral').
'**Merculest**' *see* Chlormerodrin.
Mercumallyl-theophylline *see* Mercum-
atilin sodium.
MERCUMATILIN SODIUM*** (mixture o
8-(3-hydroxymercuri-2-methoxypropyl)-3-
coumarincarboxylic acid sodium salt with
theophylline; mercumallyl-theophylline;
'cumertilin').
MERCURAN (tr) (lindane with ethylmercuric chloride).
Mercurescein-Na *see* Merbromin.
'**Mercurex**' *see* Meralein sodium.
MERCURIC CHLORIDE (HgCl$_2$; mercury
bichloride; mercury perchloride; corrosive
sublimate).
**MERCURIC SODIUM PHENOLDI-
SULFONATE** ('hermophenyl').
MERCUROBUTOL*** (4-*tert*-butyl-2-
chloromercuriphenol; chloromercuriiso-
butylphenol; 'mercryl').
Mercurochrome *see* Merbromin.
'**Mercuron**' *see* Chlormerodrin-theophylline.
MERCUROPHYLLINE*** (3-(3-hydroxy-
mercuri-2-methoxypropyl)camphoramic
acid sodium salt with theophylline).
Mercurothiolate* *see* Thiomersal.
MERCUROUS CHLORIDE (HgCl;
mercury monochloride; mercury proto-
chloride; mercury subchloride; mild
mercury chloride; calomel; précipité blanc;
French white precipitate; 'calogreen',
'calotabs', 'cyclosan').
Mercury bichloride *see* Mercuric chloride.
Mercurylurée* *see* Chlormerodrin.
Mercury monochloride *see* Mercurous
chloride.
Mercury perchloride *see* Mercuric chloride.
Mercury subchloride *see* Mercurous
chloride.
MERCUSAL (tr) (mersalyl-barbital com-
plex).
'**Mereprine**' *see* Doxylamine succinate.
'**Meretran**' *see* Pipradrol.
Merfalan *see* Sarcolysin.
'**Merfen**' *see* Phenylmercuric acetate.
Meridil (tr) *see* Methylphenidate.
'**Merinax**' *see* Hexapropymate.
MERISOPROL (^{197}**Hg**)***** (1-hydroxy-
mercuri(^{197}Hg)-2-propanol; merisoprol
Hg-197; 'merprane').

'Meritin' *see* Ambucetamide.
Merkaptofos (tr) *see* Demeton-O.
Merkaptofos tiolovyj (tr) *see* Demeton-S.
'Merodicein' *see* Meralein sodium.
Merpanit (tr) *see* Caramiphen.
Merphalan *see* Sarcolysin.
'Merphene' *see* Benzalkonium.
'Merphenyl' *see* Phenylmercuric acetate.
'Merphos' *see* Tributyl phosphorotrithioite.
'Merprane' *see* Merisoprol (^{197}Hg).
'Mersagel' *see* Phenylmercuric nitrate.
MERSALYL** (*o*-[*N*-(3-hydroxymercuri-
   2-methoxypropyl)carbamyl]phenoxyacetic
   acid sodium salt theophylline derivative).
Mersalyl-barbital complex *see* Mercusal.
'Mersolite 8' *see* Phenylmercuric acetate.
'Mersolite 19' *see* Phenylmercuric salicylate.
'Mertect' *see* Tiabendazole.
'Merthiolate' *see* Thiomersal.
'Mertricone' *see* Phenylmercuric acetate.
'Mervacycline' *see* Tetracycline bitartrate-
   nucleic acid complex.
'Mervan' *see* Alclofenac.
MESABOLONE*** (17β-methoxycyclo-
   hexyloxy)-5α-androst-1-en-3-one).
'Mesalphene' *see* Xenysalate.
'Mesantoin' *see* Mephenytoin.
Mesaton *see* Phenylephrine.
MESCALINE (3,4,5-trimethoxyphenethyl-
   amine; mezcaline).
'Mesconit' *see* Scopolamine methyl nitrate.
'Mescophil' *see* Scopolamine methyl bromide.
Mesdicaine *see* Trimecaine.
'Mesentol' *see* Ethosuximide.
MESFENAL (tr) (3-diethylaminopropyl
   2,2-diphenylacetate methyl methosulfate;
   mesphenal).
MESIDINE (2,4,6-trimethylaniline).
MESILATE(S)** (methanesulfonate(s);
   mesylate(s)).
'Mesitol' *see* Inositol.
MESITYLENE (1,3,5-trimethylbenzene).
MESNA*** (sodium 2-mercaptoethane-
   sulfonate; UCB-3983; 'mistabron').
Mesocaine (tr) *see* Trimecaine.
MESOCARB** (3-(α-methylphenethyl)-
   N-(phenylcarbamoyl)sydnone imine).
Mesoinosite *see* Inositol.
Mesoinositol *see* Inositol.
Mesomucinase *see* Hyaluronidase.
'Mesonex' *see* Inositol nicotinate.
'Mesonitrol' *see* Inositol hexanitrate.
'Mesopin' *see* Homatropine methyl bromide.
'Mesopren' *see* Methylprednisolone.
'Mesoranil' *see* Aziprotryne.
Mesorgydine *see* Lisuride.
MESORIDAZINE*** (10-[2-(1-methyl-
   piperid-2-yl)ethyl]-2-(methylsulfinyl)-
   phenothiazine; thioridazine oxide; NC-123;
   TPS-23; 'lidanar', 'lidanil', 'serentil').
MESOXALIC ACID (dihydroxymalonic
   acid; ketomalonic acid; oxomalonic acid).
Mesphenal *see* Mesfenal.
MESTANOLONE*** (17-methyl-5α-
   androstan-17β-ol-3-one; 17β-hydroxy-
   17-methyl-5α-androstan-3-one; 17-methyl-
   androstanolone; 'androstalone').

MESTEROLONE** (1α-methyl-5α-andros-
   tan-17β-ol-3-one; 17β-hydroxy-1α-methyl-
   5α-androstan-3-one; SH-723; 'mestoran',
   'proviron').
MESTILBOL* (α,α'-diethyl-4-hydroxy-
   4-methoxystilbene; stilbestrol monomethyl
   ether; 'monomestrol').
'Mestinon' *see* Pyridostigmine.
'Mestoran' *see* Mesterolone.
MESTRANOL*** (17-ethynyl-3-methoxy-
   1,3,5(10)-estratrien-17β-ol; 3-methoxy-
   19-nor-17α-pregna-1,3,5(10)-trien-20-yn-
   17-ol; 17-hydroxy-3-methoxy-19-nor-
   17α-pregna-1,3,5(10)-trien-10-yne; ethinylestradiol 3-methyl ether; EE₃ME; L-33355).
   See also Anagestone acetate with mestranol;
   Chlormadinone acetate with mestranol;
   6-Chloro-17α-hydroxy-16-methylenepregna-
   4,6-diene-3,20-dione acetate with mestranol;
   Ethynerone with mestranol; Etynodiol diacetate with mestranol; 17α-Hydroxy-16-
   methylenepregna-4,6-diene-3,20-dione
   acetate with mestranol; Lynestrenol with
   mestranol; Megestrol acetate with
   mestranol; Norethisterone with mestranol;
   Noretynodrel with mestranol.
'Mesulene' *see* Diaveridine with sulfadimethoxine.
MESULFEN** (2,7-dimethylthianthrene;
   mesulphene; 'cutilen', 'mitabol', 'mitigal',
   'neosulfine', 'odylen', 'sudermo').
Mesulphene* *see* Mesulfen.
MESUPRINE** (2'-hydroxy-5'-[1-hydroxy-
   2-(*p*-methoxyphenethylamino)propyl]-
   methanesulfonanilide; *N*-[2-hydroxy-2-[4-
   hydroxy-5-(methylsulfonamido)phenyl]-
   1-methylethyl]-*p*-methoxyphenethylamine;
   4-hydroxy-α-[1-(*p*-methoxyphenethyl-
   amino)ethyl]-5-(methylsulfonamido)benzyl
   alcohol; mesuprine hydrochloride; MJ-
   1987).
'Mesurol' *see* Methiocarb.
MESUXIMIDE*** (*N*,2-dimethyl-2-phenyl-
   succinimide; 1,3-dimethyl-3-phenyl-2,5-
   pyrrolidinedione; methsuximide; α-methyl-
   phensuximide; PM-396; 'celontin',
   'petinutin').
Mesylate(s)* *see* Mesilate(s).
MESYLCHOLINE (choline bromide
   methanesulfonate; choline methanesulfonate bromide).
'Metabolan' *see* Xantinol nicotinate with
   B-group vitamins.
METABROMSALAN** (3,5-dibromosalicyl-
   anilide).
   See also Dibromsalan; Tribromsalan.
METABUTOXYCAINE* (2-diethylamino-
   ethyl 3-amino-2-butoxybenzoate; meta-
   butoxycaine hydrochloride; 'primacaine').
'Metacaine' *see* Ethyl *m*-aminobenzoate.
Metacaraphen *see* Metcaraphen.
'Metace' *see* Chlorotrianisene.
METACETAMOL*** (*m*-acetamidophenol;
   3-acetamidophenol; 3'-hydroxyacetanilide;
   N-acetyl-*m*-aminophenol; BS-479).
'Metacide' *see* Parathion-methyl.
Metacin (tr) *see* Oxyphenonium.

Metacortandracin *see* Prednisone.
Metacortandralone *see* Prednisolone.
Metacresylacetate* *see* *m*-Cresyl acetate.
METACYCLINE** (4-dimethylamino-1,4,4a,5,5a,6,11,12a-octahydro-3,5,10,12,12a-pentahydroxy-6-methylene-1,11-dioxonaphthacene-2-carboxamide; 5-hydroxy-6-methylenetetracycline; 6-methyleneoxytetracycline; 6-deoxy-6-demethyl-6-methylene-5-oxytetracycline; methacycline; methylenecycline; GS-2876; 'optimycin', 'rondomycin').
'Metadelphene' *see* Diethyltoluamide.
Metadiazine *see* Pyrimidine.
Metadrenaline *see* Metanephrine.
Metafos (tr) *see* Parathion-methyl.
'Metagin' *see* Methyl paraben.
METAGLYCODOL*** (2-(*m*-chlorophenyl)-3-methyl-2,3-butanediol).
METAHEXAMIDE*** (1-(3-amino-*p*-toluenesulfonyl)-3-cyclohexylurea; 1-(3-amino-4-methylbenzenesulfonyl)-3-cyclohexylurea; glyhexylamide; meta-hexanamide; S-1600; 'euglycin', 'melanex', 'melonex').
Metahexanamide *see* Metahexamide.
'Metahydrin' *see* Trichlormethiazide.
'Metaisosystox' *see* Demeton-O-methyl plus demeton-S-methyl.
'Metaisosystox(i)' *see* Demeton-S-methyl.
'Metaisosystox R' *see* Oxydemeton-methyl.
'Metaisosystoxsulfon' *see* Demeton-S-methylsulfon.
Metaisosystoxsulfoxide *see* Oxydemeton-methyl.
Metakson (tr) *see* Chlorfenson.
β-Metal-binding globulin *see* Transferrin.
'Metalcaptase' *see* Penicillamine.
METALLIBURE*** (1-(1-methylallyl-thiocarbamoyl)-2-(methylthiocarbamoyl)-hydrazine; 1-methyl-6-(1-methylallyl)-2,5-dithiobiurea; methallibure; AY-61122; ICI-33828; 'aimax', 'alimax', 'turi-synchron').
METALLIBURE ZINC COMPLEX ('suisynchron', 'turisynchron Z').
METALOL* (4'-(1-hydroxy-2-methylamino-propyl)methanesulfonanilide; metalol hydrochloride; MJ-1998).
METAMFAZONE*** (4-amino-6-methyl-2-phenyl-3(2H)-pyridazinone; metham-phazone).
METAMFEPRAMONE** (2-dimethyl-aminopropiophenone; 'dimepropion').
'Metamine' *see* Trolnitrate.
METAMIZIL (tr) (2-(diethylamino)propyl benzilate; methyldiazil; methyl-benactyzine; methamizil).
Metamizole *see* Novaminsulfon.
METAMPICILLIN*** (6-(2-methylene-amino-2-phenylacetamido)penicillanic acid; α-(methyleneamino)benzylpenicillin; methyleneampicillin; 'magnipen', 'pravacilin', 'suvipen').
METAM-SODIUM* (sodium methylcarba-modithioate; sodium methyl dithiocarba-mate; metham-sodium; karbation;

'carbathion', 'nematin', 'SMOC', 'tri-maton', 'vapam', 'VPM').
'Metamucil' *see* Ispagula.
METANDIENONE** (17α-methyl-1,4-androsta-1,4-dien-17β-ol-3-one; 17β-hydroxy-17-methylandrosta-1,4-dien-3-one; metandrostenolone; methandienone; methandrostenolone; C-17309; 'abirol', 'dianabol', 'geabol', 'NBL', 'nerobol', 'neroboletta', 'vanabol').
Metandrostenolone *see* Metandienone.
METANEPHRINE (4-hydroxy-3-methoxy-α-methylaminomethylbenzyl alcohol; 3-*o*-methyladrenaline; 3-*o*-methylepine-phrine; metadrenaline).
METANILAMIDE (*m*-aminobenzenesulfon-amide).
'Metanite' *see* Atropine methonitrate.
METANIXIN** (2-(2,6-xylidino)nicotinic acid; 2-(2,6-dimethylanilino)nicotinic acid).
α-Metaoxedrine *see* Phenylephrine.
Metaphos (tr) *see* Parathion methyl.
Metaphoxide *see* Metepa.
METAPRAMINE** (10,11-dihydro-5-methyl-10-(methylamino)-5H-dibenz(b,f)-azepine).
'Metaprel' *see* Orciprenaline.
Metaproterenol* *see* Orciprenaline.
Metaradrine* *see* Metaraminol.
METARAMINOL*** ((−)-α-(1-amino-ethyl)-*m*-hydroxybenzyl alcohol; (−)-2-amino-1-(*m*-hydroxyphenyl)-1-propanol; isophenylephrine; metaradrine).
METARAMINOL TARTRATE (metara-minol bitartrate; metaraminol hydrogen tartrate; 'aramine', 'levicor', 'pressonex').
'Metarsen' *see* Oxophenarsine.
'Metasan' *see* Ziram.
Metasarcolysin *see* *m*-Sarcolysin.
'Metaspas' *see* Dihexyverine.
Metasynephrine *see* Phenylephrine.
'Metasystox' *see* Demeton-O-methyl plus demeton-S-methyl.
'Metasystox(i)' *see* Demeton-S-methyl.
'Metasystox R' *see* Oxydemeton-methyl.
'Metatensin' *see* Reserpine with trichlor-methiazide.
'Metathion' *see* Fenitrothion.
METAXALONE*** (5-(3,5-xylyloxymethyl)-oxazolidin-2-one; 5-(3,5-dimethylphenoxy-methyl)-2-oxazolidinone; metaxolone; AHR-438; 'skelaxin').
Metaxolone* *see* Metaxalone.
Metaxon *see* (4-Chloro-2-methylphenoxy)-acetic acid.
METAZAMIDE*** (1-(*p*-methoxyphenyl)-5-methyl-4-imidazolin-2-one).
Metazepium iodide* *see* Buzepide metiodide.
METAZIDE** ($N^2,N^{2'}$-methylenebisiso-niazid; isonicotinic acid 2,2'-methylene-dihydrazide; methazide).
METAZOCINE** (1,2,3,4,5,6-hexahydro-8-hydroxy-3,6,11-trimethyl-2,6-methano-3-benzazocine; 2'-hydroxy-2,5,9-trimethyl-6,7-benzomorphan).
METCARAPHEN (2-diethylaminoethyl 1-(*o*-xylyl)cyclopentanecarboxylate; di-

289

methylcaramiphen; metacaraphen; G-3012; 'netrin').

METEMBONATE(S)** (4,4'-methylenebis-(3-methoxy-2-naphthoate(s))).

METENOLONE*** (1-methyl-5α-androst-1-en-17β-ol-3-one; 17β-hydroxy-1-methyl-5α-androst-1-en-3-one; methylandrostenolone; 1-methyl-1-androstenolone; methenolone; SQ-16374).

METENOLONE ACETATE (SH-567; SQ-16496; 'nibal' ,'primobolan S').

METENOLONE ACETATE WITH CALCIUM PHOSPHATE (SH-60931).

METENOLONE ENANTATE (metenolone heptanoate; metenolone enanthate; methenolone oenanthate; SH-601; SQ-16374; 'nibal injection', 'primobolan depot')

Metenolone heptanoate *see* Metenolone enantate.

'Meteorex' *see* Dimeticone.

METEPA (N,N',N''-tris(2-methyl-1-aziridinyl)phosphine oxide; 1,1',1''-phosphinylidynetris(2-methylaziridine); MAPO; metaphoxide; methaphoxide; methyl aphoxide).

Meterazine (tr) *see* Prochlorperazine.

METERGOLINE*** ((+)-N-carboxy-1-methyl-9,10-dihydrolysergamine benzyl ester; benzyl 9,10-dihydro-1-methyl-(+)-lysergamine-N-carboxylate; N-carbobenzyloxy-9,11-dihydro-1-methyllysergamine; 8β-carbobenzyloxyaminomethyl-1-methyl-10α-ergoline; MCE).

METERGOTAMINE** (1-methylergotamine).

'Meterox' *see* Merbiurelidin.

METESCUFYLLINE*** (7-(2-diethylaminoethyl)theophylline (7-hydroxy-4-methyl-2-oxo-2H-1-benzopyran-6-yloxy)acetate; etamiphylline (7-hydroxy-4-methyl-2-oxo-1-benzopyran-6-yloxy)acetate; methescufylline; 'veinartan').

'Metet' *see* 7-[2-(Methylthio)ethyl]theophylline.

METETHOHEPTAZINE*** (4-ethoxycarbonyl-1,3-dimethyl-4-phenylhexamethylenimine; ethyl hexahydro-1,3-dimethyl-4-phenylazepine-4-carboxylate; hexahydro-1,3-dimethyl-4-phenylazepine-4-carboxylic acid ethyl ester; Wy-535).

METETOIN*** (5-ethyl-1-methyl-5-phenylhydantoin; methetoin; N-3; 'deltoin').

Metflorylthiadiazine *see* Hydroflumethiazide.

METFORMIN** (1,1-dimethylbiguanide; N,N-dimethylguanylguanidine; N,N-dimethyldiguanide; NNDG; LA-6023; 'deltamine', 'flumamine', 'glucophage', 'haurymellin', 'meguan', 'metiguanide').

METFORMIN p-CHLOROPHENOXYACETATE ('glucinan').

METFORMIN WITH TOLBUTAMIDE ('glucosulfa').
See also Chlorpropamide with metformin; Glycyclamide with metformin.

Methabarbital *see* Metharbital.

METHABENZTHIAZURON* (1-benzothia-zol-2-yl-1,3-dimethylurea; 'tribunil').

METHACHOLINE CHLORIDE*** ((2-hydroxypropyl)trimethylammonium chloride acetate; acetyl-β-methylcholine).

'Methacin' *see* Methocidin.

'Methacolimycin' *see* Colistin mesilate.

METHACRYLIC ACID (2-methylacrylic acid; 2-methyl-2-propenoic acid).

Methacrylic acid polymers *see* Crofilcon; Dimefilcon; Hefilcon; Polacrilin; Vifilcon.

Methacycline* *see* Metacycline.

Methadol *see* Dimepheptanol.

METHADONE** (6-dimethylamino-4,4-diphenyl-3-heptanone; amidone; methadone hydrochloride; phenadon; AN-148; Hö-10820; WIN-1766).

'Methadren' *see* N-Methylepinephrine.

Methadyl acetate *see* Acetylmethadol.

'Methaform' *see* Chlorbutol.

METHAFURYLENE* (N-furfuryl-(N',N'-dimethyl-N-pyrid-2-ylethylenediamine; methafurylene hydrochloride; dihydrogen citrate or fumarate; F-151; 'foralamin').

Methalamic acid *see* Iotalamic acid.

METHALLATAL (5-ethyl-5-(2-methylallyl)-2-thiobarbituric acid; V-12; 'mosidal').

METHALLENESTRIL*** (3-(6-methoxynaphth-2-yl)-2,2-dimethylvaleric acid; β-ethyl-6-methoxy-α,α-dimethyl-2-naphthalenepropionic acid; methallenoestril; 'novestrine', 'vallestril').

Methallenoestril* *see* Methallenestril.

Methallibure* *see* Metallibure.

METHALTHIAZIDE* (3-(allylthiomethyl)-6-chloro-3,4-dihydro-2-methyl-7-sulfamoyl-(2H)-1,2,4-benzothiadiazine 1,1-dioxide; P-2530).

METHAMIDOPHOS* (O,S-dimethyl phosphoramidothioate; 'monitor', 'tamaron').

Methaminodiazepoxide *see* Chlordiazepoxide.

Methamizil (tr) *see* Metamizil.

Methamphazone* *see* Metamfazone.

METHAMPHETAMINE*** ((+)-N,α-dimethylphenethylamine; N-methylamphetamine; 2-methylamino-1-phenylpropane; desoxyephedrine; methamphetamine hydrochloride; methamphetamine sulfate; methamphetaminium chloride; phenylmethylaminopropane).

METHAMPHETAMINE WITH MEPROBAMATE ('euphoramin').

Methamphetaminium chloride *see* Methamphetamine.

'Methampyrone' *see* Novaminsulfon.

Metham-sodium *see* Metam-sodium.

Methanal *see* Formaldehyde.

Methandienone* *see* Metandienone.

METHANDRIOL*** (17α-methyl-5-androstene-3β,17β-diol; methyldihydrotestosterone).

Methandrostenolone *see* Metandienone).

METHANEARSONIC ACID (methylarsinic acid; methylarsonic acid; monomethylarsinic acid).
See also Disodium methanearsonate.

Methanedicarboxylic acid *see* Malonic acid.

Methanesulfonic acid, esters and salts *see* Mesilate(s).

METHANIAZIDE*** (isonicotinic acid-2-sulfomethylhydrazide; *N'*-sulfomethyl-isoniazid; 1-isonicotinoyl-2-sulfomethyl-hydrazine).

Methanimidamide *see* Formamidine.

METHANOL (methyl alcohol; carbinol; wood alcohol).

'Methanopyranorin' *see* Cyclocoumarol.

METHANTHELINE BROMIDE** (2-di-ethylaminoethyl ester methobromide of 9-xanthenecarboxylic acid; diethyl(2-hy-droxyethyl)methylammonium bromide 9-xanthenecarboxylate; dixamon bromide; mantheline; MTB-51; SC-2910).

METHAPHENILENE*** (*N,N*-dimethyl-*N'*-phenyl-*N'*-(2-thenyl)ethylenediamine; W-50).

Methaphoxide *see* Metepa.

Methapyrapone *see* Metyrapone.

METHAPYRILENE*** (*N,N*-dimethyl-*N'*-(2-pyridyl)-*N'*-(2-thenyl)ethylenedi-amine; thenylpyramine; AH-42; PM-262; W-33).

Methapyrone *see* Novaminsulfon.

METHAQUALONE*** (2-methyl-3-*o*-tolyl-4(3H)-quinazolinone; orthonal; metha-qualone hydrochloride; methylquinazolone; B-100; R-148; TR-495; QZ-2; 'cateudyl', 'certonal', 'citexal', 'dobrizon', 'dormogen', 'dormutil', 'hyminal', 'hyptor', 'melsedin', 'motolon', 'mozambin', 'nobedorm', 'noxybel', 'optimil', 'parest', 'quaalude', 'revonal', 'somnofac', 'sopor', 'toquilone', 'tuazole', 'tuazolone').

METHAQUALONE WITH DIPHEN-HYDRAMINE ('mandrax', 'metodril', 'toquilone compositum').

METHAQUALONE WITH ETODROXI-ZINE MALEATE (UCB-1414M; 'isonox', 'somnibel').

METHAQUALONE WITH PROMAZINE ('eatan').

METHARBITAL*** (5,5-diethyl-1-methyl-barbituric acid; endiemal; methabarbital; metharbitone; 'gemonil').

Metharbitone* *see* Metharbital.

METHASTYRIDONE*** (2,2-dimethyl-5-styryloxazolidin-4-one).

'Methatropine' *see* Homatropine methyl bromide.

Methazide *see* Metazide.

METHAZOLAMIDE*** (*N*-(4-methyl-2-sulfamoyl-△²-1,3,4-thiadiazolin-5-yl-idene)acetamide; 5-acetylimino-4-methyl-2-sulfamoyl-1,3,4-thiadiazoline; CL-8490; 'neptazane').

Methazole *see* Chlormethazole.

Methbipyrapone *see* Metyrapone.

METHDILAZINE*** (10-(1-methylpyrrol-idin-3-ylmethyl)phenothiazine; methdil-azine hydrochloride; MJ-5022; 'dilosyn', 'disyncran', 'tacaryl', 'tacazyl').

'Methedrine' *see* Methamphetamine.

METHEMOGLOBIN (methaemoglobin; hemiglobin).

Methenamide *see* Formamide.

METHENAMINE*** (hexamethylenetetra-mine; aminoform; aminoformaldehyde; formamine; formin; hexamethylenamine; hexamine; urisol; uritone; urotropin; 'antihydral', 'cystamin', 'cystogen', 'hexa-loid', 'metramine', 'mictasol', 'naphth-amine', 'uralysol', 'uraseptine', 'urogenine', 'utropine', 'vesalvine').

METHENAMINE ANHYDROMETHYL-ENECITRATE (citrohexal; citrohexamine; formamol; hexacitramine; 'citramin', 'citroformin', 'formanol', 'helmitol', 'new urotropin', 'uropurgol', 'uropuryl').

METHENAMINE BORATE (borohex-amine; uroboramine; 'borovertin').

Methenamine bromoform complex *see* Brometenamine.

Methenamine camphorate *see* Hexa-camphamine.

METHENAMINE ETHOBROMIDE (bromethylformin; 'bromalin', 'bromo-formin').

METHENAMINE HIPPURATE (hexamine hippuric acid complex; methenamine hippurate; 'hippramine', 'hiprex', 'urex').

METHENAMINE MANDELATE (hexy-daline; 'cedopurin', 'cedulamin', 'hexa-mandelate', 'hexydal', 'mandamina', 'mandamine', 'mandelamine', 'mantro-pine', 'reflux', 'urocedulamin', 'uro-mandelin', 'uronamin').

METHENAMINE SALICYLATE ('sali-formin', 'solurine', 'urazine', 'vesalvine-S').

METHENAMINE SULFOSALICYLATE ('hexal', 'hexalet', 'neohexal').

METHENAMINE THIOCYANATE ('aminoweidnerit', 'otrhomin', 'rhodan-hexamine', 'rhodovet').

Methenolone* *see* Metenolone.

N,N'-**Methenyl-*o*-phenylenediamine see** Benzimidazole.

'Metheph' *see* *N*-Methylephedrine.

METHEPTAZINE*** (4-carbomethoxy-1,2-dimethyl-4-phenylhexamethylenimine; methyl 1,2-dimethyl-4-phenylhexamethyl-enimine-4-carboxylate; methyl 1,2-di-methyl-4-phenylhexahydroazepine-4-carboxylate; hexahydro-1,2-dimethyl-4-phenylazepine-4-carboxylic acid methyl ester).

'Methergen' *see* Methylergometrine tartrate.

'Methergin' *see* Methylergometrine maleate.

Methescufylline* *see* Metescufylline.

METHESTROL*** (4,4'-(1,2-diethyl-ethylene)di-*o*-cresol; α,α'-diethyl-4,4'-di-hydroxy-3,3'-dimethylbibenzyl; 3,4-bis(*p*-hydroxy-*m*-methylphenyl)hexane; di-methylhexestrol; methoestrol).

METHESTROL DIPROPIONATE* (3,4-bis(*m*-methyl-*p*-propionoxyphenyl)hexane; promethestrol; promethoestrol; 'meprane').

Methetharimide *see* Bemegride.

Methetoin* *see* Metetoin.

Methexenyl *see* Hexobarbital.

Methicillin* *see* Meticillin.
METHIDATHION* (*S*-(2-methoxy-5-oxo-1,3,4-thiadiazol-4-ylmethyl) *O,O*-dimethyl phosphorodithioate; 4-[[(dimethoxyphosphinothioyl)thio]methyl]-2-methoxy-1,3,4-thiadiazol-5-one; 'supracid', 'ultracid(e)').
Methimazole* *see* Thiamazole.
METHINDETHYRIUM* ([3-[4-(2-(1-methylindol-3-yl)ethyl)pyrid-1-yl]propyl]-trimethylammonium dibromide; 1-(3-dimethylaminopropyl)-4-[2-(1-methylindol-3-yl)ethyl]pyridine dimethobromide; IN-391; 'isotensen').
Methindione *see* Metindione.
METHIOCARB (3,5-dimethyl-4-(methylthio)phenyl methylcarbamate; 4-(methylthio)-3,5-xylyl methylcarbamate; mercaptodimethur; metmercapturan; Bayer-37344; MXMC; OMS-93; 'draza', 'mesurol', 'slug guard').
METHIODAL SODIUM*** (sodium iodomethanesulfonate; sergosin; metiodol).
METHIOFLURANE (2,2-dichloro-1,1-difluoroethyl methyl sulfide).
METHIOMEPRAZINE** (DL-10-(3-dimethylamino-2-methylpropyl)-2-(methylthio)phenothiazine; SKF-6270; 'vontac').
(−)-**Methiomeprazine** *see* Levometiomeprazine.
'Methionamine' *see* Acetylmethionine.
METHIONINE*** ((+)-2-amino-4-(methylthio)butyric acid; 'acimetion', 'lobamine', 'menine', 'meonine', 'metione', 'neomethidin', 'oradash', 'pedameth').
Methionine acetate *see* Acetylmethionine.
Methionine hydroxy analogue *see* 2-Hydroxy-4-(methylthio)butyric acid.
Methionine methylsulfonium methylsulfate *see* Vitamin U.
Methionine selenium analogue *see* Selenomethionine (^{75}Se).
METHIONINE SULFONE (2-amino-4-(methylsulfonyl)butyric acid).
METHIONINE SULFOXIDE (DL-2-amino-4-(methylsulfinyl)butyric acid; NSC-3084).
Méthioplégium *see* Trimetaphan camsilate.
METHIOPRIM (4-amino-2-(methylthio)-5-pyrimidinemethanol; MAHP; NSC-3431).
Methiothepin *see* Metitepine.
METHIOTRIAZAMINE (4,6-diamino-1,2-dihydro-2,2-dimethyl-1-[*p*-(methylthio)phenyl]-*s*-triazine.
Methioturiate *see* Methitural.
Methisazone* *see* Metisazone.
METHISOPRINOL (inosine dimethylamino-2-propanol *p*-acetamidobenzoate complex; NPT-10381; 'inosiplex', 'isoprinosine').
METHITURAL*** (5-(1-methylbutyl)-5-[2-(methylthio)ethyl]-2-thiobarbituric acid; methioturiate; methiurate; thiomethibumal).
METHITURAL SODIUM (AM-109; Sch-3132; 'neraval', 'thiogenal').
Methiurate *see* Methitural.

Methixene* *see* Metixene.
METHOCARBAMOL*** (3-(*o*-methoxyphenoxy)-1,2-propanediol 1-carbamate; guaifenesin carbamate; guaiphenesin carbamate; AHR-85; 'lumirelax', 'neuraxin', 'robaxin').
Methocarbolane *see* Mephosfolan.
METHOCIDIN** (hydroxymethylgramicidin; methylolgramicidin; 'argicillin', 'methacin').
Methodichlorophen *see* Metodiclorofen.
Methoestrol* *see* Methestrol.
'Methofazine' *see* Sulfametomidine.
METHOHEXITAL*** (α-DL-5-allyl-1-methyl-5-(1-methyl-2-pentenyl)barbituric acid; methohexitone; methohexital sodium; L-25398; 'brevital', 'brietal').
Methohexitone* *see* Methohexital.
Methoin *see* Mephenytoin.
'Metholone' *see* Drostanolone.
METHOMYL* (methyl *N*-[[(methylamino)carbonyl]oxy]ethanimidothioate; methyl *N*-[[(methylamino)carbonyl]oxy]-acetimidothioate; *S*-methyl *N*-(methylcarbamoyloxy)thioacetimidate; 'lannate').
Methophenazine* *see* Metofenazate.
Methopholine* *see* Metofoline.
METHOPRENE (isopropyl (2*E*,4*E*)-11-methoxy-3,7,11-trimethyl-2,4-dodecadienoate; 'altosid').
METHOPROMAZINE*** (10-(3-dimethylaminopropyl)-2-methoxyphenothiazine; methoxypromazine).
METHOPROMAZINE MALEATE (FI-5631; RP-4632; 'mopazine', 'tentone', 'vetomazin').
METHOPROTRYN* (2-isopropylamino-4-(3-methoxypropylamino)-6-(methylthio)-*s*-triazine; *N*-(3-methoxypropyl)-*N*'-(1-methylethyl)-6-(methylthio)-1,3,5-triazine-2,4-diamine; methoprotryne; 'gesaran 25').
METHOPROTRYN PLUS SIMAZINE ('gesaran 207', 'gesaran 211', 'gesaran 2079').
Methoprotryne *see* Methoprotryn.
'Methopyranorin' *see* Cyclocoumarol.
Methopyrimazole *see* Epirizole.
Methorphan *see* Racemethorphan.
Methorphinan *see* Racemorphan.
'Methosarb' *see* Calusterone.
METHOSERPIDINE*** (10-methoxydeserpidine; 11-desmethoxy-10-methoxyreserpine; 'decaserpyl').
METHOSERPIDINE WITH BENZTHIAZIDE AND POTASSIUM CHLORIDE ('tensimic').
METHOTREXATE*** (*N*-[*p*-[(2,4-diamino-6-pteridylmethyl)methylamino]benzoyl]-L-(+)-glutamic acid; 4-amino-4-desoxy-*N*[10]-methylfolic acid; methylaminopterin; CL-14377; NSC-740; MTX; 'amethopterin', 'ledertrexate').
Methotrimeprazine* *see* Levomepromazine.
'Methoxa-dome' *see* Methoxsa'en.
Methoxamedrine* *see* Methoxamine.
METHOXAMINE** (α-(1-aminoethyl)-

2,5-dimethoxybenzyl alcohol; 2-amino-1-(2,5-dimethoxyphenyl)-1-propanol; methoxamedrine; methoxamine hydrochloride; 'pressomin', 'vasoxine', 'vasoxyl', 'vasylox').

Methoxiflurane* *see* Methoxyflurane.
METHOXINE (2-amino-4-methoxybutyric acid; oxymethionine).
Methoxiphenadrin* *see* Methoxyphenamine.
'Methoxone' *see* (4-Chloro-2-methylphenoxy)acetic acid.
METHOXSALEN* (9-methoxy-7H-furo-(3,2-g)(1)benzopyran-7-one; 9-methoxy-7H-furo(3,2-g)chromen-7-one; δ-lactone of 6-hydroxy-7-methoxy-5-benzofuranacrylic acid; 8-methoxypsoralen; 9-methoxypsoralen; ammoidin; xanthotoxin; 8-MOP; 'meladinin', 'meloxine', 'methoxa-dome', 'oxsoralen', 'pigmentigen 8-MOP').
Methoxyaniline *see* Anisidine.
3-Methoxy-8-aza-19-nor-17α-pregna-1,3,5-trien-20-yn-17-ol *see* Estrazinol.
Methoxybenzene *see* Anisole.
2-(p-Methoxybenzhydryloxy)-N,N-dimethylethylamine *see* Medrylamine.
p-Methoxybenzoic acid *see* Anisic acid.
1-(6-Methoxybenzothiazol-2-yl)-3-phenylurea *see* Frentizole.
3-(p-Methoxybenzoyl)-6-methoxy-2-methylindole-1-acetic acid *see* Duometacin.
1-[3-(p-Methoxybenzoyl)propyl]-4-phenylpiperidine *see* Anisoperidone.
2-[(p-Methoxybenzyl)(2-dimethylaminoethyl)amino]thiazole *see* Zolamine.
N-(p-Methoxybenzyl)-N',N'-dimethyl-N-pyrid-2-ylethylenediamine *see* Mepyramine.
N-(p-Methoxybenzyl)-N',N'-dimethyl-N-pyrimid-2-ylethylenediamine *see* Thonzylamine.
N-(p-Methoxybenzyl)-N',N'-dimethyl-N-thiazol-2-ylethylenediamine *see* Zolamine.
α-(α-Methoxybenzyl)-4-(β-methoxyphenethyl)-1-piperazineethanol *see* Zipeprol.
6-Methoxy-N,N'-bis(1-methylethyl)-1,3,5-triazine-2,4-diamine *see* Prometon.
3-[(Methoxycarbonyl)amino]phenyl m-tolylcarbamate *see* Phenmedipham.
METHOXYCHLOR* (1,1'-(2,2,2-trichloroethylene)bis(4-methoxybenzene); 1,1,1-trichloro-2,2-bis(p-methoxyphenyl)-ethane; 2,2-di-p-anisyl-1,1,1-trichloroethane; dimethoxy-DT; DMDT; methoxy-DDT; 'marlate', 'metox').
2-Methoxy-5-chloroprocainamide *see* Metoclopramide.
6-Methoxycinchonine *see* Quinine.
p-Methoxycinnamic acid 2-ethoxyethyl ester *see* Cinoxate.
2-Methoxy-p-cresol *see* Creosol.
17β-(1-Methoxycyclohexyloxy)-5α-androst-1-en-3-one *see* Mesabolone.
Methoxy-DDT *see* Methoxychlor.
10-Methoxydeserpidine *see* Methoserpidine.
1-(8-Methoxydibenz(b,f)oxepin-10-yl)-4-methylpiperazine *see* Metoxepin.

10-Methoxy-1,6-dimethylergoline-8β-methanol 5-bromonicotinate *see* Nicergoline.
o-Methoxy-N,α-dimethylphenethylamine *see* Methoxyphenamine.
7-Methoxy-α,10-dimethylphenothiazine-2-acetic acid *see* Protizinic acid.
7-Methoxy-2,4-dimethyl-3-quinolyl methyl ketone *see* Acequinoline.
2-Methoxy-N,N-dimethyl-△9,γ-xanthenepropylamine *see* Dimeprozan.
Methoxydiuron *see* Linuron.
Methoxydone *see* Mephenoxalone.
3-Methoxyestra-1,3,5(10)-triene-16α,17α-diol *see* Epimestrol.
2-METHOXYETHANOL ('methylcellosolve').
2-[[2-(2-Methoxyethoxy)ethyl]aminomethyl]-1,4-benzodioxan *see* Ambenoxan.
N-[2-(2-Methoxyethoxy)ethyl]-1,4-benzodioxan-2-methylamine *see* Ambenoxan.
[N-[5-(2-Methoxyethoxy)pyrimidin-2-yl]-benzenesulfonamido] sodium *see* Glymidine.
S-[2-[(2-Methoxyethyl)amino]-1-oxoethyl] O,O-dimethyl phosphorodithioate *see* Amidithion.
3,3'-(2-Methoxyethylidene)bis-(4-hydroxycoumarin) *see* Coumetarol.
2-(2-Methoxyethyl)pyridine *see* Metyridine.
METHOXYFLURANE* (2,2-dichloro-1,1-difluoro-1-methoxyethane; 2,2-dichloro-1,1-difluoroethyl methyl ether; methoxiflurane; 'ingalan', 'inhalan', 'penthrane', 'pentrane').
9-Methoxy-7H-furo(3,2-g)chromen-7-one *see* Methoxsalen.
Methoxyhydrastine *see* Noscapine.
N-[2-(5-Methoxyindol-3-yl)ethyl]acetamide *see* Melatonin.
Methoxymarc *see* Anisuron.
4-Methoxy-2-(5-methoxy-3-methylpyrazol-1-yl)-6-methylpyrimidine *see* Epirizole.
7-Methoxy-8-(p-methoxyphenoxy)-2-methylisoquinoline *see* Cularine.
3-Methoxy-2-methylaminobenzoic acid methyl ester *see* Damascenine.
4'-Methoxy-2-methylaminopropiophenone *see* Methoxyphedrine.
o-Methoxy-N-methylamphetamine *see* Methoxyphenamine.
7-Methoxy-3-methyl-8-dimethylaminomethylflavone *see* Dimefline.
2-Methoxy-10-(2-methyl-3-dimethylaminopropyl)phenothiazine *see* Levomepromazine.
8-Methoxy-3,4-methylenedioxy-10-nitrophenanthrene-1-carboxylic acid *see* Aristolochic acid.
3-Methoxy-16-methyl-1,3,5(10)-estratriene-16β,17β-diol *see* Mytatrienediol.
3-Methoxy-N-methylmorphinan *see* Dextromethorphan; Levomethorphan; Racemethorphan.
(+)-6-Methoxy-α-methyl-2-naphthaleneacetic acid *see* Naproxen.

(−)-6-Methoxy-β-methyl-2-naphthalene-ethanol *see* Naproxol.

5-Methoxy-2-methyl-1-nicotinoylindole-3-acetic acid *see* Niometacin.

2-Methoxymethyl-5-nitrofuran *see* 5-Nitrofurfuryl methyl ether

[2-(9-Methoxy-7-methyl-5-oxo-5H-furo-(3,2-g)(1)benzopyran-4-yloxy)ethyl]tri-methylammonium theophylline deri-vative *see* Visnafylline.

2-Methoxy-4-methylphenol *see* Creosol.

9-Methoxy-3-methyl-9-phenyl-3-azabi-cyclo(3.3.1)nonane *see* Anazocine.

9-Methoxy-3-methyl-9-phenylisograna-tanine *see* Anazocine.

4β-Methoxy-1-methyl-4α-phenyl-3α,5α-propanopiperidine *see* Anazocine.

4-Methoxy-5-methyl-o-phthalaldehyde-3-carboxylic acid *see* Gladiolic acid.

8-Methoxy-10-(4-methylpiperazin-1-yl)-dibenz(b,f)oxepin *see* Metoxepin.

2-Methoxy-10-[2-(1-methylpiperid-2-yl)-ethyl]phenothiazine *see* Oxyridazine.

1-(4-Methoxy-6-methylpyrimidin-2-yl)-5-methoxy-3-methylpyrazole *see* Epirizole.

N¹-(6-Methoxy-2-methylpyrimidin-4-yl)-sulfanilamide *see* Sulfametomidine.

β-Methoxy-N-methyl-m-trifluoromethyl-phenethylamine *see* Fludorex.

7-Methoxy-8-methyltropinium bromide benzilate *see* Tropenziline bromide.

3-(4-Methoxy-1-naphthoyl)propionic acid *see* Menbutone.

3-(6-Methoxy-2-naphthyl)-2,2-dimethyl-valeric acid *see* Methallenestril.

(+)-2-(6-Methoxynaphth-2-yl)propionic acid *see* Naproxen.

endo-1-[[4-[2-(2-Methoxynicotinamido)-ethyl]piperid-1-yl]sulfonyl]-3-(5-nor-bornen-2-ylmethyl)urea *see* Gliamilide.

3-(2-Methoxy-4-nitrophenyl)-2-methyl-quinazolin-4-one *see* Nitromethaqualone.

4-Methoxy-α′-nitro-α-[p-(2-pyrrolidin-1-ylethoxy)phenyl]stilbene *see* Nitromifene.

11β-Methoxy-19-nor-17α-pregna-1,3,5(10)-trien-20-yne-3,17-diol *see* Moxestrol.

3-Methoxy-19-nor-17α-pregna-1,3,5(10)-trien-20-yn-17-ol *see* Mestranol.

2-Methoxyoctaethyleneoxyethyl *p*-butyl-aminobenzoate *see* Benzonatate.

S-(5-Methoxy-4-oxo-4H-pyran-2-ylmethyl)-O,O-dimethyl phosphorothioate *see* Endothion.

S-(2-Methoxy-5-oxo-1,3,4-thiadiazol-4-yl-methyl) O,O-dimethyl phosphorodi-thioate *see* Methidathion.

6-Methoxy-6-pentyl-*p*-benzoquinone *see* Primin.

METHOXYPHEDRINE*** (1-(*p*-methoxy-phenyl)-2-methylamino-1-propanone; 4′-methoxy-2-methylaminopropiophenone).

METHOXYPHENAMINE*** (α-(2-methoxyphenyl)-β-methylaminopropane; 1-(*o*-methoxyphenyl)-N-methyl-2-propyl-amine; *o*-methoxy-N,α-dimethylphenethyl-amine; *o*-methoxy-N-methylamphetamine; methoxiphenadrin; methoxyphenamine

hydrochloride; mexyphamine; U-0433; 'orthoxine', 'ortodrinex').

6-Methoxy-1-phenazinol 5,10-dioxide *see* Myxin.

4-(β-Methoxyphenethyl)-α-phenyl-1-piper-azinepropanol *see* Eprozinol.

p-Methoxyphenol *see* Mequinol.

Methoxyphenoserpine *see* Mefeserpine.

1-[3-(2-Methoxyphenothiazin-10-yl)-2-methylpropyl]-4-piperidinol *see* Perimetazine.

p-Methoxyphenoxyacetic acid methyl-reserpate ester *see* Mefeserpine.

1-[2-[2-(2-(*o*-Methoxyphenoxy)ethoxy)-ethoxy]ethyl]piperidine *see* Guaiapate.

5-(*o*-Methoxyphenoxymethyl)-2-oxazolid-inone *see* Mephenoxalone.

3-(*o*-Methoxyphenoxy)-N-methyl-3-phenylpropylamine *see* Nisoxetine.

3-(*o*-Methoxyphenoxy)-1,2-propanediol *see* Guaifenesin.

N-[2-(*m*-Methoxyphenoxy)propyl]-*m*-tolylacetamidine *see* Xylamidine.

2-(*o*-Methoxyphenoxy)triethylamine *see* Guaiactamine.

2-(*p*-Methoxy-α-phenylbenzyloxy)-N,N-dimethylethylamine *see* Medrylamine.

6-Methoxy-2-[(phenylcarbamoyl)amino]-benzothiazole *see* Frentizole.

2-(*o*-Methoxyphenyl)-3,3-diphenylacrylic acid *see* Anisacril.

1-(*p*-Methoxyphenyl)-4,5-dithia-1-cyclo-pentene-3-thione *see* Anethole trithione.

5-(*p*-Methoxyphenyl)-1,2-dithiole-3-thione *see* Anethole trithione.

1-(*o*-Methoxyphenyl)-4-(3-methoxyprop-yl)piperazine *see* Dimetholizine.

1-(*p*-Methoxyphenyl)-5-methyl-4-imid-azolin-2-one *see* Metazamide.

1-[2-[4-[1-(4-Methoxyphenyl)-2-nitro-2-phenylethenyl]phenoxy]ethyl]pyrro-lidine *see* Nitromifene.

1-(*p*-Methoxyphenyl)-2-nitro-1-[*p*-(2-pyrrolidin-1-ylethoxy)phenyl]ethylene *see* Nitromifene.

1-[2-[*p*-[α-(*p*-Methoxyphenyl)-β-nitro-styryl]phenoxy]ethyl]pyrrolidine *see* Nitromifene.

7-[2-[4-(*o*-Methoxyphenyl)piperazin-1-yl]-ethyl](5H)-1,3-dioxolo(4,5-f)indole *see* Solypertine.

6-[[3-[4-(*o*-Methoxyphenyl)piperazin-1-yl]propyl]amino]-1,3-dimethyluracil *see* Urapidil.

4′-Methoxy-4-(4-phenylpiperid-1-yl)-butyrophenone *see* Anisoperidone.

p-Methoxyphenylpropenetrithione *see* Anethole trithione.

p-Methoxyphenyltrithiopropene *see* Anethole trithione.

Methoxypromazine *see* Methopromazine.

1-Methoxy-4-propenylbenzene *see* Ane-thole.

Methoxypropiocin *see* Naproxen.

3-(*o*-Methoxy-*p*-propionylphenoxy)-1,2-propanediol *see* Meprophenidol.

17β-Methoxy-3-propoxyestra-1,3,5(10)-

294

triene see Promestriene.
N-(3-Methoxypropyl)-*N'*-(1-methylethyl)-6-(methylthio)-1,3,5-triazine-2,4-diamine see Methoprotryn.
Methoxypsoralen see Methoxsalen.
N[1]-(3-Methoxypyrazin-2-yl)sulfanilamide see Sulfalene.
N[1]-(6-Methoxypyridazin-3-yl)-*N*[4]-salicylazosulfanilamide see Salazodine.
5-[[*p*-(6-Methoxypyridazin-3-yl)sulfamoyl]phenylazo]salicylic acid see Salazodine.
N[1]-(6-Methoxypyridazin-3-yl)sulfanilamide see Sulfamethoxypyridazine.
N[1]-(5-Methoxypyrimidin-2-yl)sulfanilamide see Sulfametoxydiazine.
N[1]-(6-Methoxypyrimidin-4-yl)sulfanilamide see Sulfamonomethoxine.
4-[6-(6-Methoxyquinolin-8-ylamino)-hexyl]-α-methyl-1-piperazinepropanol see Moxipraquine.
4-[4-[6-(6-Methoxyquinolin-8-ylamino)-hexyl]piperazin-1-yl]-2-butanol see Moxipraquine.
1-(6-Methoxyquinolin-4-yl)-3-(3-vinyl-piperid-4-yl)-1-propanone see Viquidil.
5-Methoxyresorcinol see Flamenol.
Methoxyserpidine see Methoserpidine.
5-Methoxy-2-sulfanilamidopyrimidine see Sulfametoxydiazine.
N[1]-(4-Methoxy-1,2,5-thiadiazol-3-yl)sulfanilamide see Sulfametrole.
Methoxytipepidine methobromide see Timepidium bromide.
5-Methoxy-4'-(trifluoromethyl)valerophenone (*E*)-*O*-(2-aminoethyl)oxime see Fluvoxamine.
11-Methoxy-3,9,11-trimethyldodeca-2,4-dienethioic acid *S*-ethyl ester see Triprene.
11-Methoxy-3,7,11-trimethyl-2,4-dodecadienoic acid isopropyl ester see Methoprene.
5-METHOXYTRYPTAMINE (serotonin methyl ether; mexamine).
6-Methoxyumbelliferone see Scopoletin.
'Methral' see Fluperolone.
Methscopolamine* see Scopolamine methyl bromide.
Methsuximide see Mesuximide.
'Methural' see 1,3-Bis(hydroxymethyl)-urea.
METHYCLOTHIAZIDE* (6-chloro-3-chloromethyl-3,4-dihydro-2-methyl-7-sulfamoyl-1,2,4-benzothiadiazine 1,1-dioxide; methylchlorothiazide; 'aquatensen', 'enduron').
Methyl 4-acetamido-2-ethoxybenzoate see Ethopabate.
N-**METHYLACETANILIDE** (methylantifebrin; 'exalgin').
Methylacetopyronone see Dehydroacetic acid.
Methyl-2-acetoxyethyl-2'-chloroethylamine see Acetylcholine mustard.
METHYL ACETYLSALICYLATE (methyl ester of acetylsalicylic acid; 'analjol').

2-Methylacrylic acid see Methacrylic acid.
3-Methylacrylic acid see Crotonic acid.
α-Methyl-1-adamantanemethylamine see Rimantadine.
METHYLADIPHENINE (2-diethylaminoisopropyl 2,2-diphenylacetate; methyldifacil).
3-*O*-Methyladrenaline see Metanephrine.
N-**Methyladrenaline** see *N*-Methylepinephrine.
METHYLAL (dimethoxymethane; formal).
Methylalacetamide see Formicin.
Methyl alcohol see Methanol.
Methyl aldehyde see Formaldehyde.
1-(1-Methylallylthiocarbamoyl)-2-(methylthiocarbamoyl)hydrazine see Metallibure.
METHYLAMINACRIN* (9-amino-4-methylacridine; 5-amino-4-methylacridine; neomonacrin).
METHYLAMINE (carbinamine).
Methylaminoacetic acid see Sarcosine.
Methylaminoantipyrine see Noramidopyrine.
N-[[(Methylamino)carbonyl]oxy]acetimidothioic acid methyl ester see Methomyl.
N-[[(Methylamino)carbonyl]oxy]-ethanimidothioic acid 2-cyanoethyl ester see Thiocarboxim.
N-[[(Methylamino)carbonyl]oxy]-ethanimidothioic acid methyl ester see Methomyl.
1-Methylamino-1-deoxy-D-glucitol see Meglumine.
6-Methylamino-4,4-diphenyl-3-heptanol acetate see Noracymethadol.
4-(2-Methylaminoethyl)-1,2-methylenedioxybenzene see Homarylamine.
2-(2-Methylaminoethyl)pyridine see Betahistine.
Methyl 4-amino-3-hydroxybenzoate see Orthocaine.
Methylaminoisobornane see Mecamylamine.
Methylaminoisocamphane see Mecamylamine.
Methylaminoisooctane see Isometheptene.
Methyl 2-amino-3-mercaptopropionate see Mecysteine.
1-Methylaminomethyldibenzo(b,e)bicyclo(2.2.2)octadiene see Benzoctamine.
2-Methylamino-6-methylhept-5-ene see Isometheptene.
Methylaminonaphthol see Vitamin K_5.
4-Methylaminophenazone see Noramidopyrine.
2-Methylamino-1-phenyl-1-propanol see Pseudoephedrine.
2-[3-(Methylamino)-1-phenylpropoxy]-anisole see Nisoxetine.
Methyl [(*p*-aminophenyl)sulfonyl]carbamate see Asulan.
3β-Methylaminopregn-5-ene-18,20-diol see Paravallarinol.
1-(3-Methylaminopropyl)dibenzo(b,e)-bicyclo(2.2.2)octadiene see Maprotiline.

5-(3-Methylaminopropyl)dibenzo(a,d)-cycloheptene see Protriptyline.
(3-Methylaminopropylidene)cyclohepta-diene see Nortriptyline.
5-(3-Methylaminopropylidene)(5H)-dibenzo(a,d)cycloheptene see Dihydro-amitriptyline.
Methylaminopterin see Methotrexate.
N-**Methylamphetamine** see Methamphet-amine.
2-Methylamphetamine see Ortetamine.
o-**Methylamphetamine** see Ortetamine.
p-**METHYLAMPHETAMINE** (1-(*p*-tolyl)-2-propylamine; 'aptrol').
17-Methylandrosta-3,5-diene-3,17β-diol 3-cyclopentyl ether see Penmesterol.
17α-Methylandrosta-1,4-diene-4,17-diol-3-one see Enestebol.
16α-Methylandrosta-1,4-dien-17β-ol-3-one see Metandienone.
17α-Methyl-5α-androstano(2,3-c)furazan-17β-ol see Furazabol.
2α-Methylandrostan-15β-ol-3-one see Drostanolone.
1α-Methyl-5α-androstan-17β-ol-3-one see Mesterolone.
17-Methyl-5α-androstan-17β-ol-3-one see Mestanolone.
17α-Methyl-5α-androstano(3,2-e)pyrazol-17β-ol see Stanozolol.
17α-Methyl-5-androstene-3β,17-diol see Methandriol.
17-Methyl-3-androstene-4,17β-diol-3-one see Oxymesterone.
1-Methyl-5α-androst-1-en-17β-ol-3-one see Metenolone.
2-Methyl-5α-androst-1-en-17β-ol-3-one see Stenbolone.
N-**METHYLANILINE** (extralin).
Methylantifebrin see Methylacetanilide.
Methylantipyrine see Tolpyrine.
METHYLARSINE BIS(DIMETHYLTHIO-CARBAMATE) ('urbazid').
'Methylaspriodine' see Methyl iodoacetyl-salicylate.
Methylatropine bromide* see Atropine methobromide.
Methylatropine nitrate* see Atropine methonitrate.
8-Methylatropinium bromide see Atropine methobromide.
8-Methylatropinium nitrate see Atropine methonitrate.
METHYLAZOXYMETHANOL (MAM).
Methylazoxymethanol glucoside see Cycasin.
Methylazoxymethanol primeveroside see Macrozamin.
Methylbenactyzine see Metamizil.
METHYLBENACTYZIUM BROMIDE** (diethyl(2-hydroxyethyl)methylammonium bromide benzilate; benactyzine metho-bromide; 'paragone').
METHYLBENZETHONIUM CHLORIDE*** (benzyldimethyl[2-[2-(*p*-1,3,3-tetramethylbutyltoloxy)ethoxy]-ethyl]ammonium chloride; benzyldi-

methyl(octylcresoxyethoxyethyl)am-monium chloride monohydrate; 'am-morid', 'diaparene chloride', 'hyamine 10X').
Methylbenzoic acid see Toluic acid.
Methyl benzoquate* see Nequinate.
2-METHYL-*p*-BENZOQUINONE (*p*-tolu-quinone; 2,5-toluquinone).
2-(2-Methylbenzo(b)thien-3-ylmethyl)-2-imidazoline see Metizoline.
Methyl 5-benzoyl-2-benzimidazolecar-bamate see Mebendazole.
Methylbenztropine see Etybenzatropine.
N-**(*o*-Methylbenzyl)adenosine** see Metrifudil.
6-(*o*-Methylbenzylamino)-9-β-D-ribofur-anosyl-9H-purine see Metrifudil.
N-**(α-Methylbenzyl)-3,3-diphenyl-1-propylamine** see Fendiline.
α-Methylbenzylhydrazine see Mebanazine.
2-(α-Methylbenzyl)hydrazine-1-carboxylic acid ethyl ester see Carbenzide.
α-Methylbenzyl 3-hydroxycrotonate dimethyl phosphate see Crotoxyphos.
3-(*p*-Methylbenzylideneamino)-4-phenyl-4-thiazoline-2-thione see Fezatione.
1-(α-Methylbenzyl)imidazole-5-carboxylic acid ethyl ester see Etomidate.
1-(α-Methylbenzyl)imidazole-5-carboxy-lic acid methyl ester see Metomidate.
N-**(α-Methylbenzyl)linoleamide** see Melinamide.
Methyl 7-benzyloxy-6-butyl-1,4-dihydro-4-oxo-3-quinolinecarboxylate see Nequinate.
Methyl 7-benzyloxy-6-butyl-4-hydroxy-quinoline-3-carboxylate see Nequinate.
2-[1-(*p*-Methylbenzyl)piperid-4-yl]-2-phenylglutarimide see Meletimide.
4-Methylbicyclo(2.2.2)oct-2-ene-1-car-boxylic acid, esters and salts see Ciclotate(s).
Methylbis-β-chloroethylamine see Chlormethine.
Methyl 2-[*p*-[bis(2-chloroethyl)amino]-phenylacetamido]-3-imidazol-4-ylpro-pionate see Hisphen.
Methyl *N*-[*p*-[bis(2-chloroethyl)amino]-phenylacetyl]-L-histidinate see Hisphen.
2-METHYL-2-BUTANOL (*tert*-amyl alcohol; amylene hydrate).
2-Methyl-2-butanol carbamate see Amyl carbamate.
2-Methyl-2-butenoic acid see Tiglic acid.
3-Methyl-2-butenoic acid see Senecioic acid.
3-METHYL-2-BUTEN-1-OL (prenol).
2-Methyl-2-butenoyltropine see Tropigline.
N-**(3-Methyl-2-butenyl)adenosine** see Riboprine.
4-(3-Methyl-2-butenyl)-1,2-diphenyl-3,5-pyrazolidinedione see Feprazone.
9-(3-Methyl-2-butenyloxy)-7H-furo-(3,2-g)(1)benzopyran-7-one see Pento-salen.
'Methyl butex' see Methyl paraben.
1-[2-(3-Methylbutoxy)-2-phenylethyl]-

pyrrolidine see Amixetrine.
Methyl butter yellow see 4-Dimethylamino-3'-methylazobenzene.
3-Methylbutylamine see Isopentylamine.
Methyl 5-butyl-2-benzimidazolecarbamate see Parbendazole.
Methyl 1-(butylcarbamoyl)benzimidazole-2-carbamate see Benomyl.
5-(1-Methylbutyl)-5-(2-methylthioethyl)-2-thiobarbiturate see Methitural.
5-(1-Methylbutyl)-5-vinylbarbituric acid see Vinylbital.
3-Methylbutyric acid see Isovaleric acid.
METHYL CARBAMATE (methyl urethan; 'urethylane').
Methylcarbamic acid esters see Bendiocarb; Carbofuran; Dioxacarb; Promecarb.
2-(Methylcarbamido)benzothiazole see Benzthiazuron.
Methylcarbamodithioic acid sodium salt see Metam-sodium.
1-(Methylcarbamoyl)-3-[3-(5-nitro-2-furyl)allylideneamino]-2-imidazolinone see Nifurizone.
1-Methyl-N-carbobenzyloxydihydrolysergamine see Metergoline.
Methyl-CCNU see Semustine.
'Methylcellosolve' see 2-Methoxyethanol.
METHYLCELLULOSE*** (cellulose methyl ether).
   See also Sodium carboxymethylcellulose.
Methylcephaeline see Emetine.
β-Methylchalcone see Dypnone.
Methyl chloride see Chloromethane.
16α-Methylchlormadinone see Clomegestone.
Methyl 2-(4'-chlorobiphenyl-1-yloxy)-2-methylpropionate see Methyl clofenapate.
Methyl 3-chloro-3-(p-chlorophenyl)-propionate see Chlorfenprop-methyl.
Methyl 6-chloro-3,4-dihydro-2-methyl-7-sulfamoyl-2H-1,2,4-benzothiadiazine-3-carboxylate 1,1-dioxide see Carmetizide.
Methylchloroform see 1,1,1-Trichloroethane.
Methyl N'-(p-chlorophenyl)-N-N-dimethylcarbamimidate see Trimeturon.
Methyl α-[p-(p-chlorophenyl)phenoxy]-isobutyrate see Methyl clofenapate.
Methyl 2-[p-(p-chlorophenyl)phenoxy]-2-methylpropionate see Methyl clofenapate.
Methylchlorothiazide see Methyclothiazide.
Methyl 7-chloro-6,7,8-trideoxy-6-(trans-**1-methyl-4-propyl-L-2-pyrrolidinecarboxamido)-1-thio-L-**threo-α-D-galacto-**octopyranoside** see Clindamycin.
Methyl 7-chloro-6,7,8-trideoxy-6-(4-pentyl-L-2-pyrrolidinecarboxamido)-1-thio-L-threo-D-galacto-**octopyranoside** see Mirincamycin.
Methylchlorphenoxamine see Mecloxamine.
Methylchol see Methacholine.
3-METHYLCHOLANTHRENE (20-methylcholanthrene; NSC-21970).
20-Methylcholanthrene see 3-Methylcholanthrene.
β-METHYLCHOLINE ((2-hydroxypropyl)-trimethylammonium ion or salts).
β-Methylcholine acetate see Methacholine.
β-Methylcholine carbamate see Bethanechol.
β-Methylcholine xylyl ether see β-Methylxylocholine.
3-Methylchromen-4-one see Methylchromone.
METHYLCHROMONE*** (3-methylchromen-4(4H)-one; 'crodimyl', 'diacromone').
Methylchrysazin see Chrysophanic acid.
METHYL CLOFENAPATE (methyl 2-(4'-chlorobiphenyl-1-yloxy)-2-methylpropionate; methyl α-[p-(p-chlorophenyl)phenoxy]-isobutyrate; methyl 2-[p-(p-chlorophenyl)-phenoxy]-2-methylpropionate; clofenapate; CDIB; ICI-55695).
2-Methylcrotonic acid see Tiglic acid.
3-Methylcrotonic acid see Senecioic acid.
Methyl cyanide see Acetonitrile.
Methyl 2-cyanoacrylate see Mecrilate.
METHYL CYANOFORMATE ('cyclon A').
Methylcyclobarbital see Hexobarbital.
β-Methylcyclohexaneacrylic acid see Cicrotoic acid.
p-(trans-**2-Methylcyclohexyl)hydratropic acid** see Mexoprofen.
2-[4-(trans-**2-Methylcyclohexyl)phenyl]-propionic acid** see Mexoprofen.
1-(2-Methylcyclohexyl)-3-phenylurea see Siduron.
Methyl 5-cyclopropylcarbonyl-2-benzimidazolecarbamate see Ciclobendazole.
Methyl cysteine* see Mecysteine.
3'-MethylDAB see 4-Dimethylamino-3'-methylazobenzene.
Methyldamascenine see Damascenine.
Methyl demeton see Demeton-O-methyl plus demeton-S-methyl.
Methyl demeton methyl see Demephion-S.
Methyl demeton-O-sulfoxide see Oxydemeton-methyl.
6-Methyl-△⁶-deoxymorphine see Methyldesorphine.
N-Methyldeptropine see Deptropine methobromide.
METHYLDESORPHINE*** (3-hydroxy-6,N-dimethyl-4,5-epoxymorphin-6-ene; 6-methyl-△⁶-deoxymorphine; MK-57).
Methyldiazepinone see Diazepam.
Methyldiazil (tr) see Methylbenactyzine.
N-Methyl-5H-dibenzo(a,d)cycloheptene-5-propylamine see Protriptyline.
6-Methyl-4H-dibenzo(de,g)quinoline see Aporphine.
Methyl α,4-dichlorobenzenepropanoate see Chlorfenprop-methyl.
Methyl 3,4-dichlorocarbanilate see Swep.
Methyl 2,10-dichloro-12H-dibenzo(d,g)-(1,3)dioxocin-6-carboxylate see Treloxinate.
Methyl 3,6-dichloro-2-methoxybenzoate

see Dicamba-methyl.

Methyl 6,8-dideoxy-6-(1-methyl-*trans*-4-propyl-L-2-pyrrolidinecarboxamido)-1-thio-D-erythro-α-D-galactoocto-pyranoside *see* Lincomycin.

Methyl 2-(2-diethylaminoacetamido)-*m*-toluate *see* Tolycaine.

Methyl 7-diethylamino-4-hydroxy-6-propyl-3-quinolinecarboxylate *see* Amquinate.

Methyl diethyl carbinol urethan *see* Emylcamate.

Methyldifacil (tr) *see* Methyladiphenine.

β-Methyldigoxin *see* Medigoxin.

METHYLDIHYDROMORPHINE* (dihydro-6-methylmorphine; 3,6-dihydroxy-6,N-dimethyl-4,5-epoxymorphinan).

6-Methyldihydromorphinone *see* Metopon.

Methyldihydrotestosterone *see* Methandriol.

Methyl 7-[3,5-dihydroxy-2-(3-hydroxy-3-methyl-1-octenyl)cyclopentyl]-4,5-heptadienoate *see* Prostalene.

Methyl 12,13-dimethoxyibogamine-18-carboxylate *see* Conopharyngine.

Methyl 3-(dimethoxyphosphinyloxy)-2-butenoate *see* Mevinphos.

Methyl 2-(dimethylamino)-N-[[(methylamino)carbonyl]oxy]-2-oxoethanimidothioate *see* Oxamyl.

Methyl 1,2-dimethyl-4-phenylhexamethylenimine-4-carboxylate *see* Metheptazine.

2-Methyl-3,5-dinitrobenzene *see* Dinitolmide.

3-(2-Methyl-1,3-dioxo-2,8-diazaspiro(4.5)-decan-8-yl)-4'-fluorobutyrophenone *see* Roxoperone.

N-Methyldiphenethylamine *see* Demelverine.

α-Methyldiphenhydramine *see* Moxastin.

p-METHYLDIPHENHYDRAMINE (N,N-dimethyl-2-(p-methylbenzhydryloxy)ethylamine; 'neobenodine', 'oxyvermin', 'toladryl').

3-Methyl-5,5-diphenylhydantoin *see* Methylphenytoin.

γ-Methyl-α,α-diphenyl-1-piperidine-propanol *see* 1,1-Diphenyl-3-piperid-1-yl-1-butanol).

5-Methyl-4,4-diphenyl-6-piperid-1-yl-3-hexanone *see* Pipanone.

3-Methyl-1,2-diphenyl-4-pyrrolidin-1-yl-2-butanol acetate *see* Pyrrolifene.

2-Methyl-1,2-dipyrid-3-yl-1-propanone *see* Metyrapone.

1-Methyl-3,3-dithien-2-ylallylamine *see* Thiambutene.

(4-Methyl-1,3-dithiolan-2-ylidene)phosphoramidic acid diethyl ester *see* Mephosfolan.

6-Methyl-1,3-dithiolo(4,5-b)quinoxalin-2-one *see* Chinomethionat.

N-Methyldithio-1-naphthalenecarbamic acid 2-benzoxazolyl ester *see* Naftoxate.

Methyl dodecahydro-2α,11-dimethoxy-3β-(3,4,5-trimethoxybenzoyloxy)-benz(g)indolo(2,3-a)quinolizine-1β-

carboxylate *see* Reserpine.

Methyl dodecahydro-2α,11-dimethoxy-3β-(3,4,5-trimethoxycinnamoyloxy)-benz(g)indolo(2,3-a)quinolizine-1β-carboxylate *see* Rescinnamine.

METHYLDOPA* ((−)-3-(3,4-dihydroxyphenyl)-2-methylalanine; (−)-2-amino-3-(3,4-dihydroxyphenyl)-2-methylpropionic acid; alpha methyl dopa; MK-351; 'aldomet', 'aldometil', 'dopamet', 'dopegyt', 'hyperpax', 'mulfasin', 'presinol', 'sedometil', 'sembrina'). *See also* Guanacline with methyldopa.

α-Methyldopa-hydrazine *see* Carbidopa.

METHYLDOPA WITH HYDROCHLOROTHIAZIDE ('aldoril').

METHYLDOPA WITH MEFRUSIDE ('sali-presinol').

METHYLDOPATE* (ethyl 2-amino-3-(3,4-dihydroxyphenyl)-2-methylpropionate; ethyl ester of methyldopa; methyldopate hydrochloride; 'aldomet ester', 'aldomet injection').

α-(Methyleneamino)benzylpenicillin *see* Metampicillin.

6-[2-(Methyleneamino)-2-phenylacetamido]penicillanic acid *see* Metampicillin.

Methyleneampicillin *see* Metampicillin.

2,2'-Methylenebis(4-chlorophenol) *see* Dichlorophen.

2,2'-Methylenebis(6-chlorothymol) *see* Biclotymol.

4,4'-Methylenebis(cyclohexyltrimethylammonium iodide) *see* Mebezonium iodide.

3,3'-Methylenebis(4-hydroxycoumarin) *see* Dicoumarol.

4,4'-Methylenebis(3-hydroxy-2-naphthoic acid), esters and salts *see* Embonate(s).

N,N'-Methylenebisisoniazid *see* Metazide.

4,4'-Methylenebis(3-methoxy-2-naphthoic acid), esters and salts *see* Metembonate(s).

3,3'-Methylenebis(2-naphthalenesulfonic acid) phenylmercuric salt *see* Hydrargaphen.

4,4'-Methylenebis(tetrahydro-1,2,4-thiadiazine 1,1-dioxide) *see* Taurolin.

2,2'-Methylenebis(3,4,6-trichlorophenol) *see* Hexachlorophene.

METHYLENE BLUE* (3,7-bis(dimethylamino)phenazathionium chloride; methylthioninium chloride; tetramethylthionine chloride; Swiss blue; CI-922; Schultz-1038; 'chromosmon', 'desmoid').

Methylene chloride *see* Dichloromethane.

Methylenechlormadinone *see* Cyproterone.

Methylenecitrodisalicylic acid *see* Citrodisalyl.

Methylenecycline* *see* Metacycline.

p,p'-METHYLENEDIANILINE (4,4'-diaminodiphenylmethane).

Methylene dichloride *see* Dichloromethane.

METHYLENEDI(m-CRESOLSULFONIC ACID) POLYMER (m-cresolsulfonic acid formaldehyde condensation product;

298

'albothyl', 'lotagen', 'negatan', 'negatol', 'nelex').

(Methylenedi-1,4-cyclohexylene)bis(trimethylammonium iodide) see Mebezonium iodide.

3,4-METHYLENEDIOXYAMPHETAMINE ((3,4-methylenedioxyphenyl)isopropylamine; 1-piperonylethylamine; MDA).

3,4-Methylenedioxybenzaldehyde see Piperonal.

1,2-Methylenedioxybenzene see 1,3-Benzodioxole.

3,4-Methylenedioxybenzoic acid see Piperonylic acid.

1-(3,4-Methylenedioxybenzyl)-4-pyrimid-2-ylpiperazine see Piribedil.

3,4-Methylenedioxymandelamidine see Olmidine.

1,2-Methylenedioxy-4-[2-(octylsulfinyl)-propyl]benzene see Sulfoxide.

3,4-Methylenedioxyphenol see Sesamol.

2-(3,4-Methylenedioxyphenoxy)-6-(3,4-methylenedioxyphenyl)-cis-3,7-dioxabicyclo(3.3.0)octane see Sesamolin.

(3,4-Methylenedioxyphenyl)isopropylamine see 3,4-Methylenedioxyamphetamine.

1-(3,4-Methylenedioxyphenyl)-3,6,9-trioxaundecane see Sesamex.

3,3'-Methylenedithiobis(2-aminopropionic acid) see Djenkolic acid.

3,3'-Methylenedithiodialanine see Djenkolic acid.

Methylene oxide see Formaldehyde.

5-Methylene-2-oxodihydrofuran see Protoanemonin.

6-Methyleneoxytetracycline see Metacycline.

16-Methyleneprednisolone see Prednylidene.

16-Methylenepregnadiene-17α-ol-3,20-dione see 17α-Hydroxy-16-methylene-pregna-4,6-diene-3,20-dione.

16-Methylenepregna-1,4-diene-11β,17α,21-triol-3,20-dione see Prendylidene.

16-Methylenepregna-4,6-diene-11β,17α,21-triol-3,20-dione see Isoprednidene.

Methylenesuccinic acid see Itaconic acid.

S,S'-Methylene-O,O,O',O'-tetraethyl phosphorodithioate see Ethion.

N-METHYLEPHEDRINE ('metheph').

Methyl-18-epi-O-methylreserpate see Metoserpate.

N-METHYLEPINEPHRINE (α-dimethyl-aminomethyl-3,4-dihydroxybenzyl alcohol; N-methyladrenaline; 'methadren').

3-O-Methylepinephrine see Metanephrine.

Methyl 18-epireserpate methyl ether see Metoserpate.

Methylergobasine see Methylergometrine.

'Methylergobrevine' see Methylergometrine.

(+)-N-(6-Methylergolin-8β-ylmethyl)-acetamide see Acetergamine.

METHYLERGOMETRINE*** (N-(1-hydroxymethylpropyl)-(+)-lysergamide; lysergic acid butanolamide; methylergo-

basine; methylergonovine; 'methylergobrevine').

METHYLERGOMETRINE MALEATE ('methergin').

METHYLERGOMETRINE TARTRATE ('basofortina', 'methergen', 'partergin').

METHYLERGOMETRINE WITH OXYTOCIN (SYNTHETIC) ('syntometrin').

1-Methylergotamine see Metergotamine.

7α-Methylestra-1,3,5-(10)trien-3-ol-17-one see Almestrone.

17-Methylestra-4-9,11-trien-17β-ol-3-one see Metribolone.

7α-Methylestr-4-en-3-one-17β-ol see Trestolone.

METHYLESTRENOLONE (17α-methyl-4-estren-17-ol-3-one; 17α-methyl-19-nortestosterone; normethandrolone; 'orgasteron').

[[(1-Methyl-1,2-ethanediyl)bis(carbamodithioato)](2-)]zinc homopolymer see Propineb.

1,1'-[(Methylethanediylidene)dinitrilo]-diguanide see Mitoguazone.

N-Methyl-9,10-ethanoanthracene-9(10H)-methylamine see Benzoctamine.

N-Methyl-9,10-ethanoanthracene-9(10H)-propylamine see Maprotiline.

2-(1-Methylethoxy)phenyl methylcarbamate see Propoxur.

3-(1-Methylethyl)-1H-2,1,3-benzothiadiazin-4(3H)-one 2,2-dioxide see Bentazon.

1-Methylethyl 4-bromo-α-(4-bromophenyl)-α-hydroxybenzeneacetate see Bromopropylate.

1-Methylethyl 4-chloro-α-(4-chlorophenyl)-α-hydroxybenzeneacetate see Chloropropylate.

1-Methylethyl 3-chlorophenylcarbamate see Chlorpropham.

Methylethyldimethylaminoindole see Medmain.

4-(1-Methylethyl)-2,6-dinitro-N,N-dipropylbenzenamine see Isopropalin.

1-Methylethyl [2-(1-methylpropyl)-4,6-dinitrophenyl] carbonate see Dinobuton.

O-Methyl 2-[(2-ethyl-5-nitroimidazol-1-yl)ethyl]carbamothioate see Sulnidazole.

1-Methylethyl phenylcarbamate see Propham.

2-(1-Methylethyl)phenyl methylcarbamate see Isoprocarb.

Methyletynodiol see Metynodiol.

Methylflavone-8-carboxylic acid piperidylethyl ester see Flavoxate.

METHYLFLUDROCORTISONE (9α-fluoro-2-methylhydrocortisone; methylfluorocortisol).

α-Methylfluorene-2-acetic acid see Cicloprofen.

Methyl 5-(p-fluorobenzoyl)-2-benzimidazolecarbamate see Flubendazole.

Methylfluorocortisol see Methylfludrocortisone.

Methylflurether see Enflurane.

299

5-Methylfurazolidone *see* Furmethoxadone.
(Methylfurfurylideneethylidene)iso-
niazid *see* Larusan.
Methyl-GAG *see* Mitoguazone.
***N*-Methylglucamine** *see* Meglumine.
Methylglucamine iodipamide *see* Adipio-
done meglumine.
***N*-Methylglycine** *see* Sarcosine.
1-(*N*-Methylglycine)-5-L-valine-L-alanine
angiotensin II *see* Saralasin.
1-Methylglycocyamidine *see* Creatinine.
Methylglycocyamine *see* Creatine.
Methyl glycol *see* Propylene glycol.
***N*-[1-[*N*-[*N*-[*N*-[*N*-[*N*²-(*N*-Methyl-**
glycyl)-L-arginyl]-L-valyl]-L-tyrosyl]-
L-valyl]-L-histidyl]prolyl]-L-alanine
see Saralasin.
METHYLGLYOXAL (2-ketopropional-
dehyde; 2-oxopropanal; 2-oxopropional-
dehyde; acetylformaldehyde; pyruvaldehyde; MSC-79019).
Methylglyoxal bisguanylhydrazone *see*
Mitoguazone.
4-Methylguaiacol *see* Creosol.
Methylguanidoacetic acid *see* Creatine.
'Methyl guthion' *see* Azinphos-methyl.
***N*-METHYLHEPTAMINOL** (2-methyl-
6-methylamino-2-heptanol; EA-83;
'aranthol').
1-(1-Methylheptyl)hydrazine *see* Octa-
moxine.
Methylhexabital *see* Hexobarbital.
Methyl hexahydro-1,2-dimethyl-4-phenyl-
azepine-4-carboxylate *see* Meheptazine.
2-Methyl-3-(3,7,11,15,19,23-hexamethyl-
2,6,10,14,18,22-tetracosahexaenyl)-
1,4-naphthoquinone *see* Farnoquinone.
Methylhexanamine *see* Dimethylamylamine.
Methylhexobarbital *see* Hexobarbital.
1-Methylhexylamine *see* Tuaminoheptane.
1-METHYLHISTAMINE (4-(2-amino-
ethyl)-1-methylimidazole).
Methylhydantoin *see* Mephenytoin.
1-Methylhydantoin-2-imide *see* Creatinine.
'Methylhydrazine' *see* Procarbazine.
Methyl *p*-hydroxybenzoate *see* Methyl
paraben.
Methyl 3-hydroxy-*cis*-crotonate dimethyl
phosphate *see* Mevinphos.
Methyl 4-hydroxy-6,7-diisopropoxy-
3-quinolinecarboxylate *see* Proquinolate.
***N*-Methylhyoscine methyl sulfate** *see*
Scopolamine methyl methosulfate.
1-Methylimidazole-3,5-dicarboxylic acid
diethylamide *see* Antithemine.
1-Methyl-2-imidazolethiol ethyl carbo-
nate *see* Carbimazole.
2-Methyl-2-imidazoline *see* Lysidine.
[(Methylimino)diethylene]bis(ethyldi-
methylammonium bromide) *see*
Azamethonium bromide.
3-Methylindole *see* Skatole.
1-Methylindole-2,3-dione thiosemicarb-
azone *see* Metisazone.
[3-[4-(2-(1-Methylindol-3-yl)ethyl)pyrid-
1-yl]propyl]trimethylammonium di-
bromide *see* Methindethyrium.

METHYL IODOACETYLSALICYLATE
('methylaspriodine').
METHYLISACONITINE (mellictine;
alkaloid from *Delphinium dictiocarpum*).
Methylisatin thiosemicarbazone *see*
Metisazone.
Methyl isodemeton *see* Demeton-S-methyl.
***N*-Methylisooctenylamine** *see* Isomethep-
tene.
Methylisosystox *see* Demeton-S-methyl.
Methylisosystoxsulfon *see* Demeton-S-
methylsulfon.
Methylisosystox sulfoxide *see* Oxydemeton-methyl.
***N*¹-(3-Methylisothiazol-2-yl)sulfanil-**
amide *see* Sulfasomizole.
4-[4-[3-(5-Methylisoxazole-3-carbox-
amido)ethyl]benzenesulfonyl]-1,1-hexa-
methylenesemicarbazide *see* Glisoxepide.
5-Methyl-3-isoxazolecarboxylic acid
2-benzylhydrazide *see* Isocarboxazid.
***N*¹-(5-Methylisoxazol-3-yl)sulfanilamide**
see Sulfamethoxazole.
Methyllysergic acid butanolamide *see*
Methysergide.
METHYLLYSERGIDE (*N,N*-diethyl-1-
methyllysergamide; diethylamide of
1-methyllysergic acid; MLD-41).
Methylmaleic acid *see* Citraconic acid.
Methylmecamylamine *see* Dimecamine.
Methylmelubrin *see* Novaminsulfon.
'Methylmercadone' *see* Nifuratel.
Methylmercaptoimidazole *see* Thiamazole.
Methylmercaptophos *see* Demeton-O-
methyl.
Methylmercaptophos oxide *see* Oxy-
demeton-methyl.
METHYL MESILATE (methyl methane-
sulfonate; methyl mesylate; CB-1540;
NSC-50256).
Methyl methacrylate polymer *see*
Polymethyl methacrylate.
Methyl methacrylate polymer with
2,3-dihydroxypropyl methacrylate *see*
Crofilcon A.
Methyl methacrylate polymer with 2-
hydroxyethyl methacrylate and ethyl-
enebis(oxyethylene) dimethacrylate *see*
Dimefilcon A.
Methyl methanesulfonate *see* Methyl
mesilate.
Methylmethionine sulfonium chloride
see Vitamin U.
Methyl 3-methoxy-2-methylamino-
benzoate *see* Damascenine.
Methyl 3-methoxy *N*-methylanthra-
nilate *see* Damascenine.
1-Methyl-6-(1-methylallyl)-2,5-dithio-
biurea *see* Metallibure.
Methyl *N*-[[(methylamino)carbonyl]oxy]-
acetimidothioate *see* Methomyl.
Methyl *N*-[[(methylamino)carbonyl]oxy]-
ethanimidothioate *see* Methomyl.
2-Methyl-6-methylamino-2-heptanol *see*
Methylheptaminol.
3-Methyl-3-(3-methylaminopropyl)-1-
phenylindoline *see* Daledalin.

3-Methyl-3-(3-methylaminopropyl)-1-phenyl-2-indolinone *see* Amedalin.

N-Methyl-2-(*o*-methylbenzhydryloxy)-ethylamine *see* Tofenacin.

Methyl 1-(α-methylbenzyl)imidazole-5-carboxylate *see* Metomidate.

S-Methyl *N*-(methylcarbamoyloxy)thio-acetimidate *see* Methomyl.

(−)-6-Methyl-2-(4-methyl-3-cyclohexen-1-yl)-5-hepten-2-ol *see* Levomenol.

6-Methyl-5-(2-methylenebutyryl)-2-benzofurancarboxylic acid *see* Furacrinic acid.

N-Methyl-3,4-methylenedioxyphenethyl-amine *see* Homarylamine.

1-(α-Methyl-3,4-methylenedioxyphen-ethyl)-4-(4-methylthiazol-2-yl)piper-azine *see* Podilfen.

6-Methyl-16-methylenepregna-4,6-diene-17α-ol-3,20-dione *see* Melengestrol.

Methyl *O*-methyl-18-epireserpate *see* Metoserpate.

(1-Methyl)methylergometrine *see* Methysergide.

2-Methyl-3-(1-methylethyl)-4,6-dinitro-phenol *see* Dinoprop.

3-Methyl-5-(1-methylethyl)phenyl methylcarbamate *see* Promecarb.

1-Methyl-3-[2-(5-methylimidazol-4-yl-methylthio)ethyl]guanidine-2-carbo-nitrile *see* Cimetidine.

1-Methyl-3-[2-[(5-methylimidazol-4-ylmethyl)thio]ethyl]-2-thiourea *see* Metiamide.

O-Methyl [2-(2-methyl-5-nitroimidazol-1-yl)ethyl]thiocarbamate *see* Carnida-zole.

1-Methyl 3-[2-methyl-4-oxo-2-(2,4-penta-dienyl)-2-cyclopenten-1-yl]chrysanthe-mumdicarboxylate *see* Pyrethrin II.

α-Methyl-*N*-(1-methyl-2-phenoxyethyl)-phenethylamine *see* Dextrofemine; Race-femine.

10-Methyl-2-(4-methylpiperazin-1-yl)-3,4-diazaphenoxazine *see* Azafen.

2-Methyl-11-(4-methylpiperazin-1-yl)-dibenzo(b,f)(1,4)thiazepine *see* Metiap-ine.

D-(+)-1-Methyl-1-(1-methylpiperid-2-yl)-ethyl diphenylacetate *see* Pinolcaine.

Methyl 4-methyl-3-(2-propylaminopro-pionamido)-2-thiophenecarboxylate *see* Carticaine.

N-Methyl-*N*-(3-methylpyridyl)tropamide *see* Pimetremide.

Methyl 2-methyl-5-[D-*arabino*-1,2,3,4-tetra-(nicotinoyloxy)butyl]-3-furoate *see* Nicofuroate.

1-Methyl-1-[2-(*N*-methyl-α-thien-2-yl-mandelamido)ethyl]pyrrolidinium bromide *see* Dotefonium bromide.

2-Methyl-2-(methylthio)propanal *O*-[(methylamino)carbonyl]oxime *see* Aldicarb.

2-Methyl-2-(methylthio)propionaldehyde *O*-(methylcarbamoyl)oxime *see* Aldi-carb.

Methylmitomycin *see* Porfiromycin.

Methylmorphine *see* Codeine.

4-Methyl-7-(4-morpholinecarboxamido)-3-(2-morpholinoethyl)coumarin *see* Morocromen.

3-Methyl-4-morpholinobutyryl-2,2-di-phenylpyrrolidine *see* Dextromoramide; Levomoramide; Racemoramide.

1-(3-Methyl-4-morpholino-2,2-diphenyl-butyryl)pyrrolidine *see* Dextromoramide; Levomoramide; Racemoramide.

4-Methyl-3-[(2-morpholinoethyl)amino]-6-phenylpyridazine *see* Minaprine.

1-Methyl-2-[[[5-(morpholinomethyl)-2-oxooxazolidin-3-yl]imino]methyl]-5-nitroimidazole *see* Moxnidazole.

2-Methyl-*N*-(morpholinomethyl)-2-phenylsuccinimide *see* Morsuximide.

2-Methyl-4-(morpholinomethyl)-2-(3,4,5-trimethoxyphenyl)-1,3-dioxolane *see* Trioxolane.

1-Methyl-3-morpholinopropyl tetra-hydro-4-phenyl-2H-pyran-4-carboxylate *see* Fedrilate.

7α-Methylnandrolone *see* Trestolone.

α-Methyl-1-naphthaleneacetic acid ester with 1,4-piperazinediethanol *see* Nafiverine.

2-Methyl-1,4-naphthalenediamine *see* Vitamin K$_6$.

2-Methyl-1,4-naphthalenediol *see* Menadiol.

2-Methyl-1,4-naphthalenedione *see* Menadione.

2-Methyl-1,4-naphthoquinone *see* Menadione.

N-Methyl-*N*-naphth-1-yldithiocarbamic acid 2-benzoxazolyl ester *see* Naftoxate.

N-Methyl-*N*-naphth-1-ylfluoroacetamide *see* *N*-(2-Fluoroacetyl)-*N*-methyl-1-naphth-ylamine.

O-(2-Methylnaphth-1-ylmethyl)hydroxyl-amine *see* Nafomine.

*N*¹-METHYLNICOTINAMIDE (3-car-bamoyl-1-methylpyridinium hydroxide or salts).

4-Methyl-1-(5-nitrofurfurylideneamino)-2-imidazolidinone *see* Nifurimide.

5-Methyl-3-(5-nitro-2-furfurylidene-amino)-2-oxazolidinone *see* Furmethox-adone.

2-Methyl-6-[2-(5-nitro-2-furyl)vinyl]-4-pyrimidinol *see* Nifurvidine.

2-Methyl-5-nitroimidazole-1-ethanol *see* Metronidazole.

2-Methyl-4-nitroimidazole-1-propanol *see* Ternidazole.

4-[2-(2-Methyl-5-nitroimidazol-1-yl)-ethyl]pyridine *see* Panidazole.

[2-(2-Methyl-5-nitroimidazol-1-yl)ethyl]-thiocarbamic acid methyl ester *see* Carnidazole.

1-Methyl-5-nitroimidazol-5-ylmethyl carbamate *see* Ronidazole.

3-[[(1-Methyl-5-nitroimidazol-2-yl)-methylene]amino]-5-(morpholino-methyl)-2-oxazolidinone *see* Moxnida-zole.

2-[(1-Methyl-5-nitroimidazol-2-ylmethyl)-thio]pyridine *see* Pirinidazole.

1-(2-Methyl-5-nitroimidazol-1-yl)-2-propanol *see* Secnidazole.

6-(1-Methyl-4-nitroimidazol-5-ylthio)-guanine *see* Tiamiprine.

6-(1-Methyl-4-nitroimidazol-5-ylthio)-purine *see* Azathioprine.

5-Methyl-5-(*p*-nitrophenylazo)rhodanine *see* Nitrodan.

3-Methyl-5-(4-nitrophenylazo)thiazolidin-4-one-2-thione *see* Nitrodan.

Methylnitrophos (tr) *see* Fenitrothion.

2-Methyl-5-nitro-1-(2-pyrid-4-ylethyl)-imidazole *see* Panidazole.

1-Methyl-5-nitro-2-[(pyrid-2-ylthio)-methyl]imidazole *see* Pirinidazole.

1-METHYL-1-NITROSOUREA (NSC-23909).

2-Methyl-4′-nitro-3′-(trifluoromethyl)-propionanilide *see* Flutamide.

9-Methylnon-6-enoic acid vanillylamide *see* Capsaicin.

2-Methyl-2-nonyl-1,3-dioxolan-4-ylmethyl carbamate *see* Dioxolan.

α-Methylnoradrenaline *see* Corbadrine.

3-*O*-Methylnoradrenaline *see* Normetane-phrine.

17α-Methylnorandrosta-4,9,11-trien-17β-ol-3-one *see* Metribolone.

17-Methyl-B-norandrost-4-en-17β-ol-3-one *see* Benorterone.

α-Methylnorepinephrine *see* Corbadrine.

3-*O*-Methylnorepinephrine *see* Normetane-phrine.

7α-Methylnoretynodrel *see* Tibolone.

17-Methyl-19-norpregna-4,9-diene-3,20-dione *see* Demegestone.

11β-Methyl-19-norpregn-4-en-17-ol-3,20-dione acetate *see* Norgestomet.

11β-Methyl-19-nor-17α-pregn-4-en-20-yne-3β,17-diol *see* Metynodiol.

17α-Methyl-△⁹-19-norprogesterone *see* Demegestone.

Methylnortestosterone *see* Methylestre-nolone.

7α-Methyl-19-nortestosterone *see* Trestolone.

17α-Methyl-B-nortestosterone *see* Benorterone.

Methyloestrenolone *see* Methylestrenolone.

Methylolchlortetracycline *see* Clomocycline.

Methylolgramicidin *see* Methocidin.

METHYLOL RIBOFLAVIN* (mixture of hydroxymethyl derivatives of riboflavin; 'hyflavin').

17-Methyl-2-oxa-5α-androstan-17β-ol-3-one *see* Oxandrolone.

6-Methyl-1,2,3-oxathiazin-4(3H)-one 2,2-dioxide *see* Acesulfame.

Methyloxazepam *see* Temazepam.

4-(2-Methyl-4-oxo-3,3-diphenyl-4-pyrrol-idin-1-ylbutyl)morpholine *see* Dextro-moramide; Levomoramide; Racemor-amide.

2-Methyl-4-oxo-2-(2,4-pentadienyl)-

2-cyclopenten-1-yl chrysanthemate *see* Pyrethrin I.

5-Methyl-3-oxo-6-phenylmorpholine *see* Fenmetramide.

3-Methyl-4-oxo-5-piperid-1-ylthiazolid-inylidene-2-acetic acid ethyl ester *see* Etozolin.

2-Methyl-4-oxo-3-(2-propenyl)-2-cyclo-penten-1-yl 2,2-dimethyl-3-(2-methyl-1-propenyl)cyclopropanecarboxylate *see* Allethrin; Bioallethrin.

1-Methyl-2-oxo-6-trifluoromethyl-quinoline *see* Flucarbril.

4-METHYL-2-OXOVALERIC ACID (α-ketoisocaproic acid).

METHYL PARABEN (methyl *p*-hydroxy-benzoate; 'metagin', 'methyl parasept', 'methyltegosept', 'nipagin M', 'methyl-butex', 'solbrol').

Methylparafynol* *see* Methylpentynol.

'Methyl parasept' *see* Methyl paraben.

Methyl parathion *see* Parathion methyl.

Methyl partricin *see* Mepartricin.

3-Methyl-2,4-pentanediol dicarbamate *see* Pentabamate.

4-Methyl-3-penten-2-one (1-phthalazinyl)-hydrazone *see* Budralazine.

N-Methyl-*p*-pentylamphetamine *see* Amfepentorex.

3-Methyl-3-pentyl carbamate *see* Emyl-camate.

METHYLPENTYNOL* (3-methyl-1-pentyn-3-ol; ethyl ethynyl methyl car-binol; 2-ethynyl-2-butanol; 1-ethyl-1-methyl-2-propyn-1-ol; (1-hydroxy-1-methylpropyl)acetylene; methylpara-fynol; meparfynol).

Methylpentynol phthalate *see* Ftalofyne.

Methylperidide *see* Meperidide.

Methylperidol *see* Moperone.

Methylperone* *see* Melperone.

10-Methylphenazin-1-one *see* Pyocyanine.

α-Methylphenethylamine *see* Amphetamine; Dexamphetamine; Levamfetamine.

9-[2-(α-Methylphenethylamino)ethyl]-acridine *see* Acridorex.

4-[2-(α-Methylphenethylamino)ethyl]-morpholine *see* Morforex.

7-[2-(α-Methylphenethylamino)ethyl]-theophylline *see* Fenetylline.

2-(α-Methylphenethylamino)-2-phenyl-acetonitrile *see* Amphetaminil.

3-(α-Methylphenethylamino)propio-nitrile *see* Fenproporex.

N-[2-(*N*-Methylphenethylamino)propyl]-propionanilide *see* Diampromide.

N-(α-Methylphenethyl)formamide *see* Formetorex.

α-Methylphenethylhydrazine *see* Pheni-prazine.

(3α-Methylphenethyl)-*N*-(phenylcarba-moyl)sydnone imine *see* Mesocarb.

N-(α-Methylphenethyl)thioxanthene-9-ethylamine *see* Tixadil.

(−)-1-(α-Methylphenethyl)-3-(*p*-tolyl-sulfonyl)urea *see* Tosifen.

302

Methylphenetoin *see* Mephenytoin.
METHYLPHENIDATE*** (methyl α-phenyl-2-piperidineacetate; methyl 2-phenyl-2-piperid-2-ylacetate; methylphenidylacetate; phenidylate; methylphenidate hydrochloride; C-4311/b; meridil; 'ritalin').
Methylphenidylacetate* *see* Methylphenidate.
METHYLPHENOBARBITAL*** (5-ethyl-1-methyl-5-phenylbarbituric acid; *N*-methylphenobarbital; methylphenobarbitone; mephobarbital; enphenemal; phemitone; 'isonal', 'mebaral', 'prominal').
Methylphenol(s) *see* Cresol(s).
10-Methylphenothiazin-2-ylacetic acid *see* Metiazinic acid.
1-Methyl-1-(1-phenothiazin-2-ylcarbonylethyl)pyrrolidinium bromide *see* Propyromazine.
[1-Methyl-2-(phenothiazin-10-yl)ethyl]-trimethylammonium ion *see* Thiazinamium.
N-(1-Methyl-2-phenoxyethyl)amphetamine *see* Dextrofemine; Racefemine.
1-(1-Methyl-2-phenoxyethyl)hydrazine *see* Fenoxypropazine.
(1-Methyl-1-phenoxyethyl)penicillin *see* Isopropicillin.
(α-Methylphenoxymethyl)penicillin *see* Pheneticillin.
3-(o-Methylphenoxy)-1,2-propanediol *see* Mephenesin.
2-METHYL-2-PHENOXYPROPIONIC ACID (2-phenoxyisobutyric acid).
2-Methyl-2-phenoxypropionic acid 2-morpholinoethyl ester *see* Promolate.
Methylphensuximide *see* Mesuximide.
2-Methyl-2-phenylacetic acid *see* Hydratropic acid.
1-Methyl-4-phenylazacycloheptane-4-carboxylic acid ethyl ester *see* Ethoheptazine.
5-Methyl-5-phenylbarbituric acid *see* Mephebarbital.
3-Methyl-4-phenyl-3-butenoic acid *see* 3-Benzylidenebutyric acid.
METHYL PHENYLDIAZENECARBOXYLATE (azoester).
Methyl phenyl ether *see* Anisole.
7-[2-(1-Methyl-2-phenylethylamino)-ethyl]theophylline *see* Fenetylline.
2-[(1-Methyl-2-phenylethyl)amino]-2-phenylacetonitrile *see* Amphetaminil.
1-Methyl-4-phenylhexamethylenimine-4-carboxylic acid ethyl ester *see* Ethoheptazine.
(5-Methyl-3-phenyl-4-isoxazolyl)penicillin *see* Oxacillin.
3-Methyl-2-phenylmorpholine *see* Phenmetrazine.
2-(Methylphenylmorpholino)ethyl phenylbutyrate *see* Fenbutrazate.
4-(3-Methyl-2-phenylmorpholinomethyl)-antipyrine *see* Morazone.
4-(3-Methyl-2-phenylmorpholinomethyl)-phenazone *see* Morazone.

5-Methyl-6-phenyl-3-morpholinone *see* Fenmetramide.
(−)-N-(p-Methyl-α-phenylphenethyl)-linoleamide *see* Moctamide.
Methyl α-phenyl-2-piperidineacetate *see* Methylphenidate.
5-Methyl-4-phenyl-1-piperid-1-yl-3-hexanol *see* Piperphenidol.
N-Methyl-N-(1-phenylprop-2-yl)-2-furfurylamine *see* Furfenorex.
1-(1-Methyl-3-phenylpropyl)hydrazine *see* Phenylisobutylhydrazine.
3-Methyl-5-phenylpyrazole *see* Phemerazole.
3-METHYL-1-PHENYLPYRAZOL-5-YL DIMETHYLCARBAMATE (G-22008; 'pyrolan').
N¹-(3-Methyl-1-phenylpyrazol-5-yl)-sulfanilamide *see* Sulfapyrazole.
N¹-(5-Methyl-2-phenylpyrazol-3-yl)-sulfanilamide *see* Sulfapyrazole.
4-[2-[(4-Methyl-6-phenylpyridazin-3-yl)-amino]ethyl]morpholine *see* Minaprine.
5-Methyl-1-phenylpyridin-2(1H)-one *see* Pirfenidone.
N-Methyl-2-phenylsuccinimide *see* Phensuximide.
Methyl 5-(phenylsulfinyl)-2-benzimidazolecarbamate *see* Oxfendazole.
Methyl-5-(phenylthio)-2-benzimidazolecarbamate *see* Fenbendazole.
1-Methyl-5-phenyl-7-trifluoromethyl-1H-1,5-benzodiazepine-2,4-(3H,5)-dione *see* Triflubazam.
N-Methyl-3-phenyl-3-[p-(trifluoromethyl)-phenoxy]propylamine *see* Fluoxetine.
N-Methyl-3-phenyl-3-[(α,α,α-trifluoro-p-tolyl)oxy]propylamine *see* Fluoxetine.
METHYLPHENYTOIN (3-methyl-5,5-diphenylhydantoin; 'melantoin').
Methylphosphoramidic acid [2-chloro-4-(1,1-dimethylethyl)phenyl] methyl ester *see* Crufomate.
Methyl phthalate *see* Dimethyl phthalate.
2-Methyl-3-phytyl-1,4-naphthalenediol *see* Phytonadiol.
2-Methyl-3-phytyl-1,4-naphthalenedione *see* Phytomenadione.
2-Methyl-3-phytyl-1,4-naphthoquinone *see* Phytomenadione.
N-Methyl-N-(3-picolyl)tropamide *see* Pimetremide.
4-Methyl-1-piperazineacetic acid (5-nitrofurfurylidene)hydrazide *see* Nifurpipone.
1-[2-(4-Methylpiperazin-1-yl)acetyl]-2-(5-nitrifurfurylidene)hydrazine *see* Nifurpipone.
(4-Methylpiperazin-1-ylcarbonyl)cyclohexane *see* Pexantel.
21-(4-Methylpiperazin-1-yl)deprodone *see* Mazipredone.
6-(4-Methylpiperazin-2-yl)dibenz(b,e)-azepine *see* Perlapine.
2-(4-Methylpiperazin-1-yl)ethyl 2-trifluoromethylphenothiazin-10-yl ketone *see* Ftormetazine.
3-(4-Methylpiperazin-1-yliminomethyl)-

303

rifamycin SV *see* Rifampicin.
6-(4-Methylpiperazin-1-yl)morphanthridine *see* Perlapine.
10-[3-(4-Methylpiperazin-1-yl)propionyl]-2-trifluoromethylphenothiazine *see* Ftormetazine.
10-[3-(4-Methylpiperazin-1-yl)propyl]-phenothiazine *see* Perazine.
10-[3-(4-Methylpiperazin-1-yl)propyl]-2-propionylphenothiazine *see* Propionylperazine.
1-[10-[3-(4-Methylpiperazin-1-yl)propyl]-phenothiazin-2-yl]-1-butanone *see* Butaperazine.
10-[3-(4-Methylpiperazin-1-yl)propyl]-2-trifluoromethylphenothiazine *see* Trifluperazine.
2-Methylpiperidine *see* 2-Pipecoline.
2-Methyl-1-piperidinepropanol benzoate *see* Piperocaine.
1-Methyl-4-piperidinol ester of 2,2-bis-(p-chlorophenoxy)acetic acid *see* Lifibrate.
5-(1-Methyl-4-piperidinylidene)-5H-(1)-benzopyrano(2,3-b)pyridine *see* Azanator.
1-Methylpiperid-3-yl benzilate methobromide *see* Mepenzolate.
1-Methylpiperid-4-yl p-butylaminobenzoate *see* Paridocaine.
1-Methylpiperid-3-yl cyclohexaneglycolate *see* Oxyclipine.
1-Methylpiperid-3-yl cyclohexylmandelate *see* Propenzolate.
2-Methyl-3-[p-(2-piperid-1-ylethoxy)-anilino]phthalimidine *see* Omidoline.
Methyl o-[p-(2-piperid-1-ylethoxy)-benzoyl]benzoate *see* Pitofenone.
2-(4-Methylpiperid-1-yl)ethyl 6-ethyl-2,3,6,9-tetrahydro-3-methyl-2,9-dioxo-thiazolo(5,4-f)quinoline-8-carboxylate *see* Metioxate.
10-[2-(1-Methylpiperid-2-yl)ethyl]-2-(methylsulfinyl)phenothiazine *see* Mesoridazine.
10-[2-(1-Methylpiperid-2-yl)ethyl]-2-methylsulfonylphenothiazine *see* Sulforidazine.
10[2-(1-Methylpiperid-2-yl)ethyl]-2-(methylthio)phenothiazine *see* Thioridazine.
N-**[2-(1-Methylpiperid-2-yl)ethyl]propion-anilide** *see* Phenampromide.
N-**(1-Methyl-2-piperid-1-ylethyl)-N-pyrid-2-ylpropionamide** *see* Propiram.
Methylpiperid-4-yl glyoxylate 2-[bis-(p-chlorophenyl)acetal] *see* Lifibrate.
5-(1-Methyl-4-piperidylidene)-5H-(1)-benzopyrano(2,3-b)pyridine *see* Azanator.
1-Methylpiperid-3-ylidenedithien-2-yl-methane *see* Tipepidine.
9-(N-Methyl-4-piperidylidene)thioxanthene *see* Pimethixene.
1-Methylpiperid-4-yl 3-methyl-2-phenyl-valerate *see* Pentapiperide.
10-(1-Methylpiperid-3-ylmethyl)phenothiazine *see* Pecazine.

9-(1-Methylpiperid-3-ylmethyl)thioxanthene *see* Metixene.
2-Methyl-3-(β-piperid-1-yl-p-phenetidino)-phthalimidine *see* Omidoline.
N-**(1-Methylpiperid-4-yl)-N-phenyl-benzylamine** *see* Bamipine.
1-Methylpiperid-3-yl α-phenylcyclohex-aneglycolate *see* Oxyclipine.
D-(+)-**2-(1-Methylpiperid-2-yl)-2-propanol diphenylacetate** *see* Pinolcaine.
3-(2-Methylpiperid-1-yl)propyl benzoate *see* Piperocaine.
3-(2-Methylpiperid-1-yl)propyl p-cyclo-hexylbenzoate *see* Cyclomethycaine.
2-Methyl-3-piperid-1-ylpyrazine *see* Modaline.
2-Methyl-3-piperid-1-yl-1-(p-tolyl)-1-propanone *see* Tolperisone.
Methylpolysiloxane *see* Dimeticone.
7-Methyl 21-potassium 17-hydroxy-3-oxo-17α-pregn-4-ene-7α,21-dicarboxylate *see* Mexrenoate potassium.
METHYLPREDNISOLONE* (6α-methyl-prednisolone; 6α-methylpregna-1,4-diene-11β,17α,21-triol-3,20-dione; 11β,17α,21-tri-hydroxy-6α-methylpregna-1,4-diene-3,20-dione; NSC-19987; 'medrol', 'medrone', 'mesopren', 'metrisone', 'urbason').
6α-Methylprednisolone *see* Methylpredni-solone.
METHYLPREDNISOLONE ACETATE ('depo-medrol', 'depo-medrone').
METHYLPREDNISOLONE SODIUM SUCCINATE ('solu-medrol').
16β-Methylprednisone *see* Meprednisone.
16β-Methylpregna-1,4-diene-17α,21-diol-3-one *see* Meprednisone.
6α-Methylpregna-1,4-diene-11β,17α,21-triol-3,20-dione *see* Methylprednisolone.
6α-Methylpregna-1,4-dien-11β-ol-3,20-dione *see* Endrisone.
6-Methylpregna-4,6-dien-17α-ol-3,20-dione *see* Megestrol.
6α-Methylpregn-4-en-11β-ol-3,20-dione *see* Medrysone.
6α-Methylpregn-4-en-17α-ol-3,20-dione *see* Medroxyprogesterone.
6α-Methylpregn-4-en-17-ol-20-one *see* Anagestone.
Methylpregnone *see* Medroxyprogesterone.
N-**Methylproline choline ester iodide methiodide** *see* Trepirium iodide.
Methylpromazine *see* Alimemazine.
2-METHYL-1-PROPANOL (isobutyl alcohol).
2-METHYL-2-PROPANOL (tert-butyl alcohol).
N-**Methyl-N-propargylbenzylamine** *see* Pargyline.
2-Methyl-2-propenoic acid *see* Methacrylic acid.
p-(1-Methylpropenyl)phenyl acetate *see* Fenabutene.
Methylpropiolic acid *see* Tetrolic acid.
2-Methylpropionic acid *see* Isobutyric acid.
Methyl 5-propoxy-2-benzimidazole-carbamate *see* Oxibendazole.

N-**Methylpropranolol methochloride** *see*
Pranolium chloride.
2-Methyl-2-propylamino-*o*-acetotoluidide
see Prilocaine.
α-**(1-Methylpropylaminomethyl)-5,6,7,8-**
tetrahydro-2-naphthalenemethanol
see Butidrine.
4-Methyl-3-(2-propylaminopropion-
amido)-2-thiophenecarboxylic acid
methyl ester *see* Carticaine.
o-**Methyl-α-propylaminopropionanilide**
see Prilocaine.
2′-Methyl-2-propylaminopropionanilide
see Prilocaine.
2-Methyl-2-propylamino-*o*-propionotol-
uidide *see* Quatacaine.
2-Methyl-2-propylaminopropyl benzoate
see Meprylcaine.
2-(1-Methylpropylamino)-1-(5,6,7,8-tetra-
hydronaphth-2-yl)ethanol *see* Butidrine.
Methyl propyl carbinol carbamate *see*
Hedonal.
N-**[1-Methyl-2-(*N*-propylcarboxamido)-**
ethyl]-*p*-phenetidine *see* Etapromide.
6-(1-Methylpropyl)-2,4-dinitrophenol *see*
Dinoseb.
2-(1-Methylpropyl)-4,6-dinitrophenyl
3-methyl-2-butenoate *see* Binapacryl.
METHYL PROPYL ETHER ('metopryl',
'neothyl').
2-METHYL-2-PROPYL-1,3-PROPANE-
DIOL (2-hydroxymethyl-2-methyl-1-
pentanol).
m-**(1-Methyl-3-propylpyrrolidin-3-yl)-**
phenol *see* Profadol.
6-METHYL-2-PROPYLPYRIMID-4-YL
N,*N*-**DIMETHYLCARBAMATE**
('pyramat').
Methyl 5-(propylthio)benzimidazole-2-
carbamate *see* Albendazole.
5-Methyl-5-propyl-2-*p*-tolyl-1,3,2-dioxa-
borinane *see* Tolboxane.
8-Methyl-*O*-(2-propylvaleryl)tropinium
bromide *see* Octatropine methyl bromide.
N-**Methyl-*N*-(2-propynyl)benzylamine**
see Pargyline.
1-Methylprop-2-ynyl *m*-chlorocarbanilate
see Chlorbufam.
1-Methyl-2-propynyl 3-chlorophenyl-
carbamate *see* Chlorbufam.
[2-Methyl-5-(2-propynyl)furan-3-yl]-
methyl 2,2-dimethyl-3-(2-methyl-1-
propenyl)cyclopropanecarboxylate
see Prothrin.
2-Methyl-5-prop-2-ynyl-3-furylmethyl
chrysanthemate *see* Prothrin.
4′-*O*-Methylproscillaridin *see* Rambufaside.
5-Methylpyrazinecarboxylic acid 4-oxide
see Acipimox.
1-[2-(5-Methylpyrazol-3-yl)ethyl]-4-*m*-
tolylpiperazine *see* Tolpiprazole.
Methylpyridine *see* Picoline.
1-Methyl-5-pyrid-3-ylpyrrolidin-2-one
see Cotinine.
N[1]-**(4-Methylpyrimidin-2-yl) sulfanil-**
amide *see* Sulfamerazine.
N[1]-**(5-Methylpyrimidin-2-yl) sulfanil-**

amide *see* Sulfaperin.
1-Methylpyrrolidine-2-carboxylic acid
dimethylaminoethyl ester dimeth-
iodide *see* Hygronium.
1-Methyl-3-pyrrolidinemethanol benzilate
ester *see* Triclazate.
2-Methyl-2-pyrrolidin-1-yl-*o*-acetotolui-
dide *see* Aptocaine.
1-Methylpyrrolidin-3-ylmethyl benzilate
see Triclazate.
1-Methylpyrrolidin-2-ylmethyl benzilate
methosulfate *see* Poldine metilsulfate.
1-Methylpyrrolidin-2-ylmethyl bis(*p*-
chlorophenoxy)acetate *see* Biclofibrate.
1-(2-Methylpyrrolidin-3-ylmethyl)-3-
phenylindan *see* Pyrophendane.
10-(1-Methylpyrrolidin-3-yl)phenothi-
azine *see* Methdilazine.
2′-Methyl-2-pyrrolidin-1-ylpropion-
anilide *see* Aptocaine.
10-[2-(1-Methylpyrrolidin-1-yl)propion-
yl]phenothiazine *see* Propyromazine.
3-(1-Methylpyrrolidin-2-yl)pyridine *see*
Nicotine.
4′-Methyl-2-pyrrolidin-1-ylvalerophenone
see Pyrovalerone.
Methylquinazolone *see* Methaqualone.
6-Methyl-8-quinolinol bismuth hydroxide
compound *see* Mebiquine.
3-Methylquinoxaline-2-carboxylic acid
2,4-dioxide 2-hydroxyethyl ester *see*
Temodox.
3-Methylquinoxaline-2-carboxylic acid
hydrazide 1,4-dioxide *see* Drazidox.
6-Methyl-2,3-quinoxalinedithiol cyclic
S,*S*-**dithiocarbonate** *see* Chinomethionat.
3-Methyl-2-quinoxalinemethanol 1,4-di-
oxide *see* Mequidox.
Methyl 3-(2-quinoxalinylmethylene)-
carbazoate *N*[1],*N*[4]-**dioxide** *see* Carbadox.
Methyl reserpate esters *see* Mefeserpine;
Rescinnamine; Reserpine; Syrosingopine.
5-Methylresorcinol *see* Orcinol.
Methylrosaniline chloride*** *see* Crystal
violet.
3-Methylsalicylamide *see* Cresotamide.
METHYL SALICYLATE (Betula oil;
Gaultheria oil; oil of wintergreen; sweet
birch oil; teaberry oil).
3-Methylsalicylic acid *see* Hydroxytoluic
acid.
5-Methylsalicylic acid *see* 2,5-Cresotic acid.
Methyl scopolamine nitrate* *see* Scopolamine methyl nitrate.
24-Methyl-9,10-secocholesta-5,7,10(19),22-
tetraen-3β-ol *see* Ergocholesterol.
24-Methyl-9,10-secocholesta-5,7,22-trien-
3β-ol *see* Dihydrotachysterol.
Methyl serpentinate *see* Serpentine.
Methylstanazole *see* Stanozolol.
10-Methylstearic acid *see* Tuberculostearic
acid.
Methyl styryl ketone *see* Benzylideneacetone.
2-Methylsulfadiazine *see* Sulfamerazine.
5-Methylsulfadiazine *see* Sulfaperin.
Methyl sulfanilylcarbamate *see* Asulam.

Methylsulfapyrimidine *see* Sulfamerazine.
Methyl sulfate(s) *see* Metilsulfate(s).
Methylsulfazine (tr) *see* Sulfamerazine.
2-(Methylsulfinylacetyl)pyridine *see* Oxisuran.
Methylsulfinylmethyl 2-pyridyl ketone *see* Oxisuran.
METHYLSULFONAL (2,2-bis(ethylsulfonyl)butane; bis(ethylsulfonyl)ethylmethylmethane; sulfonethylmethane; ethylsulfonal; 'trional').
4-Methylsulfonyl-2,6-dinitro-*N*,*N*-dipropylaniline *see* Nitralin.
6-[(*R*)-2-[3-(Methylsulfonyl)-2-oxo-1-imidazolidinecarboxamido]-2-phenylacetamido]penicillanic acid *see* Mezlocillin.
1-[3-(2-Methylsulfonylphenothiazin-10-yl)propyl]isonipecotamide *see* Metopimazine.
2-[*p*-(Methylsulfonyl)phenyl]imidazole-(1,2-a)pyridine *see* Zolimidine.
Methyl sulfoxide *see* Dimethyl sulfoxide.
'Methylsympatol' *see* *p*-Hydroxyephedrine.
Methyl-systox (tr) *see* Demeton-O-methyl plus demeton-S-methyl.
'Methyl tegosept' *see* Methyl paraben.
METHYLTESTOSTERONE*** (17β-hydroxy-17α-methylandrost-4-en-3-one; 17α-methylandrost-4-en-17β-ol-3-one; 17-methyltestosterone).
(−)-2-Methyl-3′-(2,3,5,6-tetrahydroimidazo(2,1-b)thiazol-6-yl)propionanilide *see* Butamisole.
trans-**3-Methyl-2-[2-(1,4,6-tetrahydro-1-methylpyrimid-2-yl)vinyl]thiophene** *see* Morantel.
2-Methyl-2-[*p*-(1,2,3,4-tetrahydronaphth-1-yl)phenoxy]propionic acid *see* Nafenopin.
Methyl tetrahydronicotinate *see* Guvacoline.
3-Methyl-7-[2-[*p*-(1,4,5,6-tetrahydropyrimidin-2-yl)phenyl]acetamido]-2-cephem-2-carboxylic acid *see* Cefrotil.
2-Methyl-3-(3,7,11,15-tetramethylhexadecatetraenyl)-1,4-naphthoquinone *see* Menatetrenone.
2-Methyl-3-*all-trans*-tetraprenyl-1,4-naphthoquinone *see* Farnoquinone.
N¹-(5-Methyl-1,3,4-thiadiazol-2-yl)-sulfanilamide *see* Sulfamethizole.
3-[[(5-Methyl-1,3,4-thiadiazol-2-yl)thio]-methyl]-7-[2-(1H-tetrazol-1-yl)acetamido]-2-cephem-2-carboxylic acid *see* Cefazolin.
1-(4-Methylthiazol-2-yl)-4-(3-piperonylprop-2-yl)piperazine *see* Podilfen.
N¹-(4-Methylthiazol-2-yl)sulfanilamide *see* Sulfamethylthiazole.
Methylthiazothion *see* Azinphos-methyl.
α-Methyl-4-(2-thienylcarbonyl)benzeneacetic acid *see* Suprofen.
6-Methylthiochroman-7-sulfonamide 1,1-dioxide *see* Meticrane.
7-[2-(METHYLTHIO) ETHYL]THEOPHYLLINE ('metet').

3-Methyl-2-thioimidazoline-1-carboxylic acid ethyl ester *see* Carbimazole.
5-(Methylthiomethyl)-3-(5-nitrofurfurylideneamino)-2-oxazolidinone *see* Nifuratel.
Methylthioninium chloride*** *see* Methylene blue.
Methyl thiophanate *see* Thiophanate methyl.
6-(METHYLTHIO)PURINE (6-methyl-MP; NSC-20105).
6-(METHYLTHIO)PURINE RIBOSIDE (6-methylmercaptopurine riboside; NSC-40774).
3-(Methylthio)-5-(4,5,6-trichlorobenzimidazol-2-ylthio)-1,2,4-thiadiazole *see* Subendazole.
METHYLTHIOURACIL*** (6-methyl-2-thiouracil; 4-methyl-2-thiouracil; MTU).
4(5)-[4-(3-Methylthioureido)butyl]-imidazole *see* Burimamide.
5-Methyl-4-[[[2-(2-thioureido)ethyl]-thio]methyl]imidazole *see* Metiamide.
α-Methyl-*N*-(2-thioxanthen-9-ylethyl)-phenethylamine *see* Tixadil.
1-Methyl-4-(thioxanthen-9-ylidene)-piperidine *see* Pimethixene.
1-Methyl-3-thioxanthen-9-ylmethyl-piperidine *see* Metixene.
4-Methylthio-3,5-xylyl methylcarbamate *see* Methiocarb.
α-Methyl-DL-thyroxine ethyl ester *see* Etiroxate.
1-Methyl-5-*p*-toluoylpyrrole-2-acetic acid *see* Tolmetin.
1-Methyl-2-*o*-tolylethylamine *see* Ortetamine.
5-Methyl-3-[2-(4-*m*-tolylpiperazin-1-yl)-ethyl]pyrazole *see* Tolpiprazole.
β-Methyl-γ-(*p*-tolyl)-1-piperidinepropanone *see* Tolperisone.
2-Methyl-3-(*o*-tolyl)-4-quinazolinone *see* Methaqualone.
(−)-α-Methyl-*N*-[(*p*-tolylsulfonyl)carbamoyl]phenethylamine *see* Tosifen.
N-Methyl-*N*-(*m*-tolyl)thionocarbamic acid 2-naphthyl ester *see* Tolnaftate.
Methyl 3,5,6-tri-*O*-benzyl-D-glucofuranoside *see* Mebenoside.
α-Methyl-*N*-(2,2,2-trichloroethylidene)-phenethylamine *see* Amfechloral.
2-Methyl-4-(2,2,2-trichloro-1-hydroxyethoxy)-2-pentanol *see* Chloralodol.
1-Methyl-3-(2,2,2-trichloro-1-hydroxyethyl)urea *see* Mecloralurea.
Methyltrienolone *see* Metribolone.
2-(2-Methyl-3-trifluoromethylanilino)-nicotinic acid *see* Flunixin.
2-[[α-Methyl-*m*-(trifluoromethyl)phenethyl]amino]ethanol benzoate *see* Benfluorex.
α-[[α-Methyl-*m*-(trifluoromethyl)phenethyl]carbamoyl]-*p*-acetanisidide *see* Flucetorex.
p-[[[α-Methyl-*m*-(trifluoromethyl)phenethyl]carbamoyl]methoxy]acetanilide *see* Flucetorex.

2-[[2-Methyl-3-(trifluoromethyl)phenyl]-amino]-3-pyridinecarboxylic acid *see* Flunixin.

1-Methyl-2-trifluoromethyl-6-quinolinone *see* Flucarbril.

4-[[2-Methyl-2-(3,4,5-trimethoxyphenyl)-1,3-dioxolan-4-yl]methyl]morpholine *see* Trioxolane.

Methyl 11,17α,18α-trimethoxy-3β,20α-yohimban-16β-carboxylate *see* Metoserpate.

2-Methyl-2-(4′,8′,12-trimethyltrideca-3,7,11-trienyl)-6-chromanol *see* Tocotrienol.

'Methyltrithion' *see* Carbofenotion methyl.

Methyltropic acid tropine ester *see* Levomepate.

Methyltropinium bromide propylvalerate *see* Octatropine methyl bromide.

8-Methyltropinium bromide xanthene-9-carboxylate *see* Trantelinium bromide.

2-METHYLTRYPTAMINE (α-methyltryptamine: indopan).

N-METHYLTRYPTOPHAN (abrine).

'Methyl tuads' *see* Thiram.

α-Methyltyramine *see* Hydroxyamphetamine.

α-METHYL-m-TYRAMINE (m-(2-aminopropyl)phenol).

(−)-α-Methyl-L-tyrosine *see* Metirosine.

4-Methylumbelliferone *see* Hymecromone.

5-Methyluracil *see* Thymine.

Methyl urethan *see* Methyl carbamate.

Methyl vinyl ether polymer with maleic acid, iron salt *see* Ferropolimaler.

METHYL VIOLET* (mixture of hydrochlorides of (chiefly)tetra-, penta- and hexamethylparasosanilines). *See also* Crystal violet.

Methyl viologen *see* Paraquat.

β-METHYLXYLOCHOLINE ([2-(2,6-dimethylphenoxy)propyl]trimethylammonium chloride hydrate; β-methylcholine 2,6-xylyl ether chloride; β-TM-10; SK&F-6890).

1-Methyl-2-(2,6-xylylcarbamoyl)piperidine *see* Mepivacaine.

1-Methyl-2-(2,6-xylyloxy)ethylamine *see* Mexiletine.

1-Methylyohimbane *see* Mimbane.

Methyl yohimbate *see* Yohimbine.

Methynodiol diacetate* *see* Metynodiol diacetate.

Methypregnone* *see* Medroxyprogesterone.

METHYPRYLON*** (3,3-diethyl-5-methyl-2,4-piperidinedione; dimerin; Ro-1-6463; 'doseval', 'noctan', 'noludar').

Methyridine* *see* Metyridine.

'Methyrit' *see* Chlorpheniramine maleate.

METHYSERGIDE*** (N-(1-hydroxymethylpropyl)-1-methyl-D-lysergamide; 1-methyllysergic acid butanolamide; dimethylergometrine; dimethylergonovine; methysergide tartrate; UML-491; 'deseril', 'desernil', 'sansert').

METHYSTICIN (5,6-dihydro-4-methoxy-6-(3,4-methylenedioxystyryl)-2-pyrone; methylenedioxykavain; kavahin; kavatin).

Methyzazone* *see* Metisazone.

METIAMIDE** (1-methyl-3-[2-[(5-methylimidazol-4-ylmethyl)thio]ethyl]-2-thiourea; 5-methyl-4-[[[2-(2-thioureido)ethyl]thio]methyl]imidazole).

METIAPINE*** (2-methyl-11-(4-methylpiperazin-1-yl)dibenzo(b,f)(1,4)thiazepine).

METIAZINIC ACID*** (2-(carboxymethyl)-10-methylphenothiazine; 10-methylphenothiazin-2-ylacetic acid; 10-methylphenothiazine-2-acetic acid; FI-6642; 'soridermal', 'soripal').

METICILLIN** (6-(2,6-dimethoxybenzamido)penicillanic acid; dimethoxyphenyl penicillin; dimethoxyphenecillin; methicillin; sodium methicillin; meticillin sodium; penicillin X-1497; BRL-1241; SQ-16123; 'belfacillin', 'celbenin', 'cepillina', 'cinopenil', 'dimocillin', 'flabellin', 'lucopenin', 'penistaph', 'stafylopenin', 'staphcillin', 'synticillin').

Meticillin 2-diethylaminoethyl ester *see* Tameticillin.

Meticlorpindol *see* Clopidol.

METICRANE*** (6-methylthiochroman-7-sulfonamide 1,1-dioxide; thiachromane; 'fontilix').

'Metifex' *see* Ethacridine lactate.

'Metiguanide' *see* Metformin.

'Metilar' *see* Paramethasone.

Metil-merkaptofos (tr) *see* Demeton-O-methyl.

Metilmerkaptosoksid (tr) *see* Oxydemeton-methyl.

Metil-merkaptofos tiolovyj (tr) *see* Demeton-S-methyl.

METILSULFATE(S)** (methyl sulfate(s)).

Metiltriazotion (tr) *see* Azinphos-methyl.

METINDIONE (tr) (2-ethyl-2-methylaminoindan-1,3-dione; methindione; metindione hydrochloride).

METINDIZATE*** (2-(hexahydro-1-methylindolin-3-yl)ethyl benzilate).

'Metindol' *see* Indometacin.

Metiodol* *see* Methiodal.

'Metione' *see* Methionine.

METIOXATE** (2-(4-methylpiperid-1-yl)-ethyl 6-ethyl-2,3,6,9-tetrahydro-3-methyl-2,9-dioxothiazolo(5,4-f)quinoline-8-carboxylate; tioxacin 2-(4-methylpiperid-1-yl)-ethyl ester).

METIPIROX*** (1-hydroxy-4,6-dimethylpyridin-2-(1H)-one).

METIPRENALINE*** (4-hydroxy-α-isopropylaminomethyl-3-methoxybenzyl alcohol; α-isopropylaminomethylvanillyl alcohol).

METIROSINE** ((−)-α-methyl-L-tyrosine; H 9/88).

METIROSINE METHYL ESTER (H 44/68).

METISAZONE*** (N-methylisatin thiosemicarbazone; 1-methylindolin-2,3-dione 3-thiosemicarbazone; methisazone; methyzazone; BW-33T57; 'marboran').

METITEPINE** (1-[10,11-dihydro-8-(methylthio)dibenzo(b,f)thiepin-10-yl]-4-methylpiperazine; 10,11-dihydro-10-(4-methylpiperazin-1-yl)-8-(methylthio)-dibenzo(b,f)thiepin; methiothepin).

METIXENE*** (9-(1-methylpiperid-3-yl-methyl)thioxanthene; 1-methyl-3-(thio-xanthen-9-ylmethyl)piperidine; methixene; methixene hydrochloride; SJ-1977; 'tremaril', 'tremonil', 'trest').

METIXINE WITH NOVAMINSULFON ('dorsedin').

'Metizol' *see* Thiamazole.

METIZOLINE*** (2-(2-methylbenzo(b)-thien-3-ylmethyl)imidazoline; 3-(2-imida-zolin-2-ylmethyl)-2-methylbenzo(b)thio-phene; benazoline; benazoline hydro-chloride; metyzoline; EX-10-781; 'elsyl', 'eunasin').

Metmercapturan *see* Methiocarb.

METOBROMURON (1-(p-bromophenyl)-3-methoxy-3-methylurea; 'patoron').

METOCHALCONE*** (2′,4,4′-trimethoxy-chalcone; CB-1314; 'neocolan', 'vesidryl').

METOCINIUM IODIDE** ((2-hydroxy-ethyl)trimethylammonium iodide benzilate; choline iodide benzilate; choline benzilate).

METOCLOPRAMIDE*** (4-amino-5-chloro-N-(2-diethylaminoethyl)-2-methoxy-benzamide; 4-amino-5-chloro-N-(2-diethyl-aminoethyl)-o-anisamide; 5-chloro-2-methoxyprocainamide; metoclopramide di-hydrochloride; AHR-3070-C; MK-745; 'maxolon', 'paspertin', 'plasil', 'primperan', 'reglan', 'rimetin', 'sinemet').

METOCLOPRAMIDE WITH MEDAZEPAM ('randum').

METODICLOROFEN (2,4-diamino-5-(3,4-dichlorophenyl)-6-methylpyrimidine; methodichlorophen; DDMP; BW-50197; NSC-19494; SK-5265).

'Metodril' *see* Methaqualone with di-phenhydramine.

METOFENAZATE*** (2-chloro-10-[3-[4-(2-(3,4,5-trimethoxybenzoyloxy)ethyl)piper-azin-1-yl]propyl]phenothiazine; 2-[4-[3-(2-chlorophenothiazin-10-yl)propyl]piper-azin-1-yl]ethyl 3,4,5-trimethoxybenzoate; 1-[3-(2-chlorophenothiazin-10-yl)propyl]-4-[2-(3,4,5-trimethoxybenzoyloxy)ethyl]-piperazine; methophenazine; 'frenolon').

METOFOLINE** (1-(p-chlorophenethyl)-1,2,3,4-tetrahydro-6,7-dimethoxy-2-methyl-isoquinoline; methopholine; ARC-I-K-1; I-K-1; NIH-7672; Ro-4-1778/1; 'versid-yne').

Metofurone* *see* Nifurmerone.

METOGEST*** (17β-hydroxy-16,16-di-methylestr-4-en-3-one; 16,16-dimethylestr-4-en-17β-ol-3-one; SC-14207.

METOLAZONE*** (7-chloro-1,2,3,4-tetra-hydro-2-methyl-4-oxo-3-o-tolyl-6-quin-azolinesulfonamide; SR-720-22; 'zaroxo-lyn').

METOMIDATE*** (methyl 1-(α-methyl-benzyl)imidazole-5-carboxylate; R-7315; 'hypnodil').

METOPIMAZINE*** (1-[3-(2-methyl-sulfonylphenothiazin-10-yl)propyl]isonipe-cotamide; 10-[3-(4-carboxamidopiperid-4-yl)propyl]-2-methylsulfonylphenothiazine; 10-[3-(4-carbamoylpiperid-1-yl)propyl]-2-methanesulfonylphenothiazine; EXP-999; RP-9965; 'vogalene').

'Metopirone' *see* Metyrapone.

METOPON** (5-methyldihydromorphinone; 4,5-epoxy-3-hydroxy-5,N-dimethyl-6-oxo-morphinan; metopon hydrochloride; methopon).

METOPROLOL** ((±)-1-isopropylamino-3-[p-(2-methoxyethyl)phenoxy]-2-propan-ol; H-93/26; 'beloc', 'betaloc', 'lopresor', 'seloken').

METOPROLOL TARTRATE (metoprolol L-(+)-tartrate; CGP-2175).

'Metopryl' *see* Methyl propyl ether.

'Metopyrone' *see* Metyrapone.

METOQUIZINE*** (3,5-dimethyl-N-(4,6,6a,7,8,9,10,10a-octahydro-4,7-di-methylindolo(4,3-fg)quinolin-9-yl)pyrazole-1-carboxamide; 4,7-dimethyl-9-(3,5-di-methylpyrazole-1-carboxamido)-4,6,6a,7,8,9,10,10a-octahydroindolo(4,3-fg)quin-oline; L-42406).

Metorin (tr) *see* Fluanisone.

METOSERPATE*** (methyl O-methyl-18-epireserpate; methyl 18-epi-O-methyl-reserpate; methyl 18-epireserpate methyl ether; methyl 11,17α,18α-trimethoxy-3β,20α-yohimban-16β-carboxylate mono-hydrochloride; metoserpate hydrochloride; Su-9064; 'mepiserpate', 'pacitran').

'Metosine' *see* Fluocinonide.

'Metosyn' *see* Fluocinonide.

'Metox' *see* Methoxychlor.

METOXEPIN*** (1-(8-methoxydibenz(b,f)-oxepin-10-yl)-4-methylpiperazine; 8-meth-oxy-10-(4-methylpiperazin-1-yl)dibenz-(b,f)oxepin).

'Metoxon' *see* Chlorpropham.

Metoxuran *see* Metoxuron.

METOXURON* (1-(3-chloro-4-methoxy-phenyl)-3,3-dimethylurea; metoxuran; 'dosanex').

Metoxymarc *see* Anisuron.

METRAFAZOLINE*** (2-[(1,2,3,4-tetra-hydro-7-methyl-1,4-ethanonaphth-6-yl)-methyl]-2-imidazoline; 1,2,3,4-tetrahydro-6-(2-imidazolin-2-ylmethyl)-1,4-ethano-naphthalene).

'Metramas' *see* Amiton.

'Metramine' *see* Methenamine.

'Metrazole' *see* Pentetrazole.

Metriben *see* Tricamba.

METRIBOLONE*** (17-methylestra-4,9,11-trien-17β-ol-3-one; 17β-hydroxy-17-methylestra-4,9,11-trien-3-one; 17α-methyl-19-norandrosta-4,9,11-trien-17β-ol-3-one; 17β-hydroxy-17α-methyl-19-norandrosta-4,9,11-trien-3-one; methyltrienolone).

METRIBUZIN* (4-amino-6-tert-butyl-3-(methylthio)-1,2,4-triazin-5(4H)-one; 4-amino-6-(1,1-dimethylethyl)-3-(methyl-thio)-as-triazin-5(4H)-one; Bay-94337;

'sencor').

METRIFONATE*** (dimethyl (2,2,2-trichloro-1-hydroxyethyl)phosphonate; chlorofos; chlorophos; DETF; klorofos; phoschlorin; phosclorine; trichlorphon; trichlorophone; triclorfon; Bayer L-13/59; Bayer-2349; 'bilarcil', 'dipterex', 'dylox', 'foschlor', 'fosgran', 'fosgren', 'tugon').

Metrifonate butyrate *see* Butonate.

METRIFONATE PLUS OXYDEMETON-METHYL ('dipterex-ER').

METRIFONATE WITH ATROPINE ('neguvon').

METRIFONATE WITH ATROPINE AND PRALIDOXIME ('bubulin').

METRIFUDIL*** (6-(*o*-methylbenzylamino)-9-β-D-ribofuranosyl-9H-purine; *N*-(*o*-methylbenzyl)adenosine; 6-(*o*-methylbenzylamino)purine riboside).

'Metrisone' *see* Methylprednisolone.

METRIZAMIDE*** (2-[3-acetamido-2,4,6-triiodo-5-(*N*-methylacetamido)benzamido]-2-deoxy-D-glucose; 'amipaque').

METRIZOIC ACID* (3-acetamido-2,4,6-triiodo-5-(*N*-methylacetamido)benzoic acid).
See also Meglumine metrizoate; Sodium metrizoate.

METRIZOIC ACID SALTS WITH MEGLUMINE METRIZOATE ('ronpacon 440').

Metrogestone *see* Medrogestone.

'Metromin' *see* *N,N*-Dimethylamphetamine.

'Metron' *see* Parathion-methyl *and* Pheniramine.

METRONIDAZOLE*** (1-(2-hydroxyethyl)-2-methyl-5-nitroimidazole; 2-methyl-5-nitroimidazole-1-ethanol; Bayer-5360; RP-8823; 'clont', 'elyzol', 'flagyl', 'fossyol', 'klion', 'sanatrichom', 'trichex', 'trichomol', 'trichomonacid', 'trichopol').

METRONIDAZOLE BENZOATE (benzoylmetronidazole; RP-9712; 'benzoyl-flagyl').

METRONIDAZOLE WITH LYSOZYME ('deflamon').

METRONIDAZOLE WITH SPIRAMYCIN ('rodogyl').

'Metropine' *see* Atropine methonitrate.

'Metrotonin' *see* *N,N*-Dimethylamphetamine.

'Metrulen' *see* Etynodiol diacetate with mestranol.

'Metubine' *see* Dimethyltubocurarine.

METUREDEPA*** (ethyl [bis(2,2-dimethyl-1-aziridinyl)phosphinyl]carbamate; dimethylurethamide; dimethylurethimine; AB-132; NSC-51325; 'turloc').

Metylperone *see* Melperone.

METYNODIOL*** (11β-methyl-19-nor-17α-pregn-4-en-20-yne-3β,17-diol; 17α-ethynyl-3β,17β-dihydroxy-11β-methylestr-4-ene; 17α-ethynyl-11β-methylestr-4-ene-3β,17-diol; 17α-ethynyl-11β-methyl-19-norandrost-4-ene-3β,17-diol; methyletynodiol; methynodiol).

METYNODIOL DIACETATE (methynodiol diacetate; SC-19198).

METYRAPONE*** (2-methyl-1,2-dipyrid-3-yl-1-propanone; methapyrapone; methbipyrapone; methopyrapone; metyrapone hydrochloride; Su-8874; 'metopirone', 'metopyrone').

METYRAPONE TARTRATE (Su-4885).

METYRIDINE** (2-(2-methoxyethyl)-pyridine; methyridine; 'dekelmin', 'prominthic').

Metyzoline* *see* Metizoline.

MEVALONIC ACID (3,5-dihydroxy-3-methylvaleric acid; hiochic acid; MK-91).

'Mevasine' *see* Mecamylamine.

MEVINPHOS* ((1-carbomethoxy-1-propen-3-yl) dimethyl phosphate; 2-carbomethoxy-1-methylvinyl dimethyl phosphate; 3-(dimethoxyphosphinyloxy)-*cis*-crotonic acid methyl ester; methyl 3-hydroxy-*cis*-crotonate dimethyl phosphate; methyl 3-(dimethoxyphosphinyloxy)-2-butenoate; PD-5; 'phosdrin').

MEXACARBATE* (4-dimethylamino-3,5-dimethylphenyl methylcarbamate; 4-dimethylamino-3,5-xylyl methylcarbamate; OMS-47; 'zectran').

'Mexaform' *see* Clioquinol with phanquinone and oxyphenonium bromide.

Mexamine *see* 5-Methoxytryptamine.

MEXENONE** (2-hydroxy-4-methoxy-4'-methylbenzophenone; 'uvistat 2211').

MEXILETINE*** (1-methyl-2-(2,6-xylyl-oxy)ethylamine; 2-(2-aminopropoxy)-*m*-xylene; 1-(2,6-dimethylphenoxy)-2-propylamine; mexiletine hydrochloride; Kö-1173; 'mexitil').

'Mexitil' *see* Mexiletine.

'Mexocine' *see* Demeclocycline.

MEXOPROFEN*** (*p*-(*trans*-2-methylcyclohexyl)hydratropic acid; 2-[4-(*trans*-2-methylcyclohexyl)phenyl]propionic acid).

MEXRENOATE POTASSIUM*** (7-methyl 21-potassium 17-hydroxy-3-oxo-17α-pregn-4-ene-7α,21-dicarboxylate dihydrate; 17-hydroxy-3-oxo-17α-pregn-4-ene-7,21-dicarboxylic acid 7-methyl ester 21-potassium salt dihydrate).

Mexyphamine *see* Methoxyphenamine.

Mezaton (tr) *see* Phenylephrine.

Mezcaline *see* Mescaline.

MEZEPINE*** (5,6-dihydro-5-(3-methylaminopropyl)-11H-dibenz(b,e)azepine).

MEZLOCILLIN** ((2S,5R,6R)-6-[(R)-2-[3-(methylsulfonyl)-2-oxo-1-imidazolidinecarboxamido]-2-phenylacetamido]-penicillanic acid; mezlocillin sodium; BAY f-1353).

MF-10 *see* Doxepin.

MFQ *see* Morfamquat.

Mg-46 *see* Clofibride.

Mg-137 *see* Diethylstilbestrol disulfate.

Mg-1480 *see* Salinazid.

Mg-1559 *see* Xenbucin.

Mg-5771 *see* Butixirate.

MG-42799 *see* Trospium chloride.

2M-4H-M (tr) *see* 4-(4-Chloro-2-methylphenoxy)butyric acid.

MH-532 *see* Phenprobamate.

MHIP *see* Toliprolol.
Mi-85 *see* Azapropazone.
MI-217 *see* Ecothiopate iodide.
MI-860 *see* Anagestone acetate with mestranol.
MIANSERIN** (1,2,3,4,10,14b-hexahydro-2-methyldibenzo(c,f)(pyrazino-1,2-a)-azepine; GB-94; 'tolvin', 'tolvon').
Miazine *see* Pyrimidine.
Miazole *see* Imidazoline.
MIBOLERONE*** (17β-hydroxy-7α,17-dimethylestr-4-en-3-one; 7α,17-dimethylestr-4-en-17β-ol-3-one; 7α,17-dimethylnandrolone; 7α,17-dimethyl-19-nortestosterone; U-10997).
'Micasin' *see* Chlorfenethol.
'Micatin' *see* Miconazole.
Mico... *see also* Myco...
'Micol' *see* Cetrimonium.
MICONAZOLE*** (1-[2,4-dichloro-β-(2,4-dichlorobenzyloxy)phenethyl]imidazole; miconazole nitrate; R-14889; 'dactarin', 'daktarin', 'dermonistat', 'epi-monistat', 'gynodaktarin', 'gyno-monistat', 'micatin', 'monistat').
'Micoren' *see* Prethcamide.
'Microcillin' *see* Carbenicillin.
'Microgynon' *see* Levonorgestrel with ethinylestradiol.
Microlut' *see* Levonorgestrel.
'Microluton' *see* Levonorgestrel.
Micromonospora purpurea, antibiotic *see* Gentamicin.
Micromonospora rosaria, antibiotic *see* Rosamicin.
'Micronor' *see* Norethisterone.
Micronovum *see* Norethisterone.
'Micropenin' *see* Oxacillin.
'Microval' *see* Levonorgestrel.
'Mictasol' *see* Methenamine.
'Mictine' *see* Aminometradine.
MIDAFLUR** (4-amino-2,2,5,5-tetrakis-(trifluoromethyl)-3-imidazoline; 5-imino-2,2,4,4-tetrakis(trifluoromethyl)imidazolidine; EXP-338).
'Midalgyl' *see* Proxyfenone with cresotamide.
MIDAMALINE* (N-(5-chloro-2-benzimidazolylmethyl)-N',N'-dimethyl-N-phenylethylenediamine).
'Midamor' *see* Amiloride.
'Midantane' *see* Amantadine.
MIDECAMYCIN** (7-(formylmethyl)-4,10-dihydroxy-5-methoxy-9,16-dimethyl-2-oxooxacyclohexadeca-11,13-dien-6-yl 3,6-dideoxy-4-O-(2,6-dideoxy-3-C-methyl-α-L-ribo-hexopyranosyl)-3-dimethylamino-β-D-glucopyranoside 4,4''-dipropionate ester; mydecamycin; SF-837; 'medemycin').
'Midicel' *see* Sulfamethoxypyridazine.
'Midikel' *see* Sulfamethoxypyridazine.
MIDODRINE*** (2-amino-N-(β-hydroxy-2,5-dimethoxyphenethyl)acetamide; N-(2-aminoacetyl)-β-hydroxy-2,5-dimethoxyphenethylamine; ST-1085; 'gutron').
'Midol' *see* Cinnamedrine.
'Midosal' *see* Carbutamide.

'Midoxin' *see* Doxycycline.
'Midronal' *see* Cinnarizine.
'Mielucin' *see* Busulfan.
'Miglucan' *see* Glibenclamide.
'Migristene' *see* Dimetotiazine mesilate.
MIH *see* Procarbazine.
MIKAMYCIN*** (antibiotic from *Str. mitakaensis*; mikamycin B; ostreogrycin B).
'Mikedimide' *see* Bemegride.
'Mikro-30' *see* Levonorgestrel.
'Milbam' *see* Ziram.
'Milbex' *see* Chlorfenethol plus chlorfensulfide.
'Milcurb' *see* Dimethirimol.
'Mildex' *see* Dinocap.
'Milid' *see* Proglumide.
MILIPERTINE*** (5,6-dimethoxy-3-[2-[4-(o-methoxyphenyl)piperazin-1-yl]-ethyl]-2-methylindole; 1-[2-(5,6-dimethoxy-2-methylindol-3-yl)ethyl]-4-(o-methoxyphenyl)piperazine).
'Milkinol' *see* Sodium dioctyl sulfosuccinate.
'Millicaine' *see* Betoxycaine.
'Millicorten' *see* Dexamethasone.
'Millophylline' *see* Etamiphyllin camsilate.
'Milogard' *see* Antu.
'Milontin' *see* Phensuximide.
'Milonton' *see* Phensuximide.
'Milstem' *see* Ethirimol.
'Milton' *see* Sodium hypochlorite.
'Mil-U-cal' *see* Calcium levulinate.
'Milurit' *see* Allopurinol.
MIMBANE*** (1,2,3,4,4a,5,7,8,13,13b,14,14a-dodecahydro-13-methylbenz(g)indolo-(2,3a)quinolizine; 1-methylyohimbane; mimbane hydrochloride; W-2291-A).
MIMOSINE ((−)-2-amino-3-(3-hydroxy-4-oxopyrid-1-yl)propionic acid; (−)-α-amino-(3-hydroxy-4-pyridinone)propionic acid; 3-hydroxy-4-oxo-1(4H)-pyridine-alanine; (−)-leucenol).
See also Leucenol.
MINA *see* Isonitrosoacetone.
'Minacide' *see* Promecarb.
'Minanine' *see* Tosylchloramide.
MINAPRINE** (4-[2-[(4-methyl-6-phenylpyridazin-3-yl)amino]ethyl]morpholine; 4-methyl-3-[(2-morpholinoethyl)amino]-6-phenylpyridazine; Agr-1240).
'Mincard' *see* Aminometradine.
'Minelcin' *see* Benzilonium bromide.
MINEPENTATE*** (2-(2-dimethylaminoethoxy)ethyl 1-phenylcyclopentanecarboxylate; UCB-1549).
'Minidiab' *see* Glipizide.
'Minifage' *see* Fenfluramine.
'Minifom' *see* Dimeticone.
'Minikel' *see* Sulfamethoxypyridazine.
'Minilyn' *see* Ethinylestradiol with lynestrenol.
'Minipress' *see* Prazosin.
'Minirin' *see* Desmopressin diacetate.
'Minocin' *see* Minocycline.
'Minocine' *see* Minocycline.
'Minocrin' *see* Aminoacridine.
MINOCYCLINE*** (4,7-bis(dimethyl-amino)-1,4,4a,5,5a,6,11,12a-octahydro-

3,10,12,12a-tetrahydroxy-1,11-dioxo-2-naphthacenecarboxamide; 6-demethyl-6-deoxy-7-dimethylaminotetracycline; 'klinomycin', 'minocin', 'minocine', 'minocyn', 'minomax', 'minomycin', 'mynocine').
'Minocyn' *see* Minocycline.
'Minodiab' *see* Glipizide.
'Minomax' *see* Minocycline.
'Minomycin' *see* Minocycline.
MINOXIDIL*** (2,4-diamino-6-piperid-1-ylpyrimidine 3-oxide; 6-piperidino-2,4-pyrimidine 3-oxide).
(*Previously described as* 6-amino-1,2-dihydro-1-hydroxy-2-imino-4-piperid-1-ylpyrimidine).
'Minovlar' *see* Norethisterone acetate with ethinylestradiol.
'Minozinan' *see* Levomepromazine.
'Mintacol' *see* Paraoxon.
'Mintezol' *see* Tiabendazole.
'Mintussin' *see* Atropine methobromide.
'Minuric' *see* Benzbromarone.
'Minurin' *see* Desmopressin diacetate.
'Minus' *see* Sodium alginate.
'Minzil' *see* Chlorothiazide.
'Minzol' *see* Tiabendazole.
Mio... *see also* Myo...
'Miocarpine' *see* Pilocarpine.
'Miokon' *see* Sodium diprotrizoate.
'Miorelax' *see* Guaifenesin.
'Miostat' *see* Carbachol.
'Mioticol' *see* Diisopropyl *p*-nitrophenyl phosphate.
'Miotisal' *see* Paraoxon.
MIPAFOX* (bis(isopropylamino)fluoro-phosphine oxide; *N,N'*-diisopropylphos-phorodiamidic fluoride; *N,N'*-bis(1-methylethyl) phosphorodiamidic fluoride; isopestox; 'pestox XV').
'Mipax' *see* Dimethyl phthalate.
MIPC *see* Isoprocarb.
'Mipicin' *see* Isoprocarb.
'Miracil-D' *see* Lucanthone.
'Miracol' *see* Lucanthone.
'Miradon' *see* Anisindione.
'Mirapront' *see* Phentermine resin.
'Mirbedal' *see* Sulfatolamide.
MIREX (1,1a,2,2,3,3a,4,5,5,5a,5b,6-dodeca-chlorooctahydro-1,3,4-metheno-1H-cyclo-buta(cd)pentalene).
MIRINCAMYCIN** (mixture of *cis* and *trans* forms of methyl 7-chloro-6,7,8-tri-deoxy-6-(4-pentyl-L-2-pyrrolidinecarbox-amido)-1-thio-L-*threo*-α-D-*galacto*-octo-pyranoside; mirincamycin hydrochloride; U-24729A).
'Mirion' *see* Methenamine tetraiodide.
'Mirvan' *see* Alclofenac.
'Miscleron' *see* Clofibrate.
'Mistabron' *see* Mesna.
'Misulban' *see* Busulfan.
'Mitabol' *see* Mesulfen.
'Mitarson' *see* Defosfamide.
'Mitenyl' *see* Dibromsalan with tribromsalan.
'Mithracin' *see* Mithramycin.
MITHRAMYCIN*** (antibiotic from *Str. tanashiensis*; A-2371; NSC-24559; PA-144;

'mithracin').
'Mitigal' *see* Mesulfen.
MITOBRONITOL*** (1,6-dibromo-1,6-di-deoxy-D-mannitol; dibromomannitol; DBM; NSC-94100; 'myelobromol').
MITOCARCIN** (antibiotic from a Strep-tomyces (Mich. Dept. Publ. Hlth No. 24281)).
MITOCLOMINE*** (*N,N*-bis(2-chloro-ethyl)-4-methoxy-3-methyl-1-naphthyl-amine).
MITOCROMIN* (antibiotic from *Str. viridochromogenes*; B-35251; NSC-77471).
MITOGILLIN*** (antibiotic from *Aspergil-lus restrictus*).
MITOGUAZONE*** (1,1'-[(methylethane-diylidene)dinitrilo]diguanidine; methyl-glyoxal bisguanylhydrazone; methyl-GAG; NSC-32946).
MITOLACTOL*** (1,6-dibromo-1,6-di-deoxy-D-galactitol; 1,6-dibromo-1,6-dide-oxydulcitol; dibromodulcitol; dibrom-dulcit; DBD; NSC-104800; 'elobromo').
MITOMALCIN*** (antibiotic from *Str. malayensis*; NSC-2992).
'Mitomen' *see* Chlormethine *N*-oxide.
MITOMYCIN*** (6-amino-1,1a,2,8,8a,8b-hexahydro-8-hydroxymethyl-8a-methoxy-5-methylazirino(2',3':3,4)pyrrolo(1,2-a)-indole-4,7-dione carbamate ester; mito-mycin C; NSC-26980; 'amecytine' 'ametycin', 'mutamycin').
Mitomycin C *see* Mitomycin.
MITOPODOZIDE*** (podophyllic acid 2-ethylhydrazide; *N'*-ethylpodophyllo-hydrazide; SP-I; 'proresid').
Mitoquinone *see* Ubiquinone.
MITOSPER*** (antibiotic from *Aspergillus glaucus*).
'Mitostan' *see* Busulfan.
MITOTANE*** (1,1-dichloro-2-(*o*-chloro-phenyl)-2-(*p*-chlorophenyl)ethane; *o,p'*-DDD; *o,p'*-TDE; chloditan; NSC-38721; 'lysodren').
MITOTENAMINE*** (5-bromo-3-[(2-chloroethyl)ethylaminomethyl]benzo(b)-thiophene; 5-bromo-*N*-(2-chloroethyl)-*N*-ethylbenzo(b)thiophene-3-methylamine; AGN-1414).
'Mitox' *see* Chlorbenside.
'Mitoxine' *see* Chlormethine.
'Mitronal' *see* Cinnarizine.
MIXIDINE*** (2-(3,4-dimethoxyphenethyl-imino)-1-methylpyrrolidine; McN-1589).
'Mixtencillin' *see* Dihydrostreptomycin with procaine penicillin.
MJ-12 *see* Carbocisteine with theophylline.
MJ-217 *see* Ecothiopate iodide.
MJ-505 *see* Fenyramidol.
MJ-1987 *see* Mesuprine.
MJ-1988 *see* Quazodine.
MJ-1992 *see* Soterenol.
MJ-1998 *see* Metalol.
MJ-1999 *see* Sotalol.
MJ-5022 *see* Methdilazine.
MJ-5190 *see* Amidefrine mesilate.
MK-02 *see* Benzatropine mesilate.

MK-7 *see* Homarylamine.
MK-53 *see* Glaucarubin.
MK-56 *see* Pyrazinamide.
MK-57 *see* Methyldesorphine.
MK-65 *see* Cycloserine.
MK-89 *see* Anileridine.
MK-91 *see* Mevalonic acid.
MK-125 *see* Dexamethasone.
MK-128 *see* Ubiquinone.
MK-130 *see* Cyclobenzaprine.
MK-135 *see* Benzmalecene.
MK-185 *see* Halofenate.
MK-240 *see* Protriptyline.
MK-250 *see* Emylcamate.
MK-351 *see* Methyldopa.
MK-356 *see* Pivampicillin probenecid ester.
MK-360 *see* Tiabendazole.
MK-486 *see* Carbidopa.
MK-595 *see* Etacrynic acid.
MK-665 *see* Ethynerone with mestranol.
MK-745 *see* Metoclopramide.
MK-870 *see* Amiloride.
MK-905 *see* Cambendazole.
MK-915 *see* Flunidazole.
MK-950 *see* Timolol maleate.
MLD-41 *see* Methyllysergide.
MnEDB *see* Maneb.
MNFA *see* N-(2-Fluoroacetyl)-N-methyl-1-naphthylamine.
MO-911 *see* Pargyline.
MO-1255 *see* Encyprate.
'Mobam' *see* 4-Benzothienyl N-methylcarbamate.
'Moban' *see* Molindone.
MO-BAY 950 *see* Penicillamine.
MOBECARB*** (phenacyl 4-morpholineacetate).
MOBECARB WITH PIBECARB ('afragil', 'ciergin', 'C-total').
'Mobenate' *see* Sodium benzyl succinate.
'Mobenol' *see* Tolbutamide.
'Mobilene' *see* Sodium o-pyrocatechuate.
'Mobutazon' *see* Mofebutazone.
'Mobuzon' *see* Mofebutazone.
'Mocap' *see* Ethoprop.
'Moccasin' *see* Snake venom.
MOCTAMIDE** ((−)-N-(p-methyl-α-phenylphenethyl)linoleamide; N-linoleamido-p-methyl-α-phenylphenethylamine).
'Modacor' *see* Oxyfedrine.
MODALINE*** (2-methyl-3-piperid-1-ylpyrazine; modaline monosulfate; modaline sulfate; W-3207-B).
'Modamide' *see* Amiloride.
'Modecate' *see* Fluphenazine decanoate.
'Moderil' *see* Rescinnamine.
'Modirax' *see* Hexapropymate.
'Moditen' *see* Fluphenazine.
'Modumate' *see* Arginine glutamate.
'Moduretic' *see* Amiloride with hydrochlorothiazide.
Moenomycin *see* Bambermycin.
MOFEBUTAZONE*** (4-butyl-1-phenyl-3,5-pyrazolidinedione; monophenylbutazone; 'arcobutine', 'arcomonol', 'mobutazon', 'mobuzon', 'monazan', 'monazone', 'monobutazon', 'monofen',

'monomex', 'monomil', 'monoprine', 'mozol').
Mofedione *see* Oxazidione.
MOFLOVERINE*** (2,4,6-trimethoxybenzoic acid 2-morpholinoethyl ester; 2-morpholinoethyl 2,4,6-trimethoxybenzoate).
MOFOXIME** (4-[(p-acetylphenoxy)acetyl]morpholine p-oxime; 4-[[p-[1-(hydroxyimino)ethyl]phenoxy]acetyl]morpholine).
'Mogadan' *see* Nitrazepam.
'Mogadon' *see* Nitrazepam.
'Molevac' *see* Pyrvinium embonate.
MOLINATE* (S-ethyl hexahydro-1H-azepine-1-carbothioate; 'ordram').
MOLINAZONE*** (3-morpholino-1,2,3-benzotriazin-4(3H)-one).
MOLINDONE*** (3-ethyl-6,7-dihydro-2-methyl-5-morpholinomethylindol-4(5H)-one; molindone hydrochloride; EN-1733A; 'moban').
Molinuron *see* Monolinuron.
'Molofac' *see* Sodium dioctyl sulfosuccinate.
MOLSIDOMINE*** (N-ethoxycarbonyl-3-morpholinosydnone imine; N-carboxy-3-morpholinosydnone imine ethyl ester; SIN-10).
'Molucid' *see* Isobutyltritylamine.
MOMA *see* Vanilmandelic acid.
Monacrine *see* Aminoacridine.
MONALIDE* (N-(4-chlorophenyl)-2,2-dimethylpentanamide; N-(p-chlorophenyl)-2,2-dimethylvaleramide; chlorvalamide).
'Monalium hydrate' *see* Magaldrate.
'Monase' *see* Etryptamine.
'Monazan' *see* Mofebutazone.
'Monazone' *see* Mofebutazone.
MONENSIN*** (2-[5-ethyltetrahydro-5-[tetrahydro-3-methyl-5-(tetrahydro-6-hydroxy-6-hydroxymethyl-3,5-dimethylpyran-2-yl)-2-furyl]-2-furyl]-9-hydroxy-β-methoxy-α,γ,2,8-tetramethyl-1,6-dioxaspiro(4.5)decane-7-butyric acid; 2-[5-[5-(3,5-dimethyl-6-hydroxy-6-hydroxymethyl-2-tetrahydropyranyl)-3-methyl-2-tetrahydrofuryl]-5-ethyl-2-tetrahydrofuryl]-9-hydroxy-β-methoxy-α,γ,2,8-tetramethyl-1,6-dioxaspiro(4.5)decane-7-butyric acid; L-67314; 'coban').
'Monistat' *see* Miconazole.
'Monitan' *see* Polysorbate 80.
'Monitor' *see* Methamidophos.
MONOAMINE OXIDASE (amine oxidase; amino oxidase; adrenaline oxidase; MAO; tyraminase).
MONOBENZONE*** (monobenzyl ether of hydroquinone; p-benzyloxyphenol; 'agerite alba', 'benoquin', 'depigman').
'Monobutazon' *see* Mofebutazone.
'Monocaine' *see* Butethamine.
Monocalcium tetrasodium bis[pentaaqua-[D-gluconato(4-)]tetra-μ-hydroxydioxotriferrate(3-)] *see* Calcium sodium ferriclate.
Monochlorimipramine *see* Clomipramine.
Monochlorphenamide* *see* Clofenamide.
'Monocortin' *see* Paramethasone.
MONOCROTOPHOS* (3-(dimethoxyphos-

phinyloxy)-*N*-methyl-*cis*-crotonamide; dimethyl 1-methyl-3-methylamino-3-oxo-1-propenyl phosphate; 3-hydroxy-*N*-methyl-*cis*-crotonamide dimethyl phosphate; *O,O*-dimethyl *O*-(1-methylcarboxamido-1-propen-2-yl) phosphate; 1-methyl-2-(methylcarboxamido)vinyl phosphate; dimethyl (2-methylcarbamoyl-1-methylvinyl)phosphate; 'azodrin', 'nuvacron').

'**Monoderm**' *see* Fluocinolone acetonide.

'**Monodorm**' *see* Butethal.

'**Monodral**' *see* Penthienate.

MONOETHANOLAMINE OLEATE*** (2-aminoethanol oleate; ethanolamine oleate; ethaminol).

'**Monofen**' *see* Mofebutazone.

Monoglycol salicylate *see* Glycol salicylate.

'**Monolene**' *see* Propylene glycol monostearate.

MONOLINURON* (1-(*p*-chlorophenyl)-3-methoxy-3-methylurea; molinuron; 'aresin', 'arezine').

'**Monomestrol**' *see* Mestilbol.

MONOMETACRINE*** (9,9-dimethyl-10-(3-methylaminopropyl)acridan).

'**Monomex**' *see* Mofebutazone.

'**Monomil**' *see* Mofebutazone.

'**Monopar**' *see* Stilbazium.

'**Monophen**' *see* 2-(4-Hydroxy-3,5-diiodobenzyl)cyclohexanecarboxylic acid.

Monophenylbutazone *see* Mofebutazone.

'**Monophosaden**' *see* Adenosine phosphate.

MONOPHOSPHOTHIAMINE*** (thiamine monophosphate; thiamine phosphate).

'**Monoprine**' *see* Mofebutazone.

MONOSTEARIN (stearic acid monoglyceryl ester).

MONOSULFIRAM* (tetraethylthiuram monosulfide; bis(diethylthiocarbamyl) sulfide; sulfiram; 'sanigal', 'tetmosol').

Monothioglycol *see* 2-Mercaptoethanol.

MONOXERUTIN** (7-*O*-(2-hydroxyethyl)rutoside; Z-3011; Z-12007; 'venoruton').

Monoxychlorosene *see* Oxychlorosene.

MONURON* (1-(*p*-chlorophenyl)-3,3-dimethylurea; CMU; CMV; chlorfenidim; klorfenidim; 'telvar').

MONURON TRICHLOROACETATE (monuron-TCA; 'urox').

8-MOP *see* Methoxsalen.

'**Mopazine**' *see* Methopromazine.

MOPERONE** (1-[3-(*p*-fluorobenzoyl)-propyl]-4-(*p*-tolyl)-4-piperidinol; 4'-fluoro-4-[4-hydroxy-4-(*p*-tolyl)piperid-1-yl]-butyrophenone; methylperidol; mopiperone; R-1658; 'luvatren'). *See also* Hexadiphane with moperone.

Mopiperone* *see* Moperone.

MOQUIZONE** (2,3-dihydro-1-(morpholinoacetyl)-3-phenyl-4-(1H)-quinazolinone; 1,2,3,4-tetrahydro-1-morpholinoacetyl-3-phenylquinazolin-4-one; Rec-14/0127).

MORACIZINE*** (ethyl 10-(3-morpholinopropionyl)phenothiazine-2-carbamate; ethmozine; etmozine).

MORANTEL** (*trans*-1,4,5,6-tetrahydro-1-methyl-2-[2-(3-methylthien-2-yl)vinyl]-pyrimidine; *trans*-3-methyl-2-[2-(1,4,5,6-tetrahydro-1-methylpyrimid-2-yl)vinyl]thiophene).

MORANTEL TARTRATE ('banminth II', 'pyrequan').

'**Moranyl**' *see* Suramin.

MORAZINE (10-(3-morpholinopropyl)-phenothiazine).

MORAZONE*** (2,3-dimethyl-4-(3-methyl-2-phenylmorpholinomethyl)-1-phenyl-3-pyrazolin-5-one; 4-(3-methyl-2-phenylmorpholinomethyl)antipyrine; 4-(3-methyl 2-phenylmorpholinomethyl)phenazone; 'novartrine', 'pirisal', 'tarugan').

'**Morbasin**' *see* Aminothiazole.

'**Morbicid**' *see* Formaldehyde.

MORCLOFONE*** (4'-chloro-3,5-dimethoxy-4-(2-morpholinoethoxy)benzophenone; K-3712).

'**Morestan**' *see* Chinomethionat.

'**Morestin**' *see* Estrone sulfate.

Morfamoquat *see* Morfamquat.

MORFAMQUAT* (1,1'-bis[2-(3,5-dimethylmorpholino)-2-oxoethyl]-4,4'-bipyridinium dichloride; 1,1'-bis(3,5-dimethylmorpholinocarbonylmethyl)-4,4'-bipyridinium dichloride; morfamoquat; MFQ; 'morfoxone').

Morficon *see* Hydromorphone.

'**Morfolep**' *see* Morsuximide.

MORFOREX** (4-[2-(α-methylphenethyl-amino)ethyl]morpholine; *N*-(2-morpholinoethyl)amphetamine).

'**Morfoxone**' *see* Morfamquat.

'**Morgalin**' *see* Moroxydine.

MORIN (2',3,4',5,7-pentahydroxyflavone).

MORINAMIDE** (*N*-morpholinomethyl-pyrazinamide; *N*-morpholinomethyl-pyrazine-2-carboxamide; morphazinamide; 'diazolina', 'nicoprazine', 'piafolina', 'piazol', 'piazolina').

'**Mornidine**' *see* Pipamazine.

Morocide' *see* Binapacryl.

MOROCROMEN*** (4-methyl-7-(4-morpholinecarboxamido)-3-(2-morpholino-ethyl)coumarin).

'**Moronal**' *see* Nystatin.

MOROXYDINE*** (*N*-(guanidinoformi-midoyl)morpholine; 4-morpholinecarboxi-midoylguanidine; N^1,N^1-cyclo-3-oxapenta-methylenebiguanide; N^1,N^1-anhydrobis-(2-hydroxyethyl)biguanide; biguamor; ABOB; 'flumidin', 'morgalin', 'spenitol', 'virobis', 'virugon', 'virustat').

Morphacetinum *see* Diamorphine.

MORPHANTHRIDINE (11H-dibenz-(b,e)azepine).

Morphazinamide *see* Morinamide.

MORPHERIDINE*** (ethyl ester of 1-(2-morpholinoethyl)-1-phenylisonipecotic acid; morpholinylethylnorpethidine).

Morphethylbutyne* *see* Promolate.

Morphicon *see* Hydromorphone.

MORPHINAN (1,2,3,9,10,10a-hexahydro-10,4a(4H)iminoethanophenanthrene).

MORPHINE (5,6-dihydroxy-*N*-methyl-4,5-epoxy-7-morphinene).

Ψ-Morphine *see* Pseudomorphine.

Morphine benzyl ether *see* Benzylmorphine.

Morphine diacetate *see* Diamorphine.

Morphine dinicotinate *see* Nicomorphine.

Morphine ethyl ether *see* Ethylmorphine.

Morphine methyl ether *see* Codeine.

Morphine morpholinoethyl ether *see* Pholcodine.

MORPHINE NOSCAPINE MECONATE (double salt of morphine and noscapine with meconic acid; 'narcophine', 'narphin').

MORPHINE *N*-OXIDE (morphine aminoxide; 'genomorphine').

MORPHOL (3,4-dihydroxyphenanthrene).

'Morpholep' *see* Morsuximide.

MORPHOLINE (tetrahydro-1,4(2H)-oxazine; diethylene imidoxide; diethylene oximide).

1-(Morpholinoacetyl)-3-phenyl-2,4-dihydro-4(1H)-quinazolinone *see* Moquizone.

3-Morpholino-1,2,3-benzotriazin-4(3H)-one *see* Molinazone.

4-Morpholinocarboximidoylguanidine *see* Moroxydine.

4-Morpholino-2,2-diphenylbutyric acid ethyl ester *see* Dioxaphetyl butyrate.

1-(4-Morpholino-2,2-diphenylbutyryl)-pyrrolidine *see* Desmethylmoramide.

6-Morpholino-4,4-diphenyl-3-heptanone *see* Phenadoxone.

***N*-(2-Morpholinoethyl)amphetamine** *see* Morforex.

2-Morpholinoethyl 2-methyl-2-phenoxypropionate *see* Promolate.

Morpholinoethylmorphine *see* Pholcodine.

1-(2-Morpholinoethyl)-5-nitroimidazole *see* Nimorazole.

Morpholinoethylnorpethidine *see* Morpheridine.

2-Morpholinoethyl 2-phenoxyisobutyrate *see* Promolate.

Morpholinoethylrutoside *see* Ethoxazorutoside.

2-Morpholinoethyl 2,4,6-trimethoxybenzoate *see* Mofloverine.

4-Morpholinomethylesculetin *see* Folescutol.

5-Morpholinomethylfurazolidone *see* Furaltadone.

3-Morpholinomethyl-1-(5-nitrofurfurylideneamino)hydantoin *see* Nifurfoline.

5-(4-Morpholinomethyl)-3-(5-nitrofurfurylideneamino)-2-oxazolidinone *see* Furaltadone.

2-(Morpholinomethyl)-2-phenyl-1,3-indandione *see* Oxazidone.

10-(3-Morpholinopropionyl)phenothiazine-2-carbamic acid ethyl ester *see* Moracizine.

4-(3-Morpholinopropyl)benzyl phenyl ether *see* Fomocaine.

10-(3-Morpholinopropyl)phenothiazine *see* Morazine.

10-(3-Morpholinopropyl)-2-propionylphenothiazine *see* Propionylmorazine.

MORPHOTHEBAINE (apomorphine 10-methyl ether).

MORPHOTHION* (*O*,*O*-dimethyl *S*-(2-morpholino-2-oxoethyl)phosphorodithioate; *O*,*O*-dimethyl *S*-(2-morpholin-4-ylacetyl) phosphorodithioate; 'ekatin F', 'ekatin M', 'morphotox').

'Morphotox' *see* Morphothion.

MORSUXIMIDE* (2-methyl-*N*-morpholinomethyl-2-phenylsuccinimide; 'morfolep', 'perlepsin').

'Moryl' *see* Carbachol.

'Mosatil' *see* Sodium calcium edetate.

'Mosegor' *see* Pizotifen maleate.

'Mosidal' *see* Methallatal.

'Motilyn' *see* Dexpanthenol.

'Motival' *see* Fluphenazine with nortriptyline.

'Motolon' *see* Methaqualone.

MOTRAZEPAM** (1,3-dihydro-1-(methoxymethyl)-7-nitro-5-phenyl-2H-1,4-benzodiazepin-2-one).

'Motrin' *see* Ibuprofen.

'Motylkopielik' *see* Dinoprop.

Mould fibrinolysin *see* Brinase.

'Movellan' *see* Strychnine *N*-oxide.

'Movirene' *see* Dipyrocetyl.

'Mowiol' *see* Polyvinyl alcohol.

MOXASTINE* (2-(1,1-diphenylethoxy)-*N*,*N*-dimethylethylamine; *N*,*N*-dimethyl-2-(α-methylbenzhydryloxy)ethylamine; α-methyldiphenhydramine; mephenhydramine; Spofa-325; 'alfadryl', 'alphadryl').

MOXAVERINE*(1-benzyl-3-ethyl-6,7-dimethoxyisoquinoline; 'eupaverin').

MOXESTROL* (11β-methoxy-19-nor-17α-pregna-1,3,5(10)-trien-20-yne-3,17-diol; 3,17-dihydroxy-11β-methoxy-19-nor-17α-pregna-1,3,5-trien-20-yne; 17-ethynyl-11β-methoxyestradiol; 'surestryl').

MOXICOUMONE* (5,7-bis(2-morpholinoethoxy)-4-methylcoumarin; Rec-15/0019; 'moxile').

'Moxile' *see* Moxicoumone.

MOXIPRAQUINE* (8-[6-[4-(3-hydroxybutyl)piperazin-1-yl]hexylamino]-6-methoxyquinoline; 4-[4-[6-(6-methoxyquinolin-8-ylamino)hexyl]piperazin-1-yl]-2-butanol; moxypraquine; BW-349C59).

MOXISYLYTE* ([2-(4-acetoxy-2-isopropyl-5-methylphenoxy)ethyl]dimethylamine; 2-(4-acetoxythymoxy)-*N*,*N*-dimethylethylamine; 4-acetoxythymol dimethylaminoethyl ether; 4-(2-dimethylaminoethoxy)-5-isopropyl-2-methylphenyl acetate; 2-(4-hydroxy-2-isopropyl-5-methylphenoxy)-*N*,*N*-dimethylethylamine acetate ester; 4-acetoxy-β-dimethylamino-2-isopropyl-5-methylphenetole; 4-(2-dimethylaminoethoxy)carvacrol acetate; thymoxamine; moxisylyte hydrochloride; 'arlytene', 'carlytene', 'opilon').

MOXNIDAZOLE* (3-[[(1-methyl-5-nitroimidazol-2-yl)methylene]amino]-5-

314

(morpholinomethyl)-2-oxazolidinone;
1-methyl-2-[[[5-(morpholinomethyl)-2-
oxooxazolidin-3-yl]imino]methyl]-5-
nitroimidazole).
Moxypraquine *see* Moxipraquine.
'Mozambin' *see* Methaqualone.
'Mozol' *see* Mofebutazone.
6-MP *see* Mercatopurine.
MP-11 *see* Perlapine.
MP-267 *see* *m*-Sarcolysin.
MP-271 *see* Iosefamic acid.
MP-506 *see* Formylsarcolysin.
MP-1051 *see* Simaldrate.
MPD *see* Meprophenidol.
MRD-108 *see* Pipradrol.
MRD-125 *see* Phenythilone.
MRL-41 *see* Clomifene.
MS-53 *see* Sulfamethoxazole.
MS-222 *see* Ethyl *m*-aminobenzoate.
MS-752 *see* Lucanthone.
MSH *see* Intermedin.
MTB-51 *see* Methantheline.
MTS-263 *see* Tropenzilium.
MTU *see* Methylthiouracil.
MTX *see* Methotrexate.
'Mucantil' *see* (2-Iodopropylidenedioxy)-
propanol.
MUCIC ACID (tetrahydroadipic acid;
saccharolactic acid; Schleimsäure).
'Mucilose' *see* Ispagula.
'Mucitux' *see* Eprazinone.
'Mucodyne' *see* Carbocisteine.
MUCOITIN POLYSULFATE ESTERS
('eleparon', 'elheparin', 'elheparon').
'Mucomyst' *see* Acetylcysteine.
'Muco-polycid' *see* Chlormidazole.
'Mucosolvin' *see* Acetylcysteine.
'Mudeka' *see* Amobarbital.
'Mugia' *see* Dimethyl phthalate.
'Mulfasin' *see* Methyldopa.
'Mulsopaque' *see* Iofendylate.
'Multergan' *see* Thiazinamium.
'Multezin' *see* Thiazinamium.
'Multifuge' *see* Piperazine citrate.
'Multimycin' *see* Colistin.
'Mundiquin' *see* Quinidine polygalacturonate.
'Mundisal' *see* Choline salicylate.
MURAMIC ACID (3-*O*-(1-carboxyethyl)-
D-glucosamine).
'Murbetol' *see* Propham plus endothal
sodium.
'Murel' *see* Valethamate.
MUREXINE (choline salt of urocanic acid;
[2-(β-imidazol-4(5)-ylacryloyloxy)ethyl]-
trimethylammonium chloride hydro-
chloride; imidazoleacryloylchloline;
urocanoylcholine).
'Murfotox' *see* Mecarbam
Muriatic ether *see* Chloroethane.
'Murotox' *see* Mecarbam.
'Murvesco' *see* Fenson.
'Muscaran' *see* Bethanechol.
'Muscatox' *see* Coumafos.
MUSCIMOL (5-aminomethyl-3-isoxazolol;
agarin; pantherin).
'Musculamine' *see* Spermine.
Mussel poison *see* Saxitoxin.

MUSTARD GAS (bis(2-chloroethyl)sulfide;
H; HS; Kampfstoff; Lost; sulfur mustard;
yperite; 'psoriasin').
Mustard oil *see* Allyl isothiocyanate.
'Mustargen' *see* Chlormethine.
Mustine *see* Chlormethine.
'Mustron' *see* Chlormethine *N*-oxide.
'Mutabase' *see* Diazoxide.
'Mutabon' *see* Amitriptyline with perphen-
azine.
'Mutamycin' *see* Mitomycin.
'Mutanxion' *see* Amitriptyline with per-
phenazine.
'Mutaspline' *see* Amitriptyline with per-
phenazine.
'Mutox' *see* Dichlorvos.
MW-274115 *see* Dichlozoline.
MXMC *see* Methiocarb.
MY-33-7 *see* Prilocaine.
MY-41-6 *see* Parsalamide.
My-301 *see* Guaifenesin.
'Myagen' *see* Bolasterone.
'Myalex' *see* Fenclozic acid.
'Myambutol' *see* Ethambutol.
Myarsenol (tr) *see* Sulfarsphenamine.
'Myasul' *see* Sulfamethoxypyridazine.
'Myavan' *see* Toloxychlorinol.
'My-B-Den' *see* Adenosine phosphate.
MYC-1080 *see* Stercuronium iodide.
'Mycal' *see* Dodecyltriphenylphosphonium
bromide.
'Mycanden' *see* Haloprogin.
'Mycaptine' *see* Mercaptopurine.
Mycerin (tr) *see* Neomycin.
'Mycil' *see* Chlorphenesin.
'Mycivin' *see* Lincomycin.
'Mycobactyl' *see* Gluconiazone.
'Mycoban(s)' *see* Calcium propionate;
Sodium propionate.
'Mycocten' *see* Ethyl paraben.
'Mecodecyl' *see* Undecenoic acid.
MYCOMYCIN (3,5,7,8-tridecatetraene-
10,12-diynoic acid).
MYCOPHENOLIC ACID* ((*E*)-6-(4-
hydroxy-6-methoxy-7-methyl-3-oxophtha-
lan-5-yl)-4-methyl-4-hexenoic acid; 6-(5-
carboxy-3-methylpent-2-enyl)-7-hydroxy-
5-methoxy-4-methylphthalide; NSC-
129185).
'Mycoplex' *see* Sulbentine.
'Myco-polycid' *see* Chlormidazole.
'Mycosin' *see* Undecenoic acid.
'Mycosporin' *see* Clotrimazole.
'Mycostatin' *see* Nystatin.
'Mycota' *see* Undecenoic acid.
'Mycozol' *see* Chlorobutol.
Mydecamycin *see* Midecamycin.
'Mydeton' *see* Tolperisone.
'Mydocalm' *see* Tolperisone.
'Mydriacyl' *see* Tropicamide.
'Mydrial' *see* Tyramine.
'Mydriatin' *see* Norephedrine.
'Mydrilate' *see* Cyclopentolate.
'Mydrin' *see* Tropicamide.
'Myelobromol' *see* Mitobronitol.
Myelosan (tr) *see* Busulfan.
'Myelucin' *see* Busulfan.

MYFADOL*** (1-benzoylmethyl-2,3-di-
methyl-3-(*m*-hydroxyphenyl)piperidine;
2-[3-(*m*-hydroxyphenyl)-2,3-dimethyl-
piperid-1-yl]acetophenone; 3-(*m*-hydroxy-
phenyl)-2,3-dimethyl-1-phenacylpiperidine
TA-306).
'Mykestron' *see* Amoxydramine undecenate.
'Mykomed' *see* Benzyl benzoate.
'Mylanta' *see* Dimeticone.
'Mylaxen' *see* Hexafluronium.
'Mylecytan' *see* Busulfan.
'Mylepsin' *see* Primidone.
'Myleran' *see* Busulfan.
'Mylicon' *see* Dimeticone.
'Mylone' *see* Dazomet.
'Mynocine' *see* Minocycline.
Myoarsenobenzol *see* Sulfarsphenamine.
'Myocaine' *see* Guaifenesin.
'Myocholine' *see* Bethanechol.
'Myochrysin' *see* Sodium aurothiomalate.
'Myocrisin' *see* Sodium aurothiomalate
'Myocuran' *see* Mephenesin.
'Myodil' *see* Iofendylate.
'Myofedrin' *see* (±)-Oxyfedrine.
Myohematin *see* Cytochrome c.
Myoinositol *see* Inositol.
'Myolastan' *see* Tetrazepam.
'Myordil' *see* Aminoxytriphene.
'Myoscaine' *see* Guaifenesin.
'Myoston' *see* Adenosine phosphate.
'Myotonine' *see* Bethanechol.
'Myprozine' *see* Natamycin.
MYRALACT** (2-tetradecylaminoethanol
lactate; *N*-(2-hydroxyethyl)tetradecylamine
lactate; *N*-(2-hydroxyethyl)tetradecyl-
ammonium lactate; myristylethanolamine
lactate.)
'Myriamycin' *see* Tetracycline dodecylsulfa-
mate.
MYRICETIN (3,3',4',5,5',7-hexahydroxy-

flavone; cannabiscetin).
MYRISTIC ACID (tetradecanoic acid).
See also Myrophine.
MYRISTICIN (1-allyl-3-methoxy-4,5-methyl-
enedioxybenzene).
Myristylethanolamine lactate *see* Myralact.
MYRISTYLPICOLINIUM CHLORIDE
(*N*-tetradecylpicolinium chloride;
'quatrasan').
Myristyltrimethylammonium bromide
see Tetradonium bromide.
'Myrj 45' *see* Macrogol stearate 8.
'Myrj 52' *see* Macrogol stearate 40.
MYROPHINE*** (myristyl ester of benzyl-
morphine; 3-benzyloxy-*N*-methyl-6-myrist-
yloxy-4,5-epoxymorphin-7-ene; 3-benzyl-
oxy-6-hydroxy-*N*-methyl-4,5-epoxymor-
phin-7-ene tetradecanoate ester).
MYRTECAINE*** (2-[2-(6,6-dimethyl-
2-norpinen-2-yl)ethoxy]trimethylamine;
2-[2-(6,6-dimethylbicyclo(3.1.1)hept-2-en-
2-yl)ethoxy]trimethylamine; homomyrtenyloxytriethylamine; 'algesal suractive',
'nopoxamine').
Myrticolorin *see* Rutoside.
'Mysoline' *see* Primidone.
'Mysteclin V' *see* Tetracycline with
amphotericin B.
'Mysuran' *see* Ambenonium.
MYTATRIENEDIOL (3-methoxy-16α-
methyl-1,3,5(10)-estratriene-16β,17β-diol;
SC-6924; 'anvene', 'manvene').
'Mytelase' *see* Ambenonium.
'Mytolon' *see* Benzoquinonium.
'Myxal' *see* Dodecyltriphenylphosphonium
bromide.
MYXIN (6-methoxy-1-phenazinol-5,10-di-
oxide).
MZ-144 *see* Rimazolium metilsulfate.

N

N-3 *see* Metetoin.
N-68 *see* Captodiame.
N-399 *see* Xenytropium.
N-640 *see* Trantelinium bromide.
N-714 *see* Chlorprothixene.
N-750 *see* Amitriptyline.
N-1113 *see* Pipoctanone.
N-7001 *see* Melitracen.
N-7020 *see* Meprotixol.
N-7048 *see* Nortriptyline.
N-7049 *see* Litracen.
NA-66 *see* Pimeclone.
NA-97 *see* Pancuronium bromide.
NA-274 *see* Bromhexine.
NA-872 *see* Ambroxol.
NA-III *see* 2-Ethyl-3,3-diphenylpropen(2)-

ylamine.
NAB-365 *see* Clenbuterol.
NABAM* (disodium 1,2-ethanediylbis-
(carbamodithioate); sodium *N*,*N*'-ethyl-
enebis(dithiocarbamate); DSE; 'dithane
D14', 'dithane 1740', 'parzate', 'parzate
liquid').
'NAC' *see* Acetylcysteine.
'Nacenyl' *see* Chlormadinone acetate.
'Naclex' *see* Hydroflumethiazide.
'Nacom' *see* Levodopa with carbidopa.
'Nactate' *see* Poldine.
'Nacton' *see* Poldine.
NAD *see* Nadide.
'Nadeine' *see* Dihydrocodeine.
NADIDE*** (3-carbamoyl-1-β-D-ribofurano-

sylpyridinium hydroxide 5'-ester with adenosine 5'-pyrophosphate inner salt; nicotinamide adenine dinucleotide; CO-I; codehydrogenase I; coenzyme I; cozymase; diphosphopyridine nucleotide; DPN; NAD; 'enzopride').

NADIDE PHOSPHATE (nicotinamide adenine dinucleotide phosphate; CO-II; codehydrogenase II; coenzyme II; triphosphopyridine nucleotide; TPN; NADP).

'Nadisan' *see* Carbutamide.

Nadizan (tr) *see* Carbutamide.

NADOLOL** (1-(*tert*-butylamino)-3-[(5,6,7,8-tetrahydro-*cis*-6,7-dihydroxynaphth-1-yl)oxy]-2-propanol; 1-(3-*tert*-butylamino-2-hydroxypropoxy)-5,6,7,8-tetrahydro-*cis*-6,7-naphthalenediol; (2*R*,3*S*)-5-(3-*tert*-butylamino-2-hydroxypropoxy)-1,2,3,4-tetrahydronaphthalene-2,3-diol; SQ-11725).

NADOXOLOL** (3-hydroxy-4-naphth-1-yloxybutyramidoxime; 1-[4-amino-2-hydroxy-4-(hydroxyimino)butoxy]naphthalene; LL-1530; 'bradyl 250').

NAEPAINE (2-amylaminoethyl ester of *p*-aminobenzoic acid; 'amylcaine', 'amylsine').

NAFARIN (tr) (4-hydroxy-3-(1-phenyl-2-propionylethyl)coumarin sodium salt; napharin).

NAFCAPROIC ACID** (2-ethyl-2-naphtha-1-ylbutyric acid; α,α-diethyl-1-naphthaleneacetic acid; DA-808).

NAFCILLIN** (6-(2-ethoxy-1-naphthamido)-3,3-dimethyl-7-oxo-4-thia-1-azabicyclo(3.2.0)heptane-2-carboxylic acid; 6-(2-ethoxy-1-naphthamido)penicillanic acid; 2-ethoxynaphth-1-ylpenicillin; nafcillin sodium; Wy-3277; 'naftopen', 'unipen').

Nafenoic acid *see* Nafenopin.

NAFENOPIN** (2-methyl-2-[*p*-(1,2,3,4-tetrahydronaphth-1-yl)phenoxy]propionic acid; nafenoic acid; C-13437-Su; Su-13437).

NAFIVERINE** (1,4-piperazinediethanol α-methyl-1-naphthaleneacetate ester; 1,4-bis(2-hydroxyethyl)piperazine bis-(2-naphth-1-ylpropionate); 1,4-[2-(2-naphth-1-ylpropionyloxy)ethyl]piperazine nafiverine hydrochloride; naftimipezine; naphthiepazine; DA-914; 'naftidan').

NAFOMINE** (*O*-(2-methylnaphth-1-yl-methyl)hydroxylamine).

NAFOXIDINE** (1-[2-[*p*-(3,4-dihydro-6-methoxy-2-phenylnaphth-1-yl)phenoxyl]-ethyl]pyrrolidine; nafoxidine hydrochloride; U-11100A).

'Nafrine' *see* Oxymetazoline.

NAFTALOFOS** (*N*-hydroxynaphthylimide diethyl phosphate; *N*-hydroxynaphthalimide diethyl phosphate; diethyl (*N*-hydroxynaphthylimido) phosphate; diethyl naphthyloximido phosphate; phthalophos; Bay-9002; Bayer-9002; E-9002; ENT-25567; S-940; 'maretin').

Naftamon (tr) *see* Bephenium hydroxynaphthoate.

NAFTAZONE** (1,2-naphthoquinone 2-semicarbazone; β-naphthoquinone monosemicarbazone; SCBN; 'haemostop', 'karbinone').

'Naftidan' *see* Nafiverine.

Naftidon (tr) *see* Menadiol sodium phosphate.

NAFTIDROFURYL** (2-diethylaminoethyl tetrahydro-α-(1-naphthylmethyl)-2-furanpropionate ester; LS-121; 'dusodril', 'iridus', 'praxilene').

NAFTIDROFURYL OXALATE (IS-121; LS-121).

Naftimepezine *see* Nafiverine.

Naftipramide *see* Naftypramide.

Naftizin (tr) *see* Naphazoline.

'Naftopen' *see* Nafcillin.

NAFTOXATE** (2-benzoxazolyl *N*-methyldithio-1-naphthalenecarbamate; *N*-methyldithio-1-naphthalenecarbamic acid 2-benzoxazolyl ester; *N*-methyl-*N*-naphth-1-yldithiocarbamic acid 2-benzoxazolyl ester).

NAFTYPRAMIDE** (α-(2-dimethylaminoethyl)-α-isopropyl-1-naphthaleneacetamide; naftipramide; naphthypramide; DA-992).

'Naganin' *see* Suramin.

'Naganol' *see* Suramin.

'Nagarse' *see* Subtilisin BPN[1].

NALBUPHINE** (17-cyclobutylmethyl-4,5α-epoxymorphinan-3,6α,14-triol; 12-cyclobutylmethyl-7,7a,8,9-tetrahydro-3,7a-dihydroxy-6H-8,9c-iminoethanophenanthro(4,5-bcd)furan-5(4aH)-ol; nalbuphine hydrochloride; EN-2234-A).

NALED* (1,2-dibromo-2,2-dichloroethyl dimethyl phosphate; bromchlophos; 'bromex', 'dibrom').

'Nalfon' *see* Fenoprofen.

Nalidixan* *see* Nalidixic acid.

NALIDIXIC ACID** (1-ethyl-1,4-dihydro-7-methyl-4-oxo-1,8-naphthyridine-3-carboxylic acid; 1-ethyl-7-methyl-1,8-naphthyridine-4-one-3-carboxylic acid; nalidixan; nalidixin; WIN-18320; 'neggram', 'negram', 'nevigramon', 'unstetic', 'wintomylon').

See also Sodium nalidixate.

Nalidixin *see* Nalidixic acid.

'Nalline' *see* Nalorphine.

NALMEXONE** (7,7a,8,9-tetrahydro-3,7a-dihydroxy-12-(3-methyl-2-butenyl)-6H-8,9c-iminoethanophenanthro(4,5-bcd)-furan-5(4aH)-one; 7,8-dihydro-14-hydroxy-*N*-(3-methyl-2-butenyl)normorphinone; nalmexone hydrochloride; EN-1620A).

NALORPHINE** (*N*-allylnormorphine; *N*-allyl-*N*-desmethylmorphine; allorphine; antorfin; antorphine; allylmorphine; NANM; nalorphine hydrobromide; 'anarcon', 'lethidrone', 'nalline').

NALORPHINE DINICOTINATE ('nimelan').

See also Nicomorphine with nalorphin dinicotinate.

NALOXONE** (12-allyl-7,7a,8,9-tetrahydro-3,7a-dihydroxy(4aH)(8,9-c)imino-ethanophenanthro(4,5-bcd)furan-5(6H)-one; L-N-allyl-14-hydroxynordihydromorphinone; N-allylnoroxymorphone; N-naloxone hydrochloride; EN 1530; 'narcan', 'narcon').

'Nalpen' see Azidocillin.
NALTREXONE*** ((−)-17-(cyclopropylmethyl)-3,5α-epoxy-3,4-dihydroxymorphinan-6-one; naltrexone hydrochloride; EN-1639A).
NALTROPINE (N-allylnoratropine).
'Namestin' see Clonidine.
Namol xenyrate see Namoxyrate.
NAMOXYRATE*** (2-dimethylaminoethanol 2-(p-biphenylyl)butyrate salt; deanol salt with 2-xenylbutyric acid; deanol xenbucin salt; namol xenyrate; W-1760-A).
'Nanbacin' see Xibornol.
NANDROLONE** (19-nortestotserone; 19-norandrost-4-en-17β-ol-3-one; 17β-hydroxyestr-4-en-3-one; 4-estren-17β-ol-3-one; norandrostenolone; nortestosterone; SG-4341; 'nortestonate').
Nandrolone adamantane-1-carboxylate see Bolmantalate.
NANDROLONE CIPIONATE (nandrolone 17-(3-cyclopentanepropionate); nandrolone cypionate; 'depo-nortestonate').
NANDROLONE CYCLOHEXANECAR-BOXYLATE (nandrolone hexahydrobenzoate; NSC-3351; 'durabol', 'nordurandron', 'anorlongandron').
NANDROLONE CYCLOHEXANEPRO-PIONATE (nandrolone 17-cyclohexylpropionate; 'sanabolic').
Nandrolone cyclopentanepropionate see Nandrolone cipionate.
NANDROLONE CYCLOTATE* (nandrolone 4-methylbicyclo(2.2.2)oct-2-ene-1-carboxylate; RS-3268R).
Nandrolone cypionate see Nandrolone cipionate.
NANDROLONE DECANOATE* ('decadurabolin', 'retabolil').
Nandrolone dodecanoate see Nandrolone laurate.
Nandrolone hexahydrobenzoate see Nandrolone cyclohexanecarboxylate.
NANDROLONE (p-HEXYLOXY)HYDRO-CINNAMATE (nandrolone 3-(p-hexyloxyphenyl)propionate; PNS; 'anadur').
Nandrolone 3-(p-hexyloxyphenyl)propionate see Nandrolone (p-hexyloxy)hydrocinnamate.
Nandrolone hydrocinnamate see Nandrolone phenpropionate.
NANDROLONE LAURATE (nandrolone dodecanoate; 'clinibolin').
Nandrolone 4-methylbicyclo(2.2.2)oct-2-2-ene-1-carboxylate see Nandrolone cyclotate.
NANDROLONE PHENPROPIONATE* (nandrolone 17-(3-phenylpropionate); nandrolone hydrocinnamate; NSC-23162; 'durabolin', 'nerobolil').

NANDROLONE PHENPROPIONATE WITH DESOXYCORTONE PHEN-PROPIONATE ('docabolin').
Nandrolone phenylpropionate see Nandrolone phenpropionate.
Naniopin* see Nanofin.
'Nankor' see Fenclofos.
NANM see Nalorphine.
NANOFIN*** (2,6-dimethylpiperidine; 2,6-lupetidine; naniopin; nanophyn).
Nanophyn see Nanofin.
'Naotin' see Sodium nicotinate.
NAPADISILATE(S)** (naphthalene-1,5-disulfonate(s); napadisylate(s)).
See also Mebhydrolin napadisilate.
Napadisylate(s)* see Napadisilate(s).
'Napafen' see Paracetamol.
'Napaltan' see Mafenide acetate.
Napharin (tr) see Nafarin.
NAPHAZOLINE*** (2-(1-naphthylmethyl)-2-imidazoline; naphazoline hydrochloride; naphazoline nitrate; naftizin; naphthyzine).
Naphthacaine see Naphthocaine.
Naphthalenecarboxylic acid(s) see Naphthoic acid(s).
NAPHTHALENE 1,5-DIISOCYANATE ('desmodure 15').
1,8-Naphthalenediol-3,6-disulfonic acid see Chromotropic acid.
Naphthalenedione see Naphthoquinone.
Naphthalene-1,5-disulfonic acid, esters and salts see Napadisilate(s).
2-Naphthalenesulfonic acid, esters and salts see Napsilate(s).
'Naphthamine' see Methenamine.
Naphthazoline see Naphazoline.
Naphthiepazine see Nafiverine.
'Naphthiomate-T' see Tolnaftate.
NAPHTHIONIC ACID (4-aminonaphthalene-1-sulfonic acid; α-naphthylamine-4-sulfonic acid).
NAPHTHOCAINE (2-diethylaminoethyl 4-amino-1-naphthoate; naphthocaine hydrochloride; naphthacaine).
Naphthohydroquinone see 1,4-Naphthalenediol.
NAPHTHOIC ACID(S) (naphthalenecarboxylic acid(s)).
1-NAPHTHOL (α-naphthol).
2-NAPHTHOL (β-naphthol).
NAPHTHONONE*** (2-(2-hydroxynaphth-1-yl)cyclohexanone; 1-(2-oxocyclohexyl)-2-naphthol).
1,2-Naphthoquinone 2-semicarbazone see Naftazone.
β-Naphthoquinone semicarbazone see Naftazone.
Naphthydrofuryl see Naftidrofuryl.
1-NAPHTHYLAMINE (α-naphthylamine).
2-NAPHTHYLAMINE (β-naphthylamine).
Naphthylamine blue see Trypan blue.
1-Naphthylamine-4-sulfonic acid see Naphthionic acid.
2-[(Naphth-1-ylamino)carbonyl]benzoic acid see Naptalam.
1-(Naphth-1-ylazo)-2-naphthol-3,6-di-

318

sulfonic acid *see* Bordeaux B.
2-NAPHTHYL BENZOATE (benzonaphthol).
1-(2-Naphthyl)-2-isopropylaminoethanol
see Pronetalol.
2-NAPHTHYL LACTATE (lactonaphthol;
'lactol').
1-Naphthyl *N*-methylcarbamate *see*
Carbaril.
2-(1-Naphthylmethyl)-2-imidazoline *see*
Naphazoline.
**2-Naphthyl *N*-methyl-*N*-(*m*-tolyl) thiono-
carbamate** *see* Tolnaftate.
1-NAPHTHYL SALICYLATE (alphol).
2-NAPHTHYL SALICYLATE (betol;
salinaphthol).
α-**Naphthylthiourea** *see* Antu.
1-Naphth-1-yl-2-thiourea *see* Antu.
Naphthypramide *see* Naftypramide.
Naphthyzine (tr) *see* Naphazoline.
'**Naphuride**' *see* Suramin.
'**Napoton**' *see* Chlordiazepoxide.
Napriline (tr) *see* Propranolol.
'**Naproc**' *see* Procaine-penicillin.
NAPROPAMIDE (*N*,*N*-diethyl-2-(naphth-
1-yloxy)propionamide; 1-[1-(diethyl-
carbamoyl)ethoxy]naphthalene; 'devrinol').
'**Napropion**' *see* Sodium propionate.
'**Naprosine**' *see* Naproxen.
'**Naprosyn**' *see* Naproxen.
NAPROXEN*** ((+)-6-methoxy-α-methyl-
2-naphthaleneacetic acid; (+)-2-(6-meth-
oxynaphth-2-yl)propionic acid; meth-
oxypropiocin; CG-3117; RS-3540; 'napros-
ine', 'naprosyn', 'proxen', 'synaxsyn').
NAPROXOL*** ((−)-6-methoxy-β-methyl-
2-naphthaleneethanol).
'**Naprylate**' *see* Sodium octanoate.
NAPSILATE(S)** (naphthalene-2-sulfo-
nate(s); napsylate(s)).
See also Dextropropoxyphene napsilate.
Napsylate(s)* *see* Napsilate(s).
NAPTALAM* (2-[(naphth-1-ylamino)-
carbonyl]benzoic acid; 1-(2-carboxy-
benzamido)naphthalene; APA; 'alanap').
'**Naqua**' *see* Trichlormethiazide.
'**Naquival**' *see* Reserpine with trichlormethiazide.
'**Naramycin**' *see* Cycloheximide.
NARANOL*** (8,9,10,11,11a,12-hexahydro-
8,10-dimethyl-7aH-naphtho(1',2':5,6)-
pyrano(3,2-c)pyridin-7a-ol).
NARASIN** (α-ethyl-6-[5-[3-(5-ethyltetra-
hydro-5-hydroxy-6-methyl-2H-pyran-2-yl)-
15-hydroxy-2,10,12-trimethyl-1,6,8-
trioxadispiro(4.1.5.3)pentadec-13-en-9-yl]-
2-hydroxy-1,3-dimethyl-4-oxoheptyl]tetra-
hydro-3,5-dimethyl-2H-2-pyran-2-acetic
acid).
'**Narcan**' *see* Naloxone.
Narcobarbital *see* Enibomal.
'**Narcodorm**' *see* Enibomal.
'**Narcogen**' *see* Trichloroethylene.
'**Narcolo**' *see* Dextromoramide.
'**Narcompren**' *see* Noscapine.
'**Narcon**' *see* Naloxone.
'**Narconumal**' *see* Enallylpropymal.

'**Narcophine**' *see* Morphine noscapine
meconate.
Narcosine *see* Noscapine.
'**Narcotal**' *see* Enibomal.
'**Narcotile**' *see* Chloroethane.
DL-**Narcotine** *see* Gnoscopine.
L-**Narcotine** *see* Noscapine.
'**Narcovene**' *see* Enibomal.
'**Narcyl**' *see* Ethylnarceine.
'**Narcylene**' *see* Acetylene.
'**Nardelzine**' *see* Phenelzine.
'**Nardil**' *see* Phenelzine.
'**Naridan**' *see* Oxyphencyclimine.
NARINGENIN (4',5,7-trihydroxyflavanone;
'asahina', 'inubuse').
Naringenin 5-rhamnoglucoside *see*
Aurantiin.
Naringenin 7-rutoside *see* Aurantiin.
Naringin *see* Aurantiin.
Naringoside *see* Aurantiin.
'**Narkogen**' *see* Buthalital.
'**Narkolan**' *see* Bromethol.
'**Narkotal**' *see* Enibomal.
'**Narkothion**' *see* Thiobutabarbital.
'**Narodrine**' *see* Noradrenaline.
'**Narphen**' *see* Phenazocine.
'**Narphin**' *see* Morphine noscapine meconate.
'**Nasan**' *see* Tetryzoline.
'**Nasivin**' *see* Oxymetazoline.
NAT-324 *see* Quindecamine acetate.
NAT-327 *see* Trimoxamine.
'**Nataba**' *see* Sodium *p*-aminobenzoate.
NATAMYCIN*** (antibiotic from *Str.*
natalensis; pimaricin; myprozine;
'pimafucin').
'**Natirose**' *see* Glyceryl trinitrate.
'**Natisedine**' *see* Quinidine ethylphenyl-
barbiturate.
'**Natorexic**' *see* Amfepramone.
'**Natrionex**' *see* Acetazolamide.
Natrog (tr) *see* Sodium trihydroxyglutarate.
'**Natrol**' *see* Bismuth tartrate.
'**Natulan**' *see* Procarbazine.
'**Natulanar**' *see* Procarbazine.
'**Naturetin**' *see* Bendroflumethiazide.
'**Naturine**' *see* Bendroflumethiazide.
'**Natusan**' *see* Benzalkonium chloride.
'**Nausidol**' *see* Pipamazine.
'**Nautamine**' *see* Diphenhydramine theo-
phyllinate.
'**Nautisan**' *see* Chlorbutol.
'**Navadel**' *see* Dioxation.
'**Navane**' *see* Tiotixene.
'**Navicalm**' *see* Meclozine.
'**Navidrex**' *see* Cyclopenthiazide.
'**Navidrix**' *see* Cyclopenthiazide.
'**Naxogin**' *see* Nimorazole.
'**N.B.L.**' *see* Metandienone.
NC-123 *see* Mesoridazine.
NC-150 *see* Phenazopyridine.
NC-1264 *see* Tonzonium.
NC-1968 *see* Fungimycin.
NC-2983 *see* Chlorflurazole.
NC-5016 *see* Fenazaflor.
NC-6897 *see* Bendiocarb.
NC-7197 *see* Esproquine.
ND-50 *see* Octopamine.

319

NDGA *see* Nordihydroguaiaretic acid.
NDR-263 *see* Oxyclipine.
NDR-304 *see* Ethyl dibunate.
NDR-5061A *see* Alfetamine.
NDR-5523A *see* Trimoxamine.
'N.E.A.' *see* Norethisterone acetate.
NEALBARBITAL*** (5-allyl-5-(2,2-di-methylpropyl)barbituric acid; allyl-neopentylbarbituric acid; nealbarbitone; neallymal; 'censedal', 'nevental').
Neallymal* *see* Nealbarbital.
'Neazolin' *see* Sulfafurazole.
'Nebcin' *see* Tobramycin.
NEBRAMYCIN** (antibiotic complex from *Str. tenebrarius*; tenemycin; A-12253A).
Nebramycin factor 6 *see* Tobramycin.
'Nebs' *see* Paracetamol.
Nebularine *see* Purine riboside.
Nebuline *see* Purine riboside.
Neburea *see* Neburon.
NEBURON* (1-butyl-3-(3,4-dichlorophenyl)-1-methylurea; neburea; 'kloben').
'Necatorina' *see* Carbon tetrachloride.
'Nectadon' *see* Noscapine.
'Nedeltran' *see* Alimemazine.
NEFOPAM*** (3,4,5,6-tetrahydro-5-methyl-1-phenyl-1H-2,5-benzoxazocine; Riker-738).
'Nefrix' *see* Hydrochlorothiazide.
'Nefrolan' *see* Clorexolone.
'Negatan' *see* Methylenedi(*m*-cresolsulfonic acid) polymer.
'Negatol' *see* Methylenedi(*m*-cresolsulfonic acid) polymer.
'Neggram' *see* Nalidixic acid.
'Negram' *see* Nalidixic acid.
'Neguvon' *see* Metrifonate with atropine.
'Neirotrast' *see* Iofendylate.
'Nelex' *see* Methylenedi(*m*-cresolsulfonic acid) polymer.
'Nema' *see* Tetrachloroethylene.
'Nemacide' *see* Dichlofenthion.
'Nemacur P' *see* Fenamiphos.
'Nemafos' *see* Thionazin.
'Nemaphos' *see* Thionazin.
'Nematin' *see* Metam-sodium.
'Nematolyt' *see* Papain.
'Nemazine' *see* Phenothiazine.
'Nembutal' *see* Pentobarbital sodium.
NEMOTIN (4-hydroxy-5,6-undecadiene-8,10-diynoic acid γ-lactone).
'Nemural' *see* Arecoline-acetarsol.
Nendrin *see* Endrin.
'Neo-absentol' *see* Ethadione.
'Neo-alfasol' *see* Algestone acetofenide.
'Neoantimosan' *see* Stibophen.
NEOARSPHENAMINE*** (sodium 3,3'-diamino-4,4'-dihydroxyarsenobenzene-*N*-formaldehydesulfoxylate; arsphenamine methylenesulfoxylic acid sodium salt; 'neosalvarsan').
'Neo-arsycodile' *see* Disodium methane-arsonate.
'Neoatromidin' *see* Clofibrate.
'Neobenodine' *see p*-Methyldiphenhydramine.
'Neobicin salicyl' *see* Salinazid.

'Neocalcin' *see* Calcium levulinate.
NEOCARZINOSTATIN (polypeptide from *Str. carzinostaticus*; NSC-69856).
'Neo-cebicure' *see* Isoascorbic acid.
'Neo-cebitate' *see* Sodium isoascorbate.
'Neocide' *see* DDT.
'Neocidol' *see* Dimpylate.
NEOCINCHOPHEN** (ethyl 6-methyl-2-phenyl-4-quinolinecarboxylate; ethyl ester of 6-methyl-2-phenylcinchoninic acid).
'Neo-citrullamon' *see* Phenytoin valerate.
'Neo-cobefrin' *see* (−)-Corbadrine.
'Neocolan' *see* Metochalcone.
'Neoconserviet' *see* Propham.
'Neocortef' *see* Hydrocortisone.
'Neodecyllin' *see* Neomycin undecenate.
'Neo-dema' *see* Chlorothiazide.
'Neo-diacid' *see* Bromisoval.
Neodicumarin (tr) *see* Ethyl biscoumace-tate.
'Neo-distol' *see* Bithionol sulfoxide.
'Neodorm' *see* Pentobarbital.
'Neodrast' *see* Oxyphenisatine.
'Neodrol' *see* Androstanolone.
NEODYMIUM PYROCATECHOLDI-SULFONATE COMPLEX ('phlogodym').
NEODYMIUM 3-SULFOISONICOTIN-ATE ('thrombodym').
'Neodyne' *see* Ethyl dibunate.
Neoeserine *see* Neostigmine.
'Neofemergen' *see* Ergometrine.
'Neogel' *see* Carbenoxolone.
'Neogest' *see* Norgestrel.
'Neo-gilurtymal' *see* Prajmalium bitartrate.
'Neogynon' *see* Levonorgestrel with ethinyl-estradiol.
'Neohexal' *see* Methenamine sulfosalicylate.
'Neo-hibernex' *see* Promazine.
'Neo-hollaxans' *see* Phenisatin.
'Neo-hydrazid' *see* Cyacetacide.
'Neohydrin' *see* Chlormerodrin.
'Neo-iopax' *see* Iodoxyl.
Neoisocodeine *see* Pseudocodeine.
'Neo-istafene' *see* Meclozine.
'Neoisuprel' *see* Isoetarine.
'Neokompensan' *see* Povidone.
'Neolin' *see* Benzathine penicillin.
'Neolutin' *see* Hydroxyprogesterone caproate.
'Neomercazole' *see* Carbimazole.
'Neo-methidin' *see* Methionine.
Neomonacrin *see* Methylaminacrin.
NEOMYCIN** (antibiotic from *Str. fradiae*; colimycin; framycin; mycerin; neomycin sulfate).
See also Berberine with neomycin; Clostebol acetate with neomycin.
Neomycin B *see* Framycetin.
NEOMYCIN UNDECENATE (neomycin undecylenate; 'neodecyllin').
Neomycin undecylenate* *see* Neomycin undecenate.
NEOMYCIN WITH BACITRACIN (by-komycin).
NEOMYCIN WITH OXYTETRACY-CLINE ('neotarchocin', 'neoterramycin').
NEOMYCIN WITH SULFAMETHIZOLE (By-123; 'uro-nebacetin').

'Neomyson G' *see* Thiamphenicol glycinate.
'Neo-naclex' *see* Bendroflumethiazide.
'Neonal' *see* Butethal.
'Neoniagar' *see* Mebutizide.
'Neoniazide' *see* Gluconiazone.
Neonicotine *see* Anabasine.
'Neo-oxedrine' *see* Phenylephrine.
'Neo-oxypate' *see* Pyrvinium embonate.
'Neopenil' *see* Penethamate hydriodide.
NEOPENTANE (2,2-dimethylpropane; tetramethylmethane).
1,1',1'',1'''-(Neopentanetetryltetraoxy)-tetrakis(2,2,2-trichloroethanol) *see* Petrichloral.
'Neo-penyl' *see* Clemizole penicillin.
'Neophylline' *see* Diprophylline with 7-(2-hydroxypropyl)theophylline.
Neopinamine *see* Tetramethrin.
NEOPINE (β-codeine).
'Neoprontosil' *see* Azosulfamide.
'Neopsicaine' *see* Pseudococaine.
NEOPTERIN (2-amino-4-hydroxy-6-(tri-hydroxypropyl)pteridine).
'Neo-pynamin' *see* Tetramethrin.
Neopyrithiamine *see* Pyrithiamine.
'Neoron' *see* Bromopropylate.
'Neorontyl' *see* Bendroflumethiazide.
'Neosalvarsan' *see* Neoarsphenamine.
'Neo-scabicidol' *see* Lindane.
'Neosedyl' *see* Thalidomide.
'Neosoralen' *see* Trioxysalen.
'Neostam' *see* Stibamine glucoside.
NEOSTANOX* (hexakis(1-methyl-2-phenyl-propyl)distannoxane; 'torque', 'vendex').
'Neostibosan' *see* Ethylstibamine.
NEOSTIGMINE BROMIDE** ((*m*-hydroxy-phenyl)trimethylammonium bromide dimethylcarbamate; neoeserine; proserine; synstigmine).
'Neoston' *see* Alclofenac.
'Neosulfine' *see* Mesulfen.
'Neotarchocin' *see* Neomycin with oxyte-tracycline.
'Neoterramycin' *see* Neomycin with oxytetracycline.
NEOTETRAZOLIUM (*p,p*'-biphenylene-2,2'-bis(3,5-diphenyltetrazolium chloride)).
'Neothiate' *see* *m*-Chlorophenyl dimethyl phosphorothioate.
'Neothyl' *see* Methyl propyl ether.
'Neo-thyreostat' *see* Carbimazole.
'Neotizide' *see* Isoniazid methanesulfonate.
'Neotran' *see* Bis(*p*-chlorophenoxy)methane.
NEOTROPIN (2',6'-diamino-2-butoxy-3,3'-azopyridine; 6-butoxy-3-(2,6-diamino-3-pyridylazo)pyridine; 'niazo').
'Neo-urofort' *see* Chlorazanil.
'Neoviacept' *see* Chloroquine diphosphate with glycobiarsol.
Neovitamin A *see* *cis*-Retinol.
'Neozine' *see* Levomepromazine.
Nephocarp *see* Carbofenotion.
'Nephramid' *see* Acetazolamine.
'Nephril' *see* Polythiazide.
'Nephrin' *see* Cystine.
'Nephrotest' *see* Sodium *p*-aminohippurate.
'Nepresol' *see* Dihydralazine.

'Neptal' *see* Mercuderamide.
'Neptazane' *see* Methazolamide.
NEQUINATE** (methyl 7-benzyloxy-6-butyl-1,4-dihydro-4-oxo-3-quinoline-carboxylate; methyl 7-benzyloxy-6-butyl-4-hydroxyquinoline-3-carboxylate; 7-benzyloxy-6-butyl-3-methoxycarbonyl-quinolin-4-one; methyl benzoquate; AY-20385; ICI-55052; 'statyl').
'Neratox' *see* Warfarin.
'Neraval' *see* Methitural.
'Neravan' *see* Secbutabarbital.
NEREISTOXIN (4-dimethylamino-1,2-dithiolane).
'Nerial' *see* Peruvoside.
Neriine *see* Conessine.
'Nerobol' *see* Metandienone.
'Neroboletta' *see* Metandienone.
'Nerobolil' *see* Nandrolone phenpropionate.
'Nervacton' *see* Benactyzine.
'Nervanaid B' *see* Tetrasodium edetate.
Nervic acid *see* 15-Tetracosenoic acid.
Nervonic acid *see* 15-Tetracosenoic acid.
'Nesacaine' *see* Chloroprocaine.
'Nesdonal' *see* Thiopental.
'Nesivine' *see* Oxymetazoline.
'Nesontil' *see* Oxazepam.
'Netamine' *see* Etafedrine.
Nethalide *see* Pronetalol.
'Nethamine' *see* Etafedrine.
'Netilar' *see* Paramethasone.
'Netrin' *see* Metcaraphen.
'Netropsin' *see* Congocidine.
Neuberg ester *see* Fructose 6-phosphate.
'Neugen' *see* Macrogol esters.
'Neulactil' *see* Periciazine.
'Neuleptil' *see* Periciazine.
'Neupentedrin' *see* Oxedrine.
'Neuractil' *see* Levomepromazine.
'Neuraxin' *see* Methocarbamol.
Neuridine *see* Spermine.
NEURINE (trimethylvinylammonium hydroxide).
'Neuriplege' *see* Chlorproethazine.
'Neurocil' *see* Levomepromazine.
'Neurolepsin' *see* Lithium carbonate.
'Neuroleptone' *see* Benactyzine.
'Neuroplegil' *see* Promazine.
'Neurosterone' *see* Cyclopregnol.
Neurotrast (tr) *see* Iofendylate.
'Neurotropan' *see* Choline citrate.
NEUTRAL INSULIN INJECTION* (porcine insulin solution buffered to pH 7; 'insulin novoactrapid', 'insulin actrapid', 'nuso').
'Neutralon' *see* Aluminium sodium silicate.
NEUTRAMYCIN*** (antibiotic from *Str. rimosus*; AE-705W; LL-705W).
'Neutrapen' *see* Penicillinase.
'Neutrazyme' *see* Sodium dodecyl sulfate.
'Neuvitan' *see* Octotiamine.
'Nevax' *see* Sodium dioctyl sulfosuccinate.
'Nevenal' *see* Nealbarbital.
'Nevigramon' *see* Nalidixic acid.
'Nevriton' *see* Bentiamine *and* Prosultiamin.
'New cacodyle' *see* Disodium methanearso-nate.

'New urotropin' *see* Methenamine anhydro-methylenecitrate.
'Nexagan' *see* Bromofos-ethyl.
'Nexagan G' *see* Bromofos-ethyl.
'Nexarato' *see* Warfarin.
NEXERIDINE** (1-[2-(dimethylamino)-1-methylethyl]-2-phenylcyclohexanol acetate ester).
'Nexion' *see* Bromofos.
'Nezeril' *see* Oxymetazoline.
NF-35 *see* Thiophanate.
NF-44 *see* Thiophanate methyl.
NF-67 *see* Nidroxyzone.
NF-71 *see* Nifurmerone.
NF-84 *see* Nifuraldezone.
NF-161 *see* Nifursemizone.
NF-246 *see* Nifuradene.
NF-602 *see* Levofuraltadone.
NF-902 *see* Levofuraltadone hydrochloride.
NF-963 *see* Furazolium chloride.
NF-1010 *see* Nifurdazil.
NF-1088 *see* Nifurquinazol.
NF-1120 *see* Nifurimide.
NF-1425 *see* Furazolium tartrate.
NIA-10242 *see* Carbofuran.
Niacin *see* Nicotinic acid.
Niacinamide *see* Nicotinamide.
'Niacol' *see* Nicotinyl alcohol.
'Niagar' *see* Hydrochlorothiazide.
'Niagara-1240' *see* Ethion.
'Niagara blue' *see* Trypan blue.
'Niagaramite' *see* Butylphenoxyisopropyl chloroethyl sulfite.
'Niagestin' *see* Megestrol.
NIALAMIDE*** (isonicotinic acid 2-[(2-benzylcarbamoyl)ethyl]hydrazide; *N*-(2-benzylcarbamylethyl)-*N'*-isonicotinoylhydrazine; *N'*-(2-benzylcarbamylethyl)-isoniazid; BEIH; 'niamid', 'nuredal', 'surgex').
'Nialate' *see* Ethion.
'Niallate' *see* Ethion.
'Niamid' *see* Nialamide.
NIAPRAZINE*** (*N*-[3-[4-(*p*-fluorophenyl)-piperazin-1-yl]-1-methylpropyl]nicotinamide).
'Niazo' *see* Neotropin.
'Nibal' *see* Metenolone acetate.
'Nibal injection' *see* Metenolone enantate.
'Nibiol' *see* Nitroxoline.
NIBROXANE** (5-bromo-2-methyl-5-nitro-*m*-dioxane).
NIBUFIN (tr) (dibutyl *p*-nitrophenyl phosphate).
NICAMETATE*** (2-diethylaminoethyl nicotinate).
NICAMETATE CITRATE (nicametate dihydrogen citrate; 'eucast', 'euclidan', 'provisan', 'soclidan').
'Nicamin' *see* Ethanolamine nicotinate.
'Nicarb' *see* Nicarbazin.
NICARBAZIN (equimolecular complex of 4,4'-dinitrocarbanilic acid and 4,6-dimethyl-2-pyrimidinol; 'nicarb', 'nicoxin', 'nicrazin').
'Nicastubin' *see* Ascorbic acid-nicotinamide addition compound.

NICERGOLINE*** (8β-(5-bromonicotino-yloxymethyl)-10α-methoxy-1,6-dimethyl-ergoline; 8β-hydroxymethyl-10α-methoxy-1,6-dimethylergoline 5-bromonicotinate; FI-6714; 'sermion').
NICERITROL*** (pentaerythrityl tetranicotinate; 'cardiolipol', 'perycit').
Nicethamide *see* Nikethamide.
NICEVERINE*** (4-(6,7-dimethoxyisoquinolin-1-ylmethyl)pyrocatechol dinicotinate; papaverine dinicotinate).
Nichlorfos *see* Phosnichlor.
'Nicholin' *see* Citicoline.
Niclofen *see* Nitrofen.
NICLOFOLAN*** (5,5'-dichloro-2,2'-dihydroxy-3,3'-dinitrodiphenyl; 5,5'-dichloro-3,3'-dinitro-2,2'-biphenol; 4,4'-dichloro-6,6'-dinitro-*o*,*o*-biphenol; menichlopholan; Bay-9015; Bayer-9015; Me-3635; 'bilevon', 'bilevon M', 'distolon').
NICLOSAMIDE*** (5-chloro-*N*-(2-chloro-4-nitrophenyl)salicylamide; 2',5-dichloro-4'-nitrosalicylanilide; 2',5-dichloro-2-hydroxy-4'-nitrobenzanilide; fenasal; phenasal; Bayer-2353; RP-10768; 'lintex', 'pestocid', 'sagimid', 'vermitin', 'yomesan').
Niclosamide ethanolamine salt *see* Clonitralide.
NICLOSAMIDE PIPERAZINE SALT ('mansonil').
NICOCLONATE*** (*p*-chloro-α-isopropyl-benzyl nicotinate).
NICOCODINE*** (6-nicotinoylcodeine; codeine 6-nicotinate; 'lyopect').
'Nicodan' *see* Sodium nicotinate.
NICODICODINE** (6-nicotinoyldihydrocodeine; dihydrocodeine 6-nicotinate; 7,8-dihydro-*O*³-methyl-*O*⁶-nicotinoylmorphine).
Nicofezon (tr) *see* Nifenazone.
NICOFIBRATE** (pyrid-3-ylmethyl 2-(*p*-chlorophenoxy)-2-methylpropionate; clofibric acid ester with nicotinyl alcohol).
NICOFURANOSE** (D-fructofuranose 1,3,4,6-tetranicotinate; fructose nicotinate; fructose tetranicotinate; nicofurazone; nicotinoylfructose; tetranicotinoylfructofuranose; 'bradilan', 'cardilan', 'kardylan').
NICOFURATE*** (5-(D-*arabino*-1,2,3,4-tetrahydroxybutyl)-2-methyl-3-furoic acid methyl ester tetranicotinate; methyl 2-methyl-5-[D-*arabino*-1,2,3,4-tetra(nicotinoyloxy)butyl]-3-furoate).
Nicofurazone *see* Nicofuranose.
'Nicolane' *see* Noscapine.
Nicomethanol* *see* Nicotinyl alcohol.
NICOMOL*** (2-hydroxy-1,1,3,3-cyclo-hexanetetramethanol 1,1,3,3-tetranicotinate).
NICOMORPHINE*** (3,6-dinicotinoyl-morphine; morphine 3,6-dinicotinate; nicomorphine hydrochloride; 'vilan').
NICOMORPHINE WITH NALORPHINE DINICOTINATE (morphine dinicotinate with nalorphine dinicotinate; 'vendal neu').
NICOPHOLINE*** (4-nicotinoylmorpho-line).
'Nicoprazine' *see* Morinamide.

322

'Nicopyron' see Nifenazone.
'Nicorine' see Nikethamide.
'Nicorol' see Furosemide.
'Nicoscorbine' see Ascorbic acid-nicotin-amide addition compound.
NICOSIN (tr) (ethyl 3-[p-[bis(2-chloroethyl)-amino]phenyl]-2-nicotinoylaminopropion-ate; ethyl ester of p-[bis(2-chloroethyl)-amino]-N-nicotinoylphenylalanine; N-sarcolysylnicotinamide; nicozin).
'Nicosode' see Sodium nicotinate.
Nicotafuryl* see Thurfyl nicotinate.
NICOTHIAZONE*** (nicotinaldehyde thiosemicarbazone; G-469).
NICOTINALDEHYDE (3-pyridyl aldehyde; β-pyridyl aldehyde).
Nicotinaldehyde thiosemicarbazone see Nicothiazone.
NICOTINAMIDE*** (3-pyridinecarbox-amide; niacinamide; PP factor; amide PP; vitamin B₃).
Nicotinamide adenine dinucleotide see Nadide.
2-Nicotinamidoethyl clofibrate see Picafibrate.
NICOTINE (3-(1-methyl-2-pyrrolidyl)-pyridine).
NICOTINIC ACID*** (3-pyridinecarboxylic acid; niacin; PP factor).
See also Pentifylline with nicotinic acid.
Nicotinic acid esters see Benzyl nicotinate; Butoxyethyl nicotinate; Etofibrate; Guvacoline; Hepronicate; Inositol nico-tinate; Nicametate; Nicoclonate; Nico-codine; Nicodicodine; Nicomorphine; Nicopholine; Nicofuranose; Nicofurate; Thurfyl nicotinate; Xantinol nicotinate.
Nicotinic acid N-methylbetaine see Trigonelline.
Nicotinic acid N-oxide see Oxiniacic acid.
Nicotinic acid salts see Aluminium nico-tinate; Ethanolamine nicotinate; Sodium nicotinate.
Nicotinic acid tocopheryl ester see α-Toco-pherol nicotinate.
Nicotinic acid trans-3,3,5-trimethylcyclo-hexyl ester see Ciclonicate.
Nicotinic alcohol see Nicotinyl alcohol.
p-Nicotinoylaminobenzoic acid 2-diethyl-aminoethyl ester see Nicotinoylprocaine.
N-Nicotinoylamphetamine see Phenatin.
6-Nicotinoylcodeine see Nicocodine.
6-Nicotinoyldihydrocodeine see Nicodi-codine.
Nicotinoylfructose see Nicofuranose.
Nicotinoylglycine see Nicotinuric acid.
2-(Nicotinoyloxy)ethyl clofibrate see Etofibrate.
NICOTINOYLPROCAINE (2-diethyl-aminoethyl p-nicotinoylaminobenzoate; 'sklerovitol').
NICOTINURIC ACID (nicotinoylglycine).
NICOTINYL ALCOHOL* (3-pyridine-methanol; β-pyridyl carbinol; nico-methanol; nicotinic alcohol; Nu-2121; Ro-1-5155; 'niacol', 'roniacol', 'ronicol').
Nicotinyl alcohol ester with clofibric

acid see Nicofibrate.
Nicoumalone see Acenocoumarol.
'Nicoxin' see Nicarbazin.
Nicozin (tr) see Nicosin.
'Nicrazin' see Nicarbazin.
NICTINDOLE*** (2-isopropylindol-3-yl pyrid-3-yl ketone; L-8027).
NIDROXYZONE*** (2-(2-hydroxyethyl)-semicarbazone of 5-nitro-2-furaldehyde; furaloxon; F-26; NF-67; 'furadroxyl').
NIFEDIPINE*** (dimethyl 1,4-dihydro-2,6-dimethyl-4-(2-nitrophenyl)pyridine-3,5-dicarboxylate; BAY a-1040; 'adalate').
NIFENALOL*** (α-isopropylaminomethyl-p-nitrobenzyl alcohol; N-isopropyl-p-nitrophenylethanolamine; INPEA).
NIFENAZONE*** (2,3-dimethyl-4-nicotin-amido-1-phenyl-3-pyrazolin-5-one; N-anti-pyrinylnicotinamide; nicofezon; 'nicopyron' 'thylin').
'Niflucid' see Niflumic acid.
NIFLUMIC ACID*** (2-(3-trifluoromethyl-anilino)nicotinic acid; 2-(α,α,α-trifluoro-m-toluidino)nicotinic acid; 2-(3-trifluoro-methylanilino)pyridine-3-carboxylic acid; N-(3-carboxypyridin-2-yl)-α,α,α-trifluoro-m-toluidine; JDL-37; R-368c; 'actol', 'artricid', 'forenol', 'inflaryl', 'niflucid', 'nifluril').
'Nifluril' see Niflumic acid.
'Nifos' see Tetraethyl pyrophosphate.
'Nifos T' see Tetraethyl pyrophosphate.
'Nifulidone' see Furazolidone.
NIFUNGIN*** (antibiotic from Aspergillus giganteus).
NIFURADENE*** (1-(5-nitrofurfurylidene-amino)-2-imidazolinone; oxafuradene; NF-246; 'renafur').
Nifuralazin* see Furalazine.
NIFURALDEZONE*** (5-nitro-2-fural-dehyde semioxamazone; NF-84; 'entefur', 'furamazone').
NIFURALIDE** (2-(allylamino)-4-thiazole-carboxylic acid [3-(5-nitro-2-furyl)allyl-idene]hydrazide; 1-[(2-allylamino)-1,3-thiazol-4-yl]-6-(5-nitro-2-furyl)-1-oxo-2,3-diaza-3,5-hexadiene; CB-12025).
'Nifurantin' see Nitrofurantoin.
NIFURATEL*** (5-(methylthiomethyl)-3-(5-nitrofurfurylideneamino)-2-oxazoli-dinone; SAP-113; 'inimur', 'macmiror', 'magmilor', 'omnes', 'polmiror', 'tydantil').
NIFURATRONE*** (N-(2-hydroxyethyl)-α-(5-nitro-2-furyl)nitrone).
Nifurazolidone* see Furazolidone.
NIFURDAZIL*** (1-(2-hydroxyethyl)-3-(5-nitrofurfurylideneamino)-2-imidazol-idinone; edrofuradene; NF-1010).
NIFURETHAZONE*** (2-(2-dimethyl-aminoethyl) semicarbazone of 5-nitro-2-furaldehyde).
NIFURFOLINE*** (3-morpholinomethyl-1-(5-nitrofurfurylideneamino)hydantoin).
NIFURIMIDE** (DL-4-methyl-1-(5-nitro-furfurylideneamino)-2-imidazolidinone; NF-1120).
NIFURIZONE** (1-(methylcarbamoyl)-

323

3-[3-(5-nitro-2-furyl)allylideneamino]-2-imidazolinone).

NIFURMAZOLE*** (3-(hydroxymethyl)-1-[3-(5-nitro-2-furyl)allylideneamino]-hydantoin).

NIFURMERONE*** (chloromethyl 5-nitro-2-furyl ketone; metofurone; NF-71).

NIFUROXAZIDE*** (p-hydroxybenzoic acid 5-nitro-2-furfurylidenehydrazide; p-hydroxy-N^2-(5-nitro-2-furfurylidene)benzohydrazide; 'ercefuryl').

NIFUROXIME*** (5-nitro-2-furaldehyde oxime).

NIFURPIPONE*** (4-methyl-1-piperazineacetic acid (5-nitrofurfurylidene)-hydrazide; 1-[2-(4-methylpiperazin-1-yl)-acetyl]-2-(5-nitrofurfurylidene)hydrazine; 5-nitrofuraldehyde [(4-methylpiperazin-1-yl)acetyl]hydrazone; Rec-15/0122; 'recofur').

NIFURPIRINOL*** (6-[2-(5-nitro-2-furyl)-vinyl]-2-pyridinemethanol; 6-[2-(5-nitro-2-furanyl)ethenyl]-2-pyridinemethanol; P-7138; 'furanace').

NIFURPRAZINE*** (3-amino-6-[2-(5-nitro-2-furyl)vinyl]pyridazine; furenapyridazine; furenazine; 'carofur').

NIFURQUINAZOL*** (2,2'-[2-(5-nitrofur-2-yl)quinazolin-4-ylimino]diethanol; 4-[bis(2-hydroxyethyl)amino]-2-(5-nitrofur-2-yl)quinazoline; NF-1088).

NIFURSEMIZONE*** (5-nitro-2-furaldehyde 2-ethylsemicarbazone; etafurazone; NF-161).

NIFURSOL** (3,5-dinitrosalicylic acid 2-(5-nitrofurfurylidene)hydrazide; 2-(3,5-dinitrosalicoyl)-1-(5-nitrofurfurylidene) hydrazine; RT-6912).

NIFURTHIAZOLE*** (2-(2-formylhydrazino)-4-(5-nitro-2-furyl)thiazole; AS-17665).

NIFURTIMOX*** (tetrahydro-3-methyl-4-(5-nitrofurfurylideneamino)-1,4-thiazine 1,1-dioxide; 3-methyl-4-(5-nitrofurfurylideneamino)tetrahydro-1,4-thiazine 1,1-dioxide; 4-(5-nitrofurfurylideneamino)-3-methylthiomorpholine 1,1-dioxide; 'lampit').

NIFURVIDINE** (2-methyl-6-[2-(5-nitro-2-furyl)vinyl]-4-pyrimidinol).

Nigelline see Damascenine.

'**Nigrin**' see Streptonigrin.

NIH-7519 see Phenazocine.

NIH-7667 see Noracymethadol.

NIH-7672 see Metofoline.

NIH-7856 see Etazocine.

NIHYDRAZONE*** (acetylhydrazone of 5-nitro-2-furaldehyde; acetic acid 5-nitrofurfurylidenehydrazide).

NIKETHAMIDE*** (N,N-diethylnicotinamide; betapyrimidum; cordiamin; nicethamide).

'**Nikkol HCO 50**' see Ricinomacrogol.

'**Nikoban**' see Lobeline.

'**Nilatil**' see Itramin tosilate.

'**Nilergex**' see Isothipendyl.

NILESTRIOL*** (3-cyclopentyloxy-19-nor-17α-pregna-1,3,5(10)-trien-20-yne-16α,17-diol; 3-cyclopentyloxy-16α, 17-dihydroxy-19-nor-17α-pregna-1,3,5(10)-trien-20-yne; nylestriol).

'**Nilevar**' see Norethandrolone.

'**Nilodin**' see Lucanthone.

'**Nilstat**' see Nystatin.

'**Nilverm**' see Tetramisole.

'**Nilverm GL**' see Levamisole.

'**Nimaol**' see Octamoxin.

NIMAZONE** (3-(p-chlorophenyl)-4-imino-2-oxo-1-imidazoleacetonitrile; 3-(p-chlorophenyl)-1-cyanomethyl-4-imino-imidazolidine-2-one).

'**Nimelan**' see Nalorphine dinicotinate.

NIMETAZEPAM*** (1,3-dihydro-1-methyl-7-nitro-5-phenyl-2H-1,4-benzodiazepin-2-one; ID-530; S-1530).

NIMIDANE** (cyclic methylene (4-chloro-o-tolyl)dithioimidocarbonate; 4-chloro-N-1,3-dithietan-2-ylidene-2-methylaniline; CL-84633; ENT-29106; 'abequito').

NIMORAZOLE*** (4-[2-(5-nitroimidazol-1-yl)ethyl]morpholine; 1-(2-morpholino-ethyl)-5-nitroimidazole; nitrimidazine; K-1900; 'acterol', 'naxogin', 'nulogyl').

Ninhydrin (1,2,3-indantrione hydrate).

'**Nioform**' see Clioquinol.

NIOMETACIN*** (5-methoxy-2-methyl-1-nicotinoylindole-3-acetic acid).

'**Nionate**' see Ferrous gluconate.

'**Niozymin**' see Nicotinamide.

'**Nipabenzyl**' see Benzyl paraben.

'**Nipantiox 1-F**' see Butylated hydroxyanisole.

'**Nipagin**' see Methyl paraben.

'**Nipagen E**' see Ethyl paraben.

'**Nipaphenyl**' see Phenyl paraben.

'**Nipasol**' see Butyl paraben.

'**Nipasol P**' see Propyl paraben.

'**Nipaxon**' see Noscapine.

NIPECOTIC ACID (3-piperidinecarboxylic acid).

'**Niperyt**' see Pentaerythrityl tetranitrate.

'**Nipodal**' see Prochlorperazine.

NIPROFAZONE*** (N-[(antipyrinylisopropylamino)methyl]nicotinamide; 4-[(isopropyl)(nicotinamidomethyl)amino]-2,3-dimethyl-1-phenyl-3-pyrazolin-5-one; 4-[(isopropyl)(nicotinamidomethyl)amino]-phenazone; RA-101).

'**Niran**' see Parathion.

'**Niren**' see Polychlorinated biphenyl mixture.

NIRIDAZOLE*** (1-(5-nitrothiazol-2-yl)-imidazolidin-2-one; nitrothiamidazol; Ba-32644; C-32644-Ba; 'ambilhar').

'**Nirvanil**' see Valnoctamide.

'**Nirvegil**' see Carfimate.

'**Nirvotin**' see Carfimate.

'**Nirvotinal**' see Carfimate.

'**Nisentil**' see Alphaprodine.

'**Nisidan**' see Opipramol.

'**Nisidana**' see Opipramol.

NISOBAMATE*** (2-hydroxymethyl-2,3-dimethylpentyl carbamate isopropylcarbamate; 2-sec-butyl-2-methyl-1,3-propanediol carbamate isopropylcarbamate; W-1015).

NISOXETINE** ((±)-3-(o-methoxyphenoxy)-*N*-methyl-3-phenylpropylamine; (±)-2-(3-methylamino-1-phenylpropoxy)-anisole).

'Nissol' *see* *N*-(2-Fluoroacetyl)-*N*-methyl-1-naphthylamine.

'Nisulfazole' *see* Nitrosulfathiazole.

NITARSONE*** (*p*-nitrobenzenearsonic acid; 'hep-a-stat', 'histostat').

Nithiazide *see* 1-Ethyl-3-(5-nitrothiazol-2-yl)-urea.

'Nitoman' *see* Tetrabenazine.

NITRACRINE** (9-[[3-(dimethylamino)-propyl]amino]-1-nitroacridine; C-283; 'ledacrin').

NITRALAMINE* (2-(*o*-chloro-α-nitromethylbenzylthio)ethylamine; nitralamine hydrochloride; SC-12350).

'Nitralettae' *see* Trolnitrate.

NITRALIN* (4-(methylsulfonyl)-2,6-dinitro-*N*,*N*-dipropylaniline; 'planavin').

NITRAMISOLE*** ((±)-2,3,5,6-tetrahydro-6-(*m*-nitrophenyl)imidazo(2,1-b)thiazole).

'Nitramyl' *see* Amyl nitrite.

'Nitrangin' *see* Mannityl hexanitrate.

'Nitranitol' *see* Mannityl hexanitrate.

Nitranol (tr) *see* Trolnitrate.

2-Nitratoethylamine *see* Itramin.

NITRAZEPAM*** (1,3-dihydro-7-nitro-5-phenyl-2H-1,4-benzodiazepin-2-one; 7-nitro-5-phenyl-1,3-dihydro-(2H)-1,4-benzodiazepin-2-one; LA-1; Ro-4-5360; Ro-5-3059; 'benzalin', 'dumolid', 'eunoctin', 'mogadan', 'mogadon', 'pacisyn', 'radedorm').
See also Potassium nitrazepate.

'Nitretamin' *see* Trolnitrate.

NITRICHOLINE PERCHLORATE*** (choline nitrate ester perchlorate; nitrocholine).

'Nitricide' *see* Fenson.

2-Nitrilo-*N*-*tert*-butylphenoxypropanolamine *see* Bunitrolol.

Nitrilotriacetic acid *see* Triglycollamic acid.

Nitrilotriethanol *see* Triethanolamine.

Nitrimidazine *see* Nimorazole.

NITRITOCOBALAMIN (vitamin B$_{12c}$).

3-Nitro *see* Roxarsone.

***p*-Nitrobenzenearsonic acid** *see* Nitarsone.

NITROCAPHANE (3-[2-[2-[bis(2-chloroethyl)amino]ethyl]-4-nitrophenyl]alanine; 2-[2-(2-amino-2-carboxyethyl)-4-nitrophenyl]-2',2''-dichlorotriethylamine; 2-(2-amino-2-carboxyethyl)-*N*,*N*-bis(2-chloroethyl)-4-nitrophenethylamine; AT-1258).

Nitrocellulose *see* Pyroxylin.

Nitrochloroform *see* Chloropicrin.

Nitrocholine *see* Nitricholine.

NITROCYCLINE*** (4-dimethylamino-1,4,4a,5,5a,6,11,12a-octahydro-3,10,12,12a-tetrahydroxy-7-nitro-1,11-dioxo-2-naphthacenecarboxamide; 6-demethyl-6-deoxy-7-nitrotetracycline).

NITRODAN** (3-methyl-5-(*p*-nitrophenylazo)rhodanine; 3-methyl-5-(4-nitrophenylazo)thiazolidin-4-one-2-thione; CTR-6110; 'nitroduran').

'Nitroduran' *see* Nitrodan *and* Trolnitrate.

'Nitroerythrite' *see* Erythrityl tetranitrate.

Nitroerythrol *see* Erythrityl tetranitrate.

'Nitrofar' *see* Dinitro-*o*-cresol.

NITROFEN* (2,4-dichloro-1-(*p*-nitrophenoxy)benzene; 2,4-dichloro-4'-nitrodiphenyl ether; niclofen; 'TOK E25').

'Nitrofungin' *see* 2-Chloro-4-nitrophenol.

'Nitrofuracin' *see* Nitrofurantoin.

NITROFURAL** (semicarbazone of 5-nitro-2-furaldehyde; furacilin; nitrofurazone; NSC-2100).

5-Nitro-2-furaldehyde acetylhydrazone *see* Nihydrazone.

5-Nitro-2-furaldehyde (dimethylaminoethyl)semicarbazone *see* Nifurethazone.

5-Nitro-2-furaldehyde 2-ethylsemicarbazone *see* Nifursemizone.

5-Nitro-2-furaldehyde (hydroxyethyl)-semicarbazone *see* Nidroxyzone.

5-Nitro-2-furaldehyde isonicotinoylhydrazone *see* Nitrofurfurylideneisoniazid.

5-Nitro-2-furaldehyde [(4-methylpiperazin-1-yl)acetyl]hydrazone *see* Nifurpipone.

5-Nitro-2-furaldehyde oxime *see* Nifuroxime.

5-Nitro-2-furaldehyde semicarbazone *see* Nitrofural.

5-Nitro-2-furaldehyde semioxamazone *see* Nifuraldezone.

5-NITRO-2-FURALDEHYDE THIOSEMICARBAZONE (benzazone-VII; F-8; SHCH-49).

NITROFURANTOIN*** (1-(5-nitro-2-furfurylideneamino)hydantoin; furadoine; furadonin; furazidin; NSC-2107; F-30; 'alfuran', 'berkfurin', 'chemiofuran', 'cyantin', 'cystit', 'furadantin', 'furadantoin', 'furadonine', 'furantoin', 'furatin', 'ituran', 'macrodantin', 'nifurantin', 'nitrofuracin', 'N-toin', 'parfuran', 'urosept').

NITROFURANTOIN WITH LIQUORICE ('ceduran').

6-[2-(5-Nitro-2-furanyl)ethenyl]-2-pyridinemethanol *see* Nifurpirinol.

Nitrofurazone *see* Nitrofural.

1-(5-NITRO-2-FURFURYLIDENE-AMINO)GUANIDINE SULFATE (furaguanidine; F-28; 'guanofuracin').

1-(5-Nitro-2-furfurylideneamino)hydantoin *see* Nitrofurantoin.

1-(5-Nitrofurfurylideneamino)-2-imidazolinone *see* Nifuradene.

4-(5-Nitrofurfurylideneamino)-3-methylthiomorpholine 1,1-dioxide *see* Nifurtimox.

3-(5-Nitrofurfurylideneamino)-2-oxazolidinone *see* Furazolidone.

1-(5-Nitrofurfurylidene)-2-(3,5-dinitrosalicoyl)hydrazine *see* Nifursol.

NITROFURFURYLIDENEISONIAZID (5-nitro-2-furfurylideneisoniazid; 5-nitro-2-furaldehyde isonicotinoylhydrazone; isonicotinic acid (5-nitro-2-furfurylidene)-hydrazide; furanoiozid; F-74).

NITROFURFURYL METHYL ETHER (5-nitro-2-furfuryl methyl ether; 2-methoxy-

methyl-5-nitrofuran; furamicid; F-1;
'furaspor', 'furbenal').
1-(5-Nitrofurylacrylideneamino)-1,3,4-
triazole see Furacrylin.
2,2'-[2-(5-Nitrofur-2-yl)quinazolin-4-yl-
imino]diethanol see Nifurquinazol.
6-[2-(5-Nitro-2-furyl)vinyl]-2-pyridine-
methanol see Nifurpirinol.
Nitrogen dioxide see Nitrogen peroxide.
Nitrogen monoxide see Nitrous oxide.
Nitrogen mustard see Chlormethine.
NITROGEN PEROXIDE (NO_2; N_2O_4;
nitrogen dioxide; nitrogen tetroxide).
Nitrogen protoxide see Nitrous oxide.
Nitrogen tetroxide see Nitrogen peroxide.
NITROGEN TRICHLORIDE ('agene').
Nitroglycerin see Glyceryl trinitrate.
Nitroglycerol see Glyceryl trinitrate.
'Nitrogranulogen' see Chlormethine.
NITROGUANIL (1-amidino-3-(p-nitro-
phenyl)urea; T-72; WR-25979).
4-[2-(5-Nitroimidazol-1-yl)ethyl]-
morpholine see Nimorazole.
N-[[(**2-Nitroimidazol-1-yl)methyl]-**
carbonyl]benzylamine see Benznidazole.
Nitrolin see Calcium carbimide.
'Nitroman' see Mannityl hexanitrate.
Nitromannite see Mannityl hexanitrate.
Nitromannitol see Mannityl hexanitrate.
NITROMETHAQUALONE (3-(2-methoxy-
4-nitrophenyl)-2-methylquinazolin-4-one;
'parnox').
NITROMIDE* (3,5-dinitrobenzamide).
NITROMIFENE* (1-[2-[p-[α-(p-methoxyphenyl)-β-nitrostyryl]phenoxy]ethyl]-
pyrrolidine; 4-methoxy-α'-nitro-α-[p-(2-
pyrrolidin-1-ylethoxy)phenyl]stilbene;
1-(p-methoxyphenyl)-2-nitro-1-[p-[(2-
pyrrolidin-1-yl)ethoxy]phenyl]ethylene;
1-[2-[4-[1-(4-methoxyphenyl)-2-nitro-2-
phenylethenyl]phenoxy]ethyl]pyrrolidine;
CN-55945).
'Nitromin' see Chlormethine N-oxide.
'Nitrong' see Glyceryl trinitrate.
2-Nitro-1-(p-nitrophenoxy)-4-(trifluoro-
methyl)benzene see Fluorodifen.
Nitropentaerythrite see Pentaerythrityl
tetranitrate.
Nitropenton see Pentaerythrityl tetranitrate.
p-(p-**Nitrophenoxy)phenyl isothiocyanate**
see Nitroscanate.
p-**NITROPHENYL DIBUTYLPHOSPHIN-**
ATE (nivufin; nivuphin).
7-Nitro-5-phenyl-1,3-dihydro-1,4-benzo-
diazepin-2-one see Nitrazepam.
7-Nitro-5-phenyl-1,3-dihydro-1,4-benzo-
diazepin-2-one-3-carboxylic acid
potassium salt see Potassium nitrazepate.
1-[5-(p-Nitrophenyl-2)-furfurylidene-
amino]hydantoin see Dantrolene.
4'-[(p-Nitrophenyl)sulfamoyl]acetanilide
see Sulfanitran.
5-Nitro-8-quinolinol see Nitroxoline.
NITROSCANATE* (p-(p-nitrophenoxy)-
phenyl isothiocyanate).
'Nitrositol' see Inositol hexanitrate.
N-**Nitrosodiethylamine** see Diethylnitros-

amine.
N-**Nitrosodimethylamine** see Dimethylnitrosamine.
Nitrostigmine* see Parathion.
NITROSULFATHIAZOLE* (p-nitro-
N-(2-thiazolyl)benzenesulfonamide;
2-(p-nitrophenylsulfonamido)thiazole;
'nisulfazole').
'Nitro-tabletten' see Trolnitrate.
Nitrothiamidazol see Niridazole.
1-(5-Nitrothiazol-2-yl)imidazolidin-2-one
see Niridazole.
1-(2-Nitro-p-tolylazo)-2-naphthol see
Toluidine red.
4'-Nitro-3'-(trifluoromethyl)isobutyr-
anilide see Flutamide.
NITROUS OXIDE (nitrogen monoxide;
nitrogen protoxide; N_2O; laughing gas;
dinitrogen monoxide; hyponitrous acid
anhydride; factitious air).
NITROVIN (1,5-bis(5-nitro-2-furyl)-1,4-
pentadien-3-one amidinohydrazone;
'payzone').
p-**[2-(5-Nitro-1-vinylimidazol-2-yl)vinyl]-**
benzoic acid see Stirimazole.
'Nitrox' see Parathion-methyl.
Nitroxanthic acid see Picric acid.
NITROXINIL* (4-hydroxy-3-iodo-5-nitro-
benzonitrile; 4-cyano-2-iodo-6-nitrophenol;
nitroxynil; 'dovenix').
NITROXINIL MEGLUMINE (methylglucamine salt of nitroxinil; 'trodax').
NITROXOLINE ** (5-nitro-8-quinolinol;
8-hydroxy-5-nitroquinoline; 5-NOK;
'nibiol').
Nitroxynil see Nitroxinil.
NIUIF-1 (tr) see Ethyl mercuriphosphate.
NIUIF-100 (tr) see Parathion.
NIVACORTOL* (2'-(p-fluorophenyl)-2'H-
17α-pregna-2,4-dien-20-yno(3,2-c)pyrazol-
17-ol; nivazol; WIN-27914).
NIVALENOL (3α,4β,7α,15-tetrahydroxy-
scirp-9-en-8-one).
Nivaline see Galantamine.
'Nivaquine B' see Chloroquine.
'Nivaquine C' see Sontoquine.
Nivazol* see Nivacortol.
'Nivelona' see Diphemanil metilsulfate.
'Nivembin' see Chloroquine sulfate with
diiodohydroxyquin.
'Nivitin' see Sorbitol.
'Nivoman' see Triflupromazine.
Nivufin (tr) see p-Nitrophenyl dibutyl-
phosphinate.
Nivuphin (tr) see p-Nitrophenyl dibutyl-
phosphinate.
NIXYLIC ACID* (2-(2,3-xylidino)nicotinic
acid; 2-(2,3-dimethylanilino)nicotinic acid;
2-(2,3-xylidino)pyridine-3-carboxylic acid).
'Nizin' see Zinc sulfanilate.
N-Lost see Chlormethine.
NNDG see Metformin.
'Noan' see Diazepam.
'Nobacid' see Salsalate.
'Nobacter' see Triclocarban.
'Nobamide' see Malonylbis(procainamide).
'Nobecutane' see Thiram.

'Nobedon' *see* Paracetamol.
'Nobedorm' *see* Methaqualone.
'Nobrium' *see* Medazepam.
Nocardia lurida, antibiotic *see* Ristocetin.
'Nocertone' *see* Oxetorone fumarate.
'Noctal' *see* Propallylonal.
'Noctan' *see* Methyprylone.
'Noctenal' *see* Propallylonal.
'Noctinal' *see* Secbutabarbital.
'Nocu' *see* Diazepam.
'Nodapton' *see* Glycopyrronium bromide.
'Noflamol' *see* Polychlorinated biphenyl
mixture.
NOGALAMYCIN* (antibiotic from *Str.*
nogalater; U-15167).
'Nogest' *see* Medroxyprogesterone acetate
with ethinylestradiol.
'Nogos' *see* Dichlorvos.
'Nogos G50' *see* Dichlorvos.
5-NOK *see* Nitroxoline.
'Nokhel' *see* Amikhellin.
'No-kotin' *see* Lobeline.
'Nolamine' *see* Phenindamine tartrate.
'Noleptan' *see* Fominoben.
'Noltran' *see* Dicapthon.
'Noludar' *see* Methyprylone.
'Nolvadex' *see* Tamoxifen.
'Nolvasan' *see* Chlorhexidine.
'Nomersan' *see* Thiram.
'Nometan' *see* Piperazine adipate.
'Nometine' *see* Pipamazine.
NOMIFENSINE* (8-amino-1,2,3,4-tetra-
hydro-2-methyl-4-phenylisoquinoline;
'alival').
NOMIFENSINE MALEATE (HOE-36984).
**Nonaethylene glycol methyl *p*-butyl-
aminobenzoate** *see* Benzonatate.
Nonaethylene glycol monododecyl ether
see Polidocanol.
**3,5,7,9,11,13,15,26,27-Nonahydroxy-
2-(1-hydroxyhexyl)-16-methyl-16,18,20,
22,24-octacosapentaenoic acid 1,27-
lactone** *see* Filipin.
NONAMETHYLENE DIMESILATE
(1,9-nonanediol di(methanesulfonate); 1,9-
di(methanesulfonyloxy)nonane; CB-2067;
NSC-3052).
1,9-Nonanediol di(methanesulfonate) *see*
Nonamethylene dimesilate.
NONANOIC ACID (*n*-nonylic acid; 1-oc-
tanecarboxylic acid; pelargonic acid).
NONAPYRIMINE* (4-nonylamino(7H)-
pyrrolo(2,3-d)pyrimidine).
Nonasodium phytate *see* Sodium phytate.
'Nonex' *see* Macrogol esters.
'Nonframin' *see* Tinoridine.
'Nonidet' *see* Tyloxapol.
'Nonipol' *see* Nonoxinol.
'Non-ovlon' *see* Norethisterone acetate with
ethinylestradiol.
**2,5,8,11,14,17,20,23,26-Nonoxaoctacosan-
28-ol *p*-butylaminobenzoate** *see* Benzo-
natate.
NONOXINOL(S)* (α-(*p*-nonylphenyl)-ω-
hydroxypoly(oxyethylene); poly(ethylene-
glycol) *p*-nonylphenyl ether(s); nonyl-
phenoxypolyethoxyethanol(s); polyoxy-

ethylene nonylphenyl ether(s); nonoxyn-
ol(s); 'nonipol(s)').
NONOXINOL 4* (2-[2-[2-[2-(*p*-nonyl-
phenoxy)ethoxy]ethoxy]ethoxy]ethanol;
α-(*p*-nonylphenyl)-ω-hydroxytetra(oxyethylene); 'igepal CO-430').
NONOXINOL 9* (α-(*p*-nonylphenyl)-
ω-hydroxynona(oxyethylene); 'conceptrol',
'delfen', 'orthodelfen', 'orthoform').
NONOXINOL 15* (44-(*p*-nonylphenoxy)-
3,6,9,12,15,18,21,24,27,30,33,36,39,42-
tetradecaoxatetratetracontan-1-ol; α-(*p*-
nonylphenyl)-ω-hydroxypentadeca(oxyethylene); 'igepal CO-730').
NONOXINOL 30* (89-(*p*-nonylphenoxy)-
3,6,9,12,15,18,21,24,27,30,33,36,39,42,45,
48,51,54,57,60,63,66,69,72,75,78,81,84,87-
nonacosaoxanonaoctacontan-1-ol; α-(*p*-
nonylphenyl)-ω-hydroxytriaconta(oxyethylene); 'igepal CO-880').
Nonoxynol* *see* Nonoxinol.
Non-staining scarlet *see* Aminoazotoluene.
**4-Nonylamino(7H)pyrrolo(2,3-d)pyri-
midine** *see* Nonapyrimine.
Nonylic acid *see* Nonanoic acid.
Nonylic acid vanillamide *see* Vanillylnonamide.
Nonylphenoxypolyethoxyethanol *see*
Nonoxinol(s).
**α-(*p*-Nonylphenyl)-ω-hydroxypoly(oxy-
ethylene)** *see* Nonoxinol(s).
'Nootropyl' *see* Piracetam.
'Nopenol' *see* Procaine-penicillin.
'Nopoxamine' *see* Myrtecaine.
NOPRYLSULFAMIDE (disodium salt of
N^4-(3-phenyl-1,3-disulfopropyl)sulfathia-
zole; thiasolucin; 'soluthiazole').
'Noracycline' *see* Lynestrenol with mestranol.
NORACYMETHADOL* ((±)-6-methyl-
amino-4,4-diphenyl-3-heptanol acetate;
(±)-α-4-acetoxy-1,*N*-dimethyl-3,3-diphen-
ylhexylamine; (±)-α-3-acetoxy-6-methyl-
amino-4,4-diphenylheptane; noracymethadol hydrochloride; L-30109; NIH-7667).
'Noradin' *see* Methamphetamine.
NORADNAMINE (5-aminomethyl-2,3,7,8-
tetrahydroxydibenzo(a,e)cycloheptatriene).
NORADRENALINE* (L-α-aminomethyl-
3,4-dihydroxybenzyl alcohol; arterenol;
levarterenol; norepinephrine; noradrenaline bitartrate; sympathin; 'narodrine').
Noradrenaline-theophylline *see* Theodrenaline.
NORADRENALONE (2-amino-3',4'-di-
hydroxyacetophenone).
'Noral' *see* Norgestrel with ethinylestradiol.
Noramidazophen *see* Novaminsulfon.
NORAMIDOPYRINE (4-methylamino-
phenazone; 2,3-dimethyl-4-methylamino-
1-phenyl-3-pyrazolin-5-one; methylaminoantipyrine).
**Noramidopyrine methanesulfonate
sodium** ** *see* Novaminsulfon.
19-Norandrostane *see* Estrane.
19-Norandrosta-4,9,11-trien-17β-ol-3-one
see Trienolone.
19-Norandrost-4-en-17β-ol-3-one *see*

327

Nandrolone.

'Norbiogest' *see* Norethisterone with mestranol.

NORBIOTIN (hexahydro-2-oxo(1H)thieno-(3,4)imidazole-4-butyric acid).

Norbolethone* *see* Norboletone.

NORBOLETONE* (13-ethyl-17-hydroxy-18,19-dinor-17α-pregn-4-en-3-one; 13-ethyl-18,19-dinor-17α-pregn-4-en-17-ol-3-one; DL-13,17α-diethyl-17-hydroxygon-4-en-3-one; norbolethone; Wy-3475; 'genabol').

'Norboral' *see* Carbutamide.

NORBORMIDE* (5-(α-hydroxy-α-pyrid-2-ylbenzyl)-7-(α-pyrid-2-ylbenzylidene)-norborn-5-ene-2,3-dicarboximide; 3a,4,7,7a-tetrahydro-5-(hydroxyphenyl-2-pyridinyl-methyl)-7-(phenyl-2-pyridinylmethylene)-4,7-methano-1H-isoindole-1,3(2H)-dione; McN-1025; 'raticate', 'shoxin').

NORBORNANAMINE (norcamphanamine).

NORBORNANE (bicyclo(2.2.1)heptane; 1,4-*endo*-methylenecyclohexane; norcamphane).

NORBORNENE (bicyclo(2.2.1)hept-2-ene; 1,4-*endo*-methylene-2-cyclohexane; norcamphene).

5-NORBORNENE-2,3-DICARBOXYLIC ACID (3,6-endomethylene-1,2,3,6-tetra-hydrophthalic acid; 1,4-endomethylene-△⁵-cyclohexene-2,3-dicarboxylic acid). *See also* Dimethyl 5-norbornene-2,3-di-carboxylate.

2-(1-Norbornen-5-yl-1-phenylethoxy)-triethylamine methobromide *see* Ciclonium bromide.

α-(5-Norbornen-2-yl)-α-phenyl-1-piper-idinepropanol *see* Biperiden.

NORBUDRINE* (2-cyclobutylamino-1-(3,4-dihydroxyphenyl)ethanol; α-cyclo-butylaminomethyl-3,4-dihydroxybenzyl alcohol; N-cyclobutylnoradrenaline; norbutrine; RD-9338).

Norbutrine* *see* Norbudrine.

Norcaine *see* Benzocaine.

Norcamphanamine *see* Norbornanamine.

Norcamphane *see* Norbornane.

Norcamphene *see* Norbornene.

NORCAPERATIC ACID (α-tetradecylcitric acid).

NORCLOSTEBOL* (4-chloro-17β-hydroxyestr-4-en-3-one; 4-chloro-19-nor-testosterone; 4-chloroandrolone; CP-73; SK&F-6611).

NORCODEINE* (4,5-epoxy-6-hydroxy-3-methoxymorphin-7-ene; N-desmethyl-codeine).

(−)-Norcoralydine *see* Xylopinine.

Nordefrin *see* Corbadrine.

'Norden' *see* Octopamine.

NORDIHYDROGUAIARETIC ACID (1,4-bis(3,4-dihydroxyphenyl)-2,3-di-methylbutane; 2,3-bis(3,4-dihydroxy-benzyl)butane; 4,4′-(2,3-dimethyltetra-methylene)dipyrocatechol; NSC-4291; NDGA).

NORDINONE* (11α-hydroxy-17,17-di-methyl-18-norandrosta-4,13-dien-3-one;

17,17-dimethyl-18-norandrosta-4,13-dien-11α-ol-3-one).

Nordopan (tr) *see* Uramustine.

'Nor-durandron' *see* Nandrolone cyclo-hexanecarboxylate.

Norea *see* Noruron.

NOREPHEDRINE (α-(1-aminoethyl)-benzyl alcohol; 2-amino-1-phenyl-1-propa-nol; apoephedrine; phenylpropanolamine; 'apodrine', 'apophedrine', 'mydriatin', 'pressedrine', 'procol', 'propadrine').

Norephedrine-theophylline *see* Cafedrine.

Norepinephrine* *see* Noradrenaline.

NORETHANDROLONE* (17α-ethyl-4-estren-17-ol-3-one; 17α-ethyl-17-hydroxy-19-norandrost-4-en-3-one; 17-ethyl-19-nor-testosterone; 'nilevar').

Norethindrone *see* Norethisterone.

NORETHISTERONE ** (17α-ethynyl-19-nortestosterone; 17α-ethynyl-4-estren-17β-ol-3-one; 17α-ethynyl-17-hydroxy-19-norandrost-4-en-3-one; 17β-hydroxy-19-norpregnen-4-en-20-yn-3-one; anhydro-hydroxynorprogesterone; ethinylnor-testosterone; norethindron; norethyndron; norpregneninolone; NSC-9564; 'micronor', 'micronovum', 'noriday', 'norlutin', 'norluton', 'primolut N').

NORETHISTERONE ACETATE ('nor-lutate', 'orlutate').

NORETHISTERONE ACETATE WITH ETHINYLESTRADIOL (J66; ORF-1557-BA; SH-420; 'anovlar', 'gynophase', 'gynovlar', 'minovlar', 'non-ovlon', 'norlestrin', 'orlest', 'orlestrin').

NORETHISTERONE WITH MESTRA-NOL ('conlumin', 'enidrel', 'norbiogest', 'norinyl', 'ortho 1557-0', 'orthonovin', 'ortho-novum', 'regovar', 'sophia').

Norethyndron *see* Norethisterone.

Norethynodrel* *see* Noretynodrel.

NORETYNODREL* (17α-ethynyl-5(10)-estren-17-ol-3-one; 17β-hydroxy-19-nor-17α-pregn-5(10)-en-20-yn-3-one; norethyn-odrel; SC-4642).

NORETYNODREL WITH MESTRANOL ('conovid', 'enavid', 'enovid', 'feminor sequential', 'infecundin').

'Nor-evipal' *see* Norhexobarbital.

NORFENEFRINE* (2-amino-1-(3-hydroxyphenyl)ethanol; α-aminomethyl-m-hydroxybenzyl alcohol; 2-(m-hydroxy-phenyl)ethanolamine; norfenefrine hydro-chloride; norphenylephrine; 'novadral', 'stagural').
See also Octodrine camsilate with nor-fenefrine and adenosine.

'Norflex' *see* Orphenadrine.

NORFLURANE* (1,1,1,2-tetrafluoro-ethane).

'Norgesic' *see* Orphenadrine citrate with paracetamol.

NORGESTERONE ** (17α-vinyl-5(10)-estren-17β-ol-3-one; 17β-hydroxy-17-vinyl-5(10)-estren-3-one).

NORGESTIMATE ** ((+)-13-ethyl-17-hydroxy-18,19-dinor-17α-pregn-4-en-20-

yn-3-one oxime acetate; (+)-17-acetoxy-13-ethyl-18,19-dinor-17α-pregn-4-en-20-yn-3-one oxime; norgestrel oxime acetate; D-138).

NORGESTOMET*** (17-hydroxy-11β-methyl-19-norpregn-4-ene-3,20-dione acetate; 11β-methyl-19-norpregn-4-en-17-ol-3,20-dione acetate; 17-acetoxy-11β-methyl-19-norpregn-4-ene-3,20-dione; SC-21009).

NORGESTREL*** ((±)-13β-ethyl-17-hydroxy-18,19-dinor-17α-pregn-4-en-20-yn-3-one; 13β-ethyl-17α-ethynylgon-4-en-17β-ol-3-one; Wy-3707; 'neogest'). *See also* Levonorgestrel.

NORGESTREL WITH ETHINYLESTRA-DIOL ('duoluton', 'eugynon', 'follinett', 'neogynon', 'noral', 'ovral', 'stediril').

Norgestrel oxime acetate *see* Norgestimate.

NORGESTRIENONE*** (17-hydroxy-19-nor-17α-pregna-4,9,11-trien-20-yn-3-one; 19-nor-17α-pregna-4,9,11-trien-20-yn-17-ol-3-one; 17α-ethynylestra-4,9,11-trien-17-ol-3-one; ethinyltrienolone; A-301).

NORGESTRIENONE WITH ETHINYL-ESTRADIOL (R-178; 'rapitest').

Norgine *see* Alginic acid.

'**Norglycin**' *see* Tolazamide.

NORHEXOBARBITAL (5-(1-cyclohexen-1-yl)-5-methylbarbituric acid; 'nor-evipal').

Norhomoepinephrine *see* Corbadrine.

'**Noriday**' *see* Norethisterone.

Norimipramine *see* Desipramine.

'**Norinyl**' *see* Norethisterone with mestranol.

'**Noritren**' *see* Nortriptyline.

'**Norkhel**' *see* Amikhellin.

Norlaudanosoline *see* Tetrahydropapaveroline.

'**Norlax**' *see* Sodium dioctyl sulfosuccinate.

'**Norlestrin**' *see* Norethisterone acetate with ethinylestradiol.

NORLEUCINE (2-aminohexanoic acid; α-aminocaproic acid; caprine; glycoleucine).

NORLEUSACTIDE** (D-Ser¹-Nle⁴-(val-NH₂)-β¹⁻²⁵-corticotrophin; pentacosactride).

NORLEVORPHANOL*** ((−)-3-hydroxymorphinan).

'**Norlongandron**' *see* Nandrolone cyclohexanecarboxylate.

'**Norlutate**' *see* Norethisterone acetate.

'**Norlutin**' *see* Norethisterone.

'**Norluton**' *see* Norethisterone.

'**Normabrain**' *see* Piracetam.

'**Normatens**' *see* Pempidine.

'**Normatensyl**' *see* Hydracarbazine with pempidine.

'**Normenon**' *see* Chlormadinone acetate.

Normetadrenaline *see* Normetanephrine.

NORMETANEPHRINE (α-aminomethyl-4-hydroxy-3-methoxybenzyl alcohol; 3-O-methylnoradrenaline; 3-O-methyl-norepinephrine; normetadrenaline).

NORMETHADONE*** (6-dimethylamino-4,4-diphenyl-3-hexanone; Hö-10582; 'daartil').

Normethandrolone *see* Methylestrenolone.

'**Normolipem**' *see* Clofibric acid.

NORMORPHINE*** (4,5-epoxy-3,6-di-hydroxymorphin-7-ene; N-desmethyl-morphine).

'**Normoson**' *see* Ethchlorvynol.

'**Normospas**' *see* Atromepine.

Noroxedrine *see* Octopamine.

'**Norpace**' *see* Disopyramide.

NORPETHIDINE (ethyl 4-phenylisoni-pecotate).

'**Norphen**' *see* Octopamine.

Norphenylephrine *see* Norfenefrine.

Norpholedrine *see* Hydroxyamphetamine.

Norphytane *see* Pristane.

2-NORPINENE (bicyclo(3.1.1)hept-2-ene).

NORPIPANONE*** (4,4-diphenyl-6-piperid-1-yl-3-hexanone; norpipanone hydrobromide; 'hexalgon').

'**Norpramine**' *see* Desipramine.

19-NORPREGNANE (17β-ethylestrane).

19-NOR-17α-PREGNANE (17α-ethyl-estrane).

19-Norpregna-4,5-dien-17-ol-3,20-dione *see* Gestadienol.

19-NORPREGNATRIEN-20-ONE (17-acet-ylestratriene).

19-Nor-17α-pregna-4,9,11-trien-20-yn-17-ol-3-one *see* Norgestrienone.

Norpregneninolone *see* Norethisterone.

19-Nor-17α-pregn-5-en-17-ol *see* Bolenol.

19-Norpregn-4-en-17-ol-3,20-dione *see* Gestonorone.

19-Norpregn-4-en-20β-ol-3-one *see* Oxogestone.

19-Norpregn-4-en-17-ol-3-one *see* Nor-ethandrolone.

19-Nor-17α-pregn-4-en-20-yne-3β,17-diol *see* Etynodiol.

19-Nor-17α-pregn-4-en-20-yn-1-ol *see* Lynestrenol.

19-Nor-17α-pregn-5-en-20-yn-17-ol *see* Cingestol.

19-Nor-17α-pregn-5(10)-en-20-yn-17-ol *see* Tigestol.

NORPSEUDOEPHEDRINE (α-(1-amino-ethyl)benzyl alcohol; norisoephedrine; cathine; katine; 'exponcit', 'fugoa'). *See also* Phenobarbital-norpseudoephedrine.

NORPSEUDOTROPINE (3β-hydroxy-2,3-dihydronortropidine; 8-desmethyl-pseudotropine).

NORPSEUDOTROPINE BENZOATE (nortropacocaine).

Norsulfazole (tr) *see* Sulfathiazole.

'**Norsympathol**' *see* Octopamine.

'**Norsynephrine**' *see* Octopamine.

'**Nortensin**' *see* Reserpine with furosemide.

'**Nortestonate**' *see* Nandrolone.

Nortestosterone *see* Nandrolone.

19-Nortestosterone *see* Nandrolone.

NORTETRAZEPAM*** (7-chloro-5-cyclo-hexen-1-yl-1,3-dihydro-2H-1,4-benzo-diazepin-2-one).

NORTHIADENE (6,11-dihydro-11-(3-methylaminopropylidene)dibenzo(b,e)-thiepine hydrochloride; desmethyl-prothiadene).

329

'Nortran' *see* Ethofumesate.
'Nortrilen' *see* Nortriptyline.
NORTRIPTYLINE*** (10,11-dihydro-5-
(3-methylaminopropylidene)-5H-dibenzo-
(a,d)-cycloheptene; 10,11-dihydro-*N*-
methyl-5H-dibenzo(a,d)cycloheptene-
$\triangle^{5,\gamma}$-propylamine; 3-(3-methylamino-
propylidene)-1,2:4,5-dibenzocyclohepta-
1,4-diene; desmethylamitriptyline; desitriptyline; nortriptyline hydrochloride;
L-38489; N-7048; 'acetexa', 'allegron',
'arentyl', 'aventyl', 'noritren', 'nortrilen',
'psychostyl', 'sensaval').
See also Fluphenazine with nortriptyline.
Nortropacocaine *see* Norpseudotropine
benzoate.
NORTROPANE (8-azabicyclo(3.2.1)octane;
2,3-dihydronortropidine).
2-Nortropene *see* Nortropidine.
NORTROPIDINE (2-nortropene).
NORTROPINE (3α-hydroxy-2,3-dihydro-
nortropidine; 8-desmethyltropine; 3α-
nortropanol).
NORURON* (1-(3a,4,5,6,7,7a-hexahydro-
4,7-methanoindan-5-yl)-3,3-dimethylurea;
1,1-dimethyl-3-(octahydro-4,7-methano-
1H-inden-5-yl)urea; 'herban', 'norea').
'Norval' *see* Sodium dioctyl sulfosuccinate.
NORVALINE (2-aminovaleric acid;
2-aminopentanoic acid).
'Norvedan' *see* Fentiazac.
NORVINISTERONE*** (17α-vinylestr-4-en-
17β-ol-3-one; 17β-hydroxy-17α-vinylestr-
4-en-3-one; 17α-vinyl-19-nortestosterone).
'Noscapal' *see* Noscapine.
'Noscapect' *see* Noscapine.
NOSCAPINE** ((−)-1-(6,7-dimethoxy-
3-phthalidyl)-8-methoxy-2-methyl-
6,7-methylenedioxy-1,2,3,4-tetrahydroiso-
quinoline; 5-(6,7-dimethoxyphthalidyl)-
5,6,7,8-tetrahydro-4-methoxy-6-methyl-
1,3-dioxolo(4,5-g)isoquinoline; narcosine;
narcotine; (−)-α-narcotine; methoxyhydrastine; opian; opianine; 'coscopine',
'coscotabs', 'longamex', 'narcompren',
'nectadon', 'nicolane', 'nipaxon', 'noscapal',
'noscapect', 'respilyt', 'sinecod', 'tuscapine',
'tussils').
DL-**Noscapine** *see* Gnoscopine.
NOSCAPINE EMBONATE (noscapine
pamoate; 'teletux').
Noscapine pamoate *see* Noscapine em-
bonate.
See also Clofedanol noscapine succinate;
Morphine noscapine meconate.
NOSCAPINE WITH GUAIFENESIN
('tuscalman').
NOSIHEPTIDE** (antibiotic from *Str.*
actuosus 40037).
'No-spa' *see* Drotaverine.
Nospanum (tr) *see* Drotaverine.
'Nostal' *see* Propallylonal.
'Nostral' *see* Propallylonal.
'Nostyn' *see* Ectylurea.
'Notec' *see* Chloral hydrate.
'Notensil' *see* Acepromazine.
'Nothiazine' *see* Pecazine.

'Notyol' *see* Ammonium sulfobituminate.
'Nourical' *see* Calcium gluconate.
'Nourilax N' *see* Bisacodyl.
'Nourycid' *see* Lindane.
'Novabsorb' *see* Magnesium trisilicate.
'Novactyl' *see* Magnesium acetylsalicylate.
'Novacrysin' *see* Sodium aurotiosulfate.
'Novacyl' *see* Magnesium acetylsalicylate.
'Novadral' *see* Norfenefrine.
'Novafed' *see* Pseudoephedrine.
'Novahistex' *see* Phenylephrine with
diphenylpyraline.
'Novaine' *see* Carnitine.
'Novaldin' *see* Novaminsulfon.
'Novalgetol' *see* Novaminsulfon.
'Novalgin' *see* Novaminsulfon.
'Novamidon' *see* Aminophenazone.
'Novamin' *see* Dimenhydrinate.
NOVAMINSULFON (sodium salt of [[(2,3-
dimethyl-5-oxo-1-phenyl-3-pyrazolin-4-yl)-
methyl]amino]methanesulfonate; 4-methyl-
aminophenazone methanesulfonic acid
sodium salt; noramidopyrine methane-
sulfonate sodium; sodium (antipyrinyl-
methylamino)methanesulfonate; meta-
mizole; analgin; dipyrone; methampyrone;
methapyrone; methylmelubrin; noramidaz-
ophen; sulpyrin).
See also Chlormezanone with novaminsulfon;
Metixene with novaminsulfon.
'Novarscodyle' *see* Disodium methane-
arsonate.
'Novartrine' *see* Morazone.
'Novaspirin' *see* Citrodisalyl.
'Novastat' *see* Aklomide with sulfanitran.
'Novasurol' *see* Merbaphen.
'Novatoxyl' *see* Tryparsamide.
'Novatrine' *see* Homatropine methyl
bromide.
Novatropine *see* Homatropine methyl
bromide.
Novaurantium *see* Orange G.
'Novdimal' *see* Malonylbis(procaine).
'Novedrin' *see* Etafedrine.
NOVEMBICHIN (tr) (2-chloro-*N*,*N*-bis(2-
chloroethyl)-1-propylamine hydrochloride;
embichin 7).
'Noveril' *see* Dibenzepin.
'Novesin' *see* Oxybuprocaine.
'Novestrin' *see* Methallenestril.
'Novex' *see* Fenticlor.
'Novicodin' *see* Dihydrocodeine.
'Novidium' *see* Ethidium chloride.
'Noviform' *see* Bibrocathol.
'Novivermol' *see* Piperazine.
NOVOBIOCIN*** (7-carbamoyltetra-
hydro(3-hydroxy-5-methoxy-6,6-dimethyl-
pyran-2-yloxy)-4-hydroxy-3-[4-hydroxy-3-
(3-methylbut-2-enyl)benzamido]-8-methyl-
2H-chromen-2-one; glucoside of 3-[4-
hydroxy-3-(3-methyl-2-butenyl)benz-
amido]-4,7-dihydroxy-8-methylcoumarin;
crystallinic acid; streptonivicin; novobiocin
sodium; novobiocin calcium; PA-93;
'albamycin', 'biotexin', 'cardelmycin',
'cathocin', 'cathomycin', 'inamycin',
'spheromycin', 'vulcamycin', 'vulkamycin').

See also Tetracycline dihydronovobiocin
sodium phylate.
'**Novocaine**' *see* Procaine.
'**Novocell**' *see* Oxidized cellulose.
Novocephalgin (tr) *see* APC.
Novocillin (tr) *see* Procaine-penicillin.
'**Novocodon**' *see* Thebacon.
'**Novodigal**' *see* β-Acetyldigoxin.
Novoembichin *see* Novembichin.
'**Novoform**' *see* Bibrocathol.
'**Novofosfan**' *see* Sodium 4-dimethylamino-
o-toluenephosphonate.
'**Novofur**' *see* Furazolium chloride.
'**Novohydrin**' *see* Ambuside.
'**Novolaudon**' *see* Hydromorphone.
'**Novon**' *see* Erbon.
'**Novonal**' *see* 2,2-Diethyl-4-pentenoic amide.
'**Novophone**' *see* Dapsone.
'**Novoquens**' *see* Megestrol acetate with
ethinylestradiol.
'**Novoscabian**' *see* Benzyl benzoate.
'**Novoscabin**' *see* Benzyl benzoate.
'**Novoseptale**' *see* Sulfamethylthiazole.
'**Novosparol**' *see* Bietamiverine.
'**Novospasmin**' *see* Camylofin.
'**Novostat**' *see* Aklomide.
'**Novotrone**' *see* Aldesulfone.
'**Novrad**' *see* Levopropoxyphene napsilate.
'**Novutox**' *see* Procaine.
'**Noxfish**' *see* Rotenone.
NOXIPTILINE*** (10,11-dihydro-5H-di-
benzo(a,d)cyclohepten-5-one-*O*-(2-di-
methylaminoethyl)oxime; 3-(2-dimethyl-
aminoethyloxyimino)-1,2:4,5-dibenzocyclo-
hepta-1,4-diene; noxiptyline hydrochloride;
dibenzoxine; BAY-1521; 'agedal').
Noxiptyline* *see* Noxiptiline.
'**Noxiron**' *see* Glutethimide.
'**Noxiurotan**' *see* Piperazine tartrate.
'**Noxybel**' *see* Methaqualone.
N-oxyd-Lost *see* Chlormethine *N*-oxide.
'**Noxyflex**' *see* Noxytiolin.
'**Noxyron**' *see* Glutethimide.
Noxythiolin* *see* Noxytiolin with tetracaine.
NOXYTIOLIN*** (1-hydroxymethyl-
3-methyl-2-thiourea; noxythiolin).
NOXYTIOLIN WITH TETRACAINE
('noxyflex').
'**Nozinan**' *see* Levomepromazine.
NP-13 *see* Bemegride.
NP-297 *see* Mefexamide.
NPA *see* Naptalam.
NPH insulin *see* Isophane insulin.
NPT-10381 *see* Methisoprinol.
NRDC-104 *see* Resmethrin.
NRDC-107 *see* Bioresmethrin.
NRDC-119 *see* Cisresmethrin.
NSC-185 *see* Cycloheximide.
NSC-660 *see* Diacetyl monoxime.
NSC-739 *see* Aminopterin.
NSC-740 *see* Methotrexate.
NSC-741 *see* Hydrocortisone acetate.
NSC-742 *see* Azaserine.
NSC-746 *see* Urethan.
NSC-749 *see* Azaguanine.
NSC-750 *see* Busulfan.
NSC-751 *see* Ethionine.

NSC-752 *see* Tioguanine.
NSC-753 *see* Purine.
NSC-755 *see* Mercaptopurine.
NSC-757 *see* Colchicine.
NSC-758 *see* Glucosamine.
NSC-762 *see* Chlormethine.
NSC-1026 *see* Cycloleucine.
NSC-1390 *see* Allopurinol.
NSC-1895 *see* Guanazole.
NSC-2100 *see* Nitrofural.
NSC-2105 *see* Propham.
NSC-2107 *see* Nitrofurantoin.
NSC-3052 *see* Nonamethylene dimesilate.
NSC-3053 *see* Dactinomycin.
NSC-3055 *see* Puromycin.
NSC-3056 *see* Puromycin aminonucleoside.
NSC-3061 *see* Pyrimethamine.
NSC-3063 *see* Desoxypyridoxine.
NSC-3070 *see* Diethylstilbestrol.
NSC-3073 *see* Folic acid.
NSC-3084 *see* Methionine sulfoxide.
NSC-3085 *see* Desthiobiotin.
NSC-3086 *see* Pantoyltaurine.
NSC-3087 *see* Oxophenarsine.
NSC-3088 *see* Chlorambucil.
NSC-3096 *see* Demecolcine.
NSC-3097 *see* Arsphenamine.
NSC-3100 *see* Isoriboflavine.
NSC-3351 *see* Nandrolone cyclohexanecarb-
oxylate.
NSC-3364 *see* Filipin.
NSC-3425 *see* Azauracil.
NSC-3426 *see* Azathymine.
NSC-3431 *see* Methioprim.
NSC-3590 *see* Calcium folinate.
NSC-4280 *see* Dimethylphenanthroline.
NSC-4291 *see* Nordihydroguaiaretic acid.
NSC-4730 *see* Ethylaminothiadiazole.
NSC-4911 *see* Mercaptopurine riboside.
NSC-6135 *see* Cholic acid.
NSC-6396 *see* Thiotepa.
NSC-7365 *see* DON.
NSC-8746 *see* Cysteine.
NSC-8798 *see* Cholesterol.
NSC-8806 *see* Melphalan.
NSC-9120 *see* Prednisolone.
NSC-9166 *see* Testosterone propionate.
NSC-9168 *see* Fumagillin.
NSC-9169 *see* Oxytetracycline.
NSC-9170 *see* *N*-Deacetylthiocolchicine.
NSC-9369 *see* Methylnitronitrosoguanidine.
NSC-9564 *see* Norethisterone.
NSC-9566 *see* Estradiol benzoate.
NSC-9698 *see* Mannomustine.
NSC-9700 *see* Testosterone.
NSC-9702 *see* 11-Dehydrocorticosterone.
NSC-9703 *see* Cortisone.
NSC-9704 *see* Progesterone.
NSC-9705 *see* Corticosterone.
NSC-9706 *see* Tretamine.
NSC-9717 *see* Tepa.
NSC-9894 *see* Hexestrol.
NSC-10023 *see* Prednisone.
NSC-10107 *see* Chlormethine *N*-oxide.
NSC-10108 *see* Chlorotrianisene.
NSC-10270 *see* Ambomycin.
NSC-10481 *see* Fosfestrol.

NSC-10483 *see* Hydrocortisone.
NSC-11319 *see* Desoxycortone.
NSC-12165 *see* Fluoxymesterone.
NSC-12169 *see* Estriol.
NSC-12198 *see* Drostalone.
NSC-13252 *see* Chlortetracycline.
NSC-13875 *see* Hexamethylmelamine.
NSC-14083 *see* Streptomycin.
NSC-14210 *see* Sarcolysin.
NSC-14347 *see* 2-Methylene-3-oxocyclopen-
tanecarboxylic acid.
NSC-14574 *see* Lucanthone.
NSC-17261 *see* Inproquone.
NSC-17590 *see* Estradiol valerate.
NSC-18016 *see* Chloroethyl mesilate.
NSC-18334 *see* Cinerubin A.
NSC-18429 *see* Aniline mustard.
NSC-19494 *see* Metodiclorofen.
NSC-19892 *see* Hydrogen peroxide.
NSC-19893 *see* Fluorouracil.
NSC-19962 *see* Carbestrol.
NSC-19987 *see* Methylprednisolone.
NSC-20105 *see* Methylthiopurine.
NSC-21206 *see* Aminonicotinamide.
NSC-21970 *see* Methylcholanthrene.
NSC-22877 *see* (Aminoethyl)isothiuronium.
NSC-23162 *see* Nandrolone phenpropionate.
NSC-23759 *see* Testolactone.
NSC-23909 *see* Methylnitrosourea.
NSC-24559 *see* Mithramycin.
NSC-24818 *see* Podophyllotoxin.
NSC-24819 *see* β-Peltatin.
NSC-25154 *see* Pipobroman.
NSC-26198 *see* Oxymetholone.
NSC-26271 *see* Cyclophosphamide.
NSC-26386 *see* Medroxyprogesterone acetate.
NSC-26805 *see* Ethyl mesilate.
NSC-26812 *see* Apholate.
NSC-26980 *see* Mitomycin C.
NSC-27381 *see* m-Sarcolysin.
NSC-27640 *see* Floxuridine.
NSC-29215 *see* Triaziquone.
NSC-29422 *see* Thioguanosine.
NSC-30211 *see* Trichlormethine.
NSC-31083 *see* Actinobolin.
NSC-31717 *see* Tetrakis(1-aziridinyl)benzo-
quinone.
NSC-32065 *see* Hydroxycarbamide.
NSC-32074 *see* Azauridine.
NSC-32946 *see* Mitoguazone.
NSC-33012 *see* Acetoxydihydrocycloheximide.
NSC-33669 *see* Emetine.
NSC-34462 *see* Uramustine.
NSC-34521 *see* Dexamethasone.
NSC-34533 *see* Griseofulvin.
NSC-35051 *see* Medphalan.
NSC-37024 *see* Formylmelphalan.
NSC-37095 *see* Uredepa.
NSC-37096 *see* Benzodepa.
NSC-37538 *see* Mannityl dimesilate.
NSC-37917 *see* Streptozocin with zedalan.
NSC-38297 *see* Broxuridine.
NSC-38721 *see* Mitotane.
NSC-38887 *see* Tiamiprine.
NSC-39068 *see* D-Dihydroxybusulfan.
NSC-39069 *see* Treosulfan.
NSC-39070 *see* Erythrityl dimesilate.

NSC-39084 *see* Azathioprine.
NSC-39147 *see* Hydroxycycloheximide.
NSC-39274 *see* Formylsarcolysin.
NSC-39661 *see* Idoxuridine.
NSC-40774 *see* 6-(Methylthio)purine riboside.
NSC-44175 *see* Dihydroxydiphenylbenzo-
quinone.
NSC-44629 *see* Dopan.
NSC-45383 *see* Streptonigrin.
NSC-45384 *see* Streptonigrin methyl ester.
NSC-45388 *see* Dacarbazine.
NSC-45624 *see* Sodium thiosulfate.
NSC-47438 *see* Fluorometholone acetate.
NSC-47774 *see* Piposulfan.
NSC-49000 *see* 5α-Androstane.
NSC-49842 *see* Vinblastine.
NSC-50256 *see* Methyl mesilate.
NSC-50257 *see* Chloroethyl esilate.
NSC-51097 *see* Duazomycin.
NSC-51325 *see* Meturedepa.
NSC-52142 *see* Fluoroethyl dimesilate.
NSC-52947 *see* Pactamycin.
NSC-55202 *see* Roseolic acid.
NSC-56308 *see* Epipropidine.
NSC-56410 *see* Porfiromycin.
NSC-56423 *see* Melatonin.
NSC-56654 *see* Azotomycin.
NSC-57199 *see* o-Sarcolysin.
NSC-58368 *see* Fumagillin dicyclohexylamine
salt.
NSC-58514 *see* Chromomycin A₃.
NSC-59727 *see* Sparsomycin.
NSC-61586 *see* Phleomycin.
NSC-62709 *see* Isopropylideneazastrep-
tonigrin.
NSC-62786 *see* Epinephrine.
NSC-63878 *see* Cytarabine.
NSC-64393 *see* Spiramycin.
NSC-67574 *see* Vincristine.
NSC-67934 *see* Glyceraldehyde.
NSC-69856 *see* Neocarzinostatin.
NSC-70968 *see* Melengestrol.
NSC-71795 *see* Ellipticine.
NSC-71964 *see* Chlorphenacyl.
NSC-76455-D *see* Peliomycin.
NSC-77213 *see* Procarbazine.
NSC-77471 *see* Mitocromin.
NSC-77622 *see* Estradiol valerate with
progesterone hydroxyhexanoate.
NSC-79019 *see* Methylglyoxal.
NSC-79037 *see* Lomustine.
NSC-80087 *see* 1-(4-Dimethylaminobenzyl-
idene)indene.
NSC-82116 *see* Gloxazone.
NSC-82151 *see* Daunorubicin.
NSC-82260 *see* Benzathine tenuazonate.
NSC-83142 *see* Daunorubicin.
NSC-83265 *see* Tritylthioalanine.
NSC-83799 *see* Simtrazene.
NSC-85680 *see* Zedalan.
NSC-85998 *see* Streptozocin.
NSC-89199 *see* Estramustine.
NSC-94100 *see* Mitobronitol.
NSC-95441 *see* Semustine.
NSC-97925 *see* Glutamine.
NSC-100880 *see* Camptothecin.
NSC-102498 *see* Carbamoylcysteine.

NSC-102627 *see* Improsulfan.
NSC-102816 *see* 5-Azacytidine.
NSC-104469 *see* Phenesterin.
NSC-104800 *see* Mitolactol.
NSC-109229 *see* L-Asparaginase.
NSC-109724 *see* Ifosfamide.
NSC-111180 *see* Acetylcysteine.
NSC-112259 *see* Estradiol mustard.
NSC-112846 *see* Quinaspar.
NSC-116785 *see* Phenester.
NSC-119875 *see* cis-Platinum (II) diamino-
    dichloride.
NSC-120949 *see* Poly I:C.
NSC-122819 *see* Teniposide.
NSC-123127 *see* Doxorubicin.
NSC-125066 *see* Bleomycin.
NSC-129185 *see* Mycophenolic acid.
NSC-129220 *see* Ancitabine acetate.
NSC-129943 *see* Razoxane.
NSC-130678 *see* Buthiopurine.
NSC-132313 *see* 1,2:5,6-Dianhydrogalactitol.
NSC-133100 *see* Rifamycin.
NSC-134679 *see* Carboquone.
NSC-140781 *see* Daunosaminyldaunorubicin.
NSC-141540 *see* Etoposide.
NSC-143114 *see* Daunorubicin semicarb-
    azone.
NSC-143491 *see* Daunorubicin oxime.
NSC-143969 *see* Tilorone.
NSC-169774 *see* Bromocriptine.
NSC-172755 *see* Butocin.
NSC-400018 *see* Paraxanthine.
NSC-400978 *see* Iludin M.
NSC-400979 *see* Iludin S.
NSC-402815 *see* Penicillin G.
NSC-409962 *see* Carmustine.
NSC-525816 *see* Sodium tenuazonate.
NSC-529860 *see* Deazaaminopterin.
NSC-529861 *see* Chlorasquin.
NSC-B-2992 *see* Mitomalcin.
NSD-1055 *see* Brocresine.
NTD-2 *see* Cartap.
'N-toin' *see* Nitrofurantoin.
Nu-455 *see* Sulfafurazole.
Nu-903 *see* Pyrithyldione.

Nu-1196 *see* Alphaprodine.
Nu-1504 *see* Phenindamine.
Nu-1510 *see* Dihyprylone.
Nu-2121 *see* Nicotinyl alcohol.
Nu-2206 *see* Racemorphan.
Nu-2222 *see* Trimetaphan camsilate.
'Nuarsol' *see* Sodium arsanilate.
'Nucidol' *see* Dimpylate.
'Nucidrina' *see* Adrenaline.
Nucin *see* Juglone.
Nucite *see* Inositol.
NUCLOTIXENE** (3-[(2-chlorothioxan-
    then-9-ylidene)methyl]quinuclidine;
    2-chloro-9-(quinuclidin-3-ylmethylene)-
    thioxanthene).
'Nulans' *see* Oxazepam hemisuccinate.
'Nullapon' *see* Tetrasodium edetate.
'Nulogyl' *see* Nimorazole.
'Nulsa' *see* Proglumide.
'Numorphan' *see* Oxymorphone.
'Numotac' *see* Isoetarine.
'Nuncital' *see* Emylcamate.
'Nupa-sal' *see* Salinazid.
'Nupercaine' *see* Cinchocaine.
'Nuprin' *see* Sulfamoxole.
'Nuran' *see* Cyproheptadine.
'Nuredal' *see* Nialamide.
'Nuso' *see* Neutral insulin injection
'Nutinal' *see* Benactyzine.
'Nuvacron' *see* Monocrotophos.
'Nuvacron N' *see* Iodofenphos.
'Nuvan' *see* Dichlorvos.
'Nuvanol'M *see* Iodofenphos.
'Nycoline' *see* Macrogols.
'Nydrane' *see* Beclamide.
Nylestriol* *see* Nilestriol.
Nylidrin* *see* Buphenine.
'Nylmerate' *see* Phenylmercuric borate.
'Nyloxin' *see* Cobra venom.
'Nystan' *see* Nystatin.
NYSTATIN*** (antibiotic from *Str. noursei*;
    fungicidin; 'moronal', 'mycostatin',
    'nilstat', 'nystan', 'stamicin', 'stamycin').
    See also Oxytetracycline with nystatin.
'Nyxolan' *see* 8-Quinolinol aluminium sulfate.

O

OAAT (tr) *see* Aminoazotoluene.
'Obesin' *see* Propylhexedrine.
'Obesitex' *see* Amfepramone.
OBIDOXIME CHLORIDE** (1,1'-oxydi-
    methylenebis(4-formylpyridinium chloride)
    dioxime; bis(4-hydroxyimino-1-methyl-
    pyridinium methyl ether) dichloride;
    pralidoxime methyl ether dichloride;
    LüH6; 'toxogenin', 'toxogonin').
'Obiturin' *see* Fluorescein disodium salt.

'Obracine' *see* Tobramycin.
'Obsidan' *see* Propranolol.
'Obston' *see* Sodium dioctyl sulfosuccinate.
OBTUSASTYRENE (*p*-cinnamylphenol).
OCAPHANE (3-[*o*-[2-[bis(2-chloroethyl)ami-
    no]ethyl]phenyl]alanine; 2-[2-(2-amino-2-
    carboxyethyl)phenyl]-2',2''-dichlorotri-
    ethylamine; 2-(2-amino-2-carboxyethyl)-
    N,N-bis(2-chloroethyl)phenethylamine;
    AT-581).

'Ocestrol' *see* Benzestrol.
OCRASE*** (fibrinolytic enzyme from *Aspergillus ochraceus*).
OCRILATE*** (octyl 2-cyanoacrylate).
OCTABENZONE*** (2-hydroxy-4-octyloxy-benzophenone; 'spectrasorb UV-531').
OCTACAINE** (3-diethylaminobutyranilide; 'amplicaine').
Octachlor *see* Chlordane.
1,3,4,5,6,7,8,8,-Octachloro-1,3,3a,4,7,7a-hexahydro-4,7-methanoisobenzofuran *see* Isobenzan.
1,3,4,5,6,7,8,8-Octachloro-3a,4,7,7a-tetra-hydro-4,7-methanophthalan *see* Isobenzan.
'Octacide 264' *see* *N*-(2-Ethylhexyl)bicyclo-(2.2.1)hept-5-ene-2,3-dicarboximide.
Octacosactrin* *see* Tosactide.
cis,cis-**9,12-Octadecadienoic acid** *see* Linoleic acid.
Octadecanoic acid *see* Stearic acid.
1-OCTADECANOL (octodecyl alcohol; stearyl(ic) alcohol; 'stenol').
9,12,15-Octadecatrienoic acid *see* Linolenic acid.
cis,cis,cis-**Octadeca-6,9,12-trienoic acid** *see* Gamolenic acid.
cis-**6-Octadecenoic acid** *see* Petroselinic acid.
trans-**6-Octadecenoic acid** *see* Petroselaidic acid.
cis-**9-Octadecenoic acid** *see* Oleic acid.
trans-**9-Octadecenoic acid** *see* Elaidic acid.
trans-**11-Octadecenoic acid** *see* Vaccenic acid.
9-Octadecenylamine hydrofluoride *see* Dectaflur.
3-Octadecyloxy-1,2-propanediol *see* Batilol.
Octadine (tr) *see* Guanethidine.
'Octaflex' *see* Octafonium.
OCTAFLUOROCYCLOBUTANE (per-fluorocyclobutane; 'freon C-318').
OCTAFONIUM CHLORIDE*** (benzyldi-ethyl[2-[*p*-(1,1,3,3-tetramethylbutyl)-phenoxy]ethyl]ammonium chloride; octa-phonium chloride; phenoctide; 'octaflex', 'octaphen').
Octahydroazocine *see* Heptamethylenimine.
1-(Octahydroazocin-2-ylmethyl)-guanidine *see* Guanazodine.
2,3,4,4a,8,9,13b,14-Octahydro-1H-benzo-(6,7)cyclohepta(1,2,3-de)pyrido(2,1-a)-isoquinoline *see* Taclamine.
Octahydro-5,8-dihydroxy-4,6,9,10-tetra-methyl-6-vinyl-3a,9-propano-3aH-cyclopentacycloocten-1(4H)-one esters *see* Pleuromulin; Tiamulin.
1,3,3a,5,6,11,12,12a-Octahydro-8-hydroxy-1H-benzo(a)cyclopenta(f)quinolizi-nium bromide *see* Quindonium bromide.
(+)-**2,3,4,4aβ,8,9,13bα,14-Octahydro-3α-isopropyl-1H-benzo(6,7)cyclohepta-(1,2,3-de)pyrido(2,1-a)isoquinolin-3-ol** *see* Dexclamol.
1,2,3,4,6,7,7a,11c-Octahydro-9-methoxy-2-methylbenzofuro(4,3,2-efg)benzazocin-6-ol *see* Galantamine.
Octahydro-1-(3,4,5-trimethoxybenzoyl)-azocine *see* Trocimine.
Octahydro-1-(3,4,5-trimethoxycinnam-oyl)-azocine *see* Cinoctramide.
4,6,8,10,12,14,16,27-Octahydroxy-3-(1-hydroxyhexyl)-17,28-dimethyloxa-cyclooctacosa-17,19,21,23,25-pentaen-2-one *see* Filipin.
'Octa-klor' *see* Chlordane.
'Octalene' *see* Aldrin.
'Octalox' *see* Dieldrin.
Octamethyl (tr) *see* Schradan.
Octamethyldiphosphoramide *see* Schradan
Octamethylpyrophosphoramide *see* Schradan.
OCTAMOXIN*** (1-(1-methylheptyl)-hydrazine; 2-hydrazinooctane; D-15-14; 'nimaol').
OCTAMYLAMINE*** (*N*-isoamyl-1,5-di-methyl-1-hexylamine; 2-isoamylamino-6-methylheptane; *N*-(1,5-dimethylhexyl)-isopentylamine; *N*-isopentyl-1,5-dimethyl-hexylamine).
1-Octanecarboxylic acid *see* Nonanoic acid.
1,8-Octanedicarboxylic acid *see* Sebacic acid.
Octanedioic acid *see* Suberic acid.
'Octanil' *see* Isometheptene.
OCTANOIC ACID (1-heptanecarboxylic acid; caprylic acid; octoic acid; octylic acid).
See also Calcium octanoate; Sodium octanoate; Zinc octanoate.
1-OCTANOL (octyl alcohol; caprylic alcohol).
2-OCTANOL (hexyl methyl carbinol).
'Octaphen' *see* Octafonium.
Octaphonium* *see* Octafonium.
'Octapressin' *see* Felypressin.
Octasodium tetrakis(gluconato)bis-(salicylato) μ-diacetodialuminate III dihydrate *see* Sodium glucaspaldrate.
Octatensin (tr) *see* Guanethidine.
OCTATROPINE METHYLBROMIDE*** (*N*-methyl-*O*-(2-propylpentanoyl)tropi-nium bromide; 8-methyl-*O*-(2-propyl-valeryl)tropinium bromide; 8-methyl-tropinium bromide 2-propylvalerate; 8-methyltropinium bromide 2-propylpenta-noate; anisotropine methylbromide; 'valpin').
OCTAVERINE*** (6,7-dimethoxy-1-(3,4,5-triethoxyphenyl)isoquinoline).
OCTAZAMIDE** (5-benzoylhexahydro-1H-furo(3,4-c)pyrrole).
Octestrol (tr) Benzestrol.
OCTICIZER* (2-ethylhexyl diphenyl phos-phate; 'santicizer 141').
'Octin' *see* Isometheptene.
'Octinum' *see* Isometheptene.
Octoclothepin *see* Clorotepine.
Octodecyl alcohol *see* 1-Octadecanol.
OCTODRINE*** (1,5-dimethylhexylamine; 2-amino-6-methylheptane; SK&F-51; 'heptamine').
OCTODRINE CAMSILATE (octodrine camphorsulfonate; octodrine camsylate).

334

OCTODRINE CAMSILATE WITH NORFENEFRINE AND ADENOSINE ('ordinal').

Octoestrol see Benzestrol.

'Octofollin' see Benzestrol.

'Octon' see Isometheptene.

OCTOPAMINE*** (L-α-aminomethyl-*p*-hydroxybenzyl alcohol; 2-(*p*-hydroxyphenyl)ethanolamine; β,4-dihydroxyphenethylamine; noroxedrine; *p*-hydroxymandelamine; ND-50; WV-569; 'norden', 'norphen', 'norsympathol', 'norsynephrine').

OCTOTIAMINE*** (3-(3-acetylthio-7-methoxycarbonylheptyldithio)-4-[*N*-(4-amino-2-methylpyrimid-5-ylmethyl)formamido]pent-3-en-1-ol; 8-[2-[*N*-(4-amino-2-methylpyrimidin-5-ylmethylformamido)-1-(2-hydroxyethyl)propenyl]dithio]-6-mercaptooctanoic acid methyl ester acetate; thiamine acetylthiooctyl disulfide; TATD; 'neuvitan').

OCTOXINOL** (α-[*p*-(1,1,3,3-tetramethylbutyl)phenyl]-ω-hydroxypoly(oxyethylene).

OCTRIPHENATE (octadecyltrimethylammonium pentachlorophenate; 'hyamine 3528').

OCTRIPTYLINE*** (dihydro-*N*-methyldibenzo(a,e)cyclopropa(c)cyclohepten-△⁶⁽¹ᴴ⁾,γ-propylamine; dihydro-6-(3-methylaminopropylidene)dibenzo(a,e)cyclopropa(c)cycloheptene).

Octyl alcohol see 1-Octanol.

Octylatropinium bromide see Atropine octyl bromide.

N-**Octylbicycloheptenedicarboximide** see *N*-(2-Ethylhexyl)bicyclo(2.2.1)hept-5-ene-2,3-dicarboximide.

Octyl 2-cyanoacrylate see Ocrilate.

tert-**Octylguanidine** see Guanoctine.

Octylphenoxyethoxyethyl ether sulfonate sodium see Sodium octylphenoxyethoxyethyl ether sulfonate.

4'-Octyl-3-piperid-1-ylpropiophenone see Pipoctanone.

Octylphenoxypolyethoxyethanol* see Tyloxapol.

Octyl sulfate see Sodium octyl sulfate.

5-[2-(Octylsulfinyl)propyl]-1,3-benzodioxole see Sulfoxide.

'Ocuseptine' see Sodium propionate.

Ocytocin see Oxytocin.

ODA-914 see Demoxytocin.

'Oddibil' see Fumaria officinalis.

O-Dimethoate see Omethoate.

'Odiston' see Diatrizoic acid.

'Odylen' see Mesulfen.

Oenanthaldehyde see Heptyl aldehyde.

Oenanthic acid see Enanthic acid.

Oestr.... see Estr....

'Off' see Diethyl-*m*-toluamide.

'Ogostal' see Capreomycin.

'Ohton' see Dimethylthiambutene.

OIL SCARLET (1-(*p*-phenylazophenylazo)-2-naphthol; cerasine red; Sudan III).

Oil of wintergreen see Methyl salicylate.

'Oilzo' see Triolein ozonide.

Okt.... see also Oct....

Oktadin (tr) see Guanethidine.

Oktametil (tr) see Schradan.

OL-1 see Tioxolone.

OL-110 see Tioxolone.

OLAFLUR*** (2,2'-[[3-(2-hydroxyethyl)-octadecylaminopropyl]imino]diethanol dihydrofluoride; SK&F-38095).

Olamine* see Ethanolamine.

OLAQUINDOX** (*N*-(2-hydroxyethyl)-3-methyl-2-quinoxalinecarboxamide 1,4-dioxide).

'Oleanbel' see Troleandomycin.

OLEANDOMYCIN*** (antibiotic from *Str. antibioticus*; 'amimycin', 'matromycin', 'romicil').
See also Chloramphenicol with oleandomycin; Tetracycline with oleandomycin.

Oleandomycin 4',11-dipropionate see Diproleandomycin.

Oleandomycin triacetate ester see Troleandomycin.

OLEANDOPEN (oleandomycin salt of penicillin G).

OLEIC ACID (*cis*-9-octadecenoic acid). See also Calcium oleate.

Oleocid (tr) see Sodium morrhuate.

'Oleosorbate(s)' see Polysorbate(s).

'Oleothorb' see Polysorbate 80.

Oleovitamin A see Retinol.

Oleovitamin D₂ see Ergocalciferol.

Oleovitamin D₃ see Colecalciferol.

'Oletetrin' see Tetracycline with oleandomycin.

Oleum iodatum see Iodinated poppyseed oil.

Oleum iodisatum see Iodinated poppyseed oil.

OLIVOMYCIN*** (antibiotic from *Actinomyces olivoreticuli*).

OLMIDINE** (3,4-methylenedioxymandelamidine; 2-hydroxy-2-(3,4-methylenedioxyphenyl)acetamidine; α-hydroxypiperonylformamidine; LL-1418).

'Olympax' see Difencloxazine.

OM-518 see Mephenoxalone.

'Omadine' see Pyrithione.

'Omadine disulfide' see Dipyrithione.

'Omadine zinc' see Zinc pyrithione.

Omain (tr) see Demecolcine.

'Omal' see Trichlorophenol(s).

'Omca' see Fluphenazine.

OMDS see Dipyrithione.

'Omega' see Adrenochrome.

'Omeril' see Mebhydrolin napadisilate.

OMETHOATE* (*O,O*-dimethyl *S*-(methylcarbamoylmethyl) phosphorothioate; *O,O*-dimethyl *S*-[2-(methylamino)-2-oxoethyl] phosphorothioate; dimethoxon; O-dimethoate; 'folimat').

OMIDOLINE** (2-methyl-3-(β-piperid-1-yl-*p*-phenetidino)phthalimidine; 2-methyl-3-[*p*-(2-piperid-1-ylethoxy)anilino]phthalimidine; tamidoline).

'Omite' see Propargite.

'Omnes' see Nifuratel.

'Omni-passin' see Dithiazanine iodide.

'Omnipen' see Ampicillin.

335

OMPA *see* Schradan.
OMS-1 *see* Malathion.
OMS-2 *see* Fenthion.
OMS-32 *see* Isoprocarb.
OMS-33 *see* Propoxur.
OMS-43 *see* Fenitrothion.
OMS-47 *see* Mexacarbate.
OMS-93 *see* Methiocarb.
OMS-198 *see* Isodrin.
OMS-479 *see* Dimetilan.
OMS-597 *see* Trimethylphenyl methyl-carbamate.
OMS-708 *see* Benzo(b)thienyl methylcarb-amate.
OMS-736 *see* Temefos.
OMS-971 *see* Chlorpyrifos.
OMS-1394 *see* Bendiocarb.
OMS-1438 *see* Leptophos.
OMS-1800 *see* Cismethrin.
OMU *see* Cycluron.
'Omyl' *see* Lindane with DDT.
'Oncotiotepa' *see* Thiotepa.
'Oncovin' *see* Vincristine.
'Ondasil' *see* Glutethimide.
'Ondena' *see* Daunorubicin.
'Ondogyne' *see* Cyclofenil.
'Ondonid' *see* Cyclofenil.
'Onix-BTC' *see* Benzalkonium.
'Onkotin' *see* Dextran.
Ononein *see* Formonetin.
'Onservan' *see* Procyclidine.
ONTIANIL** (4'-chloro-2,6-dioxocyclo-hexanecarbothioanilide).
'Ontosein' *see* Orgotein.
OOSPONOL (8-hydroxyisocoumarin-4-yl hydroxymethyl ketone).
'Opalene' *see* Trimetozine.
'Operidene' *see* Phenoperidine.
'Opertil' *see* Oxypertine.
OPHIDINE (*N*-(β-alanyl)-2-methyl-histidine).
'Ophtalmokalixan' *see* Kanamycin.
'Ophtamedine' *see* Hexamidine isetionate.
'Ophthaine' *see* Proxymetacaine.
Ophthalin *see* Retinol.
'Ophthetic' *see* Proxymetacaine.
'Ophthochlor' *see* Chloramphenicol.
'Ophticor' *see* Cortisone.
Opial *see* Opium alkaloids.
Opian *see* Noscapine.
OPIANIC ACID (5,6-dimethoxyphthalalde-hydic acid).
Opianic acid isonicotinoylhydrazone *see* Opiniazide.
Opianine *see* Noscapine.
Opianyl *see* *m*-Meconin.
'Opilon' *see* Moxisylyte.
OPINIAZIDE*** (isonicotinoylhydrazone of 5,6-dimethoxyphthalaldehydic acid; carb-oxyverazid; isonicotinic acid (2-carboxy-3,4-dimethoxybenzylidene)hydrazide; 2-carboxy-3,4-dimethoxybenzaldehyde isonicotinoylhydrazone; *N*'-2-carboxy-veratrylideneisoniazid; opianic acid isonicotinoylhydrazone; saluzid).
See also Streptomycin opiniazide salt.
'Opino' *see* Buphenine.

OPIPRAMOL*** (4-[3-(5H-dibenz(b,f)-azepin-5-yl)propyl]-1-piperazineethanol; 5-[3-[4-(2-hydroxyethyl)piperazin-1-yl]-propyl]-5H-dibenzo(b,f)azepine; opipra-mol dihydrochloride; G-33040; RP-8307; 'ensidon', 'eusidon', 'insidon', 'nisidan', 'pramolan').
'Opiran' *see* Pimozide.
OPIUM ALKALOIDS (laudanum; meco-nium; opial; papaveretum; tetrapon). *See also* Codeine; Meconin; Morphine; Narceine; Noscapine; Papaverine; Pare-goric; Thebaine.
Opromazine *see* Chlorpromazine sulfoxide.
'Optamine' *see* Dihydroergotoxine mesilate.
'Optanox' *see* Vinylbital.
'Opticortenol' *see* Dexamethasone pivalate.
'Opticortenol-S' *see* Dexamethasone pivalate with prednisolone.
'Optiform' *see* Formaldehyde.
'Optimax' *see* Tryptophan with pyridoxine.
'Optimil' *see* Methaqualone.
'Optimycin' *see* Metacycline.
'Optojod' *see* 2,6-Diiodo-1-phenol-4-sulfonic acid.
'Orabet' *see* Tolbutamide.
'Orabetic' *see* Carbutamide.
'Orabilex' *see* Bunamiodyl.
'Orabilix' *see* Bunamiodyl.
'Orabolin' *see* Ethylestrenol.
'Oracaine' *see* Meprylcaine.
'Oracef' *see* Cefalexin.
'Oracon' *see* Dimethisterone with ethinyl-estradiol
'Oraconal' *see* Megestrol acetate with ethinylestradiol.
'Oradash' *see* Methionine.
'Oradexon' *see* Dexamethasone.
'Oradian' *see* Chlorhexamide.
'Oragest' *see* Medroxyprogesterone.
'Oragrafin-Na' *see* Sodium iodopate.
'Oragulant' *see* Diphenadione.
'Oralcon' *see* Diclofenamide.
'Oraldene' *see* Hexetidine.
'Oralin' *see* Tolbutamide.
'Oralopen' *see* Pheneticillin.
'Oral turinabol' *see* 4-Chloro-17β-hydroxy-17-methyl-1,4-androstadien-3-one.
'Oramercur' *see* Chlormerodrin.
'Oramyl' *see* α-Amylase.
'Oranabol' *see* Oxymesterone.
ORANGE G* (chiefly the di-Na salt of 1-phenylazo-2-naphthol-6,8-disulfonic acid; novaurantium).
ORANGE RN (sodium 1-phenylazo-2-naphthol-6-sulfonate; croceine orange; C.I.No. 15970).
'Oranil' *see* Carbutamide.
'Orap' *see* Pimozide.
'Orasulin' *see* Carbutamide.
'Ora-testryl' *see* Fluoxymesterone.
'Oratrol' *see* Diclofenamide.
ORAZAMIDE*** (5-aminoimidazole-4-carb-oxamide orotate; 'aicamide').
'Orbenin' *see* Cloxacillin.
'Orbinamon' *see* Tiotixene.
Orcin *see* Orcinol.

ORCINOL (5-methylresorcinol; 1,3-di-hydroxy-5-methylbenzene; 3,5-dihydroxy-toluene; orcin).
Orcinol dimethyl ether *see* Elemicin.
ORCIPRENALINE*** (3,5-dihydroxy-α-(isopropylaminomethyl)benzyl alcohol; 1-(3,5-dihydroxyphenyl)-2-isopropyl-aminoethanol; orciprenaline sulfate; metaproterenol sulfate; Th-152; 'alotec', 'alupent', 'metaprel').
ORCIPRENALINE WITH OXAZEPAM ('tranquo-alupent').
'Ordimel' *see* Acetohexamide.
'Ordinal' *see* Octodrine camsilate with norfenefrine and adenosine.
'Ordinator' *see* Fenozolone.
'Ordram' *see* Molinate.
'Orencil' *see* Benzhydrylamine penicillinate.
'Oresol' *see* Guaifenesin.
'Oreson' *see* Guaifenesin.
ORESTRATE** (17β-cyclohexen-1-yloxy-estra-1,3,5(10)-trien-3-ol propionate; estradiol 17-cyclohexen-1-yl ether 3-propionate).
'Oretic' *see* Hydrochlorothiazide.
OREXIN (3,4-dihydro-3-phenylquinazoline; cedrarin; phenzoline).
ORF-1557-BA *see* Norethisterone acetate with ethinylestradiol.
ORF-8063 *see* Triflubazam.
Orferon (tr) *see* Ferroglycine sulfate complex.
Org.817 *see* Epimestrol.
Org.NA97 *see* Pancuronium bromide.
Org.OD-14 *see* Tibolone.
'Orgabolin' *see* Ethylestrenol.
'Orgametil' *see* Lynestrenol.
'Orgametril' *see* Lynestrenol.
'Organidin' *see* Iodinated glycerol.
'Orga-phenkapton' *see* Phenkapton.
'Orgasteron' *see* Methylestrenolone.
ORGOTEIN** (soluble metalloproteins from liver, red blood cells and other mammalian tissues; ormetein; 'ontosein', 'palosein').
'Oricillin' *see* Propicillin.
'Oricur' *see* Chlormerodrin.
'Orientomycin' *see* Cycloserine.
'Orinase' *see* Tolbutamide.
'Orion' *see* Triamcinolone.
'Orisul' *see* Sulfaphenazole.
'Orisulf' *see* Sulfaphenazole.
'Orlest' *see* Norethisterone acetate with ethinylestradiol.
'Orlestrin' *see* Norethisterone acetate with ethinylestradiol.
'Orlutate' *see* Norethisterone acetate.
Ormetein *see* Orgotein.
ORMETOPRIM*** (2,4-diamino-5-(6-methylveratryl)pyrimidine; 2,4-diamino-5-(3,4-dimethoxy-6-methylbenzyl)pyrimidine).
ORMETOPRIM WITH SULFADIMETH-OXINE ('rofenaid').
'Ornicetil' *see* Ornithine oxoglurate.
Ornid (tr) *see* Bretylium tosilate.
ORNIDAZOLE*** (α-(chloromethyl)-2-

methyl-5-nitroimidazole-1-ethanol; 1-(3-chloro-2-hydroxypropyl)-2-methyl-5-nitroimidazole; Ro 7-0207; 'tiberal').
ORNIPRESSIN*** (8-ornithine vasopressin; orpressin; POR-8).
ORNITHINE (2,5-diaminovaleric acid; 2,5-diaminopentanoic acid).
ORNITHINE ASPARTATE ('hepa-Merz').
ORNITHINE CARBAMYL TRANS-FERASE ('preortan').
ORNITHINE OXOGLURATE (ornithine 2-oxoglutarate; ornithine α-keto-glutarate; 'ornicetil').
Ornithine 2-oxoglutarate *see* Ornithine oxoglurate.
8-Ornithine vasopressin *see* Ornipressin.
'Ornitrol' *see* Azacosterol.
'Oronol' *see* Aurothioglucose.
OROTIC ACID (6-uracilcarboxylic acid; 1,2,3,6-tetrahydro-2,6-dioxo-4-pyrimidine-carboxylic acid; animal glucose factor; whey factor).
See also Choline orotate; Magnesium orotate.
Orotic acid salt of 5-amidoimidazole-4-carboxamide *see* Orazamide.
ORPHENADRINE*** (N,N-dimethyl-2-(o-methylbenzhydryloxy)ethylamine; N,N-dimethyl-2-(α-o-tolylbenzyloxy)ethyl-amine; N,N-dimethyl-2-(o-methyl-α-phenylbenzyloxy)ethylamine; o-methyldi-phenhydramine; benhexol; orphenadrine hydrochloride; BS-5930; 'brocadisipal', 'brocasipal', 'disipal', 'mephenamine').
ORPHENADRINE CITRATE ('norflex').
ORPHENADRINE CITRATE WITH APC ('orphenisal').
ORPHENADRINE CITRATE WITH PARACETAMOL ('norgesic').
'Orphenisal' *see* Orphenadrine citrate with APC.
'Orpidan' *see* Chlorazanil.
'Orpizin' *see* Chlorazanil.
Orpressin *see* Ornipressin.
'Orsin' *see* p-Phenylenediamine.
'Orstanorm' *see* Dihydroergotamine maleate.
'Ortal' *see* Hexethal.
ORTETAMINE*** (o-α-dimethylphenethyl-amine; 2,α-dimethylphenethylamine; o-methylamphetamine; 1-methyl-2-(o-tolyl)-ethylamine).
ORTHANILAMIDE (o-aminobenzenesulfon-amide).
'Orthene' *see* Acephate.
'Orthesin' *see* Benzocaine.
'Orthiourea' *see* Sodium auroallylthioureido-benzoate.
Ortho 1557-0 *see* Norethisterone with mestranol.
ORTHOCAINE* (methyl ester of 3-amino-4-hydroxybenzoic acid; 'aminobenz', 'orthoform').
'Orthocide-406' *see* Captan
'Orthocol' *see* Sulfogaiacol.
'Ortho crabgrass killer' *see* Disodium methanearsonate.

'**Orthodelfen**' *see* Nonoxinol 9.
Orthodiazine *see* Pyridazine.
'**Ortho dibrom**' *see* Naled.
Orthoferulic acid *see* o-Ferulic acid.
'**Orthoform**' *see* Nonoxinol 9 *and* Orthocaine.
'**Orthoiodine**' *see* Sodium o-iodohippurate.
'**Ortho-klor**' *see* Chlordane.
'**Ortho-mite**' *see* Butylphenoxyisopropyl chloroethyl sulfite.
'**Orthonal**' *see* Methaqualone.
'**Orthonovin**' *see* Norethisterone with mestranol.
'**Ortho-novum**' *see* Norethisterone with mestranol.
'**Orthoparaquat**' *see* Paraquat.
Orthophosphoric acid *see* Phosphoric acid.
ORTHOPROCAINAMIDE (o-amino-N-(2-diethylaminoethyl)benzamide).
Orthosarcolysin *see* o-Sarcolysin.
'**Orthoxenol**' *see* Phenylphenol.
'**Orthoxine**' *see* Methoxyphenamine.
'**Ortin**' *see* Trolnitrate.
'**Ortizon**' *see* Hydrogen peroxide-urea.
'**Ortodrine**' *see* Methoxyphenamine.
'**Ortol**' *see* Ethylhexylbarbituric acid.
'**Orudis**' *see* Ketoprofen.
ORYZALIN* (4-(dipropylamino)-3,5-dinitrobenzenesulfonamide; 3,4-dinitro-N^4,N^4-dipropylsulfanilamide; 'ryzelan').
'**Oryzanin**' *see* Thiamine.
'**Osadrin**' *see* Aminophenazone with diphenylpyrazolidinedione.
OSALMID*** (4'-hydroxysalicylanilide; N-(p-hydroxyphenyl)salicylamide; oxafenamide; L-1718; 'driol', 'endiran', 'enidran', 'salmidochol').
Osarsol (tr) *see* Acetarsol.
'**Osbil**' *see* Iobenzamic acid.
'**Oscine**' *see* Scopolamine.
OSMADIZONE*** ([2-(phenylsulfinyl)-ethyl]malonic acid mono(1,2-diphenyl-hydrazide).
'**Osmitrol**' *see* Mannitol.
'**Osmofundin**' *see* Mannitol.
'**Ospolot**' *see* Sultiame.
'**Ossiamina**' *see* Chlormethine N-oxide.
'**Ossiclorin**' *see* Chlormethine N-oxide.
'**Ossitetra**' *see* Oxytetracycline.
'**Ostamer**' *see* Polyurethane foam.
'**Ostensin**' *see* Trimethidinium.
'**Osthol**' *see* 8-Isopentenyl-7-methoxycoumarin.
'**Ostreocin**' *see* Ostreogrycin.
OSTREOGRYCIN*** (antibiotic from *Str. ostreogriseus*; 'ostreocin').
Ostreogrycin B *see* Mikamycin B.
'**Ostrocilline**' *see* Benzathine penicillin V.
OSTRUTHIN (6-geranyl-7-hydroxycoumarin).
'**Osvan**' *see* Benzalkonium.
Osyritin *see* Rutoside.
Osyritrin *see* Rutoside.
'**Otocones**' *see* Benzododecinium.
'**Otokalixan**' *see* Kanamycin.
'**Otrhomin**' *see* Methenamine thiocyanate.
'**Otrivine**' *see* Phenamazoline *and* Xylometazoline.

'**OTS 68**' *see* Oxytocin synthetic analogue(s).
Ouabagenin L-rhamnoside *see* Ouabain.
OUABAIN ($1\beta,3\beta,5,11\alpha,14,19$-hexahydroxy-$5\beta$-card-20($22$)-enolide 3-L-rhamnoside; ouabagenin L-rhamnoside; g-strophanthin; acocantherin; gratus strophanthin; 'purostrophan').
'**Ovanon**' *see* Lynestrenol with mestranol.
'**Ovaribran**' *see* Conjugated estrogens with oxazepam.
'**Ovariostat**' *see* Lynestrenol with mestranol.
'**Ovatran**' *see* Chlorfenson.
Ovex *see* Chlorfenson.
'**Ovitrol**' *see* Fenticlor.
Ovochlor *see* Chlorfenson.
Ovoflavin *see* Riboflavine.
'**Ovosiston**' *see* Chlormadinone acetate with mestranol.
'**Ovotran**' *see* Chlorfenson.
'**Ovral**' *see* Norgestrel with ethinylestradiol.
'**Ovran**' *see* Levonorgestrel with ethinylestradiol.
'**Ovranette**' *see* Levonorgestrel with ethinylestradiol.
'**Ovulen**' *see* Etynodiol diacetate with mestranol.
'**Owadofos**' *see* Fenitrothion.
m-(**1-Oxa-4-azaspiro(4,6)undec-2-yl)phenol** *see* Ciclafrine.
'**Oxabel**' *see* Oxacillin.
endo-endo-**7-Oxabicyclo(2.2.1)heptane-2,3-dicarboxylic acid disodium salt** *see* Endothal sodium.
OXABOLONE CIPIONATE*** (17β-(3-cyclopentylpropionyloxy)-4-hydroxy-estr-4-en-3-one; estr-4-ene-4,17β-diol-3-one 17-cyclopentanepropionate; oxabolone cypionate; 'steranabol depot').
OXACEPROL** ((−)-1-acetyl-4-hydroxy-L-proline; N-acetylhydroxyproline; 'jonctum').
OXACILLIN** (6-[(5-methyl-3-phenyl-isoxazol-4-yl)carboxamido]penicillanic acid; 5-methyl-3-phenylisoxazol-4-ylpenicillin; oxacillin sodium; sodium oxacillin; isoxacillin; oxazacillin; P-12; SQ-16423; 'bactocill', 'bristopen', 'cryptocillin', 'micropenin', 'oxabel', 'oxastaph', 'penstapho', 'prostaphlin', 'resistopen', 'stapenor').
See also Ampicillin with oxacillin.
Oxacyclobutane *see* Oxetane.
OXADIMEDINE*** (N-benzoxazol 2-yl-N-benzyl-N,N'-dimethylethylenediamine; 2-[benzyl(2-dimethylaminoethyl)amino]-benzoxazole).
Oxadrol* *see* Dioxadrol.
7-Oxa-3,6-endomethylenehexahydro-phthalic acid disodium salt *see* Endothal sodium.
Oxafenamide *see* Osalmid.
OXAFLOZANE*** (4-isopropyl-2-(α,α,α-trifluoro-m-tolyl)morpholine).
OXAFLUMAZINE*** (10-[3-[4-(2-m-dioxanylethyl)piperazin-1-yl]propyl]-2-trifluoromethyl phenothiazine).
Oxafuradene *see* Nifuradene.

Oxagestone *see* Oxogestone phenpropionate.
17α-Oxa-D-homoandrosta-1,4-diene-3,17-dione *see* Testolactone.
'Oxaine' *see* Oxetacaine.
OXALACETIC ACID (ketosuccinic acid; oxosuccinic acid).
Oxalaldehyde *see* Glyoxal.
Oxalamide *see* Oxamide.
OXALIC ACID (ethanedioic acid).
Oxalic acid diamide *see* Oxamide.
Oxalic acid monoamide *see* Oxamic acid.
'Oxalid' *see* Oxyphenbutazone.
[Oxalylbis(iminoethylene)]bis[(o-chloro-benzyl)diethylammonium chloride] *see* Ambenonium chloride.
1,3-Oxalylurea *see* Parabanic acid.
OXAMARIN*** (6,7-bis(2-diethylamino-ethoxy)-4-methylcoumarin; ethoxarine; 'idro P-3').
OXAMIC ACID (oxalic acid monoamide; aminoglyoxylic acid; aminooxoacetic acid).
Oxamic acid hydrazide *see* Semioxamazide.
OXAMIDE (oxalic acid diamide; ethane diamide; oxalamide).
Oxammonium *see* Hydroxylamine.
OXAMNIQUINE*** (1,2,3,4-tetrahydro-2-isopropylaminomethyl-7-nitro-6-quinoline-methanol; 1,2,3,4-tetrahydro-6-hydroxy-methyl-2-isopropylaminomethyl-7-nitro-quinoline; UK-4271).
Oxamphetamine* *see* Hydroxyamphet-amine.
'Oxamycin' *see* Cycloserine.
OXAMYL* (methyl 2-(dimethylamino)-*N*-[[(methylamino)carbonyl]oxy]-2-oxoethan-imidothioate; 'vydate').
OXANAMIDE*** (2,3-epoxy-2-ethylhexan-amide; 1,2-epoxy-1-ethylpentane-1-carb-oxamide; 2,3-epoxy-2-ethyl-3-propyl-propionamide; 2-ethyl-3-propylglycid-amide; 'quiactin').
OXANDROLONE*** (dodecahydro-3-hydroxy-6-hydroxymethyl-3,3a,6-trimeth-yl(1H)benz(e)indene-7-acetic acid δ-lactone; 17-methyl-2-oxa-5α-androstan-17β-ol-3-one; 17β-hydroxy-17-methyl-2-oxa-5α-androstan-3-one; SC-11585; 'anavar').
OXANTEL** ((*E*)-*m*-[2-(1,4,5,6-tetrahydro-1-methylpyrimidin-2-yl)vinyl]phenol; *trans*-1,4,5,6-tetrahydro-2-(3-hydroxy-styryl)-1-methylpyrimidine; *trans*-1,4,5,6-tetrahydro-2-[2-(*m*-hydroxyphenyl)vinyl]-1-methylpyrimidine; *trans*-3-hydroxy-β-(1,4,5,6-tetrahydro-1-methylpyrimid-2-yl)-styrene; CP-14445).
OXANTEL EMBONATE (oxantel pamo-ate; CP-14445-16).
Oxantel pamoate* *see* Oxantel embonate.
3-Oxapentane-1,5-diol *see* Diethylene glycol.
OXAPIUM IODIDE** (1-(2-cyclohexyl-2-phenyl-1,3-dioxolan-4-ylmethyl)-1-methyl-piperidinium iodide; 'esperan').
OXAPRAZINE* (10-[3-[4-(2-*m*-dioxan-2-ylethyl)piperazin-1-yl]propyl]phenothia-zine; 2-[2-[4-(3-phenothiazin-10-ylpropyl)-piperazin-1-yl]ethyl]-*m*-dioxan; 1-(2-*m*-

dioxan-2-ylethyl)-4-(3-phenothiazin-10-ylpropyl)piperazine).
OXAPROPANIUM IODIDE*** ((1,3-di-oxolan-4-ylmethyl)trimethylammonium iodide; 4-dimethylaminomethyl-1,3-dioxa-cyclopentane methiodide; 1-dimethyl-amino-2,3-methylenedioxypropane methio-dide; 4-dimethylaminomethyl-1,3-dioxolane methiodide; formal of (dihydroxypropyl)-trimethylammonium iodide; F-2249; 'dilvasene').
OXAPROZIN** (4,5-diphenyl-2-oxazole-propionic acid; 3-(4,5-diphenyloxazol-2-yl)-propionic acid; Wy-21743).
'Oxastaph' *see* Oxacillin.
Oxaundecamethylenebis(trimethylam-monium chloride) *see* Oxydipentonium.
Oxazacillin* *see* Oxacillin.
OXAZEPAM*** (7-chloro-1,3-dihydro-3-hydroxy-5-phenyl-2H-1,4-benzodiazepin-2-one; CB-8092; Wy-3498; Z-10TR; 'adum-bran', 'praxiten', 'nesontil', 'serax', 'serenid', 'serepax', 'seresta', 'sobril', 'vaben').
See also below and Conjugated estrogen with oxazepam; Orciprenaline with oxazepam; Scopolamine butyl bromide with oxazepam.
Oxazepam dipropylacetate *see* Oxazepam valproate.
OXAZEPAM HEMISUCCINATE (Wy-4426; 'nulans') .
Oxazepam pivalate *see* Pivoxazepam.
Oxazepam 2-propylvalerate *see* Oxazepam valproate.
Oxazepam trimethylacetate *see* Pivoxa-zepam.
OXAZEPAM VALPROATE (oxazepam 2-propylvalerate; oxazepam dipropylace-tate; SAS-554).
OXAZIDIONE*** (2-(morpholinomethyl)-2-phenyl-1,3-indandione; mofedione; LD-4610; 'amplidione').
Oxazimedrine* *see* Phenmetrazine.
OXAZOLAM*** (10-chloro-2,3,7,11b-tetra-hydro-2-methyl-11b-phenyloxazolo(3,2-d)-(1,4)benzodiazepine-6(5H)-one; CS-370; 'serenal').
OXAZOLE (furo(b)monazole).
OXAZOLIDINE (tetrahydrooxazole).
OXAZOLINE (dihydrooxazole).
OXAZORONE*** (7-hydroxy-4-morpho-linomethylcoumarin).
OX BILE (fel tauri; 'anabile', 'choloplant', 'desibyl', felkreon, 'glissitol').
OXEDRINE* (*p*-hydroxy-α-methylamino-methylbenzyl alcohol; 1-(*p*-hydroxyphenyl)-2-methylaminoethanol; *N*-methyltyr-amine; aetaphen; pentedrine; synephrine; vasoton).
OXEDRINE ASCORBATE ('corva-C').
OXEDRINE TARTRATE ('analeptin', 'cardiodynamin', 'corvasymton', 'neupen-tedrin', 'parasympathol', 'simpalon', 'symcortol', 'sympathol', 'sympatol', 'synthenate', 'vasocordrin').
OXELADIN*** (2-diethylaminoethoxy-

339

ethyl ester of 2-ethyl-2-phenylbutyric acid; diethylaminoethoxyethyl diethylphenylacetate).

OXELADIN CITRATE ('dorex', 'paxeladine', 'pectamol', 'tussinol').

OXETACAINE*** (2,2'-(2-hydroxyethylimino)bis[N-(α,α-dimethylphenethyl)-N-methylacetamide]; 2-[bis(N-methyl-N-phenyl-*tert*-butylcarbamoylmethyl)-amino]ethanol; N,N-bis[N-methyl-N-(phenyl-*tert*-butyl)acetamido]-2-hydroxyethylamine; oxetacaine hydrochloride; oxethazaine; Wy-806; 'oxaine', 'tepilta').

OXETACILLIN*** ((2S,5R,6R)-6-[(R)-[4-(p-hydroxyphenyl)-2,2-dimethyl-5-oxoimidazolidin-1-yl]]penicillanic acid).

OXETANE (trimethylene oxide; oxacyclobutane; oxethane).

2-Oxetanone see β-Propiolactone.

Oxethane see Oxetane.

Oxethazaine* see Oxetacaine.

OXETORONE*** (N,N-dimethylbenzofuro-(3,2-c)(1)benzoxepin-△⁶⁽¹²ᴴ⁾,γ-propylamine; 6-(3-dimethylaminopropylidene)-(12H)benzofuro(3,2-c)(1)benzoxepine).

OXETORONE FUMARATE (L-6257; 'nocertone').

OXFENDAZOLE** (methyl 5-(phenylsulfinyl)-2-benzimidazolecarbamate).

Oxiamin see Inosine.

OXIBENDAZOLE** (methyl 5-propoxy-2-benzimidazolecarbamate; SK&F-30310).

OXIBETAINE*** ((carboxymethyl)dimethyl(2-hydroxyethyl)ammonium hydroxide inner salt).

Oxibutynin* see Oxybutynin.

Oxiclipine* see Oxyclipine.

Oxichlorochin* see Hydroxychloroquine.

Oxiconum see Oxycodone.

OXIDIZED CELLULOSE* (oxidized cellulosic acid; oxycellulose; 'hemo-pak', 'novocell', 'oxycel', 'sorbacel').

OXIDIZED REGENERATED CELLULOSE* ('surgicel', 'tabotamp').

Oxifenamate* see Oxyfenamate.

OXIFENTOREX*** (N-benzyl-N,α-dimethylphenethylamine N-oxide; N-benzyl-N-methylamphetamine N-oxide; benzphetamine oxide).

Oxilapine see Loxapine.

OXILORPHAN** ((−)-17-(cyclopropylmethyl)morphinan-3,14-diol; (−)-17-(cyclopropylmethyl)-3,4-dihydroxymorphinan).

Oximetazoline* see Oxymetazoline.

Oxin see 8-Quinolinol.

OXINDOLE (2,3-dihydro-2-oxoindole; 2(3H)-indolone; 2-indolinone).

Oxine see 8-Quinolinol.

OXINE-COPPER* (oxine-Cu; bis(8-quinolinato-N²,O⁸)copper; 8-quinolinol copper compound).

OXINIACIC ACID*** (nicotinic acid 1-oxide; nicotinic acid N-oxide).

'Oxinofen' see Oxycinchophen.

Oxipendyl* see Oxypendyl.

OXIPEROMIDE** (1-[1-(2-phenoxyethyl)-piperid-4-yl]benzimidazolin-2-one; 4-(2-oxobenzimidazolin-1-yl)-1-(2-phenoxyethyl)piperidine; 1,3-dihydro-1-[1-(2-phenoxyethyl)piperid-4-yl]-2H-benzimidazol-2-one; R-4714).

Oxipertin see Oxypertine.

OXIPURINOL*** (1H-pyrazolo(3,4-d)-pyrimidin-4,6-diol; 4,6-dihydroxypyrazolo-(3,4-d)pyrimidine; oxypurinol; BW-55-5).

Oxipyrronium* see Oxypyrronium.

OXIRAMIDE*** (N-[4-(2,6-dimethylpiperid-1-yl)butyl]-2-phenoxy-2-phenylacetamide; 1-[4-(2-phenoxy-2-phenylacetamido)butyl]-2,6-dimethylpiperidine).

Oxirane see Ethylene oxide.

Oxisone* see Oxysonium.

OXISOPRED*** (11β,17,21-trihydroxy-B-homo-A-norpregn-1-ene-3,6,20-trione).

OXISURAN*** (methylsulfinylmethyl 2-pyridyl ketone; 2-(methylsulfinylacetyl)-pyridine).

OXITEFONIUM BROMIDE*** (diethyl-(2-hydroxyethyl)methylammonium bromide α-phenyl-2-thiopheneglycolate; F-70).

OXITRIPTYLINE*** (2-(10,11-dihydro-5H-dibenzo(a,d)cyclohepten-5-yloxy)-N,N-dimethylacetamide; 5-[(dimethylcarbamoyl)-methoxy]-10,11-dihydro-5H-dibenzo(a,d)-cycloheptene; oxytriptyline).

Oxo... etc. See also Keto... etc.

Oxoacetic acid see Glyoxylic acid.

'Oxo-ate' see Amiodoxyl benzoate.

Oxo-ate-B'* see Calciodoxyl benzoate.

4-(2-Oxobenzimidazolin-1-yl)-2-(2-phenoxyethyl)piperidine see Oxiperomide.

4-Oxo-4H-1-benzopyran-2-carboxylic acid see Chromocarb.

4-Oxo-1-benzopyran-2-carboxylic acid 5,5'-diether with glycerol see Cromoglicic acid.

2-Oxo-2H-1,3-benzoxazine-3(4H)-acetamide see Caroxazone.

γ-Oxo(1,1'-biphenyl)-4-butanoic acid see Fenbufen.

2-OXO-3-BORNANECARBOXYLIC ACID (3-camphorcarboxylic acid; camphocarboxylic acid; camphocarbonic acid).

2-Oxobornane-10-sulfonic acid see Camphorsulfonic acid.

4-(3-Oxobutyl)-1,2-diphenyl-3,5-pyrazolidinedione see Kebuzone.

1-(2-Oxocyclohexylmethyl)piperidine see Pimeclone.

1-(2-Oxocyclohexyl)-2-naphthol see Naphthonone.

γ-Oxo-2-dibenzofuranbutyric acid see Furobufen.

γ-Oxo-8-fluoranthrenebutyric acid see Florantyrone.

9-Oxofluoren-2-ylglyoxal bisulfite compound see Florenal.

OXOGESTONE*** (19-norpregn-4-en-20β-ol-3-one; 20β-hydroxy-19-norpregn-4-en-3-one).

Oxogestone hydrocinnamate see Oxogestone phenpropionate.

OXOGESTONE PHENPROPIONATE*
(oxogestone 20-phenylpropionate; oxogestone hydrocinnamate; oxagestone).
OXOGLURATE(S)** (2-oxoglutarate(s);
2-ketoglutarate(s)).
See also Arginine oxoglurate; Ornithine
oxoglurate.
2-OXOGLUTARIC ACID (2-ketoglutaric
acid; α-ketoglutaric acid).
2-Oxoglutaric acid, esters and salts *see*
Oxoglurate(s).
3-Oxo-L-gulofuranolactone *see* Ascorbic
acid.
2-Oxohexamethylenimine *see* Caprolactam.
3-OXOHEXANOIC ACID (3-ketohexanoic
acid, ketocaproic acid; butyrylacetic acid).
3-Oxohexonic acid lactone *see* Isoascorbic
acid.
1-(5-Oxohexyl)theobromine *see* Pentoxifylline.
**6-[2-(2-Oxoimidazoline-1-carboxamido)-
2-phenylacetamido]penicillanic acid**
see Azlocillin.
p-**(1-Oxoisoindolin-2-yl)hydratropic acid**
see Indoprofen.
OXOLAMINE*** (5-(2-diethylaminoethyl)-
3-phenyl-1,2,4-oxadiazole).
**OXOLAMINE BENZILATE WITH
TETRACYCLINE** ('proxybron').
OXOLAMINE CITRATE (AF-438;
'bredon', 'perebron').
OXOLIN (tr) (1,2,3,4-tetrahydro-1,2,3,4-
tetraoxonaphthalene dihydrate; tetrahydro-
naphthalenetetrone dihydrate).
OXOLINIC ACID*** (5-ethyl-5,8-dihydro-
8-oxo-1,3-dioxolo(4,5-g)quinoline-7-carb-
oxylic acid; W-4565; 'urotrate').
Oxomalonic acid *see* Mesoxalic acid.
OXOMEMAZINE*** (10-(3-dimethyl-
amino-2-methylpropyl)phenothiazine
5,5-dioxide; alimemazine *S,S*-dioxide; trimeprazine *S,S*-dioxide; RP-6847; 'doxergan', 'dysedon', 'imakol').
Oxomethane *see* Formaldehyde.
OXONAZINE*** (2-diallylamino-4,6-di-
amino-*s*-triazine *N*²-oxide; *N*²,*N*²-diallyl-
melamine *N*²-oxide).
'Oxone' *see* Sodium peroxide.
OXOPHENARSINE*** (2-amino-4-arseno-
sophenol; *m*-amino-*p*-hydroxyphenylarsine
oxide; 3-amino-4-hydroxyphenylarsenoxide;
arsphenoxide; oxyphenarsine; phen-
arsoxide; oxophenarsine hydrochloride;
Ehrlich-5; NSC-3087).
**[(4-Oxo-2-phenyl-4H-1-benzopyran-
5,7-diyl)dioxy]diacetic acid** *see* Flavodic
acid.
**5-Oxo-*N*-(*trans*-2-phenylcyclopropyl)-
2-pyrrolidinecarboxamide** *see* Rolicyprine.
**4-(3-Oxo-3-phenylpropyl)-1,2-diphenyl-
3,5-pyrazolidinedione** *see* Benzopyrazone.
**2-Oxo-5-phenyl-*N*-propyloxazolidine-
3-carboxamide** *see* Profexalone.
**2-(2-Oxopiperid-3-yl)-1,2-benzisothia-
zolin-3-one 1,1-dioxide** *see* Supidimide.

11-Oxoprogesterone *see* Pregnenetrione.
5-Oxoproline *see* Pyroglutamic acid.
**5-Oxo-L-prolyl-L-glutaminyl-L-aspartyl-
L-tyrosyl-L-threonylglycyl-L-trypto-
phyl-L-methionyl-L-aspartyl-L-phenyl-
alaninamide 4-(hydrogen sulfate)
ester** *see* Ceruletide.
5-Oxo-L-prolyl-L-histidyl-L-prolinamide
see Protirelin.
**5-Oxo-L-prolyl-L-histidyl-L-tryptophyl-
L-seryl-L-tyrosylglycyl-L-leucyl-L-
arginyl-L-prolylglycinamide** *see* Gonadorelin.
2-Oxopropanal *see* Methylglyoxal.
1-Oxopropionaldehyde *see* Methylglyoxal.
N-**[1-Oxo-5(1H)-(purin-6-ylthio)pentyl]-
glycine ethyl ester** *see* Butocin.
2-Oxo-1-pyrrolidineacetamide *see* Piracetam.
5-Oxo-2-pyrrolidinecarboxylic acid *see*
Pyroglutamic acid.
**1-(2-Oxopyrrolidino)-4-pyrrolidino-
2-butyne** *see* Oxotremorine.
2-(2-Oxopyrrolidin-1-yl)acetamide *see*
Piracetam.
Oxosuccinic acid *see* Oxalacetic acid.
**8-Oxo-5-thia-1-azabicyclo(4.2.0)oct-2-ene-
2-carboxylic acid** *see* 2-Cephem-2-
carboxylic acid.
**2-[2-[4-Oxo-3-(*o*-tolyl)quinazolin-2-yl]-
vinyl]pyridine** *see* Piriqualone.
OXOTREMORINE (1-(2-oxopyrrolidino)-
4-pyrrolidino-2-butyne).
Oxpentifylline* *see* Pentoxifylline.
OXPHENERIDINE*** (ethyl ester of
1-(β-hydroxyphenethyl)-4-phenylpiperidine-
4-carboxylic acid; ethyl ester of 1-(2-hydr-
oxy-2-phenylethyl)-4-phenylisonipecotic
acid).
OXPRENOLOL*** (1-(*o*-allyloxyphenoxy)-
3-isopropylaminopropan-2-ol; 2-(*o*-allyl-
oxyphenoxy)-2-hydroxy-*N*-isopropyl-
1-propylamine; oxprenolol hydrochloride;
Ba-39089; C-39089-Ba; 'coretal', 'trasi-
cor').
'Oxsoralen' *see* Methoxsalen.
Oxtrimethylline* *see* Choline theophyllinate.
Oxtriphylline* *see* Choline theophyllinate.
'Oxucide' *see* Piperazine citrate.
'Oxurasin' *see* Piperazine adipate.
'Oxyamine' *see* Chlormethine *N*-oxide.
OXYBATE SODIUM* (sodium 4-hydroxy-
butyrate; sodium oxybate; gamma-OH;
Wy-3478; 'fisiogamma', 'somsanit').
OXYBENZONE*** (2-hydroxy-4-methoxy-
benzophenone; 'spectrasorb UV 9', 'uvinul
M-40').
'Oxy-biciron' *see* Tramazoline with oxy-
tetracycline.
β,β'-**Oxybis(*p*-acetophenetidide)** *see* Di-
amfenetide.
4',4'''-Oxybis(2-chloroacetophenone) *see*
Clofenoxyde.
Oxybis(*p*-ethoxyacetanilide) *see* Diamfenetide.
**3,3'-[Oxybis(ethyleneoxyethylenecarbon-
ylimino)]bis(2,4,6-triiodobenzoic acid)**

see Iotranic acid.

3,3′-[Oxybis(ethyleneoxymethylene-carbonylimino)]bis(2,4,6-triiodoben-zoic acid) *see* Iotroxic acid.

3,3′-[Oxybis(methylenecarbonylimino)]-bis(2,4,6-triiodobenzoic acid) *see* Ioglycamic acid.

[Oxybis(pentamethylene)]bis(trimethyl-ammoniumchloride) *see* Oxydipentonium chloride.

Oxybisphenacetin *see* Diamfenetide.

OXYBUPROCAINE*** (2-diethylamino-ethyl ester of 4-amino-3-butoxybenzoic acid; 'cébésine', 'novesin').

OXYBUTYNIN*** (4-diethylamino-2-butynyl α-phenylcyclohexaneglycolate; oxybutynin chloride; oxibutynin; oxybutynin chloride; MJ-4309-1; 'ditropan').

'Oxycaine' *see* Hydroxyprocaine.

Oxycarboxin *see* Carboxin dioxide.

'Oxycel' *see* Oxidized cellulose.

Oxycellulose *see* Oxidized cellulose.

Oxychloroquine *see* Hydroxychloroquine.

Oxychinolin *see* 8-Quinolinol.

OXYCHLOROSENE* (complex of hypochlorous acid with phenylsulfonates of aliphatic hydrocarbons; monoxychlorosene; 'clorpactin').

OXYCINCHOPHEN** (2-hydroxy-3-phenyl-cinchoninic acid; 3-hydroxy-2-phenyl-4-quinolinecarboxylic acid; HPC; 3-hydroxy-cinchophen; 'chinoxone', 'fenidrone', 'oxinofen').

OXYCLIPINE*** ((+)-1-methylpiperid-3-yl (±)-α-phenylcyclohexaneglycolate; oxiclipine; propenzolate; oxyclipine hydrochloride; JB-840; NDR-263; 'delinal').

OXYCLOZANIDE*** (3,5,6,3′,5′-penta-chloro-2,2′-dihydroxybenzanilide; 'zanil').

OXYCODONE*** (14-hydroxydihydro-codeinone; 4,5-epoxy-14-hydroxy-3-meth-oxy-N-methyl-6-oxomorphinan; dihydro-hydroxycodeinone hydrochloride; oxiconum; thecodin; tekodin; laokon).

OXYCODONE PECTINATE ('pancodone', 'pandione', 'proladone').

OXYDEMETON-METHYL* (S-(2-ethyl-sulfinyl)ethyl O,O-dimethyl phosphoro-thioate; demeton-S-methylsulfoxide; methyl demeton-O-sulfoxide; methyl-mercaptophos oxide; metilmerkaptofosok-sid; methylisosystox sulfoxide; metaiso-systox sulfoxide; 'metaisosystox R', 'meta-systox R').
See also Metrifonate plus oxydemeton-methyl.

α,α′-Oxydi(3-acetamido-2,4,6-triiodo-benzoic acid) *see* Ioglycamic acid.

Oxydiacetic acid *see* Diglycolic acid.

Oxydibenzamidine *see* Phenamidine.

1,1′-Oxydimethylenebis(4-formylpyri-dinium chloride) dioxime *see* Obidoxime.

Oxydimethylquinazine*** *see* Phenazone.

Oxydimorphine *see* Pseudomorphine.

OXYDIPENTONIUM CHLORIDE*** (5,5′-bis(trimethylammonium)dipentyl ether dichloride; 6-oxa-1,11-undecamethyl-enebis(trimethylammonium chloride); [oxybis(pentamethylene)]bis(trimethyl-ammonium chloride); UCB-5067; 'brevatonal').

OXYDISULFOTON* (O,O-diethyl S-[2-(ethylsulfinyl)ethyl] phosphorodithioate; 'disyston-S').

Oxyethyltheophylline *see* Etofylline.

OXYFEDRINE*** ((−)-3-(β-hydroxy-α-methylphenethylamino)-3′-methoxy-propiophenone; (−)-3-(2-hydroxy-1-methyl-2-phenylethylamino)-3′-methoxy-propiophenone; β-hydroxy-N-[2-(m-meth-oxybenzoyl)ethyl]amphetamine; 3-(1-hydr-oxy-1-phenylisopropylamino)-3′-methoxy-propiophenone; (−)-oxyfedrine; D-563; 'ildamen', 'modacor').

(±)-OXYFEDRINE ('myofedrin').

(−)-Oxyfedrine *see* Oxyfedrine.

OXYFENAMATE*** (β-ethyl-β-hydroxy-phenethyl carbamate; 2-hydroxy-2-phenyl-butyl carbamate; 2-phenyl-1,2-butanediol carbamate; 1-carbamoyloxy-2-phenyl-2-butanol; α-carbamoyloxymethyl-α-ethyl-benzyl alcohol; hydroxyphenamate; oxi-fenamate; AL-0361; P-301; 'listica').

Oxyflavyl *see* Efloxate.

'Oxy-kesso-tetra' *see* Oxytetracycline.

'Oxyleine' *see* 8-Quinolinol.

Oxylidine *see* Benzoclidine.

'Oxylone' *see* Fluorometholone.

OXYMESTERONE*** (4,17β-dihydroxy-17-methylandrost-4-en-3-one; 17-methyl-4-androsten-4,17β-diol-3-one; 'oranabol').

OXYMETAZOLINE*** (6-tert-butyl-3-(2-imidazolin-2-ylmethyl)-2,4-dimethyl-phenol; 2-(4-tert-butyl-3-hydroxy-2,6-dimethylbenzyl)-2-imidazoline; oxy-metazoline hydrochloride; oximetazoline; H-990; 'afrin', 'hazol', 'iliadin', 'nafrine', 'nasivin', 'nesivine', 'nezeril').

OXYMETHEBANOL (dihydro-14-hydroxy-6β-thebainol 4-methyl ether; RAM-327).

Oxymethionine *see* Methoxinine.

OXYMETHOLONE*** (17β-hydroxy-2-hydroxymethylene-17-methyl-5β-andro-stan-3-one; 2-hydroxymethylene-17α-methylandrostan-17-ol-3-one; 2-hydroxy-methylene-17α-methyldihydrotestosterone; HMD; CI-406; NSC-26198; 'adroyd', 'anadrol', 'anapolon', 'plenastril', 'synasteron', 'zenalosyn').

Oxymethylene *see* Formaldehyde.

OXYMORPHONE*** (7,8-dihydro-14-hydroxymorphinone; 4,5-epoxy-3,14-di-hydroxy-N-methyl-6-oxomorphinan; hydroxydihydromorphinone; 'numorphan').

Oxyneurine *see* Betaine.

'Oxypate' *see* Piperazine adipate.

OXYPENDYL*** (4-[3-(10H-pyrido(3,2-b)-(1,4)benzothiazin-10-yl)propyl]piperazin-1-ylethanol; 1-(2-hydroxyethyl)-4-[3-(10H-pyrido(3,2-b)(1,4)benzothiazin-10-yl)propyl]piperazine; 1-(1-azapheno-thiazin-10-yl)-4-(2-hydroxyethyl)piper-azine; 10-[3-[4-(2-hydroxyethyl)piperazin-

1-yl]propyl]-9-thia-1,2-diazanthracene; oxipendyl; perthipendyl; 'pervetral').

OXYPERTINE*** (5,6-dimethoxy-2-methyl-3-[2-(4-phenylpiperazin-1-yl)ethyl]indole; oxipertin; WIN-18501-2; 'equipertine', 'forit', 'integrin'; 'opertil').

Oxyphenarsine see Oxophenarsine.

OXYPHENBUTAZONE*** (4-butyl-1-(p-hydroxyphenyl)-2-phenyl-3,5-pyrazolidinedione; p-hydroxyphenylbutazone; G-27202; 'oxalid', 'tandacote', 'tanderil'). See also Fenyramidol oxyphenbutazone salt; Ampicillin with oxyphenbutazone; Etapromide with oxyphenbutazone.

OXYPHENBUTAZONE WITH PREDNISOLONE ('realin').

OXYPHENBUTAZONE WITH PROPETAMIDE ('binartrina').

OXYPHENCYCLIMINE*** (1,4,5,6-tetrahydro-1-methyl-2-pyrimidinemethanol α-phenylcyclohexaneglycolate ester; 1-methyl-1,4,5,6-tetrahydropyrimid-2-yl-methyl α-phenylcyclohexaneglycolate ester; SI-1236; 'cardan', 'caridan', 'daricon', 'dominil', 'naridan'). See also Meprobamate with oxyphencyclimine.

OXYPHENISATINE*** (3,3-bis(p-hydroxyphenyl)oxindole; 3,3-bis(p-hydroxyphenyl)-2-indolinone; 'dialose plus', 'neodrast', 'veripaque').

Oxyphenisatine acetate see Acetphenolisatin.

Oxyphenisatine dehydrocholate see Cofisatin.

'Oxyphenon duplex' see Oxyphenonium bromide.

OXYPHENONIUM BROMIDE*** (2-diethylaminoethyl ester methobromide of α-phenylcyclohexaneglycolic acid; diethyl-(2-hydroxyethyl)methylammonium bromide α-phenylcyclohexaneglycolate; metacin; Ba-5473; C-5473; 'antrenyl', 'oxyphenon duplex'). See also Clioquinol with phanquinone and oxyphenonium bromide.

'Oxyphylline' see Etofylline.

Oxypolyethoxydodecane see Polidocanol.

Oxyprocaine see Hydroxyprocaine.

OXYPROTHEPINE (10,11-dihydro-10-[4-(3-hydroxypropyl)piperazin-1-yl]-8-(methylthio)dibenzo(b,f)thiepin).

OXYPROTHEPINE DECANOATE (VUFB-9977).

Oxypurinol* see Oxipurinol.

OXYPYRRONIUM BROMIDE*** (2-(hydroxymethyl)-1,1-dimethylpyrrolidinium bromide α-phenylcyclohexaneglycolate; 1,1-dimethyl-2-(hydroxymethyl)-pyrrolidinium bromide α-phenylcyclohexaneglycolate; oxipyrronium; BRL-556).

Oxyquinoline see 8-Quinolinol.

OXYQUINOTHEINE (compound of quinine and caffeine; oxychinotheine).

OXYRIDAZINE*** (2-methoxy-10-[2-(1-methylpiperid-2-yl)ethyl]phenothiazine).

OXYSONIUM IODIDE*** ((2-hydroxyethyl)dimethylsulfonium iodide α-phenylcyclohexaneglycolate ester; oxisone; 'thiospasmin').

OXYTETRACYCLINE*** (5-hydroxytetracycline; oxytetracycline hydrochloride; NSC-9169; 'berkmycen', 'biostat', 'clinimycin', 'imperacin', 'macocyn', 'ossitetra', 'oxy-kesso-tetra', 'riomitsin', 'ryomycin', 'terrafungine', 'terramycin', 'terra-tablinen', 'terravenos', 'tetran', 'ursocyclin', 'vendarcin'). See also Bromhexine with oxytetracycline; Hydrocortisone with oxytetracycline; Neomycin with oxytetracycline; Tramazoline with oxytetracycline.

OXYTETRACYCLINE WITH NYSTATIN ('terrastatin').

OXYTHIAMINE (4-desamino-4-hydroxythiamine).

OXYTOCIN*** (α-hypophamine; ocytocin).

OXYTOCIN SYNTHETIC (OTS-68; 'syntocinon'). See also Argiprestocin; Demoxytocin; Methylergometrine with oxytocin (synthetic); Vasotocin.

Oxytriptyline see Oxitriptyline.

'Oxyvermin' see p-Methyldiphenhydramine.

'Oxyzin' see Piperazine adipate.

'Oy' see Carbutamide.

'Ozothine' see Turpentine oil oxidation product.

P

P-2-S see Pralidoxime mesilate.
P-4 see Dipiproverine.
P-12 see Oxacillin.
P-15 see Cloxacillin.
P-21 see Trigentisic acid.
P-23 see 2,6-Pyridinedimethanol bis-

(methylcarbamate).
P-50 see Ampicillin.
P-113 see Saralasin acetate.
P-201-1 see Caroverine.
P-204 see Polyvinylpyridine N-oxide.
P-241 see Phenylbutazone-calcium.

P-248 see Levopropicillin.
P-253 see Diphenylpyraline.
P-301 see Oxyfenamate.
P-391 see Pecazine.
P-463 see Fenamole.
P-501 see Glucosulfone.
P-607 see Chlorpropamide.
P-652 see Fomocaine.
P-683 see Puromycin.
P-725 see Perazine.
P-841 see Barbexaclone.
P-845 see Phenobarbital-norpseudoephedrine.
P-1003 see Guanoxan.
P-1011 see Dicloxacillin.
P-1029 see Guanoclor.
P-1048 see Pecazine sulfoxide.
P-1306 see Glyparamide.
P-1393 see Benzthiazide.
P-1496 see Zeranol.
P-1742 see Fluperolone.
P-1779 see Altizide.
P-2105 see Epithiazide.
P-2525 see Polythiazide.
P-2530 see Methalthiazide.
P-2647 see Benzquinamide.
P-3693A see Doxepin.
P-3896 see Guanisoquin.
P-4385B see Clotixamide.
P-4599 see Cidoxepin.
P-4657B see Tiotixene.
P-5227 see Pinoxepin.
P-7138 see Nifurpirinol.
P-9295 see Azamethonium.
P-17922 see Sulfaphenazole.
PA-93 see Novobiocin.
PA-94 see Cycloserine.
PA-106 see Anisomycin.
PA-144 see Mithramycin.
PA-248 see Propicillin.
PAA-155 see Indolmycin.
PAA-701 see Bialamicol.
PAA-3854 see Clamoxyquin.
'Paarlan' see Isopropalin.
PAB see p-Aminobenzoic acid.
PABA see p-Aminobenzoic acid.
Pabacidum see p-Aminobenzoic acid.
'Pabialgin' see Aminophenazone with
  allobarbital.
PABP see Piperazine p-aminobenzoate.
PABS see Sulfanilamide.
'PAC' see Calcium aminosalicylate and Para-
  thion.
'Pacatal' see Pecazine.
'Pacatol' see Pecazine.
'Pacilan' see Calcium carbamoylaspartate.
'Pacinol' see Flufenazine.
'Pacinox' see Capuride.
'Pacisyn' see Nitrazepam.
'Pacitran' see Metoserpate.
'Pactal' see Pecazine.
PACTAMYCIN (antibiotic from Str. pactum;
  NSC-52947).
'Pactol' see Pecazine.
PAD see Pralidoxime dodecyl iodide.
'Padan' see Cartap.
PADIMATE*** (pentyl p-dimethylamino-
  benzoates; mixture of pentyl, isopentyl and

2-methylbutyl p-dimethylaminobenzoates).
PADIMATE A* (pentyl p-dimethylamino-
  benzoate; 'escalol 506').
PADIMATE O* (2-ethylhexyl p-dimethyl-
  aminobenzoate; 'escalol 507').
'Padisal' see Thiazinamium.
'Padophene' see Phenothiazine.
'Padreatin' see Kallidinogenase.
'Padrin' see Prifinium bromide.
'Padutin' see Kallidinogenase.
Paecillomyces varioti banier var. anti-
  bioticus, antibiotic see Pecilocin.
'Paediathrocin' see Erythromycin ethyl
  succinate.
Paeonol see Peonol.
'Pagitane' see Cycrimine.
PAH see p-Aminohippuric acid.
'Palacos' see Polymethyl methacrylate.
'Palaprin' see Aloxiprin.
'Palatinol M' see Dimethyl phthalate.
'Palerol' see Tropenzilium.
'Palfium' see Dextromoramide.
'Palitrex' see Cefalexin.
Pallethrine see Allethrin.
'Pallidin' see Sulfaperin.
PALMIDROL*** (N-(2-hydroxyethyl)-
  palmitamide).
PALMITAMIDE (hexadecanamide).
PALMITIC ACID (hexadecanoic acid;
  cetylic acid).
'Palohex' see Inositol nicotinate.
'Palosein' see Orgotein.
'Paloxin' see Aloxiprin.
'Palphium' see Dextromoramide.
'Paludrine' see Proguanil.
'Palusil' see Proguanil.
PAM see Melphalan; Pralidoxime; Procaine-
  penicillin aluminium monostearate.
PAM-780 see Amopyroquine.
Pamachin see Pamaquine.
'Pamacyl' see Aminosalicylic acid.
Pamaquin see Pamaquine.
PAMAQUINE*** (8-(4-diethylamino-1-
  methylbutylamino)-6-methoxyquinoline
  salt of 4,4'-methylenebis(3-hydroxy-2-
  naphthoic acid); pamaquine embonate;
  pamaquine naphthoate; pamaquine
  pamoate; gametocidum; pamachin; plas-
  mochin; plasmoquin; F-710; SN-971;
  'aminoquin', 'beprochin', 'gamefar',
  'pamaquin', 'panaquine', 'plasmocide',
  'plasmozid', 'praequine', 'prequine',
  'quipenyl').
Pamaquine embonate* see Pamaquine.
Pamaquine naphthoate* see Pamaquine.
Pamaquine pamoate* see Pamaquine.
PAMBA see p-Aminomethylbenzoic acid.
'Pameion' see Papaverine.
'Pamine' see Scopolamine methyl bromide.
PAM-MR-807-23a see Cycloguanil embonate
'PAMN' see Prampine methyl nitrate.
Pamoate(s)* see Embonate(s).
'Panabolide' see Ginseng extract in trome-
  tamol buffer.
'Panacaine' see Fomocaine.
'Panacur' see Fenbendazole.
'Panadol' see Paracetamol.

344

'Panalba' *see* Tetracycline with novobiocin.
'Panangin' *see* Potassium magnesium aspartate.
'Panaquine' *see* Pamaquine.
Panax ginseng *see* Ginseng.
'Panbesy' *see* Phentermine.
'Pancal' *see* Calcium pantothenate.
'Panclar' *see* Deanol phosphate.
'Pancodone' *see* Oxycodone pectinate.
'Pancreabil' *see* Fenocinol.
PANCREATIC DORNASE* (pancreatic desoxyribonuclease; 'dornavac').
PANCRELIPASE* (lipancreatin; 'cotazym', 'viokase').
Pancreozymin *see* Cholecystokinin-pancreozymin.
PANCURONIUM BROMIDE*** (2β,16β-dipiperid-1-yl-5α-androstane-3α,17β-diol diacetate dimethobromide; (3α,17β-dihydroxy-5α-androstan-2β,16β-ylene)bis-(1-methylpiperidinium bromide) 3,17-diacetate; NA-97; Org.NA97; 'pavulon').
'Pandigal' *see* Lanatoside(s).
'Pandiona' *see* Oxycodone pectinate.
'Panectyl' *see* Alimemazine.
'Panergon' *see* Papaverine.
'Panets' *see* Paracetamol.
'Panfuran S' *see* Di(hydroxymethyl)-furalazine.
'Pangametin' *see* Pangamic acid sodium salt.
PANGAMIC ACID (6-dimethylaminoacetyl-gluconic acid; 'calgam', 'sopangamine').
PANGAMIC ACID SODIUM SALT (vitamin B₁₅; 'pangametin').
'Panhepin' *see* Heparin potassium.
PANIDAZOLE*** (4-[2-(2-methyl-5-nitro-imidazol-1-yl)ethyl]pyridine; 2-methyl-5-nitro-1-(2-pyrid-4-ylethyl)imidazole).
'Panitrin' *see* Papaverine nitrate.
'Panjopaque' *see* Iopanoic acid.
'Panklar' *see* Deanol phosphate.
'Panlanat' *see* Lanatoside(s).
'Panolid' *see* Etybenzatropine.
'Panparnit' *see* Caramiphen.
Pantaphene (tr) *see* Caramiphen.
PANTETHEINE (N-pantothenylmercapt-amine; 2-pantothenylaminoethanethiol; LBF thiol form).
PANTETHINE (bis(2-pantothenylamino-ethyl)disulfide; LBF disulfide form).
PANTHENOL*** (2,4-dihydroxy-N-(3-hydroxypropyl)-3,3-dimethylbutyramide; pantothenyl alcohol; pantothenol; panto-thenylol; 'bepanthen', 'panthoderm').
See also Dexpanthenol.
Pantherin *see* Muscimol.
'Panthesine' *see* Leucinocaine mesilate.
'Panthoderm' *see* Panthenol.
'Pantocaine' *see* Tetracaine.
Pantocide (tr) *see* Halazone.
'Pantofenicol' *see* Chloramphenicol panto-thenate complex.
PANTOIC ACID (2,4-dihydroxy-3,3-di-methylbutyric acid).
See also Pantolactone; Sodium dipantoyl ferrate.
PANTOLACTONE (3-hydroxy-4,4-di-

methyl-4,5-dihydro-2(3H)-furanone; pantoic acid γ-lactone; pantoyl lactone).
'Pantomicina' *see* Erythromycin.
'Pantomycin' *see* Erythromycin ethyl succinate.
PANTONINE (2-amino-4-hydroxy-3,3-di-methylbutyric acid).
'Pantopaque' *see* Iofendylate.
'Pantosept' *see* Halazone.
'Pantothaxin' *see* Calcium pantothenate.
PANTOTHENIC ACID (N-(2,4-dihydroxy-3,3-dimethylbutyryl)-β-alanine; chick antidermatitis factor; vitamin B₅).
See also Calcium pantothenate; Chloram-phenicol pantothenate complex.
Pantothenol *see* Panthenol.
Pantothenyl alcohol *see* Panthenol.
Pantothenylaminoethanethiol *see* Pantetheine.
Pantothenylol *see* Panthenol.
Pantothenylmercaptamine *see* Pante-theine.
'Pantovernil' *see* Chloramphenicol panto-thenate.
'Panto-viocin' *see* Viomycin with dex-panthenol.
Pantoyl lactone *see* Pantolactone.
PANTOYLTAURINE (N-(2,4-dihydroxy-3,3-dimethylbutyryl)taurine; thiopanic acid; NSC-3086).
'Panwarfin' *see* Warfarin.
'Panzalone' *see* Pregnenolone succinate.
PAPAIN (enzyme mixture from *Carica papaya*; papayotin; vegetable pepsin; 'arbuz', 'caripeptic', 'caroid', 'nematolyt', 'papase', 'summetrin', 'velardon', 'vermizym').
See also Chymopapain; Phenylbutazone with papain.
'Papase' *see* Papain.
Papaveretum *see* Opium alkaloids.
PAPAVERINE (6,7-dimethoxy-1-veratryl-isoquinoline; 1-(3,4-dimethoxybenzyl)-6,7-dimethoxyisoquinoline; papaverine hydrochloride; 'cardioverina', 'dispamil', 'pameion', 'panergon', 'pavabid').
See also Dihydroergotoxine estilate with papaverine.
PAPAVERINE ADENYLATE (papaverine monophosadenine; CERM-3209; 'dicertan').
Papaverine dinicotinate *see* Niceverine.
PAPAVERINE MANDELATE (papaverine phenylglycolate; 'endoverine').
Papaverine monophosadenine *see* Papaverine adenylate.
PAPAVERINE NITRATE ('panitrin').
Papaverine phenylglycolate *see* Papaverine mandelate.
PAPAVEROLINE (6,7-dihydroxy-1-proto-catechuylisoquinoline; 1-(3,4-dihydroxy-benzyl)-6,7-dihydroxyisoquinoline; tetrakis(desmethyl)papaverine; 1-(3,4-dihydroxybenzyl)-6,7-isoquinolinediol).
PAPAVEROLINE MEGLUMINE (papa-veroline N-methylglucamine compound; 'udieci').

Papayotin see Papain.
'Papetherine' see Ethaverine.
'Papital' see Pecazine.
PARABANIC ACID (imidazolidinetrione; 1,3-oxalylurea).
PARABENS* (esters of *p*-hydroxybenzoic acid; 'butex', 'chemosept', 'nipa', 'parasept', 'solbrol', 'tegosept').
See also Benzyl paraben; Butyl paraben; Ethyl paraben; Methyl paraben; Phenyl paraben; Propyl paraben.
Parabenzylphenylcarbamate see Diphenan.
'Parabis' see Dichlorophen.
'Parabrom' see Mepyramine bromotheophyllinate.
Parabromdylamine* see Brompheniramine.
Paracarbinoxamine see Carbinoxamine.
Paracetaldehyde see Paraldehyde.
PARACETAMOL* (*p*-acetamidophenol; 4'-hydroxyacetanilide; *N*-acetyl-*p*-aminophenol; acetaminophen; acetomenophen; 'amadil', 'apamide', 'APAP', 'ben-U-ron 500', 'calpol', 'eneril' 'finimal', 'hedex', 'lyteca', 'nebs', 'nobedon', 'panadol', 'panets', 'paramol', 'tabalgin', 'tempra', 'termidor', 'tralgon', 'tylenol').
See also below and Acecarbromal with paracetamol; Acetylsalicylic acid with paracetamol; Chlormezanone with paracetamol; Dextropropoxyphene with paracetamol; Orphenadrine citrate with paracetamol.
Paracetamol acetate see Diacetamate.
Paracetamol acetylsalicylate see Benorilate.
PARACETAMOL WITH ASCORBIC ACID ('efferalgan').
PARACETAMOL WITH PHENYL-BUTAZONE ('parazolidine').
Paracetophentidine see Phenacetin.
Parachloralose see β-Chloralose.
Parachlotamine see Meclozine.
Parachlorocide see DDT.
Parachlorophenol see *p*-Chlorophenol.
'Paracodin' see Dihydrocodeine.
'Paractol' see Dimeticone with algeldrate.
Paradiazine see Pyrazine.
'Paradione' see Paramethadione.
'Paradrine' see Hydroxyamphetamine.
'Paraflex' see Chlorzoxazone.
PARAFLUTIZIDE* (6-chloro-3-(*p*-fluoro-benzyl)-3,4-dihydro-2H-1,2,4-benzothia-diazine-7-sulfonamide 1,1-dioxide).
See also Spirgetine with paraflutizide.
Paraform see Paraformaldehyde.
PARAFORMALDEHYDE* (polymerized formaldehyde; paraform; paraformic aldehyde; pentamethanal; trioxymethylene; 'cavoform', 'citromint', 'formamint', 'formitrol', 'marvosan', 'maryosan', 'phiangin', 'triformol').
Paraformic aldehyde see Paraformaldehyde.
'Paragone' see Methylbenactyzium bromide.
'Parahexyl' see Pyrahexyl.
Paralaudin see Diacetyldihydromorphine.
PARALDEHYDE (polymerized acetaldehyde; paracetaldehyde; 'rektidon').

Paralytic shellfish poison see Saxitoxin.
Paramandelic acid see Mandelic acid.
Parametazon see Paramethasone.
PARAMETHADIONE* (5-ethyl-3,5-dimethyloxazolidine-2,4-dione; isoethadione; 'paradione').
PARAMETHASONE* (6α-fluoro-16α-methylpregna-1,4-diene-11β,17,21-triol-3,20-dione; 6α-fluoro-11β,17,21-trihydroxy-16α-methylpregna-1,4-diene-3,20-dione; 6α-fluoro-16α-methylprednisolone; parametazon; paramezone; 'monocortin').
PARAMETHASONE ACETATE (paramethasone 21-acetate; 'dilar', 'dillar', 'haldrate', 'haldrone', 'metilar', 'netilar', 'stemex').
Paramezone see Paramethasone.
'Paramidine' see Bucolome.
'Paraminol' see *p*-Aminobenzoic acid.
'Paramol' see Paracetamol.
'Paramon' see Calcium benzyl succinate-*p*-aminobenzoate.
PARAMORPHAN (dihydromorphine hydrochloride).
Paramorphine see Thebaine.
'Paramoth' see Dichlorobenzene.
PARAMYON (tr) (*p*,*p*'-(1,2-diethylethylene)-bis(phenyltrimethylammonium iodide)).
'Paranausine' see Dimenhydrinate.
Paranyline* see Renytoline.
PARAOXON (diethyl (*p*-nitrophenyl) phosphate; phosphacol; fosfakol; E-600; 'eticol', 'mintacol', 'miotisal').
PARAPENZOLATE BROMIDE* (4-benziloyloxy-1,1-dimethylperidinium bromide; 4-hydroxy-1,1-dimethyl-piperidinium bromide benzilate; 'relanol').
'Paraphos' see Parathion.
PARAPROPAMOL (4'-hydroxypropion-anilide; *p*-propionamidophenol; 'solvodol').
PARAQUAT* (1,1'-dimethyl-4,4'-bipyridi-nium dichloride; 1,1'-dimethyl-4,4'-dipyridylium dichloride; methyl viologen; 'gramoxone W', 'orthoparaquat', 'preeglone', 'weedol').
PARAQUAT METILSULFATE (paraquat bis(methyl sulfate); 'aerial grammoxone', 'gramoxone').
PARAROSANILINE (tris(*p*-aminophenyl)-methanol).
PARAROSANILINE EMBONATE* (tris-(*p*-aminophenyl)methylium hemi[4,4'-methylenebis(3-hydroxy-2-naphthoate)] hydrate; bis[tris(*p*-aminophenyl)methyl-ium] 4,4'-methylenebis(3-hydroxy-2-naphthoate) dihydrate; pararosaniline pamoate; CI-403A).
'Parasan' see Benactyzine.
'Parasept' see Parabens.
PARASORBIC ACID (lactone of 5-hydroxy-2-hexenoic acid; δ-hexenolactone; hexenolide; sorbic oil).
Parasoxon (tr) Diethyl methylpyrazolyl phosphate.
'Parastimal' see Meprochol.
'Parasympatol' see Oxedrine.
'Paratensiol' see Reserpilene.

346

'**Parathesin**' *see* Benzocaine.
Parathiazan *see* Thiamorpholine.
PARATHIAZINE** (10-(2-pyrrolidin-1-ylethyl)phenothiazine; pyrathiazine; RP-4270; 'pyrrolazote', 'rolazote')'
PARATHIAZINE DIOXIDE (parathiazine *N*,*S*-dioxide; U-5641).
PARATHION* (*O*,*O*-diethyl *O*-(*p*-nitrophenyl) phosphorothioate; diethyl nitrophenyl thiophosphate; nitrostigmine; parathion ethyl; phosphostigmine; DNTP; E-605; NIUIF-100; T-47; 'AAT', 'alkron', 'alphamite', 'bladan', 'corthion', 'ecatox', 'etilon', 'folidol', 'folidol E', 'fosferno', 'niran', 'PAC', 'paraphos', 'phosphemol', 'rhodiatox', 'SNP', 'thiophos 3422', 'tiofos', 'tox 47').
See also Malathion with parathion.
Parathion ethyl* *see* Parathion.
PARATHION ISOMETHYL (*O*,*S*-dimethyl *O*-(*p*-nitrophenyl) phosphorothioate; isomethyl parathion; HC-8061).
PARATHION-METHYL* (*O*,*O*-dimethyl *O*-(*p*-nitrophenyl) phosphorothioate; metaphos; methyl parathion; Bayer-45515; Bayer-45545; E-605; HC-8056; 'dalf', 'folidol M', 'metacide', 'metron', 'nitrox', 'wofatox').
'**Parathorm**' *see* Parathyroid hormone.
'**Parathormone**' *see* Parathyroid hormone.
PARATHYROID HORMONE ('parathorm', 'parathormone').
PARAVALLARINE (20-hydroxy-3β-methylaminopregn-5-ene-18-carboxylic acid 18,20 lactone).
PARAVALLARINOL (18,20-dihydroxy-3β-methylaminopregn-5-ene; 3β-methylaminopregn-5-ene-18,20-diol).
PARAXANTHINE (1,7-dimethylxanthine; urotheobromine; NSC-400018).
'**Parazine**' *see* Piperazine.
'**Parazolidine**' *see* Paracetamol with phenylbutazone.
Parazoxon (tr) *see* Diethyl methylpyrazolyl phosphate.
PARBENDAZOLE** (methyl 5-butyl-2-benzimidazolecarbamate; SK&F-29044; 'worm guard').
'**Paredrine**' *see* Hydroxyamphetamine.
'**Paredrinex**' *see* Hydroxyamphetamine.
PAREGORIC (camphorated opium tincture).
'**Parenogen**' *see* Fibrinogen.
'**Parenteral**' *see* Hydroxyzine.
'**Parenzyme**' *see* Trypsin.
'**Parenzymol**' *see* Trypsin.
'**Parephylline**' *see* Etamiphylline.
'**Parest**' *see* Methaqualone.
PARETHOXYCAINE** (2-diethylaminoethyl ester of *p*-ethoxybenzoic acid; parethoxycaine hydrochloride; 'diethoxin', 'intracaine', 'maxicaine').
PARETHOXYCAINE AMIDE (*N*-(2-diethylaminoethyl)-*p*-ethoxybenzamide; 'intracaine amide', 'maxicaine amide').
'**Parfenac**' *see* Bufexamac.
Parfezin (tr) *see* Profenamine.

'**Parfuran**' *see* Nitrofurantoin.
PARGYLINE** (*N*-benzyl-*N*-methylprop-2-ynylamine; *N*-methyl-*N*-prop-2-ynylbenzylamine; *N*-methyl-*N*-propargylbenzylamine; pargyline hydrochloride; A-19120; Mo-911; 'eudatin', 'eutonyl').
'**Parid**' *see* Piperazine.
PARIDOCAINE** (1-methyl-4-piperidyl *p*-butylaminobenzoate; *p*-butylaminobenzoic ester of 1-methyl-4-piperidinol).
Parietic acid *see* Rhein.
PARINOL* (α,α-bis(*p*-chlorophenyl)-3-pyridinemethanol; *p*,*p*'-dichloro-α-pyrid-3-ylbenzhydrol; *p*-chloro-α-(*p*-chlorophenyl)-α-pyrid-3-ylbenzyl alcohol; EL-241; 'parnon').
'**Paritol**' *see* Sodium polyanhydromannuronic acid sulfate.
'**Parkemed**' *see* Mefenamic acid.
'**Parkinane**' *see* Trihexyphenidyl.
'**Parkopan**' *see* Trihexyphenidyl.
'**Parks-12**' *see* Pridinol.
'**Parlodel**' *see* Bromocriptine mesilate.
Parmaceti *see* Cetaceum.
'**Parmacetyl**' *see* Cetaceum.
'**Parmetol**' *see* Chlorocresol.
'**Parnate**' *see* Tranylcypromine.
'**Parnon**' *see* Parinol.
'**Parnox**' *see* Nitromethaqualone.
PAROMOMYCIN** (*O*-(2,6-diamino-2,6-dideoxy-β-L-idopyranosyl)-(1→3)-*O*-β-D-ribofuranosyl)-(1→5)-*O*-(2-amino-2-deoxy-α-D-glucopyranosyl)-(1→4)]-2-deoxystreptamine; aminosidin; amminosidine; catenulin; hydroxymycin; C-1488; FI-5853; paromomycin sulfate; 'aminoxidin', 'crestomicina', 'farmiglucina', 'gabbromycin', 'gabbroral', 'humatin', 'humycin').
'**Paroven**' *see* Troxerutin.
PAROXYPROPIONE** (*p*-hydroxypropiophenone; 4'-hydroxypropiophenone; 1-(*p*-hydroxyphenyl)-1-propanone; ethyl *p*-hydroxyphenyl ketone; *p*-propionylphenol; proxyfenone; POP; B-360; H-365).
'**Parpanit**' *see* Caramiphen.
'**Parpon**' *see* Benactyzine.
PARSALMIDE** (5-amino-*N*-butyl-2-prop-2-ynyloxybenzamide; MY-41-6).
'**Parsetic**' *see* Procaine.
Parsley camphor *see* Apiole.
'**Parsotil**' *see* Phenpropamine.
'**Parstelazine**' *see* Tranylcypromine with trifluoperazine.
'**Parstelin**' *see* Tranylcypromine with trifluoperazine.
'**Partel**' *see* Dithiazanine.
'**Partergin**' *see* Methylergometrine.
'**Parterol**' *see* Dihydrotachysterol.
PARTRICIN** (antibiotic from *Str. aureofaciens*; SPA-S-132).
Partricin methyl ester *see* Mepartricin.
'**Partusisten**' *see* Fenoterol.
'**Parzate**' *see* Nambam; Zineb.
'**Parzone**' *see* Dihydrocodeine.
PAS *see* Aminosalicylic acid.

PASA *see* Aminosalicylic acid.
'Pasaden' *see* Homofenazine.
'Pasalin' *see* Difenamizole.
Pascain (tr) *see* Hydroxyprocaine.
'Pascorbic' *see* Aminosalicylic acid with ascorbic acid.
'Pasdrazide' *see* Aminosalicylic acid hydrazide.
PASINIAZID** (isoniazid 4-aminosalicylate; P-106; 'dipasic', 'fintozid', 'GEWO 339', 'INHA-PÁS').
'PASIT' *see* Glyprothiazole.
PASK *see* Aminosalicylic acid.
'Paskalium' *see* Potassium aminosalicylate.
'Paskate' *see* Potassium aminosalicylate.
'Pasomycin' *see* Dihydrostreptomycin aminosalicylate.
'Pasoyl' *see* Calcium benzamidosalicylate.
'Paspertin' *see* Metoclopramide.
PAT *see* Antimonyl potassium tartrate.
PATENT BLUE (anhydro-4,4'-bis(diethyl-amino)-5''-hydroxytriphenylmethanol-2'',4''-disulfonic acid sodium salt; 'alphazurine 2G').
Patent blue V *see* Sulfan blue.
'Pathilon' *see* Tridihexethyl iodide.
'Pathocil' *see* Dicloxacillin.
'Pathomycin' *see* Sisomicin.
'Patoron' *see* Metobromuron.
'Patrovina' *see* Adiphenine.
'Pavabid' *see* Papaverine.
'Paveril' *see* Dimoxyline.
'Pavulon' *see* Pancuronium bromide.
PAXAMATE*** (4-biphenylyl methyl-carbamate).
'Paxeladine' *see* Oxeladin citrate.
'Paxistil' *see* Hydroxyzine embonate.
'Paxital' *see* Secbutabarbital *and* Pecazine.
'Payzone' *see* Nitrovin.
'Pazidet' *see* Tyloxapol.
PAZOXIDE** (6,7-dichloro-3-(3-cyclopen-ten-1-yl)-2H-1,2,4-benzothiadiazine 1,1-dioxide).
PB-89 *see* Fominoben.
PB-106 *see* Pipethanate ethobromide.
PC-1 *see* Fenipentol.
PC-63-1 *see* Piperidine caffeate.
PC-1421 *see* Piperacetazine.
PCA *see* Pyrazon.
PCB *see* Polychlorinated biphenyl mixture.
PCBS *see* Fenson.
PCI *see* Fenson.
PCM *see* Trichloromethane sulfenyl chloride.
PCMX *see* Chloroxylenol.
PCNB *see* Quintozene.
PCPBS *see* Fenson.
PCPCBS *see* Chlorfenson.
PCT *see* Polychlorinated terphenyl mixture.
PD-5 *see* Mevinphos.
PDDB *see* Domiphen bromide.
PDX *see* Polidexide.
PEBC *see* Pebulate.
PEBULATE* (*S*-propyl butylethylcarbamo-thioate; PEBC; 'tillam').
PECAZINE** (10-[1-methylpiperid-3-yl)-methyl]phenothiazine; mepazine; mepasin; pecazine hydrochloride; pecazine acetate;

P-391; W-1224; 'lacumin', 'nothiazine', 'pacatal', 'pacatol', 'pactal', 'pactol', 'papital', 'paxital').
PECAZINE SULFOXIDE (P-1048).
PECILOCIN*** (antibiotic from *Paecillo-myces varioti banier* var. *antibioticus*; 'leofungin', 'supral', 'variotin').
PECOCYCLINE** (*N*-tetracyclinylmethyl-nipecotic acid).
'Pectamol' *see* Oxeladin.
'Pectan' *see* 8-Quinolinol potassium sulfate.
'Pedaform' *see* Formaldehyde.
'Pedameth' *see* Methionine.
PEDG *see* Phenformin.
'Pediathrocin' *see* Erythromycin ethyl succinate.
'Pedilaxin' *see* Acetphenolisatin.
Pedinex *see* Dinex.
'Pedyol' *see* Cetylpyridinium *o*-thymotate.
'Pedzyl' *see* Undecenoic acid.
PEG *see* Marcogols.
'Peganone' *see* Ethotoin.
PEGLICOL 5 OLEATE* (mixture of partial mixed esters of glycerol and polyethylene glycols of mol. wt. 200-400, with average number of ethylene glycol units = 5; glycérides oléiques polyoxy-éthylénés; 'labrafil M-1944CS').
PEGOTERATE** (poly(oxyethyleneoxy-terephthaloyl)); condensation polymer between terephthalic acid and ethylene glycol; poly(oxy-1,2-ethanediyloxy-carbonyl-1,4-phenylenecarbonyl); 'aviester').
PEGOXOL 7 STEARATE* (mixture of mono- and distearic esters of ethylene glycol and of polyoxyethylene glycol (average mol. wt. 450) with average number of ethylene glycol units = 7; 'tefose 63').
'Pehanorm' *see* Trometamol.
Pelargonic acid *see* Nonanoic acid.
'Pelentan' *see* Ethyl biscoumacetate.
PELIOMYCIN*** (antibiotic from *Str. luteogriseus*; NSC-76455-D).
PELLETIERINE (punicine; 1-(2-pyridyl)-2-propanone).
'Pellidol' *see* Diacetazotol.
Pelosine *see* Bebeerine.
'Pelpica' *see* Promethazine.
PELS *see* Erythromycin estolate.
β-PELTATIN (5,6,7,8-tetrahydro-7-(hydr-oxymethyl)-5-(3,4,5-trimethoxyphenyl)-naphtho(2,3-d)-1,3-dioxole-6-carboxylic acid; NSC-24819).
PEMERID*** (4-(3-dimethylaminopropoxy)-1,2,2,6,6-pentamethylpiperidine).
PEMOLINE*** (2-amino-5-phenyl-2-oxazolin-4-one; 2-imino-5-phenyloxazoli-din-4-one; phenylisohydantoin; azoxodone fenoxazol; phenoxazole; LA-956; PW/135; 'deltamine', 'dentromin', 'hyton', 'kethamed', 'pioxol', 'ronyl', 'sofro', 'tradon', 'volital').
PEMOLINE WITH MAGNESIUM HYDROXIDE (magnesium pemoline; A-30400; A-31528; 'cylert').

PEMPIDINE*** (1,2,2,6,6-pentamethyl-
piperidine; pempidine hydrogen tartrate;
pempidine bitartrate; M&B-4486; Th-
2131; 'normatens', 'perolysen', 'rivon',
'tenormal').
See also Hydracarbazine with pempidine.
PEMPIDINE TOSILATE (pempidine *p*-
toluenesulfonate; pempidine tosylate;
pirilene; 'pyrilene', 'synaplege').
'Penadur' *see* Benzathine penicillin.
PENAMECILLIN*** (acetoxymethyl 6-
phenylacetamidopenicillanate; acetoxymethyl ester of penicillin G; acetate ester
of hydroxymethyl ester of benzylpenicillin).
'Penbristol' *see* Ampicillin.
'Penbritin' *see* Ampicillin.
'Penbritin-S' *see* Ampicillin sodium.
'Penbrock' *see* Ampicillin.
Penbutalol *see* Penbutolol.
PENBUTOLOL*** (1-*tert*-butylamino-3-
(*o*-cyclopentylphenoxy)-2-propanol;
penbutalol; HOE-893d).
'Pen-colistin' *see* Penicillin with colistin.
PENDECAMAINE*** ((carboxymethyl)di-
methyl(3-palmitamidopropyl)ammonium
hydroxide inner salt; *N,N*-dimethyl(3-
palmitamidopropyl)acetic acid; betaine;
'tego-betaine').
Pendepon *see* Benzathine penicillin.
'Pendex' *see* Penicillin G.
'Pen-di-ben' *see* Benzathine penicillin.
'Pendine' *see* Pentolonium.
'Pendiomid' *see* Azamethonium.
'Penditan' *see* Benzathine penicillin.
'Penduran' *see* Benzathine penicillin.
'Penemvé' *see* Pheneticillin.
'Penetek' *see* Pentaerythritol.
PENETHAMATE HYDRIODIDE
(2-diethylaminoethyl ester hydriodide of
penicillin G; 'bronchopen', 'deripen',
'estopen', 'leocillin', 'neopenil', 'pulmo 500').
'Penetracyne' *see* Penimepicycline.
'Penetradol' *see* Phenylbutazone with
papain.
PENFLURIDOL*** (4-(4-chloro-α,α,α-tri-
fluoro-*m*-tolyl)-1-[4,4-bis(*p*-fluorophenyl)-
butyl]-4-piperidinol; R-16341; 'longoperidol', 'semap').
PENFLUTIZIDE*** (3,4-dihydro-3-pentyl-
6-trifluoromethyl-2H-1,2,4-benzothiadia-
zine-7-sulfonamide 1,1-dioxide; 3,4-dihydro-
3-pentyl-7-sulfamoyl-6-trifluoromethyl-2H-
1,2,4-benzothiadiazine 1,1-dioxide).
PENGITOXIN*** (gitoxin pentaacetate;
pentaacetylgitoxin; 'carnacid-cor',
'pentagit').
'Penglobe' *see* Bacampicillin.
'Penhexamin' *see* Tetramethylcyclohexyl-
amine.
PENICILLAMINE*** (D-3-mercaptovaline;
β,β-dimethylcysteine; 3,3-dimethyl-
cysteine; MO-BAY 950; 'artamin', 'beracillin', 'cuprimine', 'distamine', 'kelatin',
'metalcaptase', 'sulredox', 'trolovol').
PENICILLANIC ACID (3,3-dimethyl-7-
oxo-4-thia-1-azabicyclo(3.2.0)heptane-2-
carboxylic acid).

Penicillin 152 *see* Pheneticillin.
PENICILLINASE*** (enzyme obtained by
fermentation from cultures of *Bac. cereus*;
'neutrapen').
Penicillin B *see* Pheneticillin.
Penicillin benzatin* *see* Benzathine
penicillin.
PENICILLIN WITH COLISTIN ('pen-
colistin').
PENICILLIN F (amylpenicillin; 2-pen-
tenylpenicillin; gigantic acid; penicillin I).
PENICILLIN G (6-(phenylacetamido)-
penicillanic acid; benzylpenicillin;
penicillin; penicillin sodium; penicillin
potassium; bacinol).
See also Benethamine penicillin; Benzathine
penicillin; Benzhydrylamine penicillin;
Clemizole penicillin; Ephenamine penicillin
Hydrabamine penicillin; Hydroxyprocaine
penicillin; Kanamycin with penicillin;
Oleandopen; Penethamate-HI; Procaine-
penicillin.
Penicillin G acetoxymethyl ester *see*
Penamecillin.
PENICILLIN G, PURIFIED (BRL-3000;
'purapen G').
Penicillin I *see* Penicillin F.
PENICILLIN K (heptylpenicillin).
Penicillin MV *see* Pheneticillin.
Penicillin N *see* Adicillin.
Penicillin O *see* Almecillin.
Penicillin P-12 *see* Oxacillin.
Penicillin-procaine *see* Procaine-penicillin.
PENICILLIN S (γ-chlorocrotylmercapto-
methylpenicillin).
PENICILLIN T (*p*-aminobenzylpenicillin).
PENICILLIN V (phenoxymethylpenicillin;
fenoxypen; phenomycillin; penicillin V
potassium).
See also Penimepicycline.
Penicillin V pipacycline salt *see* Penimepi-
cycline.
PENICILLIN X (*p*-hydroxybenzylpenicillin).
Penicillin X-1497 *see* Meticillin.
**2-(Penicillin-6-ylaminomethyl)tetracy-
cline** *see* Penimocycline.
Penicillium notatum, antibiotic *see*
Xantocillin.
Penicillium stoloniferum, antibiotic *see*
Vistatolon.
Penicinate *see* Hetacillin.
'Penicline' *see* Ampicillin.
'Penidryl' *see* Benzhydrylamine penicillinate.
'Penidural' *see* Benzathine penicillin.
'Penidure' *see* Benzathine penicillin.
PENIMEPICYCLINE*** (phenoxymethyl-
penicillinate of [4-(2-hydroxyethyl)-
piperazin-1-ylmethyl]tetracycline; pipa-
cycline phenoxymethylpenicillinate;
penicillin V pipacycline salt; 'cyclipen',
'penetracyne', 'ultrabiotic').
PENIMOCYCLINE*** (6-(tetracyclin-2-yl-
methylamino)penicillin G; 2-(penicillin-6-
ylaminomethyl)tetracycline; 'intraxium').
'Penistaph' *see* Meticillin.
PENMESTEROL*** (3-cyclopentyloxy-17-
methylandrosta-3,5-dien-17β-ol; 17-methyl-

androsta-3,5-diene-3,17β-diol 3-cyclopentyl
ether).
PENOCTONIUM BROMIDE*** (diethyl
(2-hydroxyethyl)octylammonium bromide
dicyclopentylacetate; (2-dicyclopentylacet-
oxyethyl)diethyloctylammonium bromide;
Ug-767).
'Pen-oral' *see* Penicillin V.
'Penorsin' *see* Ampicillin.
'Penplenum' *see* Hetacillin.
'Penspek' *see* Fenbenicillin.
'Penstapho' *see* Oxacillin.
'Penstapho N' *see* Cloxacillin.
'Pensyn' *see* Ampicillin.
Pentaacetylgitoxin *see* Pengitoxin.
PENTABAMATE*** (3-methyl-2,4-pentane-
diol dicarbamate).
'Pentac' *see* Dienochlor.
Pentacemin* *see* Pentetic acid.
Pentachlorin *see* DDT.
**3,3′,5,5′,6-Pentachloro-2,2′-dihydroxy-
benzanilide** *see* Oxyclozanide.
Pentachloronitrobenzene *see* Quintozene.
Pentacine (tr) *see* Calcium trisodium
pentetate.
Pentacosactride* Norleusactide.
PENTACYNIUM CHLORIDE*** (4-[2-[(5-
cyano-5,5-diphenylpentyl)methylamino]-
ethyl]-4-methylmorpholinium chloride
methochloride; N-(5-cyano-5,5-diphenyl-
pentyl)-N,N,N′-trimethyl-1-ammonium-2-
2-morpholinium chloride; BW-139C55;
'presidal').
Pentaerithrityl tetranitrate*** *see* Pentaerythrityl tetranitrate.
PENTAERYTHRITOL (2,2-bis(hydroxymethyl)-1,3-propanediol; tetrakis(hydroxymethyl)methane; tetramethylolmethane;
'penetek', 'pentek').
Pentaerythritol-chloral *see* Petrichloral.
**Pentaerythritol tetrakis(2-phenylbutyr-
ate)** *see* Feneritrol.
Pentaerythritol tetranitrate *see* Pentaery-
thrityl tetranitrate.
Pentaerythritol trinitrate *see* Pentrinitrol.
Pentaerythrityl tetranicotinate *see*
Niceritrol.
PENTAERYTHRITYL TETRANITRATE
(pentaerythritol tetranitrate; pentaerithrityl
tetranitrate; pentanitrol; nitropenton;
niperyt; penthrit; PETN; erinit).
See also Butidrine with pentaerythrityl
tetranitrate.
Pentaerythrityl trinitrate *see* Pentrinitrol.
'Pentafen' *see* Caramiphen.
Pentaformylgitoxin *see* Gitoformate.
PENTAGASTRIN*** (N-(tert-butoxy-
carbonyl)-β-alanyl-L-tryptophyl-L-methion-
yl-L-aspartyl-L-phenylalanine amide;
gastrin-like pentapeptide; AY-6608; ICI-
50123; 'gastrodiagnost', 'peptavlon').
PENTAGESTRONE*** (3-cyclopentyloxy-
17-hydroxypregna-3,5-dien-20-one; pregna-
3,5-diene-3,17-diol-20-one 3-clycopentyl
ether).
PENTAGESTRONE ACETATE* (pentagestrone 17-acetate).

'Pentagin' *see* Pentazocine.
'Pentagit' *see* Pengitoxin.
3,3′,4′,5,7-Pentahydroxyflavan *see*
Catechol.
3,3′,4′,5,7-Pentahydroxyflavanone *see*
Taxifolin.
Pentahydroxyhexanoic acid *see* Gluconic
acid.
Pentakis(N-sulfomethyl)polymyxin B
see Sulfomyxin.
PENTALAMIDE*** (o-pentyloxybenzamide;
O-pentylsalicylamide).
Pentamethazene *see* Azamethonium.
Pentamethazol *see* Pentetrazole.
PENTAMETHONIUM BROMIDE***
(pentamethylene-1,5-bis(trimethylammo-
nium bromide); C 5).
**Pentamethylenebis(1-methylpyrrolidi-
nium bitartrate)** *see* Pentolonium tartrate.
**Pentamethylenebis(trimethylammo-
nium bromide** *see* Pentamethonium
bromide).
Pentamethylenediamine *see* Cadaverine.
Pentamethylenedioxydibenzamidine *see*
Pentamidine.
**β,β-Pentamethylene-γ-hydroxybutyric
acid** *see* Hexacyclonic acid.
Pentamethylene-1,5-tetrazole *see*
Pentetrazole.
**N,N,2,3,3-Pentamethyl-2-norbornan-
amine** *see* Dimecamine.
Pentamethylpiperidine *see* Pempidine.
PENTAMIDINE*** (4,4′-pentamethylene-
dioxydibenzamidine).
Pentamidine diisethionate *see* Pentamidine isetionate.
PENTAMIDINE ISETIONATE (pentamidine di(ethanol-2-sulfonate); pentamidine
bis(2-hydroxyethanesulfonate); pentamidine diisethionate; M&B-800; RP-2512;
'lomidine').
Pentamine (tr) *see* Azamethonium.
PENTAMOXANE*** (2-isopentylamino-
methyl-1,4-benzodioxan).
1-Pentanecarboxylic acid *see* Hexanoic
acid.
Pentanedial *see* Glutaral.
1,5-Pentanediamine *see* Cadaverine.
1,5-Pentanedicarboxylic acid *see* Pimelic
acid.
2,4-Pentanediol dimethanesulfonate *see*
Dimethyltrimethylene dimesylate.
2,4-Pentanedione *see* Acetylacetone.
Pentanitrol* *see* Pentaerythrityl tetranitrate.
PENTANOCHLOR* (N-(3-chloro-4-
methylphenyl)-2-methylpentanamide;
N-(3-chloro-4-methylphenyl)-2-methyl-
valeramide; 3′-chloro-2,4′-dimethyl-
valeranilide; 'solan').
Pentanoic acid *see* Valeric acid.
2-PENTANOL (methyl propyl carbinol).
'Pentaphene' *see* Caramiphen.
PENTAPIPERIDE*** (1-methylpiperid-4-
yl ester of 3-methyl-2-phenyl valeric acid).
PENTAPIPERIDE FUMARATE (pentapiperide hydrogen fumarate; C-4675;
'lyspafen').

PENTAPIPERIDE HYDROCHLORIDE (C-4245).
Pentapiperide methylsulfate* *see* Pentapiperium metilsulfate.
Pentapiperium methylsulfate* *see* Pentapiperium metilsulfate.
PENTAPIPERIUM METILSULFATE***
(4-hydroxy-1,1-dimethylpiperidinium methylsulfate 3-methyl-2-phenylvalerate ester; pentapiperide methylsulfate; pentapiperium methylsulfate; AY-5810; 'crillin', 'crylene', 'quilene').
Pentapyrrolidinium *see* Pentolonium.
PENTAQUINE***(8-(5-isopropylamino-pentylamino)-6-methoxyquinoline; 6-methoxy-8-(5-isopropylaminoamylamino)-quinoline; 6-methoxy-8-(5-isopropylamino-pentylamino)quinoline; SN-13276).
'Pentastib' *see* p-Aminobenzenestibonic acid.
PENTAZOCINE***(1,2,3,4,5,6-hexahydro-6,11-dimethyl-3-(3-methyl-2-butenyl)-2,6-methano-3-benzazocin-8-ol; 2'-hydroxy-5,9-dimethyl-2-(3-methyl-2-butenyl)-6,7-benzomorphan; WIN-20228; 'fortal', 'fortalgesic', 'fortral', 'fortralin', 'pentagin', 'sosegon', 'sosenyl', 'talwin').
Pentazol(e) *see* Pentetrazole.
Pentedrine *see* Oxedrine.
'Pentek' *see* Pentaerythritol.
2-Pentenylpenicillin *see* Penicillin F.
PENTETIC ACID (2,2'-carboxymethyl-iminobis(ethyleniminodiacetic acid); carboxymethyliminobis(ethylenenitrilo-diacetic acid); diethylenetriaminepenta-acetic acid; pentacemin; DTPA; 'chel DTPA', 'penthanil').
See also Calcium trisodium pentetate.
PENTETRAZOLE***(6,7,8,9-tetrahydro-azepotetrazole; 6,7,8,9-tetrahydro-5H-tetrazoloazepine; pentamethylene-1,5-tetrazole; tetrazolo(1,5)perhydroazepine; corazol; leptazol; pentamethazol; pentazol(e); pentylenetetrazole).
'Penthamil' *see* Calcium trisodium pentetate.
Penthanil *see* Pentetic acid.
PENTHIENATE* (2-diethylaminoethyl ester methobromide of α-cyclopentyl-2-thiophene-glycolic acid; WIN-4369; 'monodral').
Penthiobarbital* *see* Thiopental.
'Penthrane' *see* Methoxyflurane.
PENTHRICHLORAL***(5,5-bis(hydroxy-methyl)-2-trichloromethyl-1,3-dioxane; 5,5-di(hydroxymethyl)-2-trichloromethyl-1,3-dioxane; 2-trichloromethyl-m-dioxane-5,5-dimethanol).
Penthrit *see* Pentaerythrityl tetranitrate.
'Penticidum' *see* DDT.
PENTIFYLLINE* (1-hexyl-3,7-dimethyl-xanthine; 1-hexyltheobromine; SK-7).
'Pentilium' *see* Pentolonium.
PENTOBARBITAL***(5-ethyl-5-(1-methyl-butyl)barbituric acid; mebubarbital; pento-barbital sodium; pentobarbital soluble; ethaminal; mebumal; pentobarbital calcium).
Pentolinium* *see* Pentolonium.
PENTOLONIUM TARTRATE***(1,1'-

pentamethylenebis(1-methylpyrrolidinium bitartrate); pentapyrrolidinium bitartrate; pentolinium tartrate; pentolonium hydro-gen tartrate; pyrroplégium; M&B-2050A; 'ansolysen', 'pendine', 'pentilium', 'recuryl', 'tensilest').
PENTOREX***(α,α,β-trimethylphenethyl-amine).
PENTOREX TARTRATE (pentorex acid tartrate; pentorex bitartrate; RD-354; 'liprodene').
PENTOSALEN*(9-(3-methyl-2-butenyloxy)-7H-furo(3,2-g)(1)benzopyran-7-one; 9-(3-methylbut-2-enyloxy)furo(3,2-g)-chromen-7-one; isoamylenoxypsoralen; imperatorin; 'ammidin').
PENTOSAN POLYSULFATE (SP-54; 'fibrase', 'tavan').
PENTOSAN POLYSULFATE WITH XANTINOL NICOTINATE ('pervium').
'Pentostam' *see* Sodium stibogluconate.
'Pentothal' *see* Thiopental.
Pentothiobarbital *see* Thiopental.
'Pentovis' *see* Quinestradol.
PENTOXIFYLLINE***(1-(5-oxohexyl)-theobromine; 3,7-dimethyl-1-(5-oxohexyl)-xanthine; oxpentifylline; BL-191; 'torental', 'trental').
Pentoxil (tr) *see* Pentoxyl.
PENTOXYL (tr) (5-hydroxymethyl-6-methyluracil; pentoxil).
PENTOXYVERINE***(2-diethylamino-ethoxyethyl ester of 1-phenylcyclopentane-carboxylic acid; carbetapentane).
PENTOXYVERINE CITRATE (UCB-2543; 'sedotussin', 'toclase', 'tuclase').
'Pentrane' *see* Methoxyflurane.
'Pentrexyl' *see* Ampicillin.
PENTRINITROL*(pentaerythritol trinitrate; W-2197).
'Pentritol' *see* Pentaerythrityl tetranitrate.
'Pentrofane' *see* Desipramine.
Pentyl carbamate *see* Hedonal.
6-Pentyl-m-cresol *see* Amylmetacresol.
Pentyl p-dimethylaminobenzoates *see* Padimate.
Pentylenetetrazole *see* Pentetrazole.
p-Pentylmethamphetamine *see* Amfepen-torex.
o-Pentyloxybenzamide *see* Pentalamide.
Pentyl phenyl ketone *see* Hexanophenone.
2-Pentyl-6-phenyl-1H-pyrazolo(1,2-a)-cinnolin-1,3(2H)-dione *see* Cinno-pentazone.
O-Pentylsalicylamide *see* Pentalamide.
Pentymal* *see* Amobarbital.
PEONOL (2'-hydroxy-4'-methoxyaceto-phenone; resacetophenone 4-methyl ether; paeonol).
Peppermint camphor *see* Menthol.
PEPSTATIN***(isovaleryl-L-valyl-L-valyl-4-amino-3-hydroxy-6-methylheptanoyl-L-alanyl-4-amino-3-hydroxy-6-methyl-heptanoic acid).
'Peptavlon' *see* Pentagastrin.
PEPTICHEMIO (complex of peptides of L-3-[m-[bis(2-chloroethyl)amino]phenyl]-

alanine with amino acids).

PEPTIDE 67-82 (alanylglycylisoleucinyl-valylserine; 'solvosterol').

Peptonized iron see Ferric peptonate.

'Peracon' see Isoaminile.

'Peralga' see Barbipyrine.

PERAQUINSIN** (6,7-dimethoxy-2-[2-[4-(o-methoxyphenyl)piperazin-1-yl]-ethyl]-4(3H)-quinazolinone; 1-(6,7-dimethoxy-4(3H)-oxoquinazolin-2-yl)-4-(o-methoxyphenyl)piperazine).

PERASTINE** (1-(2-diphenylmethoxyethyl)-piperidine; 1-(2-benzhydryloxyethyl)-piperidine; 'benzperidine').

PERATHIEPINE (10,11-dihydro-10-(4-methylpiperazin-1-yl)benzo(b,f)thiepin).

PERATIZOLE** (1-[4-(2-dimethylthiazol-5-yl)butyl]-4-(4-methylthiazol-2-yl)-piperazine; EMD-19698).

PERAZINE* (10-[3-(1-methylpiperazin-4-yl)-propyl]phenothiazine; P-725; 'taxilan').

'Percarbamid' see Hydrogen peroxide.

Perchlorethylene see Tetrachloroethylene.

Perchlorobenzene see Hexachlorobenzene.

Perchloroethane see Hexachloroethane.

'Perclene' see Tetrachloroethylene.

'Perclusone' see Clofezone.

'Percorten' see Desoxycortone.

'Perdilatal' see Buphenine.

'Perebron' see Oxolamine.

'Perfanazin' see Perphenazine.

'Perfekthion' see Dimethoate.

Perfenazine see Perphenazine.

Perfluorocyclobutane see Octafluorocyclo-butane.

'Pergalen' see Sodium apolate.

'Pergonal' see Human menopausal gonado-trophin.

PERHEXILINE** (2-(2,2-dicyclohexyl-ethyl)piperidine).

PERHEXILINE MALEATE* (perhexilene hydrogen maleate; WSM-3978G; 'pexid').

'Perhydrit' see Hydrogen peroxide-urea.

Perhydroazepine see Hexamethylenimine.

6-(Perhydroazepin-1-ylmethyleneamino)-penicillanic acid see Mecillinam.

Perhydroazocine see Heptamethylenimine.

'Perhydrol' see Hydrogen peroxide.

'Periactin' see Cyproheptadine.

'Periactinol' see Cyproheptadine.

'Pericel' see Flavodic acid sodium salt.

'Perichlor' see Petrichloral.

PERICIAZINE* (2-cyano-10-[3-(4-hydroxy-piperid-1-yl)propyl]phenothiazine; 10-[3-(4-hydroxypiperid-1-yl)propyl]pheno-thiazine-2-carbonitrile; pericyazine; propericiazine; RP-8909; 'aolept', 'aolet', 'neulactil', 'neuleptil').

'Periclor' see Petrichloral.

Pericyazine* see Periciazine.

'Perilax' see Bisacodyl.

PERIMETAZINE** (10-[3-(4-hydroxy-piperid-1-yl)-2-methylpropyl]-2-methoxy-phenothiazine; 1-[3-(2-methoxypheno-thiazin-10-yl)-2-methylpropyl]-4-piperid-inol; AN-1317; RP-9159; 'leptryl').

Perimycin see Fungimycin.

'Perin' see Piperazine calcium edetate.

'Peripherin' see Etofylline with theophylline ephedrine.

Periphermium see Diacetazotol.

PERISOXAL** (α-(5-phenylisoxazol-3-yl)-1-piperidineethanol; 3-(1-hydroxy-2-piperid-1-ylethyl)-5-phenylisoxazole; S-31252).

'Peristim' see Casanthranol.

'Periston' see Povidone.

PERITHIADENE (6,11-dihydro-11-(1-methyl-4-piperidylidene)dibenzo(b,e)-thiepine; perithiadene hydrochloride).

'Peritol' see Cyproheptadine.

'Peritonan' see Chlorocresol.

'Perivar' see Sparteine.

'Perklone' see Tetrachloroethylene.

PERLAPINE* (6-(4-methylpiperazin-1-yl)-morphanthridine; 6-(4-methylpiperazin-1-yl)dibenz(b,e)azepine; AW-142333; HF-2333; MP-11).

'Perlepsin' see Morsuximide.

'Perlutex' see Medroxyprogesterone acetate.

'Permapen' see Benzathine penicillin.

'Permitil' see Fluphenazine.

'Permonid' see Desomorphine.

'Pernazene' see Tymazoline.

'Perneuron' see Mefexamide.

'Pernocton' see Butallylonal.

'Pernoston' see Butallylonal.

'Perocan' see Isoaminile.

'Peroidin' see Potassium perchlorate.

'Perolysen' see Pempidine.

'Peronine' see Benzylmorphine.

'Perparin' see Ethaverine.

'Perphenan' see Perphenazine.

PERPHENAZINE** (2-chloro-10-[3-[4-(2-hydroxyethyl)piperazin-1-yl]propyl]-phenothiazine; chlorpiprozine; chlorper-phenazine; chlorpiprazine; ethaperazine; etaperazine; perfenazine; Sch-3940; 'decentan', 'dezentan', 'etapirazin', 'etha-pirazine', 'fentazin', 'grenolon', 'perfanazin', 'perphenan', 'PZC', 'thilatazin', 'tran-quisan', 'trilafan', 'trilafon').
See also Amitriptyline with perphenazine; Fentonium bromide with perphenazine.

Perphenazine-prednisolone succinate see Prednazate.

'Persantin' see Dipyridamole.

'Persedon' see Pyrithyldione.

'Persistol Höl/193' see Tretamine.

'Perspex' see Polymethyl methacrylate.

Perstoff see Diphosgene.

'Pertestis' see Testosterone cipionate.

'Perthane' see 1,1-Dichloro-2,2-bis(p-ethyl-phenyl)ethane.

Perthipendyl see Oxypendyl.

'Pertofran' see Desipramine.

'Pertofrina' see Desipramine.

'Peruol' see Benzyl benzoate.

Peruscabin see Benzyl benzoate.

PERUSITIN (cannogenic acid L-thevetoside).

PERUVOSIDE (cannogenin α-L-thevetoside; 'encordin', 'nerial').

'Pervetral' see Oxypendyl.

'Pervincamine' see Vincamine.

'Pervit' see Tetrachloroethylene.

'Pervitin' *see* Methamphetamine.
'Pervium' *see* Pentosan polysulfate with xantinol nicotinate.
'Perycit' *see* Niceritrol.
PES *see* Sodium polyethylene sulfonate.
'Peson' *see* Sodium apolate.
'Pestan' *see* Mecarbam.
'Pestocid' *see* Niclosamide.
'Pestox III' *see* Schradan.
'Pestox XIV' *see* Dimefox.
'Pestox XV' *see* Mipafox.
Pethanol *see* Pethidine.
PETHIDINE*** (ethyl ester of 1-methyl-4-phenylisonipecotic acid; ethyl ester of 1-methyl-4-phenylpiperidine-4-carboxylic acid; isonipecaine; meperidine; pethanol; piridosal).
PETHIDINE WITH LEVALLORPHAN ('pethilorfan').
'Pethilorfan' *see* Pethidine with levallorphan.
'Petidon' *see* Trimethadione.
'Petinutin' *see* Mesuximide.
PETN *see* Pentaerythrityl tetranitrate.
'Petnidan' *see* Ethosuximide.
PETRICHLORAL*** (1,1',1'',1'''-(neo-pentanetetryltetraoxy)tetrakis(2,2,2-trichloroethanol); pentaerythritol-chloral; 'perichlor', 'periclor').
PETROSELAIDIC ACID (*trans*-6-octa-decenoic acid).
PETROSELINIC ACID (*cis*-6-octadecenoic acid).
PEUCEDANIN (5-isopropyl-4-methoxy(7H)-furo(3,2-g)(1)benzopyran-7-one; 5-iso-propyl-4-methoxyfuro-2,3,6,7-coumarin; peutsedanin).
Peutsedanin (tr) *see* Peucedanin.
'Pevaryl' *see* Econazole.
'Pe-ve-gel' *see* Polyvinyl alcohol.
PEXANTEL*** (1-(cyclohexylcarbonyl)-4-methylpiperazine; cyclohexyl 4-methyl-piperazin-1-yl ketone; (4-methylpiperazin-1-ylcarbonyl)cyclohexane).
'Pexid' *see* Perhexilene maleate.
'Pezavin' *see* Tetrachloroethylene.
PFA-186 *see* Meglumine salicylate.
PFU *see* Phenformin.
PGA *see* Polyglycolic acid.
PGF$_\alpha$THAM *see* Dinoprost trometamol.
Ph-218 *see* Edogestrone.
Ph-1503 *see* Hexachlorophene mono-phosphate.
PHACETOPERAN* (L-α-phenyl-2-piperid-inemethanol acetate; acetate ester of α-piperid-2-ylbenzyl alcohol; acetoxy-(piperid-2-yl)phenylmethane; aceto-pherane; phacetoperan hydrochloride; levophacetoperane; RP-8228; 'lidepran').
'Phaldrone' *see* Chloral hydrate.
'Phaltan' *see* Folpet.
PHANQUINONE** (4,7-phenanthroline-5,6-dione; 4,7-phenanthroline-5,6-quinone; phanquone; fankinon; C-11925; 'entobex'). *See also* Clioquinol with phanquinone and oxyphenonium bromide.
Phanquone* *see* Phanquinone.
'Phanurane' *see* Canrenone.

'Pharmaethyl 114' *see* Cryofluorane.
'Pharmocaine' *see* Diethylaminoethyl *p*-butylaminobenzoate.
'Pharmodex' *see* Dextran.
'Pharmotal' *see* Thiopental.
Pharnoquinone *see* Farnoquinone.
'Phasal' *see* Lithium carbonate.
Phaseolosaxin *see* Phytohemagglutinin.
Phaseomannitol *see* Inositol.
PHB *see* Phenylmercuric borate.
Phebutazine *see* Febuverine.
PHEDRAZINE (2-(3,4,5-trimethoxybenzyl)-2-imidazoline).
PHEMERAZOLE (tr) (3-methyl-5-phenyl-pyrazole).
'Phemeride' *see* Benzethonium.
'Phe-mer-nite' *see* Phenylmercuric nitrate.
'Phemerol' *see* Benzethonium.
Phemitone *see* Methylphenobarbital.
Phen.... *see also* Fen....
PHENACAINE** (*N,N'*-di-*p*-phenethyl-acetamidine; *N,N'*-bis(*p*-ethoxyphenyl)-acetamidine; phenetidylphenacetin; phenacaine hydrochloride; 'holocaine', 'polocaine').
Phenacal* *see* Phenacemide.
Phenacarbamide *see* Fencarbamide.
PHENACEMIDE*** (1-(2-phenylacetyl)-urea; phenacetylurea; phenacal).
PHENACETIN*** (*N*-(*p*-ethoxyphenyl)-acetamide; *p*-ethoxyacetanilide; 4'-ethoxy-acetanilide; *N*-acetyl-*p*-phenetidine; *p*-acetophenetidide; acetophenetidin; acetparaphenalide; acetylphenetidine; paracetophenetidine).
See also APC; Phenapyrine.
Phenacetylurea *see* Phenacemide.
'Phenacide' *see* Campheclor.
Phenacon (tr) *see* Fenaclon.
PHENACRIDAN CHLORIDE* (9-(*p*-hexyl-oxyphenyl)-10-methylacridinium chloride; 'acrizane').
PHENACTROPINIUM CHLORIDE*** (*N*-phenacylhomatropinium chloride; homatropine phenacyl chloride; 'trophenium').
Phenacyl chloride *see* Chloroacetophenone.
Phenacylhomatropinium chloride *see* Phenactropinium chloride.
Phenacyl 4-morpholineacetate *see* Mobecarb.
Phenacyl pivalate *see* Pibecarb.
'Phenadone' *see* Methadone.
PHENADOXONE*** (6-morpholino-4,4-diphenyl-3-heptanone; phenodoxone; CB-11; Hö-10600).
PHENAGLYCODOL*** (2-(*p*-chlorophenyl)-3-methyl-2,3-butanediol).
Phenalzine *see* Phenelzine.
PHENAMAZOLINE*** (2-anilinomethyl-2-imidazoline; 'otrivine').
PHENAMET (tr) (ethyl 2-[*p*-[bis(2-chloro-ethyl)amino]phenylacetamido]-4-(methyl-thio)butyrate; ethyl ester of *N*-[*p*-[bis-(2-chloroethyl)amino]phenylacetyl]-methionine; fenamet).
PHENAMIDINE (4,4'-oxydibenzamidine;

353

4,4'-diamidinodiphenyl ether).
Phenamine *see* Phenocoll.
Phenamine (tr) *see* Amphetamine.
Phenamizole *see* Amiphenazole.
PHENAMPROMIDE*** (*N*-[2-(1-methyl-piperid-2-yl)ethyl]propionanilide).
PHENANTHRIDINE (benzo(c)quinoline).
4,7-Phenanthroline-5,6-dione *see* Phan-quinone.
4,7-Phenanthroline-5,6-quinone *see* Phan-quinone.
Phenantoin *see* Mephenytoin.
PHENAPHAN (tr) (ethyl 2-acetamido-3-[*p*-[bis(2-chloroethyl)amino]phenyl]propion-ate; ethyl ester of *N*-acetyl-*p*-[bis(2-chloro-ethyl)amino]phenylalanine; fenafan).
PHENAPYRINE (condensation product of phenacetin, phenazone and caffeine).
PHENARSAZINE CHLORIDE (5-aza-10-arsenaanthracene chloride; 10-chloro-5,10-dihydrophenarsazine chloride; 10-chloro-5,10-dihydroarsacridine; diphenylamine chlorarsine; phenazarsine; adamsite; DM).
PHENARSONE SULFOXYLATE** (com-pound of 4-hydroxy-*m*-arsanilic acid with sodium formaldehydesulfoxylate; sodium salt of *N*-methanal sulfoxylate of 3-amino-4-hydroxybenzenearsonic acid; 'aldarsone').
Phenasal (tr) *see* Niclosamide.
PHENASTEZIN (tr) (ethyl *p*-[2-*p*-[bis(2-chloroethyl)amino]phenylacetamido]-benzoate; fenastezin).
PHENATIN (tr) (*N*-nicotinoylamphetamine diphosphate; *N*-(2-phenylisopropyl)-nicotinamide; fenatin).
'Phenatol' *see* Phenetole.
'Phenatox' *see* Campheclor.
Phenazacillin *see* Hetacillin.
Phenazarsine *see* Phenarsazine chloride.
Phenazidinium *see* Fazadinium bromide.
PHENAZINE (dibenzopyrazine; dibenzo-paradiazine; azophenylene).
PHENAZOCINE*** (2'-hydroxy-5,9-di-methyl-2-phenethyl-6,7-benzomorphan; 1,2,3,4,5,6-hexahydro-6,11-dimethyl-3-phenethyl-2,6-methano-3-benzazocin-8-ol; phenazocine hydrochloride; fenethylazo-cine; NIH-7519; SK&F-6574; 'narphen', 'prinadol').
'Phenazodine' *see* Phenazopyridine.
'Phenazol' *see* Pentetrazole.
Phenazoline *see* Antazoline.
PHENAZONE*** (2,3-dimethyl-1-phenyl-3-pyrazolin-5-one; analgésine; antipyrine; azophenum; dimethyloxchinizin; di-methyloxyquinazine; oxydimethylquin-azine).
Phenazone acetylsalicylate *see* Acetopyr-ine.
Phenazone benzoate *see* Benzopyrine.
PHENAZONE MANDELATE ('tussol').
PHENAZONE SALICYLACETATE ('pyrosal').
PHENAZONE SALICYLATE (capellin; saliphenazone; 'salazolon', 'salipyrazolon', 'salipyrin').
PHENAZONE SODIUM SULFONATE

('phesin').
PHENAZOPYRIDINE*** (2,6-diamino-3-phenylazopyridine; phenazopyridine hydrochloride; NC-150; W-1655; 'azo-dyne', 'bisteril', 'gastracid-test', 'gastrazid', 'gastrotest', 'mallophene', 'phenazodine', 'pyridacil', 'pyridium', 'pyripyridium', 'uromide').
Phenbenicillin* *see* Fenbenicillin.
PHENBENZAMINE* (*N*-benzyl-*N'*,*N'*-dimethyl-*N*-phenylethylenediamine; PM-245; RP-2339; 'antergan', 'bridal', 'dimetina', 'lergitin').
PHENBENZAMINE *N'*-**ETHOBROMIDE** ([2-(benzylpropylamino)ethyl]dimethyl-ammonium bromide; 'dispasmol').
Phenbutrazate* *see* Fenbutrazate.
Phencapton *see* Phenkapton.
Phencarbamide *see* Fencarbamide.
Phenchlorphos *see* Fenclofos.
PHENCYCLIDINE*** (1-(1-phenylcyclo-hexyl)piperidine; phencyclidine hydro-chloride; CI-395; GP-121; 'hog', 'sernyl', 'sernylan').
PHENDIMETRAZINE** ((+)-3,4-dimethyl-2-phenylmorpholine; 'anovan', 'antapen-tan', 'bacarate', 'dietrol', 'sedafamen').
PHENDIMETRAZINE EMBONATE (phendimetrazine pamoate; 'fringanor').
PHENDIMETRAZINE TARTRATE (phendimetrazine bitartrate; phendimetr-azine hydrogen tartrate; 'plegine').
Phenecyclamine *see* Phenetamine.
'Phenegic' *see* Phenothiazine.
'Phénégol' *see* Mercuric potassium dinitro-phenolsulfonate.
PHENELZINE** (β-phenethylhydrazine; 1-(2-phenylethyl)hydrazine; fenizin; phenal-zine; phenelzine sulfate; W-1544; 'MAO-rem', 'nardelzine', 'nardil', 'stinerval').
Phenemal *see* Phenobarbital.
(**Phenenyltrisoxyethylene**)**tris**(**trimethyl-ammonium iodide**) *see* Gallamine tri-ethiodide.
'Phenergan' *see* Promethazine.
PHENERIDINE** (ethyl 1-phenethyl-4-phenylisonipecotate).
PHENESTER (2-[*p*-(bis(2-chloroethyl)-amino)phenyl]ethyl acetate; NSC-116785).
PHENESTERIN (tr) (cholesteryl *p*-[bis(2-chloroethyl)amino]phenylacetate; chlorphenacyl cholesteryl ester; fenesterin; phenestrin; NSC-104469).
Phenestrin *see* Phenesterin.
PHENETAMINE* (2-(α-cyclohexylbenzyl)-*N*,*N*,*N'*,*N'*-tetraethyl-1,3-propanediamine; 1-cyclohexyl-2,2-bis(diethylaminomethyl)-1-phenylethane; phenecyclamine; UCB-1545; 'licaran').
Phenetazine *see* Fenethazine.
'Phenethamid' *see* 2-Phenylbutyramide.
Phenethanolamine *see* Phenylethanolamine.
Phenethazine *see* Fenethazine.
Phenethicillin* *see* Pheneticillin.
PHENETHYL ALCOHOL* (2-phenyl-ethanol; benzyl carbinol; phenethylol).
PHENETHYLAMINE (2-phenylethylamine).

Phenethylbiguanide see Phenformin.
Phenethyldiguanide see Phenformin.
Phenethylene see Styrene.
Phenethylhydrazine see Phenelzine.
Phenethylol see Phenethyl alcohol.
8-Phenethyl-1-oxa-3,8-diazaspiro(4.5)-decan-2-one see Fenspiride.
N-**Phenethylphenethylamine** see Diphenethylamine.
1-Phenethyl-4-phenylisonipecotic acid ethyl ester see Pheneridine.
3-[2-(1-Phenethylpiperid-4-yl)ethyl] indole see Indopine.
1-Phenethyl-4-(*N*-propionylanilino)-piperidine see Fentanyl.
1-Phenethyl-4-(2-propynyl)-4-piperidinol propionate see Propinetidine.
PHENETICILLIN*** (6-(2-phenoxypropionamido)penicillanic acid; 1-phenoxyethylpenicillin; penicillin B; penicillin 152; α-methylphenoxymethylpenicillin; phenethicillin; phenethicillin potassium; BL P-152; BRL-152; K-MV; penicillin-MV; 'alpen', 'bendralan', 'broxil', 'chemipen', 'darcil', 'maxipen', 'oralopen', 'penemvé', 'ro-cillin', 'semopen', 'semophen', 'syncillin').
'Phenetidin' see Phenacetin.
p-**PHENETIDINE** (*p*-ethoxyaniline).
2-*p*-Phenetidino-*N*-propylpropionamide see Propetamide.
Phenetidylphenacetin see Phenacaine.
PHENETOLE (ethoxybenzene; ethyl phenyl ether; 'phenatol').
Phenetolurea see Phenetylurea.
'Phenetsal' see Acetaminosalol.
'Pheneturide' see Ethylphenacemide.
4-(*p*-Phenetylazo)-*m*-phenylenediamine see Etoxazene.
PHENETYLSUCCINIMIDE (*N*-(*p*-ethoxyphenyl)succinimide; *N*-phenetylsuccinimide; 'phenosuccin', 'pyrantin').
PHENETYLUREA (1-(*p*-ethoxyphenyl)-urea; *p*-phenetylurea; phenetolurea; 'dulcin', 'sucrol', 'valzin').
Phenfluoramine* see Fenfluramine.
PHENFORMIN** (1-phenethylbiguanide; 1-(2-phenylethyl)biguanide; *N'*-(*β*-phenethyl)formamidinyliminourea; phenethyldiguanide; phenformin hydrochloride; DBI; PEDG; PFU; W-32; 'betoral', 'cronoformin', 'DB-retard', 'debinyl', 'dibein', 'dibotin', 'dipar', 'feguanide', 'glucopostin', 'insoral', 'meltrol').
See also Carbutamide with phenformin; Glibenclamide with phenformin.
PHENFORMIN PLUS TOLBUTAMIDE ('tolbutaphen').
PHENGLUTARIMIDE*** (α-(2-diethylaminoethyl)-α-phenylglutarimide; 2-(2-diethylaminoethyl)-2-phenylglutarimide; phenglutarimide hydrochloride; 'aturbal', 'aturbane').
'Phenhydan' see Phenytoin.
Phenic acid see Phenol.
PHENICARBAZIDE*** (phenylsemicarbazide; 'cryogenin', 'febrimin', 'rayogenin').

PHENIDIUM CHLORIDE (8-amino-6-(*p*-aminophenyl)-5-methylphenanthridinium chloride).
Phenidylate see Methylphenidate.
PHENINDAMINE*** (2,3,4,9-tetrahydro-2-methyl-9-phenyl-1H-indeno(2,1-c)pyridine; 1,2,3,4-tetrahydro-2-methyl-9-phenyl-2-pyridindene; 1,2,3,4-tetrahydro-2-methyl-9-phenyl-2-azafluorene).
PHENINDAMINE TARTRATE (phenindamine bitartrate; phenindamine hydrogen tartrate; Nu-1504; PM-254; 'nolamine', 'thephorin').
'Phenindan' see Phenindione.
PHENINDIONE* (2-phenyl-1,3-indandione; phenyllin; PID).
PHENIODOL SODIUM*** ((sodium 4-hydroxy-3,5-diiodophenyl)-2-phenylpropionate; sodium 3,5-diiodo-α-phenylphloretate; iodoalphionic acid sodium salt; bilitrast; feniodol).
'Phenipan' see Broxyquinoline with broxaldine.
PHENIPRAZINE** (α-methylphenethylhydrazine; 1-(1-methyl-2-phenylethyl)-hydrazine; 1-phenyl-2-hydrazinopropane; phenylisopropylhydrazine; PIH; pheniprazine hydrochloride; Hm-11; JB-516; 'castron', 'catran', 'catron', 'catromazid', 'cavodil').
PHENIRAMINE*** (2-[α-(2-dimethylaminoethyl)benzyl]pyridine; *N*,*N*-dimethyl-3-phenyl-3-(2-pyridyl)propylamine; prophenpyridamine; histapyridamine).
PHENIRAMINE AMINOSALICYLATE (pheniramine 4-aminosalicylate; pheniramine *p*-aminosalicylate; 'avil', 'daneral').
PHENIRAMINE MALEATE (Hö-11513; PM-241; 'inhiston', 'metron', 'trimeton', 'tripoton').
PHENISATIN* (3,3-bis(*p*-acetoxyphenyl)-1-acetyloxindole; triacetyldihydroxydiphenylisatin; 'neo-hollaxans', 'laxatin').
Phenisobromolate see Bromopropylate.
PHENISONONE (3',4'-dihydroxy-2-isopropyl; aminopropiophenone; phenisonone hydrobromide; bronchodilator 1313; 'dapanone').
'Phenitol' see Phenylmercuric nitrate.
Phenitron see Fenitron.
'Phenixin' see Carbon tetrachloride.
PHENKAPTON* (*S*-[(2,5-dichlorophenylthio)methyl] *O*,*O*-diethyl phosphorodithioate; phencapton; przedziorkofos; 'orga-phenkapton').
PHENMEDIPHAM* (3-[(methoxycarbonyl)amino]phenyl *m*-tolylcarbamate; fenmedifam; 'betanal').
'Phenmerzyl' see Phenylmercuric nitrate.
Phenmethylol see Benzyl alcohol.
Phenmetralin* see Phenmetrazine.
Phenmetramide see Fenmetramide.
PHENMETRAZINE** (3-methyl-2-phenylmorpholine; dexphenmetrazine; oxazimedrine; phenmetralin; A-66; 'gracidin', 'ikapharm', 'marsin', 'preludin', 'psychamine').

355

PHENMETRAZINE TEOCLATE (phen-
metrazine 8-chlorotheophyllinate; phen-
metrazine theoclate; R-382).
**PHENMETRAZINE TEOCLATE WITH
N-(2-HYDROXYETHYL)PHENMETR-
AZINE 2-PHENYLBUTYRATE**
('cafilon').
PHENOBARBITAL*** (5-ethyl-5-phenyl-
barbituric acid; phenobarbitone; phen-
emal; phenobarbital sodium).
See also Bromisoval with phenobarbital;
Diniprofylline with phenobarbital;
Phenytoin with phenobarbital.
**PHENOBARBITAL-ETHYLENEDI-
AMINE** ('lavasyl').
**PHENOBARBITAL-NORPSEUDOEPHE-
DRINE** (P-845; 'falepsin').
Phenobarbital-propylhexedrine *see*
Barbexaclone.
Phenobarbitone* *see* Phenobarbital.
PHENOBENZURON* (1-benzoyl-1-(3,4-
dichlorophenyl)-3,3-dimethylurea; *N*-(3,4-
dichlorophenyl)-*N*-[(dimethylamino)-
carbonyl]benzamide).
PHENOBUTIODIL*** (2-(2,4,6-triiodo-
phenoxy)butyric acid; Th-4114; 'biliodyl',
'felotrast', 'vesipaque').
'Phenoclor' *see* Polychlorinated biphenyl
mixture.
PHENOCOLL (*N*-aminoacetyl-*p*-pheneti-
dine; glycine-*p*-phenetidine; phenamine).
Phenocoll salicylate *see* Salocoll.
Phenoctide *see* Octafonium.
'Phenoctyl' *see* Propiomazine.
'Phenodianisyl'* *see* Guanicaine.
'Phenodin' *see* Hematin.
Phenododecinium bromide *see* Domiphen
bromide.
Phenodoxone *see* Phenadoxone.
PHENOL (hydroxybenzene; carbolic acid;
phenic acid).
PHENOLPHTHALEIN (3,5-bis(*p*-hydroxy-
phenyl)phthalide; dihydroxyphthalophen-
one; purgenum).
PHENOLPHTHALOL (*o*-[bis(*p*-hydroxy-
phenyl)methyl]benzyl alcohol; dihydroxy-
phenylmethenylbenzyl alcohol; 'egmol').
Phenol red *see* Phenolsulfonphthalein.
Phenol rubrum *see* Phenolsulfonphthalein.
PHENOLSULFAZOLE (*N*-(2-thiazolyl)-*p*-
phenolsulfonamide; 'darvisul', 'virazene').
2-PHENOLSULFONIC ACID (phenylsulf-
onic acid; sulfocarbolic acid; sozolic acid;
'aseptol').
See also Cupric phenolsulfonate.
PHENOLSULFONPHTHALEIN* (3,3-bis-
(*p*-hydroxyphenyl)-2,1(3H)-benzoxathiole
1,1-dioxide; phenol red; phenol rubrum;
PSP; 'sulfenthal', 'sulfonthal').
Phenoltetraiodophthalein *see* Iodophthal-
ein.
Phenomerbor *see* Phenylmercuric borate.
Phenomitur *see* Barbexaclone.
PHENOMORPHAN*** (3-hydroxy-*N*-
phenethylmorphinan; 3-hydroxy-*N*-(2-
phenylethyl)morphinan).
Phenomycillin* *see* Penicillin V.

PHENOPERIDINE*** (ethyl ester of 1-(3-
hydroxy-3-phenylpropyl)-4-phenylpiperid-
ine-4-carboxylic acid; ethyl 1-(3-hydroxy-
3-phenylpropyl)-4-phenylisonipecotate;
fenoperidine; R-1406; 'lealgin', 'operidine').
'Phenopromin' *see* Amphetamine.
Phenopropazine *see* Prophenamine.
'Phenopropyl' *see* Alverine.
'Phenopyrazone' *see* 1,2-Diphenyl-3,5-
pyrazolidinedione.
'Phenosuccin' *see* Phenetylsuccinimide.
Phenosulfazole *see* Phenolsulfazole.
PHENOTHIAZINE*** (dibenzoparathiazine; thiodiphenylamine; 'fenoverm',
'nemazine', 'padophene', 'phénégic',
'phenovis', 'souframine').
(3H)PHENOTHIAZIN-3-ONE (phenothiazone).
Phenothiazinylethylenediamine *see*
Diethazine.
**(Phenothiazinylethyl)triethylammonium
iodide** *see* Diethazine ethiodide.
**1-(Phenothiazin-10-ylmethylcarbonyl)-4-
piperonylpiperazine** *see* Fenoverine.
**3-(Phenothiazin-10-ylmethyl)quinuclid-
ine** *see* Mequitazine.
**Phenothiazin-10-yl 4-piperonylpiperazin-
1-ylmethyl ketone** *see* Fenoverine.
**2-[2-[4-(3-Phenothiazin-10-ylpropyl)-
piperazin-1-yl]ethyl]-*m*-dioxan** *see*
Oxaprazine.
Phenothiazone *see* Phenothiazin-3-one.
'Phenovis' *see* Phenothiazine.
'Phenoxadrine' *see* Phenyltoloxamine.
'Phenoxalid' *see* Aconiazide.
'Phenoxazole' *see* Pemoline.
'Phenoxene' *see* Chlorphenoxamine.
'Phenoxethol' *see* 2-Phenoxyethanol.
'Phenoxetol' *see* 2-Phenoxyethanol.
'Phenoxin' *see* Carbon tetrachloride.
'Phenoxine' *see* Chlorphenoxamine.
2-PHENOXYACETIC ACID (*O*-phenyl-
glycolic acid; 'phenylium').
PHENOXYBENZAMINE*** (*N*-(2-chloro-
ethyl)-*N*-(1-methyl-2-phenoxyethyl)benzyl-
amine; *N*-(2-chloroethyl)-*N*-(2-phenoxy-
isopropyl)benzylamine; bensylyt; SKF-
688-A; 'dibenyline', 'dibenzyline',
'dibenzyran').
Phenoxybenzylpenicillin *see* Fenbenicilllin.
**6-(2-Phenoxybutyramido)penicillanic
acid** *see* Propicillin.
**6-(α-Phenoxycarbonylphenylacetamido)-
penicillinac acid** *see* Carfecillin.
2-PHENOXYETHANOL (ethylene glycol
monophenyl ether; 'endifasept', 'phenoxethol', 'phenoxetol', 'phenyl cellosolve',
'solvent P').
**2-Phenoxyethyl 1-(3-cyano-3,3-diphenyl-
propyl)-4-phenylisonipecotate** *see*
Fetoxilate.
2-Phenoxyethyl difenoxilate *see* Fetoxilate.
1-Phenoxyethylpenicillin *see* Pheneticillin.
**1-[1-(2-Phenoxyethyl)piperid-4-yl]-
benzimidazolin-2-one** *see* Oxiperomide.
(±)-*m*-Phenoxyhydratropic acid *see*
Fenprofen.

2-Phenoxyisobutyric acid *see* 2-Methyl-2-phenoxypropionic acid.

'Phenoxyisopropylnorsuprifen' *see* Isoxsuprine.

Phenoxymethylpenicillin*** *see* Penicillin V.

4-[3-(4-Phenoxymethylphenyl)propyl]-morpholine *see* Fomocaine.

1-[4-(2-Phenoxy-2-phenylacetamido)-butyl]-2,6-dimethylpiperidine *see* Oxiramide.

2-(3-Phenoxyphenyl)propionic acid *see* Fenprofen.

Phenoxypropazine* *see* Fenoxypropazine.

6-(2-Phenoxypropionamido)penicillanic acid *see* Pheneticillin.

1-(3-Phenoxypropyl)guanidine *see* Guanoxyfen.

(1-Phenoxypropyl)penicillin *see* Propicillin.

4-Phenoxy-3-pyrrolidin-1-yl-5-sulfamoyl-benzoic acid *see* Piretanide.

'Phenphene' *see* Campheclor.

Phenpiazine *see* Quinoxaline.

Phenpiperazole *see* Zolertine.

PHENPROBAMATE*** (3-phenylpropyl carbamate; proformiphen; MH-532; 'actozine', 'gamaquil', 'quilil').

PHENPROBAMATE WITH ACETYL-SALICYLIC ACID ('diaflexol').

Phenprocoumarol *see* Phenprocoumon.

PHENPROCOUMON*** (3-(α-ethylbenzyl)-4-hydroxycoumarin; 4-hydroxy-3-(1-phenylpropyl)coumarin; phenylpropylhydroxycoumarin; phenprocoumarol; 'liquamar', 'marcoumar', 'marcumar').

PHENPROMETHAMINE*** (N,β-dimethylphenethylamine; N-methyl-β-phenylpropylamine; phenylpropylmethylamine; 1-methylamino-2-phenylpropane; 'vonedrine').

Phenpropamine* *see* Alverine.

PHENSUXIMIDE*** (N-methyl-2-phenyl-succinimide; N-methyl-α-phenylsuccinimide; PM-334; 'epimide', 'lifene', 'milontin', 'milonton', 'succitimal').

Phentanyl *see* Fentanyl.

PHENTERMINE*** (α,α-dimethylphenethylamine; 1,1-dimethyl-2-phenylethylamine; 2-benzyl-2-propylamine; β-phenyl-*tert*-butylamine; phentermine hydrochloride; terbutylamine; 'ex-adipos', 'panbesy', 'reducyl', 'wilpo').

PHENTERMINE RESIN* (complex of phentermine with an ion-exchange resin; 'adipex neu', 'duromine', 'ionamin', 'linyl', 'mirapront').

Phenthiazine *see* Phenothiazine.

PHENTHOATE* (ethyl α-[(dimethoxyphosphinothioyl)thio]benzeneacetate; ethyl 2-[(dimethoxyphosphinothioyl)thio]-2-phenylacetate; S-(α-ethoxycarbonyl-benzyl) O,O-dimethyl phosphorodithioate; dimethenthoate; 'cidial', 'elsan', 'tanone').

PHENTOLAMINE*** (2-[N-(m-hydroxyphenyl)-N-(p-tolyl)aminomethyl]-2-imidazoline; 2-[[N-(m-hydroxyphenyl)-p-toluidino]methyl]-2-imidazoline).

PHENTOLAMINE MESILATE (phentolamine methanesulfonate; phentolamine mesylate; C-7337; 'imidaline', 'regitin', 'rogitine').

PHENTRIAZOPHOS* (O,O-diethyl O-(1-phenyl-1H-1,2,4-triazol-3-yl) phosphorothioate; 3-[(diethoxyphosphinothioyl)oxy]-1-phenyl-1H-1,2,4-triazole; 'hostathion').

PHENTYDRONE (1,2,3,4-tetrahydro-9-fluorenone).

'Phenurone' *see* Phenacemide.

'Phenychol' *see* 1-Phenyl-1-propanol.

7-Phenylacetamidocephalosporanic acid *see* Cefaloram.

6-Phenylacetamidopenicillanic acid *see* Penicillin G.

6-Phenylacetamidopenicillanic acid acetoxymethyl ester *see* Penamecillin.

α-Phenylacetophenone *see* Desoxybenzoin.

Phenyl acetylsalicylate *see* Acetylsalol.

1-(2-Phenylacetyl)urea *see* Phenacemide.

Phenylacrylic acid *see* Cinnamic acid.

PHENYLALANINE (2-amino-3-phenyl-propionic acid; α-amino-β-phenylpropionic acid; 3-phenylalanine; β-phenylalanine; α-aminohydrocinnamic acid).

Phenylalanine-lysine vasopressin *see* Felypressin.

D-Phenylalanine mustard *see* Medphalan.

DL-Phenylalanine mustard *see* Sarcolysin.

L-Phenylalanine mustard *see* Melphalan.

Phenylallyl alcohol *see* Cinnamyl alcohol.

Phenylamine *see* Aniline.

Phenyl 4-aminosalicylate* *see* Fenamisal.

Phenylamyl camphorate *see* Fenipentol camphorate.

Phenylarsinic acid *see* Benzenearsonic acid.

Phenylarsonic acid *see* Benzenearsonic acid.

Phenylazoaniline *see* Aminoazobenzene.

Phenylazoformic acid phenylhydrazide *see* Diphenylcarbazone.

1-Phenylazo-2-naphthol-6,8-disulfonic acid *see* Orange G.

1-Phenylazo-2-naphthol-6-sulfonic acid sodium salt *see* Orange RN.

1-(p-Phenylazophenylazo)-2-naphthol *see* Oil scarlet.

4-Phenylazo-m-phenylenediamine *see* Chrysoidine.

Phenylazothionoformic acid phenyl-hydrazide *see* Dithizone.

N-Phenylbarbital *see* Phetharbital.

N-Phenylbenzamide *see* Benzanilide.

2-Phenylbenzimidazole *see* Phenzidole.

α-Phenylbenzylamine *see* Benzhydrylamine.

8-(p-Phenylbenzyl)atropinium bromide *see* Xenytropium bromide.

2-Phenylbicyclo(2.2.1)heptane-2-carboxylic acid *see* 2-Phenylnorbornane-2-carboxylic acid.

Phenylbutanamide *see* Phenylbutyramide.

2-Phenyl-1,2-butanediol 1-carbamate *see* Oxyfenamate.

PHENYLBUTAZONE*** (4-butyl-1,2-diphenyl-3,5-pyrazolidinedione; butadion; diphenylbutazone; diphebuzol; fenbutazone; phenylbutazone sodium; G-13871).

See also below and Aminophenazone with phenylbutazone; 4-Isopropylaminophenazone with phenylbutazone; Paracetamol with phenylbutazone.

Phenylbutazone 2-amino-2-thiazoline compound *see* Thiazolinobutazone.

PHENYLBUTAZONE CALCIUM (P-241).

Phenylbutazone clofexamide compound *see* Clofezone.

Phenylbutazone dextropropoxyphene compound *see* Proxifezone.

Phenylbutazone-5-enolate of benzydamine *see* Benzydamine phenylbutazone-5-enolate.

Phenylbutazone piperazine* *see* Pyrazinobutazone.

PHENYLBUTAZONE 3,4,5-TRIMETHOXYBENZOATE (phenylbutazone trimethylgallate; LH-150; 'ditrone').

PHENYLBUTAZONE WITH PAPAIN ('penetradol').

PHENYLBUTAZONE WITH PREDNISOLONE ('delta-elmedal', 'rheosolon').

PHENYLBUTAZONE WITH PREDNISONE ('delta-butazolidine').

4-Phenyl-3-buten-2-one *see* Benzylideneacetone.

β-Phenyl-*tert*-butylamine *see* Phentermine.

'Phenyl-*sec*-butylnorsuprifen' *see* Buphenine.

2-PHENYLBUTYRAMIDE (2-ethyl-2-phenylacetamide; 2-phenylbutanamide; phenylethylacetamide; TH-4128; 'hyposterol', 'phenethamid', 'redusterol').

2-PHENYLBUTYRIC ACID (2-ethyl-2-phenylacetic acid; phenylethylacetic acid; α-phenylbutyric acid).
See also Butamirate; Butetamate; Cetamifen; Febuverine; Fenbutrazate; Feneritrol; Fenetradil.

1-(2-Phenylbutyryl)urea *see* Ethylphenacemide.

Phenylcarbamic acid *see* Carbanilic acid.

4-(Phenylcarbamoyl)butyric acid *see* Glutaranilic acid.

Phenyl carbinol *see* Benzyl alcohol.

'Phenyl cellosolve' *see* 2-Phenoxyethanol.

2-Phenylchroman *see* Flavan.

2-Phenylchromone *see* Flavone.

3-Phenylchromone *see* Isoflavone.

2-Phenylcinchoninic acid *see* Cinchophen.

Phenylcinnamic acid *see* Diphenylacrylic acid.

α-Phenyl-*o*-cresol *see* *o*-Benzylphenol.

Phenyl cyanide *see* Benzonitrile.

α-Phenylcyclohexaneacetic acid diethylaminoethyl ester *see* Drofenine.

α-PHENYLCYCLOHEXANEGLYCOLIC ACID (cyclohexylmandelic acid).
See also Ibuverine; Oxybutynin; Oxyclipine; Oxyphencyclimine; Oxyphenonium; Oxypyrronium; Oxysonium.

[2-(Phenylcyclohexylacetoxy)ethyl]-dimethylsulfonium iodide *see* Hexasonium.

trans-**4-Phenylcyclohexylamine 2-(*p*-biphenylyl)butyrate** *see* Butixirate.

trans-**4-Phenylcyclohexylamine α-ethyl-4-biphenylacetic acid compound** *see* Butixirate.

trans-**4-Phenylcyclohexylamine xenbucin salt** *see* Butixirate.

1-(1-Phenylcyclohexyl)piperidine *see* Phencyclidine.

1-Phenylcyclopentanecarboxylic acid esters *see* Caramiphen; Minepentate; Pentoxyverine; Tropentane.

2-Phenylcyclopentylamine *see* Cypenamine.

trans-**2-Phenylcyclopropylamine** *see* Tranylcypromine.

Phenyldiallylacetic acid *see* 2-Allyl-2-phenyl-4-pentenoic acid.

Phenyl 5,6-dichloro-2-(trifluoromethyl)-1H-benzimidazole-1-carboxylate *see* Fenazaflor.

6-Phenyl-5,6-dihydroimidazo(2,1-b)-thiazole *see* Antafenite.

3-Phenyl-3,4-dihydroquinazoline *see* Orexin.

Phenyldimethylpyrazolone *see* Phenazone.

1,1'-*o*-Phenylenebis[3-(ethoxycarbonyl)-2-thiourea] *see* Thiophanate.

p-**Phenylene bis(isothiocyanate)** *see* Bitoscanate.

1,1-*o*-Phenylenebis[(3-methoxycarbonyl)-2-thiourea] *see* Thiophanate methyl.

4,4'-(*p*-Phenylene)bis(methyleneamino)-di(isoxazolidin-3-one) *see* Terizidone.

$N^4,N^{4'}$-(*p*-**Phenylene)bis(methylene)di-(cycloserine)** *see* Terizidone.

4,4'-[*m*-Phenylene(oxyethylene)]bis-[hexahydro-1-hydroxy-7-(hydroxymethyl)pyrrolizinium chloride] *see* Diplacin.

Phenylenebis(oxypropylene)bis(dimethylethylammonium iodide) *see* Dipropamine.

4,4'-*o*-Phenylenebis(3-thioallophanic acid) diethyl ester *see* Thiophanate.

4,4'-*o*-Phenylenebis(3-thioallophanic acid) dimethyl ester *see* Thiophanatemethyl.

α,β-Phenylenebutyrolactone *see* Phthalide.

β,γ-Phenylenebutyrolactone *see* 2-Coumaranone.

PHENYLENEDIAMINE(S) (diaminobenzene(s); 'ursol').

Phenylene diisothiocyanate *see* Bitoscanate.

N,N'-(*p*-**Phenylenedimethylene)bis[2,2-dichloro-*N*-(2-ethoxyethyl)acetamide]** *see* Teclozan.

Phenylenedioxybis[ethylhydroxy(hydroxymethyl)hexahydropyrrolopyrrole] *see* Diplacin.

PHENYLEPHRINE** ((−)-*m*-hydroxy-α-(methylaminomethyl)benzyl alcohol; L-*m*-synephrine; mesaton; mezaton; metaoxedrine; neo-oxedrine; phenylephrine hydrochloride).

PHENYLEPHRINE WITH DIPHENYLPYRALINE ('novahistex').

PHENYLEPHRINE WITH ZINC SULFATE ('zincfrin').

PHENYLETHANOLAMINE (α-amino-methylbenzyl alcohol; 2-amino-1-phenyl-ethanol; β-hydroxyphenethylamine; phenethanolamine).
PHENYL ETHER (diphenyl ether; diphenyl oxide; phenoxybenzene).
Phenylethylacetamide see 2-Phenylbutyramide.
Phenylethylacetylurea see Ethylphenacemide.
2-Phenylethylamine see Phenethylamine.
1-Phenylethyl 3-(dimethoxyphosphinyl-oxy)-2-butenoate see Crotoxyphos.
1-(1-Phenylethyl)hydrazine see Mebanazine.
Phenylethylmalonic acid monoethyl ester diethylaminoethylamide see Fenalamide.
N-**Phenylformamide** see Formanilide.
Phenylformic acid see Benzoic acid.
N-**Phenylglutaramic acid** see Glutaranilic acid.
N-**Phenylglycinamide-*p*-arsonic acid sodium salt** see Tryparsamide.
α-**Phenylglycolic acid** see Mandelic acid.
O-**Phenylglycolic acid** see Phenoxyacetic acid.
Phenylglyoxylnitrile oxime *O*,*O*-diethyl phosphorothioate see Phoxim.
2-Phenylhydracrylic acid see Tropic acid.
1-Phenyl-2-hydrazinopropane see Pheniprazine.
Phenyl *p*-hydroxybenzoate see Phenyl paraben.
2-Phenyl-1,3-indandione see Phenindione.
PHENYLISOBUTYLHYDRAZINE (1-(1-methyl-3-phenylpropyl)hydrazine; 1-(4-phenylbut-2-yl)hydrazine; JB-835).
Phenylisohydantoin see Pemoline.
β-**Phenylisopropylamine** see Amphetamine.
Phenylisopropylhydrazine see Pheniprazine.
PHENYLISOPROPYLISONIAZID (*N*′-(2-phenylisopropyl)isoniazid; isonicotinic acid (α-methylphenethyl)hydrazide; 1-isonicotinoyl-2-(phenylisopropyl)hydrazine; JB-821).
N-(**2-Phenylisopropyl)nicotinamide** see Phenatin.
N-(**2-Phenylisopropyl)nicotinthioamide** see Thiophenatin.
3-(2-Phenylisopropyl)sydnone imine see Sydnofen.
3-(2-Phenylisopropyl)sydnone imine *N*-phenylcarbamoyl derivative see Sydnocarb.
α-(**5-Phenylisoxazol-3-yl)-1-piperidine ethanol** see Perisoxal.
'Phenylium' see Phenoxyacetic acid.
Phenyllin (tr) see Phenindione.
N-**Phenylmaleamic acid** see Maleanilic acid.
6-(Phenylmalonamido)penicillanic acid disodium salt see Carbenicillin.
α-**Phenylmandelic acid** see Benzilic acid.
6-Phenylmercaptoacetamidopenicillanic acid see Tifencillin.

PHENYLMERCURIC ACETATE ('merfen', 'merphenyl', 'mersolite 8', 'mertricone', 'sanmicron', 'volpar').
PHENYLMERCURIC BORATE (PHB; phenomerbor; 'aderman', 'exomycol', 'hydromerfene', 'nylmerate').
See also Dexamethasone pivalate with phenylmercuric borate.
PHENYLMERCURIC LACTATE ('lactophenymer').
PHENYLMERCURIC NITRATE ('aeroped', 'calped', 'epido', 'mersagel', 'phemer-nite', 'phenitol', 'phenmerzyl', 'phenymer', 'scleromerfen', 'spidox').
PHENYLMERCURIC SALICYLATE ('mersolite 19').
Phenylmethylaminopropane see Methamphetamine.
Phenylmethylaminopropanol see Ephedrine.
Phenylmethylimidazoline see Tolazoline.
2-PHENYLNORBORNANE-2-CARB-OXYLIC ACID (2-phenylbicyclo(2.2.1)-heptane-2-carboxylic acid).
2-Phenylnorbornane-2-carboxylic acid esters see Bicyclophenamine; Bornaprine.
PHENYL PARABEN (phenyl *p*-hydroxy-benzoate; 'nipaphenyl').
Phenyl-PAS see Fenamisal.
1-Phenyl-1-pentanol see Fenipentol.
Phenylpentyl camphorate see Fenipentol camphorate.
α-**Phenylphenacylamine** see Desylamine.
α-**Phenylphenethylamine** see Stilbylamine.
o-**PHENYLPHENOL** (2-hydroxybiphenyl; *o*-phenyl phenol sodium; 'dowicide', 'loyrthol', 'orthoxenol', 'rotoline').
2-Phenyl-2-(phenylisopropylamino)-acetonitrile see Amphetaminil.
Phenylphosphonothioic acid *O*-(4-bromo-2,5-dichlorophenyl) *O*-methyl ester see Leptophos.
Phenylphosphonothioic acid *O*-(*p*-cyanophenyl) *O*-ethyl ester see Cyanofenphos.
Phenylphosphonothioic acid *O*-ethyl *O*-(*p*-nitrophenyl) ester see Ethyl (*p*-nitrophenyl) phenylphosphonothioate.
Phenylphosphonothioic acid *O*-ethyl *O*-quinolin-8-yl ester see Quintiofos.
N-**Phenylphthalamic acid** see Phthalanilic acid.
3-(4-Phenylpiperazin-1-yl)-1,2-propane-diol see Dropropizine.
α-**PHENYL-1-PIPERIDINEACETIC ACID** (2-phenyl-2-piperid-1-ylacetic acid).
See also Bietamiverine; Dipiproverine; Piprocurarium.
α-**PHENYL-2-PIPERIDINEACETIC ACID** (2-phenyl-2-piperid-2-ylacetic acid).
See also Butopiprine.
α-**Phenyl-2-piperidinemethanol acetate** see Phacetoperan.
1-Phenyl-1-piperid-1-ylcyclohexane see Phencyclidine.
2-[(*N*-Phenyl)[*N*-(2-piperid-1-ylethyl)]-aminomethyl]pyridine see Picoperine.

5-Phenyl-5-piperid-2-ylmethylbarbituric acid see Prazitone.
3-Phenyl-3-piperid-1-ylpropionic acid butyl ester see Butaverine.
N-Phenyl-2-piperid-1-yl-N-pyrid-2-yl-methylethylamine see Picoperine.
1-Phenyl-3-piperid-1-ylpyrrolidin-2-one see Felipyrine.
Phenylprenazone see Feprazone.
1-PHENYL-1-PROPANOL (α-ethylbenzyl alcohol; 'felicur', 'phenychol').
Phenylpropanolamine* see Norephedrine.
Phenylpropenoic acid see Cinnamic acid.
3-Phenyl-2-propen-1-ol see Cinnamyl alcohol.
2-Phenyl-2-prop-2-enyl-4-penten-1-oic acid see 2-Allyl-2-phenyl-4-pentenoic acid.
2-Phenylpropionic acid see Hydratropic acid.
3-Phenylpropionic acid see Hydrocinnamic acid.
1-Phenyl-2-propylamine see Amphetamine.
1-PHENYLPROPYL CARBAMATE ('alphaquil').
2-PHENYLPROPYL CARBAMATE ('betaquil').
3-Phenylpropyl carbamate see Phenprobamate.
Phenylpropylhydroxycoumarin see Phenprocoumon.
Phenyl propyl ketone see Butyrophenone.
Phenylpropylmethylamine see Phenpromethamine.
1-Phenyl-2-propynyl carbamate see Carfimate.
N¹-(2-Phenylpyrazol-3-yl)sulfanilamide see Sulfaphenazole.
2-PHENYL-2-PYRID-2-YLTHIOACET-AMIDE (antigastrin; SC-15396).
5-Phenylpyrimido(4,5-d)pyrimidine-2,4,7-triamine see Ampyrimine.
Phenylpyrrolidinopentane see Prolintane.
2-Phenyl-N-(2-pyrrolidin-1-ylethyl)-glycine isopentyl ester see Camiverine.
N-Phenyl-N-(2-pyrrolid-1-ylethyl)benzyl-amine see Histapyrrodine.
1-Phenyl-2-pyrrolid-1-ylpentane see Prolintane.
N-Phenylsalicylamide see Salicylanilide.
Phenyl salicylate see Salol.
3-Phenylsalicylic acid diethylaminoethyl ester see Xenysalate.
Phenylsemicarbazide see Phenicarbazide.
Phenylstibonic acid see Benzenestibonic acid.
Phenyl styryl ketone see Chalcone.
N-Phenylsuccinamic acid see Succinanilic acid.
N¹-Phenylsulfanilamide see Sulfabenz.
Phenylsulfapyrazole see Sulfaphenazole.
5-(Phenylsulfinyl)-2-benzimidazole-carbamic acid methyl ester see Oxfendazole.
[2-(Phenylsulfinyl)ethyl]malonic acid mono(1,2-diphenylhydrazide)see Osmadizone.
6-(2-Phenyl-2-sulfoacetamido)penicil-

lanic acid see Sulbenicillin.
6-[2-Phenyl-D-(sulfoamino)acetamido]-penicillanic acid see Suncillin.
Phenyl sulfone see Diphenyl sulfone.
4-Phenyl-1-(tetrahydrofurfuryloxyethyl)-isonipecotic acid ethyl ester see Furethidine.
6-[2-Phenyl-2-[2-[p-(1,4,5,6-tetrahydro-pyrimidin-2-yl)phenyl]acetamido]-acetamido]penicillanic acid see Rota-micillin.
1-Phenyl-1-(2-tetrazol-5-ylethyl)piper-azine see Zolertine.
6-Phenylthioacetamidopenicillanic acid see Tifencillin.
5-(Phenylthio)-2-benzimidazolecarbamic acid methyl ester see Fenbendazole.
Phenylthiocarbamide see Phenylthiourea.
Phenylthiomethyl penicillin see Tifencillin.
α-Phenyl-2-thiopheneglycolic acid ester with diethyl(2-hydroxyethyl)methyl-ammonium bromide see Oxitefonium bromide.
PHENYLTHIOUREA (1-phenyl-2-thiourea; phenylthiocarbamide; PTC).
PHENYLTHIOURETHAN (ethyl thiono-carbanilate; Et ester of phenylthionocarb-amic acid).
PHENYLTOLOXAMINE*** (N,N-di-methyl-2-(α-phenyl-o-toloxy)ethylamine; 2-(2-benzylphenoxy)-N,N-dimethylethyl-amine).
PHENYLTOLOXAMINE CITRATE (phenyltoloxamine dihydrogen citrate; C-5581-H; PRN; 'antin', 'bistrimin', 'bristain', 'bristamine', 'phenoxadrine').
2-(α-Phenyl-o-toloxy)triethylamine see Etoloxamine.
2-Phenyl-4-(trichloromethyl)-△²-1,3,4-oxadiazolin-5-one see Clotioxone.
PHENYLURETHAN (ethyl carbanilate; Et ester of phenylcarbamic acid).
2-Phenylvaleric acid diethylaminoethyl ester see Propivane.
Phenyl vinyl ketone see Acrylophenone.
'Phenymer' see Phenylmercuric nitrate.
'Pheny-pas-tebamin' see Fenamisal.
PHENYRACILLIN*** (2,5-diphenylpiper-azine salt of penicillin G; 2,5-diphenyl-piperazine 1,4-bis[(6-phenylacetamido)-penicillanate]).
'Phenyral' see 5-Allyl-5-phenylbarbituric acid.
Phenyramidol* see Fenyramidol.
PHENYTHILONE*** (2-ethyl-2-phenyl-thiamorpholine-3,5-dione; 2-ethyltetra-hydro-2-phenyl-1,4-thiazine-3,5-dione; MRD-125; 'dolitrone').
PHENYTOIN*** (5,5-diphenylhydantoin; 5,5-diphenylimidazoline-2,4-dione; diphenin; difenin; phenytoin sodium).
PHENYTOIN WITH DIAZEPAM (A-124).
PHENYTOIN WITH PHENOBARBITAL ('garoin').
PHENYTOIN VALERATE (phenytoin 3-valerate; 'neo-citrullamon').
PHENZIDOLE (2-phenylbenzimidazole).

Phenzoline see Orexin.
Phepracet (tr) see Fepracet.
'Phesin' see Phenazone sodium sulfonate.
Phetenylate see Thyphenytoin.
Phethanol (tr) see Etilefrine.
PHETHARBITAL*** (5,5-diethyl-1-phenyl-barbituric acid; *N*-phenylbarbital; 'pyrictal').
Phethenylate* see Thyphenytoin.
'Phiangin' see Paraformaldehyde.
'Phiniphos' see Sodium 4-dimethylamino-*o*-toluenephosphonite.
'pHisoderm' see Sodium octylphenoxy-ethoxyethyl ether sulfonate.
'Phisohex' see Hexachlorophene.
'Phlebolan' see Dimethyl sulfoxide.
PHLEOMYCIN (antibiotic from *Str. verticillus*; NSC-61586).
'Phlogodym' see Neodymium pyrocatechol-disulfonate.
'Phlogosam' see Samarium-sulfosalicylic acid complex.
PHLORETIC ACID (*p*-hydroxyhydrocinn-amic acid; 3-(*p*-hydroxyphenyl)propionic acid).
PHLORETIN (2',4',6'-trihydroxy-3-(*p*-hydroxyphenyl)propiophenone; 3-(*p*-hydroxyphenyl)phloropropiophenone; asebogenol; phloretol).
Phlorhizin see Phlorizin.
Phloridzin see Phlorizin.
Phlorimycin (tr) see Viomycin.
PHLORIZIN (phloretin 2'-β-glucoside; phlorhizin; phloridzin; asebotin; 'kalmin').
Phlorizoside see Phlorizin.
PHLOROGLUCINOL (1,3,5-trihydroxy-benzene; phloroglucin; 'dilospan').
PHLOROGLUCINOL WITH 1,3,5-TRI-METHOXYBENZENE (phloroglucinol with trimethylphloroglucinol; LL-172; 'dilexan', 'spasfon').
Phloropropiophenone see Flopropione.
PHNB (tr) see Quintozene.
'Phobex' see Benactyzine.
'Phoebex' see Benactyzine.
'Phoenixin' see Carbon tetrachloride.
PHOLCODINE*** ((morpholinylethyl)-morphine; M.E.M.; 3-(2-morpholino-ethyl) ether of morphine; homocodeine; pholcodine citrate or tartrate).
PHOLEDRINE***(*p*-(2-methylaminopropyl)-phenol; *N*,α-dimethyl-*p*-hydroxyphenethyl-amine; *N*-methylparedrine; isodrin; pro-methin).
PHORATE* (*O*,*O*-diethyl *S*-ethylthiomethyl phosphorodithioate; L-11-6; timet; 'thimet').
PHOSACETIM* (*O*,*O*-bis(*p*-chlorophenyl) (1-iminoethyl)phosphoramidothioate).
'Phosaden' see Adenosine phosphate.
PHOSALONE* (*S*-[(6-chloro-2-oxobenz-oxazol-3(2H)-yl)methyl] *O*,*O*-diethyl phosphorodithioate; 6-chloro-3(2H)-[[(diethoxyphosphinothioyl)thio]methyl]-benzoxazol-2-one; 'zolone').
'Phosarbin' see Pyrophos.
Phoschlorin see Metrifonate.

Phosclorine see Metrifonate.
'Phosdrin' see Mevinphos.
Phosethoprop see Ethoprop.
PHOSFOLAN* (diethyl 1,3-dithiolan-2-ylidenephosphoramidate; 2-(diethoxy-phosphinylimino)-1,3-dithiolane; carbo-lane; 'cylan', 'cyolane').
PHOSGENE (COCl$_2$; carbonyl chloride; chloroformyl chloride; collongite).
PHOSMET* (*S*-[(1,3-dihydro-1,3-dioxo-2H-isoindol-2-yl)methyl] *O*,*O*-dimethyl phosphorodithioate; 2-[[(dimethoxy-phosphinothioyl)thio]methyl]phthalimidyl; ftalofos; phthalofos).
PHOSNICHLOR* (*O*-(4-chloro-3-nitro-phenyl) *O*,*O*-dimethyl phosphorothioate; nichlorfos).
'Phosodyl' see Sodium 4-dimethylamino-*o*-toluenephosphonite.
Phosphacol (tr) see Paraoxon.
Phosphagen see Creatinephosphoric acid.
'Phosphalgel' see Aluminium phosphate.
Phosphamide (tr) see Dimethoate.
PHOSPHAMIDON* (2-chloro-*N*,*N*-diethyl-3-hydroxycrotonamide dimethyl phosphate; (2-chloro-2-(diethylcarbamoyl)-1-methyl-vinyl) dimethyl phosphate; (2-chloro-1-diethylaminocroton-3-yl) dimethyl phos-phate; (2-chloro-3-diethylamino-1-methyl-3-oxo-1-propenyl) dimethyl phosphate; 'dimecron', 'liromidon').
PHOSPHANILIC ACID (*p*-aminobenzene-phosphonic acid).
PHOSPHATIDYLCHOLINE (lecithin; 'lexinol-cal').
Phosphemol see Parathion.
2,2'-Phosphinicodilactic acid see Foscolic acid.
1,1',1''-Phosphinylidynetris(2-methyl-aziridine) see Metepa.
Phosphocreatine see Creatinephosphoric acid.
'Phosphoestrol' see Fosfestrol.
'Phospholine' see Ecothiopate.
'Phosphonefrin' see Epinephrine phosphate.
Phosphonoacetic acid disodium salt monohydrate see Fosfonet sodium.
Phosphonodithioimidocarbonic acid ethylene dibenzyl *P*,*P*,*P*',*P*'-tetraethyl ester see Zilantel.
Phosphonomycin see Fosfomycin.
Phosphoramide(s) see Phosphoramidic acid; Phosphoric triamide; Phosphorodi-amidic acid.
PHOSPHORAMIDIC ACID (phosphoric acid monoamide; phosphoramide).
PHOSPHORIC ACID (orthophosphoric acid).
Phosphoric acid amide see Phosphoramidic acid.
Phosphoric acid diamide see Phosphoro-diamidic acid.
Phosphoric acid monoamide see Phosphoramidic acid.
Phosphoric acid triamide see Phosphoric triamide.
Phosphoric acid triethylenimide see Tepa.

PHOSPHORIC TRIAMIDE (phosphoric acid triamide; phosphoramide).
PHOSPHORODIAMIDIC ACID (phosphoric acid diamide).
Phosphorodiamidic anhydride see Pyrophosphoramide.
PHOSPHORODIAMIDIC FLUORIDE (phosphorofluoridic diamide).
PHOSPHORODITHIOIC ACID (dithiophosphoric acid).
Phosphorofluoridic acid isopropyl ester see Dyflos.
Phosphorofluoridic diamide see Phosphorodiamidic fluoride.
PHOSPHOROTHIOIC ACID (thiophosphoric acid).
PHOSPHOROTHIOIC TRIAMIDE (triaminophosphine sulfide; phosphorothioic acid triamide; thiophosphoramide).
Phosphorylcreatine see Creatinephosphoric acid.
Phosphoryldimethylaminoethanol see Deanol phosphate.
Phosphostigmine* see Parathion.
'Phostoxin' see Aluminium phosphide with ammonium carbamate.
'Phosvel' see Leptophos.
'Photodyn' see Hematoporphyrin.
PHOXIM*** (phenylglyoxylnitrile oxime *O,O*-diethyl phosphorothioate; *O,O*-diethyl *O*-(α-nitrilobenzylimino) phosphorothioate; *O*-(α-cyanobenzylimino) *O,O*-diethyl phosphorothioate; α-[[(diethoxyphosphinothioyl)oxy]imino]benzeneacetonitrile; 'baython', 'valexon').
Phrenosin* see Cerebrin.
'Phrenotropin' see Prothipendyl.
PHTHALALDEHYDIC ACID (*o*-formylbenzoic acid; benzaldehyde-2-carboxylic acid).
'Phthalamaquin' see Quinetalate.
PHTHALAMIC ACID (*o*-carbamoylbenzoic acid; phthalic acid monoamide).
See also Ammonium phthalamate.
PHTHALAMIDE (phthalic acid diamide).
Phthalamudine see Chlortalidone.
PHTHALAN (1,3-dihydroisobenzofuran).
PHTHALANILIC ACID (*N*-phenylphthalamic acid).
PHTHALAZINE (2,3-benzodiazine; β-phenodiazine).
Phthalazino(2,3-b)phthalazine-5,12(7H, 14H)-dione see Diftalone.
3-Phthalazin-1-ylcarbazic acid ethyl ester see Todralazine.
Phthalazole see Phthalylsulfathiazole.
PHTHALHYDRAZIDE (2,3-dihydro-1,4-phthalazinedione; phthalic acid hydrazide; phthalhydrazine).
PHTHALIC ACID (*o*-benzenedicarboxylic acid).
Phthalic acid amides see Phthalamic acid; Phthalamide.
Phthalic acid esters see Calcium benzyl phthalate; Dibutyl phthalate; Dimethyl phthalate.
Phthalic acid hydrazide see Phthalhydr-azide.
Phthalic acid imide see Phthalimide.
PHTHALIDE (1-(3H)isobenzofuranone; 1-isocoumaranone; α,β-phenylenebutyrolactone; S-3).
Phthalidyl 6-(D(—)-α-aminophenylacetamido)penicillinate see Talampicillin.
Phthalidylampicillin see Talampicillin.
PHTHALIMIDE (1,3-isoindoledione).
PHTHALIMIDINE (1-isoindolinone).
3-(*N*-Phthalimido)glutarimide see Thalidomide.
Phthalofos see Phosmet.
Phthalofyne* see Ftalofyne.
Phthalophos see Naftalofos.
Phthalthrin see Tetramethrin.
PHTHALYLSULFACETAMIDE* (*N*¹-acetyl-*N*⁴-phthaloylsulfanilamide; 4'-acetylsulfamoylphthalanilic acid; ftalicetimida).
PHTHALYLSULFAMETHIZOLE*** (*N*¹-(5-methyl-1,3,4-thiadiazol-2-yl)-*N*⁴-phthaloylsulfanilamide; 4'-[(5-methyl-1,3,4-thiadiazol-2-yl)sulfamoyl]phthalanilic acid).
PHTHALYLSULFATHIAZOLE*** (*N*¹-thiazol-2-yl-*N*⁴-phthaloylsulfanilamide; 4'-(thiazol-2-ylsulfamoyl)phthalanilic acid; phthalazole; phthalylsulfonazole).
Phthalylsulfonazole see Phthalylsulfathiazole.
PHTHIOCOL (2-hydroxy-3-methyl-1,4-naphthoquinone).
Phthivazid see Ftivazide.
Phycite see Erythritol.
Phycitol see Erythritol.
'Phygon' see Dichlone.
'Phyllocormin-N' see Etofylline.
α-Phyllohydroquinone see Phytonadiol.
PHYLLOKININ (bradykinylisoleucyltyrosine *O*-sulfate).
Phylloquinone see Phytomenadione.
'Physiolax' see Sodium dioctyl sulfosuccinate.
'Physoscorbate' see Physostigmine ascorbate.
PHYSOSTIGMINE (2,3,3a,8a-tetrahydro-5-hydroxy-1,3a,8-trimethylpyrrolo(2,3-b)-indole methylcarbamate ester; eserine; eseroline methylcarbamate; physostigmine sulfate or salicylate; 'physostol').
PHYSOSTIGMINE ASCORBATE ('physoscorbate').
PHYSOSTIGMINE *N*-OXIDE (eseridine; 'geneserine').
'Physostol' see Physostigmine.
PHYTANIC ACID (3,7,11,15-tetramethylhexadecanoic acid; tetramethylpalmitic acid).
PHYTIC ACID (inositolhexaphosphoric acid; cyclohexanehexol hexaphosphate; fytic acid; phytinic acid).
See also Calcium magnesium phytate; Sodium phytate.
'Phytin' see Calcium magnesium phytate.
'Phytobiase' see Calcium magnesium phytate.
Phytocalcine see Calcium magnesium phytate.
PHYTOHEMAGGLUTININ (phaseolosaxin; 'difco M').

PHYTOL (3,7,11,15-tetramethyl-2-hexa-decen-1-ol).

Phytomelin see Rutin.

PHYTOMENADIONE*** (2-methyl-3-phytyl-1,4-naphthoquinone; 3-phytyl-menadione; phylloquinone; phytonadione; vitamin K$_1$; antihemorrhagic vitamin).

PHYTONADIOL (2-methyl-3-phytyl-1,4-naphthalenediol; α-phyllohydroquinone; dihydrovitamin K$_1$; vitamin K$_1$ hydro-quinone).

PHYTONADIOL SODIUM DIPHOS-PHATE*** (phytonadiol 1,4-di(sodium hydrogen phosphate)).

Phytomenadione* see Phytomenadione.

'Phytosol' see Trichloronat.

'Piafolina' see Morinamide.

'Piarine' see Promazine.

Pi-A-T see Piperazine diantimonyl tartrate.

Piazine see Pyrazine.

'Piazol' see Morinamide.

'Piazolina' see Morinamide.

PIBECARB*** (phenacyl pivalate).
See also Mobecarb with pibecarb.

PICAFIBRATE** (2-(p-chlorophenoxy)-2-methylpropionic acid ester with N-(2-hydroxyethyl)nicotinamide; 2-nicotin-amidoethyl clofibrate).

'Picfume' see Chloropicrin.

PICLOPASTINE*** (2-[2-[4-(p-chloro-α-pyrid-2-ylbenzyl)piperazin-1-yl]ethoxy]-ethanol; 1-(p-chloro-α-pyrid-2-ylbenzyl)-4-[2-(2-hydroxyethoxy)ethyl]piperazine).

PICLORAM* (4-amino-3,5,6-trichloro-picolinic acid; 4-amino-3,5,6-trichloro-2-pyridinecarboxylic acid; 'tordon').

PICLOXYDINE*** (1,1'-[1,4-piperazinediyl-bis(imidocarbonyl)]bis[3-(p-chlorophenyl)-guanidine]; 1,4-bis[N^1-[N^1-(p-chloro-phenyl)amidino]amidino]piperazine).

PICODRALAZINE*** (1-hydrazino-4-pyrid-4-ylmethylphthalazine).

PICOLAMINE*** (3-(aminomethyl)-pyridine).

PICOLINALDEHYDE (2-pyridinaldehyde; 2-formylpyridine).

Picolinaldoxime see Pralidoxime.

2-PICOLINE (2-methylpyridine; α-picoline).

4-PICOLINE (4-methylpyridine; γ-picoline).

PICOLINIC ACID (α-picolinic acid; 2-pyridinecarboxylic acid).

β-Picolinic acid see Nicotinic acid.

γ-Picolinic acid see Isonicotinic acid.

4,4'-(2-Picolylidene)bis(phenylsulfuric acid)disodium salt see Sodium pico-sulfate.

Picoperidamine see Picoperine.

PICOPERINE*** (1-[2-(N-pyrid-2-yl-methylanilino)ethyl]piperidine; 2-[(N-phenyl)(N-piperid-1-ylethyl)amino-methyl]pyridine; N-(2-piperid-1-ylethyl)-N-pyrid-2-ylmethylaniline; N-phenyl-2-piperid-1-yl-N-pyrid-2-ylmethylethyl-amine; picoperidamine; picoperine hydro-chloride; 'coben').

Picosulfol see Sodium picosulfate.

PICRIC ACID (2,4,6-trinitrophenol; carb-

azotic acid; nitroxanthic acid; picronitric acid; 'trinitrophenon', 'trinophenon').

Picronitric acid see Picric acid.

PICROTOXIN (cocculin).

PID see Diphenadione and Phenindione.

'Pielik' see (2,4-Dichlorophenoxy)acetic acid.

PIFENATE*** (ethyl 2,2-diphenyl-3-piperid-2-ylpropionate; ethyl α,α-diphenyl-2-piperidinepropionate; AGN-197).

PIFEXOLE*** (5-(o-chlorophenyl)-3-pyrid-4-yl-1,2,4-oxadiazole; 4-[5-(o-chloro-phenyl)-1,2,4-oxadiazol-3-yl]pyridine; RJ-64).

PIFLUTIXOL** (1-[3-[6-fluoro-2-(trifluoro-methyl)thioxanthen-9-ylidene]propyl]-4-piperidineethanol; 6-fluoro-9-[3-[4-(2-hydroxyethyl)piperid-1-yl]propylidene]-2-(trifluoromethyl)thioxanthene).

PIFOXIME** (1-[(p-acetylphenoxy)acetyl]-piperidine p-oxime; 1-[[p-[1-(hydroxy-imino)ethyl]phenoxy]acetyl]piperidine; LF-77; 'flamanil').

'Pigmentigen 8-MOP' see Methoxsalen.

PIH see Pheniprazine.

Piknolepsin (tr) see Ethosuximide.

PILOCARPINE (5-[(4-ethyl-2,3,4,5-tetra-hydrofuran-5-on-3-yl)methyl]-1-methyl-imidazole; 'borocarpine', 'miocarpine', 'pilocarpol', 'syncarpine', 'vitacarpine').

'Pilocarpol' see Pilocarpine.

'Pimafucin' see Natamycin.

Pimaricin see Natamycin.

PIMECLONE*** (2-piperid-1-ylmethyl-cyclohexanone; 1-(2-oxocyclohexylmethyl)-piperidine; Na-66; 'karion', 'spiractin').

PIMEFYLLINE*** (7-[2-[(pyrid-3-yl-methyl)amino]ethyl]theophylline).

PIMEFYLLINE NICOTINATE (ES-902; 'teonicon').

PIMELIC ACID (heptanedioic acid; 1,5-pentanedicarboxylic acid).

PIMETHIXENE*** (1-methyl-4-(thio-xanthen-9-ylidene)piperidine; 9-(N-methyl-piperid-4-ylidene)thioxanthene; BP-400).

PIMETINE*** (4-benzyl-1-(2-dimethyl-aminoethyl)piperidine; pimetine hydro-chloride; IN-379).

PIMETREMIDE*** (N-methyl-2-phenyl-N-pyrid-3-ylmethylhydracrylamide; tropic acid N-methyl-N-(β-picolyl)amide HBr; N-methyl-N-(3-picolyl)tropicamide-HBr; pimetremide hydrobromide).

PIMINODINE*** (ethyl ester of 1-(3-anilino-propyl)-4-phenylisonipecotic acid; 4-carbethoxy-1-(3-phenylaminopropyl)-4-phenylpiperidine).

PIMINODINE ESILATE (piminodine ethansulfonate; piminodine esylate; 'alvodine').

PIMOZIDE*** (1-[1-[4,4-bis(p-fluorophenyl)-butyl]piperid-4-yl]-2-benzimidazolinone; 1-[4,4-bis(p-fluorophenyl)butyl]-4-(2-oxo-benzimidazolin-1-yl)piperidine; R-6238; 'opiran', 'orap').

Pinacoloxy methyl phosphoryl fluoride see Soman.

PINACOLYL ALCOHOL (3,3-dimethyl-

2-butanol).

Pinacolyl methylphosphonofluoridate
see Soman.

PINAVERIUM BROMIDE*** (4-(6-bromo-
veratryl)-4-[2-[2-(6,6-dimethyl-2-norpinyl)-
ethoxy]ethyl]morpholinium bromide;
4-(2-bromo-4,5-dimethoxybenzyl)-4-[2-[2-
(6,6-dimethylbicyclo(3.1.1)hept-2-yl)-
ethoxy]ethyl]morpholinium bromide).

PINAZEPAM*** (7-chloro-1,3-dihydro-
5-phenyl-1-prop-2-ynyl-2H-1,4-benzo-
diazepin-2-one; Z-905).

PINDOLOL*** (4-(2-hydroxy-3-isopropyl-
aminopropoxy)indole; 1-indol-4-yloxy-
3-isopropylamino-2-propanol; prinodolol;
LB-46).

PINDONE* (2-(2,2-dimethyl-1-oxopropyl)-
1H-indene-1,3(2H)-dione; 2-pivaloyl-
1,3-indandione; 2-(2,2,2-trimethylacetyl)-
1,3-indandione; pivalylindandione; pivaldione; 'pival', 'pivalyl valone').

PINDONE SODIUM ('pivalyn').

PINENE (α-pinene; 2,6,6-trimethylbicyclo-
(3.1.1)-2-heptene).

Pinite *see* Pinitol.

PINITOL (*meso*-inositol methyl ether; matecite; matezite; pinite; sennite).

PINOLCAINE*** (D-(+)-1-methyl-1-
(1-methylpiperid-2-yl)ethyl diphenylacetate; D-(+)-2-(1-methylpiperid-2-yl)-
2-propanol diphenylacetate; D-(+)-2-
(1-hydroxy-1-methylethyl)-
piperidine diphenylacetate (ester)).

PINOXEPIN*** (*cis*-4-[3-(2-chlorodibenz-
(b,e)oxepin-11(6H)-ylidene)propyl]-
1-piperazineethanol; *cis*-4-[3-(2-chloro-
dibenz(b,e)oxepin-11(6H)-ylidene)propyl]-
1-(2-hydroxyethyl)piperazine; pinoxepin
hydrochloride; pinoxepin dihydrochloride;
P-5227).

'Piostacin' *see* Pristinamycin.

'Pioxol' *see* Pemoline.

PIPACYCLINE*** (4-dimethylamino-1,4,4a,
5,5a,6,11,12a-octahydro-3,6,10,12,12a-
pentahydroxy-N-[[4-(2-hydroxyethyl)-
1-piperazinyl]methyl]-6-methyl-1,11-dioxo-
2-naphthacenecarboxamide; N-[4-
(2-hydroxyethyl)piperazin-1-ylmethyl]-
tetracycline; piperazinoethyltetracycline;
mepicycline; 'ambravein', 'mepilon',
'valtomicina').

Pipacycline penicillin V salt *see* Penimepicycline.

Pipacycline phenoxymethylpenicillanate
see Penimepicycline.

'Pipadone' *see* Dipipanone.

'Pipadox' *see* Piperazine adipate.

PIPAMAZINE*** (10-[3-(4-carbamoyl-
1-piperidyl)propyl]-2-chlorophenothiazine;
'mornidine', 'nausidol').

PIPAMPERONE*** (1-[3-(*p*-fluorobenzoyl)-
propyl]-4-piperid-1-ylisonipecotamide;
1'-[3-(*p*-fluorobenzoyl)propyl]-1,4'-bipi-
peridine-4'-carboxamide; 4'-carbamoyl-
1-[3-(*p*-fluorobenzoyl)propyl]-1,4'-bipi-
peridine; 4-(4-carbamoyl-4-piperid-
1-ylpiperidino)-4'-fluorobutyrophenone;

4-(4-carbamoyl-4-piperid-1-ylpiperid-1-yl)-
4'-fluorobutyrophenone; R-3345; fluoro-
pipamide; 'dipiperon', 'piperonyl',
'propitan').

PIPANONE (5-methyl-4,4-diphenyl-
6-piperid-1-yl-3-hexanone; pipanone
hydrochloride; BW-29C48; 'pipidone').

'Piparsine' *see* Piperazine glycolylarsanilate.

PIPAZETATE*** (2-(2-piperid-1-ylethoxy)-
ethyl ester of 10H-pyrido(3,2-b)(1,4)benzo-
thiazine 10-carboxylic acid; 2-(2-piperid-
1-ylethoxy)ethyl ester of 9-thia-1,10-diazan-
thracene-10-carboxylic acid; 2-(2-piperid-
1-ylethoxy)ethyl ester of 1-azapheno-
thiazine-10-carboxylic acid; pipazethate;
thiophenylpyridylamine; pipazetate hydrochloride; D-254; SK&F-70230-A; SQ-
15874; 'leuropect', 'selvigon', 'theratuss').

Pipazethate* *see* Pipazetate.

PIPEBUZONE*** (4-butyl-4-(4-methyl-
piperazin-1-ylmethyl)-1,2-diphenyl-
3,5-pyrazolidinedione; 'elarzone').

PIPECOLIC ACID (2-piperidinecarboxylic
acid; hexahydropicolinic acid; dihydrobaikiaine; homoproline).

2-PIPECOLINE (2-methylpiperidine).

PIPECOLINIC ACID (1-piperidine-
carboxylic acid).

PIPEMIDIC ACID*** (8-ethyl-5,8-dihydro-
5-oxo-2-piperazin-1-ylpyrido(2,3-d)-
pyrimidine-6-carboxylic acid).

PIPENDYL METHANE (1-ethylpiperid-
4-ylidene-1,1'-dithienylmethane; Sch-2747;
'prantal-dithienyl').

'Pipenin' *see* Piperazine.

PIPENZOLATE BROMIDE*** (1-ethyl-
piperid-3-yl benzilate methobromide;
1-ethyl-3-hydroxy-1-methylpiperidinium
bromide benzilate; JB-323; 'piptal').

PIPERACETAZINE*** (2-acetyl-10-[3-[4-
(2-hydroxyethyl)piperid-1-yl]propyl]pheno-
thiazine; 10-[3-[4-(2-hydroxyethyl)piperid-
1-yl]propyl]phenothiazin-2-yl methyl
ketone; PC-1421; 'psymod', 'quide').

PIPERAMIDE*** (4'-[4-(3-dimethylamino-
propyl)piperazin-1-yl]acetanilide; 1-acet-
amidophenyl-4-(3-dimethylaminopropyl)-
piperazine).

PIPERAMIDE MALEATE* (piperamide
dimaleate; CL-54131).

'Piperate' *see* Piperazine tartrate.

'Piperazate' *see* Piperazine phosphate.

Piperazidine *see* Piperazine.

PIPERAZINE (diethylenediamine; piperazidine; hexahydropyrazine; piperazine
hexahydrate; 'anthalazine', 'antipar',
'arpezine', 'arthriticin', 'dispermin',
'helmicid', 'lumbrical', 'novivermol',
'oxyzin', 'parid', 'pipenin', 'telmin',
'thelmin', 'uricida', 'uvilon', 'vermisol').

PIPERAZINE ADIPATE ('adiprazine',
'entacyl', 'eravern', 'helminthex', 'mapiprin', 'nometan', 'oxurasin', 'oxypate',
'oxyzin', 'pipadox', 'toxivers', 'vermicompren').

Piperazine calcium edathamil *see*
Piperazine calcium edetate.

PIPERAZINE CALCIUM EDETATE***
(piperazine calcium edathamil; chelate of
piperazine with edetic acid and calcium;
'perin').

PIPERAZINE CITRATE ('antepar', 'arpezine', 'ascarex', 'exelmin', 'helmezine',
'multifuge', 'oxucide', 'oxyzin', 'parazine',
'pipizan', 'rhomex', 'tasnon', 'ta-verm').

PIPERAZINE CITROSALICYLATE
('urazine').

**PIPERAZINE DIANTIMONYL TAR-
TRATE** (Pi-A-T; 'bilharcid').

1,4-PIPERAZINEDIETHANOL (1,4-bis-
(2-hydroxyethyl)piperazine).

**1,4-Piperazinediethanol di(2-phenyl-
butyrate**) see Febuverine.

**1,4-Piperazinediethanol α-methyl-
1-naphthaleneacetate** see Nafiverine.

**Piperazine-1,4-diphosphoric acid tetra-
ethylenimide** see Dipin.

PIPERAZINE DITHIOCARBAMATE
('choisine').

**1,4-Piperazinediylbis[bis(1-aziridinyl)-
phosphine oxide]** see Dipin.

**1,4-Piperazinediylbis[bis(1-aziridinyl)-
phosphine sulfide]** see Thiodipin.

**1,1'-(Piperazinediyl(1,4)dicarbonimidoyl)-
bis[3-(p-chlorophenyl)guanidine]** see
Picloxydine.

Piperazine edetate see Piperazine calcium
edetate.

PIPERAZINE ESTRONE SULFATE
(sulestrex piperazine; 'harmogen').

PIPERAZINE GLUCONATE ('vermizene').

PIPERAZINE GLYCOLYLARSANILATE
('piparsine').

PIPERAZINE PHOSPHATE ('piperazate',
'pripsen', 'urodan').

PIPERAZINE QUINATE ('sidonal').

PIPERAZINE TARTRATE ('noxiurotan',
'piperate', 'veroxil').

Piperazine theophyllin-7-ylacetate see
Acefylline piperazine.

Piperazinoethyltetracycline see Pipacycline.

2-Piperazin-1-ylquinoline see Quipazine.

PIPERIDINE (hexahydropyridine).

PIPERIDINE CAFFEATE (piperidine
3,4-dihydroxycinnamate; PC-63-1).

1-Piperidinecarboxylic acid see Pipecolinic
acid.

2-Piperidinecarboxylic acid see Pipecolic
acid.

3-Piperidinecarboxylic acid see Nipecotic
acid.

4-Piperidinecarboxylic acid see Isonipecotic acid.

2,6-Piperidinedione see Glutarimide.

1-Piperidineethanol benzilate see Pipethanate.

1-PIPERIDINEPROPANOL (3-piperid-
1-yl-1-propanol).

Piperidinomethylcyclohexane see Leptacline.

**1-Piperidino-3-(p-octylphenyl)-3-propa-
none** see Pipoctanone.

Piperidione see Dihyprylone.

PIPERIDOLATE*** (1-ethylpiperid-3-yl
diphenylacetate; JB-305; 'dactil').

Piperidyl amidone see Dipipanone.

α-Piperid-2-ylbenzhydrol see Pipradrol.

α-Piperid-4-ylbenzhydrol see Azacyclonol.

α-Piperid-2-ylbenzyl acetate see Phacetoperan.

**α-Piperid-2-yl-2,8-bis(trifluoromethyl)-
4-quinolinemethanol** see Mefloquin.

**o-[p-(2-Piperid-1-ylethoxy)benzoyl]-
benzoic acid methyl ester** see Pitofenone.

**2-Piperid-1-ylethyl α-acetoxy-α-benzyl-
hydrocinnamate** see Fenperate.

**2-Piperid-1-ylethoxyethyl 1-azapheno-
thiazine-10-carboxylate** see Pipazetate.

2-Piperid-2-ylethyl o-aminobenzoate see
Piridocaine.

2-Piperid-1-ylethyl benzilate see Pipethanate.

**2-Piperid-1-ylethyl α-benzyl-α-hydroxy-
hydrocinnamate acetate** see Fenperate.

**2-Piperid-1-ylethyl bicyclohexylcarboxyl-
ate** see Dihexyverine.

2-Piperid-1-ylethyl 2,2-diphenylacetate
see Anicaine.

**2-Piperid-1-ylethyl 8-methylflavone-
carboxylate** see Flavoxate.

**2-Piperid-1-ylethyl 3-methyl-2-phenyl-
4-oxo(4H)-1-benzopyran-8-carboxylate**
see Flavoxate.

**2-Piperid-1-ylethyl phenylpiperidyl-
acetate** see Dipiproverine.

**2-Piperid-1-ylethyl p-propoxyphenyl
ketone** see Propipocaine.

**N-(2-Piperid-1-ylethyl)-N-pyrid-2-yl-
methylaniline** see Picoperine.

2-Piperid-1-ylmethyl-1,4-benzodioxan
see Piperoxan.

Piperid-1-ylmethylcyclohexane see
Leptacline.

2-Piperid-1-ylmethylcyclohexanone
see Pimeclone.

**Piperid-1-ylmethyl α-phenylcyclohexane-
glycolate** see Oxyclipine.

3-Piperid-1-yl-1-propanol see 1-Piperidine-
propanol.

1-Piperid-2-yl-2-propanone see Isopelletierine.

β-Piperid-1-yl-4-propoxypropiophenone
see Propipocaine.

3-Piperid-1-ylpropyl m-anisate see
Pribecaine.

3-Piperid-1-ylpropyl 1,2-dicarbanilate
see Diperodon.

3-Piperid-1-ylpropyl m-methoxybenzoate
see Pribecaine.

**6-Piperid-1-yl-2,4-pyrimidinediamine
3-oxide** see Minoxidil.

Piperilate see Pipethanate.

Piperilone see Piperylone.

PIPERINE (1-piperoylpiperidine).

PIPEROCAINE*** (3-(2-methylpiperid-
1-yl)propyl benzoate; benzoate of
3-(2-methylpiperid-1-yl)-1-propanol;
piperocaine hydrochloride).

PIPERONAL (3,4-methylenedioxybenz-
aldehyde).

PIPERONAL BIS[2-(2-BUTOXY-ETHOXY)ETHYL]ACETAL (5-[bis-[2-(2-butoxyethoxy)ethoxy]methyl]-1,3-benzodioxole; 'tropital').

'Piperonyl' see Pipamperone.

PIPERONYL BUTOXIDE* (α-[2-(2-butoxyethoxy)ethoxy]-4,5-methylene-dioxy-2-propyltoluene; O-(4,5-methylene-dioxy-2-propylbenzyl)-O'-butyl diethylene-glycol; 5-[[2-(2-butoxyethoxy)ethoxy]-methyl]-6-propyl-1,3-benzodioxole; 'butacide').

PIPERONYLIC ACID (3,4-methylenedioxy-benzoic acid).

Piperonylic acid 2-(2-butoxyethoxy)ethyl ester see 2-(2-Butoxyethoxy)ethyl piper-onylate.

1-[(4-Piperonylpiperazin-1-yl)acetyl]-phenothiazine see Fenoverine.

2-(4-Piperonylpiperazin-1-yl)pyrimidine see Piribedil.

1-Piperonyl-4-pyrimid-2-ylpiperazine see Piribedil.

PIPEROXAN*** (2-piperid-1-ylmethyl-1,4-benzodioxan hydrochloride; benzo-dioxane; F-933).

1-Piperoylpiperidine see Piperine.

PIPERPHENAMINE* (5-methyl-4-phenyl-1-piperid-1-yl-3-hexanol methobromide; 1-(3-hydroxy-5-methyl-4-phenylhexyl)-1-methylpiperidinium bromide; piperphen-idol methobromide; mepiperphenidol; compound 1575; 'darstine').

PIPERPHENIDOL* (5-methyl-4-phenyl-1-piperid-1-yl-3-hexanol; piperphenidol-hydrochloride; 'reltine').

Piperphenidol methobromide see Piper-phenamine.

PIPERYLONE** (4-ethyl-1-(1-methyl-piperid-4-yl)-3-phenyl-3-pyrazolin-5-one; piperilone; PR-66).

PIPETHANATE*** (2-piperid-1-ylethyl benzilate; 1-piperidineethanol benzilate; piperilate; pipethanate hydrochloride; 'sycotrol').

PIPETHANATE ETHOBROMIDE (1-ethyl-1-(2-hydroxyethyl)piperidinium bromide benzilate; PB-106).

'Pipidone' see Pipanone.

'Pipizan' see Piperazine citrate.

PIPOBROMAN** (1,4-bis(3-bromo-propionyl)piperazine; di(bromopropionyl)-piperazine; A-8103; NSC-25154; 'vercyte').

PIPOCTANONE*** (4'-octyl-3-piperid-1-ylpropiophenone; 1-piperidino-3-(p-octyl-phenyl)-3-propanone; pipoctanone hydro-chloride; N-1113).

'Piportil' see Pipotiazine.

PIPOSULFAN*** (1,4-dihydracryloyl-piperazine dimethanesulfonate; 1,4-bis-(3-hydroxypropionyl)piperazine dimesilate; A-20968; NSC-47774; 'ancyte').

Pipothiazine* see Pipotiazine.

PIPOTIAZINE*** (10-[3-[4-(2-hydroxy-ethyl)piperid-1-yl]propyl]-N,N-dimethyl-phenothiazine-2-sulfonamide; 4-(2-hydroxy-ethyl)-1-[3-(2-dimethylsulfamoylpheno-thiazin-10-yl)propyl]piperidine; pipo-thiazine; RP-19366; 'piportil').

PIPOTIAZINE PALMITATE* (2-[1-[3-[2-(dimethylaminosulfonyl)-10H-phenothiazin-10-yl]propyl]piperidin-4-yl]ethyl hexa-decanoate; FI-6927; IL-19552; RP-19552).

PIPOTIAZINE UNDECENATE (RP-19551).

PIPOXIZINE*** (2-[2-[2-(4-diphenyl-methylenepiperid-1-yl)ethoxy]ethoxy]-ethanol; 4-diphenylmethylene-1-[2-[2-(2-hydroxyethoxy)ethoxy]ethyl]piperidine).

PIPOXOLAN** (5,5-diphenyl-2-(2-piperid-1-ylethyl)-1,3-dioxolan-4-one; BR-18; 'rowapraxin').

PIPRADROL*** (α-piperid-2-ylbenzhydrol; α,α-diphenyl-2-piperidinemethanol; piri-drol; pipradrol hydrochloride; MRD-108; 'alertol', 'gadexyl', 'gerodyl', 'leptidrol', 'meratonic', 'meratran', 'meretran').

PIPRATECOL*** (α-(3,4-dihydroxyphenyl)-4-(2-methoxyphenyl)-1-piperazineethanol; 1-[2-(3,4-dihydroxyphenyl)-2-hydroxy-ethyl]-4-(o-methoxyphenyl)piperazine; 3,4-dihydroxy-α-[4-(o-methoxyphenyl)-piperazin-1-ylmethyl]benzyl alcohol; SE-711).

See also Raubasine with pipratecol.

Piprazine see Piribedil.

PIPRINHYDRINATE*** (4-benzhydryloxy-1-methylpiperidine salt of 8-chlorotheo-phylline; diphenylpyraline teoclate; 'kolton', 'mepedyl', 'sea-legs').

PIPROCURARIUM IODIDE*** (2-(2-diethylaminoethoxy)ethyl ester dimethio-dide of α-phenyl-1-piperidineacetic acid; 1-α-carboxybenzyl-1-methylpiperidinium iodide diethyl-[2-(2-hydroxyethoxy)ethyl]-methylammonium iodide ester; LD-2480; 'brevicurarium').

PIPROFUROL** (α-(p-hydroxyphenethyl)-4,7-dimethoxy-6-(2-piperid-1-ylethoxy)-5-benzofuranmethanol).

PIPROZOLIN*** (ethyl 3-ethyl-4-oxo-5-piperid-1-yl-△²,ˣ-thiazolidineacetate; Gö-919; W-3699; 'probilin').

'Piptal' see Pipenzolate.

PIQUIZIL*** (isobutyl 4-(6,7-dimethoxy-quinazolin-4-yl)-1-piperazinecarboxylate; piquizil hydrochloride; CP-12521-1).

PIR-353 see Indometacin arginine salt.

PIRACETAM** (2-oxo-1-pyrrolidineacet-amide; 1-carbamoylmethyl-2-pyrrolidinone; 2-(2-oxopyrrolidin-1-yl)acetamide; UCB-6215; 'ideaxan', 'nootropyl', 'normabrain').

PIRANDAMINE*** (1,3,4,9-tetrahydro-N,N-1-trimethylindeno(2,1-c)pyran-1-ethylamine; 1-(2-dimethylaminoethyl)-1,3,4,9-tetrahydro-1-methylindeno(2,1-c)-pyran; pirandamine hydrochloride; AY-23713).

Pirazocillin see Prazocillin.

PIRAZOFURIN** (4-hydroxy-5-β-D-ribo-furanosyl-1H-pyrazole-3-carboxamide; 4-hydroxypyrazole-3-carboxamide 5-riboside; 4-hydroxypyrazole-5-carbox-amide 3-riboside; pyrazofurin; L-47599).

PIRBENICILLIN** ((2S, 5R, 6R)-6-[(R)-2-

[2-(isonicotinimidoylamino)acetamido]-2-phenylacetamido]penicillanic acid).

PIRBUTEROL** (α^6-(*tert*-butylamino-methyl)-3-hydroxy-2,6-pyridinedimethanol; 6-(2-*tert*-butylamino-1-hydroxyethyl)-3-hydroxy-2-(hydroxymethyl)pyridine; 2-*tert*-butylamino-1-(5-hydroxy-6-hydroxy-methylpyrid-2-yl)ethanol; pirbuterol dihydrochloride; CP-24314-1).

PIRDONIUM BROMIDE*** (1,1-dimethyl-2-[(*p*-methyl-α-phenylbenzyloxy)methyl]-piperidinium bromide; 1,1-dimethyl-2-(*p*-methylbenzhydryloxymethyl)-piperidinium bromide).

Piref (tr) *see* Diethyl pyrocarbonate.

PIRENZEPINE** (5,11-dihydro-11-[(4-methylpiperazin-1-yl)acetyl]-6H-pyrido(2,3-b)(1,4)benzodiazepin-6-one; 1-[[(5,11-dihydro-6-oxo-6H-pyrido(2,3-b)-(1,4)benzodiazepin-11-yl)carbonyl]-methyl]-4-methylpiperazine; 5,11-dihydro-6-oxo-6H-pyrido(2,3-b)(1,4)benzodiazepin-11-yl 4-methylpiperazin-1-ylmethyl ketone).

PIRETANIDE*** (4-phenoxy-3-pyrrolidin-1-yl-5-sulfamoylbenzoic acid).

'Pirevan' *see* Quinuronium.

'Pirexyl' *see* Benproperine.

PIRFENIDONE*** (5-methyl-1-phenyl-pyrrolidin-2(1H)-one).

PIRIBEDIL*** (2-(4-piperonylpiperazin-1-yl)pyrimidine; 1-piperonyl-4-pyrimid-2-ylpiperazine; 1-(3,4-methylenedioxy-benzyl)-4-pyrimid-2-ylpiperazine; piprazine; piribendyl; pyrimidylpiperonyl-piperazine; ET-495; EU-4290; 'trivastal').

Piribendyl* *see* Piribedil.

Piribenzil *see* Bevonium metilsulfate.

PIRIDOCAINE*** (2-piperidineethanol anthranilate; *o*-aminobenzoate of 2-(2-piperidyl)ethanol; piridocaine hydrochloride; 'lucaine').

'Piridol' *see* Aminophenazone.

'Piridolan' *see* Piritramide.

Piridosal *see* Pethidine.

PIRIDOXILATE*** (2-[(5-hydroxy-4-hydroxymethyl-6-methylpyrid-3-yl)-methoxy]glycolic acid compound with [4,5-bis(hydroxymethyl)-2-methylpyrid-3-yloxy]glycolic acid (1:1); 'glyo 6').

Piridrol (tr) *see* Pipradrol.

Pirilene (tr) *see* Pempidine tosilate.

PIRIMICARB* (2-dimethylamino-5,6-di-methylpyrimidin-4-yl dimethylcarbamate; 'pirimor').

PIRIMIPHOS ETHYL* (*O*-(2-diethylamino-6-methylpyrimidin-4-yl) *O*,*O*-diethyl phosphorothioate).

PIRIMIPHOS METHYL* (*O*-(2-diethyl-amino-6-methylpyrimidin-4-yl) *O*,*O*-dimethyl phosphorothioate; 'actellic').

'Pirimor' *see* Pirimicarb.

PIRINIDAZOLE*** (2-[(1-methyl-5-nitro-imidazol-2-yl)thio]pyridine; 1-methyl-5-nitro-2-[(pyrid-2-ylthio)methyl]-imidazole).

Pirinitramide* *see* Piritramide.

PIRIQUALONE** (2-(2-pyrid-2-ylvinyl)-3-

(*o*-tolyl)quinazolin-4(3H)-one; 2-[2-[4-oxo-3-(*o*-tolyl)quinazolin-2-yl]vinyl]pyridine).

'Pirisal' *see* Morazone.

'Pirissal' *see* Aminophenazone gentisate.

PIRITRAMIDE*** (1'-(3-cyano-3,3-diphen-ylpropyl)-1,4'-bipiperidine-4'-carbox-amide; 1-(3-cyano-3,3-diphenylpropyl)-4-piperid-1-ylpiperidine-4-carboxamide; 4-(4-carbamoyl-4-piperid-1-ylpiperid-1-yl)-2,2-diphenylbutyronitrile; pirinitramide; R-3365; 'dipidolor'; 'piridolan', 'pirium').

'Pirium' *see* Piritramide.

'Pirocrid' *see* Protizinic acid.

'Pirocyl' *see* Quinuronium.

PIROHEPTINE*** (3-(10,11-dihydro-5H-dibenzo(a,d)cyclohepten-5-ylidene)-1-ethyl-2-methylpyrrolidine; piroheptine hydrochloride; 'trimol').

PIROLAZAMIDE*** (hexahydro-α,α-di-phenylpyrrolo(1,2-a)pyrazine-2(1H)-butyramide).

PIROMIDIC ACID*** (5,8-dihydro-8-ethyl-5-oxo-2-pyrrolidin-1-ylpyrido(2,3-d)pyri-midine-6-carboxylic acid).

'Pirothesin' *see* Aptocaine.

PIROXICAM*** (4-hydroxy-2-methyl-*N*-pyrid-2-yl-2H-1,2-benzothiazine-3-carbox-amide 1,1-dioxide).

PIROZADIL*** (2,6-pyridinediyldimethylene bis(3,4,5-trimethoxybenzoate).

PIRPROFEN*** (3-chloro-4-(3-pyrrolin-1-yl)hydratropic acid; 2-[3-chloro-4-(3-pyrrolin-1-yl)phenyl]propionic acid; 1-[4-(1-carboxyethyl)-2-chlorophenyl]-3-pyrroline; Su-21524).

PIRRALKONIUM BROMIDE*** (bis[3-(2,5-dimethylpyrrolidin-1-yl)propyl]hexa-decylmethylammonium bromide).

'Pistocaine' *see* Polidocanol.

Pitayine *see* Quinidine.

PITOFENONE*** (methyl *o*-[*p*-(2-piperid-1-ylethoxy)benzoyl]benzoate).

'Pitressin' *see* Lypressin tannate.

'Pival' *see* Pindone.

Pivaldione *see* Pindone.

PIVALIC ACID* (2,2-dimethylpropionic acid; 2,2,2-trimethylacetic acid).
See also Clocortolone pivalate; Flumeta-sone pivalate; Fluocortolone pivalate; Prednisolone pivalate.

2-Pivaloyl-1,3-indandione *see* Pindone.

Pivaloyloxymethyl (2*S*,5*R*,6*R*)-**6-(per-hydroazepin-1-ylmethyleneamino)-penicillanate** *see* Pevmecillinam.

Pivalylindandione *see* Pindone.

'Pivalyl valone' *see* Pindone.

'Pivalyn' *see* Pindone sodium.

PIVAMPICILLIN*** (hydroxymethyl 6-(D-(−)-α-aminophenylacetamido)penicillinate pivalate; ampicillin hydroxymethyl ester pivalate (ester); pivampicillin hydro-chloride; 'berocillin', 'maxifen', 'pivatil', 'pondocillin').

Pivampicillin *p*-(**dipropylsulfamoyl**)-**benzoate** *see* Pivampicillin probenecid ester.

PIVAMPICILLIN PROBENECID ESTER

367

(pivampicillin *p*-(dipropylsulfamoyl)-benzoate (1:1); pivampicillin probenicidate; MK-356).
'Pivatil' *see* Pivampicillin.
Pivazide *see* Pivhydrazine.
PIVHYDRAZINE* (1-benzyl-2-pivaloylhydrazine; 1-benzyl-2-(trimethylacetyl)-hydrazine; betamezid; pivazide; Ro 4-1634; 'tersavid').
PIVMECILLINAM*** ((2*S*,5*R*,6*R*)-6-[(hexahydroazepin-1-ylmethylene)amino]penicillanic acid pivaloyloxymethyl ester; mecillinam hydroxymethyl ester pivalate; pivaloyloxymethyl (2*S*,5*R*,6*R*)-6-(perhydroazepin-1-ylmethyleneamino)penicillanate; FL-1039).
PIVOXAZEPAM** (oxazepam pivalate ester; oxazepam trimethylacetate).
PIZOTIFEN*** (9,10-dihydro-4-(1-methylpiperid-4-ylidene)-4H-benzo(4,5)cyclohepta-(1,2-b)thiophene; 4-(9,10-dihydro-4H-benzo(4,5)cyclohepta(1,2-b)thien-4-ylidene)-1-methylpiperidine; pizotyline; BC-105; 'litec', 'mosegor', 'sandomigran').
Pizotyline* *see* Pizotifen.
'Placidyl' *see* Ethchlorvynol.
'Planavin' *see* Nitralin.
'Planoform' *see* Butylcaine.
'Planor' *see* Etynodiol diacetate with mestranol.
'Planovin' *see* Megestrol acetate with ethinylestradiol.
PLANTAGO OVATA (psyllium).
See also Ispagula; Sodium psylliate.
'Plantavax' *see* Carboxin dioxide.
'Plaquenil' *see* Hydroxychloroquine.
'Plasdone' *see* Povidone.
'Plasil' *see* Metoclopramide.
'Plasin' *see* Proguanil.
PLASMIN* (fibrinolysin; serum tryptase; 'actase', 'thrombolysin').
PLASMINOGEN* (profibrinolysin; plasma trypsinogen).
Plasmochin *see* Pamaquine.
PLASMOCID (tr) (8-(3-diethylaminopropylamino)-6-methoxyquinoline; plasmozid; plasmocid dihydrochloride; plasmocid diphosphate; plasmocid methylenebis(salicylate); F-710; SN-3115; 'antimalarine', 'rhodoquine').
'Plasmodex' *see* Dextran.
Plasmokinase *see* Streptokinase.
Plasmoquine *see* Pamaquine.
Plasmoquinum *see* Pamaquine.
'Plasmosan' *see* Povidone.
'Plasmozid' *see* Plasmocide.
'Plastenan' *see* Acexamic acid.
cis-**PLATINUM (II) DIAMINODICHLORIDE** (*cis*-dichloridiammine platinum (II); NSC-119875).
PLATYNECINE (2,3,5,6,7,7a*α*-hexahydro-7*β*-hydroxy-1H-pyrrolizine-1*β*-methanol).
'Plavolex' *see* Dextran.
'Plazmoid' *see* Oxypolygelatin.
'Plegicil' *see* Acepromazine.
'Plegicin' *see* Acepromazine.
'Plegicyl' *see* Acepromazine.

'Plegine' *see* Phendimetrazine.
'Pleiatensin' *see* Bietaserpine with hydrochlorothiazide.
'Plenastril' *see* Oxymetholone.
'Pleocide' *see* Aminitrozole.
'Plesmet' *see* Ferroglycine sulfate complex.
'Plethorit-C' *see* Hydralazine.
PLEUROMULIN** (glycolic acid 8-ester with octahydro-5,8-dihydroxy-4,6,9,10-tetramethyl-6-vinyl-3a,9-propano-3aH-cyclopentacycloocten-1(4H)-one).
'Plexiglas' *see* Polymethyl methacrylate.
'Plexochrom' *see* Trisodium edetate.
'Plexombrine' *see* Meglumine acetrizoate.
'Plictran' *see* Cyhexatin.
'Plitrexyl' *see* Ampicillin.
PLUMBAGIN (5-hydroxy-2-methyl-1,4-naphthoquinone).
'Plurine' *see* Hydroflumethiazide.
'Pluronic' *see* Poloxamer.
'Pluryl' *see* Bendroflumethiazide.
PLV-2 *see* Felypressin.
PM-241 *see* Pheniramine.
PM-245 *see* Phenbenzamine.
PM-254 *see* Phenindamine.
PM-255 *see* Diphenhydramine.
PM-262 *see* Methapyrilene.
PM-265 *see* Antazoline.
PM-273 *see* Mepyramine.
PM-284 *see* Promethazine.
PM-297 *see* Glaziovine.
PM-334 *see* Phensuximide.
PM-396 *see* Mesuximide.
PM-671 *see* Ethosuximide.
PM-1807 *see* Fenimide.
PMC *see* Leptacline.
PMP *see* Tolperisone.
PMS *see* Serum gonadotrophin.
PMSG *see* Serum gonadotrophin.
'Pneumorel' *see* Fenspiride.
PNS *see* Nandrolone (*p*-hexyloxy)hydrocinnamate.
PODILFEN*** (1-(*α*-methyl-3,4-methylenedioxyphenethyl)-4-(4-methylthiazol-2-yl)-piperazine; 1-(4-methylthiazol-2-yl)-(3-piperonylprop-2-yl)-4-piperazine).
Podophyllic acid ethylhydrazide *see* Mitopodozide.
PODOPHYLLOTOXIN (5,6,7,8-tetrahydro-8-hydroxy-7-(3,4,5-trimethoxyphenyl)naphtho(2,3-d)-1,3-dioxole-6-carboxylic acid *γ*-lactone; NSC-24818).
PODOPHYLLOTOXIN BENZYLIDENE GLUCOSIDE (SP-G).
POF *see* Protogen.
POISONOAK EXTRACT* (extract of *Toxicodendron quercifolium*; 'anergex').
POLACRILIN*** (divinylbenzene-methacrylic acid polymer).
'Polamidone' *see* Methadone.
'Polaramine' *see* Dexchlorpheniramine.
'Polase' *see* Potassium magnesium aspartate.
'Polawax' *see* Polysorbate 80.
POLDINE METILSULFATE** (2-benzilyloxymethyl-1,1-dimethylpyrrolidinium methosulfate; 2-hydroxymethyl-1,1-dimethylpyrrolidinium methyl sulfate benzilate;

poldine methosulfate; 1-methyl-2-pyrrol-idinemethanol benzilate methylsulfate; poldonium methylsulfate; poldone IS-499; McN-R-726-47; 'nactate', 'nacton').

Poldone* *see* Poldine.

'Polfamycine' *see* Tetracycline.

'Polibutin' *see* Trimebutin.

POLICAPRAM** (poly(iminocarbonyl-pentamethylene); caprolactam polymer; poly[imino(1-oxo-1,6-hexanediyl)]; 'aviamide-6').

POLIDEXIDE*** (dextran cross-linked with epichlorohydrin and O-substituted with 2-diethylaminoethyl groups, some quatern-ized with diethylaminoethyl chloride; dextran 2-(diethylaminoethyl) 2-[2-(di-ethylaminoethyl)diethylammonio]ethyl ether chloride, hydrochloride, epichloro-hydrin cross-linked; PDX; 'secholex').

POLIDOCANOL*** (polyethylene glycol monododecyl ether (av. polymer n=9); oxypolyethoxydodecane; nonaethylene glycol monododecyl ether; hydroxypoly-ethoxydodecane; 'aethoxysklerol', 'ethoxysclerol', 'pistocaine').

POLIGEENAN*** (3,6-anhydro-4-O-β-D-galactopyranosyl-α-D-galactopyranose 2,4'-bis(potassium/sodium sulfate)(1→3')poly-saccharide; polygalactosulfate; carrageenan degradation product; carrageenin depoly-merization product; *Euchema spinosum* degradation product; C-16; 'ebimar').

POLIHEXANIDE*** (poly(iminoimidocar-bonyliminoimidocarbonyliminohexamethyl-ene monohydrochloride)).

Poliklorkamfen (tr) *see* Campheclor.

'Polinalin' *see* Aminopyrine.

POLISAPONIN*** (total steroid saponins from *Dioscorea polystachya*).

'Polistine' *see* Carbinoxamine maleate.

POLITEF** (poly(tetrafluoroethylene); ftoroplast; PTFE; 'fluon', 'teflon').

'Poliuron' *see* Bendroflumethiazide.

'Polival' *see* Tiabendazole.

'Polmiror' *see* Nifuratel.

'Polocaine' *see* Phenacaine.

'Pologols' *see* Macrogols.

POLOXALENE** (polymer containing 67% polyoxypropylene; SK&F-18665; 'bloat guard', 'therabloat').

POLOXALKOL (polymer of ethylene oxide, propylene oxide and propylene glycol; 'magcyl', 'polykol').
See also Dantron with poloxalkol.

POLOXAMER** (α-hydro-ω-hydroxypoly-(oxyethylene)poly(oxypropylene); poly-(oxyethylene) block copolymer; 'pluronic').

Polyanetholesulfonate *see* Sodium polyane-tholesulfonate.

POLYBENZARSOL*** (mixture of polymers from reaction of formaldehyde with 4-hy-droxybenzenearsonic acid; poly(methylene-4-hydroxy-benzenearsonic acid); 'benzoral').

'Polybrene' *see* Hexadimethrine bromide.

Poly(butyl vinyl ether) *see* Polyvinox.

POLYCARBOPHIL CALCIUM*** (calcium polycarbophil; 'quival').

Polychlorcamphene (tr) *see* Camphechlor.

POLYCHLORINATED BIPHENYL MIXTURE (PCB; 'aroclor', 'chlorhextol', 'clophen', 'dykanol', 'inerteen', 'kanechlor', 'niren', 'noflamol', 'phenoclor', 'pyranol', 'therminol').

POLYCHLORINATED TERPHENYL MIXTURE (PCT; 'aroclor').

Polychrome *see* Esculin.

'Polycid' *see* Xantocillin.

'Polycillin' *see* Ampicillin.

'Polycillin-N' *see* Ampicillin sodium.

Polydimethylsiloxane *see* Dimeticone.

POLYESTRADIOL PHOSPHATE* (polyester of estradiol and phosphoric acid; SEP; Leo-114; 'estradurin').

POLYETADENE*** (1,2:3,4-diepoxybutane ethylenimine polymer; 1,2:3,4-diepoxy-butane aziridine polymer; erythritol anhy-dride polyethylenimine polymer; poly-ethadene; L-30639).

Polyethadene* *see* Polyetadene.

Polyethoxyquinoline *see* Ethoxyquin.

Polyethylene glycol monododecyl ether *see* Polidocanol.

Polyethylene glycol p-nonylphenyl ether *see* Nonoxinol.

Polyethylene glycols *see* Macrogols.

Polyethylene polyamine polymer with (chloromethyl)oxirane *see* Colestipol.

Polyethylene sodium sulfonate *see* Sodium polyethylenesulfonate.

POLY(ETHYLENETHIURAM DISUL-FIDE) ('polyram').

POLYFEROSE* (iron chelate of polymerized sucrose derivative; 'jefron').

Polygalactosulfate *see* Poligeenan.

POLYGELINE** (polymer of urea and poly-peptides from denatured gelatin; repoly-merized gelatin; 'haemaccel').

POLYGLACTIN* (glycolic-lactic acid polyester; poly[(oxycarbonyl methylene)m co-(oxycarbonylethylidene)n]; XLG; polyglactin 910; 'vicryl').

Polyglucin (tr) *see* Dextran.

Polyglukina (tr) *see* Dextran.

POLYGLYCOLIC ACID*** (poly(oxycar-bonylmethylene); PGA; 'dexon').

Poly(2-hydroxyethyl methacrylate) *see* Hefilcon A.

Poly(2-hydroxyethyl methacrylate-co-ethylene dimethacrylate-co-methacrylic acid-co-1-vinylpyrrolidin-2-one) *see* Vifilcon A.

POLY I:C (polyinosinic acid polycytidylic acid complex; In:Cn; poly I:poly C; NSC-120949).

Poly(iminoimidocarbonyliminoimido-carbonyliminohexamethylene mono-hydrochloride) *see* Polihexanide.

Poly[imino(1-oxo-1,6-hexanediyl)] *see* Policapram.

Polyinosinic polycytidylic acid complex *see* Poly I:C.

Poly(iminocarbonylpentamethylene) *see* Policapram.

Poly I:poly C *see* Poly I:C.
'Polykol' *see* Poloxalkol.
'Polymal' *see* Macrogols.
Poly[methi[bis(hydroxymethyl)]-
ureylene]amer *see* Polynoxylin.
POLY(1-METHYLENEPIPERAZINE)
('viruseen').
POLYMETHYL METHACRYLATE
(polymerized methyl methacrylate;
'palacos', 'perspex', 'plexiglas').
POLYMYXIN B*** (antibiotic from *Bac.*
polymyxa; bacillosporin; 'aerosporin').
Polymyxin E *see* Colistin.
POLYNOXYLIN*** (poly[methi[bis(hydro-
xymethyl)]ureylene]amer; polymer of
methylenebis(hydroxymethyl)urea; poly-
oxymethyleneurea; 'anaflex', 'larex',
'ponoxylan').
Polyoestradiol *see* Polyestradiol.
Poly(oxycarbonylmethylene) *see* Polyglycolic acid.
Poly[(oxycarbonylmethylene)$_m$ co-(oxy-
carbonylethylidene)$_n$] *see* Polyglactin.
Poly(oxy-1,2-ethanediyloxycarbonyl-1,4-
phenylenecarbonyl) *see* Pegoterate.
Polyoxyethylene nonylphenyl ether(s)
see Nonoxinol(s).
Poly(oxyethyleneoxyterephthaloyl) *see*
Pegoterate.
POLYOXYETHYLENE 20 SORBITAN
(tris(polyethylene glycol 300) sorbitan
ethers).
Polyoxyethylene 20 sorbitan esters *see*
Polysorbate(s).
POLYOXYL LANOLIN* (polyoxyethylene
condensation products of anhydrous
lanolin; 'aqualose').
Polyoxyl 8 stearate* *see* Macrogol
stearate 8.
Polyoxyl 40 stearate* *see* Macrogol
stearate 40.
POLYOXYMETHYLENE GLYCOL
(mixture of polymers of di- and trioxy-
methylene glycols; 'merapid').
Polyoxymethyleneurea *see* Polynoxylin.
Polyporic acid *see* 2,5-Dihydroxy-3,6-di-
phenyl-*p*-benzoquinone.
Polyporin *see* 2,5-Dihydroxy-3,6-diphenyl-*p*-
benzoquinone.
'Polyram' *see* Poly(ethylenethiuram disulfide).
'Polysan' *see* Magnesium hydroxide.
Polysilane* *see* Dimeticone.
Polysiloxane *see* Dimeticone.
POLYSORBATE 20*** (polyoxyethylene 20
sorbitan monolaurate; sorbimacrogol
laurate 300; sorethytan 20 monolaurate;
'emasol', 'tween 20').
POLYSORBATE 40*** (polyoxyethylene 20
sorbitan monopalmitate; sorbimacrogol
palmitate 300; 'tween 40').
POLYSORBATE 60*** (polyoxyethylene 20
sorbitan monostearate; sorbimacrogol
stearate 300; 'tween 60').
POLYSORBATE 65*** (polyoxyethylene 20
sorbitan tristearate; sorbimacrogol tristearate 300; 'tween 65').
POLYSORBATE 80*** (polyoxyethylene 20

sorbitan monooleate; sorbimacrogol oleate
300; sorethytan 20 monooleate; 'monitan',
'oleosorbate 89', 'oleothorb', 'polawax',
'rybadet', 'sorbester', 'sorlate 80', 'tween
80').
POLYSORBATE 85*** (polyoxyethylene 20
sorbitan trioleate; sorbimacrogol trioleate
300; 'tween 85').
Poly(tetrafluoroethylene) *see* Politef.
POLYTHIAZIDE*** (6-chloro-3,4-dihydro-
2-methyl-7-sulfamoyl-3-(2,2,2-trifluoro-
ethylthiomethyl)2H-1,2,4-benzothiadiazine
1,1-dioxide; P-2525; 'drenusil', 'nephril',
'renese').
POLYURETHANE FOAM* ('ostamer').
Polyvidone** *see* Povidone.
POLYVINOX* (poly(butyl vinyl ether);
'Shostakovsky balsam', 'vinilin', 'vinylene').
POLYVINYL ALCOHOL (PV-17; 'alvyl',
'elvanol', 'gelvatol', 'ivalon', 'mowiol',
'pe-ve-gel', 'polyviol', 'resistoflex', 'rhodo-
viol', 'solvar', 'vibatex S', 'vinarol', 'vinol').
POLYVINYLPYRIDINE N-OXIDE
(PVNO; P-204; Bayer 3504).
Polyvinylpyrrolidone *see* Povidone.
'Polyviol' *see* Polyvinyl alcohol.
'Pomarsol' *see* Thiram.
'Pomasol' *see* Thiram.
'Ponalid' *see* Etybenzatropine.
PONCEAU MX (disodium salt of 1-(2,4-
xylylazo)-2-naphthol-3,6-disulfonic acid;
Ponceau R; Ponceau 2R; C.I.No. 16150).
Ponceau R *see* Ponceau MX.
Ponceau 2R *see* Ponceau MX.
PONCEAU SX (disodium salt of 2-(5-sulfo-
2,4-xylylazo)-1-naphthol-4-sulfonic acid;
FD&C Red No. 4; Food red 1; CI-14700).
'Ponderal' *see* Fenfluramine.
'Ponderax' *see* Fenfluramine.
'Ponderex' *see* Fenfluramne.
'Pondinil' *see* Mefenorex.
'Pondocillin' *see* Pivampicillin.
'Ponoxylan' *see* Polynoxylin.
'Ponsital' *see* Imiclopazine.
'Ponstan' *see* Mefenamic acid.
'Ponstel' *see* Mefenamic acid.
'Ponstyl' *see* Mefenamic acid.
'Pontal' *see* Mefenamic acid.
'Pontalin' *see* Chlorbetamide.
'Pontocaine' *see* Tetracaine.
'POP' *see* Paroxypropione.
Populin *see* Salicin benzoate.
'Poquil' *see* Pyrvinium.
POR-8 *see* Ornipressin.
PORFIROMYCIN*** (carbamic acid ester
with 6-amino-1,1a,2,8,8a,8b-hexahydro-8-
(hydroxymethyl)-8a-methoxy-1,5-dimethyl-
azirino(2′,3′:3,4)pyrrolo(1,2-a)indole-4,7-
dione; 6-amino-8-carbamoyloxymethyl-1,
1a,2,8,8a,8b-hexahydro-8a-methoxy-1,5-
dimethylazirino(2′,3′:3,4)pyrrolo(1,2-a)-
indole-4,7-dione; methylmitomycin; NSC-
56410; U-14743).
'Porfyron' *see* Hematoporphyrin.
PORPHOBILINOGEN (2-(aminomethyl)-
4-(2-carboxyethyl)-3-(carboxymethyl)-
pyrrole).

'Portamycin' see Streptolydigin.
'Portyn' see Benzilonium.
'Posedrine' see Beclamide.
'Positol' see Sitosterols.
POSKINE*** (3-[2-phenyl-2-(propionyloxy-
methyl)acetoxy]-6,7-epoxytropane; pro-
pionylscopolamine; propionylhyoscine;
poskine hydrobromide; 'proscopine').
'Postafene' see Meclozine.
'Postonal' see Macrogols.
'Potaba' see Potassium p-aminobenzoate.
POTASSIUM p-AMINOBENZOATE
('potaba').
POTASSIUM 4-AMINOSALICYLATE
('paskalium', 'paskate').
Potassium ascorbate flavonoid complex
see Galascorbin.
POTASSIUM ASPARTATE (Wy-2837).
See also Magnesium aspartate with potas-
sium aspartate; Potassium magnesium
aspartate.
Potassium bitartrate see Potassium
hydrogen tartrate.
Potassium canrenoate see Canrenoate
potassium.
Potassium clorazepate see Dipotassium
clorazepate.
Potassium dichloroisocyanurate see
Troclosene potassium.
Potassium 6,7-dihydro-17-hydroxy-3-oxo-
3'H-cyclopropa(6,7)-17α-pregna-4,6-
diene-21-carboxylate see Prorenoate
potassium.
Potassium 2,3-dihydro-7-nitro-5-phenyl-
1H-1,4-benzodiazepin-2-one-3-carbo-
xylate see Potassium nitrazepate.
Potassium dihydroxy gluconatoaluminate see Potassium glucaldrate.
POTASSIUM DIIODOPHENOL-
SULFONATE (potassium 2,6-diiodo-1-
phenol-4-sulfonate; potassium 3,5-diiodo-
p-phenolsulfonate; potassium soziodolate;
'quimbo', 'quimbosan').
POTASSIUM GLUCALDRATE***
(potassium dihydroxy gluconatoaluminate;
potassium dihydroxy(gluconato)diaquo-
aluminate; glucaldrate potassium; McN-R
1162; 'aciquel').
POTASSIUM GLUCONATE ('kaon').
Potassium guaiacol sulfonate see Sulfogaiacol.
POTASSIUM HYDROGEN TARTRATE
(cream of tartar; K bitartrate; K acid
tartrate).
Potassium levopropylcillin* see
Levopropicillin.
POTASSIUM MAGNESIUM ASPARTATE
('conditio', 'delassine veride', 'elozell',
'healthus D', 'inzellon', 'inzolen', 'intraion',
'panangin' 'polase', 'spartase', 'trophicard').
Potassium menadiol disulfate see
Menadiol potassium sulfate.
Potassium mexrenoate see Mexrenoate
potassium.
POTASSIUM NITRAZEPATE*** (potassium 2,3-dihydro-7-nitro-5-phenyl-1H-1,4-
benzodiazepin-2-one-3-carboxylate).

POTASSIUM PERCHLORATE ('astru-
mal', 'irenat', 'periodin', 'thyrochlorate').
Potassium prorenoate see Prorenoate
potassium.
POTASSIUM SODIUM TARTRATE
(Rochette salt; Seignette salt).
Potassium soziodolate see Potassium di-
iodophenolsulfonate.
Potassium thiophencillin* see Tifencillin.
Potassium 2-(2,4,5-trichlorophenoxy)
propionate see Fenoprop potassium.
Potassium troclosene* see Troclosene
potassium.
'Poteseptyl' see Sulfadimidine with tri-
methoprim.
'Povan' see Pyrvinium embonate.
POVIDONE* (polyvinylpyrrolidone;
PVP; RP-143; 'colidon', 'gemodez',
'hemodyn', 'kollidon', 'neokompensan',
'periston', 'plasdone', 'plasmosan', 'PVP-
macrose', 'protagent', 'subtosan', 'vinisil').
See also Povidone-iodine; Tolpovidone.
POVIDONE-IODINE* (complex of povidone
with iodine; 'betadine', 'bevidine',
'disadine', 'isodine').
PP-036 see Chloramphenicol pantothenate.
PP-4420 see Hexamethonium.
PPCF see Proaccelerin.
PPD see p-Phenylenediamine.
PP-factor see Nicotinamide; Nicotinic acid.
PR-66 see Piperylone.
PR-3847 see Teroxalene.
PRACTOLOL** (4'-(2-hydroxy-3-isopropyl-
aminopropoxy)acetanilide; 1-(p-acetamido-
phenoxy)-3-isopropylamino-2-propanol;
AY-21011; ICI-50172; 'dalzic', 'eraldin').
'Praenitrona' see Trolnitrate.
'Praequine' see Pamaquine.
'Pragmacort' see Prednisone with triam-
cinolone.
'Pragman' see Tolpropamine.
PRAJMALIUM BITARTRATE*** (N-
propylajmalinium hydrogen tartrate;
'neo-gilurtymal').
PRALIDOXIME (2-pyridinaldoxime;
picolinaldoxime; PAM; 2-PAM).
PRALIDOXIME CHLORIDE* (2-pyridin-
aldoxime methochloride).
PRALIDOXIME DODECYL IODIDE
(PAD).
PRALIDOXIME IODIDE*** (2-pyridin-
aldoxime methiodide; 2-formyl-1-methyl-
pyridinium iodide oxime; 2-(hydroxy-
iminomethyl)-1-methylpyridinium iodide;
pralidoxime methiodide; picolinaldoxime
methiodide; 2-PAM iodide; 'protopam').
PRALIDOXIME MESILATE (pralidoxime
methanesulfonate; pralidoxime mesylate;
P2S; RP-7676; 'contrathion').
Pralidoxime methanesulfonate see
Pralidoxime mesilate.
Pralidoxime methiodide see Pralidoxime
iodide.
Pralidoxime methyl ether see Obidoxime.
PRALIDOXIME PHENACYL CHLORIDE
(FAOP).
'Pramidex' see Tolbutamide.

Pramindole see Iprindole.
PRAMIVERINE*** (4,4-diphenyl-*N*-iso-propylcyclohexylamine; *N*-isopropyl-4,4-diphenylcyclohexylamine; Hsp-2986; 'sintaverin').
PRAMOCAINE*** (4-butoxy-1-[3-(4-morpholino)propoxy]benzene; 4-[3-(*p*-butoxyphenoxy)propyl]morpholine; *p*-butoxyphenyl 3-morpholinopropyl ether; pramoxine; pramocaine hydrochloride; 'anugesic', 'tronothane').
'Pramolan' see Opipramol.
Pramoxine' see Pramocaine.
PRAMPINE*** (*O*-propionylatropine; propionate ester of atropine).
PRAMPINE METHONITRATE (PAMN).
PRANOLIUM CHLORIDE*** ((2-hydroxy-3-naphth-1-yloxypropyl)isopropyldimethyl-ammonium chloride; *N*-methylpropranolol methochloride; 2-hydroxy-*N*,*N*-dimethyl-*N*-(1-methylethyl)-3-(1-naphthalenyloxy)-1-propanaminium chloride; SC-27761).
PRANOLIUM IODIDE (*N*-methylpro-pranolol methiodide; UM-272).
PRANOSAL*** (2,5-dimethyl-1-pyrrolidine-propanol salicylate (ester)).
'Prantal' see Diphemanil metilsulfate.
'Prantal-dithienyl' see Pipendyl methane.
PRASTERONE** (3*β*-hydroxyandrost-5-en-17-one; androst-5-en-3*β*-ol-17-one; dehydroepiandrosterone; dehydroandro-sterone; DHA; 'chetovis', 'diandrone', 'hormoformin').
PRASTERONE ENANTATE WITH ESTRADIOL VALERATE (SH-70833 D).
PRATOL (7-hydroxy-4'-methoxyflavone).
'Pravacillin' see Metampicillin.
'Pravocaine' see Propoxycaine.
PRAXADINE*** (pyrazole-1-carboxa-midine).
'Praxilene' see Naftidrofuryl.
'Praxinor' see Cafedrine with theodrenaline.
'Praxiten' see Oxazepam.
PRAZEPAM*** (7-chloro-1-(cyclopropyl-methyl)-1,3-dihydro-5-phenyl-2H-1,4-benzodiazepin-2-one; W-4020; 'demetrim', 'demetrin', 'reapam').
PRAZEPINE** (5-(3-dimethylaminopropyl)-5,6-dihydro-11H-dibenz(b,e)azepine; 5-(3-dimethylaminopropyl)5,6-dihydro-morphanthridine).
'Prazil' see Chlorpromazine.
'Prazine' see Promazine.
PRAZIQUANTEL** (2-(cyclohexylcarbo-nyl)-1,2,3,6,7,11b-hexahydro-4H-pyrazino-(2,1-a)isoquinolin-4-one; EMBAY 8440).
PRAZITONE** (5-phenyl-5-piperid-2-ylmethylbarbituric acid; prazitone hydro-chloride; AGN-511).
PRAZOCILLIN** (6-[1-(2,6-dichlorophen-yl)-4-methylpyrazol-5-ylcarboxamido]-penicillanic acid; pyrazocillin; pirazocillin; prazocillin sodium; F-75).
PRAZOSIN*** (1-(4-amino-6,7-dimethoxy-quinazolin-2-yl)4-(2-furoyl)piperazine; 4-amino-2-[4-(2-furoyl)-6,7-dimethoxy-piperazin-1-yl]quinazoline; furazosin

hydrochloride; CP-12299-1; 'hypovase', 'minipress', 'sinetens').
'Prebane' see Terbutryn.
Prebediolone see Pregnenolone.
Précipité blanc see Mercurous chloride.
Preconsol (tr) see 8-Quinolinol.
Prednacinolone acetonide see Desonide.
PREDNAZATE*** (compound of predniso-lone 21-hydrogen succinate with perphena-zine).
PREDNAZOLINE*** (prednisolone 21-dihy-drogen phosphate compound with 2-(2-iso-propylphenoxymethyl)-2-imidazoline; fenoxazoline prednisolone compound; 'deturgylone').
PREDNIMUSTINE** (prednisolone 21-[4-[*p*-[bis(2-chloroethyl)amino]phenyl]-butyrate]; chlorambucil prednisolone 21-ester).
PREDNISOLAMATE*** (prednisolone 21-diethylaminoacetate; prednisolone 21-(*N*,*N*-diethylglycine ester); prednisolamate hydrochloride; 'deltacortril DA').
PREDNISOLONE*** (pregna-1,4-diene-11*β*,17*α*,21-triol-3,20-dione; 11*β*,17*α*,21-trihydroxypregna-1,4-diene-3,20-dione; dehydrocortisol; △¹-dehydrohydrocortisone; delta F; deltahydrocortisone; metacortan-dralone; NSC-9120; prednisolone alcohol or acetate).
See also Oxyphenbutazone with predniso-lone; Phenylbutazone with prednisolone.
Prednisolone acetamidocaproate see Prednisolone acexamate.
Prednisolone acetate see Prednisolone.
PREDNISOLONE ACEXAMATE (pred-nisolone 6-acetamidohexanoate; predniso-lone acetamidocaproate).
Prednisolone 21-[4-[*p*-[bis(2-chloroethyl)-amino]phenyl]butyrate] see Predni-mustine.
PREDNISOLONE *tert*-**BUTYLACETATE** ('codelcortone-TBA').
Prednisolone 21-diethylaminoacetate see Prednisolamate.
Prednisolone 21-(*N*,*N*-diethylglycine ester) see Prednisolamate.
Prednisolone 21-dihydrogen phosphate compound with fenoxazoline see Prednazoline.
PREDNISOLONE PIVALATE (predniso-lone trimethylacetate; 'ultracortenol').
PREDNISOLONE SODIUM PHOSPHATE (prednisolone 21-phosphoric acid disodium salt; 'codelsol', 'hydeltrasol', 'predsol').
PREDNISOLONE SODIUM SUCCINATE ('soludacortin').
PREDNISOLONE SODIUM *m*-**SULFO-BENZOATE** (R-812; 'solucort').
PREDNISOLONE STEAGLATE*** (prednisolone 21-stearoylglycolate; stearate ester of prednisolone 21-glycolate; 'glistel-one', 'sintisone').
PREDNISOLONE *m*-**SULFOBENZOATE** ('solupred').
Prednisolone trimethylacetate see Prednisolone pivalate.

PREDNISOLONE TRIMETHYLOCTA-NOATE ('mecortolone').
Prednisolone valerate *see* Prednival.
PREDNISONE**** (pregna-1,4-diene-17α, 21-diol-3,11,20-trione; 17α,21-dihydroxy-pregna-1,4-diene-3,11,20-trione; $\triangle^1$-dehydrocortisone; 1,2-dehydrocortisone; deltacortisone; metacortandracin; delta E; NSC-10023; prednisone alcohol or acetate).
See also Chloramphenicol with prednisone; Phenylbutazone with prednisone.
PREDNISONE WITH TRIAMCINOLONE ('pragmacort').
PREDNIVAL* (prednisolone 17-valerate; W-4869).
PREDNYLIDENE**** (11β,17,21-trihydroxy-16-methylenepregna-1,4-diene-3,20-dione; 16-methyleneprednisolone; ST-104; 'decortilen').
'Predsol' *see* Prednisolone sodium phosphate.
'Preeglone' *see* Paraquat.
'Prefar' *see* Bensulide.
'Prefix' *see* Chlorthiamid.
'Prefox' *see* Ethiolate.
'Preforan' *see* Fluorodifen.
Pregna-1,4-diene-11β,17α-diol-3,20-dione *see* Deprodone.
Pregna-3,5-diene-3,17-diol-20-one 3-cyclopentyl ether *see* Pentagestrone.
Pregna-1,4-diene-17,21-diol-3,11,20-trione *see* Prednisone.
9β,10α-Pregna-4,6-diene-3,20-dione *see* Dydrogesterone.
Pregna-1,4-diene-11β,16α,17,21-tetrol-3,20-dione cyclic acetal with acetone *see* Desonide.
Pregna-1,4-diene-11β,17α,21-triol-3,20-dione *see* Prednisolone.
17α-Pregna-2,4-dien-20-yno(2,3-d)isoxazol-17-ol *see* Danazol.
Pregnancy urine extract *see* Chorionic gonadotrophin.
Pregnane *see* 5β-Pregnane.
5α-PREGNANE (17β-ethyl-5α-androstane; 17β-ethyletioallocholane; allopregnane).
5β-PREGNANE (17β-ethyl-5β-androstane; 17β-ethyletiocholane; pregnane).
5α-Pregnane-3α,21-diol-11,21-dione *see* Alfadolone.
Pregnan-3α-ol-11,20-dione *see* Renanolone.
5α-Pregnan-3α-ol-11,20-dione *see* Alfaxalone.
Pregnan-21-ol-3,20-dione *see* Hydroxydione.
PREGNAN-20-ONE (17-acetylandrostane).
Pregnant mare serum gonadotrophin *see* Seric gonadotrophin.
4-Pregnen-18-al-11β,21-diol-3,20-dione *see* Aldosterone.
PREGN-20-ENE (17β-vinylandrostane).
4-Pregnene-3,20-dione *see* Progesterone.
4-Pregnene-11,21-diol-3,20-dione *see* Corticosterone.
4-Pregnene-16α,17-diol-3,20-dione *see* Algestone.
4-Pregnene-17α,21-diol-3,20-dione *see*

Cortodoxone.
4-Pregnene-14,17-diol-3,20-dione cyclic acetal with propionaldehyde *see* Proligestone.
4-Pregnen-21-ol-3,20-dione *see* Desoxycortone.
4-Pregnen-17β-ol-3,20-dione *see* Hydroxyprogesterone.
4-Pregnene-17α-21-diol-3,11,20-trione *see* Cortisone.
4-Pregnene-11β,16α,21-triol-3,20-dione *see* Hydrocortisone.
Pregneninolone *see* Ethisterone.
Pregneninonol *see* Ethisterone.
PREGNENOLONE**** (5-pregnen-3β-ol-20-one; 5-pregnen-3-ol-20-one; 3β-hydroxy-pregn-5-en-20-one; 3-hydroxy-20-oxo-5-pregnene; prebediolone).
PREGNENOLONE ACETATE (acetoxy-pregnenolone).
PREGNENOLONE SUCCINATE* (pregnenolone hydrogen succinate; 'panzalone').
5-Pregnen-3β-ol-20-one *see* Pregnenolone.
4-Pregnen-21-ol-3,11,20-trione *see* 11-Dehydrocorticosterone.
Pregnocin *see* Hydroxydione.
'Pregnon 28' *see* Ethinylestradiol with lynestrenol.
'Pregnyl' *see* Chorionic gonadotrophin.
PREGN-20-YNE (17-ethynylandrostane).
'Pregova' *see* Human menopausal gonadotrophin.
'Preludin' *see* Phenmetrazine.
'Premarin' *see* Conjugated estrogens.
'Premerge' *see* Dinoseb trolamine.
'Preminex' *see* Mebutamate.
'Prempar' *see* Ritodrine.
Prenazone *see* Feprazone.
Prenol *see* 3-Methyl-2-buten-1-ol.
'Prensols' *see* Hexylresorcinol.
'Prentif' *see* Hexylresorcinol.
PRENYLAMINE**** (N-(3,3-diphenyl-propyl)-α-methylphenethylamine; N-(3,3-diphenylpropyl)-1-phenyl-2-propylamine; 3,3-diphenyl-N-(3-phenylprop-2-yl)-1-propylamine; N-(3,3-diphenylpropyl)-amphetamine; B-346; FPDFPA).
PRENYLAMINE LACTATE ('corontin', 'falicor', 'hostaginan', 'sedolatan', 'segontin', 'synadrin').
4-Prenyl-1,2-diphenyl-3,5-pyrazolidine-dione *see* Feprazone.
'Preortan' *see* Ornithine carbamyl transferase.
'Pre-par' *see* Ritodrine.
'Preparin' *see* Ethaverine.
'Prequine' *see* Pamaquine.
'Pre-sate' *see* Chlorphentermine.
'Presidal' *see* Pentacynium.
'Presidal' *see* Pentacynium.
'Presidon' *see* Pyrithyldione.
'Presinol' *see* Methyldopa.
'Presomen' *see* Conjugated estrogens.
'Pressedrine' *see* Norephedrine.
'Pressomin' *see* Methoxamine.
'Pressonex' *see* Metaraminol.
'Pressoton' *see* Etilefrine.

'**Prestonal**' *see* Dioxahexadekanium bromide.
'**Presuren**' *see* Hydroxydione.
'**Presyn**' *see* Allethrin.
PRETAMAZIUM IODIDE*** (4-(4-bi-phenylyl)-3-ethyl-2-(*p*-pyrrolidin-1-ylstyryl)thiazolium iodide).
PRETHCAMIDE* (cropropamide plus crotethamide; mixture of 2-(crotonyl-propylamino)-*N*,*N*-dimethylbutyramide and 2-(crotonylethylamino)-*N*,*N*-di-methylbutyramide; G-5668; 'microen').
PRETIADIL*** (6,11-dihydro-6-methyl-11-[3-[methyl(α-methylphenethyl)amino]propyl]dibenzo(1,2,5)thiadiazepine 5,5-dioxide; *N*-[3-(6,11-dihydro-6-methyl-5,5-dioxidobibenzo(1,2,5)thiadiazepin-11-yl)propyl]-*N*,α-dimethylphenethylamine; *N*-[3-(6,11-dihydro-6-methyl-5,5-dioxido-dibenzo(1,2,5)thiadiazepin-11-yl)propyl]-*N*-methylamphetamine).
'**Prevenol**' *see* Bithionol.
'**Preventa**' *see* Anagestone acetate with mestranol.
'**Preventol-G-D**' *see* Dichlorophen.
'**Prevepen**' *see* Propicillin.
'**Priadel**' *see* Lithium carbonate.
'**Priamide**' *see* Isopropamide.
PRIBECAINE*** (3-piperid-1-ylpropyl *m*-anisate; 3-piperid-1-ylpropyl *m*-methoxy-benzoate).
PRIDINOL*** (α,α-diphenyl-1-piperidine-propanol; 1,1-diphenyl-3-piperid-1-yl-1-propanol; diphenylpiperidinopropanol; 'ParKS 12').
PRIDINOL MESILATE (pridinol methane-sulfonate; 'lyseen', 'ridinol').
PRIFINIUM BROMIDE*** (3-benzhydryl-idene-1,1-diethyl-2-methylpyrrolidinium bromide; 3-(diphenylmethylene)-1,1-diethyl-2-methylpyrrolidinium bromide; prodifenium bromide; 'padrin', 'riabal').
PRILOCAINE*** (*N*-(2-propylaminopro-pionyl)-*o*-toluidine; 2-methyl-2-propyl-amino-*o*-acetotoluidide; 2′-methyl-2-pro-pylaminopropionanilide; 2-propylamino-*o*-propionotoluidide; prilocaine hydrochlor-ide; propitocaine; Astra-1512; L-67; MY-33-7; 'bledocaine', 'citanest', 'xylonest').
'**Primacaine**' *see* Metabutoxycaine.
Primaclone *see* Primidone.
'**Primamycin**' *see* Hamycin.
PRIMAPERONE** (4′-fluoro-4-piperid-1-ylbutyrophenone; 4′-fluoro-4-piperidino-butyrophenone; 1-[3-(*p*-fluorobenzoyl)-propyl]piperidine).
PRIMAQUINE*** (8-(4-amino-1-methyl-butylamino)-6-methoxyquinoline; SN-13272).
PRIMIDONE** (5-ethyldihydro-5-phenyl-4,6(1H,5H)-pyrimidinedione; desoxypheno-barbitone; 2-desoxyphenobarbital; hexa-midine; primaclone; 'lepsiral', 'liskantin', 'mylepsin', 'mysoline', 'sertan').
PRIMIN (6-methoxy-6-pentyl-*p*-benzo-quinone).
'**Primin**' *see* 1-Isopropyl-3-methylpyrazol-5-

yl dimethylcarbamate.
'**Primobolan**' *see* Metenolone.
'**Primobolan depot**' *see* Metenolone enan-tate.
'**Primobolan S**' *see* Metenolone acetate.
'**Primolut depot**' *see* Hydroxyprogesterone caproate.
'**Primolut N**' *see* Norethisterone.
'**Primperan**' *see* Metoclopramide.
PRIMULETIN (5-hydroxyflavone).
'**Prinadol**' *see* Phenazocine.
'**Prinalgin**' *see* Alclofenac.
'**Principen**' *see* Ampicillin.
Prinodolol* *see* Pindolol.
'**Prioderm**' *see* Malathion.
'**Priscol**' *see* Tolazoline.
'**Prisilidene**' *see* Alphaprodine.
PRISTANE (2,6,10,14-tetramethylpentade-cane; norphytane).
PRISTINAMYCIN*** (antibiotic from *Str. pristina spiralis*; RP-7293; 'piostacin', 'pyostacin', 'stapyocine').
'**Privine**' *see* Naphazoline.
PRN *see* Phenyltoloxamine.
'**Pro-actidil**' *see* Triprolidine.
PROADIFEN*** (2-diethylaminoethyl 2,2-diphenylvalerate; diethylaminoethyl diphenylpropylacetate; proadifen hydro-chloride; SK&F-525-A).
Proazamine *see* Promethazine.
'**Proban**' *see* Cythioate.
PROBARBITAL SODIUM*** (sodium derivative of 5-ethyl-5-isopropylbarbituric acid; 'ipral').
'**Probe**' *see* Chlormethazole.
'**Probecid**' *see* Probenecid.
PROBENECID*** (*p*-(dipropylsulfamoyl)-benzoic acid; etamid; ethamid; 'benemid', 'probecid', 'probenid', 'prolongine', 'uricosid').
See also Pivampicillin probenecid ester.
'**Probenid**' *see* Probenecid.
'**Probilin**' *see* Piprozolin.
'**Probon**' *see* Rimazolium metilsulfate.
PROBUCOL*** (acetone bis(3,5-di-*tert*-butyl-4-hydroxyphenyl)mercaptole; isopropylidenedithiobis(2,6-di-*tert*-butyl-phenol); 4,4′-isopropylidenedithiobis(2,6-di-*tert*-butylphenol); DH-581; 'biphena-bid').
Probunafon *see* Levopropoxyphene dibudi-nate.
'**Procacillin**' *see* Procaine-penicillin.
PROCAINAMIDE*** (*p*-amino-*N*-(2-di-ethylaminoethyl)benzamide; procaine amide; procainamide hydrochloride).
PROCAINAMIDE WITH QUINIDINE ('rhythmochin').
PROCAINE*** (2-diethylaminoethyl *p*-aminobenzoate; procaine hydrochloride; H-3).
Procaine amide *see* Procainamide.
PROCAINE-CAFFEINE COMPLEX ('impletol').
Procaine 8-chlorotheophyllinate *see* Procaine teoclate.
PROCAINE-PENICILLIN (compound of 2

374

mol. procaine with 1 mol. penicillin G; novocillin).
See also Dihydrostreptomycin with procaine-penicillin.

PROCAINE-PENICILLIN ALUMINIUM MONOSTEARATE (PAM).

PROCAINE TEOCLATE (procaine 8-chlorotheophyllinate; procaine theoclate; 'francaine').

PROCAINE WITH VITAMINS ('aslavital')

'Procalm' *see* Benactyzine.

Procalmadiol *see* Meprobamate.

PROCARBAZINE*** (*N*-isopropyl-α-(2-methylhydrazino)-*p*-toluamide; 1-(4-isopropylcarbamoylbenzyl)-2-methylhydrazine; *N*-isopropyl-*p*-(2-methylhydrazinomethyl)benzamide; ibenzmethyzin; procarbazine hydrochloride; MIH; NSC-77213; Ro-4-6467; 'methylhydrazine', 'matulane', 'natulan', 'natulanar').

Prochlorpemazine *see* Prochlorperazine.

PROCHLORPERAZINE*** (2-chloro-10-[3-(4-methylpiperazin-1-yl)propyl]phenothiazine; chlormeprazine; chlorperazine; meterazine; prochlorpemazine; RP-6140; SK&F-4657; 'capazine', 'compazine', 'dicopal', 'nipodal', 'stemetil', 'tementil', 'temetil', 'vertigon').

PROCINOLOL*** (1-(*o*-cyclopropylphenoxy)-3-isopropylamino-2-propanol.

'Proclival' *see* Bufeniode.

PROCLONOL*** (α,α-bis-(*p*-chlorophenyl)-cyclopropanemethanol; R-8284).

'Procoagulo' *see* Menadiol sodium phosphate.

'Procol' *see* Norephedrine.

'Procortolon' *see* Triamcinolone.

'Procto-glyvenol' *see* Tribenoside.

PROCYCLIDINE*** (α-cyclohexyl-α-phenyl-1-pyrrolidinepropanol; 1-cyclohexyl-1-phenyl-3-pyrrolidin-1-yl-1-propanol; procyclidine hydrochloride; 'kemadrin', 'onservan').

Procyclidine methochloride *see* Tricyclamol.

PROCYMATE** (1-cyclohexylpropyl carbamate; 'equipax').

'Procytox' *see* Cyclophosphamide.

PRODECONIUM BROMIDE*** (dipropyl ester of [decamethylenebis(oxymethylene)]-bis[(carboxymethyl)dimethylammonium bromide]; 2,13-dioxatetradecamethylene-1,14-bis[dimethyl(carbopropoxymethyl)-ammonium bromide]).

'Prodermide' *see* Sodium dodecyl sulfate

'Pro-diaban' *see* Glisoxepide.

'Prodiaben' *see* Chlorpropamide.

PRODILIDINE*** (1,2-dimethyl-3-phenyl-3-pyrrolidyl propionate; prodilidine hydrochloride; A-1981-12; CI-427; Wy-1359; 'cogesic').

PRODOLIC ACID*** (1,3,4,9-tetrahydro-1-propylpyrano(3,4-b)indole-1-acetic acid; AY-23289).

'Prodox' *see* Hydroxyprogesterone.

'Produral' *see* Procaine-penicillin.

PROFADOL*** (*m*-(1-methyl-3-propyl-

pyrrolidin-3-yl)phenol; 3-(*m*-hydroxyphenyl)-1-methyl-3-propylpyrrolidine; profadol hydrochloride; A-2205; CI-572).

PROFENAMINE*** (10-(2-diethylaminopropyl)phenothiazine; ethopropazine; isothazine; isothiazine; parfezin; phenopropazine; prophenamine; profenamine hydrochloride; RP-3356; SC-2538).

'Profenid' *see* Ketoprofen.

'Profenil' *see* Alverine.

'Profenone' *see* Paroxypropione.

PROFEXALONE*** (2-oxo-5-phenyl-*N*-propyloxazolidine-3-carboxamide).

Profibrinolysin *see* Plasminogen.

PROFLAVINE** (3,6-diaminoacridine).

PROFLAVINE HEMISULFATE (neutral proflavine sulfate; 'isoflav').

PROFLAZEPAM** (7-chloro-1-(2,3-dihydroxypropyl)-5-(*o*-fluorophenyl)-1,3-dihydro-2H-1,4-benzodiazepin-2-one).

'Proformiphen' *see* Phenprobamate.

'Progallin' *see under* Gallic acid.

'Progeril' *see* Dihydroergotoxine esilate with papaverine.

'Progeryl' *see* Dihydroergotoxine esilate with papaverine.

PROGESTERONE*** (pregn-4-ene-3,20-dione; corpus luteum hormone; luteohormone; NSC-9704).

Progesterone hydroxycaproate *see* Progesterone hydroxyhexanoate.

PROGESTERONE HYDROXYHEXANO-ATE (progesterone hydroxycaproate).
See also Estradiol valerate with progesterone hydroxyhexanoate.

'Proglicem' *see* Diazoxide.

PROGLUMETACIN** (3-[4-(2-hydroxyethyl)piperazin-1-yl]propyl DL-4-benzamido-*N*,*N*-dipropylglutaramate 1-(*p*-chlorobenzoyl)-5-methoxy-2-methylindole-3-acetate (ester); indometacin ester with 3-[4-(2-hydroxyethyl)piperazin-1-yl]propyl DL-4-benzamido-*N*,*N*-dipropylglutaramate).

PROGLUMIDE** (DL-4-benzamido-*N*,*N*-dipropylglutaramic acid; xilamide; KXM; 'milid', 'nulsa', 'xyde', 'xylamide').

PROGLUMIDE WITH SCOPOLAMINE BUTYL BROMIDE (CR-242-B; 'buscalide').

'Proguanide' *see* Proguanil.

PROGUANIL*** (1-(*p*-chlorophenyl)-5-isopropylbiguanide; bigumal; chloriguane; chlorguanide; chloroguanil; diguanyl; proguanil hydrochloride; M-4888; RP-3359; SN-12837; 'balusil', 'drinupal', 'guanatol', 'paludrine', 'palusil', 'plasin', 'proguanide', 'tirian').

Proguanil metabolite *see* Cycloguanil.

'Progynova' *see* Estradiol valerate.

'Prohalone' *see* Haloprogesterone.

Proheptadiene *see* Amitriptyline.

PROHEPTATRIENE (5-(3-dimethylaminopropylidene)(5H)-dibenzo(a,d)cycloheptene).

PROHEPTAZINE*** (1,3-dimethyl-4-phenyl-4-propionoxyazacycloheptane; hexahydro-1,3-dimethyl-4-phenylazepin-4-

ol propionate ester; 1,3-dimethyl-4-phenyl-4-propionoxyhexamethylenimine).

'Prokarbol' *see* Dinitro-*o*-cresol.
'Proketazine' *see* Carfenazine maleate.
'Proladyl' *see* Pyrrobutamine.
'Prolan' *see* Chorionic gonadotrophin.
'Prolate' *see* Dimethyl phthalimidomethyl phosphorodithioate.
'Prolergic' *see* Cycliramine.
PROLIGESTONE*** (14,17-dihydroxy-pregn-4-ene-3,20-dione cyclic acetal with propionaldehyde; 14,17-dihydroxyprogesterone cyclic acetal with propionaldehyde; pregn-4-ene-14,17-diol-3,20-dione cyclic acetal with propionaldehyde).
'Proligne' *see* Amfepentorex.
PROLINE (2-pyrrolidinecarboxylic acid).
PROLINTANE*** (1-(α-propylphenethyl)-pyrrolidine; 1-phenyl-2-pyrrolidino-pentane; prolintane hydrochloride; Sp-732; 'catovit', 'katovit').
'Prolixan 300' *see* Azapropazone.
'Prolixene' *see* Fluphenazine.
'Proloid' *see* Levothyroxine sodium.
'Prolongine' *see* Probenecid.
PROLONIUM IODIDE*** (2-hydroxytri-methylene-1,3-bis(trimethylammonium iodide); bismethiodide of 1,3-bis(dimethylamino)-2-propanol; hydroxytrimethonium iodide; propiodal; 'dovine', 'endoiodine', 'endoton', 'endoyodina', 'entodon', 'esoiodine', 'hexayodina', 'iodisan', 'yodanodia').
'Prolosan' *see* Serum gonadotrophin.
Proluton C *see* Ethisterone.
'Proluton depot' *see* Hydroxyprogesterone caproate.
'Proma' *see* Promazine.
'Promacetin' *see* Sulfadiasulfone.
'Promactil' *see* Chlorpromazine.
'Promantine' *see* Promazine.
'Promanyl' *see* Promazine.
'Promaquid' *see* Dimetotiazine mesilate.
PROMAZINE** (10-(3-dimethylaminopropyl)phenothiazine; propazin; promazine hydrochloride; A-145; RP-3276; Wy-1094; 'alofen', 'ampazine', 'centractyl', 'esparin', 'lete', 'liranol', 'neo-hibernex', 'neuroplegil', 'piarine', 'prazine', 'proma', 'promantine', 'promanyl', 'promilene', 'promwill', 'protactil', 'protactyl', 'pro-tan', 'sediston', 'sparine', 'tomil', 'varophen', 'verophen').
See also Methaqualone with promazine.
'Promazol' *see* Chlorpromazine.
PROMECARB* (3-isopropyl-5-methyl-phenyl methylcarbamate; 3-methyl-5-(1-methylethyl)phenyl methylcarbamate; 'carbamult', 'minacide').
Promedol (tr) *see* Trimeperidine.
Promeran (tr) *see* Chlormerodrin.
PROMESTRIENE** (17β-methoxy-3-propoxyestra-1,3,5(10)-triene; estradiol 17β-methyl ether 3-propyl ether; 'colpo-trophin').
PROMETHAZINE*** (10-(2-dimethyl-aminopropyl)phenothiazine; diprazine; proazamine; promethazine hydrochloride; difasin; difazin; diphasin; diphazin;

L-01516; PM-284; RP-3277; RP-3389; RP-4460; 'Fen-bridal').
Promethazine 8-chlorotheophyllinate *see* Promethazine teoclate.
PROMETHAZINE *S,S*-DIOXIDE (promethazine 5,5-dioxide; 9,9-dioxopromethazine; 'prothanon').
PROMETHAZINE HYDROXYETHYL CHLORIDE (dimethyl(2-hydroxyethyl)-[1-(phenothiazin-10-ylmethyl)ethyl] ammonium chloride; *N*-hydroxyethyl-promethazine; 'aprobit').
Promethazine methochloride *see* Thiazinamium.
PROMETHAZINE TEOCLATE*** (promethazine-8-chlorotheophyllinate; promethazine teoclate; 'avomine').
Promethestrol *see* Methestrol dipropionate.
Promethin (tr) *see* Pholedrine.
Promethoestrol *see* Methestrol dipropionate.
PROMETON* (4,6-bis(isopropylamino)-2-methoxy-*s*-triazine; 6-methoxy-*N*,*N*'-bis-(1-methylethyl)-1,3,5-triazine-2,4-diamine)
PROMETRYN* (4,6-bis(isopropylamino)-2-(methylthio)-*s*-triazine; *N*,*N*'-bis(1-methylethyl)-6-(methylthio)-1,3,5-triazine-2,4-diamine; 'caparol', 'gesagard').
'Promiben' *see* Imipramine.
'Promilene' *see* Promazine.
'Prominal' *see* Methylphenobarbital.
'Prominthic' *see* Metyridine.
'Promizole' *see* Thiazosulfone.
PROMOLATE*** (2-morpholinoethyl 2-methyl-2-phenoxypropionate; 2-morpholinoethyl 2-phenoxyisobutyrate; morphethylbutyne).
PROMOXOLANE*** (2,2-diisopropyl-1,3-dioxolane-4-methanol; diisopropyl-methanoldioxolane; 'dimethylane', 'dimethylyn').
'Promwill' *see* Promazine.
'Pronarcon' *see* Enibomal.
'Prondol' *see* Iprindole.
PRONETALOL*** (2-isopropylamino-1-naphth-2-ylethanol; α-(isopropylaminomethyl)-2-naphthalenemethanol; nethalide; pronethalol; pronetalol hydrochloride; 'alderlin').
Pronethalol* *see* Pronetalol.
'Prontosil' *see* Sulfachrysoidine; Sulfamido-chrysoidine.
'Prontosil album' *see* Sulfanilamide.
'Prontosil soluble' *see* Azosulfamide.
'Prontylin' *see* Aminophenazone with bamethan.
PROPACHLOR* (2-chloro-*N*-(1-methyl-ethyl)-*N*-phenylacetamide; 2-chloro-*N*-isopropylacetanilide; 'ramrod').
'Propaderm' *see* Beclometasone.
'Propadrine' *see* Norephedrine.
'Propaesin' *see* Risocaine.
PROPAFENONE*** (2'-(2-hydroxy-3-propylaminopropoxy)-3-phenylpropio-phenone; SA-79; fenoprain; 'baxarytmon')
'Propagin' *see* Propyl paraben.
PROPALLYLONAL* (5-(2-bromoallyl)-5-isopropyl barbituric acid; bromoaprobar-

bital; 'noctal', 'noctenal', 'nostal', 'nostral', 'quietal').

PROPAMIDINE*** (*p,p'*-trimethylenedioxy-dibenzamidine; 4',4'-diamidinodiphenoxy-propane).

Propamidine diisethionate *see* Propamidine isetionate.

Propamidine isethionate* *see* Propamidine isetionate.

PROPAMIDINE ISETIONATE (propamidine di(ethanol-2-sulfonate); propamidine diisethionate; propamidine isethionate; M&B-782).

Propanal *see* Propionaldehyde.

'Propanal' *see* Dipropylbarbituric acid.

1,3-PROPANEDIAMINE (propylenediamine).

Propanedioic acid *see* Malonic acid.

1,2-Propanediol *see* Propylene glycol.

1,3-Propanediol bis[2-(*p*-chlorophenoxy)-isobutyrate] *see* Simifibrate.

1,2-PROPANEDITHIOL (1,2-dimercaptopropane).

2,3-Propanedithiol-1-sulfonic acid sodium salt *see* Unithiol.

Propane nitrile *see* Propionitrile.

Propanid (tr) *see* Propanil.

PROPANIDID*** (propyl 4-diethylcarbamoylmethoxy-3-methoxyphenylacetate; 2-(4-carbopropoxymethoxy-2-methoxyphenoxy)-*N*,*N*-diethylacetamide; [4-[(diethylcarbamoyl)methoxy]-3-methoxyphenyl]acetic acid propyl ester acetate; B-1420; Bayer-1420; FBA-1420; 'epontol', 'fabantol', 'sombrevin').

PROPANIL* (*N*-(3,4-dichlorophenyl)-propionamide; 3',4'-dichloropropionanilide; DPA; propanid; 'rogue', 'stam F-34', 'surcopur').

PROPANOCAINE*** (α-(2-diethylaminoethyl)benzyl benzoate; 3-diethylamino-1-phenylpropyl benzoate; benzoate of α-(2-diethylaminoethyl)benzyl alcohol).

1-PROPANOL (propyl alcohol).

2-PROPANOL (isopropyl alcohol; 'avantin').

Propanolide *see* Propiolactone.

2-Propanone *see* Acetone.

3,5-Propanopiperidine *see* 3-Azabicyclo-(3.3.1)nonane.

PROPANTHELINE BROMIDE*** (2-diisopropylaminoethyl ester methobromide of 9-xanthenecarboxylic acid; (2-hydroxyethyl)diisopropylmethylammonium bromide xanthene-9-carboxylate; SC-3171).

Proparacaine *see* Proxymetacaine.

PROPARGITE* (2-(*p-tert*-butylphenoxy)-cyclohexyl 2-propynyl sulfite; 2-[4-(1,1-dimethylethyl)phenoxy]cyclohexyl 2-propynyl sulfite; 'omite').

Propargylamine *see* 2-Propynylamine.

Propargylcyclohexanol carbamate *see* Hexapropymate.

'Proparthrin' *see* Prothrin.

PROPATYLNITRATE*** (2-ethyl-2-(hydroxymethyl)-1,3-propanediol trinitrate 1,1,1-trisnitratomethylpropane; 1,1,1-tris-(hydroxymethyl)propane trinitrate; 2,2-bis(hydroxymethyl)-1-hydroxybutane trinitrate; ettriol trinitrate; ETTN; WIN-9317; 'atrilon 5', 'etrynit', 'gina', 'ginapect', 'vasangor').

'Propavan' *see* Propiomazine.

'Propaxoline' *see* Proxazole.

Propazepine *see* Prazepine.

Propazin (tr) *see* Promazine.

PROPAZINE* (2-chloro-4,6-bis(isopropylamino)-*s*-triazine; 6-chloro-*N*,*N*-bis-(1-methylethyl)-1,3,5-triazine-2,4-diamine; 'gesamil').

PROPAZOLAMIDE*** (5-propionamido-1,3,4-thiadiazole-2-sulfonamide; 5-propionamido-2-sulfamoyl-1,3,4-thiadiazole).

'Propazone' *see* Dimethadione.

Propenal *see* Acrolein.

Propene nitrile *see* Acrylonitrile.

Propenoic acid *see* Acrylic acid.

2-Propen-1-ol *see* Allyl alcohol.

2-Propenylamine *see* Allylamine.

p-(1-Propenyl)phenol *see* Anol.

1-Propenyl-2,4,5-trimethoxybenzene *see* Asarone.

Propenzolate* *see* Oxyclipine.

Propericiazine* *see* Periciazine.

PROPERIDINE*** (isopropyl ester of 1-methyl-4-phenylisonipecotic acid; properidine hydrochloride; 'gevelina').

'Propesin' *see* Propylcaine.

PROPETAMIDE*** (2-*p*-phenetidino-*N*-propylpropionamide; *N*-[1-(propylcarbamoyl)ethyl]-*p*-phenetidine; etampromide). *See also* Oxyphenbutazone with propetamide.

PROPETANDROL*** (3-propionyloxy-19-nor-17α-pregn-4-en-17-ol; 19-nor-17α-pregn-4-ene-3,17-diol 3-propionate; 17α-ethylestr-4-ene-3β,17β-diol 3-propionate; 'solevar').

Propethon* *see* Tridihexethyl.

PROPHAM* (isopropyl carbanilate; isopropyl phenylcarbamate; 1-methylethyl phenylcarbamate; B-22; IFK; INPC; IPC; isoPC; NSC-2105; 'conservasept', 'Denka antisprout' 'neoconserviet' 'septon', 'tuberlite').

PROPHAM PLUS ENDOTHAL SODIUM ('murbetol').

'Prophenal' *see* 5-Allyl-5-phenylbarbituric acid.

Prophenamine* *see* Profenamine.

Prophenpyridamine *see* Pheniramine.

Prophos *see* Ethoprop.

PROPICILLIN** (1-phenoxypropylpenicillin; 6-(2-phenoxybutyramido)penicillanic acid; propicillin potassium; 'baycillin', 'bayercillin', 'brocillin', 'delprosyn', 'oricillin', 'prevepen', 'synthepen', 'trescillin', 'ultrapen'). *See also* Levopropicillin.

'Propicol' *see* Diisopropyl *p*-nitrophenyl phosphate.

PROPIDINE (1-isopropyl-4,4-diphenylpiperidine).

PROPINAL (*N*,*N*-diethyl-2-(3-methoxy-4-propylphenoxy)acetamide).

377

PROPINEB* ([[(1-methyl-1,2-ethanediyl)-bis(carbamodithioato)](2-)]zinc homopolymer; zineb methyl derivative polymer; 'antracol').

PROPINETIDINE*** (propionate of 1-phenethyl-4-(2-propynyl)-4-piperidinol).

Propinox *see* Deanol propynyloxybenzilate.

'Propiocin' *see* Erythromycin propionate.

Propiodal *see* Prolonium iodide.

PROPIOLACTONE*** (hydracrylic acid β-lactone; 2-oxetanone; propanolide; β-propiolactone; β-propionolactone; 'BPL', 'bepaprone').

PROPIOLIC ACID (acetylenecarboxylic acid).

PROPIOMAZINE*** (1-[10-(2-dimethylaminopropyl)phenothiazin-2-yl]-1-propanone; 10-(2-dimethylaminopropyl)-2-propionylphenothiazine; 10-(2-dimethylaminopropyl)phenothiazin-2-yl ethyl ketone; CB-1678).

PROPIOMAZINE MALEATE (propiomazine acid maleate; Wy-1359; 'dorevane', 'indorm', 'largon', 'phenoctyl', 'propavan').

PROPIONALDEHYDE (propanal).

*p***-Propionamidophenol** *see* Parapropamol.

3-(Propionamidosulfonyl)-4-[*m*-(trifluoromethyl)anilino]pyridine *see* Galosemide.

5-Propionamido-1,3,4-thiadiazole-2-sulfonamide *see* Propazolamide.

PROPIONATE-CAPRYLATE MIXTURE* (Ca, Na and Zn salts of propionic and octanoic acids; 'sopronol').

PROPIONATE COMPOUND* (Ca and Na salts of propionic acid; 'propion gel').

Propionate lauryl sulfate(s) *see* Estolate(s).

Propionic acid salts *see* Calcium propionate; Sodium propionate; Zinc propionate.

PROPIONITRILE (ethyl cyanide; 2-cyanoethane; propane nitrile).

Propionolactone *see* Propiolactone.

*O***-Propionylatropine** *see* Prampine.

Propionylbenzaldehyde *see* Cumaldehyde.

Propionylhyoscine *see* Poskine.

PROPIONYLMORAZINE (10-(3-morpholinopropyl)-2-propionylphenothiazine).

3-Propionyloxy-19-nor-17α-pregn-4-en-17-ol *see* Propetandrol.

PROPIONYLPERAZINE (10-[3-(4-methylpiperazin-1-yl)propyl]-1-propionylphenothiazine).

*p***-Propionylphenol** *see* Paroxypropione.

Propionylpromazine *see* Propiopromazine.

Propionylscopolamine *see* Poskine.

PROPIOPHENONE (1-phenyl-1-propanone; ethyl phenyl ketone).

PROPIOPROMAZINE (10-(3-dimethylaminopropyl)-2-propionylphenothiazine; propionylpromazine).

PROPIOPROMAZINE MALEATE ('combelan', 'tranvet').

PROPIPOCAINE*** (2-piperid-1-ylethyl *p*-propoxyphenyl ketone; 3-piperid-1-yl-4'-propoxypropiophenone; 'falicaine').

PROPIRAM** (*N*-(1-methyl-2-piperid-1-ylethyl)-*N*-pyrid-2-ylpropionamide).

PROPIRAM FUMARATE* (BAY-4503; FBA-4503; 'algeril').

PROPISERGIDE** (9,10-didehydro-*N*-[(*S*)-2-hydroxy-1-methylethyl]-1,6-dimethylergoline 8β-carboxamide).

'Propitan' *see* Pipamperone.

Propitocaine *see* Prilocaine.

PROPIVANE (2-diethylaminoethyl 2-phenylvalerate; 2-diethylaminoethyl phenylpropylacetate; 2-diethylaminoethyl α-propyltoluate; propivane hydrochloride; RP-177; 'prospasmine').

PROPIZEPINE*** (6,11-dihydro-6-(2-dimethylamino-2-methylethyl)-5H-pyrido-(2,3-b)(1,5)benzodiazepin-5-one; 6-(2-dimethylamino-2-methylethyl)-6,11-dihydro-5H-pyrido(2,3-b)(1,5)benzodiazepin-5-one).

PROPOCTAMINE (*N*¹,*N*³-bis(2-ethylhexyl)-2-methyl-1,2,3-propanetriamine).

'Proponal' *see* Dipropylbarbituric acid.

'Proponesin' *see* Tolpronine.

'Propoquin' *see* Amopyroquine.

PROPOXATE*** (propyl DL-1-(1-phenylethyl)imidazole-5-carboxylate; propyl 1-(α-methylbenzyl)imidazole-5-carboxylate; R-7464).

PROPOXUR* (*o*-isopropoxyphenyl methylcarbamate; 2-(1-methylethoxy)-phenyl methylcarbamate; arprocarb; Bayer-39007; IPMC; OMS-33; Z-100; 'apacarb', 'baygon', 'blattanex', 'bolfo', 'unden').

*o***-PROPOXYBENZAMIDE** (salicylamide propyl ether; *O*-propylsalicylamide; 'reuprosal').

5-Propoxy-2-benzimidazolecarbamic acid methyl ester *see* Oxibendazole.

PROPOXYCAINE*** (2-diethylaminoethyl ester of 4-amino-2-propoxybenzoic acid; propoxycaine hydrochloride; WIN-3459; 'blockaine', 'pravocaine', 'ranocaine', 'ravocaine').

(+)-Propoxyphene* *see* Dextropropoxyphene.

(−)-Propoxyphene *see* Levopropoxyphene.

Propoxyphene napsylate *see* Dextropropoxyphene napsilate.

PROPRANOLOL*** (1-isopropylamino-3-(1-naphthyloxy)propan-2-ol; 1-(2-hydroxy-3-isopropylaminopropoxy)naphthalene; propranolol hydrochloride; anaprilin; proprasylyte; AY-64043; ICI-45520; 'avlocardyl', 'beta-neg', 'betares', 'dociton', 'inderal', 'obsidan', 'sumial'). *See also* Dexpropranolol.

Proprasylyte* *see* Propranolol.

Propylacetic acid *see* Valeric acid.

*N***-Propylajmalinium hydrogen tartrate** *see* Prajmalium bitartrate.

1-Propylamine (propylamine).

2-Propylamine (isopropylamine).

Propyl *p*-aminobenzoate *see* Risocaine.

2-Propylamino-*o*-propionotoluidide *see* Prilocaine.

*N***-(2-Propylaminopropionyl)-*o*-toluidine** *see* Prilocaine.

Propylbarbital see Dipropylbarbituric acid.
Propyl 1,3-bis(clofibrate) see Simfibrate.
'Propyl butex' see Propyl paraben.
Propylcaine see Risocaine.
S-**Propyl butylethylcarbamothioate** see Pebulate.
N-[1-**(Propylcarbamoyl)ethyl**]-*p*-**phenetidine** see Propetamide.
Propyl 3-diacetylamino-2,4,6-triiodobenzoate see Propyl docetrizoate.
Propyl diatrizoate see Propyl docetrizoate.
Propyl 4-diethylcarbamoylmethoxy-2-methoxyphenylacetate see Propanidid.
Propyl 3,5-diiodo-4-oxo-1-piperidineacetate see Propyliodone.
S-**Propyl dipropylcarbamothioate** see Vernolate.
PROPYL DOCETRIZOATE*** (propyl ester of 3-diacetylamino-2,4,6-triiodobenzoic acid; propyl 3-diacetamido-2,4,6-triiodobenzoate; propyl diatrizoate; 'pulmidol').
2-Propyldopacetamide see 2-(3,4-Dihydroxyphenyl)valeramide.
Propylene bis(2-chloroethyl)phosphorodiamidate see Cyclophosphamide.
Propylenediamine see Propanediamine.
PROPYLENE GLYCOL* (1,2-propanediol; methylglycol).
PROPYLENE GLYCOL MONOSTEARATE (1,2-propanediol monostearate; 'monolene', 'prostearin', tegen-P')
PROPYLENE GLYCOL 1-PHOSPHATE (1,2-propanediol 1-phosphate; 2-hydroxypropyl phosphate).
PROPYLENE GLYCOL SALICYLATE (1,2-propanediol salicylate; methylglycol salicylate).
PROPYL GALLATE ('tenox PG').
PROPYLHEXEDRINE*** (*N*,α-dimethylcyclohexaneethylamine; 1-cyclohexyl-2-methylaminopropane; (cyclohexylisopropyl)methylamine; hexahydrodesoxyephedrine; E-111; 'benzedrex', 'eventin', 'obesin').
Propylhexedrine-phenobarbital see Barbexaclone.
Propyl *p*-hydroxybenzoate see Propyl paraben.
4,4'-Propylidenedi(2,6-piperazinedione) see Razoxane.
PROPYLIODONE*** (propyl 3,5-diiodo-4-oxo-1(4H)-pyridineacetate; propyl ester of 3,5-diiodo-4-oxo-1-piperidineacetic acid).
Propylisonicotinthioamide see Prothionamide.
Propyl DL-1-(α-methylbenzyl)imidazole-5-carboxylate see Propoxate.
19-Propylnorvinol see Etorphine.
'Propylon' see Isoprenaline.
PROPYL PARABEN (propyl *p*-hydroxybenzoate; 'nipasol P', 'propagin', 'propyl butex', 'solbrol P').
2-Propylpentanoic acid see Valproic acid.
Propylphenazone see Propyphenazone.
1-(α-Propylphenethyl)pyrrolidine see Prolintane.

Propyl DL-1-(1-phenylethyl)imidazole-5-carboxylate see Propoxate.
2-Propylpiperidine see Coniine.
O-**Propylsalicylamide** see *o*-Propoxybenzamide.
2-Propyl-5-thiazolecarboxylic acid see Tizoprolic acid.
5-(Propylthio)benzimidazole-2-carbamic acid methyl ester see Albendazole.
2-Propylthioisonicotinamide see Protionamide.
PROPYLTHIOURACIL*** (6-propyl-2-thiouracil; 4-propyl-2-thiouracil).
2-PROPYLVALERAMIDE (dipropylacetamide; 'depamide').
2-Propylvaleric acid see Valproic acid.
2-PROPYNYLAMINE (propargylamine).
1-(2-Propynyl)cyclohexyl carbamate see Hexapropymate.
Propynyloxybenzilic acid 2-dimethylaminoethyl ester see Deanol propynyloxybenzilate.
Propynyloxyphenylmandelic acid dimethylaminoethyl ester see Deanol propynyloxyphenylmandelate.
E,E-**2-Propynyl 3,7,11-trimethyldodeca-2,4-dienoate** see Kinoprene.
PROPYPERONE*** (4'-fluoro-4-(4-piperid-1-yl-4-propionylpiperid-1-yl)butyrophenone; 1'-[3-(*p*-fluorobenzoyl)propyl]-4-propionyl-1,4'-bipiperidine).
PROPYPHENAZONE*** (4-isopropyl-2,3-dimethyl-1-phenyl-3-pyrazolin-5-one; 4-isopropylantipyrine; isopyrine; 4-isopropylphenazone; propylphenazone; 'degripol' 'larodon').
See also Famprofazone with propyphenazone.
PROPYROMAZINE BROMIDE*** (1-methyl-1-(1-phenothiazin-10-ylcarbonylethyl)pyrrolidinium bromide; 10-[2-(1-methylpyrrolidin-1-yl)propionyl]phenothiazine bromide; SD-104-19; 'diaspasmyl').
'Propytal' see Dipropylbarbituric acid.
Proquamezine see Aminopromazine.
PROPYZAMIDE* (3,5-dichloro-*N*-(1,1-dimethyl-2-propynyl)benzamide; 'kerb').
PROQUAZONE*** (1-isopropyl-7-methyl-4-phenylquinazolin-2(1H)-one).
PROQUINOLATE*** (methyl 4-hydroxy-6,7-diisopropoxy-3-quinolinecarboxylate; mequinolate; U-1063).
PRORENOATE POTASSIUM*** (potassium 6,7-dihydro-17-hydroxy-3-oxo-3'H-cyclopropa(6,7)-17α-pregna-4,6-diene-21-carboxylate; potassium prorenoate; SC-23992).
'Proresid' see Mitopodozide.
'Proscabin' see Benzyl benzoate.
PROSCILLARIDIN*** (3β,14β-dihydroxybufa-4,20,22-trienolide 3-rhamnoside; 14-hydroxy-3β-rhamnosyloxybufa-4,20,22-trienolide; proscillaridin A; scillarenin 3β-rhamnoside; PSC-801; TV-274B; 'caradrin', 'protasin', 'sandoscill, 'solestril', 'stellarid', 'talucard', 'talusin', 'urgilan').

PROSCILLARIDIN WITH ETOFYLLINE ('teostellarid').
PROSCILLARIDIN WITH ISOSORBIDE DINITRATE (TV-274C).
PROSCILLARIDIN WITH THEO-PHYLLINE (BS-272; 'teo-caradrin').
'Proscomide' *see* Scopolamine methyl bromide.
'Proscopine' *see* Poskine.
'Proserine' *see* Neostigmine.
'Prosparol' *see* Arachis oil emulsion.
'Prospasmine' *see* Propivane.
Prospidin (tr) *see* Prospidium chloride.
PROSPIDIUM CHLORIDE*** (3,12-bis(3-chloro-2-hydroxypropyl)-3,12-diaza-6,9-diazoniadispiro(5.2.5.2)hexadecane dichloride; N,N^3-bis(3-chloro-2-hydroxypropyl)-N,N^2-dispirotripiperazine dichloride; prospidin).
PROSTAGLANDIN A$_1$ (15α-hydroxy-9-oxo-10,13-*trans* prostadienoic acid).
PROSTAGLANDIN B$_2$ (15-hydroxy-9-oxo-5-*cis*-8(12),13-*trans*-prostatrienoic acid).
Prostaglandin E$_2$ *see* Dinoprostone.
Prostaglandin F$_{2\alpha}$ *see* Dinoprost.
PROSTALENE** (($\pm$)-methyl-7-[(1R^*,2R^*, 3R^*,5S^*)-3,5-dihydroxy-2-[(E)-3-hydroxy-3-methyl-1-octenyl]cyclopentyl]-4,5-heptadienoate).
'Prostaphlin' *see* Oxacillin.
'Prostearin' *see* Propylene glycol mono-stearate.
'Prostigmine' *see* Neostigmine.
'Prostin F2 alpha' *see* Dinoprost.
Prosulthiamine* *see* Prosultiamine.
PROSULTIAMINE*** (N-(4-amino-2-methylpyrimidin-5-ylmethyl)-N-[4-hydroxy-1-methyl-2-(propyldithio)-1-butenyl]formamide; prosulthiamine; dithiopropylthiamine; thiamine propyl disulfide; DTP; TPD; 'alinamin', 'nevriton', 'taketron').
'Prosymasul' *see* Sulfasymazine.
'Prosympal' *see* (Diethylaminomethyl)-1,4-benzodioxan.
'Protacil' *see* Promazine.
'Protactyl' *see* Promazine.
'Protalba' *see* Protoveratrine.
'Protagent' *see* Povidone.
PROTAMINE ZINC INSULIN ('durasulin').
See also Isophane insulin.
'Pro-tan' *see* Promazine.
'Protanal' *see* Sodium alginate.
'Protasin' *see* Proscillaridin.
'Proteina' *see* Androstanolone.
'Prothanon' *see* Promethazine S,S-dioxide.
PROTHEOBROMINE*** (1-(2-hydroxy-propyl)theobromine; 'cordabromin', 'thebes', 'theocor').
'Prothiaden' *see* Dosulepin.
'Prothidium' *see* Pyritidium.
'Prothidryl' *see* Dosulepin with embramine.
'Prothil' *see* Medrogestone.
Prothionamide* *see* Protionamide.
PROTHIPENDYL*** (10-(3-dimethyl-aminopropyl)-10H-pyrido(3,2-b)(1,4)-benzothiazine; 10-(3-dimethylamino-propyl)-1-azaphenothiazine; 10-(3-di-methylaminopropyl)-9-thia-1,10-diazan-thracene; prothipendyl hydrochloride; Ay-5603; D-206; LG-206; 'azacon' 'dominal', 'largophren', 'phrenotropin', 'timovan' 'tolnate' 'tumovan').
PROTHIXENE*** (9-(3-dimethylamino-propylidene)thioxanthene; N,N-dimethyl-thioxanthene-$\Delta^{9,\gamma}$-propylamine).
PROTHOATE* (O,O-diethyl S-(isopropyl-carbomoylmethyl) phosphorodithioate; O,O-diethyl S-[2-[(1-methylethyl)amino]-2-oxoethyl] phosphorodithioate; trimetho-ate; 'aafac', 'FAC', 'fostion').
PROTHRIN ([2-methyl-5-(2-propynyl)-3-furanyl]methyl 2,2-dimethyl-3-(2-methyl-1-propenyl)cyclopropanecarboxylate; 2-methyl-5-prop-2-ynyl-3-furylmethyl chrysanthemate; D-1201; 'kikuthrin', 'proparthrin').
'Prothromadin' *see* Warfarin.
PROTIONAMIDE*** (2-propylisonicotin-thioamide; prothionamide; 2-propylthio-isonicotinamide; 'eketebin', 'tebeform', 'trevintix').
PROTIRELIN** (5-oxo-L-propyl-L-histidyl-L-prolinamide; thyrotrophin releasing hormone synthetic; TRH synthetic; lopremone; Abbott-38579; 'TRH-Roche').
PROTIZINIC ACID*** (7-methoxy-α,10-dimethylphenothiazine-2-acetic acid; 2-(1-carboxymethyl)-7-methoxy-10-methylphenothiazine; RP-17190; 'piro-crid').
PROTOANEMONIN (4-hydroxy-2,4-pen-tadienoic acid γ-lactone; γ-hydroxyvinyl-acrylic acid lactone; 5-methylene-2-oxodi-hydrofuran; 5-methylenedihydrofuran-2-one).
PROTOCATECHUIC ACID (3,4-dihydr-oxybenzoic acid).
PROTOCATECHUYL ALCOHOL (3,4-dihydroxybenzyl alcohol).
PROTOGEN (POF; pyruvate oxidation factor).
Protogen A *see* Thioctic acid.
Protoheme *see* Heme.
PROTOKYLOL *** (α[[(α-methyl-3,4-methylenedioxyphenethyl)amino]methyl]-protocatechuyl alcohol; N-[2-(3,4-methyl-enedioxy)isopropyl]noradrenaline; 1-(3,4-dihydroxyphenyl)-2-(α-methyl-3,4-methyl-enedioxyphenethylamino)ethanol; 3,4-dihydroxy-β-hydroxy-β'-methyl-3',4'-methylenedioxydiphenethylamine; 3,4-dihydroxy-α-(α-methyl-3,4-methylenedi-oxyphenethylaminomethyl)benzyl alcohol; protokylol hydrochloride; JB-251; 'caytine').
'Protopam' *see* Pralidoxime.
PROTOPINE (fumarine; macleyine).
'Protostib' *see* Meglumine antimonate.
PROTOVERATRINE A ('protalba', 'puroverine retard').
PROTOVERATRINES A AND B (PVS-295; 'provell', 'puroverine', 'veralba').

PROTRIPTYLINE*** (5-(3-methylamino-propyl)dibenzo(a,d)cycloheptene; 3-(5H-dibenzo(a,d)cyclohepten-5-yl)-N-methyl-propylamine; N-methyl-5H-dibenzo(a,d)-cycloheptene-5-propylamine; N-3-(5H-dibenzo(a,d)cyclohepten-5-yl)propyl-N-methylamine; protriptyline hydrochloride; amimethyline; MK-240; 'concordin', 'triptil', 'vivactil', 'vivactyl').

'Provamycin' see Spiramycin.

'Provasan' see Nicametate citrate.

'Provell' see Protoveratrines.

'Provera' see Medroxyprogesterone acetate.

'Provest' see Medroxyprogesterone acetate with ethinylestradiol.

'Proviron' see Mesterolone.

Provitamin D₃ see 7-Dehydrocholesterol.

PROXAZOLE*** (5-(2-diethylaminoethyl)-3-(α-ethylbenzyl)-1,2,4-oxadiazole; 'aerbron', 'propaxoline'; 'toness').

PROXAZOLE CITRATE* (AF-634).

'Proxen' see Naproxen.

PROXIBARBAL*** (5-allyl-5-(2-hydroxy-propyl)barbituric acid; 5-(2-hydroxy-propyl)-5-(2-propenyl)-2,4,6(1H,3H,5H)-pyrimidinetrione; ipronal; 'axeen', 'D₂H', 'vasalgin').

PROXIBUTENE*** (3-dimethylamino-methyl-1,2-diphenyl-3-buten-2-ol pro-pionate).

See also Dexproxibutene.

PROXIFEZONE** (dextropropoxyphene compound with phenylbutazone).

'Proxybron' see Oxolamine benzilate with tetracycline.

Proxyfenone see Paroxypropione.

PROXYMETACAINE*** (2-diethylamino-ethyl ester of 3-amino-4-propoxybenzoic acid; proparacaine; proxymetacaine hydro-chloride; 'alcaine', 'keracaine', 'ophthaine', 'ophthetic').

PROXYPHYLLINE*** (7-(2-hydroxy-propyl)theophylline; 'brontyl', 'puro-phyllin', 'spasmolysin', 'thean', 'theon').

PROZAPINE*** (1-(3,3-diphenylpropyl)-cyclohexamethylenimine; 1-(3,3-diphenyl-propyl)hexahydroazepine).

'Prozine' see Promazine.

Prunetol see Genistein.

'Pruralgin' see Quinisocaine.

PRUSSIAN BLUE (ferric cyanoferrate; ferric ferrocyanide).

'Pryleugan' see Imipramine.

PRYNACHLOR* (2-chloro-N-(1-methyl-2-propynyl)acetanilide; chloretin).

Przedziorkofos see Phenkapton.

P2S see Pralidoxime mesilate.

PS-2383 see Trimetozine.

PSC-801 see Proscillaridin.

PSEUDOATROPINE (tropine atrolactate; tropine α-methylmandelate).

Pseudobrucine see Ajmaline.

Pseudocholestane see Coprostane.

PSEUDOCOCAINE (D-cocaine; D-2-α-carbo-methoxy-3β-benzoyloxytropane; isocaine; isocaine; 'delcaine', 'depsococaine', 'dextrocaine', 'neopsicaine', 'psicaine').

PSEUDOCODEINE (neoisocodeine).

PSEUDOCUMIDINE (2,4,5-trimethyl-aniline).

Pseudodigitonin see Gitalin.

Pseudodigitoxin see Gitoxin.

PSEUDOEPHEDRINE*** (isoephedrine; Ψ-ephedrine; (+)-α-(1-methylamino-ethyl)benzyl alcohol; stereoisomer of ephedrine; (+)-2-methylamino-1-phenyl-propan-1-ol).

PSEUDOEPHEDRINE WITH CHLOR-PHENIRAMINE MALEATE ('decona-mine', 'demazin').

PSEUDOEPHEDRINE WITH TRIPRO-LIDINE ('actifed').

(3H)Pseudoindol-3-one (Ψ-indolone).

PSEUDOINDOXYL (2,3-dihydro-3-oxo-indole; 3-indolinone).

PSEUDOMECONIN (4,5-dimethoxy-phthalide).

PSEUDOMORPHINE (oxydimorphine; dehydromorphine; 2,2'-bimorphine; Ψ-morphine; 2,2'-dehydromorphine).

Pseudostilbestrol see 3,4-Bis(p-hydroxy-phenyl)-2-hexene.

PSEUDOTHIOUREA (isothiourea). See also Isothiuronium etc.

PSEUDOTROPINE (3β-hydroxy-8-methyl-2,3-dihydronortropidine; 3β-tropanol).

PSEUDOTROPINE BENZOATE (syn-benzoyltropine; tropacocaine).

PSEUDOUREA (carbamimidic acid; isourea).

'Psicaine' see Pseudococaine.

'Psichoperidol' see Trifluperidol.

'Psicofuranine' see Angustmycin C.

'Psiconal' see Pseudococaine.

'Psicosoma' see Magnesium glutamate hydrobromide.

PSILOCIN (N,N-dimethyl-4-hydroxy-tryptamine).

Psilocin phosphate ester see Psilocybine.

PSILOCYBINE*** (3-(2-dimethylamino-ethyl)indol-4-yl dihydrogen phosphate; 4-phosphoryloxydimethyltryptamine; psilocin phosphate ester; 'indocybin').

'Psocorten' see Flumetasone pivalate with salicylic acid and coal tar.

'Psoil' see Tioxolone with hydrocortisone.

PSORALEN ((7H)furo(3,2-g)(1)benzo-pyran-7-one; furano(2',3':6,7)coumarin).

'Psoriasin' see Mustard gas.

PSP see Phenolsulfonphthalein and Saxitoxin.

'Psychamine' see Phenmetrazine.

Psychoforine (tr) see Imipramine.

'Psychosan' see Azacyclonol.

'Psychostyl' see Nortriptyline.

'Psychoverlan' see Magnesium glutamate hydrobromide.

Psyllium see Ispagula; Sodium psylliate.

'Psymod' see Piperacetazine.

'Psyquil' see Triflupromazine.

PT-9 see Betahistine.

PTC see Phenylthiourea.

PTERIDINE (pyrimido(4,5-b)pyrazine; benzotetrazine; azinepurine).

Pterocarpus marsupium see Kino.

PTEROIC ACID (*p*-[(2-amino-4-hydroxy-6-pteridylmethyl)amino]benzoic acid).
PTEROPTERIN (pteroyldi-*γ*-glutamyl-glutamic acid; pteroyl-*γ*-glutamyl-*γ*-glutamylglutamic acid; pteroyltriglutamic acid; PTGA; fermentation *L. casei* factor; 'teropterin').
Pteroylglutamic acid *see* Folic acid.
Pteroyl-*γ*-glutamyl-*γ*-glutamylglutamic acid *see* Pteropterin.
Pteroyltriglutamic acid *see* Pteropterin.
PTFE *see* Politef.
PTG *see* Teniposide.
PTGA *see* Pteropterin.
'P9-Tus' *see* Bromhexine with fominoben.
PU-239 *see* Benzilonium.
'Puddmetin' *see* Genkwanin.
'Pularin' *see* Heparin.
'Pulmadil' *see* Rimiterol.
'Pulmaxil N' *see* Penethamate hydriodide.
'Pulmidol' *see* Propyl docetrizoate.
'Pulmo 500' *see* Penethamate hydriodide.
'Pulsoton' *see* Hydroxyamphetamine.
Punicine *see* Pelletierine.
'Puralin' *see* Thiram.
'Purantix' *see* Clocortolone pivalate.
'Purapen' *see* Azidocillin.
'Purapen G' *see* Penicillin G, purified.
'Purazol' *see* Sulfapyridine.
Purgenum *see* Phenolphthalein.
PURINE (7-imidazo(4,5-d)pyrimidine; NSC-753).
2,6(1H,3H)-Purinedione *see* Xanthine.
PURINE RIBOSIDE (9-*β*-D-ribofuranosyl-purine; nebularine; nebuline).
6-Purinethiol *see* Mercaptopurine.
'Puri-nethol' *see* Mercaptopurine.
6(1H)-Purinone *see* Hypoxanthine.
5-(Purin-6-ylthio)valeric acid *see* Buthiopurine.
N-**[5-(Purin-6-ylthio)valeryl]glycine ethyl ester** *see* Butocin.
PUROMYCIN** (3'-(*α*-amino-*p*-methoxy-hydrocinnamamido)-3'-deoxy-*N*,*N*-dimethyladenosine; 6-dimethylamino-9-[3'-deoxy-3'-(*p*-methoxy-L-phenylalanyl-amino)-*β*(or *α*)-ribosyl]purine; CL-13900; NSC-3055; P-683; 'stillomycin', 'stylomycin').
PUROMYCIN AMINONUCLEOSIDE (3'-amino-3'-desoxy-*N*,*N*-dimethyladeno-sine; 9-(3-amino-3-desoxy-*β*-D-ribofurano-syl)-6-dimethylaminopurine; aminonucleo-side; ARDMA; DNSC-3056).
PUROMYCIN HYDROCHLORIDE (puromycin dihydrochloride; CL-16536).
'Purophylline' *see* Proxyphylline.
'Purostrophan' *see* Ouabain.
'Puroverine' *see* Protoveratrines.
Purpurea glycoside C *see* Deslanoside.
Purpuric acid ammonium salt *see* Murexide.
'Purpurid' *see* Digitoxin.
PUTRESCINE (1,4-butanediamine; tetra-methylenediamine).
PVA *see* Polyvinyl alcohol.
PVNO *see* Polyvinylpyridine *N*-oxide.

PVP *see* Povidone.
'PVP-macrose' *see* Povidone.
PVS-295 *see* Protoveratrines.
PVTD *see* Dextran.
PW/135 *see* Pemoline.
PX-917 *see* Tricresyl phosphate.
'Pycaril' *see* Benzyl nicotinate.
'Pyelectan' *see* Iodoxyl.
'Pyelokon-R' *see* Sodium acetrizoate.
'Pyelombrine' *see* Sodium diatrizoate.
'Pyelombrine M' *see* Diodone meglumine.
'Pyelosil' *see* Iodopyridone.
Pyknolepsin (tr) *see* Ethosuximide.
'Pylostropin' *see* Atropine methonitrate.
'Pylumbrin' *see* Diodone.
PYOCYANINE (10-methylphenazin-1-one; cyanomycin).
'Pyopen' *see* Carbenicillin.
'Pyostacin' *see* Pristinamycin.
'Pyrabital' *see* Barbipyrine.
'Pyracetol' *see* Acetpyrogall.
Pyracetosal *see* Acetopyrine.
Pyracrimycin A *see* Desdanine.
'Pyradone' *see* Aminophenazone.
'Pyra-elmedal' *see* Aminophenazone with phenylbutazone.
PYRAHEXYL (3-hexyl-7,8,9,10-tetrahydro-6,6,9-trimethyl-6H-dibenzo(b,d)pyran-1-ol; parahexyl; synhexyl).
Pyraldin (tr) *see* Quinapyramine.
'Pyramat' *see* 6-Methyl-2-propylpyrimid-4-yl dimethylcarbamate.
'Pyramidon' *see* Aminophenazone.
'Pyramin' *see* Pyrazon.
'Pyraminal' *see* Aminophenazone.
'Pyramon' *see* Aminophenazone.
Pyranisamine *see* Mepyramine.
'Pyranol' *see* Polychlorinated biphenyl mixture.
PYRANTEL*** (1,4,5,6-tetrahydro-1-methyl-2-(*trans*-2-thien-2-ylvinyl) pyrimidine).
PYRANTEL EMBONATE (pyrantel com-pound (1:1) with 4,4'-methylenebis(3-hydroxy-2-naphthoic acid); pyrantel pamoate; CP-10423-16; 'antiminth', 'cobantril', 'combantrin', 'helmex').
Pyrantel pamoate* *see* Pyrantel embonate.
PYRANTEL TARTRATE* (CP-10423-18; 'banminth').
'Pyrantin' *see* Phenetylsuccinimide.
'Pyranum' *see* Sodium thymyl benzyloxy-benzoate.
'Pyrasanone' *see* Pyrazinobutazone.
Pyrathiazine* *see* Parathiazine.
Pyrazapon *see* Ripazepam.
PYRAZINAMIDE*** (pyrazine-2-carbox-amide; pyrazinoic acid amide; D-50; MK-56; 'aldinamide', 'tebrazid', 'zinamide').
PYRAZINE (1,4-diazine; paradiazine; piazine).
Pyrazine-2-carboxamide *see* Pyrazinamide.
Pyrazinecarboxylic acid *see* Pyrazinoic acid.
PYRAZINOBUTAZONE (phenylbutazone-piperazine; DB-139; 'carudol', 'pyrasa-none').

PYRAZINOIC ACID (pyrazinecarboxylic acid).

Pyrazinoic acid amide see Pyrazinamide.

N¹-Pyrazin-2-ylsulfanilamide see Sulfapyrazine.

Pyrazocillin see Prazocillin.

Pyrazofurin* see Pirazofurin.

'Pyrazogin' see Sulfamidopyrine.

PYRAZOLE (1,2-diazole).

Pyrazole-1-carboxamidine see Praxadine.

Pyrazole-3,4-dicarboxylic acid bis-(methylamide) see Ethipyrole.

PYRAZOLIDINE (tetrahydropyrazole).

PYRAZOLIDINONE (pyrazolidone).

Pyrazolidone see Pyrazolidinone.

Pyrazoline (dihydropyrazole).

2-PYRAZOLIN-5-ONE (5-pyrazolone).

3-PYRAZOLIN-5-ONE (3-pyrazolone).

3-Pyrazolone see 3-Pyrazolin-5-one.

5-Pyrazolone see 2-Pyrazolin-5-one.

PYRAZOLOPYRIMIDINE (tetraazaindene).

1H-Pyrazolo(3,4-d)pyrimidine-4,6-diol see Oxipurinol.

1H-Pyrazolo(3,4-d)pyrimidine-4-thiol see Tisopurine.

1H-Pyrazolo(3,4-d)pyrimidin-4-ol see Allopurinol.

PYRAZON* (4-amino-4-chloro-2-phenylpyridazin-3(2H)-one; PCA; 'pyramin'). See also Chlorbufan plus pyrazon.

PYRAZOPHOS* (ethyl 2-[(diethoxyphosphinothioyl)oxy]-5-methylpyrazolo(1,5-a)pyrimidine-6-carboxylate; 'afugan', 'curamil').

'Pyrbenine' see Benzilonium.

Pyrbenzindole see Benzindopyrine.

Pyrene (chemical name for a 4-ring system).

'Pyrene' see Carbon tetrachloride.

'Pyrequan' see Morantel.

PYRESMETHRIN* (trans-(±)-5-benzylfuran-3-ylmethyl 3-(3-methoxy-2-methyl-3-oxo-1-propenyl)-2,2-dimethylcyclopropanecarboxylate).

'Pyrethia' see Promethazine.

PYRETHRIN I (2-methyl-4-oxo-3-(2,4-pentadienyl)-2-cyclopenten-1-yl chrysanthemate; pyrethrolone ester of chrysanthemic acid).

PYRETHRIN II (1-methyl 3-[2-methyl-4-oxo-3-(2,4-pentadienyl)-2-cyclopenten-1-yl]chrysanthemumdicarboxylate; pyrethrolone ester of chrysanthemumdicarboxylic acid methyl ester).

PYRETHROLONE (4-hydroxy-3-methyl-2-(2,4-pentadienyl)-2-cyclopenten-1-one).

'Pyrgasol' see Lauralkonium.

'Pyribenzamine' see Tripelennamine.

'Pyrictal' see Phetharbital.

'Pyridacil' see Phenazopyridine.

PYRIDARONE** (2-pyrid-4-ylbenzofuran).

PYRIDAZINE (1,2-diazine; orthodiazine).

Pyridazone see Pyridazinone.

Pyridinaldehydes see Isonicotinaldehyde; Nicotinaldehyde; Picolinaldehyde.

2-Pyridinaldoxime see Pralidoxime.

2-PYRIDINDENE (2-azafluorene).

Pyridindole see Pyridoindole.

2-PYRIDINEACETAMIDE (2-pyrid-2-ylacetamide).

1-PYRIDINEACETIC ACID (2-pyrid-1-ylacetic acid).

3-PYRIDINEACETIC ACID (2-pyrid-3-ylacetic acid; 'lioxone').

2-Pyridinecarboxylic acid see Picolinic acid.

3-Pyridinecarboxylic acid see Nicotinic acid.

4-Pyridinecarboxylic acid see Isonicotinic acid.

2,3-Pyridinedicarboxylic acid see Quinolinic acid.

PYRIDINE-3,4-DIMETHANOL (3,4-bis-(hydroxymethyl)pyridine).

2,6-PYRIDINEDIMETHANOL BIS-(METHYLCARBAMATE) (2,6-bis-(hydroxymethyl)pyridyl bis(methylcarbamate); pyridinol carbamate; P-23; 'anginin', 'angioxin', 'aterofal', 'colesterinex', 'duvaline', 'sospitan', 'vasoverin').

3-Pyridinemethanol see Nicotinyl alcohol.

4-PYRIDINEMETHANOL (4-(hydroxymethyl)pyridine).

3-Pyridinemethanol 1-oxide see Mepiroxol.

Pyridine-2-thione 1-oxide see Pyrithione.

PYRIDINITRIL* (2,6-dichloro-4-phenyl-3,5-pyridinedicarbonitrile). See also Captafol with pyridinitril.

Pyridinol carbamate see 2,6-Pyridinedimethanol bis(methylcarbamate).

3-Pyridinol tartrate see Hydroxypyridine. tartrate.

'Pyridium' see Phenazopyridine.

'Pyridizin' see Isoniazid methanesulfonate.

10H-PYRIDO(3,2-b)(1,4)BENZOTHIAZINE (1-azaphenothiazine; 9-thia-1,10-diazanthracene; thiophenylpyridylamine).

4-[3-(Pyrido(3,2-b)(1,4)benzothiazin-10-yl)propyl]piperazin-1-ylethanol see Oxypendyl.

PYRIDOFYLLINE*** (pyridoxol salt of 7-(2-hydroxyethyl)theophylline hydrogen sulfate ester; ethofylline pyridoxol salt hydrogen sulfate ester; 5-hydroxy-3,4-bis-(hydroxymethyl)-6-methylpyridyl-2-(theophylline) ethoxysulfate; pyridoxol theophylline ethoxysulfate).

9H-PYRIDO(3,4-b)INDOLE (β-carboline).

5H-PYRIDO(4,3-b)INDOLE (γ-carboline).

4H-PYRIDO(1,2-a)PYRIMIDINE (homopyrimidazole).

'Pyridoscorbine' see Ascorbic acid-pyridoxine complex.

PYRIDOSTIGMINE BROMIDE*** (3-hydroxy-1-methylpyridinium bromide dimethylcarbamate; 'mestinon', 'regonol').

PYRIDOXAL (3-hydroxy-5-(hydroxymethyl)-2-methylisonicotinaldehyde; 4-formyl-3-hydroxy-5-hydroxymethyl-2-methylpyridine; pyridoxal hydrochloride).

PYRIDOXAL 5-PHOSPHATE (codecarboxylase).

PYRIDOXAMINE (4-(aminomethyl)-5-

hydroxy-6-methyl-3-pyridinemethanol; 4-aminomethyl-3-hydroxy-5-hydroxy-methyl-2-methylpyridine; pyridoxamine dihydrochloride).

PYRIDOXIC ACID (3-hydroxy-5-(hydroxymethyl)-2-methylisonicotinic acid; 3-hydroxy-5-hydroxymethyl-2-methylpyridine-4-carboxylic acid).

PYRIDOXINE*** (3-hydroxy-4,5-di(hydroxymethyl)-2-methylpyridine; 3-hydroxy-2-methyl-4,5-pyridinedimethanol; 5-hydroxy-6-methyl-3,4-pyridinedimethanol; 4,5-bis(hydroxymethyl)-3-hydroxy-α-picoline; 4,5-dimethylol-3-hydroxy-α-picoline; pyridoxine hydrochloride; pyridoxol; adermine; vitamin B₆).
See also Ascorbic acid-pyridoxine complex; Tryptophan with pyridoxine.

Pyridoxine-amphetamine condensation product *see* Pyridoxiphen.

PYRIDOXINE ASPARTATE ('aspardoxine').

Pyridoxine 5-disulfide *see* Pyritinol.

Pyridoxine 3-ether with glycolic acid *see* 2-[(5-Hydroxy-4-hydroxymethyl-6-methylpyrid-3-yl)methoxy]glycolic acid.

PYRIDOXIPHEN (tr) (amphetamine-pyridoxine condensation product).

Pyridoxol *see* Pyridoxine.

Pyridoxol theophylline ethoxysulfate *see* Pyridofylline.

2-Pyridylacetone *see* Pelletierine.

β-Pyridyl aldehyde *see* Nicotinaldehyde.

γ-Pyridyl aldehyde *see* Isonicotinaldehyde.

α-(2-Pyridylaminomethyl)benzyl alcohol *see* Fenyramidol.

2-Pyridyl-4-ylbenzofuran *see* Pyridarone.

β-Pyridyl carbinol *see* Nicotinyl alcohol.

α-(2-Pyrid-4-ylcyclopropyl)benzhydrol *see* Cyprolidol.

Pyrid-3-ylmethylamine *see* Picolamine.

7-[2-[(Pyrid-3-ylmethyl)amino]ethyl]-theophylline *see* Pimefylline.

4-(Pyrid-5-ylmethylaminomethyl)-pyridine *see* Gapicomine.

1-[2-(N-Pyrid-2-ylmethylanilino)ethyl]-piperidine *see* Picoperine.

Pyrid-2-ylmethyl 2-(p-chlorophenoxy)-2-methylpropionate *see* Nicofibrate.

4,4'-(Pyrid-2-ylmethylene)diphenol bis-(hydrogen sulfate) disodium salt *see* Sodium picosulfate.

4,4'-Pyrid-2-ylmethylenediphenol diacetate *see* Bisacodyl.

2-[(Pyrid-2-ylmethyl)sulfinyl]benzimidazole *see* Timoprazole.

3-Pyrid-1-ylmethyl-7-(thien-2-ylacetamido)-8-oxo-5-thia-1-azabicyclo-(4.2.0)oct-2-ene-2-carboxylic acid *see* Cefaloridine.

1-(3-Pyrid-2-yloxypropyl)-4-(o-tolyl)-piperazine *see* Toprilidine.

2-Pyrid-3-ylpiperidine *see* Anabasine.

1-Pyrid-2-yl-2-propanone *see* Pelletierine.

1-Pyrid-2-yl-3-pyrrolidin-1-yl-1-p-tolyl-1-propene *see* Triprolidene.

**5-[p-(2-Pyridylsulfamoyl)phenylazo]sali-

cylic acid *see* Salazosulfapyridine.

N¹-Pyrid-2-ylsulfanilamide *see* Sulfapyridine.

Pyrid-3-yl tartrate *see* Hydroxypyridine tartrate.

7-[2-(Pyrid-4-ylthio)acetamido]cephalosporanic acid *see* Cefapirin.

2-(2-Pyrid-2-ylvinyl)-3-(o-tolyl)quinazolin-4(3H)-one *see* Piriqualone.

'Pyrilamine' *see* Mepyramine.

'Pyrilene' *see* Pempidine tosilate.

PYRIMETHAMINE*** (2,4-diamino-5-(p-chlorophenyl)-6-ethylpyrimidine; chloridine; BW-50-63; NSC-3061; RP-4753; 'darapram', 'daraprim', 'erbaprelina', 'malocide').
See also Sulfadoxine with pyrimethamine.

PYRIMIDINE (1,3-diazine; metadiazine; miazine).

2,4(1H,3H)-Pyrimidinedione *see* Uracil.

5-PYRIMIDINEMETHANOL (5-(hydroxymethyl)pyrimidine).

Pyrimidine phosphoran *see* Pirimiphos methyl.

2,4,5,6(1H,3H)-Pyrimidinetetrone *see* Alloxan.

2,4,6(1H,3H,5H)-Pyrimidinetrione *see* Barbituric acid.

PYRIMIDINONE (pyrimidone).

α-(Pyrimidin-2-ylaminomethyl)benzyl alcohol *see* Fenyripol.

8-[4-[4-(Pyrimidin-2-yl)piperazin-1-yl]-butyl]-8-azaspiro(4.5)decane-7,9-dione *see* Buspirone.

N¹-Pyrimidin-2-ylsulfanilamide *see* Sulfadiazine.

Pyrimidone *see* Pyrimidinone.

Pyrimido(4,5-b)pyrazine *see* Pteridine.

PYRIMIDO(5,4-d)PYRIMIDINE (1,3,5,7-tetraazanaphthalene).

Pyrimidoquinoxalinedione *see* Isoalloxazine.

Pyrimidylpiperonylpiperazine *see* Piribedil.

Pyrimidyl-quinaldin *see* Quinapyramine.

PYRIMITATE*** (O,O-diethyl O-(2-dimethylamino-6-methylpyrimidin-4-yl) phosphorothioate; O-(2-dimethylamino)-6-methylpyrimidin-4-yl) O,O-diethyl phosphorothioate; pyrimithate; 'diothyl').

Pyrimithate* *see* Pyrimitate.

PYRINOLINE*** (α,α-dipyrid-2-yl-α-(β-di-pyrid-2-ylmethylenecyclopenta-1,4-dien-1-yl methanol; 3-dipyrid-2-ylmethylene-α,α-dipyrid-2-yl-1,4-cyclopentadiene-1-methanol; α,α,6,6-tetrapyrid-2-ylmethano-1,4-cyclopentadienemethanol; 'surexin').

'Pyripyridium' *see* Phenazopyridine.

'Pyrisept' *see* Cetylpyridinium.

PYRITHIAMINE (1-(4-amino-2-methyl-pyrimid-5-ylmethyl)-3-(2-hydroxyethyl)-2-methylpyridinium bromide hydrobromide; neopyrithiamine).

Pyrithidium* *see* Pyritidium.

PYRITHIONE SODIUM (pyridine-2-thione 1-oxide sodium derivative; B-907; 'fonderma').

PYRITHIONE ZINC*** (bis(1-hydroxy-2-(1H)-pyridinethionato)zinc; zinc bis-(pyridine-2-thione 1-oxide); zinc pyrithione; zinc pyridine thione; 'zinc omadine').

Pyrithioxine* see Pyritinol.

PYRITHYLDIONE (3,3-diethyl-2,4(1H,3H)-pyridinedione; 3,3-diethyl-1,2,3,4-tetrahydropyridine-2,4-dione; didropyridine; dihydropyridinium; Nu-903; tetridin; 'benedorm', 'persedon', 'presidon')

PYRITIDIUM BROMIDE** (3-amino-8-[(2-amino-6-methylpyrimid-4-yl)amino]-6-(*p*-aminophenyl)-5-methylphenanthridinium bromide 1'-methobromide; pyrithidium bromide; RD-2801; 'prothidium').

PYRITINOL*** (3,3'-(dithiodimethylene)-bis(5-hydroxy 6-methyl-4-pyridinemethanol); bis(3-hydroxy-4-hydroxymethyl-2-methylpyrid-5-ylmethyl) disulfide; pyridoxine 5-disulfide; pyritinol hydrochloride; pyrithioxine; 'bonifen', 'encephabol').

'Pyrizidin' see Isoniazid.

Pyroboric acid see Tetraboric acid.

'Pyrocat' see Dipyrocetyl.

Pyrocatechin see Pyrocatechol.

PYROCATECHOL (o-dihydroxybenzene; pyrocatechin).

Pyrocatechol-3,5-disulfonic acid salts see Neodymium pyrocatecholdisulfonate; Sodium pyrocatecholdisulfonate; Stibophen.

o-**PYROCATECHUIC ACID** (2,3-dihydroxybenzoic acid; pyrocatechol-3-carboxylic acid).
See also Sodium o-pyrocatechuate.

Pyrodifenum see Prifinium.

'Pyrodin' see Aminophenazone.

'Pyrodine' see Acetylphenylhydrazine.

Pyrogallic acid see Gallic acid; Pyrogallol.

PYROGALLOL (1,2,3-trihydroxybenzene; pyrogallic acid).

Pyrogallol-5-carboxylic acid see Gallic acid.

Pyrogallol monoacetate see Gallacetophenone.

Pyrogallol triacetate see Acetpyrogall.

Pyrogallol 1,2,3-tris(diethylaminoethyl ether) triethiodide see Gallamine triethiodide.

PYROGLUTAMIC ACID (5-oxopyrrolidine-2-carboxylic acid; glutimic acid; glutiminic acid; L-glutamic lactam; 2-pyrrolidone-5-carboxylic acid; 5-oxoproline).

Pyroglutamic acid 2-dimethylaminoethyl ester see Deanol pyroglutamate.

L-**Pyroglutamyl**-L-**histidyl**-L-**tryptophyl**-L-**seryl**-L-**tyrosylglycyl**-L-**leucyl**-L-**arginyl**-L-**prolylglycinamide** see Gonadorelin.

'Pyrolan' see Methylphenylpyrazolyl dimethylcarbamate.

Pyrolaxon (tr) see Gallamine triethiodide.

'Pyrolin' see Magnesium acetate.

Pyromucic acid see Furoic acid.

Pyromucic aldehyde see 2-Furaldehyde.

4-PYRONE (*γ*-pyrone).

'Pyronil' see Pyrrobutamine.

PYROPHENDANE*** (1-methyl-3-(3-phenyl-1-indanylmethyl)pyrrolidine; 1-(1-methylpyrrolidin-3-ylmethyl)-3-phenylindan).

PYROPHOS (tr) (tetraethyl thiopyrophosphate; ethyl pyrophosphothionate; tetraethyl monothiopyrophosphate; fosarbin; phosarbin).

PYROPHOSPHORAMIDE (phosphorodiamidic anhydride; pyrophosphorotetramide).

Pyrophosphoric acid tetraethyl ester see Tetraethyl pyrophosphate.

Pyrophosphorotetramide see Pyrophosphoramide.

Pyroracemic acid see Pyruvic acid.

Pyrosal see Acetopyrine.

'Pyrostib' see Stibophen.

PYROVALERONE*** (4'-methyl-2-pyrrolidin-1-ylvalerophenone; 2-pyrrolidin-1-yl-1-*p*-tolyl-1-pentanone; pyrovalerone hydrochloride: F-1983; 'centroton', 'thymergix').

PYROXAMINE*** (3-(*p*-chloro-α-phenylbenzyloxy)-1-methylpyrrolidine; 3-(*p*-chlorobenzhydryloxy)-1-methylpyrrolidine).

PYROXAMINE MALEATE* (AHR-224).

PYROXYLIN*** (nitrocellulose; soluble gun-cotton; fulmicoton).

'Pyrozone' see Hydrogen peroxide.

PYRROBUTAMINE* (1-(*p*-chlorophenyl)-2-phenyl-4-(1-pyrrolidyl)-2-butene; 1-[4-(*p*-chlorophenyl)-3-phenylbut-2-enyl]pyrrolidine; pyrrobutamine diphosphate; 'proladyl', 'pyronil').

PYRROCAINE** (2-pyrrolidin-1-yl-2',6'-acetoxylidide; 1-pyrrolidineaceto-2',6'-xylidide; EN-1010; 'dynacaine', 'endocaine').

Pyrrolamidole see Dextromoramide.

'Pyrrolazote' see Parathiazine.

PYRROLE (azole).

PYRROLIDINE (tetrahydropyrrole).

1-Pyrrolidineaceto-2',6'-xylidide see Pyrrocaine.

2-Pyrrolidinecarboxylic acid see Proline.

2,5-Pyrrolidinedione see Succinimide.

2,6-Pyrrolidinediyldimethylene bis(3,4,5-trimethoxybenzoate) see Pirozadil.

1-Pyrrolidineethanol 4-butoxy-3,5-dimethoxybenzoate see Burodiline.

2-PYRROLIDINONE (4-aminobutyric acid lactam; 2-pyrrolidone).

2-Pyrrolidin-1-yl-2',6'-acetoxylidide see Pyrrocaine.

1-(Pyrrolidin-1-ylcarbonylmethyl)-4-(3,4,5-trimethoxycinnamoyl)piperazine see Cinepazide.

2-Pyrrolidin-1-ylethyl 4-butoxy-3,5-dimethoxybenzoate see Burodiline.

10-(2-Pyrrolidin-1-ylethyl)phenothiazine see Parathiazine.

Pyrrolidinylmethyltetracycline see Rolitetracycline.

N-**(2-Pyrrolidin-1-ylpropionyl)**-*o*-**toluidine** see Aptocaine.

3-Pyrrolidin-1-ylpropyl 2,4,6-trimethoxyphenyl ketone *see* Buflomedil.

2-Pyrrolidin-1-yl-1-*p*-tolyl-1-pentanone *see* Pyrovalerone.

3-Pyrrolidin-1-yl-4'-(α,α,α-trifluoro-*p*-tolyl)propiophenone *see* Boxidine.

Pyrrolidone *see* Pyrrolidinone.

2-Pyrrolidone-5-carboxylic acid *see* Pyroglutamic acid.

PYRROLIFENE*** ((+)-3-methyl-1,2-diphenyl-4-pyrrolidin-1-yl-2-butanol acetate; (+)-α-benzyl-β-methyl-α-phenyl-1-pyrrolidinepropanol acetate; (+)-α-acetoxy-3-methyl-1,2-diphenyl-4-pyrrolidin-1-ylbutane; pyrroliphene hydrochloride).

PYRROLINE (dihydropyrrole).

trans-**3-(1-Pyrrolin-2-yl)acrylamide** *see* Desdanine.

Pyrroliphene* *see* Pyrrolifene.

PYRROLNITRIN*** (3-chloro-4-(3-chloro-2-nitrophenyl)pyrrole; L-52230).

Pyrroplégium *see* Pentolonium.

Pyrrovinyquinium *see* Pyrvinium.

Pyruvaldehyde *see* Methylglyoxal.

Pyruvate oxidation factor *see* Thioctic acid.

PYRUVIC ACID (2-ketopropionic acid; 2-oxopropionic acid; acetylformic acid; pyroracemic acid; Brenztraubensäure).

Pyruvic acid *o*-ethoxybenzylhydrazone *see* Ruavzone.

PYRVINIUM CHLORIDE*** (6-dimethylamino-2-[2-(2,5-dimethyl-1-phenyl-3-pyrrolyl)vinyl]-1-methylquinolinium chloride; Chemotheraphy Centre cpd. No. 715; pyrrovinyquinium cloride; viprynium chloride; 'poquil', 'vanquin').

PYRVINIUM EMBONATE (pyrvinium 4,4'-methylenebis(3-hydroxynaphthalene-2-carboxylate); pyrvinium pamoate; viprynium embonate; viprynium pamoate; SN-4395; 'molevac', 'neo-oxypate', 'povan', 'vanquin').

PYTAMINE** (2-[α-(2-dimethylaminoethoxy)-2,6-diethylbenzyl]pyridine; pytamine hydrochloride; BS-7161-D).

PZ-1511 *see* Carpipramine.

'PZC' *see* Perphenazine.

Q

Q-137 *see* 1,1-Dichloro-2,2-bis(*p*-ethylphenyl)-ethane.

Q-275 *see* Ubiquinone.

QB-1 *see* Cloquinozine tartrate.

QBH *see* Benquinox.

'Qidamp' *see* Ampicillin.

'Qidmycin' *see* Erythromycin stearate.

'Qidtet' *see* Tetracycline.

QM-6008 *see* Bentazepam.

'Quaalude' *see* Methaqualone.

'Quamonium' *see* Cetrimonium.

'Quantalan' *see* Colestyramine.

'Quantril' *see* Benzquinamide.

'Quarzan' *see* Clidinium.

'Quat' *see* Bromhexine.

QUATACAINE*** (2-methyl-2-propylamino-*o*-propionotoluidide; 2,2'-dimethyl-2-propylaminopropionanilide; LA-021; 'tanacaine').

QUATERON (tr) (triethyl(3-hydroxy-2,3-dimethylpropyl)ammonium iodide *p*-butoxybenzoate; [3-[(*p*-butoxybenzoyl)-oxy]-2,3-dimethylpropyl]triethylammonium iodide; 3-diethylamino-1,2-dimethylpropyl *p*-butoxybenzoate ethiodide).

'Quatommon' *see* Benzalkonium chloride.

'Quatrachlor' *see* Benzethonium.

'Quatrasan' *see* Myristylpicolinium chloride.

QUAZODINE*** (4-ethyl-6,7-dimethoxy-quinazoline; MJ-1988).

Quebrachine *see* Yohimbine.

QUEBRACHITOL (inositol methyl ether).

Quebrachol *see* Cinchol.

'Queleton' *see* Fenthion.

'Quemid' *see* Colestyramine.

QUERCETAGETIN (3,3',4',5,6,7-hexahydroxyflavone).

QUERCETIN (3,3',4',5,7-pentahydroxyflavone; flavin; meltin; sophoretin; quercétol; 'quertine').

Quercetin 3-galactoside *see* Hyperoside.

Quercetin 3-glucoside *see* Isoquercitrin.

Quercetin 3-rhamnoglucoside *see* Rutoside.

Quercetin 3-rhamnoside *see* Quercitrin.

Quercetol *see* Quercetin.

Quercimelin *see* Quercitrin.

QUERCITOL (1,2,3,4,5-cyclohexanepentol).

QUERCITRIN (quercetin 3-rhamnoside; quercitrinic acid; quercimelin).

Quercitrinic acid *see* Quercitrin.

'Quertine' *see* Quercetin.

'Questran' *see* Colestyramine.

'Quiactin' *see* Oxanamide.

'Quick' *see* Chlorophacinone.

'Quick-kill' *see* Thallium sulfate.

'Quide' *see* Piperacetazine.

'Quiescin' *see* Reserpine.

Quietal *see* Propallylonal.

'Quietidine' *see* Diphenazine.

'Quilan' *see* Benfluralin.

'Quilene' *see* Pentapiperide metilsulfate.

'Quilil' *see* Phenprobamate.

QUILLIFOLINE*** (2-(*p*-chlorophenyl)-1,3,4,6,7,11b-hexahydro-9,10-dimethoxy-

2H-benzo(a)quinolizine; chillifolin; killifolin).

'Quilonum' *see* Lithium acetate.

'Quimar' *see* Chymotrypsin.

'Quimbo' *see* Potassium diiodophenol-sulfonate.

'Quimbosan' *see* Potassium diiodophenol-sulfonate.

'Quimotrase' *see* Chymotrypsin.

Quin.... *See also* Chin....

QUINACETOPHENONE (2',5'-dihydroxy-acetophenone).

QUINACILLIN** (6-(3-carboxy-2-quin-oxalinecarboxamido)penicillanic acid; 3-carboxyquinoxalin-2-yl penicillin).

'Quinacrine' *see* Mepacrine.

'Quinaglute' *see* Quinidine gluconate.

Quinalbarbitone* *see* Secobarbital.

QUINALDIC ACID (2-quinolinecarboxylic acid).

QUINALDINE (2-methylquinoline).

QUINALDINE BLUE*** (1-ethyl-2-[3-(1-ethyl-2(1H)quinolylidene)propenyl]quino-linium chloride; 'vernitest').

QUINALPHOS* (O,O-diethyl O-quinoxalin-2-yl phosphorothioate; 2-[(diethoxyphos-phinothioyl)oxy]quinoxaline; diethchinal-phion; 'bayrusil').

'Quinambicide' *see* Clioquinol.

QUINAPHTHOL (quinine bis(2-naphthol-1-sulfonate); chinaphthol).

QUINAPYRAMINE* (4-amino-6-[(2-amino-1,6-dimethylpyrimid-4-yl)amino]-1,2-di-methylquinolinium dichloride or disulfate; pyraldin; pyrimidyl-quinaldin; M-7555; 'antrycide').

QUINASPAR (N-[p-[(2,4-diaminoquinazolin-6-ylmethyl)amino]benzoyl]aspartic acid; NSC-112846).

QUINAZOLINE (1,3-benzodiazine; benzo-(a)-pyrimidine; phenmiazine).

QUINAZOLINONE (quinazolone).

Quinazolone *see* Quinazolinone.

QUINAZOSIN*** (2-(4-allyliperazin-1-yl)-4-amino-6,7-dimethoxyquinazoline; quinazosin dihydrochloride; quinazosin hydrochloride; CP-11332-1).

QUINBOLONE*** (17β-(cyclopent-1-enyl-oxy)androsta-1,4-dien-3-one).

QUINCARBATE** (ethyl 10-chloro-3-ethoxymethyl-2,3,6,9-tetrahydro-9-oxo-p-dioxino(2,3-g)quinoline-8-carboxylate).

QUINDECAMINE** (4,4'-(decamethylene-diimino)diquinaldine; chindecamine; kindecamin).

QUINDECAMINE ACETATE* (quin-decamine diacetate; NAT-324; 'quin-demin').

'Quindemin' *see* Quindecamine acetate.

QUINDONIUM BROMIDE*** (1,3,3a,5,6,11,12,12a-octahydro-8-hydroxy-1H-benzo-(a)cyclopenta (f)quinolizinium bromide; W-3366A).

QUINDOXIN*** (quinoxaline 1,4-dioxide; RD-2579).

'Quinercyl' *see* Chloroquine digentisate.

QUINESTRADOL*** (3-cyclopentyloxy-

estra-1,3,5(10)triene-16α,17β-diol; estriol 3-cyclopentyl ether; 'pentovis').

QUINESTROL** (3-cyclopentyloxy-17α-ethynylestra-1,3,5(10)trien-17β-ol; 3-cyclopentyloxy-19-nor-17α-pregna-1,3,5(10)-trien-20-yn-17β-ol; ethinylestra-diol 3-cyclopentyl ether; W-3566; 'estro-vis').

QUINETALATE*** (compound of 4-[(2-di-methylaminoethyl)amino]-6-methoxy-quinoline with 6-diethylcarbamoyl-3-cyclo-hexene-1-carboxylic acid; 4-dimethylamino-ethylamino-6-methoxyquinoline diethyl-aminotetrahydrophthalate; 'aureoquin', 'emphysin', 'phthalamaquin', 'ventaire').

QUINETHAZONE*** (7-chloro-2-ethyl-1,2,3,4-tetrahydro-6-sulfamoyl-quinazolin-4-one; 7-chloro-2-ethyl-1,2,3,4-tetrahydro-4-oxo-6-quinazolinesulfonamide; 'aqua-mox', 'hydromox').

QUINETUM (mixture of quinine, cinchonine and cinchonidine).
See also Totaquine.

Quingamine (tr) *see* Chloroquine diphos-phate.

QUINGESTANOL*** (3-cyclopentyloxy-19-nor-17α-pregna-3,5-dien-20-yn-17-ol).
See also Ethinylestradiol with quingestanol.

QUINGESTANOL ACETATE (W-4540).

QUINGESTRONE*** (3-cyclopentyloxy-pregna-3,5-dien-20-one; W-3399).

QUINHYDRONE (benzoquinhydrone).

QUINIC ACID (1,3,4,5-tetrahydroxycyclo-hexanecarboxylic acid; chinic acid; kinic acid).
See also Piperazine quinate; Urea quinate.

'Quinicardine' *see* Quinidine.

'Quinidate' *see* Quinidine.

QUINIDINE (conchinine; conquinine; β-quinine; stereoisomer of quinine; quinidine acid sulfate or sulfate; pitayine; 'quinidate', 'quinicardine').

α-Quinidine *see* Cinchonidine.

QUINIDINE ARABOGALACTAN SULFATE ('longacor').

QUINIDINE 5-ETHYL-5-PHENYL-BARBITURATE (quinidine phenobarbital salt; 'natisedine', 'sedoquin').

QUINIDINE GLUCONATE ('dura-tab', 'gluquinate', 'quinaglute').

QUINIDINE POLYGALACTURONATE ('cardioquin', 'mundiquin').

QUININE (α-(6-methoxy-4-quinolyl)-5-vinyl-2-quinuclidinemethanol; 6-methoxy-cinchonine).

β-Quinine *see* Quinidine.

QUININE BISALICYLOSALICYLATE (quinine di(salicylsalicylate); 'quinisal', 'quinisan').

Quinine bis(2-naphthol-1-sulfonate) *see* Quinaphthol.

QUININE BISULFATE (quinine acid sulfate; neutral quinine sulfate).

QUININE CARBONATE (diquinine carb-onate).

QUININE CARBOPHENETIDINE (quininecarboxylic acid p-ethoxyanilide;

quinine carboxylic acid phenetidide; phenetidine quinine carbonate).

Quinine chloral derivative see Quinochloral.

QUININE DIETHYLBARBITURATE (quinine barbital salt; 'chineonal').

QUININE DIHYDROCHLORIDE (quinine acid hydrochloride).

QUININE DISALICYLATE ('rheumatin').

QUININE ETHYL CARBONATE (aecachininum; tasteless quinine).

QUININE GENTISATE ('gentochin').

QUININE GLYCEROPHOSPHATE ('kineurine').

QUININE HYDROCHLORIDE (quinine monohydrochloride; basic quinine-HCl; chininum chloratum; SN-359).

Quinine hydroxycaffeine derivative see Oxyquinotheine.

QUININE IODOBISMUTHATE (biioquinol; bijochinol).

QUININE IODOSULFATE (iodoquinine sulfate).

QUININE SULFATE (basic quinine sulfate).

Quiniodochlor see Clioquinol.

Quiniofon see Chiniofon.

QUINISOCAINE*** (3-butyl-1-(2-dimethylaminoethoxy)isoquinoline; dimethisoquin; quinisocaine hydrochloride; SKF-538-A; 'pruralgin', 'quotane').

Quinium see Totaquine.

QUINIZARINE (1,4-dihydroxyanthraquinone).

Quinocaine see Cinchocaine.

QUINOCHLORAL (compound of quinine and chloral; 'chinoral').

QUINOCIDE** (8-(4-aminopentylamino)-6-methoxyquinoline; chinocide; CN-115; WIN-10448.

Quinoform see Clioquinol.

QUINOL (4-hydroxy-2,5-cyclohexadienone). *See also* Hydroquinone.

QUINOLIN-2-AMIC ACID (2-carbamylnicotinic acid; quinolinic acid monoamide).

QUINOLINE (1-benzazine; benzo(b)-pyridine).

2-Quinolinecarboxylic acid see Quinaldic acid.

4-Quinolinecarboxylic acid see Cinchoninic acid.

2,3-Quinolinedicarboxylic acid see Acridinic acid.

QUINOLINIC ACID (2,3-pyridinedicarboxylic acid).

Quinolinic acid monoamide see Quinolin-2-amic acid.

2-Quinolinol see Carbostyril.

4-QUINOLINOL (4-hydroxyquinoline; kynurine).

8-QUINOLINOL (8-hydroxyquinoline; oxin; oxine; oxychinolin; oxyquinoline; kinozol; preconsol; 'bioquin', 'oxyleine', 'quinophenol').

8-Quinolinol benzoate ester see Benzoxiquine.

8-Quinolinol copper compound see Oxinecopper.

8-QUINOLINOL SULFATE ALUMINIUM SALT ('aloxyn', 'nyxolan').

8-QUINOLINOL SULFATE POTASSIUM SALT (chinosol; quinosol; 'cryptonal', 'idril', 'pectan', 'solquinate', 'sunoxol', 'superol').

1-Quinolin-2-ylpiperazine see Quipazine.

'Quinolor' see Halquinols.

Quinomethionate see Chinomethionat.

Quinone see Benzoquinone.

Quinophan see Cinchophen.

'Quinophenol' see 8-Quinolinol.

Quinopyrine see Chinopyrine.

'Quinosol' see 8-Quinolinol sulfate potassium salt.

QUINOXALINE (1,4-benzodiazine; benzoparadiazine; benzo(a)pyrazine; phenpipazine).

Quinoxaline-3-carboxylic acid penicillin derivative see Quinacillin.

Quinoxaline-2,3-dimethanol 1,4-dioxide see Dioxidine.

Quinoxaline-2,3-dimethanol 1,4-dioxide diacetate see Quinoxidine.

Quinoxaline 1,4-dioxide see Quindoxin.

3-(2-Quinoxalinylmethylene)carbazic acid N^1,N^4-dioxide methyl ester see Carbadox.

N^1-Quinoxal-2-ylsulfanilamide see Sulfaquinoxaline.

QUINOXIDINE (tr) (quinoxaline-2,3-dimethanol 1,4-dioxide diacetate; dioxidine diacetate (ester)).

QUINPRENALINE*** (8-hydroxy-α-isopropylaminomethyl-5-quinolinemethanol; 5-(1-hydroxy-2-isopropylaminoethyl)-8-quinolinol; quinterenol; quinterenol sulfate; CP-10308-8).

Quinterenol* see Quinprenaline.

QUINTIOFOS*** (O-ethyl-O-quinolin-8-yl phenylphosphonothioate; 'bacdip').

QUINTOZENE* (pentachloronitrobenzene; PCNB; PHNB; 'brassicol', 'terraclor', 'tiicarex', 'tritisan').

QUINUCLIDINE (1-azabicyclo(2.2.2)-octane; 1,4-ethylenepiperidine).

3-QUINUCLIDINYL BENZILATE (Ro-2-3308).

3-Quinuclidinyl benzoate see Benzoclidine.

10-(Quinuclidin-3-ylmethyl)phenothiazine see Mequitazine.

QUINUPRAMINE*** (10,11-dihydro-5-quinuclidin-3-yl-5H-dibenz(b,f)azepine; 3-(10,11-dihydro-5H-dibenz(b,f)azepin-5-yl)quinuclidine; LM-208).

QUINUREA (chinurea; mixed crystals of quinine and urea).

Quinuronium methyl sulfate see Quinuronium sulfate.

QUINURONIUM SULFATE (diquinolylurea dimethosulfate; 6,6'-ureylenebis-(1-methylquinolinium sulfate); N,N'-dimethylquinolinyl methyl sulfate urea; quinuronium methyl sulfate; SN-5870; 'acaprin', 'acapron', 'babesan', 'baburon', 'diveronal', 'ludobal', 'pirevan', 'pirocyl',

'zothelone').
QUIPAZINE*** (2-piperazin-1-ylquinoline; 1-quinolin-2-ylpiperazine).
QUIPAZINE MALEATE* (Ma-1291).
'Quipenyl' *see* Pamaquin.
'Quitaxon' *see* Doxepin.

'Quival' *see* Polycarbophil calcium.
'Quixalin' *see* Halquinols.
'Quotane' *see* Quinisocaine.
QX-314 *see* Lidocaine ethobromide.
'QZ 2' *see* Methaqualone.

R

R-14 *see* Fenpipramide.
R-47 *see* Trichlormethine.
R-48 *see* Chlornaphazine.
R-52 *see* Mannosulfan.
R-55 *see* Isopropamide iodide.
R-79 *see* Isopropamide iodide.
R-88 *see* 2-(*p-tert*.Butylphenoxy)isopropyl 2-chloroethyl sulfite.
R-100 *see* Ambutonium.
R-106 *see* Pasiniazid.
R-148 *see* Methaqualone.
R-178 *see* Norgestrienone with ethinyl-estradiol.
R-181 *see* Butadiene diepoxide.
R-192 *see* Isopropamide methosulfate.
R-239 *see* 5-(2-Bromoallyl)-5-(1-methylbutyl)-barbituric acid.
R-246 *see* Tretamine.
R-261-P *see* Deacetylthiocolchicine.
R-368c *see* Niflumic acid.
R-381 *see* (2-Hydroxyethyl)phenmetrazine 2-phenylbutyrate.
R-382 *see* Phenmetrazine teoclate.
R-516 *see* Cinnarizine.
R-548 *see* Trimeglamide.
R-658 *see* Buzepide.
R-661 *see* Buzepide metiodide.
R-720-11 *see* Fenetylline.
R-760 *see* Flazalone.
R-798 *see* Rimiterol.
R-812 *see* Prednisolone *m*-sulfobenzoate.
R-875 *see* Dextromoramide.
R-1132 *see* Diphenoxylate.
R-1406 *see* Phenoperidine.
R-1575 *see* Cinnarizine.
R-1625 *see* Haloperidol.
R-1647 *see* Anisoperidone.
R-1658 *see* Moperone.
R-1707 *see* Glafenine.
R-1829 *see* Butyropipazone.
R-1929 *see* Azaperone.
R-2028 *see* Fluanisone.
R-2055 *see* Calcium methyl polygalacturonate sulfonate complex.
R-2453 *see* Demegestone.
R-2498 *see* Trifluperidol.
R-2962 *see* Amiperone.
R-2963 *see* Meperidide.
R-3201 *see* Haloperidide.

R-3248 *see* Aceperone.
R-3345 *see* Pipamperone.
R-3365 *see* Piritramide.
R-3588 *see* Etamiphylline.
R-4082 *see* Floropipetone.
R-4263 *see* Fentanyl.
R-4584 *see* Benzperidol.
R-4714 *see* Oxiperomide.
R-4749 *see* Droperidol.
R-4845 *see* Bezitramide.
R-4929 *see* Benzetimide.
R-5046 *see* Cinperene.
R-5147 *see* Spiperone.
R-5183 *see* Meletimide.
R-6218 *see* Fluspirilene.
R-6238 *see* Pimozide.
R-6348 *see* Antazonite.
R-7158 *see* Roxoperone.
R-7315 *see* Metomidate.
R-7405 *see* Etomidate.
R-7464 *see* Propoxate.
R-7904 *see* Lidoflazine.
R-8141 *see* Antienite.
R-8284 *see* Proclonol.
R-8299 *see* Tetramisole.
R-9298 *see* Clofluperol.
R-10100 *see* Ethonam.
R-10948 *see* Diamocaine cyclamate.
R-11333 *see* Bromperidol.
R-12456 *see* Levamisole.
R-13558 *see* Fetoxilate.
R-14827 *see* Econazole.
R-14889 *see* Miconazole.
R-15403 *see* Difenoxin.
R-15454 *see* Isoconazole.
R-15497 *see* Gemazocine.
R-16341 *see* Penfluridol.
R-16470 *see* Dexetimide.
R-16659 *see* Etomidate.
R-17190 *see* Protizinic acid.
R-17635 *see* Mebendazole.
R-18553 *see* Loperamide.
R-18910 *see* Fluperamide.
R-19317 *see* Rodocaine.
R-22700 *see* Rodocaine hydrochloride.
R-23050 *see* Salantel.
R-25061 *see* Suprofen.
R-25160 *see* Cliprofen.
R-26333 *see* Deximafen.

RA-8 see Dipyridamole.
RA-101 see Niprofazone.
'Rabon' see Stirofos.
'Racedrine' see Racephedrine.
RACEFEMINE*** (($\pm$)-α-methyl-N-(1-methyl-2-phenoxyethyl)phenethylamine; ($\pm$)-N-(1-methyl-2-phenoxyethyl)-amphetamine).
See also Dextrofemine.
RACEFENICOL*** (($\pm$)-*threo*-2,2-dichloro-N-(β-hydroxy-α-hydroxymethyl-p-methyl-sulfonylphenethyl)acetamide; ($\pm$)-*threo*-N-(2,2-dichloroacetyl)-β-hydroxy-α-hydroxy-methyl-p-methylsulfonylphenethylamine).
Racemelfalan see Sarcolysin.
RACEMETHORPHAN*** (($\pm$)-3-methoxy-N-methylmorphinan; racemethorphan hydrobromide; methorphan; Ro-1-4570).
See also Dextromethorphan; Levomethorphan.
Racemic acid see Mandelic acid.
RACEMORAMIDE*** (($\pm$)-4-(2-methyl-4-oxo-3,3-diphenyl-4-pyrrolidin-1-ylbutyl)-morpholine; ($\pm$)-1-(3-methyl-4-morpho-lino-2,2-diphenylbutyryl)pyrrolidine; racemoramide bitartrate; R-610).
See also Dextromoramide; Levomoramide.
RACEMORPHAN*** (($\pm$)-3-hydroxy-N-methylmorphinan; methorphinan; race-morphan bitartrate; Nu-2206; Ro-1-5431; 'cetarin', 'citarin', 'racemic dromoran').
See also Dextrorphan; Levorphanol.
RACEPHEDRINE* (($\pm$)-α-(1-methyl-aminoethyl)benzyl alcohol; racemic ephedrine; racephedrine hydrochloride; 'cophedrine', 'ephedron', 'ephetonin', 'methylmydriatin', 'racedrine').
'Rachineocaine' see Procaine.
'Rachromate' see Sodium chromate (^{51}Cr).
'Racobalamin-57' see Cyanocobalamin (^{57}Co).
'Racumin' see Coumatetralyl.
'Racuza' see Dicamba-methyl.
'Radapon' see Dalapon sodium.
'Radedorm' see Nitrazepam.
'Radepur' see Chlordiazepoxide.
'Radikill' see Cyanazine.
Radioaurum* see Gold (^{198}Au) colloidal.
Radiocesium chloride see Cesium (^{131}Cs) chloride.
Radiocyanocobalamin see Cyanoco-balamin (^{57}Co); Cyanocobalamin (^{60}Co).
Radiocycobemin* see Cyanocobalamin (^{60}Co).
Radiogallium citrate see Gallium (^{67}Ga) citrate.
Radiogold, colloidal see Gold (^{198}Au) colloidal.
'Radiographol' see Methiodal.
Radioiodinated human serum albumin see Iodinated (^{125}I) human serum albumin; Iodinated (^{131}I) human serum albumin.
'Radiol' see Cetrimonium.
Radiomerisoprol see Merisoprol (^{197}Hg).
'Radiomiro' see Iodamide.
'Radiopol' see Iodinated poppyseed oil.
'Radioselectan' see Adipiodone meglumine.

Radioselenomethionine see Seleno-methionine (^{75}Se).
Radiotolpovidone see Tolpovidone (^{131}I).
Radioxenon see Xenon (^{133}Xe).
Radium emanation see Radon.
RADON (radium emanation; 'alphatron').
RAFOXANIDE*** (3'-chloro-4'-(p-chloro-phenoxy)-3,5-diiodosalicylanilide; 'afoxanide; 'flukanide', 'ranide').
RAM-327 see Oxymethebanol.
RAMBUFASIDE* (14-hydroxy-3-(4-O-methyl-α-L-rhamnopyranosyloxy)-14β-bufa-4,20,22-trienolide; 4'-O-methyl-proscillaridin).
'Ramrod' see Propachlor.
'Ramocillin' see Procaine-penicillin.
'Randolectil' see Butaperazine.
'Randonos' see Chorionic gonadotrophin.
'Randox' see Allidochlor.
'Randum' see Metoclopramide with medazepam.
'Ranestol' see Triclofenol piperazine.
'Ranide' see Rafoxanide.
RANIMYCIN*** (antibiotic from *Str. lincolnensis*).
'Ranitol' see Raubasine.
'Ranocaine' see Propoxycaine.
'Raovin' see Tolpovidone (^{131}I).
'Rapacodin' see Dihydrocodeine.
'Rapidosept' see Dichlorobenzyl alcohol.
'Rapitest' see Norgestrienone with ethinyl-estradiol.
'Rasprin' see Calcium acetylsalicylate.
'Rastinon' see Tolbutamide.
RATHYRONINE*** (DL-3-[4-(4-hydroxy-3-iodophenoxy)-3,5-diiodophenyl]alanine).
See also Detrothyronine; Liothyronine.
'Raticate' see Norbormide.
'Ratilan' see Coumachlor.
'Ratindan 1' see Diphenadione.
'Ratindan 3' see Chlorophacinone.
'Ratofarin' see Warfarin.
RATTLESNAKE VENOM ('crotalin', 'dicrotalin', 'epileptasid').
'Rattrack' see Antu.
RAUBASINE (ajmalicine; tetrahydroser-pentine; δ-yohimbine; 'hydrosarpan', 'lamuran', 'ranitol', 'rytmaline').
RAUBASINE WITH DIHYDROERGO-CRISTINE MESILATE (DF-69; 'defluina', 'iskedyl').
'Raunormine' see Deserpidine.
'Raurine' see Reserpine.
'Rau-sed' see Reserpine.
'Rautensin' see Alseroxylon.
'Rauwild' see Reserpine.
'Rauwiloid' see Alseroxylon.
RAUWOLFIA ALKALOIDS (alkaloids from *Rauwolfia serpentina* and/or *Rauwolfia vomitoria*; RS-51).
See also Alseroxylon; Ajmaline; Chandrine; Deserpidine; Raubasine; Raunescine; Rauwolscine; Rescinnamine; Reserpine.
Rauwolfin see Ajmaline.
RAUWOLSCINE (α-yohimbine).
'Raviac' see Chlorophacinone.
'Ravocaine' see Propoxycaine.

'Raybanol' *see* Sodium benzyl succinate.
'Rayomiro' *see* Iodamide.
'Raythesin' *see* Risocaine.
'Razebil' *see* Iobenzamic acid.
RAZOXANE*** (1,3-bis(3,5-dioxopiperazin-1-yl)propane; 4,4'-propylidenedi(2,6-piperazinedione); ICI-59118; ICRF-159; NSC-129943).
RB-1466 *see* Silymarin.
RC-172 *see* Aldioxa.
RC-173 *see* Alcloxa.
RCH-108 *see* Nitrosotropolone.
RD-292 *see* Fenpentadiol.
RD-354 *see* Pentorex tartrate.
RD-2579 *see* Quindoxin.
RD-2801 *see* Pyritidium.
RD-3803 *see* Diloxanide.
RD-9338 *see* Norbudrine.
RD-11654 *see* Ibufenac.
RD-13621 *see* Ibuprofen.
RD-17435 *see* Fluprofen.
RD-20000 *see* Deprodone propionate.
'Reacid' *see* Cyacetacide.
'Readcillin' *see* Penicillin G.
'Realin' *see* Oxyphenbutazone with prednisolone.
'Reapam' *see* Prazepam.
'Reasec' *see* Diphenoxylate with atropine.
'Reazide' *see* Cyacetacide.
Rec-7-0040 *see* Flavoxate.
Rec-7-0052 *see* Flavamine.
Rec-7-0267 *see* Dimefline.
Rec-7-0518 *see* Ketocaine.
Rec-14/0127 *see* Moquizone.
Rec-15/0019 *see* Moxicoumone.
Rec-15/0122 *see* Nifurpipone.
Rec-15/0691 *see* Tibezonium iodide.
'Recanescine' *see* Deserpidine.
'Recetan' *see* Butidrine.
'Recofur' *see* Nifurpipone.
'Recolip' *see* Clofibrate.
'Recordil' *see* Efloxate.
'Recrein' *see* Deanol.
'Rectanol' *see* Bromethol.
'Rectidon' *see* 5-(2-Bromoallyl)-5-(1-methylbutyl)barbituric acid.
'Recton' *see* 5-(2-Bromoallyl)-5-(1-methylbutyl)barbituric acid.
'Rectormone' *see* Testosterone propionate.
'Rectules' *see* Chloral hydrate.
'Recuryl' *see* Pentolonium.
'Redeptin' *see* Fluspirilene.
Redergam (tr) *see* Dihydroergotoxine.
'Redimyl' *see* Glutethimide.
'Redomex' *see* Amitriptyline.
'Redouline' *see* Reserpilene.
Red tetrazolium *see* 2,3,5-Triphenyl tetrazolium chloride.
'Reducdyn' *see* Acetylhomocysteine thiolactone with L-cysteine and fructose.
REDUCTIC ACID (2,3-dihydroxy-2,3-cyclopenten-1-one; 2-cyclopenta-2,3-diol-1-one).
'Reducyl' *see* Phentermine.
'Redul' *see* Glymidine.
'Redusterol' *see* 2-Phenylbutyramide.
Ref-185 *see* Cortivazol.
'Reflux' *see* Methenamine mandelate.

'Refobacin' *see* Gentamicin.
'Refugal' *see* Clofedanol.
'Refungine' *see* Sulbentine.
'Refusal' *see* Disulfiram.
'Regadrin' *see* Clofibrate.
'Regasprin' *see* Calcium acetylsalicylate.
'Regelan' *see* Clofibrate.
'Regenon' *see* Amfepramone.
'Regitin' *see* Phentolamine mesilate.
'Reglan' *see* Metoclopramide.
'Réglisse' *see* Liquorice extract.
'Reglone' *see* Diquat.
'Regonol' *see* Pyridostigmine bromide.
'Regovar' *see* Norethisterone with mestranol.
'Regroton' *see* Reserpine with chlortalidone.
'Regutol' *see* Sodium dioctyl sulfosuccinate.
'Rehibin' *see* Trigentisic acid.
'Rektidon' *see* Paraldehyde.
'Rela' *see* Carisoprodol.
'Relane' *see* Dexoxadrol.
'Relanium' *see* Diazepam.
'Relanol' *see* Parapenzolate bromide.
RELAXIN (*the hormone*) ('cervilaxin', 'releasin').
'Relaxin' *see* Magnesium gluconate.
'Releasin' *see* Relaxin.
'Relefact LH-RH' *see* Gonadorelin.
RELOMYCIN*** (antibiotic from *Str. hygroscopicus*; AM-684-Beta).
'Relovis' *see* Ethinylestradiol with quingestanol.
'Reltine' *see* Piperphenidol.
'Remanex' *see* Hexachlorophene with phenylmercuric borate.
'Remeflin' *see* Dimefline.
'Remiderm' *see* Triamcinolone with halquinols.
'Renacidin' *see* Citric acid.
Renactide *see* Giractide.
'Renafur' *see* Nifuradene.
'Renamid' *see* Acetazolamide.
RENANOLONE** (3α-hydroxy-5α-pregnane-11,20-dione; 5β-pregnane 3α-ol-11,20-dione).
'Renarcol' *see* Bromethol.
'Renascin' *see* Tocopherol nicotinate.
'Rencal' *see* Sodium phytate.
'Renese' *see* Polythiazide.
'Reno 60' *see* Meglumine diatrizoate.
'Reno 76' *see* Meglumine diatrizoate with sodium diatrizoate.
'Renoform' *see* Epinephrine.
'Renografin' *see* Meglumine diatrizoate with sodium diatrizoate.
'Renolon' *see* Calcium acetylsalicylate.
'Renopac' *see* 2,6-Diiodo-1-phenol-4-sulfonic acid.
'Renovist' *see* Meglumine diatrizoate with sodium diatrizoate.
'Renselin' *see* Undecenoic acid.
RENYTOLINE*** (α-fluoren-9-ylidene-*p*-toluamidine; 9-(*p*-aminobenzylidene)-fluorene; renytoline hydrochloride; paranyline hydrochloride).
Reoisodex (tr) *see* Dextran(s).
Reopoliglukin (tr) *see* Dextran 40.
'Reorganin' *see* Guaifenesin.

'**Reoxyl**' *see* Hexobendine.
'**Reparil**' *see* Escin.
'**Repeltin**' *see* Alimemazine.
'**Repocal**' *see* Pentobarbital.
'**Repodral**' *see* Stibophen.
'**Repoise**' *see* Butaperazine.
Repolymerized gelatin *see* Polygeline.
'**Reprodal**' *see* Stibophen.
REPROTEROL** (7-[3-[(β,3,5-trihydroxy-phenethyl)amino]propyl]theophylline; β,3,5-trihydroxy-N-(3-theophyllin-7-yl-propyl)phenethylamine).
'**Reptilase**' *see* Hemocoagulase.
RESACETOPHENONE (2′,4′-dihydroxy-acetophenone).
Resacetophenone 4-methyl ether *see* Peonol.
'**Resactin A**' *see* Hydroxycyclohexide.
'**Resantin**' *see* Fenpipramide.
RESCINNAMINE*** (methyl 1α,2β,3α,4, 4aα,5,7,8,13,13bβ,14,14aα-dodecahydro-2α,11-dimethoxy-3β-(3,4,5-trimethoxy-cinnamoyloxy)benz(g)indolo(2,3-a)quino-lizine-1β-carboxylate; 3,4,5-trimethoxycin-namate ester of methyl reserpate; reser-pinine; 'anaprel', 'moderil', 'rescisan', 'triraupin').
'**Rescisan**' *see* Rescinnamine.
'**Resercen**' *see* Reserpine.
Reserpene *see* Reserpine.
RESERPIC ACID (1α,2β,3α,4,4aα,5,7,8,13, 13bβ,14,14aα-dodecahydro-3β-hydroxy-2α,11-dimethoxybenz(g)indolo(2,3-a)quino-lizine-1β-carboxylic acid; reserpinic acid; reserpinolic acid; reserpionic acid).
See also Methyl reserpate; Rescinnamine; Reserpine; Syrosingopine.
RESERPILENE (alkaloid(s) from *R. vomi-toria* and *R. canescens*; 'paratensiol', 'redouline').
RESERPINE*** (methyl 1α,2β,3α,4,4aα,5,7, 8,13,13bβ,14,14aα-dodecahydro-2α,11-di-methoxy-3β-(3,4,5-trimethoxybenzoyloxy)-benz(g)indolo(2,3-a)quinolizine-1β-carb-oxylate; 3,4,5-trimethoxybenzoate ester of methyl reserpate; reserpene).
RESERPINE WITH BENDROFLU-METHIAZIDE ('abicol', 'tensionorme').
RESERPINE WITH CHLORTALIDONE ('darebon', 'regroton').
RESERPINE WITH CLOPAMIDE AND DIHYDROERGOCRISTINE (DCR-515; 'brinerdine', 'briserin').
RESERPINE WITH FUROSEMIDE (E-121-C; 'nortensin', 'terbolan', 'tenserlix').
RESERPINE WITH TRICHLORME-THIAZIDE ('metatensin', 'naquival').
RESERPINE WITH XIPAMIDE ('durotan').
Reserpinic acid *see* Reserpic acid.
Reserpinine *see* Rescinnamine.
Reserpinolic acid *see* Reserpic acid.
'**Reserpoid**' *see* Reserpine.
'**Resil**' *see* Guaifenesin.
'**Resistoflex**' *see* Polyvinyl alcohol.
'**Resistomycin**' *see* Kanamycin.
'**Resistopen**' *see* Oxacillin.

'**Resitan**' *see* Valethamate bromide.
'**Resitox**' *see* Coumafos.
'**Resivit**' *see* Leucocianidol.
RESMETHRIN* (*cis-trans-*(±)-5-benzyl-furan-3-ylmethyl 2,2-dimethyl-3-(2-methyl-1-propenyl)cyclopropanecarboxylate; 5-benzyl-3-furylmethyl chrysanthemate; benzylfuroline; NRDC-104; SBP-1382; 'chryson', 'synthrin').
See also Bioresmethrin; Cismethrin.
'**Resochin**' *see* Chloroquine.
'**Resochin S**' *see* Chloroquine silicate.
'**Resoquine**' *see* Chloroquine.
RESORANTEL*** (4′-bromo-γ-resorcyl-anilide; 4′-bromo-2,6-dihydroxybenzani-lide; 'terenol').
RESORCINOL (*m*-dihydroxybenzene; 1,3-benzenediol; resorcin).
RESORCINOL ACETATE (resorcinol monoacetate; 3-acetoxyphenol; 'euresol').
Resorcinol butyl ether *see* *m*-Butoxyphenol.
Resorcinolphthalein *see* Fluorescein.
Resorcinolphthalin *see* Fluorescin.
α-**RESORCYLIC ACID** (3,5-dihydroxyben-zoic acid).
β-**RESORCYLIC ACID** (2,4-dihydroxy-benzoic acid).
γ-**RESORCYLIC ACID** (2,6-dihydroxy-benzoic acid).
'**Resorptol**' *see* 16-Acetylgitoxin.
'**Resotren**' *see* Cloquinate with chloroquine diphosphate and diiodohydroxyquin.
'**Respectol**' *see* Dibromsalicil.
'**Respenyl**' *see* Guaifenesin.
'**Respigon**' *see* Bufogenin.
'**Respilyt**' *see* Noscapine.
'**Resteclin**' *see* Tetracycline with ascorbic acid.
'**Restovar**' *see* Lynestrenol with mestranol.
'**Resyl**' *see* Guaifenesin.
'**Retabolil**' *see* Nandrolone decanoate.
'**Retamin**' *see* Buclizine.
RETAMINE (α-hydroxyisosparteine).
'**Retandrol**' *see* Testosterone phenylpropio-nate.
'**Retardin**' *see* Diphenoxylate plus atropine.
'**Retenema**' *see* Betamethasone valerate.
'**Retentin**' *see* Carinamide.
'**Reticus**' *see* Desonide.
'**Retin-A**' *see* Tretinoin.
RETINAL (3,7-dimethyl-9-(2,6,6-trimethyl-1-cyclohexen-1-yl)nona-2,4,6,8-tetraenal; axerophthal; retinene; vitamin A aldehyde).
Retinene *see* Retinal.
Retinic acid *see* Glycyrrhizic acid.
Retinoic acid *see* Tretinoin.
RETINOL*** (3,7-dimethyl-9-(2,6,6-tri-methyl-1-cyclohexen-1-yl)nona-2,4,6,8-tetraen-1-ol; axerophthol; axerophthylium; antiinfective vitamin; antixerophthalmic vitamin; biosterol; oleovitamin A; oph-thalin; vitamin A; vitamin A alcohol).
RETINOL ACETATE (vitamin A acetate).
'**Retrangor**' *see* Benziodarone.
'**Retroid**' *see* Trengestone.
Retroprogestagen *see* 16α-Ethylthio-6-dehydroretroprogesterone.

RETROPROGESTERONE (19-retropro-
gesterone; 9β,10α-progesterone; 9β,
10α-pregn-4-ene-3,20-dione).
RETRORSINE N-OXIDE (isatidine).
'**Reublonil**' see Benzpiperylone.
'**Reuprosal**' see o-Propoxybenzamide.
'**Revasa**' see Aminoquinuride.
'**Reverin**' see Rolitetracycline.
'**Revertina**' see Mecamylamine.
'**Revivan**' see Dopamine.
'**Revivon**' see Diprenorphine.
'**Revonal**' see Methaqualone.
'**Revoxyl**' see Dibemethine.
'**Rezifilm**' see Thiram.
RG-270 see Iomeglamic acid.
Rhabarberone see Aloe-emodin.
'**Rhaetocaine**' see Benzocaine.
RHAMNETIN (3,3',4',5-tetrahydroxy-7-
methoxyflavone; β-rhamnocitrin; 7-methyl-
quercetin).
β-**Rhamnocitrin** see Rhamnetin.
Rhamnol see Cinchol.
Rhamnoxanthin see Frangulin.
RHAPONTIZIN (2,3,3'-trihydroxy-4'-
methoxystilbene 2-glucoside).
Rheic acid see Rhein.
RHEIN (4,5-dihydroxyanthraquinone-2-car-
boxylic acid; 1,8-dihydroxyanthraquinone-
3-carboxylic acid; chrysazin-3-carboxylic
acid; cassic acid; parietic acid; rheic acid;
rhubarb yellow).
'**Rhematin**' see Cinchophen.
'**Rhenocaine**' see Hydroxytetracaine.
'**Rheomacrodex**' see Dextran 40.
'**Rheosolon**' see Phenylbutazone with
prednisolone.
'**Rheotran**' see Dextran 40.
Rheum see Frangula emodin.
'**Rheumacyl**' see Glycol salicylate.
'**Rheumasit**' see Dexamethasone with benzyl
nicotinate.
'**Rheumatin**' see Quinine disalicylate.
'**Rheumox**' see Azapropazone.
'**Rhinogutt**' see Tramazoline.
'**Rhinoptil**' see Cafaminol.
'**Rhinosan**' see Oxymetazoline.
'**Rhinospray**' see Tramazoline.
'**Rhizoctol**' see Benquinox plus methyl-
thioxoarsine.
Rhizopus arhizus var. Delmar, lipase see
Rizolipase.
'**Rhodallin**' see Thiosinamine.
Rhodan see Thiocyanogen.
'**Rhodanhexamine**' see Methenamine thio-
cyanate.
Rhodanic acid see Rhodanine; Thiocyanic
acid.
RHODANINE (thiazolidin-4-one-2-thione;
rhodanic acid).
'**Rhodiacid**' see Ziram.
'**Rhodiatox**' see Parathion.
Rhodochromium see Merbromin.
RHODOPSIN (visual purple).
'**Rhodoquine**' see Plasmocide.
'**Rhodovet**' see Methenamine thiocyanate.
'**Rhodoviol**' see Polyvinyl alcohol.
'**Rhomex**' see Piperazine citrate.

'**Rhonal**' see Acetylsalicylic acid.
'**Rhothane**' see DDD.
Rhubarb yellow see Rhein.
'**Rhythmochin**' see Procainamide with
quinidine.
'**Rhythmodan**' see Disopyramide.
'**Rhythmodul**' see Disopyramide.
'**Riabal**' see Prifinium bromide.
RIBAMINOL*** (2-diethylaminoethyl ribonucleate; 2-diethylaminoethanol ribonucleate; ribonucleic acid compound with
2-diethylaminoethanol; 2-hydroxytriethyl-
amine ribonucleate; ICN-542).
RIBAVIRIN** (1-β-D-ribofuranosyl-1H-
1,2,4-triazole-3-carboxamide; 1H-1,2,4-
triazole-3-carboxamide riboside; ICN-
1229; 'viramid', 'virazole').
α-**RIBAZOLE** (5,6-dimethyl-1-(α-D-ribo-
furanosyl)benzimidazole).
Riboazauracil see Azaribine.
RIBOFLAVIN*** (7,8-dimethyl-10-(1-D-
ribityl)isoalloxazine; lactoflavin; ovoflavin;
vitamin B₂; vitamin G; riboflavine).
2-(β-D-**Ribofuranosyl)maleimide** see
Showdomycin.
2-β-D-**Ribofuranosyl-as-triazine-3,5-(2H,
4H)dione** see Azauridine.
2-β-D-**Ribofuranosyl-as-triazine-3,5-(2H,
4H)dione 2',3',5'-triacetate** see Azaribine.
1-β-D-**Ribofuranosyl-1,2,4-triazole-3-
carboxamide** see Ribavirin.
RIBOPRINE*** (N-(3-methyl-2-butenyl)-
adenosine; IPA).
RIBOSTAMYCIN*** (O-2,6-diamino-2,6-
dideoxy-α-D-glucopyranosyl-(1→4)-O-
[β-D-ribofuranosyl-(1→5)]-2-deoxystrepta-
mine).
RICINOLEIC ACID (2-hydroxy-9-octa-
decenoic acid).
See also Sodium ricinoleate; Zinc
ricinoleate.
RICINOMACROGOL* (castor oil polyoxy-
ethylene ether; 'nikkol HCO5').
'**Ridazole**' see Ronidazole.
'**Ridinol**' see Pridinol mesilate.
'**Rido rato**' see Warfarin.
'**Riedemil**' see Calusterone.
'**Rifa**' see Rifampicin.
'**Rifadin**' see Rifampicin.
RIFAMIDE** (N,N-diethylrifamycin B
amide; rifamycin B diethylamide; 'rifocin-
M').
RIFAMPICIN*** (3-(4-methylpiperazin-1-
yl-iminomethyl)rifamycin SV; rifampin;
AMP; 'rifa', 'rifadin', 'rifoldin',
'rimactane').
Rifampin* see Rifampicin.
RIFAMYCIN*** (5,6,9,17,19,21-hexa-
hydroxy-23-methoxy-2,4,12,16,18,20,22-
heptamethyl-2,7-(epoxypentadeca(1,11,13)-
trienimino)naphtho(2,1-b)furan-1,11(2H)-
dione 21-acetate; rifamycin SV; rifomycin;
NSC-133100; 'rifocine', 'rifocyne').
Rifamycin SV see Rifamycin.
'**Rifocine**' see Rifamycin.
'**Rifocin-M**' see Rifamide.
'**Rifocyne**' see Rifamycin.

'Rifoldin' see Rifampicin.
Rifomycin see Rifamycin.
'Rigakin' see Levodopa.
'Rigitrem' see Levodopa.
'Rigedal' see Isosorbide dinitrate.
Riker-548 see Trimeglamide.
Riker-594 see Sultiame.
Riker-595 see Butaperazine.
Riker-601 see Triaziquone.
Riker 738 see Nefopam.
'Rimactane' see Rifampicin.
RIMANTADINE*** (α-methyl-1-adamantanemethylamine; rimantadine hydrochloride; EXP-126).
'Rimaon' see Ethacridine.
RIMAZOLIUM METILSULFATE*** (3-(ethoxycarbonyl)-6,7,8,9-tetrahydro-1,6-dimethyl-4-oxo-4H-pyrido(1,2-a)pyrimidinium methyl sulfate; 3-carboxy-6,7,8,9-tetrahydro-1,6-dimethyl-4-oxo-4H-pyrido-(1,2-a)pyridinium methyl sulfate ethyl ester; 3-carbethoxy-6,7,8,9-tetrahydro-1,6-dimethyl-4-oxohomopyrimidazole methyl sulfate; MZ-144; 'probon').
'Rimetin' see Metoclopramide.
'Rimidol' see Naphazoline.
'Rimifon' see Isoniazid.
RIMITEROL*** (α-(3,4-dihydroxyphenyl)-2-piperidinedimethanol; erythro-3,4-dihydroxy-α-piperid-2-ylbenzyl alcohol; rimiterol hydrobromide; R-798; WG-253; 'pulmadil').
'Rinderon' see Betamethasone.
'Riodine' see Glyceryl iodoricinoleate.
'Riogon' see Chorionic gonadotrophin.
'Riomitsin' see Oxytetracycline.
'Riomycin' see Fluvomycin.
'Riopan' see Magaldrate.
RIPAZEPAM*** (1-ethyl-4,6-dihydro-3-methyl-8-phenylpyrazolo(4,3-e)(1,4)-diazepin-5(1H)-one; pyrazapon; CI-683).
'Ripercol' see Tetramisole.
'Risatarun' see Deanol aceglumate.
'Riself' see Mephenoxalone.
'Riseptin' see Dichlorobenzododecinium.
RISOCAINE** (propyl p-aminobenzoate; propylcaine; 'propaesin', 'raythesin').
'Risolid' see Chlordiazepoxide.
'Risordan' see Isosorbide dinitrate.
RISTOCETIN*** (antibiotic from *Nocardia lurida*; ristocetins A and B; 'riston', 'spontin').
'Riston' see Ristocetin.
RIT-1140 see Apicycline.
'Ritalin' see Methyl phenidate.
'Ritmodan' see Disopyramide.
RITODRINE*** (p-hydroxy-α-[1-(p-hydroxyphenethylamino)ethyl]benzyl alcohol; β,4,4′-trihydroxy-α-methyldiphenethylamine; erythro-2-(p-hydroxyphenethylamino)-1-(p-hydroxyphenyl)propan-1-ol; Du-21220; 'prempar', 'pre-par').
RITROPIRRONIUM BROMIDE*** (erythro-3-hydroxy-1,1-dimethylpyrrolidinium bromide α-cyclopentylmandelate).
RITROSULFAN*** (1,4-dideoxy-1,4-bis[(2-hydroxyethyl)amino]erythritol 1,4-di-

methanesulfonate (ester)).
'Rivanol' see Ethacridine.
'Rivon' see Pempidine.
'Rivotril' see Clonazepam.
'Rixapen' see Clometocillin.
RIZOLIPASE*** (lipase from *Rhizopus arhizus* var. *Delmar*).
RJ-64 see Pifexole.
Ro 0783/B see 5-Hydroxytryptophan.
Ro 1-5155 see Nicotinyl alcohol.
Ro 1-5431 see Racemorphan.
Ro 1-5470 see Racemethorphan.
Ro 1-5470/5 see Dextromethorphan.
Ro 1-5470/6 see Levomethorphan.
Ro 1-5479 see Dextromethorphan.
Ro 1-6463 see Methyprylone.
Ro 1-6794 see Dextrorphan.
Ro 1-7700 see Levallorphan.
Ro 1-7788 see Levomethorphan.
Ro 1-7929 see Levallorphan.
Ro 1-7977 see Dimercaptosuccinic acid.
Ro 1-9334 see Dehydroemetine.
Ro 1-9569 see Tetrabenazine.
Ro 2-0015 see Fluorocytosine.
Ro 2-2222 see Trimetaphan camsilate.
Ro 2-2453 see Dimazole.
Ro 2-2985 see Lasalocid.
Ro 2-3053 see Mepesulfate.
Ro 2-3198 see Edrophonium chloride.
Ro 2-3248 see Azapetine.
Ro 2-3308 see 3-Quinuclidinyl benzilate.
Ro 2-3773 see Clidinium.
Ro 2-7113 see Allylprodine.
Ro 2-9757 see Fluorouracil.
Ro 2-9915 see Flucytosine.
Ro 3-4787 see Bufuralol.
Ro 4-0403 see Chlorprothixene.
Ro 4-1575 see Amitriptyline.
Ro 4-1634 see Pivhydrazine.
Ro 4-1778/1 see Metofoline.
Ro 4-2130 see Sulfamethoxazole.
Ro 4-3816 see Alcuronium.
Ro 4-4393 see Sulfadoxine.
Ro 4-4602 see Benserazide.
Ro 4-5282 see Mefenorex.
Ro 4-5360 see Nitrazepam.
Ro 4-6467 see Procarbazine.
Ro 4-8347 see Trengestone.
Ro 5-0690 see Chlordiazepoxide.
Ro 5-0810/1 see Triclobisonium.
Ro 5-0831/1 see Isocarboxazid.
Ro 5-2092 see Demoxazepam.
Ro 5-2807 see Diazepam.
Ro 5-3059 see Nitrazepam.
Ro 5-3307/B1 see Debrisoquine.
Ro 5-3350 see Bromazepam.
Ro 5-4023 see Clonazepam.
Ro 5-4200 see Flunitrazepam.
Ro 5-4556 see Medazepam.
Ro 5-4645/10 see Coumamycin A₁.
Ro 5-5807 see Trimethoprim.
Ro 5-6846 see Flurazepam.
Ro 5-6901 see Flurazepam.
Ro 5-9110/1 see Dorastine.
Ro 6-2580/11 see Co-trimoxazole.
Ro 6-3129 see 16α-Ethylthio-6-dehydroretroprogesterone.
Ro 6-4563 see Glibornuride.

Ro 7-0207 *see* Ornidazole.
Ro 7-1051 *see* Benznidazole.
Ro 7-1554 *see* Ipronidazole.
Ro 7-4488/1 *see* Cuprimyxin.
Ro 8-0576 *see* Levodopa with benserazide.
Ro 10-7453 *see* Bromazepam with clidinium bromide.
'Robalate' *see* Aluminium glycinate.
'Robaxin' *see* Methocarbamol.
ROBENIDINE*** (1,3-bis(*p*-chlorobenzylideneamino)guanidine; robenzidine).
Robenzidine *see* Robenidine.
'Robimycin' *see* Erythromycin.
Robinson ester *see* Glucose 6-phosphate.
'Robinul' *see* Glycopyrronium.
'Robitrin' *see* Diethylaminoethyl 9-fluorenecarboxylate.
'Robitussin' *see* Guaifenesin.
'Roccal' *see* Benzalkonium.
Rochelle salt *see* Potassium sodium tartrate.
'Ro-cillin' *see* Pheneticillin.
ROCIVERINE*** (2-(diethylamino)-1-methylethyl *cis*-1-hydroxy(bicyclohexyl)-2-carboxylate).
'Rocmaline' *see* Arginine malate.
'Rocornal' *see* Trapidil.
'Rodallin' *see* Thiosinamine.
'Rodalon' *see* Benzalkonium.
'Rodameb' *see* Difetarsone.
'Rodavan' *see* Chlorphenoxamine teoclate.
'Rodilone' *see* Acedapsone.
'Rodiuran' *see* Hydroflumethiazide.
RODOCAINE** (*trans*-6'-chloro-2,3,4,4a,5,6,7,7a-octahydro-1H-pyrindine-1-propiono-*o*-toluidide; *trans*-1-[2[*N*-(6-chloro-*o*-tolyl)carboxamido]ethyl]-1H-1-pyrindine; *trans*-*N*-(6-chloro-2-methylphenyl)-3-(1H-1-pyrindin-1-yl)propionamide; R-19317).
RODOCAINE HYDROCHLORIDE (R-22700).
'Rodogyl' *see* Metronidazole with spiramycin.
'Rofenaid' *see* Ormetoprim with sulfadimethoxine.
'Rofenid' *see* Ketoprofen.
ROFLURANE*** (2-bromo-1,1,2-trifluoroethyl methyl ether; DA-893).
'Rogitine' *see* Phentolamine mesilate.
'Rogor' *see* Dimethoate.
'Rogue' *see* Propanil.
'Rohypnol' *see* Flunitrazepam.
'Rolazote' *see* Parathiazine.
ROLETAMIDE*** (3',4',5'-trimethoxy-3-(3-pyrrolin-1-yl)acrylophenone; CL-59112).
'Rolicton' *see* Amisometradine.
Rolicypram* *see* Rolicyprine.
ROLICYPRINE*** ((+)-5-oxo-*N*-(*trans*-2-phenylcyclopropyl)-L-2-pyrrolidinecarboxamide; rolicypram; EX-4883; 'cypromin').
'Rolinex' *see* 2-6-Diiodo-1-phenol-4-sulfonic acid.
ROLITETRACYCLINE*** (*N*-(pyrrolidin-1-ylmethyl)tetracycline; rolitetracycline nitrate; SQ-15659; 'bristacin', 'reverin', 'syntetrine', 'tetraverine', 'tetrin', 'tetriv',

'transcycline', 'velacycline').
ROLODINE** (4-benzylamino-2-methyl-7H-pyrrolo(2,3-d)pyrimidine; BW-58-271).
'Rometin' *see* Clioquinol.
'Romicil' *see* Oleandomycin.
ROMIFENONE** (2'-hydroxy-3-morpholinopropiophenone; *o*-hydroxyphenyl 2-morpholinoethyl ketone).
'Romilar' *see* Dextromethorphan.
'Romosol' *see* Aurothioglucose.
'Romotal' *see* Tacrine.
'Rompun' *see* 2-(2,6-Xylidino)-5,6-dihydro-1,3-thiazine.
'Rondimen' *see* Mefenorex.
'Rondomycin' *see* Metacycline.
'Ro-neet' *see* Cycloate.
'Rongalite' *see* Sodium formaldehyde sulfoxylate.
'Roniacol' *see* Nicotinyl alcohol.
'Ronicol' *see* Nicotinyl alcohol.
RONIDAZOLE** ((1-methyl-5-nitroimidazol-2-yl)methyl carbamate; 'dugro', 'ridazole').
Ronnel *see* Fenclofos.
'Ronpacon' *see* Meglumine metrizoate with sodium, calcium and magnesium metrizoates.
'Ronpacon cerebral' *see* Meglumine metrizoate with calcium metrizoate.
'Ronton' *see* Ethosuximide.
'Rontyl' *see* Hydroflumethiazide.
'Ronyl' *see* Pemoline.
'Rophene' *see* Adiphenine.
'Rophynal' *see* Flunitrazepam.
Roquessine *see* Conessine.
'Roquine' *see* Quinine valerate.
ROSAMICIN** (3-ethyl-7-hydroxy-2,8,12,16-tetramethyl-5,13-dioxo-9-(3,4,6-trideoxy-3-dimethylamino-β-D-*xylo*-hexapyranosyloxy)-4,17-dioxabicyclo(14.1.0)heptadec-14-ene-10-acetaldehyde; Sch-14947).
ROSAMICIN PROPIONATE* (rosamicin 2'-propionate; Sch-17894).
ROSAMICIN STEARATE* (rosamicin stearate salt; Sch-14947 stearate).
ROSANILINE (bis(*p*-aminophenyl)aminotolylmethanol).
ROSE BENGAL (4,5,6,7-tetrachloro-2',4',5',7'-tetraiodofluorescein).
ROSE BENGAL (^{131}I) SODIUM*** (disodium rose bengal labelled with radioiodine).
Rosein *see* Fuchsine.
ROSEOLIC ACID (4-[bis(*p*-hydroxyphenyl)methylene]-2,5-cyclohexadien-1-one; *p*-roseolic acid; NSC-55202).
'Rospin' *see* Chloropropylate.
ROTAMICILLIN** ((2S,5R,6R)-6-[(R)-2-phenyl-2-[2-[*p*-(1,4,5,6-tetrahydropyrimidin-2-yl)phenyl]acetamido]-acetamido]penicillanic acid).
ROTENONE ((2R(2α,6aα,12aα))-1,2,12,12a-tetrahydro-8,9-dimethoxy-2-(1-methylethenyl)(1)benzopyrano(3,4-b)furo(2,3-h)-(1)benzopyran-6-(6aH)-one; 1,2,12,12a-tetrahydro-2-isopropenyl-8,9-dimethoxy(1)benzopyrano(3,4-b)furo(2,3-h)(1)benzo-

pyran-6(6aH)-one; tubatoxin; 'noxfish').

'Rotersept' *see* Chlorhexidine

'Rotoline' *see* o-Phenylphenol.

ROTOXAMINE*** ((−)-2-[p-chloro-α-(2-dimethylaminoethoxy)benzyl]pyridine; levocarbinoxamine; McN-R-73-Z). *See also* Carbinoxamine.

ROTOXAMINE TARTRATE*** (rotoxamine D-tartrate; 'twiston').

'Rovamycin' *see* Spiramycin.

'Rovan' *see* Fenclofos.

'Rowapraxin' *see* Pipoxlan.

'Rowmate' *see* Dichlormate.

ROXARSONE*** (4-hydroxy-3-nitrobenzenearsonic acid; 3-nitro).

'Roxilon' *see* Mebolazine.

'Roxion' *see* Dimethoate.

ROXOLONIUM METILSULFATE***
(2-(hydroxymethyl)-1,1-dimethylpyrrolidinium methylsulfate 3β-hydroxy-11-oxoolean-12-en-30-oate; (3β,20β)-2-[[(3-hydroxy-11,29-dioxoolean-12-en-29-yl)-oxy]methyl]-1,1-dimethylpyrrolidinium methylsulfate.)

ROXOPERONE*** (8-[3-(p-fluorobenzoyl)-propyl]-2-methyl-2,8-diazaspiro(4.5)-decane-1,3-dione; 3-(2-methyl- 1,3-dioxo-2,8-diazaspiro(4.5)decan-8-yl)-4'-fluoro-butyrophenone; FR-33; R-7158).

RP 40 (tr) *see* Sulfasolucin.

RP 46 (tr) *see* Benzylsulfamide.

RP-50 (tr) *see* Dimethyl 5-norbornen-2,3-dicarboxylate.

RP 143 *see* Povidone.

RP 177 *see* Propivane.

RP 245 *see* Thiopental.

RP 866 *see* Mepacrine.

RP 2090 *see* Sulfathiazole.

RP 2168 *see* Meglumine antimonate.

RP 2224 *see* Melarsen.

RP 2254 *see* Glyprothiazole.

RP 2255 *see* Sulfathiourea.

RP 2259 *see* Glybuthiazole.

RP 2275 *see* Sulfaguanidine.

RP 2339 *see* Phenbenzamine.

RP-2512 *see* Pentamidine isetionate.

RP-2535 *see* Hexamidine isetionate.

RP 2591 *see* Dichlorophenarsine.

RP 2632 *see* Sulfamerazine.

RP 2786 *see* Mepyramine.

RP 2831 *see* Heptaminol.

RP 2856 *see* Amoxecaine.

RP 2921 *see* Aminothiazole.

RP 2987 *see* Diethazine.

RP 3015 *see* Fenethazine.

RP 3038 *see* Sontoquine.

RP 3203 *see* Diodone.

RP 3227 *see* Tetrabromsalicil.

RP 3276 *see* Promazine.

RP 3277 *see* Promethazine

RP 3356 *see* Prophenamine.

RP 3359 *see* Proguanil.

RP 3377 *see* Chloroquine.

RP 3389 *see* Promethiazine.

RP 3554 *see* Thiazinamium.

RP 3580 *see* Diethazine ethiodide.

RP 3602 *see* Mephenesin.

RP 3668 *see* Solasulfone.

RP 3697 *see* Gallamine triethiodide.

RP 3799 *see* Diethylcarbamazine.

RP 3828 *see* Aminopromazine.

RP 3854 *see* Melarsoprol.

RP 4207 *see* Thiacetazone.

RP 4270 *see* Parathiazine.

RP 4460 *see* Promethazine.

RP 4482 *see* 4-Sulfamido-o-arsanilic acid.

RP 4560 *see* Chlorpromazine.

RP 4632 *see* Methopromazine.

RP 4753 *see* Pyrimethamine.

RP 4763 *see* Difetarsone.

RP 4891 *see* Suramin pentamidine salt.

RP 4909 *see* Chlorproethazine.

RP 5015 *see* Isoniazid.

RP 5278 *see* Rufocromomycin.

RP 5337 *see* Spiramycin.

RP 6140 *see* Prochlorperazine.

RP 6484 *see* Etymemazine.

RP 6549 *see* Alimemazine.

RP 6847 *see* Oxomemazine.

RP 6870 *see* Inproquone.

RP 7044 *see* Levomepromazine.

RP 7162 *see* Trimipramine.

RP 7204 *see* Cyamemazine.

RP 7293 *see* Pristinamycin.

RP 7405 *see* Etomidate.

RP 7452 *see* Ethanolamine acetylleucinate.

RP 7522 *see* Sulfamethoxypyridazine.

RP 7676 *see* Pralidoxime mesilate.

RP 7843 *see* Thioproperazine.

RP 7891 *see* Glybuzole.

RP 8228 *see* Phacetoperan.

RP 8307 *see* Opipramol.

RP 8357 *see* Triamcinolone diacetate.

RP 8595 *see* Dimetridazole.

RP 8599 *see* Dimetotiazine.

RP 8823 *see* Metronidazole.

RP 8909 *see* Periciazine.

RP 9153 *see* Pipamazine.

RP 9159 *see* Perimetazine.

RP 9712 *see* Metronidazole benzoate.

RP 9715 *see* Cyclobenzaprine.

RP-9921 *see* Aprotinin.

RP 9965 *see* Metopimazine.

RP 10284 *see* Sultiame.

RP 10768 *see* Niclosamide.

RP 11589 *see* Acetylsulfalene.

RP 11614 *see* Canrenone.

RP 13057 *see* Daunorubicin.

RP 13097 *see* Floropipone.

RP 16091 *see* Metiazinic acid.

RP 19366 *see* Pipotiazine.

RP-19551 *see* Pipotiazine undecenate.

RP-19552 *see* Pipotiazine palmitate.

RP-19560 *see* Metapramine.

RP-19583 *see* Ketoprofen.

RP-21679 *see* Carpipramine.

RP-22050 *see* Daunorubicin benzoylhydrazone.

RP 22410 *see* Glisoxepide.

RR-32705 *see* Rutamycin.

RS-51 *see* Rauwolfia alkaloids.

RS-410 FAPG *see* Fluocinonide.

RS-1301 *see* Delmadinone acetate.

RS-1320 *see* Flunisolide acetate.

RS-1401 AT *see* Fluocinolone acetonide.
RS-2177 *see* Flumethasone.
RS-2252 *see* Fluclorolone acetonide.
RS-3268R *see* Nandrolone cyclotate.
RS-3540 *see* Naproxen.
RS-3694R *see* Cormetasone acetate.
RS-4464 *see* Triclonide.
RS-4691 *see* Cloprednol.
RS-6245 *see* Tazolol.
R&S 218-M *see* Alletorphine.
R&S 5205-M *see* Homprenorphine.
RT *see* 2,3,5-Triphenyltetrazolium chloride.
RT-6912 *see* Nifursol.
RU-4723 *see* Clobazam.
RU-12063 *see* Cismethrin.
RU-15750 *see* Floctafenine.
RU-19583 *see* Calcium clofibrate.
'Ruberon' *see* Ethylmercuric phosphate.
Rubidazone *see* Daunorubicin benzoyl-
hydrazone.
Rubidomycin *see* Daunorubicin.
Rubin *see* Fuchsine.
'Rubrocol' *see* Rubrophen.
RUBROPHEN (dihydroxytrimethoxyoxo-
triphenylmethane; dihydroxytrimethoxy-
fuchsone; 'rubrocol').
'Rucedal' *see* Deglycyrrhizinized liquorice.
'Rudotel' *see* Medazepam.
'Ruelene' *see* Crufomate.
RUFOCROMOMYCIN*** (antibiotic from
Str. rufochromogenes or *Str. flocculus*; 5-
amino-6-(7-amino-5,8-dihydro-6-methoxy-
5,8-dioxo-1-quinolyl)-4-(2-hydroxy-3,4-

dimethoxyphenyl)-3-methylpicolinic acid;
RP-5278).
'Rumarid' *see* Calcium acetylsalicylate.
'Rumicin' *see* Chrysophanic acid.
RUSSELL'S VIPER VENOM ('rusven',
'stypven').
'Rusven' *see* Russell's viper venom.
RUTAMYCIN*** (antibiotic from *Str.
rutgersensis*; A-272; RR-32705).
Rutgers-612 *see* Ethohexadiol.
Rutin *see* Rutoside.
'Rutonal' *see* Mephebarbital.
RUTOSIDE*** (3,3',4',5,7-pentahydroxy-
flavone 3-rhamnoglucoside; quercetin
3-rutinoside; quercetin rhamnoglucoside;
eldrin; globulariacitrin; myrticolorin;
melin; osyritin; osyritrin; phytomelin;
rutin; sophorin; violaquercitrin; vitamin P).
RUVAZONE*** (*o*-ethoxybenzoic acid (1-
carboxyethylidene)hydrazide; pyruvic acid
o-ethoxybenzylhydrazone; M6/42;
'ethoxydrazone', 'etossidrazone').
RX-67408 *see* Fenclofenac.
RYANODINE (alkaloid from *Ryania
speciosa*; ryanodol pyrrole-2-carboxylate).
Ryanodol pyrrole-2-carboxylate *see*
Ryanodine.
'Rybadet' *see* Polysorbate 80.
'Rydar' *see* Dioxadrol.
'Rynacrom' *see* Disodium cromoglicate.
'Ryomycin' *see* Oxytetracycline.
'Rytmaline' *see* Raubasine.
'Ryzelan' *see* Oryzalin.

S

S-2 *see* 2-Coumaranone.
S-3 *see* Phthalide.
S-7 *see* Fenticlor.
S-25 *see* Batroxobin.
S-46 *see* Ethylphenacemide.
S-51 *see* Diphenhydramine.
S-62 *see* Chlorphentermine.
S-78 *see* Valethamate.
S-115 *see* Sodium nicotinate.
S-167 *see* Deanol hemisuccinate.
S-222 *see* Ditazole.
S-567 *see* Diethylaminoethyl butylamino-
salicylate.
S-602-1 *see* Ethinylestradiol with quin-
gestanol.
S-768 *see* Fenfluramine.
S-805 *see* Loxapine.
S-940 *see* Naftalofos.
S-992 *see* Benfluorex.
S-1530 *see* Nimetazepam.
S-1600 *see* Metahexamide.
S-2957 *see* Chlorthiophos.

S-3850 *see* Chlormadinone acetate with
mestranol.
S-4004 *see* Trimetazidine.
S-4087 *see* Cyanofenphos.
S-4105 *see* Medibazine.
S-8440 *see* Betamethasone dipropionate.
S-9700 *see* Dextropropoxyphene napsilate.
S-10275 *see* Epitiostanol.
S-10364 *see* Mepitiostane.
S-31252 *see* Perisoxal.
S-55009 *see* Dichlozoline.
SA *see* Ubiquinone.
SA-1 *see* Etafenone.
SA-79 *see* Propafenone.
Sa-267 *see* Diponium bromide.
SA-504 *see* Timepidium bromide.
'Sabigal' *see* Monosulfiram.
'Sabromine' *see* Calcium dibromobehenate.
Saccharase *see* Invertase.
SACCHARIC ACID (D-glucaric acid;
D-glucosaccharic acid).
Saccharic acid 1,4:6,3-dilactone acetate

397

see Aceglatone.

SACCHARIC ACID 1,4-LACTONE (1,4-glucosaccharolactone; saccharolactone).

SACCHARIN (2,3-dihydro-3-oxobenzisosulfonazole; benzosulphimide; gluside; garantose; saccharinol; saccharoid; saccharol; saccharin and/or its sodium salt).

SACCHARIN AMMONIUM SALT ('daramin', 'sucramin').

Saccharinol *see* Saccharin.

Saccharoid *see* Saccharin.

Saccharol *see* Saccharin.

Saccharolactic acid *see* Mucic acid.

Saccharolactone *see* Saccharic acid 1,4-lactone.

Saccharose *see* Sucrose.

Saccharosonic acid *see* Isoascorbic acid.

Saccharum amylaceum *see* Glucose.

'Sadamine' *see* Xantinol nicotinate.

'S-adchnon' *see* Adrenochrome guanylhydrazone mesilate.

'Sadophos' *see* Malathion.

'Safaprin' *see* Acetylsalicylic acid with paracetamol.

'Safapryn' *see* Acetylsalicylic acid with paracetamol.

'Safprin' *see* Acetylsalicylic acid with paracetamol.

'Safpyrin' *see* Acetylsalicylic acid with paracetamol.

Safrol *see* Safrole.

SAFROLE (4-allyl-1,2-methylenedioxybenzene; allylcatechol methylene ether; allylpyrocatechol methylene ether; safrol).

'Sagimid' *see* Niclosamide.

SaH-42-348 *see* Lifibrate.

SaH-42-548 *see* Mazindol.

'Saiodine' *see* Calcium iodobehenate.

'Sajodin' *see* Calcium iodobehenate.

SALABROSE (tetraglucosan).

SALACETAMIDE*** (N-acetylsalicylamide).

'Salacetol' *see* Salicyl acetol.

'Salantal' *see* Salicyl acetol.

SALANTEL*** (3'-chloro-4'-(p-chlorobenzoyl)-3,5-diiodosalicylanilide; 2,4'-dichloro-4-(2-hydroxy-3,5-diiodobenzamido)benzophenone; R-23050).

SALAZODINE*** (5-[[p-(6-methoxypyridazin-3-yl)sulfamoyl]phenylazo]salicylic acid; N^1-(6-methoxypyridazin-3-yl)-N^4-salicylazosulfanilamide; salicylazosulfamethoxypyridazine; salazosulfamethoxypyridazine).

'Salazolon' *see* Phenazone salicylate.

'Salazopyrin' *see* Salazosulfapyridine.

SALAZOSULFADIMIDINE*** (5-[p-(4,6-dimethylpyrimidin-2-ylsulfamoyl)phenylazo]salicylic acid; 4-(4,6-dimethylpyrimid-2-ylsulfamoyl)-4-hydroxyazobenzene-3-carboxylic acid; N^4-salicylazosulfadimidine; 'azudimidine').

Salazosulfamethoxypyridazine *see* Salazodine.

SALAZOSULFAMIDE*** (5-[p-(2-pyridylsulfamoyl)phenylazo]salicylic acid; 4-sulfonamidophenylazosalicylic acid; 5-(p-sulfamoylphenylazo)salicylic acid; 'lutazol').

SALAZOSULFAPYRIDINE** (4-hydroxy-4'-(pyrid-2-ylsulfamoyl)azobenzene-3-carboxylic acid; 4-(2-pyridylaminosulfonyl)-3'-carboxy-4'-hydroxyazobenzene; N^4-salicylazosulfapyridine; sulfasalazine; 'azopyrine', 'azulfidine', 'salazopyrin').

SALAZOSULFATHIAZOLE*** (5-[p-(2-thiazolylsulfamoyl)phenylazo]salicylic acid; N^4-salicylazosulfathiazole; 4-(2-thiazolylaminosulfonyl)-4'-carboxy-3'-hydroxyazobenzene; 'salazothiazole').

'Salazothiazole' *see* Salazosulfathiazole.

SALBUTAMOL*** (α-(*tert*-butylaminomethyl)-4-hydroxy-3-hydroxymethylbenzyl alcohol; 2-*tert*-butylamino-1-(4-hydroxy-3-hydroxymethylphenyl)ethanol; α-(*tert*-butylaminomethyl)-4-hydroxy-*m*-xylene-α,α'-diol; α^1-[(1,1-dimethylethyl)-aminomethyl]-4-hydroxy-1,3-benzenedimethanol; albuterol; albuterol sulfate; AH-3365; Sch-13949W; 'broncovaleas', 'salbutan', 'sultanol', 'ventolin').

'Salbutan' *see* Salbutamol.

SALCATONIN* (Cys-Ser-Asn-Leu-Ser-Thr-Cys-Val-Leu-Gly-Lys-Leu-Ser-Gln-Glu-Leu-His-Lys-Leu-Gln-Thr-Tyr-Pro-Arg-Thr-Asn-Thr-Gly-Ser-Gly-Thr-Pro-NH$_2$; component of natural salmon calcitonin; SCT-1; 'calsynar').

SALCATONIN HYDRATED POLY-ACETATE (SMC-20-051).

'Salco' *see* Clofenamide.

SALCOLEX** (choline salicylate compound with magnesium sulfate (2:1) tetrahydrate).

'Saleral' *see* Propylene glycol salicylate.

SALETAMIDE*** (N-(2-diethylaminoethyl)-salicylamide).

'Sal-ethyl' *see* Ethyl salicylate.

'Sal-ethyl carbonate' *see* Carbethyl salicylate.

SALFLUVERINE*** (α,α,α-trifluoro-*m*-salicylotoluidide; α,α,α-trifluoro-N-salicyloyl-*m*-toluidine).

Salicain *see* Saligenin.

'Salicaine' *see* Hydroxytetracaine.

'Salicel' *see* Salicylamide.

'Saliceral' *see* Glyceryl salicylate.

SALICIL (2,2'-dihydroxybenzil; bis(2-hydroxyphenyl)glyoxal; salicyl).

SALICIN (salicoside; saligenin glucose; saligenin β-D-glucopyranoside).

SALICIN BENZOATE (benzosalicin; populin).

'Salicitrin' *see* Citrodisalyl.

'Salicoside' *see* Salicin.

Salicyl *see* Salicil.

SALICYL ACETOL (salicylate ester of 1-hydroxy-2-propanone; acetol salicylate; hydroxyacetone salicylate; 'salacetol', 'salantal').

Salicylacetone *see* Salicylideneacetone.

Salicyl alcohol *see* Saligenin.

SALICYLALDEHYDE (*o*-hydroxybenzaldehyde; 'salicylide').

SALICYLAMIDE*** (*o*-hydroxybenzamide).
Salicylamide-2-ethoxyethyl ether *see* Etosalamide.
Salicylamide ethyl ether *see* Ethenzamide.
Salicylamide pentyl ether *see* Pentalamide.
Salicylamide propyl ether *see* Propoxybenzamide.
SALICYLANILIDE (*N*-phenylsalicylamide; 'ansadol', 'salifebrin', 'salinidol', 'sanicyl', 'shirlan').
See also Zinc undecenate with salicylanilide.
Salicylazosulfadimidine *see* Salazosulfadimidine.
Salicylazosulfamethoxypyridazine *see* Salazodine.
Salicylazosulfapyridine *see* Salazosulfapyridine.
Salicylazosulfathiazole *see* Salazosulfathiazole.
N-**Salicylglycine** *see* Salicyluric acid.
SALICYLIC ACID (*o*-hydroxybenzoic acid).
Salicylic acid acetate *see* Acetylsalicylic acid.
Salicylic acid bimolecular ester *see* Salsalate.
Salicylic acid 2-diethylaminoethyl ester *see* Detanosal.
Salicylic acid ester with 2,5-dimethyl-1-pyrrolidinepropanol *see* Pranosal.
Salicylic acid esters *see above and* Acetaminosalol; Carbethyl salicylate; Chloroethyl salicylate; Ethyl salicylate; Glycol salicylate; Glyceryl salicylate; Homosalate; Methyl salicylate; Naphthyl salicylate; Propylene glycol salicylate; Salicyl acetol; Salol; Salprotoside; Salsalate; Thurfyl salicylate; Trichlorobutyl salicylate.
Salicylic acid salts *see* Aluminium salicylate; Calcium salicylate; Choline salicylate; Diethylamine salicylate; Hexamine salicylate; Lithium salicylate; Magnesium salicylate; Meglumine salicylate; Mercury salicylate; Morpholine salicylate; Phenazone salicylate; Sodium salicylate; Thiosinamine salicylate.
'Salicylide' *see* Salicylaldehyde.
SALICYLIDENEACETONE (4-(*o*-hydroxyphenyl)-3-buten-2-one; salicylacetone).
Salicylideneisoniazid *see* Salinazid.
SALICYLIDENE-*p*-PHENETIDINE (*p*-(*o*-hydroxybenzylideneimino)phenetole; 'malakin', 'saliphenin').
'Salicylix' *see* Sodium sulfosalicylate.
Salicylosalicylic acid *see* Salsalate.
Salicyl salicylate *see* Salsalate.
Salicylsulfonic acid *see* Sulfosalicylic acid.
SALICYLURIC ACID (*N*-salicoylglycine; *N*-salicylglycine).
'Salicylysin' *see* Thiosinamine salicylate.
'Salifebrin' *see* Salicylanilide.
'Saliformin' *see* Methenamine salicylate.
'Salifungin' *see* 5-Bromo-4'-chlorosalicylanilide.
SALIGENIN (*o*-hydroxybenzyl alcohol; salicyl alcohol; salicain; saligenol; 'diathesin').

Saligenin glucoside *see* Salicin.
Saligenol *see* Saligenin.
'Salimagol' *see* Magnesium salicylate with sodium salicylate.
Salinaphthol *see* Naphthyl salicylate.
SALINAZID*** (1-isonicotinoyl-2-salicylidenehydrazine; isonicotinoylhydrazone of salicylaldehyde; *N*'-salicylideneisoniazid; isonicotinic acid salicylidenehydrazide; HP-213; Mg-1480; 'INHS', 'INSH', 'neobiocin salicyl', 'nupa-sal', 'salizid').
'Salinidol' *see* Salicylanilide.
Saliphenazone *see* Phenazone salicylate.
'Saliphenin' *see* Salicylidene-*p*-phenetidine.
'Sali-presinol' *see* Methyldopa with mefruside.
'Salipyrazolon' *see* Phenazone salicylate.
'Salipyrin' *see* Phenazone salicylate.
'Salisan' *see* Chlorothiazide.
'Salisil' *see* Magnesium trisilicate.
'Salisuccyl' *see* Calcium benzyl succinate-salicylate.
'Salizid' *see* Salinazid.
SALMEFAMOL*** (1-(4-hydroxy-3-hydroxymethylphenyl)-2-(4-methoxy-α-methylphenethylamino)ethanol; 4-hydroxy-3-hydroxymethyl-α-(4-methoxy-α-methylphenethylaminomethyl)benzyl alcohol; *N*-[2-hydroxy-2-(4-hydroxy-3-hydroxymethylphenyl)ethyl]-4-methoxy-α-methylphenethylamine; 4-hydroxy-α-[(*p*-methoxy-α-methylphenethylamino)methyl]-*m*-xylene-α,α'-diol; AH-3923).
'Salmidochol' *see* Osalmid.
'Salnabrom' *see* Theobromine sodium salicylate.
SALOCOLL (salicylate of *N*-aminoacetyl-*p*-phenetidine; phenocoll salicylate).
SALOL (phenyl salicylate; salphenyl).
Salophenum *see* Acetaminosalol.
'Salostan' *see* Tin oxide.
Salphenyl *see* Salol.
'Salpix' *see* Sodium acetrizoate with povidone.
SALPROTOSIDE** (ethyl 3-*O*-propyl-glucofuranoside 5,6-disalicylate).
SALSALATE*** (salicylic acid bimolecular ester; salicyl salicylate; salicylsalicylic acid; disalicylic acid; salysal; 'dinuclan', 'diplosal', 'disalyl', 'nobacid').
Salsalate acetate *see* Acetylsalicylsalicylic acid.
SALSOLIDINE (1,2,3,4-tetrahydro-6,7-dimethoxy-1-methylisoquinoline).
SALSOLINE (1,2,3,4-tetrahydro-6-hydroxy-7-methoxy-1-methylisoquinoline).
'Saltucin' *see* Butizide.
'Salumin' *see* Aluminium salicylate.
'Salures' *see* Bendroflumethiazide.
'Saluretil' *see* Chlorothiazide.
'Saluric' *see* Chlorothiazide.
'Saluron' *see* Hydroflumethiazide.
Saluzid (tr) *see* Opiniazide.
'Salvarsan' *see* Arsphenamine.
SALVERINE** (2-(2-diethylaminoethoxy)-benzanilide; salicylanilide diethylaminoethyl ether).

'**Salvicyclin**' *see* Dequalinium acetate.
Salysal *see* Salsalate.
'**Salzen**' *see* Clofenamide.
SAMARIUM SULFOSALICYLATE
(complex of samarium with sulfosalicylic acid; 'phlogosam').
'**SAMH**' *see* Methamphetamine.
'**Samorin**' *see* Isometamidium chloride.
'**Sanabolic**' *see* Nandrolone cyclohexane-propionate.
'**Sanamycin**' *see* Cactinomycin.
'**Sanasil**' *see* Sulfadoxine.
'**Sanasthmyl**' *see* Beclometasone dipropionate.
'**Sanatrichom**' *see* Metronidazole.
SANCYCLINE*** (6-demethyl-6-deoxytetracycline; 6-demethyl-6-deoxytetracycline; GS-2147; 'bonomycin').
'**Sandocycline**' *see* Broxyquinoline with broxaldine and tetracycline.
'**Sandolanid**' *see* Acetyldigoxin.
'**Sandomigran**' *see* Pizotifen maleate.
'**Sandopart**' *see* Demoxytocin.
'**Sandoptal**' *see* Butalbital.
'**Sandoscill**' *see* Proscillaridin.
'**Sandosten**' *see* Thenalidine.
'**Sandril**' *see* Reserpine.
'**Sandrix**' *see* Scopolamine methyl methosulfate.
'**Sanegyt**' *see* Guanazodine.
'**Sanicyl**' *see* Salicylanilide.
'**Sanigal**' *see* Monosulfiram.
'**Sanisol-C**' *see* Benzalkonium.
'**Sanmicron**' *see* Phenylmercuric acetate.
'**Sanocrysin**' *see* Sodium aurotiosulfate.
'**Sanoform**' *see* Methyl diiodosalicylate.
'**Sanoma**' *see* Magnesium peroxide.
'**Sanopron**' *see* Chlorpromazine.
'**Sanoquin**' *see* Chloroquine.
'**Sanorex**' *see* Mazindol.
'**Sanotensin**' *see* Guanethidine.
'**Sansert**' *see* Methysergide.
SANTAL (7-methoxy-3′,4′,5-trihydroxyisoflavone).
Santavy's substance F *see* Demecolcine.
'**Santheose**' *see* Theobromine.
'**Santicizer 141**' *see* Octicizer.
'**Santochin**' *see* Sontoquine.
Santolactone *see* Santonin.
SANTONIN (lactone of 7-(1-carboxypropyl)-5,6,7,8-tetrahydro-8-hydroxy-1,4a-dimethyl-2(4aH)-naphthalenone; santolactone).
'**Santophen-1**' *see* Clorofene.
'**Santoquin**' *see* Ethoxyquin.
SAP-113 *see* Nifuratel.
'**Sapecron**' *see* Clofenvinfos.
'**Saphi-col**' *see* Menazon.
'**Saphizon**' *see* Menazon.
SARALASIN** (*N*-[1-[*N*-[*N*-[*N*-[*N*²-(*N*-methylglycyl)-L-arginyl]-L-valyl]-L-tyrosyl]-L-valyl]-L-histidyl]-prolyl]-L-alanine; 1-(*N*-methylglycine)-5-L-valine-8-L-alanine angiotensin II).
SARALASIN ACETATE* (saralasin acetate salt hydrate; P-113).
Sarcine *see* Hypoxanthine.
'**Sarcochlorin**' *see* Sarcolysin.

'**Sarcoclorin**' *see* Sarcolysin.
SARCOLYSIN*** (DL-3-[*p*-[bis(2-chloroethyl)amino]phenyl]alanine; merfalan; merphalan; racemelfalan; DL-phenylalanine mustard; sarcolysin hydrochloride; CB-3007; NSC-14210; 'sarcochlorin', 'sarcoclorin').
D-**Sarcolysin** *see* Medphalan.
L-**Sarcolysin** *see* Melphalan.
m-**SARCOLYSIN** (DL-3-[*m*-[bis(2-chloroethyl)amino]phenyl]alanine; *m*-sarcolysin hydrochloride; metasarcolysin; MP-267; NSC-27381).
o-**SARCOLYSIN** (DL-3-[*o*-[bis(2-chloroethyl)amino]phenyl]alanine; *o*-sarcolysin hydrochloride; orthosarcolysin; CB-1729; NSC-57199).
N-**Sarcolysylnicotinamide** *see* Nicozin.
Sarcomycin *see* 2-Methylene-3-oxocyclopentanecarboxylic acid.
SARCOSINE (*N*-methylglycine; methylaminoacetic acid).
'**Sargenor**' *see* Arginine aspartate.
SARIN (isopropyl methylphosphonofluoridate; GB).
Sarkin *see* Hypoxanthine.
Sarkolysin *see* Sarcolysin.
Sarkomycin *see* 2-Methylene-3-oxocyclopentanecarboxylic acid.
'**Sarodormin**' *see* Glutethimide.
'**Sarolex**' *see* Dimpylate.
'**Saroten**' *see* Amitriptyline.
'**Sarotex**' *see* Amitriptyline.
SAS-554 *see* Oxazepam valproate.
'**Satietyl**' *see* Amphetamine *p*-chlorophenoxyacetate.
'**Saturn**' *see* Benthiocarb.
SAXITOXIN (clam poison; mussel poison; paralytic shelfish poison; PSP).
'**Sayfos**' *see* Menazon.
Sb-58 *see* Sodium stibocaptate.
Sb-5833 *see* Camazepam.
SBP-1382 *see* Resmethrin.
SC-1627 *see* Fenethazine.
SC-1674 *see* Florantyrone.
SC-1749 *see* Menbutone.
SC-2538 *see* Profenamine.
SC-2910 *see* Methantheline.
SC-4341 *see* Nandrolone.
SC-4642 *see* Noretynodrel.
SC-6924 *see* Mytatrienediol.
SC-7031 *see* Disopyramide.
SC-7105 *see* Thiopropazate.
SC-7525 *see* Bolandiol.
SC-8470 *see* Ethisterone acetate.
SC-9376 *see* Canrenone.
SC-9420 *see* Spironolactone.
SC-9880 *see* Flugestone acetate.
SC-10363 *see* Megestrol.
SC-11585 *see* Oxandrolone.
SC-11800 *see* Etynodiol diacetate.
SC-11952 *see* 22,25-Diazacholestanol.
SC-12222 *see* Etynodiol acetate.
SC-12350 *see* Nitralamine.
SC-12937 *see* Azacosterol.
SC-14207 *see* Metogest.
SC-14266 *see* Canrenoate potassium.

SC-15396 *see* 2-Phenyl-2-pyrid-2-ylthioacetamide.
SC-16148 *see* Silandrone.
SC-19198 *see* Metynodiol diacetate.
SC-21099 *see* Norgestomet.
SC-23992 *see* Prorenoate potassium.
SC-26100 *see* Difenoximide.
SC-27761 *see* Pranolium chloride.
'Scabinol' *see* Benzyl benzoate.
'Scabintan' *see* Chloroxylenol.
'Scandicaine' *see* Mepivacaine.
SCARLET RED* (Biebrich scarlet R medicinal; Sudan IV; 1-(4-*o*-tolylazo-*o*-tolylazo)-2-naphthol; fat Ponceau R).
SCC *see* Carbamoylcysteine.
Sch-1000 *see* Ipratropium bromide.
Sch-2747 *see* Pipendyl methane.
Sch-3132 *see* Methitural.
Sch-3940 *see* Perphenazine.
Sch-5706 *see* Fenalamide.
Sch-6673 *see* Acetophenazine.
Sch-10304 *see* Clonixin.
Sch-10595 *see* Bupicomide.
Sch-11460 *see* Betamethasone dipropionate.
Sch-11527 *see* Cefaloridine.
Sch-12041 *see* Halazepam.
Sch-12169 *see* Closiramine aceturate.
Sch-12650 *see* Dazadrol maleate.
Sch-12679 *see* Trimopam maleate.
Sch-12707 *see* Clonixeril.
Sch-13475 *see* Sisomicin.
Sch-13521 *see* Flutamide.
Sch-13949W *see* Salbutamol.
Sch-14342 *see* Betamicin.
Sch-14714 *see* Flunixin.
Sch-14947 *see* Rosamicin.
Sch-15280 *see* Azanator maleate.
Sch-15427 *see* Carmantadine.
Sch-15507 *see* Dopamantine.
Sch-15698 *see* Fletazepam.
Sch-15719W *see* Labetalol.
Sch-17894 *see* Rosamicin propionate.
Sch-18020W *see* Beclometasone dipropionate.
'Scherisolon' *see* Prednisolone.
'Scherofluron' *see* Fludrocortisone acetate.
'Scherosone' *see* Cortisone.
'Scherosone-F' *see* Hydrocortisone.
Schleimsäure *see* Mucic acid.
SCHRADAN* (bis(N,N,N',N'-tetramethylphosphorodiamidic)anhydride; octamethyldiphosphoramide; octamethylpyrophosphoramide; octamethyl; oktametil; OMPA; shradan; A-15; E-3314; 'pestox III'; 'sytam').
Schultz-1038 *see* Methylene blue.
Schultz-1041 *see* Tolonium.
SCILLAREN A ($3\beta,14\beta$-dihydroxybufa-4,20,22-trienolide 3-rhamnoglucoside; 14β-hydroxy-3β-(rhamnoglucosyloxy)bufa-4,20,22-trienolide; glucoproscillaridin A).
Scillarenin 3β-rhamnoside *see* Proscillaridin.
'Scleromerfen' *see* Phenylmercuric nitrate.
'Scobenol' *see* Benzyl benzoate.
'Scolaban' *see* Bunamidine.
Scopine tropate *see* Scopolamine.
'Scopodex' *see* Scopolamine *N*-oxide.

SCOPOLAMINE (L-epoxytropine tropate; scopine tropate; atrochin; atroquin; atroscine; L-hyoscine; scopolamine hydrobromide; 'kwells', 'oscine', 'scopos', 'sereen').
See also Atropine camphorate with scopolamine camphorate.
SCOPOLAMINE BUTYL BROMIDE (hyoscine *N*-butyl bromide; SKF-1637; butylscopolamine; 'buscapine', 'buscolysin', 'buscopan').
SCOPOLAMINE BUTYL BROMIDE WITH OXAZEPAM (Bwy20; 'buscopax').
See also Proglumide with scopolamine butyl bromide.
SCOPOLAMINE METHYL BROMIDE (hyoscine *N*-methyl bromide; methscopolamine bromide; epoxymethamine bromide; U-0382; 'diopal', 'holopon', 'lescopine', 'mescopil', 'pamine', 'proscomide', 'scopolate').
SCOPOLAMINE METHYL METHOSULFATE (*N*-methylhyoscine methyl sulfate; CERM-1290; DD-234; 'sandrix').
SCOPOLAMINE METHYL NITRATE (hyoscine *N*-methyl nitrate; methscopolamine nitrate; 'mesconit', 'scopolin', 'scopovyl', 'scopyl', 'skopal', 'skopyl').
See also Amobarbital with scopolamine methyl nitrate.
SCOPOLAMINE *N*-OXIDE (hyoscine amine oxide; 'genoscopolamine', 'scopodex').
'Scopolate' *see* Scopolamine methyl bromide.
SCOPOLETIN (7-hydroxy-6-methoxycoumarin; 6-methoxyumbelliferone; chrysatropic acid).
'Scopolin' *see* Scopolamine methyl nitrate.
'Scopos' *see* Scopolamine.
'Scopovyl' *see* Scopolamine methyl nitrate.
'Scopyl' *see* Scopolamine methyl nitrate.
'Scotine' *see* Cotinine fumarate.
SCS *see* Serotonin creatinine sulfate.
SCT-1 *see* Salcatonin.
'SCTZ' *see* Clomethiazole edisilate.
'Scuroform' *see* Butylcaine.
Scyllite *see* Inositol.
SD-100-2 *see* Di(hydroxymethyl)furalazine.
SD-210-37 *see* Leptacline camsilate.
SD-709 *see* Dimetacrine tartrate.
SD-1750 *see* Dichlorvos.
SD-3447 *see* Stirofos.
SD-4402 *see* Isobenzan.
SD-7859 *see* Clofenvinfos.
SD-8447 *see* Stirofos.
SD-8530 *see* Trimethylphenyl methylcarbamate.
SD-8747 *see* Stirofos.
SD-10419 *see* Propyromazine.
SD-14112 *see* Sulclamide.
SD-15418 *see* Cyanazine.
SD-15803 *see* Vincofos.
SD-27115 *see* Furfenorex cyclamate.
SD-124817 *see* Tropatepine.
'SDC' *see* Solway purple.
SDDS *see* Sulfamoyldapsone.
Sdt-91 *see* Stibophen.

Sdt-1041 *see* Thiacetazone.
SE-711 *see* Pipratecol.
SE-1702 *see* Gliclazide.
'Sea-legs' *see* Piprinhydrinate.
SEBACIC ACID (decanedioic acid; 1,8-octanedicarboxylic acid).
'Sebaclen' *see* Xenysalate.
'Seboderm' *see* Cetrimonium.
SECBUMETON* (2-*sec*-butylamino-4-ethylamino-6-methoxy-*s*-triazine; *N*-ethyl-6-methoxy-*N'*-(1-methylpropyl)-1,3,5-triazine-2,4-diamine; 'etazine').
SECBUTABARBITAL*** (5-ethyl-5-(1-methylpropyl)barbituric acid; 5-*sec*-butyl-5-ethylbarbituric acid; butabarbital; secbutobarbitone; secumal; secbutabarbital sodium derivative; 'asturidon', 'butabarpal', 'butisol', 'neravan', 'noctinal').
Secbutobarbitone* *see* Secbutabarbital.
'Secholex' *see* Polidexide.
SECLAZONE*** (7-chloro-3,3a-dihydro-2H,9H-isoxazolo(3,2-b)(1,3)benzoxazin-9-one; W-2354).
SECNIDAZOLE** (α,2-dimethyl-5-nitroimidazole-1-ethanol; 1-(2-hydroxypropyl)-2-methyl-5-nitroimidazole; 1-(2-methyl-5-nitroimidazol-1-yl)-2-propanol).
SECOBARBITAL*** (5-allyl-5-(1-methylbutyl)barbituric acid; quinalbarbitone; meballymal; secobarbital sodium; 'barbosec', 'evronal', 'hypnotrol', 'hypotrol', 'imesonal', 'immenoctal', 'immenox', 'seconal', 'suinox', 'talesco').
9,10-Secocholesta-5,7,10(19)-triene-3b,25-diol *see* Calcifediol.
9,10-Secoergosta-5,7,10(19),22-tetraen-3β-ol *see* Ergocalciferol.
9,10-Secoergosta-5,7,22-trien-3β-ol *see* Dihydrotachysterol.
'Seconal' *see* Secobarbital.
'Secotil' *see* Chlorpromazine sulfoxide.
SECRETIN** (hormone from duodenal mucosa).
'Secrosteron' *see* Dimethisterone.
SECT *see* Cetotiamine.
'Sectral' *see* Acebutolol.
Secumal* *see* Secbutabarbital.
SECURININE** ((6*S*, 11a*R*, 11b*S*)-9,10,11,11a-tetrahydro-8H-6,11b-methanofuro(2,3-c)-pyrido(1,2-a)azepin-2(6H)-one).
'Sedafamen' *see* Phendimetrazine.
'Sedaform' *see* Chlorbutol.
'Sedalande' *see* Fluanisone.
'Sedalium' *see* Hexadiphane with moperone.
'Sedathil' *see* Sulfathiadiazole.
'Sedatin' *see* Valeridin.
'Sedatussin' *see* Cephaeline.
'Sedilan' *see* Dihyprylone.
'Sedipral' *see* Allopyrine.
'Sediston' *see* Promazine.
'Sedobex' *see* Bibenzonium bromide.
'Sedocalene' *see* Hydroxyzine embonate with calcium 2-ethylbutyrate.
'Sedolatan' *see* Prenylamine lactate.
'Sedometil' *see* Methyldopa.
'Sedomuth' *see* Camylofin with bismuth nitrate.

'Sedoquin' *see* Quinidine 5-ethyl-5-phenyl-barbiturate.
'Sedormid' *see* Apronal.
'Sedothyron' *see* Thiobarbital.
'Sedotussin' *see* Pentoxyverine.
'Sedulon' *see* Dihyprylone.
'Seduxen' *see* Diazepam.
'Seedrin' *see* Aldrin.
'Sefacin' *see* Cefaloridine.
'Sefril' *see* Cefradine.
'Segontin' *see* Prenylamine.
Seignette salt *see* Potassium sodium tartrate.
'Sekundal' *see* Carbromal with bromisoval.
Selacholic acid *see* 15-Tetracosenoic acid.
Sel anglais *see* Magnesium sulfate.
Sel de Seidlitz *see* Magnesium sulfate.
'Selectomycin' *see* Spiramycin.
'Selenex' *see* Selenium disulfide.
SELENIUM DISULFIDE (selenium sulfide; 'selenex', 'selsun').
Selenocysteamine *see* Selenomercaptamine.
SELENOMERCAPTAMINE (2-amino-ethaneselenol; selenocysteamine).
SELENOMETHIONINE (2-amino-4-(methylselenyl)butyric acid).
SELENOMETHIONINE (^{75}Se)*** (radio-selenomethionine; 'sethotope').
'Seloken' *see* Metoprolol.
'Selsun' *see* Selenium disulfide.
'Selvigon' *see* Pipazetate.
'Semap' *see* Penfluridol.
'Sembrina' *see* Methyldopa.
'Semcox' *see* Hydromorphone.
'Semdoxan' *see* Cyclophosphamide.
'Semesan' *see* Chlorohydroxymercuriphenol.
SEMICARBAZIDE (aminourea; carbamic acid hydrazide).
'Semicillin' *see* Ampicillin.
SEMIOXAMAZIDE (oxamic hydrazide).
'Semopen' *see* Pheneticillin.
'Semophen' *see* Pheneticillin.
SEMUSTINE*** (1-(2-chloroethyl)-3-(4-methylcyclohexyl)-1-nitrosourea; Me-CCNU; methyl-CCNU; NSC-95441).
'Sencor' *see* Metribuzin.
'Sendoxan' *see* Cyclophosphamide.
SENECIOIC ACID (β,β-dimethylacrylic acid; 3-methyl-2-butenoic acid; 3-methyl-crotonic acid).
Senecioic acid 2-*sec*-butyl-4,6-dinitro-phenyl ester *see* Binapacryl.
SENECIOYLCHOLINE (β,β-dimethyl-acryloylcholine; SCh).
N¹-Senecioylsulfanilamide *see* Sulfa-dicramide.
Sennite *see* Pinitol.
'Sensaval' *see* Nortriptyline.
'Sensit' *see* Fendiline.
SEP *see* Polyestriol phosphate.
'Sepazon' *see* Cloxazolam.
SEPAZONIUM CHLORIDE** (1-[2,4-di-chloro-β-[(2,4-dichlorobenzyl)oxy]phen-ethyl]-3-phenethylimidazolium chloride).
'Seperidol' *see* Clofluperol.
'Sephadex' *see* Cross-linked dextran.
'Septin' *see* Benzethonium.
'Septiolan' *see* Bensulfene.

Septiphene see Clorofene.
'Septisol' see Hexachlorophene.
'Septivon' see Triclocarban.
'Septon' see Propham.
'Septra' see Co-trimoxazole.
'Septran' see Co-trimoxazole.
'Septrin' see Co-trimoxazole.
'Sequamycin' see Spiramycin.
'Sequens' see Chlormadinone acetate with mestranol.
'Sequestrene' see Trisodium edetate.
'Sequilar' see Levonorgestrel with ethinylestradiol.
SERACTIDE** (25-L-aspartic acid-26-L-alanine-27-glycine-30-L-glutamine-31-L-serine-α$^{1-39}$-corticotrophin (pig)).
SERACTIDE ACETATE (seractide acetate salt).
'Seral' see Methylpentynol.
'Serax' see Oxazepam.
Serazide see Benserazide.
'Serbose' see Glyhexamide.
'Serc' see Betahistine.
'Serenace' see Haloperidol.
'Serenal' see Oxazolam.
'Serenase' see Haloperidol.
'Serenesil' see Ethchlorvynol.
'Serenid' see Oxazepam.
'Serenium' see Etoxazene.
'Serentil' see Mesoridazine.
'Seren vita' see Chlordiazepoxide.
'Serepax' see Oxazepam.
'Seresta' see Oxazepam.
'Seretin' see Carbon tetrachloride.
SERFIBRATE** (2-acetamido-4-mercaptobutyric acid clofibrate ester; N-acetyl-homocysteine clofibrate).
'Sergetyl' see Etymemazine.
Sergosin (tr) see Methiodal.
'Serial' see Megestrol acetate with ethinylestradiol.
Seric gonadotrophin see Serum gonadotrophin.
SERINE (2-amino-3-hydroxypropionic acid; 2-aminohydracrylic acid; β-hydroxyalanine).
Serine diazoacetate see Azaserine.
1-D-Serine-17-L-lysine-18-L-lysinamide-α$^{1-18}$-**corticotrophin** see Codactide.
DL-Serine 2-(2,3,4-trihydroxybenzyl)-hydrazide see Benserazide.
'Sermaka' see Fludroxycortide.
'Sermion' see Nicergoline.
'Sernyl' see Phencyclidine.
'Sernylan' see Phencyclidine.
'Seromycin' see Cycloserine.
SEROTONIN (5-hydroxytryptamine; 3-(2-aminoethyl)-5-indolol; DS substance; enteramine; 5-HT; thrombocytin; thrombotonin).
Serotonin benzyl analogue see Benanserin.
SEROTONIN CREATININE SULFATE (double sulfate of creatinine and serotonin; SCS; 'antemovis').
Serotonin methyl ether see 5-Methoxytryptamine.
SERPENTINE (dehydro-δ-yohimbine; dehydroraubasine; methyl serpentinate).

Serpentinic acid esters see Isobutyl serpentinate; Serpentine.
SERRAPEPTASE** (proteolytic enzyme from Serratia sp. E15; serratiopeptidase; TSP).
SERRATAMIC ACID (N-(3-hydroxydecanoyl)serine).
Serratia sp. E15, proteolytic enzyme see Serrapeptase.
Serratiopeptidase see Serrapeptase.
'Sertal' see Deanol propynyloxybenzilate.
'Sertan' see Primidone.
SERUM GONADOTROPHIN*** (pregnant mare serum gonadotrophin containing chiefly FSH activity; PMS; PMSG; equine gonadotrophin; seric gonadotrophin; 'anteron', 'antex', 'antostab', 'biotropin', 'eleagol', 'equinex', 'equoman', 'gestyl', 'gonadin', 'gonadogen', 'gonadotraphon-FSH', 'gonadyl', 'gormon', 'hemoantine', 'lobulantina', 'prelobane', 'priantin', 'primantron', 'prolosan', 'serogan', 'serotropin', 'thylakentrin').
'Servo antisprout' see Propham.
1-Seryl-2-(2,3,4-trihydroxybenzyl)hydrazine see Benserazide.
'SES' see Disul.
SESAMEX (5-[1-[2-(2-ethoxyethoxy)-ethoxy]ethyl]-1,3-benzodioxole; 1-[(2-ethoxyethoxy)ethoxy]-2-(3,4-methylenedioxyphenyl)ethane; 1-(3,4-methylenedioxyphenyl)-3,6,9-trioxaundecane; 'sesoxane').
SESAMIN (2,6-bis(3,4-methylenedioxyphenyl)-3,5-dioxabicyclo(3.3.0)octane; 'asarinin').
SESAMOL (3,4-methylenedioxyphenol).
SESAMOLIN (2-(3,4-methylenedioxyphenoxy)-6-(3,4-methylenedioxyphenyl)-cis-3,7-dioxabicyclo(3.3.0)octane).
SESELIN (8,8-dimethyl-2H,8H-benzo(1,2-b:3,4-b')dipyran-2-one).
'Sesoxane' see Sesamex.
'Sestron' see Alverine.
'Sethadil' see Sulfaethidole.
'Sethotope' see Selenomethionine (^{75}Se).
'Sethyl' see Homatropine methyl bromide.
'Sevin' see Carbaril.
'Sevinal' see Fluphenazine.
'Sevinol' see Fluphenazine.
'Sevinon' see under Undecenoic acid.
SEVOFLURANE*** (fluoromethyl 2,2,2-trifluoro-1-(trifluoromethyl)ethyl ether).
'Sexovid' see Cyclofenil.
SF-837 see Midecamycin.
SH-420 see Norethisterone acetate.
SH-567 see Metenolone acetate.
SH-582 see Gestonorone caproate.
SH-601 see Metenolone enantate.
SH-613 see Sulfametoxydiazine.
SH-617-L see Ethyl iopodate.
SH-714 see Cyproterone acetate.
SH-717 see Glymidine.
SH-742 see Fluocortolone.
SH-770 see Fluocortolone caproate.
SH-818 see Clocortolone.
SH-20932 see Meglumine diatrizoate.

SH-60931 *see* Metenolone acetate with calcium phosphate.
SH-70833D *see* Prasterone enantate with estradiol valerate.
SH-71144 *see* Levonorgestrel with ethinylestradiol.
SH-71155 *see* Levonorgestrel with ethylestradiol.
SH-80881 *see* Cyproterone.
SHCH-49 (tr) *see* 5-Nitro-2-furaldehyde thiosemicarbazone.
SHCH-58 (tr) *see* Cutizone.
SHCH-66 (tr) *see* Vanillin thiosemicarbazone.
SHCH-85 (tr) *see* Amithizone.
SHCH-87 (tr) *see* Thiacetazone.
SHCH-431 (tr) *see* Subathizone.
SH E 199 *see* Etoformin.
'Shellsol A' *see* Benzoylprop-ethyl.
SHIKIMIC ACID (3,4,5-trihydroxycyclohexene-1-carboxylic acid).
'Shirlan' *see* Salicylanilide.
SH K-203 *see* Gluocortin butyl.
'Shostakovsky balsam' *see* Polyvinox.
SHOWDOMYCIN (2-(β-D-ribofuranosyl)-maleimide).
'Shoxin' *see* Norbormide.
Shradan *see* Schradan.
'S-hydril' *see* Sodium thiosulfate.
SI-1236 *see* Oxyphencyclimine.
'Sialan' *see* Endosulfan.
'Sibena' *see* Dimeticone.
SICCANIN ** ((13a*S*)-1,2,3,4,4aβ,5,6,6a,11bβ,13bβ-decahydro-4,4,6aβ,9-tetramethyl-13H-benzo(a)furo(2,3,4-mn)xanthen-11-ol).
'Sicol' *see* Dimeticone.
Siderophilin *see* Transferrin.
Sidnocarb (tr) *see* Sydnocarb.
'Sidonal' *see* Piperazine quinate.
SIDURON* (1-(2-methylcyclohexyl)-3-phenylurea; 'tupersan').
'Sifacycline' *see* Tetracycline cyclamate.
'Sigmaform' *see* Bismuth tribromophenate.
'Sigmamycin' *see* Tetracycline with oleandomycin.
'Sigmodal' *see* 5-(2-Bromoallyl)-5-(1-methylbutyl)barbituric acid.
'Sigmuth' *see* Bismuth sodium tartrate.
'Signemycin' *see* Tetracycline with oleandomycin.
'Silain' *see* Dimeticone.
SILANDRONE* (17β-(trimethylsiloxy)-androst-4-en-3-one; SC-16148).
'Silane' *see* Dimeticone.
'Silastic' *see* Silicone rubber.
'Silazulone' *see* Dimeticone.
Silica *see* Silicon dioxide.
Silicic acid *see* Silicon dioxide.
'Silicoderm' *see* Dimeticone.
SILICON DIOXIDE (silicic acid; silica; amorphous silicon dioxide; silica gel).
Silicone *see* Dimeticone.
SILICONE RUBBER ('silastic').
See also Dimeticone.
Silidone *see* Dimeticone.
'Silital' *see* Halquinols.
Silodrate* *see* Simaldrate.
'Silomat' *see* Clobutinol.

'Silphostrol' *see* Fosfestrol.
'Silpromin' *see* Xantinol nicotinate.
'Silubin' *see* Buformin.
'Silvadene' *see* Sulfadiazine silver.
'Silvederma' *see* Sulfadiazine silver.
Silver sulfadiazine *see* Sulfadiazine silver.
Silver sulfone *see under* Diathymosulfone.
Silvex *see* Fenoprop.
SILYMARIN (mixture of isomeric flavanone derivatives (silybin, silydianin and silychristin) from *Silybum marianum*; RB-1466).
SILYMARIN SODIUM ('legalon').
SIMALDRATE ** (magnesium aluminosilicate hydrate; sitodrate; MP-1051).
Simatin' *see* Ethosuximide.
SIMAZINE* (2-chloro-4,6-bis(ethylamino)-*s*-triazine; 6-chloro-*N,N'*-diethyl-1,3,5-triazine-2,4-diamine; CDT; symazin; 'amizine', 'gesatop', 'tofazine 50W').
See also Methoprotryne plus simazine.
'Simesphylline' *see* Etamiphylline.
Simethicone* *see* Dimeticone.
SIMETRIDE ** (1,4-bis(2-methoxy-4-propyl-phenoxyacetyl)piperazine).
SIMETRYNE* (4,6-diethylamino-2-(methylthio)-*s*-triazine; *N,N'*-diethyl-6-(methylthio)-1,3,5-triazine-2,4-diamine).
SIMFIBRATE* (clofibric acid trimethylene diester; 1,3-propanediol bis[2-(*p*-chloro-phenoxy)isobutyrate]; trimethylene bis-(clofibrate); clofibric acid diester with 1,3-propanediol; propyl 1,3-bis(clofibrate); CLY-503; 'cholesolvin').
'Simpalon' *see* Oxedrine.
'Simpatol' *see* Oxedrine.
'Simplotan' *see* Tinidazole.
SIMTRAZENE* (1,4-dimethyl-1,4-diphenyl-2-tetrazene; centrazene; CL-26193; NSC-83799).
SIN-10 *see* Molsidomine.
'Sinalar' *see* Fluocinolone acetonide.
'Sinalost' *see* Trichlormethine.
'Sinanomycin' *see* Congocidine.
'Sinaspril' *see* Calcium acetylsalicylate.
'Sinaxar' *see* Styramate.
'Sinbar' *see* Terbacil.
SINCALIDE* (L-aspartyl-L-tyrosyl-L-methionylglycyl-L-tryptophyl-L-methionyl-L-aspartylphenyl-L-alaninamide hydrogen sulfate (ester); 1-de(5-oxo-L-proline)-2-de-L-glutamine-5-L-methionine caerulein; SQ-19844; 'kinevac').
Sincaline *see* Choline.
'Sinderesin' *see* Iproclozide.
'Sinecod' *see* Butamirate citrate *and* Noscapine.
'Sindiatil' *see* Buformin.
'Sinemet' *see* Levodopa with carbidopa.
'Sinequan' *see* Doxepin.
Sinestrol (tr) *see* Hexestrol.
'Sinetens' *see* Prazosin.
'Singoserp' *see* Syrosingopine.
'SINH' *see* Streptonicozid.
Sinkol (tr) Dextran.
'Sinnamin' *see* Azapropazone.
Sinocurarine *see* Gallamine triethiodide.
'Sinogan' *see* Levomepromazine.
'Sinografin' *see* Meglumine diatrizoate with

diapiodone meglumine.
SINOMENINE (coculine).
'**Sinomin**' *see* Sulfamethoxazole.
'**Sinomin acetyl**' *see* Acetylsulfamethoxazole.
'**Sinovir**' *see* Cyproterone acetate.
'**Sinox**' *see* Dinitro-*o*-cresol.
'**Sinquan**' *see* Doxepin.
'**Sintaverin**' *see* Pramiverine.
'**Sintespasmil**' *see* Camylofin.
'**Sinthrome**' *see* Acenocoumarol.
'**Sintisone**' *see* Prednisolone steaglate.
Sinto.... *See also* Syntho....
'**Sintodian**' *see* Droperidol.
'**Sintrom**' *see* Acenocoumarol.
'**Sintyal**' *see* Methylpentynol.
'**Siogen**' *see* Chlorquinaldol.
'**Sionon**' *see* Sorbitol.
'**Siopel**' *see* Dimeticone.
'**Siqualone**' *see* Fluphenazine.
'**Siosteran**' *see* Chlorquinaldol.
'**Siquil**' *see* Triflupromazine.
'**Siquoline**' *see* Flufenazine.
'**Sirmate**' *see* Dichlormate.
'**Sirolin**' *see* Sulfogaiacol.
'**Sirtal**' *see* Calcium cresolsulfonate.
SISOMICIN*** (*O*-2,6-diamino-2,3,4,6-
tetradeoxy-α-D-glycerohex-4-enopyranosyl-
(1→4)-*O*-[(3-deoxy-4-*C*-methyl-3-methyl-
amino-β-L-arabinopyranosyl)-(1→6)]-2-
deoxy-D-streptamine; Sch-13475; 'extra-
mycin', 'pathomycin', 'sisomycin').
'**Sistilin**' *see* Calcium methylpolygalact-
uronate sulfonate complex.
'**Sistometril**' *see* Lynestrenol with mestranol.
'**Sistyline**' *see* Calcium methylpolygalact-
uronate sulfonate complex.
'**Sisuril**' *see* Hydroflumethiazide.
SITOFIBRATE*** (stigmast-5-en-3β-ol
2-(*p*-chlorophenoxy)-2-methylpropionate;
stigmastenol clofibrate).
β-**SITOSTEROL** (SL-10; 'harzol').
SITOSTEROL(S) (β-sitosterol plus β-di-
hydrostigmasterol; 'cytellin', 'positol').
'**Sixtysix-20**' *see* Prednazate.
SJ-1977 *see* Metixene.
SK-7 *see* Pentifylline.
SK-74 *see* Clofedanol.
SK-100 *see* Trichlormethine.
SK-101 *see* Chlormethine.
SK-331-A *see* Xantinol nicotinate.
SK-555 *see* Dichlorodiethylamine.
SK-1133 *see* Tretamine.
SK-3818 *see* Tepa.
SK-5265 *see* Metodiclorofen.
SK-18615 *see* Thioguanosine.
'**SK-Apap**' *see* Paracetamol.
SKATOLE (3-methylindole).
'**Skelaxin**' *see* Metaxalone.
'**SK-Estrogens**' *see* Conjugated estrogens.
SK&F-51 *see* Octodrine.
SK&F-385 *see* Tranylcypromine.
SK&F-478 *see* Difenidol.
SK&F-525-A *see* Proadifen.
SK&F-538-A *see* Quinisocaine.
SK&F-688-A *see* Phenoxybenzamine.
SK&F-1340 *see* Dimefadane.

SK&F-1637 *see* Scopolamine butyl bromide.
SK&F-1700-A *see* Buphenine.
SK&F-1717 *see* Anethole trithione.
SK&F-2208 *see* Hetaflur.
SK&F-2601-A *see* Chlorpromazine.
SK&F-3050 *see* Cortodoxone.
SK&F-4657 *see* Prochlorperazine.
SK&F-5116 *see* Levomepromazine.
SK&F-5137 *see* Dextromoramide.
SK&F-5345-A *see* Trifluomeprazine.
SK&F-6270 *see* Methiotrimeprazine.
SK&F-6539 *see* Flurotyl.
SK&F-6574 *see* Phenazocine.
SK&F-6611 *see* Norclostebol.
SK&F-6890 *see* β-Methylxylocholine.
SK&F-7690 *see* Benorterone.
SK&F-7988 *see* Virginiamycin.
SK&F-12866 *see* Cloretate.
SK&F-13364-A *see* Tyromedan.
SK&F-14287 *see* Idoxuridine.
SK&F-14336 *see* Clomacran.
SK&F-18666 *see* Poloxalene.
SK&F-22908 *see* Flutuazin.
SK&F-23880-A *see* Cyclooctylamine.
SK&F-24529 *see* Lobendazole.
SK&F-29044 *see* Parbendazole.
SK&F-30310 *see* Oxibendazole.
SK&F-33134-A *see* Amiodarone.
SK&F-38094 *see* Dectaflur.
SK&F-38095 *see* Olaflur.
SK&F-39186 *see* Amicloral.
SK&F-40383 *see* Carbuterol.
SK&F-41558 *see* Cefazolin.
SK&F-70230-A *see* Pipazetate.
SK&F-92334 *see* Cimetidine.
'**Skleromexe**' *see* Clofibrate.
'**Sklerovitol**' *see* Nicotinoylprocaine.
'**Skopal**' *see* Scopolamine methyl nitrate.
'**Skopolate**' *see* Scopolamine methyl nitrate.
'**Skopyl**' *see* Scopolamine methyl nitrate.
SL-10 *see* β-Sitosterol.
SL-501 *see* Clofedanol.
SL-6057 *see* Clobenztropine.
SL-6058 *see* Clobenztropine methiodide.
SLAFRAMINE (1*S*,6*S*,8a*S*-1-acetoxy-6-
aminooctahydroindolizine; 6-amino-1-
hydroxyoctahydroindolizine acetate).
'**Slam**' *see* Azothoate.
'**Slug Guard**' *see* Methiocarb.
SM-14 *see* Dimetofrine.
SMC-20-051 *see* Salcatonin hydrated
polyacetate.
'**SMOC**' *see* Metam-sodium.
SN-44 *see* Ethyldapsone.
SN-46 *see* Dinex.
SN-166 *see* Glucosulfone.
SN-263 *see* Sodium amylosulfate.
SN-359 *see* Quinine-HCl.
SN-390 *see* Mepacrine.
SN-971 *see* Pamaquin.
SN-3115 *see* Plasmocide.
SN-4395 *see* Pyrvinium.
SN-5870 *see* Quinuronium.
SN-6771 *see* Bialamicol.
SN-6911 *see* Sontoquine.
SN-7618 *see* Chloroquine.
SN-8137 *see* Hydroxychloroquine.

SN-10751 *see* Amodiaquine.
SN-12837 *see* Proguanil.
SN-13272 *see* Primaquine.
SN-13274 *see* Isopentaquine.
SN-13276 *see* Pentaquine.
SNAKE VENOMS ('hemostypt', 'moccasin', 'venene', 'venin').
See also under Cobra; Rattlesnake; Viper, etc.
'Snip' *see* Dimetilan.
'S.N.P.' *see* Parathion.
SNR-1804 *see* Clamidoxic acid.
'Sobelin' *see* Clindamycin.
'Sobiodopa' *see* Lerodopa.
'Sobita' *see* Bismuth sodium tartrate.
'Sobril' *see* Oxazepam.
'Soclidan' *see* Nicametate citrate.
'Sodar' *see* Disodium methanearsonate.
SODIUM ACEXAMATE (sodium 6-acetamidohexanoate; sodium acetamidocaproate; sodium acetylaminocaproate; 'celuton').
Sodium 5-acetamido-2,4,6-triiodo-*N*-methylisophthalamate *see* Sodium iotalamate.
Sodium acetosulfone* *see* Sulfadiasulfone.
SODIUM ACETRIZOATE*** (Na 3-acetamido-2,4,6-triiodobenzoate; triiotrast; 'acetiodone', 'bronchoselectan', 'diaginol', 'fortombrine-N', 'iodopact', 'iodopaque', 'opacoron', 'pyelokon-R', 'salpix', 'triabrodil', 'triiodyl', 'triognost', 'triopac', 'triurol', 'urokon', 'vesamin').
See also Acetrizoic acid.
SODIUM ACETRIZOATE WITH POVIDONE ('salpix').
Sodium *N*-acetylarsanilate *see* Arsacetin sodium.
SODIUM ACTINOQUINOL* (sodium-8-ethoxyquinoline-5-sulfonate; actinoquinol sodium; sodium etoquinol; sodium tequinol; 'corodenin', 'uviban').
SODIUM ALGINATE (sodium polymannuronate; 'algin', 'kelgin', 'minus', 'protanal').
See also Calcium alginate.
Sodium aluminium phosphate basic *see* Kasal.
Sodium amidotrizoate *see* Sodium diatrizoate.
Sodium aminoauromercaptobenzoate *see* Sodium 4-amino-2-(aurothio)salicylate.
Sodium *p*-aminobenzenearsonate *see* Sodium arsanilate.
Sodium *p*-aminobenzenestibonate *see* Stibamine.
SODIUM *p*-AMINOBENZOATE ('nataba').
SODIUM AMINOCAPROATE (sodium 6-aminohexanoate; 'celuton').
Sodium 2-aminoethylthio phosphate *see* Cystafos.
Sodium 6-aminohexanoate *see* Sodium aminocaproate.
SODIUM *p*-AMINOHIPPURATE ('nephrotest').
SODIUM AMYLOSULFATE* (sodium salt of sulfonated amylopectin from *Solanum*

tuberosum (potato) tubers; SN-263; 'depepsen').
Sodium anazolene *see* Anazolene sodium.
SODIUM ANHYDROMETHYLENE-CITRATE ('citarin', 'goutin', 'transren').
Sodium anilarsonate *see* Sodium arsanilate.
Sodium anoxynaphthonate* *see* Anazolene sodium.
Sodium antimony dimercaptosuccinate *see* Sodium stibocaptate.
SODIUM ANTIMONYL GLUCONATE* (sodium salt of a trivalent antimony derivative of gluconic acid; TSAG; 'triostam', 'triostib').
See also Sodium stibogluconate.
SODIUM ANTIMONYL TARTRATE (antimony sodium tartrate; 'emeto-Na', 'stibunal').
'Sodium antimosan' *see* Stibophen.
Sodium (antipyrinylisobutylamino)-methanesulfonate *see* Dibupyrone.
Sodium (antipyrinylmethylamino)-methanesulfonate *see* Novaminsulfon.
SODIUM APOLATE*** (sodium ethenesulfonate polymer; poly(sodium ethylenesulfonate); sodium lyapolate; 'pergalen', 'peson').
SODIUM ARSANILATE (sodium *p*-aminobenzenearsonate; sodium anilarsonate).
SODIUM ASCORBATE*** (sodium derivative of 3-oxo-L-gulofuranolactone).
SODIUM AUROALLYLTHIOUREIDO-BENZOATE (sodium salt of *S*-gold derivative of *m*-[[(allylimino)mercaptomethyl]amino]benzoic acid; sodium 3-[1-(3-allyl-*S*-auropseudothioureido)]benzoate; sodium salt of *m*-auroallylthioureabenzoic acid; aurothiosinamine-*m*-benzoate sodium; C-2924; 'lopion', 'orthioura').
SODIUM AUROTHIOMALATE*** (*S*-gold derivative of thiomalic acid disodium salt; *S*-gold derivative of mercaptosuccinic acid; disodium salt; disodium aurothiomalate; 'myocrisin', 'myocrysin', 'tauredon').
Sodium aurothiosulfate *see* Sodium aurotiosulfate.
SODIUM AUROTIOSULFATE*** (gold sodium thiosulfate; sodium aurothiosulfate; sodium dithiosulfatoaurate; sel de Fordos et Gélis; 'auricidin', 'aurocidin', 'aurolin', 'auropex', 'auropin', 'aurothion', 'crisalbine', 'novacrysin', 'sanocrysin', 'solfocrisol', 'thiochrysine').
SODIUM 4-BENZAMIDOSALICYLATE ('benzacyl', 'B-PAS').
See also Calcium benzamidosalicylate.
SODIUM BENZYL SUCCINATE (succinic acid monobenzyl ester sodium salt; 'mobenate', 'raybanol', 'suxiphen').
Sodium biborate *see* Borax.
Sodium bis(acetato)tetrakis[gluconato-(2-)]-bis[salicylato(2-)] dialuminate dihydrate *see* Sodium glucaspaldrate.
Sodium bis(2,4-dihydroxy-3,3-dimethylbutyryl)ferrate *see* Sodium dipantoylferrate.
Sodium bithionolate* *see* Sodium bitionolate.

406

SODIUM BITIONOLATE*** (disodium 2,2′-thiobis(4,6-dichlorophenoxide); bithionolate sodium; sodium bithionolate; 'varicide-BN').
See also Bithionol.

SODIUM CALCIUM EDETATE*** (calcium chelate of disodium salt of ethylenediaminetetraacetic acid; disodium edetate calcium chelate; calcium disodium edetate; edathamil calcium disodium; calcitetramate disodique; calcium disodium versenate; edetate disodium calcium; 'antallin', 'calcium-Noury', 'chelintox', 'complexon-3-calcium', 'ledclair', 'mosatil').

SODIUM CAPOBENATE (sodium 6-(3,4,5-trimethoxybenzamido)hexanoate; TMBAC; C-3).

Sodium caprylate *see* Sodium octanoate.

Sodium N-(carbamoylmethyl)arsanilate *see* Tryparsamide.

Sodium carbenicillin *see* Carbenicillin.

SODIUM CARBOXYMETHYLCELLU-LOSE (sodium cellulose glycolate).

Sodium cellulose glycolate *see* Sodium carboxymethylcellulose.

Sodium cephalothin* *see* Cefalotin.

SODIUM 4-(4-CHLORO-2-METHYL-PHENOXY)BUTYRATE (MCPB sodium; 'tropotox').

SODIUM CHROMATE (^{51}Cr)*** (sodium radiochromate; 'chromitope sodium', 'rachromate').

Sodium cloxacillin* *see* Cloxacillin.

Sodium colistimethate *see* Colistin methanesulfonate.

Sodium cromoglycate* *see* Disodium cromoglicate.

Sodium cuproallylthioureidobenzoate *see* Allocupreide.

SODIUM CYCLAMATE*** (sodium salt of N-cyclohexylsulfamic acid; cyclamate; cyclamate sodium).
See also Calcium cyclamate.

Sodium cyclohexanehexol hexaphosphate *see* Sodium phytate.

Sodium N-cyclohexylsulfamate *see* Sodium cyclamate.

Sodium dehydrocholate*** *see under* Dehydrocholic acid.

Sodium dextrothyroxine*** *see* Dextrothyroxine sodium.

SODIUM DIATRIZOATE* (sodium 3,5-diacetamido-2,4,6-triiodobenzoate; sodium amidotrizoate; iododiazoate; 'hypaque', 'hypaque 50', 'pyelombrine').
See also Diatrizoic acid; Meglumine diatrizoate with sodium diatrizoate.

SODIUM DIBUNATE*** (sodium salt of 2,6-di-*tert*-butylnaphthalene-1(or 3)-sulfonic acid; L-1633; 'aducin', 'becantex', 'becantyl', 'keuten', 'linctussal').

Sodium dichloroisocyanurate *see* Troclosene sodium.

Sodium 2,2-dichloropropionate *see* Dalapon sodium.

Sodium dicloxacillin* *see* Dicloxacillin.

SODIUM DIETHYLDITHIOCAR-BAMATE (sodium N,N-diethyldithiocarbamate; dithiocarb).

SODIUM DIHEXYL SULFOSUCCINATE (bis(1-methylamyl) ester Na salt of sulphosuccinic acid; 'alphasol MA').

Sodium dihydroxygluconatoaluminate *see* Sodium glucaldrate.

Sodium diiodomethanesulfonate *see* Dimethiodal.

Sodium 3,5-diiodo-4-oxo-1(4H)-pyridine-acetate *see* Iodopyridone.

Sodium dimercaptopropanesulfonate *see* Unithiol.

Sodium 3-(dimethylaminomethylene-amino)-2,4,6-triiodohydrocinnamate *see* Sodium iopodate.

SODIUM 4-DIMETHYLAMINO-*o*-TOLUENEPHOSPHONITE ('novophosphan', 'phiniphos', 'phosodyl', 'tonofosfan', 'tonophosphan').

SODIUM DIOCTYL SULFOSUC-CINATE*** (sodium salt of sulfosuccinic acid bis(2-ethylhexyl)ester; dioctyl sodium sulfosuccinate; 'aerosol OT', 'alphasol OT', 'colace', 'coprol', 'defilin', 'dioctylal', 'diovac', 'disonate', 'doxinate', 'doxol', 'ilozoft', 'manoxol OT', 'milkinol', 'molofac', 'nevax', 'obston', 'physiolax', 'regutol', 'soffecine', 'softil', 'vatsol OT', 'velmol').
See also Calcium dioctyl sulfosuccinate.

Sodium dioxide *see* Sodium peroxide.

Sodium 1,3-dioxo-1H-benz(de)iso-quinoline-2(3H)-acetate *see* Alrestatin.

SODIUM DIPANTOYLFERRATE (sodium bis(2,4-dihydroxy-3,3-dimethylbutyryl)-ferrate; ferrous sodium pantoate; 'ferronascin').

Sodium dipropylacetate *see* Sodium valproate.

SODIUM DIPROTRIZOATE*** (3,5-dipropionamido-2,4,6-triiodobenzoic acid Na salt; 'miokon').

Sodium dithiosulfatoaurate *see* Sodium aurotiosulfate.

Sodium ditolyldiazobis-8-amino-1-naphthol-3,6-disulfonate *see* Trypan blue.

SODIUM DODECYL SULFATE (sodium lauryl sulfate; 'cycloryl', 'duponol C', 'empicol', 'irium', 'lorol', 'neutrazyme', 'prodermide', 'ucenol LS').

Sodium edetate *see* Disodium edetate; Tetrasodium edetate; Trisodium edetate.

SODIUM ETACRYNATE (sodium salt of etacrynic acid; ethacrynate sodium; sodium ethacrynate; 'lyovac sodium edecrin').

SODIUM ETASULFATE*** (sodium 2-ethylhexyl sulfate; 2-ethyl-1-hexanol sulfate sodium salt; ethasulfate sodium; sodium ethasulfate; 'tergemist').

Sodium ethacrynate *see* Sodium etacrynate.

Sodium ethasulfate* *see* Sodium etasulfate.

Sodium ethenesulfonate polymer *see* Sodium apolate.

Sodium 8-ethoxyquinoline-5-sulfonate *see* Sodium actinoquinol.

Sodium ethylenebis(dithiocarbamate) *see* Nabam.

Sodium ethylenesulfonate polymer *see* Sodium apolate.

Sodium 2-ethylhexyl sulfate *see* Sodium etasulfate.

Sodium α-ethyl-1-hydroxycyclohexaneacetate *see* Cyclobutyrol sodium.

Sodium *p*-(ethylmercurithio)benzenesulfonate *see* Sodium timerfonate.

Sodium (ethylmercurithio)salicylate *see* Thiomersal.

Sodium etoquinol *see* Sodium actinoquinol.

SODIUM FEREDETATE*** (iron chelate of sodium edetate; ferritetraceminnatrium; iron sodium edetate; sodium ironedetate; 'plexofer', 'styron').

SODIUM FUSIDATE (fusidic acid sodium salt; fusidate sodium; SQ-16360; 'fucidine'). *See also* Fusidic acid.

SODIUM GENTISATE*** (sodium 2,5-dihydroxybenzoate; sodium 5-hydroxysalicylate).

SODIUM GLUCALDRATE* (sodium dihydroxy gluconatoaluminate; sodium dihydroxy gluconate diaquoaluminate; 'glymaxil'). *See also* Potassium glucaldrate.

SODIUM GLUCASPALDRATE*** (sodium bis(acetato)tetrakis[gluconato(2-)]bis-[salicylato(2-)] dialuminate dihydrate; octasodium tetrakis(gluconato)bis(salicylato)-μ-diacetodialuminate III dihydrate).

SODIUM GLUTAMATE (monosodium glutamate; 'accent', 'glutavene').

Sodium 4-glycylamidobenzenearsonate *see* Tryparsamide.

Sodium glymidine* *see* Glymidine.

SODIUM GUALENATE*** (sodium 5-isopropyl-3,8-dimethyl-1-azulenesulfonate).

SODIUM HEPTADECYL SULFATE (3,9-diethyl-6-tridecanol Na sulfate; 'tergitol 7').

SODIUM HEXACYCLONATE*** (sodium 2-(1-hydroxymethylcyclohexyl)acetate; sodium 1-(hydroxymethyl)cyclohexaneacetate; sodium 4-hydroxy-3,3-pentamethylenebutyrate; sodium salt of β,β-pentamethylene-γ-hydroxybutyric acid; 'gevilon').

Sodium *o*-(3-hexyloxy-2-hydroxypropoxy)benzoate *see* Exiproben sodium.

SODIUM α-HYDROXYBENZYLPHOSPHINITE ('foselite', 'phos', 'phoselite').

Sodium 4-hydroxybutyrate *see* Oxybate sodium.

Sodium 2-(1-hydroxycyclohexyl)butyrate *see* Cyclobutyrol sodium.

Sodium hydroxymethylcyclohexaneacetate *see* Sodium hexacyclonate.

Sodium 4-hydroxy-3,3-pentamethylenebutyrate *see* Sodium hexacyclonate.

SODIUM HYPOCHLORITE SOLUTION(S) (eau de Javel; Labarraque's solution; 'antiformin', 'chloros', 'chlorox', 'deosan', 'hyposan', 'milton', 'voxsan').

Sodium inositol hexaphosphate *see* Sodium phytate.

SODIUM IODIDE (^{125}I)*** (sodium radioiodide (^{125}I)).

SODIUM IODIDE (^{131}I)*** (sodium radioiodide (^{131}I)).

Sodium iodipamide *see* Adipiodone.

SODIUM IODOHIPPURATE (sodium *o*-iodohippurate; 'hippodine', 'hippuran', 'medopaque', 'orthoiodine').

SODIUM IODOHIPPURATE (^{131}I)*** (sodium radioiodohippurate (^{131}I)).

Sodium iodomethamate *see* Iodoxyl.

Sodium iodomethanesulfonate *see* Methiodal.

SODIUM IOGLYCAMATE (sodium 3,3′-(diglycolyldiimino)bis(2,4,6-triiodobenzoate)). *See also* Ioglycamic acid; Ioglycamide; Ioglycamide with sodium ioglycamate.

SODIUM IOPODATE*** (sodium 3-(dimethylaminomethyleneamino)-2,4,6-triiodohydrocinnamate; sodium salt of 3-(3-dimethylaminomethylenamino-2,4,6-triiodophenyl)propionic acid; sodium ipodate; sodium triiodohydrocinnamate; SQ-15761; 'biloptin', 'oragrafin-Na').

SODIUM IOTALAMATE (sodium 5-acetamido-2,4,6-triiodo-*N*-methylisophthalamate; sodium iothalamate; 'angioconray', 'conray 80').

SODIUM IOTALAMATE (^{125}I)*** (iothalamate sodium I-125; sodium radioiotalamate; 'glofil-125').

SODIUM IOTALAMATE (^{131}I)*** (iothalamate sodium I-131; sodium radioiotalamate).

Sodium iothalamate *see* Sodium iotalamate.

Sodium ipodate* *see* Sodium iopodate.

Sodium ironedetate* *see* Sodium feredetate.

SODIUM ISOASCORBATE ('mercate-20', 'neocebitate').

Sodium 5-isopropyl-3,8-dimethyl-1-azulenesulfonate *see* Sodium gualenate.

SODIUM *N*-LAURYLSARCOSINATE (sodium *N*-dodecanoylsarcosinate; sodium dodecanoylmethylaminoacetate; 'gardol').

Sodium levothyroxine *see* Levothyroxine sodium.

Sodium liothyronine *see* Liothyronine sodium.

Sodium lyapolate* *see* Sodium apolate.

SODIUM MANDELATE ('mandelix').

Sodium menadiol diphosphate *see* Menadiol sodium phosphate.

Sodium menadiol disulfate *see* Menadiol sodium sulfate.

SODIUM MENADIOL-3-SULFONATE (sodium 1,4-dihydroxy-2-methylnaphthalene-3-sulfonate; 'katin').

Sodium meralein* *see* Meralein sodium.

Sodium 2-mercaptoethanesulfonate *see* Mesna.

Sodium metharsinite *see* Disodium methanearsonate.

Sodium methicillin* *see* Meticillin.

Sodium methylcarbamodithioate *see* Metam-sodium.

SODIUM METRIZOATE*** (sodium salt of 3-acetamido-2,4,6-triiodo-5-(*N*-methylacetamido)benzoic acid; metrizoate sodium; 'isopaque', 'triosil', 'triosol'). *See also* Metrizoic acid.

SODIUM METRIZOATE WITH CALCIUM AND MAGNESIUM METRIZOATES ('isopaque 400').

Sodium monomethylarsonate *see* Disodium methanearsonate.

SODIUM MORRHUATE*** (sodium salts of fatty acids of cod-liver oil; oleocid; 'varicocid', 'venotex').

Sodium nafcillin* *see* Nafcillin.

SODIUM NALIDIXATE (nalidixate sodium; WIN-18320-3). *See also* Nalidixic acid.

SODIUM NICOTINATE (S-115; 'naotin', 'nicodan', 'nicosode').

Sodium nitrilotriacetate *see* Sodium triglycollamate.

Sodium noramidopyrine methanesulfonate *see* Novaminsulfon.

SODIUM OCTANOATE (sodium caprylate; 'kaprylex', 'naprylate').

Sodium octanoate with sodium propionate and calcium and zinc octanoates and propionates *see* Propionate caprylate mixture.

Sodium octanoate with zinc octanoate *see* Caprylic compound.

SODIUM OCTYLPHENOXYETHYL ETHER SULFONATE ('fisohex', 'pHisoderm').

SODIUM OCTYL SULFATE (2-ethyl-1-hexanol sodium sulfate; 'tergitol 08').

Sodium oxacillin* *see* Oxacillin.

Sodium oxybate* *see* Oxybate sodium.

Sodium β,β-pentamethylene-γ-hydroxybutyrate *see* Sodium hexacyclonate.

SODIUM PERBORATE ($NaBO_3$; 'bocasan', 'dexol').

SODIUM PEROXIDE (sodium dioxide; sodium superoxide; 'oxone', 'solozone').

Sodium phenone acetate *see* Guaiacetin.

Sodium 1-phenylazo-2-naphthol-6-sulfonate *see* Orange RN.

SODIUM PHOSPHATE (^{32}P)*** (mixture of sodium dihydrogen phosphate and disodium hydrogen phosphate containing ^{32}P; sodium radiophosphate).

Sodium phosphate triamcinolone acetonide* *see* Triamcinolone acetonide.

SODIUM PHYTATE* (nonasodium phytate; sodium cyclohexanehexol hexaphosphate; SQ-9343; 'rencal').

SODIUM PICOSULFATE*** (4,4'-(2-pyridylmethylene)diphenol bis(hydrogen sulfate) disodium salt; 4,4'-(2-picolylidene)-bis(phenylsulfuric acid) disodium salt; disodium 4,4'-pyrid-2-ylmethylenedi-(phenyl sulfate); picosulfol; DA-1773; La-391; 'guttalax', 'laxoberal', 'laxoberon').

SODIUM POLYANETHOLESUL-FONATE(S) ('liquoid').

SODIUM POLYANHYDROMAN-NURONIC SULFATE ('hepoid', 'mannuronate', 'paritol', 'thrombocid').

SODIUM POLYETHYLENE SULFONATE (polyethylene Na sulfonate; PES; U-6812).

Sodium polymannuronate *see* Sodium alginate.

SODIUM PROPIONATE ('mycoban', 'napropion', 'ocuseptine').

Sodium propionate with calcium propionate *see* Propionate compound.

Sodium propionate with sodium octanoate and calcium and zinc octanoates and propionates *see* Propionate caprylate mixture.

Sodium 2-propylvalerate *see* Sodium valproate.

SODIUM PSYLLIATE (Na salts of fatty acids of *Plantago ovata* seeds; 'sylnasol').

Sodium pyrocatechol acetate *see* Guaiacetin.

Sodium pyrocatechol-3-carboxylate *see* Sodium *o*-pyrocatechuate.

SODIUM PYROCATECHOL-3,5-DISULFONATE (sodium-1,2-dihydroxybenzene-3,5-disulfonate; sodium 4,5-dihydroxy-*m*-benzenedisulfonate; 'tiferron', 'tiron').

SODIUM *o*-PYROCATECHUATE (sodium pyrocatechol-3-carboxylate; 'mobilene').

Sodium radiochromate *see* Sodium chromate (^{51}Cr).

Sodium radioiodide *see* Sodium iodide (^{125}I); Sodium iodide (^{131}I).

Sodium radioiotalamate *see* Sodium iotalamate (^{125}I); Sodium iotalamate (^{131}I).

Sodium radiophosphate *see* Sodium phosphate (^{32}P).

SODIUM RICINOLEATE ('colidosan', 'soricin').

SODIUM STIBOCAPTATE*** (hexasodium salt of the *S,S*-diester of the cyclic thioantimonate (III) of 2,3-dimercaptosuccinic acid; antimony sodium dimercaptosuccinate; antimony (III) sodium meso-2,3-dimercaptosuccinate; Sb-58; TwSb; 'astiban'). *See also* Stibocaptic acid.

SODIUM STIBOGLUCONATE*** (sodium salt of a pentavalent antimony derivative of gluconic acid; solusurmin; 'pentostam', 'solustibosan', 'solyusurmin', 'stibanate', 'stibanose', 'stibatin', 'stibinol'). *See also* Sodium antimonyl gluconate.

Sodium sulfaminochloride *see* Tosylchloramide.

SODIUM SULFATE (anhydrous sodium sulfate; Glauber salt).

SODIUM 5-SULFOSALICYLATE (sodium salicylsulfonate; 'arcylate', 'salicylix').

Sodium superoxide *see* Sodium peroxide.

Sodium tartrobismuthate *see* Bismuth sodium tartrate.

SODIUM TENUAZONATE (sodium derivative of 3-acetyl-5-*sec*-butyl-4-hydroxy-3-pyrrolin-2-one; NSC-525816).

Sodium tequinol see Sodium actinoquinol.
Sodium tetraborate see Borax.
SODIUM TETRADECYL SULFATE***
(sodium 7-ethyl-2-methyl-4-undecanol
sulfate; STS; 'sotradecol', 'tergitol 4',
'thrombovar').
**Sodium 1,2,3,4-tetrahydro-2-methyl-1,4-
dioxo-2-naphthalenesulfonate** see
Menadione sodium bisulfite.
**Sodium 2-[2-[2-[p-(1,1,3,3-tetramethyl-
butyl)phenoxy]ethoxy]ethoxy]ethane-
sulfonate** see Entsufon sodium.
**SODIUM THEOPHYLLIN-7-YLACET-
ATE** (glycolyltheophylline sodium;
'aminodal').
Sodium thimerfonate* see Sodium timerfonate.
SODIUM THIOSULFATE (sodium hyposulfite; NSC-45624; 'ametox', 'antichlor',
'hypo', 'hyposulfene', 'sodothiol', 'S-hydril',
'sulfothiorine').
SODIUM TIMERFONATE*** (sodium p-
(ethylmercurithio)benzenesulfonate; ethyl-
(p-sulfophenylthio)mercury sodium salt;
sodium thimerfonate; timerfon; 'sulfo-
merthiolate').
Sodium triclofos* see Triclofos.
SODIUM TRIGLYCOLLAMATE (sodium
nitrilotriacetate; 'trilon A').
**SODIUM 2,3,4-TRIHYDROXYGLUTAR-
ATE** (natrog).
**Sodium 6-(3,4,5-trimethoxybenzamido)-
hexanoate** see Sodium capobenate.
Sodium troclosene* see Troclosene sodium.
SODIUM TYROPANOATE*** (sodium salt
of 3-butyramido-α-ethyl-2,4,6-triiodohydro-
cinnamic acid; sodium 1-(3-butyramido-
2,4,6-triiodobenzyl)butanoate; sodium
2-(3-butyramido-2,4,6-triiodobenzyl)-
butyrate; WIN-8851-2; 'bilopaque').
Sodium usnate see Usnic acid sodium salt.
SODIUM VALPROATE (sodium 2-propyl-
valerate; sodium dipropylacetate; valproate
sodium; Abbott 44090; 'convulex',
'depakene', 'depakine', 'epilim', 'ergenyl').
'Sodothiol' see Sodium thiosulfate.
'Soffecine' see Sodium dioctyl sulfosuccinate.
'Soframycin' see Framycetin.
'Sofro' see Pemoline.
'Softcon' see Vifilcon A.
'Softenon' see Thalidomide.
'Softil' see Sodium dioctyl sulfosuccinate.
'Softran' see Buclizine.
'Solacen' see Tybamate.
'Solaesthesin' see Dichloromethane.
'Solaesthin' see Dichloromethane.
'Solamine' see Benzethonium.
'Solan' see Pentanochlor.
Solapsone* see Solasulfone.
SOLASULFONE** (tetrasodium salt of 1,1'-
[sulfonylbis(p-phenylimino)]bis(3-phenyl-
1,3-propanedisulfonic acid); tetrasodium
salt of 4,4'-bis(1,3-disulfo-3-phenylpropyl-
amino)diphenyl sulfone; solapsone; solu-
sulfone; RP-3668; 'cimedone', 'novotrone',
'sulfetrone', 'sulfonazine').
'Solbase' see Macrogols.

'Solbrol' see Methyl paraben.
'Solbrol P' see Propyl paraben.
'Solestril' see Proscillaridin.
'Solestrin' see Estrone.
'Solestro' see Estradiol benzoate.
'Solevar' see Propetandrol.
'Solex' see Dichlozoline.
'Solferino' see Fuchsine.
'Solfocrisol' see Sodium aurotiosulfate.
'Solganal-B' see Aurothioglucose.
Solid green see Brilliant green.
'Soliphylline' see Choline theophyllinate.
'Solitacin' see Indometacin with zolimidine.
'Solium' see Febarbamate.
'Solmethin' see Dichloromethane.
'Solnicol' see Chloramphenicol hemisuccinate.
'Solozone' see Sodium peroxide.
'Solprin' see Calcium acetylsalicylate.
'Solquinate' see 8-Quinolinol potassium sul-
fate.
'Solubacter' see Triclocarban.
Soluble guncotton see Pyroxylin.
'Solucort' see Prednisolone sodium
m-sulfobenzoate.
'Solucortef' see Hydrocortisone.
'Soludacortin' see Prednisolone sodium
succinate.
'Soludactone' see Canrenoate potassium.
'Soludiazine' see Sulfadiazine-meglumine.
'Solufontamide' see Sulfathiourea.
'Solugastril' see Algeldrate with calcium
carbonate.
'Solu-medrol' see Methylprednisolone sodium
succinate.
'Soluphylline' see Etamiphylline.
'Solupred' see Prednisolone m-sulfobenzoate.
'Soluran' see Clofenamide.
'Solurine' see Methenamine salicylate.
'Solusediv' see Fluanisone.
'Soluseptacin' see Sulfasolucin.
'Soluseptacine' see Sulfasolucin.
'Soluseptazine' see Sulfasolucin.
'Solustibosan' see Sodium stibogluconate.
Solusulfone (tr) see Solasulfone.
Solusurmin (tr) see Sodium stibogluconate.
'Solutedarol' see Triamcinolone diacetate.
'Solvar' see Polyvinyl alcohol.
'Solvat' see Benzyl thiocyanate.
'Solvecillin' see Penicillin.
'Solvent P' see 2-Phenoxyethanol.
'Solvezink' see Zinc sulfate.
'Solvodol' see Parapropamol.
'Solvosterol' see Peptide 67-82.
'Solvostrept A' see Streptoduocin.
'Solvotricin' see Tyrothricin.
SOLWAY PURPLE (1-hydroxy-4-toluidino-
anthraquinone-m-sulfonic acid; 'SDC',
'supracen violet').
SOLYPERTINE*** (7-[2-[4-(o-methoxy-
phenyl)piperazin-1-yl]ethyl]-5H-1,3-dio-
xolo(4,5-f)indole).
SOLYPERTINE TARTRATE* (solypertine
hydrogen tartrate; WIN-18413-2).
'Solyusurmin' see Sodium stibogluconate.
'Soma' see Carisoprodol.
'Somagest' see Amixetrine.
SOMAN (3,3-dimethyl-2-butyl methylphos-

410

phorofluoridate; methyl pinacolyl phosphonofluoridate; pinacolyloxymethylphosphoryl fluoride; pinacolyl methylphosphonofluoridate).

SOMATOMEDIN (growth hormone releasing hormone; GHRH; sulfation factor).

SOMATOSTATIN (growth hormone release inhibiting factor; somatotrophin release inhibiting factor; SRIF).

Somatotrophin *see* Growth hormone.

'Somben' *see* Carbromal.

'Sombrevin' *see* Propanidid.

'Sombulex' *see* Hexobarbital.

'Somilan' *see* Chloral betaine.

'Somilar' *see* Chloral betaine.

'Sominat' *see* Dichloralphenazone.

'Somnibel' *see* Methaqualone with etodroxizine maleate.

'Somnio' *see* Chloralose.

'Somnipront' *see* Dimethyl sulfoxide.

'Somnofac' *see* Methaqualone.

'Somnolens' *see* Phenobarbital.

'Somnos' *see* Chloral hydrate.

'Somsanit' *see* Oxybate sodium.

'Sonbutal' *see* Butallylonal.

'Soneryl' *see* Butethal.

Sontochin *see* Sontoquine.

SONTOQUINE* (7-chloro-4-(4-diethylamino-1-methylbutylamino)-3-methylquinoline; sontochin; RP-3808; SN-6911; 'nivaquine A', 'nivaquine C', 'santochin').

'Sopangamine' *see* Pangamic acid.

'Sophia' *see* Norethisterone with mestranol.

Sophoretin *see* Quercetin.

Sophorin *see* Rutoside.

'Sophorine' *see* Cytosine.

SOPITAZINE* (10-[(4-isopropylpiperazin-1-yl)carbonyl)]phenothiazine; 4-isopropylpiperazin-1-yl phenothiazin-10-yl ketone).

'Sopor' *see* Methaqualone.

'Soprintin' *see* Acepromazine.

'Sopronol' *see* Sodium propionate.

'Soprontin' *see* Acepromazine.

'Soraxa' *see* Warfarin.

'Sorbacel' *see* Oxidized cellulose.

'Sorbangil' *see* Isosorbide dinitrate.

'Sorbester' *see* Polysorbate 80.

SORBIC ACID (2,4-hexadienoic acid; 2-propenylacrylic acid).

Sorbic oil *see* Parasorbic acid.

Sorbide nitrate* *see* Isosorbide dinitrate.

'Sorbidilat' *see* Isosorbide dinitrate.

Sorbimacrogol(s)* *see* Polysorbate(s).

SORBINICATE* (D-glucitol hexanicotinate; sorbitol hexanicotinate).

SORBITAN(S) (sorbitol polymers).

Sorbitan esters *see below and* Polysorbate(s).

SORBITAN LAURATE* (monoesters of lauric acid and sorbitan; sorbitan monolaurate; 'span 20').

SORBITAN OLEATE* (monoesters of oleic acid and sorbitan; sorbitan monooleate; 'span 80').

SORBITAN PALMITATE* (monoesters of palmitic acid and sorbitan; sorbitan

monopalmitate; 'span 40').

SORBITAN SESQUIOLEATE* (mixture of monoesters and diesters of oleic acid and sorbitan; 'arlacel 3', 'arlacel 83').

SORBITAN STEARATE* (monoesters of stearic acid sorbitan; sorbitan monostearate; 'span 60').

SORBITAN TRIOLEATE* (triesters of oleic acid and sorbitan; 'span 85').

SORBITAN TRISTEARATE* (triesters of stearic acid and sorbitan; 'span 65').

D-SORBITOL (D-glucitol; D-glucohexitol; sorbite; 'diakarmon', 'karion', 'nivitin', 'sionon', 'sorbo', 'sorbol').

See also Iron sorbitex.

Sorbitol hexanicotinate *see* Sorbinicate.

Sorbitol polymers *see* Sorbitans.

'Sorbitrate' *see* Isosorbide dinitrate.

'Sorbo' *see* Sorbitol.

'Sorbol' *see* Sorbitol.

'Sorbolen' *see under* Macrogols.

'Sordinol' *see* Clopenthixol.

Sorethytan(s)* *see* Polysorbate(s).

'Sorexa' *see* Warfarin.

'Soricin' *see* Sodium ricinoleate.

'Soridermal' *see* Metiazinic acid.

'Soripal' *see* Metiazinic acid.

'Sorlate(s)' *see* Polysorbate(s).

'Sormodren' *see* Bornaprine.

'Sorot' *see* Dequalinium.

'Sosegon' *see* Pentazocine.

'Sosenyl' *see* Pentazocine.

'Sosol' *see* Sulfafurazole.

'Sospitan' *see* Pyridinedimethanol bis(methylcarbamate).

'Sotacor' *see* Sotalol.

SOTALOL* (4'-(1-hydroxy-2-isopropylaminoethyl)methanesulfonanilide; sotalol hydrochloride; MJ-1999; 'beta-cardone', 'sotacor').

SOTERENOL (2'-hydroxy-5'-(1-hydroxy-2-isopropylaminoethyl)methanesulfonanilide; 4-hydroxy-α-isopropylaminomethyl-3-methanesulfonamidobenzyl alcohol; soterenol hydrochloride; MJ-1992).

'Sotorni' *see* Levopropoxyphene dibudinate.

'Sotradecol' *see* Sodium tetradecyl sulfate.

'Souframine' *see* Phenothiazine.

'Soventol' *see* Bamipine.

Sovkain (tr) *see* Cinchocaine.

'Soxidyl' *see* Tiocarlide.

'Soxisol' *see* Sulfafurazole.

'Soxomide' *see* Sulfafurazole.

'Soziodol' *see* 2,6-Diiodo-1-phenol-4-acid.

Soziodolic acid *see* 2,6-Diiodo-1-phenol-4-sulfonic acid.

Sozoiodolic acid *see* 2,6-Diiodo-1-phenol-4-sulfonic acid.

Sozolic acid *see* Phenolsulfonic acid.

Sp-54 *see* Pentosan polysulfate.

SP-732 *see* Prolintane.

'Spa' *see* Lefetamine.

'α-Spa' *see* (+)-N,N-Dimethyl-α-phenylphenethylamine.

'Spacolin' *see* Alverine.

'Spans' *see under* Sorbitans.

'**Sparine**' *see* Promazine.
SPARSOMYCIN*** (antibiotic from *Str. sparsogenes*; NSC-59727; U-19183).
'**Spartase**' *see* Potassium magnesium aspartate.
SPARTEINE*** (dodecahydro-7,14-metha-nopyrido(1,2-a:1',2'-e)(1,5)diazocine; lupinidine; sparteine sulfate; 'actospar', 'depasan', 'perivar', 'spartepur', 'spartocin', 'tocosamine', 'unitocin').
SPARTEINE ADENYLATE (adenylic acid sparteine salt; 'spartopan').
'**Spartepur**' *see* Sparteine.
'**Spartocin**' *see* Sparteine.
'**Spartopan**' *see* Sparteine adenylate.
'**Spartrix**' *see* Carnidazole.
SPA-S-160 *see* Mepartricin.
'**Spasfon**' *see* Phloroglucinol with 1,3,5-trimethoxybenzene.
'**Spasmacol**' *see* Alverine.
'**Spasmadryl**' *see* Aprofene.
'**Spasmalgan**' *see* Denaverine.
'**Spasmamide**' *see* Fenalamide.
'**Spasmaverine**' *see* Alverine.
'**Spasmentral**' *see* Benzetimide.
'**Spasmex**' *see* Trospium chloride.
'**Spasmine**' *see* Dibenzyl succinate.
'**Spasmocalm**' *see* Diethyl benzyl(2-di-ethylaminoethyl)malonate.
'**Spasmocyclone**' *see* Cyclandelate.
'**Spasmodex**' *see* Dihexyverine.
'**Spasmodin**' *see* Benzyl benzoate.
'**Spastussin**' *see* Benzyl benzoate.
'**Spasmolysin**' *see* Proxyphylline.
Spasmolytin (tr) *see* Adiphenine.
'**Spasmonal**' *see* Dipiproverine.
'**Spasmoparid**' *see* Bietamiverine.
'**Spasmoparine**' *see* Bietamiverine.
'**Spazmokalm**' *see* Diethyl benzyl(2-di-ethylaminoethyl)malonate.
SPC-297D *see* Azidocillin.
'**Speciadopa**' *see* Levodopa.
'**Specillin**' *see* Penicillin.
'**Spectacillin**' *see* Epicillin.
SPECTINOMYCIN*** (antibiotic from *Str. spectabilis*; actinospectocin; M-141; U-18409-E; 'stanilo', 'togamycin', 'trobicin').
'**Spectra-sorb UV 9**' *see* Oxybenzone.
'**Spectra-sorb UV 24**' *see* Dioxybenzone.
'**Spectra-sorb UV 284**' *see* Sulisobenzone.
'**Spectra-sorb UV 531**' *see* Octabenzone.
'**Spectrobact**' *see* Troleandomycin.
'**Spectrocide**' *see* Dimpylate.
'**Speda**' *see* Vinylbital.
'**Speed**' *see* Methamphetamine.
'**Spenitol**' *see* Moroxydine.
'**Spergon**' *see* Chloranil.
Spermaceti *see* Cetaceum.
SPERMIDINE (*N*-(3-aminopropyl)putr-escine; *N*-(3-aminopropyl)-1,4-butane-diamine).
SPERMINE (*N*,*N*'-bis(3-aminopropyl)-putrescine; *N*,*N*'-bis(3-aminopropyl)-1,4-butanediamine; di(aminopropyl)tetra-methylenediamine; spermocrine; 'geron-tine', 'lotone', 'musculamine', 'neuridine',

'spermol').
Spermocrine (tr) *see* Spermine.
'**Spermol**' *see* Spermine.
SP-G *see* Podophyllotoxin benzylidene glucoside.
Sphaerophysin *see* Spherophysine.
'**Spheromycin**' *see* Novobiocin.
SPHEROPHYSINE (tr) (1-[4-(3-methyl-1-butenylamino)butyl]guanidine).
SPHINGINE (2-amino-1-octadecanol).
SPHINGOSINE (2-amino-4-octadecene-1,3-diol).
SP-I *see* Mitopodozide.
SPICLOMAZINE*** (8-[3-(2-chloropheno-thiazin-10-yl)propyl]-1-thia-4,8-diazaspiro-(4.5)decan-3-one; clospirazine; APY-606; 'disepron').
'**Spidox**' *see* Phenylmercuric nitrate.
SPINACEAMINE (4,5,6,7-tetrahydroimi-dazo(5,4-c)pyridine).
Spinacene *see* Squalene.
'**Spinocaine**' *see* Procaine.
SPIPERONE*** (8-[3-(*p*-fluorobenzoyl)-propyl]-1-phenyl-1,3,8-triazaspiro(4.5)-decan-4-one; 4'-fluoro-4-[spiro(5-oxo-3-phenylimidazolidin-4,4'-piperidin)-1'-yl]-butyrophenone; spiroperidol; R-5147; 'spiropitan').
'**Spiractin**' *see* Pimeclone.
SPIRAMIDE** (8-[3-(4-fluorophenoxy)-propyl]-1-phenyl-1,3,8-triazaspiro(4.5)-decan-4-one).
SPIRAMYCIN*** (antibiotic from *Str. ambofaciens*; IL-5902; NSC-64393; RP-5337; 'provamycin', 'rovamycin', 'selectomycin', 'sequamycin').
See also Metronidazole with spiramycin.
SPIRAZIDINE (tr) (3,12-bis(2-chloroethyl)-3,6,9,12-tetraazadispiro(5.5.5)hexadecane).
SPIRAZINE** (2,4-diamino-5-(*p*-chloro-phenyl)-9-methyl-1,3,5-triazaspiro(5.5)-undeca-1,3-diene).
SPIRGETINE*** ([2-(6-azaspiro(2.5)oct-6-yl)ethyl]guanidine; *N*-(2-guanidino-ethyl)-aza-6-spiro(2.5)octane; LD-3598).
SPIRGETINE WITH PARAFLUTIZIDE ('divimax').
SPIRILENE** (8-[4-(*p*-fluorophenyl)-3-pentenyl]-1-phenyl-1,3,8-triazaspiro(4.5)-decan-4-one).
Spirobarbital *see* Spiro(dimethylethylcyclo-pentane)barbituric acid.
Spirobarbituric acid *see* Spiro (dimethyl-ethylcyclopentane)barbituric acid.
Spirodiflamine *see* Fluspiriline.
SPIRO(3',5'-DIMETHYL-2'-ETHYL-CYCLOPENTANE)BARBITURIC ACID (spirobarbital; spirobarbituric acid).
SPIRO(3',5'-DIMETHYL-2'-ETHYL-CYCLOPENTANE)-2-THIOBAR-BITURIC ACID (spirothiobarbituric acid; 'spirothal').
'**Spiroform**' *see* Acetylsalol.
'**Spirogen**' *see* Ammonium phthalamate.
Spirolactone *see* Spironolactone.
SPIRONOLACTONE*** (17-hydroxy-7-mercapto-3-oxo-17α-pregn-4-ene-21-carbo-

xylic acid γ-lactone 7-acetate; 3-(7α-acetylthio-17β-hydroxy-3-oxoandrost-4-en-17α-yl)propionic acid γ-lactone; spirolactone; SC-9420; 'aldactone', 'dytaurese').

See also Butizide with spironolactone; Hydroflumethiazide with spironolactone.

Spiroperidol *see* Spiperone.
'Spiropitan' *see* Spiperone.
'Spirosal' *see* Glycol salicylate.
'Spirothal' *see* Spiro(dimethylethylcyclopentane)-2-thiobarbituric acid.
Spirothiobarbituric acid *see* Spiro(dimethylethylcyclopentane)-2-thiobarbituric acid.
SPIROXASONE*** (α-acetylthio-4′,5′-dihydrospiro(androst-4-ene-17,2′(3′H)-furan)-3-one acetate; 4′,5′-dihydro-7α(mercapto)spiro(androst-4-ene-17,2′(3′H)-furan)-3-one acetate).
SPIROXATRINE*** (8-(1,4-benzodioxan-2-ylmethyl)-1-phenyl-1,3,8-triazaspiro(4.5)-decan-4-one).
SPIROXEPIN*** (N,N-dimethylspiro [dibenz(b,e)oxepin-11(6H),2′-(1,3)dioxolane]-4′-methylamine).
Spofa-325 *see* Moxastin.
'Spofadiazin' *see* Sulfamethoxypyridazine.
'Spontin' *see* Ristocetin.
'Sporostacin' *see* Clodantoin.
Spreading factor *see* Hyaluronidase.
SQ-1089 *see* Hydroxycarbamide.
SQ-1489 *see* Thiram.
SQ-2128 *see* Etoxazene.
SQ-9343 *see* Sodium phytate.
SQ-9453 *see* Dimethyl sulfoxide.
SQ-9538 *see* Testolactone.
SQ-9993 *see* Estradiol undecylate.
SQ-10269 *see* Carbifene.
SQ-10496 *see* Tiazesim.
SQ-10643 *see* Cinanserin.
SQ-11302 *see* Epicillin.
SQ-11436 *see* Cefradine.
SQ-11725 *see* Nadolol.
SQ-15010 *see* Algestone acetofenide.
SQ-15659 *see* Rolitetracycline.
SQ-15761 *see* Sodium iopodate.
SQ-15860 *see* Glyhexamide.
SQ-15874 *see* Pipazetate.
SQ-16123 *see* Meticillin.
SQ-16150 *see* Estradiol enantate.
SQ-16360 *see* Sodium fusidate.
SQ-16374 *see* Metenolone enantate.
SQ-16401 *see* Halquinols.
SQ-16423 *see* Oxacillin.
SQ-16496 *see* Metenolone acetate.
SQ-18566 *see* Halcinonide.
SQ-19844 *see* Sincalide.
SQ-20009 *see* Etazolate.
SQ-20824 *see* Cicloprofen.
SQUALENE (2,6,10,15,19,23-hexamethyl-2,6,10,14,18,22-tetracosahexaene; spinacene).
SR-406 *see* Captan.
SR-720-22 *see* Metolazone.
SRG-95213 *see* Diazoxide.
SRIF *see* Somatostatin.

SS-578 *see* Diiodohydroxyquin.
ST-25 *see* Batroxobin.
ST-37 *see* Hexylresorcinol.
ST-52 *see* Fosfestrol.
ST-104 *see* Prednylidene.
ST-1085 *see* Midodrine.
ST-155 *see* Clonidine.
ST-1512 *see* Hexoprenaline.
ST-5066 *see* Iobenzamic acid.
ST-7090 *see* Hexobendine.
ST-9067 *see* Azintamide.
'Stabinol' *see* Glysobuzole.
'Stadacaine' *see* Leucinocaine.
'Stafac' *see* Virginiamycin.
'Stafylopenin' *see* Meticillin.
'Stagural' *see* Norfenefrine.
STALLIMYCIN** (N″-(2-amidinoethyl)-4-formamido-1,1′,1″-trimethyl-N,4′:N′,4″-ter(pyrrole-2-carboxamide); distamycin A).
'Stam F-34' *see* Propanil.
'Stamicin' *see* Nystatin.
'Stampen' *see* Dicloxacillin.
'Stamycin' *see* Nystatin.
'Stanaprol' *see* Androstanolone.
Stanazolol* *see* Stanozolol.
'Stangyl' *see* Trimipramine.
'Stanilo' *see* Spectinomycin.
'Stannacne' *see* Tin oxide.
'Stannoxyl' *see* Tin oxide.
Stanolone* *see* Androstanolone.
'Stanoprol' *see* Androstanolone.
STANOZOLOL*** (17β-hydroxy-17α-methylandrostano(3,2-c)pyrazole; 17α-methyl-5α-androstano(3,2-c)pyrazol-17β-ol; androstanazole; methylstanazole; stanazolol; WIN-14833; 'anasyth', 'stromba', 'winstrol').
'Stapenor' *see* Oxacillin.
'Staphcillin' *see* Meticillin.
'Staphobristol' *see* Cloxacillin.
'Staphylex' *see* Flucloxacillin.
'Staphylomycin' *see* Virginiamycin.
'Staporos' *see* Calcitonin.
'Stapyocine' *see* Pristinamycin.
Starch epichlorohydrin reaction product *see* Amilomer.
Starch sugar *see* Glucose.
'Sta-soft' *see under* Macrogols.
'Staticin' *see* Carinamide.
'Statran' *see* Emylcamate.
'Statyl' *see* Nequinate.
'Staxidin' *see* Virginiamycin.
StC-1106 *see* Fluprednidene acetate.
StC-1400 *see* Fludrocortisone acetate.
STEAGLATE(S)** (O-stearoylglycolate(s)).
See also Prednisolone steaglate.
STEARIC ACID (octadecanoic acid).
See also Magnesium stearate; Monostearin; Propylene glycol monostearate; Stearin.
STEARIN (stearic acid glyceryl triester).
O-Stearoylglycolate(s) *see* Steaglate(s).
Stearyl alcohol *see* 1-Octadecanol.
Stearylic alcohol *see* 1-Octadecanol.
STEARYLSULFAMIDE*** (stearylsulfanilamide; N-sulfanilylstearamide).
'Stediril' *see* Norgestrel with ethinylestradiol.
'Stediril-d' *see* Levonorgestrel with ethinyl-

413

estradiol.
STEFFIMYCIN*** (antibiotic from *Str. steffisburgensis*).
'Stelazine' *see* Trifluoperazine.
'Stellamycin' *see* Streptoduocin.
'Stellarid' *see* Proscillaridin.
'Stellidine' *see* Histidine.
'Stemetil' *see* Prochlorperazine.
'Stemex' *see* Paramethasone acetate.
STENBOLONE*** (2-methyl-5α-androst-1-en-17β-ol-3-one; 17β-hydroxy-2-methyl-5α-androst-1-en-3-one).
'Stenol' *see* 1-Octadecanol.
'Stenosine' *see* Disodium methanearsonate.
STEPA *see* Thiotepa.
'Stepin' *see* Tioxolone.
'Steramine' *see* Benzalkonium.
'Steranabol' *see* Clostebol acetate.
'Steranabol depot' *see* Oxabolone cipionate.
Stercorin *see* Coprostanol.
STERCURONIUM IODIDE*** ((cona-4,6-dienin-3β-yl)ethyldimethylammonium iodide; MYC-1080).
'Sterilon' *see* Chlorhexidine.
'Sterinol' *see* Benzododecinium chloride.
'Sterisil' *see* Hexetidine.
'Sterisol' *see* Hexedine.
'Sterlifix' *see* Triclosan.
'Sterogenol' *see* Cetylpyridinium bromide.
'Sterogyl' *see* Calciferol.
'Sterolibrin' *see* 6-Chloro-17α-hydroxy-16-methylenepregna-4,6-diene-3,20-dione acetate with mestranol.
'Sterolone' *see* Prednisolone.
'Sterosan' *see* Chlorquinaldol.
'Steroxin' *see* Chlorquinaldol.
'Ster-zac' *see* Hexachlorophene.
'Stesolid' *see* Diazepam.
STEVALADIL** (3β-(dimethylamino)-5α-pregnane-18,20α-diol diacetate ester).
STH *see* Growth hormone.
STIBAMINE* (sodium *p*-aminobenzenestibonate).
STIBAMINE GLUCOSIDE*** (*N*-glucoside of sodium *p*-aminobenzenestibonate; 'neostam').
'Stibanate' *see* Sodium stibogluconate.
'Stibanose' *see* Sodium stibogluconate.
'Stibatin' *see* Sodium stibogluconate.
STIBINE (SbH₃; antimony hydride).
'Stibinol' *see* Sodium stibogluconate.
Stibocaptate* *see* Sodium stibocaptate.
STIBOCAPTIC ACID (2,3-dimercaptosuccinic acid cyclic thioantimonate (III) *S,S*-diester; antimony dimercaptosuccinic acid; 'astiban acid').
STIBOPHEN* (antimony (III) sodium bispyrocatechol-2,4-disulfonate; Sdt-91; 'fantorin', 'fouadin', 'fuadin', 'neoantimosan', 'pyrostib', 'repodral', 'reprodal', 'sodium antimosan', 'trimon').
STIBOPHEN POTASSIUM (antimony (III) potassium bispyrocatechol-2,4-disulfonate; Heyden-611; 'antimosan').
Stibosamine** *see* Ethylstibamine.
'Stibunal' *see* Sodium antimonyl tartrate.
'Stiburea' *see* Urea stibamine.

Stickstofflost *see* Chlormethine.
Stigmastadienol *see* Stigmasterol.
Stigmast-5-en-3β-ol 2-(*p*-chlorophenoxy)-2-methylpropionate *see* Sitofibrate.
Stigmastenol clofibrate *see* Sitofibrate.
STIGMASTEROL (stigmasta-5,22-dien-3-ol; 24-ethyl-3β-hydroxycholesta-5,22-diene; antistiffness factor).
See also Sitosterol.
'Stigmenene' *see* Benzpyrinium.
'Stigminene' *see* Benzpyrinium.
Stilbamidine diisethionate *see* Stilbamidine isetionate.
Stilbamidine isethionate* *see* Stilbamidine isetionate.
STILBAMIDINE ISETIONATE*** (4,4'-stilbenedicarboxamidine bis(2-hydroxyethanesulfonate); stilbamidine di(ethanol-2-sulfonate); stilbamidine diisethionate; stilbamidine isethionate; M&B-744).
'Stilbarol' *see* Diethylstilbestrol.
STILBAZIUM IODIDE*** (2,6-bis(4-pyrrolidin-1-ylstyryl)-1-ethylpyridinium iodide; 1-ethyl-2,6-bis(*p*-pyrrolidin-1-ylstyryl)-pyridinium iodide; stilbazum; BW-61-32; 'monopar').
2-STILBAZOLE (α-stilbazole; 2-styrylpyridine).
4-STILBAZOLE (γ-stilbazole; 4-styrylpyridine).
Stilbazum* *see* Stilbazium.
STILBENE (1,2-diphenylethylene; styrylbenzene; toluylene).
4,4'-Stilbenedicarboxamidine *see* Stilbamidine.
'Stilbenol' *see* Diethylstilbestrol.
Stilbestrol *see* Diethylstilbestrol.
Stilbestrol dipalmitate *see* Stilpalmitate.
Stilbestrol diphosphate *see* Fosfestrol.
Stilboestrol* *see* Diethylstilbestrol.
STILBYLAMINE (α-phenylphenethylamine; α-aminodiphenylethane; 1,2-diphenylethylamine).
'Stillomycin' *see* Puromycin.
STILONIUM IODIDE*** (triethyl[2-(*p*-styrylphenoxy)ethyl]ammonium iodide; *p*-(2-diethylaminoethoxy)stilbene ethiodide).
STILPALMITATE* (diethylstilbestrol dipalmitate; stilbestrol dipalmitate).
'Stilphostrol' *see* Fosfestrol.
'Stimsen' *see* Tozalinone.
'Stimulest' *see* Deanol.
'Stimulexin' *see* Doxapram.
'Stinerval' *see* Phenelzine.
STIRIMAZOLE*** (2-(4-carboxystyryl)-5-nitro-1-vinylimidazole; *p*-[2-(5-nitro-1-vinylimidazol-2-yl)vinyl]benzoic acid).
STIRIPENTOL*** (4,4-dimethyl-1-[(3,4-methylenedioxy)phenyl]-1-penten-3-ol; 1-(1,3-benzodioxol-5-yl)-4,4-dimethyl-1-penten-3-ol; 5-(3-hydroxy-4,4-dimethyl-1-pentenyl)-1,3-benzodioxole; β-(1-hydroxy-2,2-dimethylpropyl)-3,4-methylenedioxy-styrene).
STIROFOS* (2-chloro-1-(2,4,5-trichlorophenyl)vinyl dimethyl phosphate; tetrachlorvinfos; CVMP; SD-3447; SD-8447;

414

SD-8747; 'gardona', 'rabon').
'Stop-scald' *see* Ethoxyquin.
'Stovaine' *see* Amylocaine.
'Stovarsol' *see* Acetarsol.
'Stovarsolan' *see* Acetarsol.
'Stoxil' *see* Idoxuridine.
'STP' *see* 2,5-Dimethoxy-4-methylampheta-mine.
STRAMONIUM (*Datura stramonium* and/or *Datura tatula*).
'Stratene' *see* Cetiedil.
'Strazide' *see* Streptoniazid.
'Strepantin' *see* Streptomycin pantothenate.
'Strepsils' *see* Amylmetacresol.
STREPTAMINE (1,3-diamino-2,4,5,6-tetra-hydroxycyclohexane).
'Streptase' *see* Streptokinase.
STREPTIDINE (1,3-diguanido-2,4,5,6-tetrahydroxycyclohexane).
Streptococcal desoxyribonuclease *see* Streptodornase.
Streptococcal fibrinolysin *see* Streptokinase.
STREPTODORNASE* (streptococcal desoxyribonuclease).
STREPTODORNASE WITH STREPTO-KINASE ('bistreptase', 'distreptaze', 'dornokinase', 'varidase').
STREPTODUOCIN* (equal parts of strepto-mycin and dihydrostreptomycin as sulfates and/or pantothenates).
'Streptohydrazid' *see* Streptoniazid.
STREPTOKINASE* (streptococcal fibrino-lysin; 'kabikinase', 'kinalysin', 'streptase'). *See also* Streptodornase with streptokinase.
STREPTOLYDIGIN (streptolydigin sodium; 'portamycin').
Streptomyces actuosus 40037, antibiotic' *see* Nosiheptide.
Streptomyces albus, antibiotic *see* Indolmycin.
Streptomyces ambofaciens, antibiotics *see* Ambomycin; Azotomycin; Duazomycin; Spiramycin.
Streptomyces antibioticus, antibiotic *see* Oleandomycin.
Streptomyces bambergiensis, antibiotic *see* Bambermycin.
Streptomyces bellus var. cirolerosis var. nova, antibiotic *see* Cirolemycin.
Streptomyces bikiniensis, antibiotic *see* Biniramycin.
Streptomyces bluensis, antibiotic *see* Bluensomycin.
Streptomyces candidus, antibiotic *see* Avoparcin.
Streptomyces canus, antibiotic *see* Amfomycin.
Streptomyces capreolus, antibiotic *see* Capreomycin.
Streptomyces carzinostaticus, polypep-tide *see* Neocarzinostatin.
Streptomyces chrysomallus, antibiotic *see* Cactinomycin.
Streptomyces coerulorubidus, anti-biotic *see* Daunorubicin.
Streptomyces desdanus, antibiotic *see* Desdanine.

Streptomyces distallicus, antibiotic *see* Stallimycin.
Streptomyces endus, antibiotic *see* Endomycin.
Streptomyces erythreus, antibiotic *see* Erythromycin.
Streptomyces flocculus, antibiotic *see* Rufocromomycin.
Streptomyces floridae, antibiotic *see* Viomycin.
Streptomyces fradiae, antibiotics *see* Neomycin; Tylosin.
Streptomyces fungicidicus, antibiotic *see* Enramycin.
Streptomyces griseoviridus var. atro-faciens, antibiotic *see* Actinobolin.
Streptomyces griseus, antibiotic *see* Candicidin.
Streptomyces griseus var. spiralis, antibiotic *see* Aspartocin.
Streptomyces hachijoensis, antibiotic *see* Hachimycin.
Streptomyces halstedii, antibiotic *see* Carbomycin.
Streptomyces hygroscopicus, antibiotic *see* Relomycin.
Streptomyces hygroscopicus var. azalo-myceticus, antibiotic *see* Azalomycin.
Streptomyces kanamyceticus, antibiotic *see* Kanamycin.
Streptomyces kitasatoensis, antibiotic *see* Kitasamycin.
Streptomyces kuwaitiensis, antibiotic *see* Kuwaitimycin.
Streptomyces lasaliensis, antibiotic *see* Lasalocid.
Streptomyces lincolnensis, antibiotics *see* Lincomycin; Ranimycin.
Streptomyces lomondensis, antibiotic *see* Lomofungin.
Streptomyces longissimus, antibiotic *see also* Antelmycin.
Streptomyces lucensis, antibiotic *see* Lucimycin.
Streptomyces luteogriseus, antibiotic *see* Peliomycin.
Streptomyces lydicus, antibiotic *see* Lidimycin.
Streptomyces malayensis antibiotic *see* Mitomalcin.
Streptomyces mediterranei, antibiotic *see* Rifamycin.
Streptomyces mitakaensis, antibiotic *see* Mikamycin.
Streptomyces mycarofaciens, antibiotic *see* Midecamycin.
Streptomyces narbonensis var. josamy-ceticus var. nova, antibiotic *see* Josamycin.
Streptomyces natalensis, antibiotic *see* Natamycin.
Streptomyces nodosus, antibiotic *see* Amphotericin B.
Streptomyces nogalata, antibiotic *see* Nogalamycin.
Streptomyces noursei, antibiotic *see* Nystatin.
Streptomyces orientalis, antibiotic *see*

Vancomycin.

Streptomyces ostreogriseus, antibiotic *see* Ostreogrycin.

Streptomyces pactum, antibiotic *see* Pactamycin.

Streptomyces peuceticus, antibiotic *see* Daunorubicin.

Streptomyces pimprina, antibiotic *see* Hamycin.

Streptomyces plicatus, antibiotic *see* Mithramycin.

Streptomyces pristina spiralis, antibiotic *see* Pristinamycin.

Streptomyces puniceus, antibiotics *see* Viomycin.

Streptomyces rimosus, antibiotic *see* Neutramycin; Paromomycin.

Streptomyces rufochromogenes, antibiotic *see* Rufocromomycin.

Streptomyces rutgersensis, antibiotic *see* Rutamycin.

Streptomyces sp. No. 24281 (Michigan Dept. of Public Health), antibiotic *see* Mitocarcin.

Streptomyces sparsogenes, antibiotic *see* Sparsomycin.

Streptomyces spectabilis, antibiotic *see* Spectinomycin.

Streptomyces spheroides, antibiotic *see* Novobiocin.

Streptomyces steffisburgensis var. steffisburgensis, antibiotic *see* Steffimycin.

Streptomyces tanahiensis, antibiotic *see* Mithramycin.

Streptomyces tanashiensis strain kala, antibiotic *see* Kalafungin.

Streptomyces tenebrarius, antibiotics *see* Apramycin; Nebramycin; Tobramycin.

Streptomyces variabilis, antibiotic *see* Streptovarycin.

Streptomyces verticillus, antibiotic *see* Bleomycin.

Streptomyces virginiae, antibiotic *see* Virginiamycin.

Streptomyces viridochromogenes, antibiotic *see* Mitocromin.

Streptomyces viridogriseus, antibiotic *see* Viridofulvin.

Streptomycilidene isonicotinoylhydrazone *see* Streptoniazid.

STREPTOMYCIN*** (2,4-diguanidino-3,5,6-trihydroxycyclohexyl-5-deoxy-2-*O*-(2-deoxy-2-methylamino-α-L-glucopyranosyl)-3-formyl-β-L-*lyxo*-pentanofuranoside; streptomycin A; streptomycin hydrochloride, phosphate or sulfate; NSC-14083).

STREPTOMYCIN GLUCURONOLAC-TONE SULFATE ('glucomycin').

STREPTOMYCIN OPINIAZIDE SALT (streptomycin isoniazidveratrylidenecarboxylate; streptosaluzid).

STREPTOMYCIN PANTOTHENATE ('strepantin', 'streptothenate'). *See also* Dihydrostreptomycin; Streptoduocin; Streptoniazid.

Streptomycylideneisoniazid sulfate *see* Streptoniazid.

STREPTONIAZID*** (isonicotinic acid streptomycilidenehydrazide; compound of isoniazid with streptomycin sulfate; streptomycilidene isonicotinoylhydrazone; streptomycylideneisoniazid sulfate; streptomycin isonicotinoylhydrazone; streptonicozid; streptotubazid; SINH; 'strazide', 'streptohydrazid').

Streptonicozid* *see* Streptoniazid.

STREPTONIGRIN* (5-amino-6-(7-amino-5,8-dihydro-6-methoxy-5,8-dioxo-2-quinolyl)-4-(2-hydroxy-3,4-dimethoxyphenyl)-3-methylpicolinic acid; bruneomycin; NSC-45383; 'nigrin').

STREPTONIGRIN METHYL ESTER (NSC-45384).

Streptonivicin *see* Novobiocin.

Streptosaluzid (tr) *see* Streptomycin opiniazide salt.

'Streptothenate' *see* Streptomycin pantothenate.

'Streptotibine' *see* Dihydrostreptomycin tri-isonicotinoylhydrazone.

Streptotubazid (tr) *see* Streptoniazid.

Streptovaricin *see* Streptovarycin.

STREPTOVARYCIN*** (antibiotic mixture from *Str. variabilis*; streptovaricin; B-44-P).

'Streptovitacin A' *see* Hydroxycycloheximide.

STREPTOZOCIN*** (1-D-glucos-2-yl-3-methyl-3-nitrosourea; 2-deoxy-2-(3-methyl-3-nitrosoureido)-D-glucopyranose; streptozotocin; NSC-85998).

STREPTOZOCIN WITH ZEDALAN (NSC-37917).

Streptozotocin *see* Streptozocin.

'Stresnil' *see* Azaperone.

'Streunex' *see* BHC.

'Striadyne' *see* Adenosine triphosphate.

'Striatran' *see* Emylcamate.

'Strobane' *see* Terpene polychlorinates.

'Strodival' *see* Ouabain.

'Stromba' *see* Stanozolol.

Strophanthidin cymaroside diglucoside *see* Strophanthoside.

Strophanthidin cymaroside glucoside *see* Strophanthin.

STROPHANTHIDOL D-**CYMAROSIDE** (cymarol).

STROPHANTHIDOL L-**RHAMNOSIDE** (convallatoxol).

STROPHANTHIN (3β,5,14-trihydroxy-19-oxo-5β-card-20(22)-enolide 3-D-cymaro-D-glucoside; strophanthidin cymaroside glucoside; cymarin; strophanthin k; C-197; 'alvonal', 'combetin', 'kombetin', laevostrophan').

Strophanthin g *see* Ouabain.

Strophanthin k *see* Strophanthin.

Strophanthin D-**glucoside** *see* Strophanthoside.

STROPHANTHOSIDE (strophanthin D-glucoside; strophanthidin cymaroside diglucoside; strophanthoside k; 'strophoside').

'**Strophoside**' *see* Strophanthoside.
'**Stryadine**' *see* Adenosine triphosphate.
Strychnine amine oxide *see* Strychnine
N-oxide.
STRYCHNINE N-OXIDE (strychnine
amine oxide; Z-203; 'genostrychnine',
'movellan').
STS *see* Sodium tetradecyl sulfate.
'**Stugeron**' *see* Cinnarizine.
'**Stylomycin**' *see* Puromycin.
STYPHNIC ACID (2,4,6-trinitroresorcinol).
'**Styptanon**' *see* Estriol succinate.
'**Stypticine**' *see* Cotarnine chloride.
'**Styptirenal**' *see* Epinephrine.
'**Styptol**' *see* Cotarnine chloride.
'**Styptopur**' *see* Aminomethylbenzoic acid.
'**Stypturon**' *see* Mepesulfate.
'**Stypven**' *see* Russell's viper venom.
STYRAMATE*** (2-hydroxy-2-phenylethyl
carbamate; α-(carbamoyloxymethyl)-
benzyl alcohol; β-hydroxyphenethyl
carbamate; 'sinaxar').
STYRENE (cinnamene; phenethylene;
styrol; styrolene; styron; vinylbenzene).
Styrol *see* Styrene.
Styrolene *see* Styrene.
Styron *see* Styrene.
Styrone *see* Cinnamyl alcohol.
Styrylbenzene *see* Stilbene.
Styrylpyridine *see* Stilbazole.
Su-3088 *see* Chlorisondamine.
Su-3118 *see* Syrosingopine.
Su-4885 *see* Metyrapone tartrate.
Su-5864 *see* Guanethidine.
Su-6518 *see* Dimetindene.
Su-8341 *see* Cyclopenthiazide.
Su-8874 *see* Metyrapone.
Su-9064 *see* Metoserpate.
Su-13437 *see* Nafenopin.
Su-18137 *see* Ciproquinate.
Su-21524 *see* Pirprofen.
'**Suavitil**' *see* Benactyzine.
'**Subamycin**' *see* Tetracycline.
SUBATHIZONE*** (p-ethylsulfonylbenz-
aldehyde thiosemicarbazone; sulzon;
SHCH-431; Tb III/1347).
'**Subcutin**' *see* Benzocaine.
Subecholine *see* Dicholine suberate.
SUBENDAZOLE** (4,5,7-trichloro-2-[3-
(methylthio)-1,2,4-thiadiazol-5-ylthio]-
benzimidazole; 3-(methylthio)-5-(4,5,7-
trichlorobenzimidazol-2-ylthio)-1,2,4-
thiadiazole).
'**Subenon**' *see* Calcium benzylsuccinate
benzoate.
SUBERIC ACID (octanedioic acid; 1,6-
hexanedicarboxylic acid).
Suberoylbis(choline) *see* Dicholine
suberate.
Suberyldicholine *see* Dicholine suberate.
'**Subeston**' *see* Aluminium acetate.
Sublimate *see* Mercuric chloride.
'**Sublimaze**' *see* Fentanyl.
'**Subose**' *see* Glyhexamide.
SUBTILISIN BPN′ ('nagarse').
'**Subtosan**' *see* Povidone.
'**Sucaryl-calcium**' *see* Calcium cyclamate.

Succicurarium *see* Suxamethonium.
SUCCINAMIC ACID (succinic acid mono-
amide).
SUCCINAMIDE (succinic acid diamide).
SUCCINANILIC ACID (N-phenylsuccin-
amic acid).
SUCCINCHLORIMIDE (N-chlorosuccin-
imide).
SUCCINIC ACID (butanedioic acid; amber
acid; Bernsteinsäure; 'asuccin').
**Succinic acid bis[2-(N-adamant-1-yl-N-
methylamino)ethyl] ester dimethio-
dide** *see* Diadonium iodide.
Succinic acid diamide *see* Succinamide.
Succinic acid 2,2-dimethylhydrazide *see*
Daminozide.
Succinic acid esters *see* Benzyl succinate;
Dibenzyl succinate; Dibutyl succinate;
Suxamethonium; Suxemerid; Suxetho-
nium.
Succinic acid imide *see* Succinimide.
Succinic acid monoamide *see* Succinamic
acid.
Succinic acid salts *see* Cadmium succinate,
Ferrous succinate, Sodium succinate.
SUCCINIMIDE (2,5-pyrrolidinedione;
butanimide; 2,5-dioxopyrrolidine).
SUCCINONITRILE (butanedinitrile;
ethylene cyanide; succine dinitrile
ethylene dicyanide; *sym.* dicyanoethane;
'deprelin', 'dinile', 'suxil').
'**Succinutin**' *see* Ethosuximide.
**Succinylbis(ethylenedimethylethyl-
ammonium chloride)** *see* Suxethonium.
**Succinylbis(ethylenetrimethylammo-
nium chloride)** *see* Suxamethonium.
Succinylcholine *see* Suxamethonium.
SUCCINYLDAPSONE (4-amino-4′-
succinylaminodiphenyl sulfone; succisulfone; F-1500).
Succinyldicholine *see* Suxamethonium.
SUCCINYLDISULFOCHOLINE
(succinylbis ester of dimethyl(2-hydroxy-
ethyl)sulfonium chloride; succinylsulfa-
choline).
SUCCINYL PEROXIDE ('alphozone').
SUCCINYLSALICYLIC ACID (bis(o-
carboxyphenyl) succinate; 'diasprin').
Succinylsulfacholine *see* Succinyldisulfo-
choline.
SUCCINYLSULFANILAMIDE (p-sulfa-
moylsuccinanilic acid).
SUCCINYLSULFATHIAZOLE*** (4′-
(thiazol-2-ylsulfamoyl)succinanilic acid;
N⁴-succinyl-N¹-thiazol-2-ylsulfanilamide;
2-(N⁴-3-carboxypropionylsulfanilamido)-
thiazole).
N⁴-Succinyl-N¹-thiazol-2-ylsulfanilamide
see Succinylsulfathiazole.
Succisulfone *see* Succinyldapsone.
'**Succitimal**' *see* Phensuximide.
Succus liquiritiae *see* Liquorice.
SUCLOFENIDE* (N-(2-chloro-4-sulfamoyl-
phenyl)-2-phenylsuccinimide; 'sulfalepsine').
SUCRALFATE*** (sucrose hydrogen sulfate
basic aluminium salt).

417

SUCRALOX*** (polymerized complex of sucrose and aluminium hydroxide; 'manalox AS').

'Sucramin' *see under* Saccharin.

Sucrase *see* Invertase.

Sucre de gelatine *see* Glycine.

'Sucrets' *see* Hexylresorcinol.

'Sucrol' *see* Phenetylurea.

SUCROSE (saccharose; α-D-glucopyranosyl-β-D-fructofuranoside).

Sucrose aluminium hydroxide complex *see* Sucralox.

Sucrose hydrogen sulfate basic aluminium salt *see* Sucralfate.

'Sucsan' *see* Liquorice.

Sudan III *see* Oil scarlet.

Sudan IV *see* Scarlet red.

'Sudermo' *see* Mesulfen.

SUDOXICAM*** (4-hydroxy-2-methyl-*N*-thiazol-2-yl-2H-1,2-benzothiazine-3-carboxamide 1,1-dioxide; CP-15973).

'Suicalm' *see* Azaperone.

'Suinox' *see* Secobarbital.

'Suisynchron' *see* Metallibure zinc complex.

'Suladrin' *see* Sulfafurazole diolamine.

SULAZEPAM*** (7-chloro-1,3-dihydro-1-methyl-5-phenyl-2H-1,4-benzodiazepine-2-thione; W-3676).

SULBENICILLIN*** (6-(2-phenyl-2-sulfo-acetamido)penicillanic acid; α-sulfobenzylpenicillin; sulbenicillin disodium; sulfocillin).

SULBENTINE*** (3,5-dibenzyltetrahydro-2H-1,3,5-thiadiazine-2-thione; dibenzthion; D-47; 'afungin', 'fungiplex', 'mycoplex', 'refungine').

Sulcimide *see* Sulcymide.

SULCLAMIDE*** (4-chloro-3-sulfamoylbenzamide; 3-carboxamido-2-chlorobenzenesulfonamide; SD-14112).

SULCYMIDE (tr) (*p*-aminobenzenesulfocyanamide; *N*¹-cyanosulfanilamide; sulcimide; sulfanilcyanamide).

'Suleo' *see* DDT.

'Sulestrex piperazine' *see* Piperazine estrone sulfate.

SULFABENZ*** (*N*¹-phenylsulfanilamide; sulfanilanilide; 'sulfa-vet').

SULFABENZAMIDE*** (*N*¹-benzoylsulfanilamide; sulfanilylbenzamide; 'sulfabenzide').

Sulfabenzamine *see* Mafenide.

'Sulfabenzide' *see* Sulfabenzamide.

Sulfabenzoylamide *see* Sulfadimethylbenzoylamide.

'Sulfabid' *see* Sulfaphenazole.

Sulfabutin *see* Busulfan.

SULFACARBAMIDE*** (*N*¹-carbamylsulfanilamide; sulfaurea; sulfanilylurea; urosulfan; 'euvernil', 'uramid').

See also Formophthalylsulfacarbamide. chrysoidine.

Sulfacarboxythiazole *see* Sulfacarizole.

SULFACARIZOLE (*N*¹-(carboxythiazolyl)-sulfanilamide; sulfacarboxythiazole).

SULFACECOLE** (2-ethoxy-4'-[(5-methylisoxazol-3-yl)sulfamoyl]acetanilide;

*N*⁴-(2-ethoxyacetyl)-*N*-(5-methylisoxazol-3-yl)sulfanilamide).

SULFACETAMIDE*** (*N*-sulfanilylacetamide; *N*¹-acetylsulfanilamide; acetosulfaminum; acetsulfanilamide; sulfacyl; sulfacetamide sodium).

Sulfachloropyrazine *see* Sulfaclozine.

SULFACHLORPYRIDAZINE*** (*N*¹-(6-chloropyridazin-3-yl)sulfanilamide; Ba-10370).

SULFACHRYSOIDINE*** (*N*⁴-(6-carboxy-2,4-diaminophenylazo)sulfanilamide; 3,5-diamino-2-(*p*-sulfoylphenylazo)benzoic acid; carboxysulfamidochrysoidine; diaminosulfamoylcarboxyazobenzene).

SULFACITINE** (*N*¹-(1-ethyl-1,2-dihydro-2-oxopyrimidin-4-yl)sulfanilamide; 1-ethyl-*N*-sulfanilylcytosine; sulfacytine).

SULFACLOMIDE** (*N*¹-(5-chloro-2,6-dimethylpyrimidin-4-yl)sulfanilamide; CI-636).

SULFACLORAZOLE*** (*N*¹-[1-(*m*-chlorophenyl)-3-methylpyrazol-5-yl]sulfanilamide).

SULFACLOZINE*** (*N*¹-(6-chloropyrazinyl) sulfanilamide; sulfachloropyrazine; Esb-3; 'sulfatyf').

Sulfacytine* *see* Sulfacitine.

Sulfadiamine *see* Acedapsone.

SULFADIASULFONE SODIUM*** (sodium *N*-acetyl-2-sulfamoyl-4,4'-diaminodiphenyl sulfone; acetosulfone; sodium acetosulfone; acetsulfonum; sodium derivative of *N*-(6-sulfanilylmetanilyl)acetamide; (*N*¹-acetyl-6-sulfanilylmetanilamido) sodium; CI-100; IA-307; 'promacetin').

SULFADIAZINE*** (*N*¹-pyrimid-2-ylsulfanilamide; sulfapyrimidine; sulfazine).

See also Bromhexine with sulfadiazine; Sulfadiazine silver.

SULFADIAZINE-MEGLUMINE (sulfadiazine methylglucamine derivative; 'soludiazine').

SULFADIAZINE SILVER (silver sulfadiazine; sulfadiazine silver salt; 'flammazin', 'silvadene', 'silvederma').

SULFADICRAMIDE*** (*N*¹-(3,3-dimethylacroyl)sulfanilamide; *N*¹-senecioylsulfanilamide; 'irgamide', 'sulfirgamide').

SULFADIMETHOXINE*** (*N*¹-(2,6-dimethoxy-4-pyrimidyl)sulfanilamide; *N*¹-(2,4-dimethoxy-6-pyrimidyl)sulfanilamide; sulfadimethoxypyrimidine; 'madribon', 'madroxin').

See also Diaveridine with sulfadimethoxine; Ormetoprim with sulfadimethoxine.

Sulfadimethoxypyrimidine *see* Sulfadimethoxine; Sulfamoprine.

SULFADIMETHYLBENZOYLAMIDE (*N*¹-(3,4-dimethylbenzoyl)sulfanilamide; sulfabenzoylamide; *N*-sulfanilyl-3,4-xylamide; G-867; 'irgafen').

Sulfadimethyloxazole *see* Sulfamoxole.

Sulfadimethylpyrimidine *see* Sulfadimidine.

Sulfadimetine (tr) *see* Sulfasomidine.

Sulfadimezine *see* Sulfadimidine.

SULFADIMIDINE*** (*N*¹ -(4,6-dimethyl-2-

pyrimidyl)sulfanilamide; dimethylsulfadiazine; dimethylsulfapyrimidine; sulfadimethylpyrimidine; sulfadimezine; sulfamethazine; sulfamethiazine; sulfamidine; sulfodimezine).

SULFADIMIDINE WITH TRIMETHOPRIM ('poteseptyl').

'Sulfadione' *see* Dapsone.

SULFADOXINE*** (N^1-(5,6-dimethoxypyrimidin-4-yl)sulfanilamide; N^1-(4,5-dimethoxypyrimidin-6-yl)sulfanilamide; sulforthodimethoxine; sulforthomidine; sulformethoxine; sulformetoxine; Ro-4-4393; WR-4873; 'fanasil', 'fanzil').

SULFADOXINE WITH PYRIMETHAMINE ('fansidar').

SULFADOXINE WITH TRIMETHOPRIM ('borgal', 'trivetrin').

SULFAETHIDOLE*** (N^1-(5-ethyl-1,3,4-thiadiazol-2-yl)sulfanilamide; 5-(*p*-aminobenzenesulfonamido)-2-ethyl-1,3,4-thiadiazole; etazole; ethazole; sulfaethylthiadiazole; VK-55; 'globucid', 'sethadil', 'sulspansion', 'sulspantabs', 'sulfa-perlongit').

SULFAETHIDOLE WITH SULFAMETHIZOLE ('harnosal').

SULFAETHOXYPYRIDAZINE (N^1-(6-ethoxypyridazin-3-yl)sulfanilamide).

SULFAFURAZOLE** (N^1-(3,4-dimethyl-5-isoxazolyl)sulfanilamide; sulfisoxazole; Nu-445; 'gantrisin', 'gantroson', 'neazolin', 'sosol', 'soxisol', 'soxomide' 'sulfalar', 'sulfazin', 'sulfoxol').

Sulfafurazole diethanolamine *see* Sulfafurazole diolamine.

SULFAFURAZOLE DIOLAMINE (2,2'-iminodiethanol salt of sulfafurazone; sulfafurazole diethanolamine; sulfisoxazole diolamine; 'gantrisin diolamine').

SULFAGUANIDINE*** (N^1-amidinosulfanilamide; sulfanilylguanidine; sulfamidinum; sulgin; RP-2275).

SULFAGUANOLE** (N^1-[(4,5-dimethyloxazol-2-yl)amidino]sulfanilamide; 'enterocura').

Sulfa-isodimerazine *see* Sulfasomidine.

Sulfaisodimidine *see* Sulfasomidine.

Sulfaisopropylthiadiazine *see* Glyprothiazole.

'Sulfalar' *see* Sulfafurazole.

SULFALENE** (N^1-(3-methoxypyrazin-2-yl)sulfanilamide; sulfamethoxypyrazine; sulfametopyrazine; sulfapyrazinmetoxin; WR-4629; 'dalysep', 'kelfizine', 'longum').

'Sulfalepsine' *see* Suclofenide.

'Sulfalex' *see* Sulfamethoxypyridazine.

SULFALOXIC ACID*** (2-[4-(hydroxymethylureidosulfonyl)phenylcarbamoyl]-benzoic acid; 4'-[(hydroxymethylcarbamoyl)sulfamoyl]phthalanilic acid).

SULFALOXIC ACID CALCIUM SALT ('enteromide').

'Sulfalumin' *see* Aluminium sulfanilate.

SULFAMERAZINE*** (N^1-(4-methylpyrimidin-2-yl)sulfanilamide; methylsulfadiazine; methylsulfapyrimidine; methylsulfazine; sulfamethyldiazine; sulfamethyl-

pyrimidine; sulfamonomethyldiazine; sulfamerazine sodium; RP-2632).

Sulfameter* *see* Sulfametoxydiazine.

Sulfamethazine *see* Sulfadimidine.

Sulfamethiazine *see* Sulfadimidine.

Sulfamethiazole *see* Sulfamethizole.

SULFAMETHIN (tr) (polymerized condensation product of diaminodiaphenylsulfone with *p*-dimethylaminobenzaldehyde).

SULFAMETHIZOLE** (N^1-(5-methyl-1,3,4-thiadiazol-2-yl)sulfanilamide; sulfamethylthiadiazole; sulfamethiazole; sulfathiodiazole; VK-53).
See also Neomycin with sulfamethizole; Sulfaethidole with sulfamethizole.

SULFAMETHOXAZOLE*** (N^1-(5-methylisoxazol-3-yl)sulfanilamide; 3-(*p*-aminobenzenesulfonamido)-5-methylisoxazole; sulfisomezole; MS-53; Ro-4-2130; 'gantanol', 'sinomin').

Sulfamethoxazole with trimethoprim *see* Co-trimoxazole.

Sulfamethoxine *see* Sulfametoxydiazine.

Sulfamethoxydiazine* *see* Sulfametoxydiazine.

'Sulfamethoxydin' *see* Sulfametoxydiazine.

Sulfamethoxypyrazine *see* Sulfalene.

SULFAMETHOXYPYRIDAZINE*** (N^1-(6-methoxypyridazin-3-yl)sulfanilamide; CL-13493; RP-7522; 'davosine', 'depovernil', 'kynex', 'lederkyn', 'midicel', 'midikel', 'minikel', 'myasul', 'spofadiazin', 'sulfalex', 'sultirene', 'unosulf').

Sulfamethoxypyrimidine *see* Sulfametoxydiazine.

Sulfa-5-methyldiazine *see* Sulfaperin.

Sulfamethylphenylpyrazole *see* Sulfapyrazole.

Sulfamethylpyrimidine *see* Sulfamerazine.

Sulfamethylthiadiazole *see* Sulfamethizole.

SULFAMETHYLTHIAZOLE (N^1-(4-methyl-2-thiazolyl)sulfanilamide; 'novoseptale', 'sulfazole', 'toriseptin', 'ultraseptyl').

Sulfametin *see* Sulfametoxydiazine.

SULFAMETOMIDINE*** (N^1-(6-methoxy-2-methylpyrimidin-4-yl)sulfanilamide; 'durasulf', 'methofazine').

Sulfametopyrazine* *see* Sulfalene.

SULFAMETOXYDIAZINE*** (N^1-(5-methoxypyrimidin-2-yl)sulfanilamide; 5-methoxy-2-sulfanilamidopyrimidine; sulfamethoxine; sulfamethoxydiazine; sulfamethoxypyrimidine; sulfameter; sulfametin; AHR-857; Bayer 5400; SH-613; 'bayrena', 'durenate', 'kiron', 'sulfamethoxydin', 'sulla', 'supramid', 'ultrax').

SULFAMETROLE** (N^1-(4-methoxy-1,2,5-thiadiazol-3-yl)sulfanilamide).

'Sulfamezathine' *see* Sulfadimidine.

Sulfamidine *see* Sulfadimidine.

Sulfamidinum *see* Sulfaguanidine.

SULFAMIDOCHRYSOIDINE (2,4-diamino-4'-sulfamoylazobenzene; sulfamidochrysoidine hydrochloride; N^4-(2,4-diaminophenylazo)sulfanilamide).

SULFAMIDOPYRINE SODIUM (Na salt

419

of 1,5-dimethyl-4-(methanesulfonylamino)-2-phenyl-3-pyrazolin-5-one; Na salt of 4-aminoamipyrine N^4-methanesulfonic acid; amizole; melaminsulfone; sulfamipyrine; 'melubrin', 'pyrazogin').

Sulfaminum see Sulfanilamide.

Sulfamipyrine see Sulfamidopyrine.

SULFAMONOMETHOXINE*** (N^1-(6-methoxypyrimidin-4-yl)sulfanilamide; DJ-1550; DS-36; ICI-32525; 'daimeton').

Sulfamonomethyldiazine see Sulfamerazine.

SULFAMOPRINE* (N^1-(4,6-dimethoxypyrimidin-2-yl)sulfanilamide).

SULFAMOXOLE*** (N^1-(4,5-dimethyloxazol-2-yl)sulfanilamide; sulfadimethyloxazole; 'nuprin', 'sulfune', 'sulfuno', 'tardamid').

p-**Sulfamoylbenzoic acid** see Carzenide.

p-**Sulfamoylbenzylamine** see Mafenide.

p-**Sulfamoylcarbanilic acid 2-hydroxyethyl ester** see Sulocarbilate.

SULFAMOYLDAPSONE (4,4'-diamino-2-sulfamoyldiphenyl sulfone; 2-sulfamoyldiaminodiphenyl sulfone; SDDS).

2-Sulfamoyldiaminodiphenyl sulfone see Sulfamoyldapsone.

5-(*p*-Sulfamoylphenylazo)salicylic acid see Salazosulfamide.

N-(*p*-**Sulfamoylphenyl)-1,4-butane sultam** see Sultiame.

Sulfamyxin see Sulfomyxin.

SULFAN BLUE *(Na salt of anhydro-4,4'-bis(diethylamino)-2'',4''-disulfotriphenylmethanol; food blue 3; patent blue V; 'blue VRS', 'disulfine blue VNS').

SULFANILAMIDE*** (*p*-aminobenzenesulfonamide; sulfaminum; PABS; sulfanilamide hydrochloride; F-1162).

SULFANILAMIDE SULFOSALICYLATE (sulfanilamide N^4-(5-sulfosuccinate); 'amindan').

Sulfanilamidomethanol glucose sodium bisulfite see Glucosulfamide.

Sulphanilanilide see Sulfabenz.

Sulfanilcyanamide see Sulcymide.

SULFANILIC ACID (*p*-aminobenzenesulfonic acid).

Sulfanilic acid salts see Aluminium sulfanilate; Cerium sulfanilate; Zinc sulfanilate.

3-Sulfanilyl-3-azabicyclo(3.2.2)nonane see Azabon.

N-**Sulfanilylbenzamide.**

N-(6-**Sulfanilylmetanilyl)acetamide** see Sulfadiasulfone.

N-(*p*-**Sulfanilylphenyl)glycine** see Acediasulfone.

(*p*-**Sulfanilylphenyl)urea** see Amidapsone.

SULFANITRAN*** (4'-[(*p*-nitrophenyl)-sulfamoyl]acetanilide; N^4-acetyl-N^1-(*p*-nitrophenyl)sulfanilamide).
See also Aklomide with sulfanitran.

SULFAPERIN*** (N^1-(5-methylpyrimidin-2-yl)sulfanilamide; 2-sulfanilamido-5-methylpyrimidine; 5-methylsulfadiazine; sulfa-5-methyldiazine; BT-325; 'durisan', 'pallidin').

SULFAPERIN WITH TRIMETHOPRIM ('trimlen').

'**Sulfa-perlongit**' see Sulfaethidole.

SULFAPHENAZOLE*** (N^1-(2-phenylpyrazol-3-yl)sulfanilamide; N^1-(1-phenylpyrazol-5-yl)sulfanilamide; phenylsulfapyrazole; sulfaphenylpyrazole; P-17922; 'eftolon', 'orisul', 'orisulf', 'sulfabid').

Sulfaphenylpyrazole see Sulfaphenazole.

SULFAPROXYLINE*** (N^1-(4-isopropoxybenzoyl)sulfanilamide; G-13289).

'**Sulfapyelon**' see Sulfamethizole.

SULFAPYRAZINE (N^1-(2-pyrazinyl)sulfanilamide; sulfapyrazine sodium).

Sulfapyrazinmetoxin see Sulfalene.

SULFAPYRAZOLE*** (N^1-(3-methyl-1-phenylpyrazol-5-yl)sulfanilamide; sulfamethylphenylpyrazole; Ba-18605; 'vesulong').

SULFAPYRIDINE** (N^1-pyrid-2-ylsulfanilamide; sulfidine; sulfapyridine sodium; M&B-693).

Sulfapyrimidine see Sulfadiazine.

SULFAQUINOXALINE (N^1-(2-quinoxalyl)-sulfanilamide; Cp-3-120; 'sulquin').

'**Sulfarlem**' see Anethole trithione.

'**Sulfarsan**' see Sulfarsphenamine.

Sulfarsenobenzene see Sulfarsphenamine.

'**Sulfarsenol**' see Sulfarsphenamine.

'**Sulfarside**' see 4-Sulfamido-*o*-arsanilic acid.

SULFARSPHENAMINE*** (disodium salt of 3,3'-bis(sulfomethylamino)-*p*-arsenophenol; disodium salt of N,N'-bis(methylenebisulfite) derivative of 3,3'-diamino-4,4'-dihydroxyarsenobenzene; myarsenol; myoarsenobenzol; sulfarsenobenzene; thioarsphenamine).
See also Bismuth sulfarsphenamine.

Sulfasalazine* see Salazosulfapyridine.

SULFASOLUCIN* (disodium salt of N^4-(1,3-disulfo-3-phenylpropyl)sulfanilamide; solucin; sulfasolutin; RP-40; 'soluseptacin', 'soluseptasine', 'soluseptazine').

SULFASOMIDINE* (N^1-(2,6-dimethylpyrimid-4-yl)sulfanilamide; sulfadimetine; sulfaisodimidine; sulfa-isodimerazine; sulfisomidine; L-30).

SULFASOMIZOLE*** (N^1-(3-methylisothiazol-5-yl)sulfanilamide; E-438; Th-2132; 'amidozol', 'bidizole').

SULFASYMAZINE*** (N^1-(4,6-diethyl-*s*-triazin-2-yl)sulfanilamide; 'prosymasul', 'symasul').

Sulfated glyptide see Sulglicotide.

Sulfatertiobutylthiadiazole see Glybuthiazole.

SULFATHIADIAZOLE (N^1-(1,3,4-thiadiazol-2-yl)sulfanilamide; 'sedathil').

SULFATHIAZOLE*** (N^1-thiazol-2-ylsulfanilamide; sulfathiazole sodium; norsulfazole; M&B-760; RP-2090).

SULFATHIAZOLE ALUMINIUM (M-640; 'lysothiazole').

Sulfathiodiazole see Sulfamethizole.

SULFATHIOUREA*** (N^1-thiocarbamylsulfanilamide; 1-sulfanilyl-2-thiourea; RP-

2255; 'badional', 'fontamide', 'solufont-amide').
    See also Sulfatolamide.
Sulfation factor see Somatomedin.
SULFATOLAMIDE*** (1-sulfanilyl-2-thiourea derivative of α-amino-*p*-toluene-sulfonamide; sulfathiourea salt of mafenide; 'aseptorid', 'marbadal-C', 'mirbedal').
SULFATROXAZOLE** (N^1-(4,5-di-methylisoxazol-3-yl)sulfanilamide).
SULFATROZOLE*** (N^1-(4-ethoxy-1,2,5-thiadiazol-3-yl)sulfanilamide).
'Sulfatyf' see Sulfaclozine.
Sulfaurea* see Sulfacarbamide.
'Sulfa-vet' see Sulfabenz.
'Sulfazin' see Sulfafurazole.
Sulfazine (tr) see Sulfadiazine.
'Sulfazole' see Sulfamethylthiazole.
Sulfbenzamine see Mafenide.
'Sulfenthal' see Phenolsulfonphthalein.
Sulfenytame see Sultiame.
SULFESTOL ('teepol').
'Sulfetrone' see Solasulfone.
Sulfidine (tr) see Sulfapyridine.
SULFINPYRAZONE*** (1,2-diphenyl-4-(2-phenylsulfinylethyl)-3,5-pyrazolidine-dione; sulfoxyphenylpyrazolidine; G-28315; 'anturan', 'enturen').
SULFIODIZOLE* (N^1-(4-iodo-3-methyl-isoxazol-3-yl)sulfanilamide; 3-iodosulfa-methoxazole).
Sulfiram see Monosulfiram.
'Sulfirgamide' see Sulfadicramide.
Sulfisomezole* see Sulfamethoxazole.
Sulfisomidine*** see Sulfasomidine.
Sulfisoxazole* see Sulfafurazole.
3-Sulfoalanine see Cysteic acid.
[α-(Sulfoamino)benzyl]penicillin see Suncillin.
6-(D-α-Sulfoaminophenylacetamido)-penicillanic acid see Suncillin.
o-SULFOBENZHEPARIDE (*N*-desulfo-(2-sulfobenzoyl)heparin).
Sulfobenzide see Diphenyl sulfone.
α-Sulfobenzylpenicillin see Sulbenicillin.
SULFOBROMPHTHALEIN (tetrabromo-phenolphthalein disodium sulfonate; 3,4,5,6-tetrabromo-3,3-bis(4-hydroxy-3-sulfophenyl)phthalide; bromosulfophtha-lein; bromphthalein; bromsulfophthalein; BSP; 'bromsulfalein', 'bromsulfonphtha-lein', 'bromthalin', 'brom-tetragnost', 'hepartest', 'hepatotestbrom').
Sulfocarbolic acid see Phenolsulfonic acid.
Sulfocillin see Sulbenicillin.
Sulfocyanic acid see Thiocyanic acid.
Sulfodiamine (tr) see Acedapsone.
p,p'-Sulfodianiline see Dapsone.
Sulfodimezine (tr) see Sulfadimidine.
N-(2-Sulfoethyl)-L-glutamine see Glutaurine.
SULFOGAIACOL*** (potassium guaiacol-sulfonate; potassium 4-hydroxy-3-methoxy-phenylsulfonate; thiocol; 'orthocol', 'sirolin').
'Sulfogal' see Anethole trithione.
Sulfoglycopeptide see Sulglicotide.
SULFOLANE (tetrahydrothiophene 1,1-

dioxide; thiophan sulfone).
'Sulfo-merthiolate' see Sodium timerfonate.
N^2-Sulfomethylisoniazid see Methaniazide.
SULFOMYXIN*** (pentakis(*N*-sulfomethyl)-polymyxin B; sulfomyxin sodium; sulfa-myxin; GS-6742; 'dynamyxin', 'thio-sporin').
SULFONAL (sulfonmethanum; bis(ethyl-sulfonyl)dimethylmethane).
Sulfonamidophenylazosalicylic acid see Salazosulfamide.
1-(4-Sulfonaphth-1-ylazo)-2-naphthol see Amaranth.
'Sulfonazine-SN' see Solasulfone.
p-Sulfondichloramidobenzoic acid see Halazone.
Sulfone N-acetate see Acetyldapsone.
Sulfone-mère see Dapsone.
'Sulfonet' see Sulfathiazole.
SULFONIAZID* (isonicotinic acid *m*-sulfo-benzylidenehydrazide; N^1-(*m*-sulfobenzyl-idene)isoniazid; isonicotinoylhydrazone of benzaldehyde-*m*-sulfonic acid; G-605).
'Sulfonphthal' see Phenolsulfonphthalein.
SULFONTEROL** (α-(*tert*-butylamino-methyl)-4-hydroxy-3-(methylsulfonyl-methyl)benzyl alcohol).
4',4'''-Sulfonylbis(acetanilide) see Acedap-sone.
4',4''-Sulfonylbis(cyclopentanetridecan-anilide) see Chaulmosulfone.
6,6'-[Sulfonylbis(p-phenyleneazo)]dithy-mol see Diathymosulfone.
p,p'-Sulfonyldiacetanilide see Acedapsone.
1-p-Sulfophenylazo-2-naphthol-6-sulfonic acid disodium salt see Sunset yellow FCF.
8-(3-Sulfopropyl)atropinium hydroxide inner salt see Sultroponium.
SULFORIDAZINE*** (10-[2-(1-methyl-piperid-2-yl)ethyl]-2-methylsulfonylpheno-thiazine; thioridazine dioxide; TPN-12; 'imagotan', 'inofal').
'Sulform' see Triphenylstibine sulfide.
Sulformethoxine* see Sulfadoxine.
Sulformetoxine see Sulfadoxine.
Sulforthodimethoxine see Sulfadoxine.
Sulforthomidine see Sulfadoxine.
SULFOSALICYLIC ACID (salicylsulfonic acid; 2-hydroxy-5-sulfobenzoic acid).
    See also Samarium-sulfosalicylic acid complex; Sodium sulfosalicylate; Sulfanil-amide sulfosalicylate.
SULFOTEP* (tetraethyl thiodiphosphate; tetraethyl dithiopyrophosphate; dithio; dithion; dithiophos; dithio-TEPP; sulfotepp; TEDTP; 'bladafum', 'bladan 393', 'dithione').
Sulfotepp see Sulfotep.
'Sulfothiorine' see Sodium thiosulfate.
'Sulfotrim' see Co-trimoxazole.
SULFOXIDE (5-[2-(octylsulfinyl)propyl]-1,3-benzodioxole; 1,2-methylenedioxy-4-[2-(octylsulfinyl)propyl]benzene).
'Sulfoxol' see Sulfafurazole.
Sulfoxone see Aldesulfone.
2-(5-Sulfo-2,4-xylylazo)-1-naphthol-4-

sulfonic acid disodium salt see Ponceau SX.

Sulfoxyphenylpyrazolidine see Sulfinpyrazone.

'Sulfralem' see Anethole trithione.

'Sulfune' see Sulfamoxole.

'Sulfuno' see Sulfamoxole.

Sulfuric oxyfluoride see Sulfuryl fluoride.

Sulfur mustard see Mustard gas.

SULFURYL FLUORIDE (sulfuric oxyfluoride; 'vikane').

Sulgin (tr) see Sulfaguanidine.

SULGLICOTIDE** (sulfuric polyester of a glycopeptide from pig duodenum; glyptide sulfate; sulfated glyptide; sulfoglycopeptide; GLPS; 'gliptide').

Sulimarin see Sulmarin.

SULINDAC** ((Z)-5-fluoro-2-methyl-1-[p-(methylsulfinyl)benzylidene]indene-3-acetic acid; 'clinoril').

SULISATIN** (3,3,bis(p-hydroxyphenyl)-7-methyl-2-indolinone bis(hydrogen sulfate)).

SULISOBENZONE** (5-benzoyl-4-hydroxy-1-methoxybenzenesulfonic acid; BSA; 'spectra-sorb UV 284', 'uval', 'uvinul').

'Sulla' see Sulfametoxydiazine.

SULMARIN** (6,7-dihydroxy-4-methyl-coumarin bis(hydrogen sulfate; sulimarin)).

'Sulmetine' see Magnesium sulfate.

'Sulmycin' see Gentamicin.

SULNIDAZOLE** (O-methyl 2-[(2-ethyl-5-nitroimidazol-1-yl)ethyl]carbamothioate).

SULOCARBILATE** (2-hydroxyethyl ester of p-sulfamoylcarbanilic acid; N⁴-(carbo-2-hydroxyethoxy)sulfanilamide; W-1548-1).

SULOCTIDIL** (p-isopropylthio)-α-(1-octamylaminoethyl)benzyl alcohol; 1-[p-(isopropylthio)phenyl]-2-octamylamino-1-propanol; 1-hydroxy-1-[p-(isopropylthio)-phenyl]-N-octyl-2-propylamine; β-hydroxy-p-(isopropylthio)-α-methyl-N-octyl-phenethylamine).

SULOXIFEN** (N-(2-diethylaminoethyl)-S,S-diphenylsulfoximide).

SULOXIFEN OXALATE* (Gö-1733; W6439A).

Sulph... see Sulf....

SULPIRIDE** (N-(1-ethylpyrrolidin-2-yl-methyl)-2-methoxy-5-sulfamoylbenzamide; N-(1-ethylpyrrolidin-2-ylmethyl)-5-sulfa-moyl-o-anisamide; FK-880; 'dobren', 'dogmatyl', 'eglonyl', 'equilid').

'Sulprim' see Co-trimoxazole.

Sulpyrin see Novaminsulfon.

'Sulquin' see Sulfaquinoxaline.

'Sulredox' see Penicillamine.

'Sul-spansion' see Sulfaethidole.

'Sul-spantab' see Sulfaethidole.

'Sultanol' see Salbutamol.

SULTIAME** (2-(p-sulfamoylphenyl)tetra-hydro-1,2-thiazine 1,1-dioxide; p-(tetra-hydro(2H)1,2-thiazin-2-yl)benzenesulfon-amide S,S-dioxide; N-(p-sulfamoylphenyl)-1,4-butanesultam; sulthiame; sulpheny-tame; Riker-594; RP-10284; 'conadil', 'contravul', 'elisal', 'ospolot', 'trolone').

'Sultirene' see Sulfamethoxypyridazine.

SULTOPRIDE** (N-(1-ethylpyrrolidin-2-ylmethyl)-5-(ethylsulfonyl)-o-anisamide; Lin-1418).

SULTROPONIUM** (8-(3-sulfopropyl)-atropinium hydroxide inner salt; A-118).

'Sulzol' see Sulfathiazole.

Sulzon (tr) see Subathizone.

SUM-3170 see Loxapine.

SUMETIZIDE** (6-chloro-3,4-dihydro-3-succinimidomethyl-2H-1,2,4-benzothiadia-zine-7-sulfonamide 1,1-dioxide).

'Sumetrolin' see Co-trimoxazole.

'Sumial' see Propranolol.

'Sumioxon' see Fenitrooxon.

'Sumithion' see Fenitrothion.

'Sumitox' see Malathion.

'Summetrin' see Papain.

'Sumycin' see Hexacycline.

SUNCILLIN** (6-[2-phenyl-D-2-(sulfo-amino)acetamido]penicillanic acid; 6-(D-α-sulfoaminophenylacetamido)penicil-lanic acid; [D-α-(sulfoamino)benzyl]-penicillin).

SUNCILLIN SODIUM (suncillin disodium salt; BL-P1462).

'Sun-nitt' see Bis(tributyltin) oxide.

'Sunoxol' see 8-Quinolinol potassium sulfate.

SUNSET YELLOW FCF (FD&C 6; C.I. (1956) No. 15985; chiefly the disodium salt of 1-p-sulfophenylazo-2-naphthol-6-sulfonic acid).

'Supanate' see Flopropione.

'Supavan' see Alverine.

'Superinone' see Tyloxapol.

'Superlutin' see 17α-Hydroxy-16-methylene-pregna-4,6-diene-3,20-dione acetate.

'Superol' see 8-Quinolinol potassium sulfate.

'Superoxol' see Hydrogen peroxide.

Superpalite see Diphosgene.

'Superseptyl' see Sulfadimidine.

SUPIDIMIDE** (2-(2-oxo-piperid-3-yl)-1,2-benzisothiazolin-3-one 1,1-dioxide).

'Suplexedil' see Fenoxedil.

'Supona' see Clofenvinfos.

'Supotran' see Chlormezanone.

'Suppangin' see Bismuth valproate.

'Supponeryl' see Butethal.

'Supracen violet' see Solway purple.

'Supracid' see Methidathion.

'Supral' see Pecilocin.

'Supramid' see Sulfametoxydiazine.

'Suprifen' see p-Hydroxyephedrine.

'Suprifen-Psb' see Buphenine.

'Suprimal' see Dimenhydrinate and Meclozine.

SUPROFEN** (p-2-thenoylhydratropic acid; 2-(p-thenoylphenyl)propionic acid; 2-[p-(1-carboxyethyl)benzoyl]thiophene; α-methyl-4-(2-thienylcarbonyl)benzeneace-tic acid; R-25061).

'Suractin' see Ampicillin.

Suramin see Suramin sodium.

SURAMIN PENTAMIDINE SALT (RP-4891).

SURAMIN SODIUM** (hexasodium salt of 8,8'-[ureylenebis[m-phenylenecarbonylimi-no(4-methyl-m-phenylene)carbonylimino]]-

di-(1,3,5-naphthalenetrisulfonic acid); hexasodium salt of symmetrical urea deriv. of 8-[3-(*m*-aminobenzoyl)amino]-*p*-methylbenzoylamino-1,3,5-naphthalenetrisulfonic acid; naphuride; Bayer-205; F-309; 'antrypol', 'belganyl', 'germanin', 'moranyl', 'naganin', 'naganol').
'Surcopur' *see* Propanil.
'Surecide' *see* Cyanofenphos.
'Surem' *see* Butalamine.
'Sureptil' *see* Cinnarizine with heptaminol theophyllineacetate.
'Surestryl' *see* Moxestrol.
'Surexin' *see* Pyrinoline.
'Surfacaine' *see* Cyclomethycaine.
'Surfak' *see* Calcium dioctyl sulfosuccinate.
'Surfathesin' *see* Cyclomethycaine.
'Surfen' *see* Aminoquinuride.
'Surgam' *see* Tiaprofenic acid.
'Surgex' *see* Nialamide.
SURGIBONE* ('boplant').
'Surgicel' *see* Oxidized regenerated cellulose.
'Surgi-cen' *see* Hexachlorophene.
'Surhème' *see* Butalamine.
'Surital' *see* Thiamylal.
'Surmontil' *see* Trimipramine maleate.
'Surofene' *see* Hexachlorophene.
Surpalite *see* Diphosgene.
'Surplix' *see* Imipramine.
'Surrectan' *see* S-(2-Aminoethyl)isothiuronium bromide.
'Sursum' *see* Iproclozide.
'Sustanon' *see* Testosterone esters.
'Sutan' *see* Butylate.
SUTILAINS** (proteolytic enzymes from *Bac. subtilis*; BAX-1515; 'travase').
'Suversin' *see* Mecamylamine.
'Suvipen' *see* Metampicillin.
'Suvren' *see* Captodiame.
SUXAMETHONIUM CHLORIDE** ((2-hydroxyethyl)trimethyl ammonium chloride succinate; succinylbis(ethylenetrimethylammonium chloride); bis(2-dimethylaminoethyl)succinate bismethochloride; diacetylcholine; ditilin; succicurarium; succinyldicholine; succinylcholine; IS 370; LT-1; M&B-2207).
SUXEMERID** (bis(1,2,2,6,6-pentamethylpiperid-4-yl) succinate.
SUXETHONIUM CHLORIDE** (ethyl-(2-hydroxyethyl)dimethylammonium chloride succinate; succinylbis(ethylenedimethylethylammonium chloride); bis(2-dimethylaminoethyl)succinate bisethochloride; IS-362; M-115; M&B-2210).
SUXIBUZONE** (4-butyl-4-hydroxymethyl-1,2-diphenyl-3,5-pyrazolidinedione hydrogen succinate (ester); 'calibene').
'Suxilep' *see* Ethosuximide.
'Suxinutin' *see* Ethosuximide.
'Suxiphen' *see* Sodium benzyl succinate.
'SVC' *see* Acetarsol.
Sweet birch oil *see* Methyl salicylate.
SWEP* (methyl 3,4-dichlorocarbanilate; methyl(3,4-dichlorophenyl)carbamate).
Swiss blue *see* Methylene blue.
SY-28 *see* N-(2-Bromoethyl)-N-ethyl-1-

naphthalenemethylamine.
'Sycotrol' *see* Pipethanate.
SYD-230 *see* Clioxanide.
SYDNOCARB (tr) (3-(1-methyl-2-phenylethyl)-1-(N-phenylcarbamoylimino)sydnone; sydnofen phenylcarbamoyl derivative; 3-(2-phenylisopropyl)-N-(phenylcarbamino)sydnone imine; sidnocarb).
SYDNOFEN (tr) (3-(2-phenylisopropyl)-sydnone imine; sydnophen).
Sydnofen N-phenylcarbamoyl derivative *see* Sydnocarb.
Sydnophen (tr) *see* Sydnofen.
'Syl' *see* Dimeticone.
'Sylnasol' *see* Sodium psylliate.
'Symasul' *see* Sulfasymazine.
Symazin *see* Simazine.
SYMCLOSENE** (trichloro-*s*-triazine-2,4,6-(1H,3H,5H)-trione; trichloroisocyanuric acid; ACL-85).
'Symcortol' *see* Oxedrine.
SYMETINE** (4,4'-ethylenedioxybis(N-hexyl-N-methylbenzylamine); symetine dihydrochloride; L-16726).
'Symmetrel' *see* Amantadine.
'Symoron' *see* Methadone.
Sympathin *see* Noradrenaline.
'Sympathol' *see* Oxedrine.
Sympatholytin (tr) *see* Dibenamine.
'Sympathomim' *see* Phenylephrine.
'Sympatol' *see* Oxedrine.
'Sympectothion' *see* Thioneine.
'Sympocaine' *see* Ambucaine.
'Symprocaine' *see* Procaine.
'Synacthar' *see* Tetracosactide.
'Synacthen' *see* Tetracosactide.
'Synacthen depot' *see* Tetracosactide zinc phosphate complex.
'Synadrin' *see* Prenylamine lactate.
'Synalar' *see* Fluocinolone acetonide.
'Synandone' *see* Fluocinolone acetonide.
'Synandrin' *see* Prenylamine.
'Synanthin' *see* Inulin.
'Synapause' *see* Estriol succinate.
'Synaplege' *see* Pempidine tosilate.
'Synasteron' *see* Oxymetholone.
'Synaxsyn' *see* Naproxen.
'Syncarpine' *see* Pilocarpine.
'Syncillin' *see* Pheneticillin.
'Syncl' *see* Cefalexin.
'Syncortyl' *see* Desoxycortone.
'Syncro-mate' *see* Flugestone acetate.
Synephrine* *see* Oxedrine.
***m*-Synephrine** *see* Phenylephrine.
'Syneptine' *see* Kitasamycin.
Synestrol (tr) *see* Hexestrol.
'Synhexyl' *see* Pyrahexyl.
'Synkonin' *see* Hydrocodone.
'Synmiol' *see* Idoxuridine.
Synnematin B *see* Adicillin.
Synstigmine *see* Neostigmine.
'Syntarpen 201' *see* Cloxacillin.
'Syntes-12A' *see* Tetrasodium edetate.
'Syntetrin' *see* Rolitetracycline.
'Syntexan' *see* Dimethyl sulfoxide.
'Synthenate' *see* Oxedrine.
'Synthepen' *see* Propicillin.

'Synthila' see Dianisylhexene.
Synthomycin (tr) see DL-Chloramphenicol.
'Synthrin' see Resmethrin.
'Synthroid' see Levothyroxine sodium.
'Synticillin' see Meticillin.
'Syntocinon' see Oxytocin synthetic.
'Syntometrin' see Methylergometrine with oxytocin (synthetic).
'Syntopressin' see Lypressin.
'Syntropan' see Amprotropine.
'Syraprim' see Trimethoprim.
SYRINGIC ACID (4-hydroxy-3,5-dimethoxy-benzoic acid).
SYROSINGOPINE*** (carbethoxysyringoyl methyl reserpate; 4-ethoxycarbonyl-3,5-di-
methoxybenzoic acid ester of methyl reserpate; ethoxycarbonylsyringoyl methyl reserpate; ester of syringic acid ethyl carbonate with methyl reserpate; methyl ester of 18-(4-ethoxy-3,5-dimethoxy-carbonyloxybenzoyl)reserpic acid; Su-3118; 'isotense', 'singoserp').
'Sysmeton' see Thiometon.
'Systogene' see Tyramine.
'Systox' see Demeton-O plus demeton-S.
'Systral' see Chlorphenoxamine.
'Sytam' see Schradan.
'Sytron' see Sodium feredetate.
'Sziodol' see 2,6-Diiodo-1-phenol-4-sulfonic acid.

T

2,4,5-T* see Trichlorophenoxyacetic acid.
T-3 see Liothyronine.
T-47 see Parathion.
T-72 see Nitroguanil.
T-712 see Amfepramone.
T-1384 see Congocidine.
T-1824 see Evans blue.
TA-306 see Myfadol.
'Tabard' see Diethyltoluamide.
'Tabotamp' see Oxidized regenerated cellulose.
TABUN (ethyl dimethylphosphoramidocy-anidate; dimethylamido ethoxy phosphoryl cyanide).
'Tabutrex' see Dibutyl succinate.
'Tacaryl' see Methdilazine.
'Tacazyl' see Methdilazine.
'Tace' see Chlorotrianisene.
'Tachmalin' see Ajmaline.
'Tachystin' see Dihydrotachysterol.
'Tacholiquin' see Tyloxapol.
'Tachystol' see Dihydrotachysterol.
'Tacitin' see Benzoctamine.
TACLAMINE*** (2,3,4,4a,8,9,13b,14-octahydro-1H-benzo(6,7)cyclohepta(1,2,3-de)pyrido(2,1-a)isoquinoline; taclamine hydrochloride; AY-22214).
TACRINE*** (9-amino-1,2,3,4-tetrahydro-acridine; hydroaminoacridine; tetrahydro-aminacrine; tacrine hydrochloride; THA; 'romotal').
'Tadip' see Guanacline with methyldopa.
'Taketron' see Prosultiamine.
TALAMPICILLIN** (D(−)-6-(2-amino-2-phenylacetamido)penicillanic acid ester with 3-hydroxyphthalide; 1,3-dihydro-3-oxo-1-isobenzofuranyl [2S-[2α,5α,6β(S)]]-6-[(aminophenylacetyl)amino]penicillanate; phthalidyl 6-(D(−)-α-aminophenyl-acetamido)penicillanate; ampicillin phthalidyl ester; phthalidylampicillin;
talampicillin hydrochloride; BRL-8988; CP-271B; 'talpen').
'Talanton' see Carbutamide.
TALASTINE*** (4-benzyl-2-(2-dimethyl-aminoethyl)-1(2H)-phthalazinone).
'Talatrol' see Trometamol.
Talbumal* see Talbutal.
TALBUTAL** (5-allyl-5-sec-butylbarbituric acid; 5-allyl-5-(1-methylpropyl)barbituric acid; talbumal; 'lotusate').
'Talcord' see Thiocarboxim.
TALERANOL*** ((3S,7S)-3,4,5,6,7,8,9,10,11,12-decahydro-7,14,16-trihydroxy-3-methyl-1H-2-benzoxacyclotetradecin-1-one).
'Talesco' see Secobarbital.
TALINOLOL*** ((±)-1-[p-(3-tert-butyl-amino-2-hydroxypropoxy)phenyl]-3-cyclo-hexylurea; (±)-1-tert-butylamino-3-[p-(3-cyclohexylureido)phenoxy]-2-propanol).
'Talofen' see Promazine.
TALOPRAM** (N,3,3-trimethyl-1-phenyl-1-phthalanpropylamine; 3,3-dimethyl-1-(3-methylaminopropyl)-1-phenylphthalan; talopram hydrochloride; AY-21554; Lu-3-010).
TALOXIMINE*** (4-(2-dimethylamino-ethoxy)-1,2-dihydro-1-hydroxyimino-phthalazine; 4-(2-dimethylaminoethoxy)-1(2H)-phthalazinone oxime).
'Talpen' see Talampicillin.
'Talsis' see Bisoxatin diacetate.
TALSUPRAM*** (1,3-dihydro-N,3,3-tri-methyl-1-phenylbenzo(c)thiophene-1-propylamine; 1-(3-aminopropyl)-1,3-dihydro-N,3,3-trimethyl-1-phenylbenzo(c)-thiophene; 3,3-dimethyl-1-(3-methyl-aminopropyl)-1-phenylthiophthalan; Lu-5-003).
'Talucard' see Proscillaridin.
'Talusin' see Proscillaridin.

'Talwin' see Pentazocine.
'Tamaron' see Methamidophos.
TAMETICILLIN** (2-(diethylamino)ethyl
(2S,5R,6R)-6-(2,6-dimethoxybenzamido)-
penicillanate; meticillin 2-diethylamino-
ethyl ester).
Tamidoline see Omidoline.
TAMOXIFEN*** (1-[p-(2-dimethylamino-
ethoxy)phenyl]-trans-1,2-diphenylbut-1-
ene; α-[p-(2-dimethylaminoethoxy)phenyl]-
α'-ethylstilbene; (Z)-2-[p-(1,2-diphenyl-1-
butenyl)phenoxy]-N,N-dimethylethyl-
amine; ICI-46474; 'nolvadex').
'Tanacaine' see Quatacaine.
Tanaceton see Absinthol.
'Tanakan' see Chloroquine.
'Tandacote' see Oxyphenbutazone.
TANDAMINE** (1-(2-dimethylamino-
ethyl)-9-ethyl-1,3,4,9-tetrahydro-1-methyl-
thiopyrano(3,4-b)indole; 9-ethyl-1,3,4,9-
tetrahydro-N,N,1-trimethylthiopyrano(3,4-
b)indole-1-ethanamine; tandamine hydro-
chloride; AY-23946).
'Tanderil' see Oxyphenbutazone.
'Tandex' see Karbutilate.
'Tanganil' see Ethanolamine acetylleucinate.
TANGERETIN (4',5,6,7,8-pentamethoxy-
flavone).
'Tannalbin' see Albumin tannate.
Tannalbumin see Albumin tannate.
Tannic acid see Tannin(s).
TANNIN(S) (gallotannic acid; tannic acid).
Tannyl acetate see Acetyltanninum.
'Tanone' see Phenthoate.
'Tantum' see Benzydamine.
'Tantum biotic' see Benzydamine with
tetracycline.
'Tao' see Troleandomycin.
'Taoryl' see Caramiphen edisilate.
'Taractan' see Chlorprothixene.
'Tarasan' see Chlorprothixene.
'Tardamid' see Sulfamoxole.
'Tardocillin' see Benzathine penicillin.
'Tardokrein' see Kallidinogenase.
'Tardolyt' see Aristolochic acid.
'Tardomycocel' see Benzathine penicillin.
'Tarodyl' see Glycopyrronium.
'Tarodyn' see Glycopyrronium.
'Tarpane' see Clobenzepam.
'Tarquinor' see Halquinols.
Tartar emetic see Antimonyl potassium
tartrate.
TARTARIC ACID (2,3-dihydroxysuccinic
acid).
TARTRAZINE (chiefly the trisodium salt of
5-hydroxy-1-(p-sulfophenyl)-4-(p-sulfo-
phenylazo)pyrazole-3-carboxylic acid).
'Tartrol' see Bismuth tartrate.
TARTRONIC ACID (hydroxymalonic acid).
'Tarugan' see Morazone.
'Task' see Dichlorvos.
'Tasnon' see Piperazine citrate.
'Tasto' see Aloglutamol.
TATBA see Triamcinolone hexacetonide.
TATD see Octotiamine.
'Tathion' see Glutathione.
'Tauredon' see Sodium aurothiomalate.

TAURINE (2-aminoethanesulfonic acid).
TAUROCHOLIC ACID (cholic acid taurine
conjugate; cholaic acid; choly ltaurine).
TAUROCYAMINE (N-guanyltaurine;
guanidotaurine).
'Tauroflex' see Taurultam.
TAUROLIN** (4,4'-methylenebis(tetra-
hydro-1,2,4-thiadiazine 1,1-dioxide)).
TAURULTAM*** (tetrahydro-1,2,4-thia-
diazine 1,1-dioxide; 'tauroflex').
'Tavan' see Pentosan polysulfate.
'Tavegil' see Clemastine.
'Ta-verm' see Piperazine citrate.
'Tavor' see Lorazepam.
TAXIFOLIN (3,3',4',5,7-pentahydroxy-
flavanone; 2,3-dihydroquercetin; distylin).
'Taxilan' see Perazine.
TAZOLOL** ((+)-1-isopropylamino-3-
thiazol-2-yloxy-2-propanol; (+)-2-(2-
hydroxy-3-isopropylaminopropoxy)thiazole;
tazolol hydrochloride; RS-6245).
Tb I/698 see Thiacetazone.
Tb III/1347 see Subathizone.
2,3,6-TBA* see Trichlorobenzoic acid.
TBP see Bithionol.
'T.B.T.O.' see Bis(tributyltin) oxide.
T-caine see Diethylaminoethyl p-butyl-
aminobenzoate.
TCAP see Cetrimonium pentachlorophenate.
'TCC' see Triclocarban.
TCDS see Tetradifon.
TCNB see Tecnazene.
TCP see Tricresyl phosphate.
TDE see DDD.
o,p'-TDE see Mitotane.
TDI see Toluylene diisocyanate.
TEA see Tetrylammonium.
Teaberry oil see Methyl salicylate.
TEAO see Trichlormethine N-oxide.
Tear gas see 2-Chloroacetophenone.
TEB see Tetrakis(aziridin-1-yl)-p-benzo-
quinone.
'Tebamin' see Fenamisol.
'Tebanyl' see Fenamisol.
'Tebeform' see Protionamide.
'Tebonin' see Ginkgo biloba extract.
TEBROFEN (tr) (3,3',5,5'-tetrabromo-
2,2',4,4'-tetrahydroxybiphenyl; tebrophen).
Tebrophen (tr) see Tebrofen.
TEBUTATE(S)** (tert-butylacetate(s)).
See also Hydrocortisone tebutate.
TEC see Triethyl(2-hydroxyethyl)ammonium
chloride.
'Tecesal' see Calcium thiosulfate.
Technetium labeled macroaggregated
human serum albumin see Macrosalb
(99mTc).
TECLOTHIAZIDE*** (6-chloro-3,4-di-
hydro-7-sulfamoyl-3-trichloromethyl-2H-
1,2,4-benzothiadiazine 1,1-dioxide; teclothiazide potassium; 'depleil', 'deplet').
TECLOZAN** (N,N'-(p-phenylenedimethyl-
ene)bis[2,2-dichloro-N-(2-ethoxyethyl)-
acetamide]; WIN-13146; WIN AM-13146;
'falmonox').
TECNAZENE* (1,2,4,5-tetrachloro-3-nitro-
benzene; TCNB; 'folosan', 'fumite TCNB',

425

'fusarex').
Tecodin (tr) *see* Oxycodone.
'Tecodin' *see* Codeine methyl bromide.
'Tecquinol' *see* Hydroquinone.
'Tecto' *see* Tiabendazole.
TECTORIGENIN (4',5,7-trihydroxy-6-methoxyisoflavone).
'Tedarol' *see* Triamcinolone diacetate.
'Tedegyl' *see* Thiodiglycol.
'Tedion' *see* Tetradifon.
TEDTP *see* Sulfotep.
'Teecaine' *see* Diethylaminoethyl *p*-butyl-aminobenzoate.
'Teepol' *see* Sulfestol.
TEF (tr) *see* Tepa.
TEFAZOLINE*** (2-(5,6,7,8-tetrahydro-naphth-1-ylmethyl)-2-imidazoline; 5,6,7,8-tetrahydro-1-(2-imidazolin-2-ylmethyl)-naphthalene; tenaphthoxaline; tefazoline nitrate; 'tenaphtho').
'Teflon' *see* Politef.
TEFLURANE*** (2-bromo-1,1,1,2-tetra-fluoroethane; tetraflurane; A-16900; DA-708).
TEFLUTIXOL*** (4-[3-[6-fluoro-2-(trifluoromethyl)thioxanthen-9-yl]propyl]-1-piperazineethanol; 6-fluoro-9-[3-[4-(2-hydroxyethyl)piperazin-1-yl]propyl]-2-(trifluoromethyl)thioxanthene).
'Tefose 63' *see* Pegoxol 7 stearate.
'Tego 103S' *see* Dodicin.
'Tego-betaine' *see* Pendecamaine.
'Tegopen' *see* Cloxacillin.
'Tegotin' *see* Vitamin T.
'Tegretol' *see* Carbamazepine.
TEH *see* Heptaminol theophyllineacetate.
Teichman's crystals *see* Hemin.
Tekodin (tr) *see* Oxycodone.
TEL *see* Tetraethyllead.
'Telebrix 38' *see* Meglumine ioxitalamate with sodium ioxitalamate.
'Telebrix 300' *see* Meglumine ioxitalamate.
'Telepaque' *see* Iopanoic acid.
'Telepathine' *see* Harmine.
'Teletrast' *see* Iopanoic acid.
'Teletux' *see* Noscapine embonate.
Telicherry bark *see* Kurchi.
'Telmid' *see* Dithiazanine iodide.
'Telmin' *see* Piperazine.
'Telodrin' *see* Isobenzan.
'Telvar' *see* Monuron.
TEM *see* Tretamine.
'Temanyl' *see* Alimemazine.
'Temaril' *see* Alimemazine.
'Temaryl' *see* Alimemazine.
'Temasept IV' *see* Dibromsalan with tribromsalan.
TEMAZEPAM*** (7-chloro-1,3-dihydro-3-hydroxy-1-methyl-5-phenyl-2H-1,4-benzodiazepin-2-one; methyloxazepam; A-102; ER-115; 'levanxol').
Temazepam dimethylcarbamate *see* Camazepam.
Temechin (tr) *see* 2,2,6,6-Tetramethyl-quinuclidine.
TEMEFOS** (*O,O'*-(thiodi-*p*-phenylene) *O,O,O',O'*-tetramethyl bis(phosphoro-

thioate); *O,O,O',O'*-tetramethyl *O,O'*-(thiodi-4,1-phenylene)phosphorothioate; temephos; OMS-736; 'abate', 'bithion').
Temephos* *see* Temefos.
Temequin (tr) *see* 2,2,6,6-Tetramethyl-quinuclidine.
'Temesta' *see* Lorazepam.
'Temetil' *see* Prochlorperazine.
'Temick' *see* Aldicarb.
'Temik' *see* Aldicarb.
'Temina' *see* Vitamin T.
TEMODOX** (2-hydroxyethyl 3-methyl-quinoxaline-2-carboxylate 1,4-dioxide).
'Temparin' *see* Dicoumarol.
'Tempidon' *see* 2,2,6,6-Tetramethylpiperid-4-one tosilate.
'Temposil' *see* Calcium carbimide.
'Tempra' *see* Paracetamol.
'Tenac' *see* Dichlorvos.
'Tenaphtho' *see* Tefazoline.
Tenaphthoxaline *see* Tefazoline.
'Tencilan' *see* Dipotassium clorazepate.
Tenemycin *see* Nebramycin.
'Tenfidil' *see* Thenyldiamine.
'Teniathane' *see* Dichlorophen.
'Teniatol' *see* Dichlorophen.
TENIPOSIDE** (4'-demethylepipodophylo-toxin 9-(4,6-*O*-2-thenylidene)-β-D-gluco-pyranoside; PTG; NSC-122819; VM-26).
'Tenoban' *see* Arecoline-acetarsol.
'Tenoran' *see* Chloroxuron.
'Tenormal' *see* Pempidine.
'Tenormine' *see* Atenolol.
'Tenox-BHA' *see* Butylated hydroxyanisole.
'Tenox-PG' *see* Propyl gallate.
'Tenserlix' *see* Reserpine with furosemide.
'Tensicor' *see* Dipropylamine dichloroacetate.
'Tensilest' *see* Pentolonium tartrate.
'Tensilon' *see* Edrophonium chloride.
'Tensimic' *see* Methoserpidine with benz-thiazide and potassium chloride.
'Tensionorme *see* Reserpine with bendro-flumethiazide.
'Tensofin' *see* Flufenazine.
'Tensopam' *see* Diazepam.
'Tentone' *see* Methopromazine.
'Tenuate' *see* Amfepramone.
TENUAZONIC ACID (3-acetyl-5-*sec*-butyl-4-hydroxy-3-pyrrolin-2-one; α-acetyl-*sec*-butyltetramic acid).
See also Benzathine tenuazonate; Sodium tenuazonate.
TENYLIDONE*** (2,6-bis(2-thenylidene)-cyclohexanone; 'margeryl').
'Teo-caradrin' *see* Proscillaridin with theophylline.
'Teocholine' *see* Choline theophyllinate.
TEOCLATE(S)** (8-chlorotheophyllinate(s); theoclate(s)).
See also Chlorphenoxamine teoclate; Embramine teoclate; Phenmetrazine teoclate; Procaine teoclate; Promethazine teoclate.
'Teonicon' *see* Pimefylline nicotinate.
'Teoquil' *see* Hedaquinium.
'Teostellarid' *see* Proscillaridin with etofylline.

TEP *see* Tetraethylpyrophosphate.
TEPA* (tris(1-aziridinyl)phosphine oxide; phosphoric acid triethylene imide; triethylenephosphoramide; *N,N',N''*-triethylenephosphoric triamide; triethylenepyrophosphoramide; TEF; aphoxide; ENT-24915; NSC-9717; SK-3818).
Tepa-132 *see* Hexamethyltepa.
'Tepanil' *see* Amfepramone.
'Teperin' *see* Amitriptyline.
'Tepilta' *see* Oxetacaine.
TEPP* *see* Tetraethyl pyrophosphate.
TEPROSILATE(S)** (1,2,3,6-tetrahydro-1,3-dimethyl-2,6-dioxopurine-7-propanesulfonate(s)).
Tequinol *see* Sodium actinoquinol.
'Tequinopil' *see* Clioquinol with chloroquine diphosphate and tetracycline.
'Teralen' *see* Alimemazine.
'Teralithe' *see* Lithium carbonate.
'Teramine' *see* Benzethonium.
TERBACIL* (3-*tert*-butyl-5-chloro-6-methyluracil; 5-chloro-3-(1,1-dimethylethyl)-6-methyl-2,4(1H,3H)-pyrimidinedione; 'sinbar').
'Terbolan' *see* Reserpine with furosemide.
TERBUCARB* (2,6-di-*tert*-butyl-4-methylphenyl methylcarbamate; 2,6-bis(1,1-dimethylethyl)-4-methylphenyl methylcarbamate; terbutol; 'azak').
TERBUFIBROL** (*p*-[3-(*p-tert*-butylphenoxy)-2-hydroxypropoxy]benzoic acid; 1-(*p-tert*-butylphenoxy)-3-(*p*-carboxyphenoxy)-2-propanol).
TERBUFICIN** (2,2-bis(3,5-di-*tert*-butyl-4-hydroxyphenyl)acetic acid).
TERBUMETON* (2-*tert*-butylamino-4-ethylamino-6-methoxy-*s*-triazine; *N*-(1,1-dimethylethyl)-*N'*-ethyl-6-methoxy-1,3,5-triazine-2,4-diamine; terbuthylaton; 'caragard').
TERBUPROL*** (1-*tert*-butoxy-3-methoxy-2-propanol).
TERBUTALINE*** (α-(*tert*-butylaminomethyl)-3,5-dihydroxybenzyl alcohol; 2-(*tert*-butylamino)-1-(3,5-dihydroxyphenyl)ethanol; terbutaline sulfate; KWD-2019; 'brethine', 'bricanyl', 'filair').
Terbuthylaton *see* Terbumeton.
Terbutol *see* Terbucarb.
TERBUTRYN* (2-*tert*-butylamino-4-ethylamino-6-(methylthio)-*s*-triazine; *N*-(1,1-dimethylethyl)-*N'*-ethyl-6-(methylthio)-1,3,5-triazine-2,4-diamine; terbutryne; 'igran', 'prebane').
Terbutryne *see* Terbutryn.
Terbutylamine *see* Phentermine.
'Tercian' *see* Cyamemazine.
Terebinth oil *see* Turpentine oil.
'Terenol' *see* Resorantel.
TEREPHTHALIC ACID (*p*-benzenedicarboxylic acid).
Terephthalic acid ethylene glycol polymer *see* Pegoterate.
TERFENADINE*** (α-(*p-tert*-butylphenyl)-4-(hydroxydiphenylmethyl)-1-piperidinebutanol; α-[1-[4-(*p-tert*-butylphenyl)-4-hydroxybutyl]piperid-4-yl]benzhydrol; *p-tert*-butyl α-[3-[4-(hydroxydiphenylmethyl)piperid-1-yl]propyl]benzyl alcohol).
'Terfluzine' *see* Trifluoperazine.
'Tergemist' *see* Sodium etasulfate.
'Tergitol 08' *see* Sodium octyl sulfate.
'Tergitol 4' *see* Sodium tetradecyl sulfate.
'Tergitol 7' *see* Sodium heptadecyl sulfate.
'Teriam' *see* Triamterene.
'Teridax' *see* Iophenoxic acid.
'Terivalidin' *see* Terizidone.
TERIZIDONE*** (4,4'-(*p*-phenylene)bis(methyleneamino)di(isoxazolidin-3-one); *N*⁴,*N*⁴'-(*p*-phenylene)bis(methylene)-di(cycloserine); 'terivalidin').
'Termidor' *see* Paracetamol.
'Termil' *see* Chlorothalonil.
Termitin *see* Vitamin T.
TERNIDAZOLE** (2-methyl-4-nitroimidazole-1-propanol; 1-(3-hydroxypropyl)-2-methyl-4-nitroimidazole).
TERODILINE*** (*N-tert*-butyl-1-methyl-3,3-diphenylpropylamine; 'bicor').
TEROFENAMATE*** (ethoxymethyl *N*-(2,6-dichloro-*m*-tolyl)anthranilate; ethoxymethyl meclofenamate; meclofenamic acid ethoxymethyl ester; etoclofene; A-3).
'Terolut' *see* Dydrogesterone.
'Teronac' *see* Mazindol.
'Teropterin' *see* Pteropterin.
TEROXALENE*** (1-(3-chloro-*p*-tolyl)-4-[*p*-(1,1-dimethylpropyl)phenoxyhexamethylene]piperazine; 4-[[4-*tert*-amylphenoxy)hexamethylene]-1-(3-chloro-4-methylphenyl)piperazine; 1-(3-chloro-*p*-tolyl)-4-[6-(*p-tert*-pentylphenoxy)-hexyl]piperazine; teroxalene hydrochloride; A-16612; PR-3847).
'Terraclor' *see* Quintozene.
'Terra-cortril' *see* Hydrocortisone with oxytetracycline.
'Terracur P' *see* Fensulfothion.
'Terrafungine' *see* Oxytetracycline.
'Terramycin' *see* Oxytetracycline.
'Terrastatin' *see* Oxytetracycline with nystatin.
'Terra-sytam' *see* Dimefox.
'Terravenos' *see* Oxytetracycline.
'Tersan' *see* Thiram.
'Tersan SP' *see* Chloroneb.
'Tersavid' *see* Pivhydrazine.
'Tertran' *see* Iprindole.
'Tertroxin' *see* Liothyronine sodium.
'Terulcon' *see* Carbenoxolone sodium.
TESICAM* (4'-chloro-1,2,3,4-tetrahydro-1,3-dioxo-4-isoquinolinecarboxanilide).
TESIMIDE*** (4-benzylidene-5,6,7,8-tetrahydro-1,3(2H,4H)-isoquinolinedione).
'Teslac' *see* Testolactone.
TESPA *see* Thiotepa.
'Tespamin' *see* Thiotepa.
'Tessalon' *see* Benzonatate.
Testenat (tr) *see* Testosterone.
'Testodrin prolongatum' *see* Testosterone cipionate.
TESTOLACTONE*** (1,2,3,4,4a,4b,7,9,10,

10a-decahydro-2-hydroxy-2,4b-dimethyl-7-oxo-1-phenanthrenepropionic acid δ-lactone; 17α-oxa-D-homoandrosta-1,4-diene-3,17-dione; △¹-testolactone; NSC-23759; SQ-9538; 'teslac').

△¹-Testolactone *see* Testolactone.

TESTOSTERONE*** (androst-4-en-17β-ol-3-one; 17β-hydroxyandrost-4-en-3-one; △⁴-androsten-17-ol-3-one; *trans*-testosterone; testenat; NSC-9700).

Testosterone caprate *see* Testosterone decanoate.

TESTOSTERONE CIPIONATE (testosterone cyclopentanepropionate; testosterone cypionate; 'depoviron', 'pertestis', 'testodrin prolongatum').

TESTOSTERONE CYCLOHEXANE-CARBOXYLATE ('lontanyl').

Testosterone cyclopentanepropionate *see* Testosterone cipionate.

Testosterone cypionate *see* Testosterone cipionate.

TESTOSTERONE DECANOATE (testosterone caprate).

TESTOSTERONE ENANTATE (testosterone 1-hexanecarboxylate; testosterone enanthate; testosterone heptanoate; 'delatestryl', 'testoviron-depot').
See also Estradiol valerate with testosterone enantate.

Testosterone heptanoate *see* Testosterone enantate.

TESTOSTERONE p-(HEXYLOXY)-HYDROCINNAMATE (testosterone 3-(p-hexyloxyphenyl)propionate; 'andradurin').

Testosterone 3-(p-hexyloxyphenyl)-propionate *see* Testosterone 3-p-(hexyloxy)-hydrocinnamate.

TESTOSTERONE ISOBUTYRATE ('perandren').
See also Estradiol benzoate with testosterone isobutyrate.

Testosterone isocaproate *see* Testosterone 4-methylvalerate.

TESTOSTERONE KETOLAURATE*** (testosterone 3-oxododecanoate; 'androdurin').

TESTOSTERONE 4-METHYL-VALERATE (testosterone isocaproate).

TESTOSTERONE NICOTINATE ('bolfortan').

Testosterone enanthate *see* Testosterone enantate.

Testosterone 3-oxododecanoate *see* Testosterone ketolaurate.

TESTOSTERONE PHENYLPROPION-ATE ('retandrol').

TESTOSTERONE PROPIONATE (TP; NSC-9166).

Testosterone trichlorohydroxyethyl ether *see* Cloxotestosterone.

TESTOSTERONE UNDECENATE ('deposteron').

'Testoviron-depot' *see* Testosterone enantate.

TET (tr) *see* Tretamine.

Tetamon (tr) *see* Tetrylammonium.

Tetiothalein *see* Iodophthalein.

'Tetmosol' *see* Monosulfiram.

'Tetra' *see* Tetrachloroethylene.

β-Tetra *see* 1,2,3,4-Tetrahydro-2-naphthylamine.

Tetraazaindene *see* Pyrazolopyrimidine.

1,3,5,7-Tetraazanaphthalene *see* Pyrimido-(5,4-d)pyrimidine.

Tetraaziridinyl-p-benzoquinone *see* 2,3,5,6-Tetrakis(aziridin-1-yl)-p-benzoquinone.

TETRABARBITAL*** (5-ethyl-5-(1-ethylbutyl) barbituric acid; 'butysedal').

TETRABENAZINE*** (1,3,4,6,7,11b-hexahydro-3-isobutyl-9,10-dimethoxy-2H-benzo(a)quinolizin-2-one; Ro-1-0569; 'nitoman').

TETRABORIC ACID ($B_4O_5(OH)_2$; pyroboric acid).
See also Borax.

Tetrabromobenzoquinone(s) *see* Bromanil; Isobromanil.

4,4',6,6'-Tetrabromo-2,2'-biphenyldiol 2-dihydrogen phosphate *see* Bromophenophos.

3,4,5,6-Tetrabromo-3,3-bis(4-hydroxy-3-sulfophenyl)phthalide *see* Sulfobromphthalein.

3,3',5,5'-Tetrabromo-2,2'-dihydroxy-benzil *see* Tetrabromsalicil.

Tetrabromophenolphthalein disodium sulfonate *see* Sulfobromphthalein.

Tetrabromosalicil *see* Tetrabromsalicil.

3,3',5,5'-Tetrabromo-2,2',4,4'-tetra-hydroxybiphenyl *see* Tebrofen.

TETRABROMSALICIL (3,3',5,5'-tetra-bromo-2,2'-dihydroxybenzil; tetrabromosalicil; RP-3227).

TETRAC (3,5,3',5'-tetraiodothyroacetic acid; α-[4-(4-hydroxy-3,5-diiodophenoxy)-3,5-diiodophenyl]acetic acid).

TETRACAINE*** (deanol p-butylaminobenzoate; 2-dimethylaminoethyl p-butyl-aminobenzoate; amethocaine; dicaine).

'Tetracap' *see* Tetrachloroethylene.

Tetra(carboxymethyl)ethylenediamine *see* Edetic acid.

Tetracemin *see* Edetic acid.

2,4,5,6-Tetrachloro-1,3-benzenedicarbo-nitrile *see* Chlorothalonil.

2,3,5,6-Tetrachlorobenzene-1,4-dicarb-oxylic acid *see* Chlorthal.

Tetrachlorobenzoquinone(s) *see* Chloranil; Isochloranil.

1,3,4,5-Tetrachloro-2,6-dicyanobenzene *see* Chlorothalonil.

TETRACHLORODIFLUOROETHANE ('frigen 112').

1,1,2,2-TETRACHLORO-1,2-DIFLUORO-ETHANE (difluorotetrachloroethane; 'freon-113').

Tetrachlorodihydroxydiphenyl sulfide *see* Bithionol.

4,5,6,7-Tetrachloro-2-(2-dimethylamino-ethyl)-2-methylisoindolinium chloride methochloride *see* Chlorisondamine chloride.

1,3,4,5-Tetrachloro-2,6-dinitrilobenzene
see Chlorothalonil.

2,4,4′,5-Tetrachlorodiphenyl sulfide *see*
Tetrasul.

2,4,4′,5-Tetrachlorodiphenylsulfone *see*
Tetradifon.

TETRACHLOROETHANE (1,1,2,2-tetra-
chloroethane; acetylene tetrachloride;
'bonoform', 'cellon').

TETRACHLOROETHYLENE (1,1,2,2-
tetrachloroethylene; perchlorethylene;
carbon dichloride; 'ankilostin', 'didakene',
'nema', 'perclene', 'perklone', 'pervit',
'pezavin', 'tetra', 'tetracap', 'tetrahelmin',
'tetralex').

N-[(**1,1,2,2-Tetrachloroethyl)thio**]-**4-
cyclohexenedicarboximide** *see* Captafol.

N-(**Tetrachloroethylthio)-△⁴-tetra-
hydrophthalimide** *see* Captafol.

2,3,5,6-Tetrachloro-4-hydroxyanisole *see*
Drosophilin A.

Tetrachloroisophthalonitrile *see* Chlorothalonil.

2,3,5,6-Tetrachloro-4-methoxyphenol *see*
Drosophilin A.

1,2,4,5-Tetrachloro-3-nitrobenzene *see*
Tecnazene.

Tetrachloronitromethane *see* Chloropicrin.

5,6,7,8-Tetrachloroquinoxaline *see*
Chlorquinox.

2,3,5,6-Tetrachloroterephthalic acid *see*
Chlorthal.

**4,5,6,7-Tetrachloro-2′,4′,5′,7′-tetraiodo-
fluorescein** *see* Rose bengal.

Tetrachlorvinphos* *see* Stirofos.

TETRACOSACTIDE*** (ACTH synthetic
analog; synthetic α¹⁻²⁴ corticotrophin;
cosyntropin; tetracosactrin; Ba-30920;
C-30920-Ba; 'cortrosyn', 'synacthar',
'synacthen').

**TETRACOSACTIDE ZINC PHOSPHATE
COMPLEX** (zinc tetracosactide; Ba-
42915; 'synacthen-depot').

Tetracosactrin* *see* Tetracosactide.

15-TETRACOSENOIC ACID (nervic acid;
nervonic acid; selacholic acid).

TETRACYCLINE*** (4-dimethylamino-
1,4,4a,5,5a,6,11,12a-octahydro-3,6,10,12,
12a-pentahydroxy-6-methyl-1,11-dioxo-
naphthacene-2-carboxamide; deschloro-
biomycin; tsiklomitsin; tetracycline hydrochloride).
See also below and Benzydamine with tetracycline; Broxyquinoline with broxaldine
and tetracycline; Clioquinol with chloroquine diphosphate and tetracycline;
Diiodohydroxyquin with tetracycline;
Erythromycin with tetracycline; Erythromycin estolate with tetracycline; Oxolamine benzilate with tetracycline.

**TETRACYCLINE WITH AMPHOTERI-
CIN B** ('mysteclin-V').

**TETRACYCLINE WITH ASCORBIC
ACID** ('resteclin').

TETRACYCLINE WITH BROMELAINS
('tetranase', 'traumanase-cyclin').

**TETRACYCLINE WITH CHLORTETRA-
CYCLINE AND DEMECLOCYCLINE**
(triple tetracycline; 'deteclo').

**TETRACYCLINE BITARTRATE-
NUCLEIC ACID COMPLEX** ('mervacycline').

Tetracycline colistin compound *see*
Colimecycline.

TETRACYCLINE CYCLAMATE (tetracycline cyclohexylsulfamate; 'sifacycline').

Tetracycline cyclohexylsulfamate *see*
Tetracycline cyclamate.

**Tetracycline 2-deoxy-2-methylamino-
glucose compound** *see* Meglucycline.

**TETRACYCLINE DIHYDRONOVO-
BIOCIN SODIUM PHYTATE** ('vulcacycline').

**TETRACYCLINE DODECYLSULF-
AMATE** ('myriamycin').

Tetracycline-L-methylene-lysine *see*
Lymecycline.

TETRACYCLINE WITH NOVOBIOCIN
('panalba').

**TETRACYCLINE WITH OLEANDOMY-
CIN** ('oletetrin', 'sigmamycin', 'signemycin', 'tetraolean').

Tetracycline phosphate complex *see*
Hexacycline.

**α-Tetracyclinyl-4-(2-hydroxyethyl)-
1-piperazineacetic acid** *see* Apicycline.

**6-(Tetracyclin-2-ylmethylamino)penicil-
lin G** *see* Penimocycline.

Tetradecanoic acid *see* Myristic acid.

2-Tetradecylaminoethanol lactate *see*
Myralact.

α-Tetradecylcitric acid *see* Norcaperatic
acid.

TETRADIFON* (2,4,4′,5-tetrachloro-
diphenyl sulfone; *p*-chlorophenyl 2,4,5-
trichlorophenyl sulfone; 1,2,4-trichloro-5-
(*p*-chlorophenylsulfonyl)benzene; chlorodifon; TCDS; 'akaritox', 'duphar',
'tedion').

TETRADONIUM BROMIDE* **(trimethyltetradecylammonium bromide;
myristyltrimethylammonium bromide).

Tetraethylammonium bromide *see*
Tetrylammonium.

Tetraethyl diphosphate *see* Tetraethyl
pyrophosphate.

Tetraethyl dithiopyrophosphate *see*
Sulfotep.

**Tetraethylenepentamine polymer with
1-chloro-2,3-epoxypropane** *see* Colestipol.

**Tetraethylenimide piperazine diphos-
phate** *see* Dipin.

Tetraethyleniminobenzoquinone *see*
Tetrakis(1-aziridinyl)-*p*-benzoquinone.

TETRAETHYLLEAD (TEL; 'ethyl').

**Tetraethyl methylenediphosphorodithio-
ate** *see* Ethion.

Tetraethyl monothiopyrophosphate *see*
Pyrophos.

TETRAETHYL PYROPHOSPHATE
(ethyl pyrophosphate; tetraethyl diphosphate; TEPP; tetrastigmine; 'nifos T',

'vapotone', 'tetron').

Tetraethyl thiodiphosphate *see* Sulfotep.

Tetraethyl thiopyrophosphate *see* Pyrophos.

Tetraethylthiuram disulfide *see* Disulfiram.

Tetraethylthiuram monosulfide *see* Monosulfiram.

TETRAFENPHOS (*O,O'*-thiodi(*p*-phenylene)phosphorothioate).

Tetrafluorobenzoquinone(s) *see* Fluoranil; Isofluoranil.

1,1,1,2-Tetrafluoroethane *see* Norflurane.

Tetrafluoroethylene polymer *see* Politef.

Tetraflurane *see* Teflurane.

'Tetraform' *see* Carbon tetrachloride.

TETRAGASTRIN (gastrin-like tetrapeptide).

Tetraglucosan *see* Salabrose.

'Tetrahelmin' *see* Tetrachloroethylene.

Tetrahydroaminacrin *see* Tacrine.

Tetrahydroazepotetrazole *see* Pentetrazole.

TETRAHYDROBERBERINE (L-tetrahydroberberine; canadine; hydroberberine; xanthopuccine).

3,4,5,6-Tetrahydro-2,3'-bipyridine *see* Anabaseine.

TETRAHYDROCANNABINOL (7,8,9,10-tetrahydro-6,6,9-trimethyl-3-pentyl-6H-dibenzo(b,d)pyran-1-ol).

△¹**-Tetrahydrocannabinol** *see* △⁹-Tetrahyrocannabinol.

△⁶**-Tetrahydrocannabinol** *see* △⁸-Tetrahydrocannabinol.

△⁸**-TETRAHYDROCANNABINOL** (△⁶-tetrahydrocannabinol).

△⁹**-TETRAHYDROCANNABINOL** (△¹-tetrahydrocannabinol).

Tetrahydrocyclohexanecarboxylic acid *see* Quinic acid.

Tetrahydro-1H-1,4-diazepine-1,4(5H)-dipropanol *see* Biopropazepan.

Tetrahydro-1H-1,4-diazepine-1,4(5H)-dipropanol 3,4,5-trimethoxybenzoate *see* Dilazep.

1,2,3,4-Tetrahydro-6,7-dihydroxy-1-(3,4-dihydroxybenzyl)isoquinoline *see* Tetrahydropapaveroline.

5,5a,13,13a-Tetrahydro-5,13-dihydroxy-8H,16H-7a,15a-epidithio-7H,15H-bis-oxepino(3',4':4,5)pyrrolo(1,2-a:1',2'-d)pyrazine-7,15-dione 5-acetate *see* Aranotin.

7,7a,8,9-Tetrahydro-3,7a-dihydroxy-12-(3-methyl-2-butenyl)-6H-8,9c-imino-ethanophenanthro(4,5-bcd)furan-5(4aH)-one *see* Nalmexone.

5,10,11,11a-Tetrahydro-9,11-dihydroxy-8-methyl-5-oxo-1H-pyrrolo(2,1-c)-(1,4)benzodiazepine-*trans*-2-acrylamide *see* Antramycin.

1,2,3,4-Tetrahydro-6,7-dihydroxy-1-protocatechuylisoquinoline *see* Tetrahydropapaveroline.

3,4,5,6-Tetrahydro-3,4-dihydroxyspiro-(benzofuran-2(3H),2'-oxirane)-6-methanol 6-acetate 3,4-diisovalerate *see* Didrovaltrate.

1,4a,5,7a-Tetrahydro-1,6-dihydroxyspiro-[cyclopenta(c)pyran-7(6H),2'-oxirane]-4-methanol 6-acetate 1,4-diisovalerate *see* Didrovaltrate.

1,2,3,4-Tetrahydro-6,7-dimethoxyiso-quinoline *see* Salsolidine.

1,2,12,12a-Tetrahydro-8,9-dimethoxy-2-(1-methylethenyl)(1)benzopyrano-(3,4-b)furo(2,3-h)(1)benzopyran-6-one *see* Rotenone.

2,3,4,5-Tetrahydro-7,8-dimethoxy-3-methyl-1-phenyl-1H-3-benzazepine *see* Trimopam.

1,2,3,6-Tetrahydro-1,3-dimethyl-2,6-dioxopurine-7-ethanesulfonic acid, esters and salts *see* Tofesilate(s).

1,2,3,6-Tetrahydro-1,3-dimethyl-2,6-dioxopurine-7-propanesulfonic acid, esters and salts *see* Teprosilate(s).

Tetrahydro-3,5-dimethyl-2H-1,3-thia-diazine-2-thione *see* Dazomet.

Tetrahydro-*p*-dioxin *see* 1,4-Dioxane.

Tetrahydro-9-fluorenone *see* Phentydrone.

4-Tetrahydrofurfuryl-1,2-benzo(c)cinno-lino-3,5-pyrazolinedione *see* Cinnofuradione.

2-Tetrahydrofurfuryl-1H-benzo(c)pyra-zolo(1,2-a)cinnoline-1,3(2H)-dione *see* Cinnofuradione.

Tetrahydrofurfuryl (2-carbamoyl-phenoxy)acetate *see* Fenamifuril.

Tetrahydrofurfuryl esters *see* Thurfyl *etc.*

Tetrahydroglyoxaline *see* Imidazolidine.

Tetrahydro-2-[3-hydroxy-5-(hydroxy-methyl)-2-methylpyrid-4-yl]-2H-1,3-thiazine-4-carboxylic acid *see* Tiapirinol.

5,6,7,8-Tetrahydro-8-hydroxy-7-(hydroxy-methyl)-5-(3,4,5-trimethoxyphenyl)-naphtho(2,3-d)-1,3-dioxole-6-carboxylic acid γ-lactone *see* Podophyllotoxin.

5,6,7,8-Tetrahydro-9-hydroxy-7-(hydroxy-methyl)-5-(3,4,5-trimethoxyphenyl)-naphtho(2,3-d)-1,3-dioxole-6-carboxylic acid γ-lactone *see* β-Peltatin.

2,3,3a,9a-Tetrahydro-3-hydroxy-6-imino-6H-furo(2',3':4,5)oxazolo(3,2-a)pyrim-idine-2-methanol *see* Ancitabine.

1,2,3,4-Tetrahydro-6-hydroxy-7-methoxy-1-methylisoquinoline *see* Salsoline.

6,7,8,14-Tetrahydro-7α-(1-hydroxy-1-methylbutyl)-6,14-*endo*-ethenooripav-ine *see* Etorphine.

6,7,8,14-Tetrahydro-7a-(1-hydroxy-1-methylbutyl)-6,14-*endo*-ethenooripav-ine 3-acetate *see* Acetorphine.

1,2,3,4-Tetrahydro-6-hydroxymethyl-2-isopropylaminomethyl-7-nitroquinol-ine *see* Oxamniquine.

3,4,5,6-Tetrahydro-N-(hydroxymethyl)-phthalimide 2,2-dimethyl-3-(2-methyl-1-propenyl)cyclopropanecarboxylate ester *see* Tetramethrin.

3a,4,7,7a-Tetrahydro-5-(hydroxyphenyl-2-pyridinylmethyl)-7-(phenyl-2-pyridin-ylmethylene)-4,7-methano-1H-isoin-dole-3(2H)-dione *see* Norbormide.

trans-**1,4,5,6-Tetrahydro-2-[2-(*m*-hydroxy-**

phenyl)vinyl]-1-methylpyrimidine *see* Oxantel.

2,3,3a,8a-Tetrahydro-5-hydroxy-1,3a,8-trimethylpyrrolo(2,3-b)indole *see* Physostigmine.

1,2,3,4-Tetrahydro-6-(2-imidazolin-2-ylmethyl)-7-methyl-1,4-ethanonaphthalene *see* Metrafazoline.

5,6,7,8-Tetrahydro-1-(2-imidazolin-2-ylmethyl)naphthalene *see* Tefazoline.

4,5,6,7-Tetrahydroimidazo(5,4-c)pyridine *see* Spinaceamine.

1,2,12,12a-Tetrahydro-2-isopropenyl-8,9-dimethoxy(1)benzopyrano(3,4-b)furo-(2,3-h)(1)benzopyran-6-one *see* Rotenone.

1,2,3,4-Tetrahydro-2-isopropylamino-methyl-7-nitro-6-quinolinemethanol *see* Oxamniquine.

9,10,11,11a-Tetrahydro-8H-6,11b-methanofuro(2,3-c)pyrido(1,2-a)-azepin-2-(6H)-one *see* Securinine.

O-(**1,2,3,4-Tetrahydro-1,4-methano-naphth-6-yl**) *m,N*-**dimethylthiocarb-anilate** *see* Tolciclate.

1,2,3,4-Tetrahydro-6-methoxy-1-methyl-9H-pyrido(3,4-b)indole *see* Glomerulo-trophin.

2,3,7,8-Tetrahydro-3-methylamino-1H-quino(1,8-ab)benzazepine *see* Ciclopram-ine.

1,2,3,4-Tetrahydro-2-methyl-1,4-dioxo-2-naphthalenesulfonic acid sodium salt *see* Menadione sodium bisulfite.

2-[(1,2,3,4-Tetrahydro-7-methyl-1,4-ethanonaphth-6-yl)methyl]-2-imida-zoline *see* Metrafazoline.

4,5,6,7-Tetrahydro-2-methyl-3-methyl-amino-2H-indazole *see* Tetridamine.

trans-**1,4,5,6-Tetrahydro-1-methyl-2-[2-(3-methylthien-2-yl)vinyl]pyrimidine** *see* Morantel.

Tetrahydro-3-methyl-4-(5-nitrofurfuryl-ideneamino)-1,4-thiazine 1,1-dioxide *see* Nifurtimox.

1,4,5,6-Tetrahydro-1-methyl-6-oxopyrid-azine-3-carboxamide *see* Medazomide.

1,2,3,4-Tetrahydro-2-methyl-9-phenyl-2-azafluorene *see* Phenindamine.

3,4,5,6-Tetrahydro-5-methyl-1-phenyl-1H-2,5-benzoxazocine *see* Nefopam.

2,3,4,9-Tetrahydro-2-methyl-9-phenyl-1H-indeno(2,1-c)pyridine *see* Phenindam-ine.

1,2,3,4-Tetrahydro-2-methyl-9-phenyl-2-pyridindene *see* Phenindamine.

2,3,5,6-Tetrahydro-6-[3-[(2-methyl-propionyl)amino]phenyl]imidazo(2,1-b)thiazole *see* Butamisole.

1,3,4,6-Tetrahydro-1-methyl-2-pyrimid-inemethanol α-phenylcyclohexane-glycolate *see* Oxyphencyclimine.

m-[**2-(1,4,5,6-Tetrahydro-1-methylpyrimi-din-2-yl)vinyl]phenol** *see* Oxantel.

5,6,7,8-Tetrahydro-3-methylquinoline-8-thiocarboxamide *see* Tiquinamide.

1,4,5,6-Tetrahydro-1-methyl-2-[*trans*-2-

(**thien-2-yl)vinyl]pyrimidine** *see* Pyran-tel.

1,2,3,4-Tetrahydro-1-morpholinoacetyl-3-phenylquinazolin-4-one *see* Moquizone

1,2,3,4-TETRAHYDRONAPHTHALENE ('tetralin').

1,2,3,4-TETRAHYDRO-2-NAPHTHYL-AMINE (2-aminotetralin; β-tetra).

Tetrahydronaphthylaminoimidazoline *see* Tramazoline.

1-(1,2,3,4-Tetrahydronaphth-1-yl)imid-azole-5-carboxylic acid ethyl ester *see* Etonam.

Tetrahydro-α-(1-naphthylmethyl)furan-2-propionic acid diethylaminoethyl ester *see* Naftidrofuryl.

2-(5,6,7,8-Tetrahydronaphth-1-ylmethyl)-2-imidazoline *see* Tefazoline.

Tetrahydronicotinic acid *see* Guvacine.

(±)**2,3,5,6-Tetrahydro-6-(*m*-nitrophenyl)-imidazo(2,1-b)thiazole** *see* Nitramisole.

Tetrahydronorcholenic acid lactone *see* Gitoxigenin.

Tetrahydro-1,4-oxazine *see* Morpholine.

cis-**Tetrahydro-2-oxothieno(3,4)imidazo-line-4-valeric acid** *see* Biotin.

N-(**Tetrahydro-2-oxothien-3-yl)acetamide** *see* Citiolone.

TETRAHYDROPAPAVEROLINE (1-(3,4-dihydroxybenzyl)-1,2,3,4-tetrahydro-6,7-dihydroxyisoquinoline; 1,2,3,4-tetrahydro-6,7-dihydroxy-1-protocate-chuylisoquinoline; norlaudanosoline).

1,2,3,6-Tetrahydro-1,2,2,6,6-pentamethyl-pyridine *see* Dropempine.

Tetrahydrophenobarbital *see* Cyclobar-bital.

Tetrahydro-6-(phenoxymethyl)-2H-1,3-oxazine-2-thione *see* Tifemoxone.

2,3,5,6-Tetrahydro-5-phenyl-1H-imidazo(1,2-a)imidazole *see* Deximafen; Imafen.

2,3,5,6-Tetrahydro-6-phenylimidazo-(2,1-b)thiazole *see* Dexamisole; Levami-sole; Tetramisole.

1,2,3,4-Tetrahydro-1-phenyl-1,4-naphthal-enedicarboxylic acid *see* Isatropic acid.

Tetrahydro-4-phenyl-2H-pyran-car-boxylic acid 1-methyl-3-morpholino-propyl ester *see* Fedrilate.

Tetrahydrophthalimidomethyl chrysan-themate *see* Tetramethrin.

1,3,4,9-Tetrahydro-1-propylpyrano(3,4-b)indole-1-acetic acid *see* Prodolic acid.

Tetrahydroprotoberberine *see* Berbine.

3,4,5,6-Tetrahydro-2-pyrid-3-ylpyridine *see* Anabaseine.

Tetrahydroserpentine *see* Raubasine.

3a,4,7,7a-Tetrahydro-2-[(1,1,2,2-tetra-chloroethyl)thio]-1H-isoiondole-1,3-(2H)-dione *see* Captafol.

1,2,3,4-Tetrahydro-1,2,3,4-tetraoxo-naphthalene dihydrate *see* Oxolin.

6,7,8,9-Tetrahydro-5H-tetrazoloazepine *see* Pentetrazole.

Tetrahydro-1,2,4-thiadiazine 1,1-dioxide *see* Taurultam.

TETRAHYDRO-1,3-THIAZINE (metathiazane).

Tetrahydro-1,4-thiazine *see* Thiamorpholine.

p-(Tetrahydro-1,2-thiazin-2-yl)benzenesulfonamide *see* Sultiame.

Tetrahydrothiophene, 1:1-dioxide *see* Sulfolane.

1,2,3,4-Tetrahydrothiopyrano(4,3-b)-indole-8-carboxylic acid 2-dimethylaminoethyl ester *see* Tipindole.

3a,4,7,7a-Tetrahydro-2-[(trichloromethyl)thio]-1H-isoindole-1,3(2H)-dione *see* Captan.

1,2,3,4-Tetrahydro-1-(3,4,5-trimethoxybenzyl)-6,7-isoquinolinediol *see* Tretoquinol.

1,3,4,9-Tetrahydro-N,N,1-trimethylindeno(2,1-c)pyran-1-ethylamine *see* Pirandamine.

7,8,9,10-Tetrahydro-6,6,9-trimethyl-3-pentyl-6H-dibenzo(b,d)pyran-1-ol *see* Tetrahydrocannabinol.

Tetrahydroxyadipic acid *see* Mucic acid.

2,3,7,8-Tetrahydroxy(1)benzopyrano-(5,4,3-cde)(1)benzopyran-5,10-dione *see* Ellagic acid.

Tetrahydroxy-p-benzoquinone *see* Tetroquinone.

5-(D-arabino-1,2,3,4-Tetrahydroxybutyl)-2-methyl-3-furoic acid methyl ester tetranicotinate *see* Nicofurate.

2′,3,5,7-Tetrahydroxyflavone *see* Datiscetin.

3,4′,5,7-Tetrahydroxyflavone *see* Kaempferol.

3′,4′,5,7-Tetrahydroxyflavone *see* Luteolin.

2,3,7,8-Tetrahydroxy-5-methylaminomethyldibenzo(a,e)cycloheptatriene *see* Adnamine.

β′,3′,4,5′-Tetrahydroxy-α-methyldiphenethylamine *see* Fenoterol.

Tetrahydroxyneopentane *see* Pentaerythritol.

11β,16α,17,21-Tetrahydroxypregna-1,4-diene-3,30-dione cyclic 16,17-acetal with acetone *see* Desonide.

Tetrahydroxyquinone *see* Tetroquinone.

3α,4β,7α,15-Tetrahydroxyscirp-9-en-8-one *see* Nivalenol.

Tetrahydrozolin* *see* Tetryzoline.

Tetraiodobenzoquinone(s) *see* Iodanil; Isoiodanil.

Tetraiodophthalein *see* Iodophthalein.

3,5,3′,5′-Tetraiodothyroacetic acid *see* Tetrac.

3,5,3′,5′-Tetraiodothyronine *see* Dextrothyroxine; Levothyroxine; Thyroxine.

Tetraiodum *see* Iodophthalein.

Tetraisopropylphosphorodiamidic anhydride *see* Iso-OMPA.

N,N′,N″,N‴-Tetraisopropylpyrophosphoramide *see* Iso-OMPA.

Tetraisopropylpyrophosphorotetramide *see* Iso-OMPA.

TETRAKIS(1-AZIRIDINYL)-p-BENZOQUINONE (tetraethyleniminobenzoquinone; 2,3,5,6-tetraaziridinyl-p-benzoquinone; TEB; NSC-31717).

Tetrakis(hydroxymagnesium)decahydroxydialuminate dihydrate *see* Magaldrate.

Tetrakis(methylsulfonyl)mannitol *see* Mannosulfan.

'Tetralex' *see* Tetrachloroethylene.

Tetralin *see* Tetrahydronaphthalene.

Tetrallobarbital *see* Butalbital.

'Tetralysal' *see* Lymecycline.

'Tetram' *see* Amiton.

Tetrameprozine *see* Aminopromazine.

Tetramesylmannitol *see* Mannosulfan.

Tetramethanesulfonylmannitol *see* Mannosulfan.

Tetramethoxyberbine *see* Xylopinine.

TETRAMETHRIN* ((1,3,4,5,6,7-hexahydro-1,3-dioxo-2H-isoindol-2-yl)methyl 2,2-dimethyl-3-(2-methyl-1-propenyl)-cyclopropanecarboxylate; N-[[2,2-dimethyl-3-(2-methyl-1-propenyl)cyclopropanecarbonyloxy]methyl]-3,4,5,6-tetrahydrophthalimide; tetrahydrophthalimidomethyl chrysanthemate; neopinamine; phthalthrin; 'neopynamin').

N,N,10,10-Tetramethyl-△⁹(10H),γ-anthracenepropylamine *see* Melitracen.

N,N,N′,N′-Tetramethylazoformamide *see* Diamide.

1,2,4,5-Tetramethylbenzene *see* Durene.

Tetramethyl-p-benzoquinone *see* Duroquinone.

(1,1,3,3-Tetramethylbutyl)guanidine *see* Guanoctine.

2-[2-[2-[p-(1,1,3,3-Tetramethylbutyl)-phenoxy]ethoxy]ethoxy]ethanesulfonic acid *see* Entsufon.

α-[p-(1,1,3,3-Tetramethylbutyl)phenyl]-ω-hydroxypoly(oxyethylene) *see* Octoxinol.

p-(1,1,3,3-Tetramethylbutyl)phenyl polyoxyethylene derivative *see* Tyloxapol.

N,N,2,2-TETRAMETHYLCYCLOHEXYLAMINE (2,2-dimethyl-1-dimethylaminocyclohexane; penhexamin).

2,2,9,9-Tetramethyl-1,10-decanediol *see* Gemcadiol.

TETRAMETHYLENE-1,4-BIS(1-METHYLPIPERIDINIUM IODIDE) (tetramine).

3,3′-[Tetramethylenebis[oxy(2-hydroxytrimethylene)(acetylimino)]]bis[2,4,6-triiodo-5-(N-methylacetamido)benzoic acid] *see* Iozomic acid.

1,1′-Tetramethylenebis(1,2,3,4-tetrahydro-6,7-dimethoxyisoquinoline) *see* Bisobrin.

Tetramethylenediamine *see* Putrescine.

Tetramethylene dimesilate *see* Busulfan.

1-Tetramethylene-3-p-toluenesulfonylurea *see* Tolpyrramide.

3,7,11,15-Tetramethylhexadecanoic acid *see* Phytanic acid.

3,7,11,15-Tetramethyl-2-hexadecen-1-ol *see* Phytol.

Tetramethylmethane see Neopentane.
Tetramethylolmethane see Pentaerythritol.
Tetramethylpalmitic acid see Phytanic acid.
2,6,10,14-Tetramethylpentadecane see Pristane.
Tetramethylphosphorodiamidic azide see Mazidox.
Tetramethylphosphorodiamidic fluoride see Dimefox.
1,2,2,6-Tetramethyl-4-piperidinol mandelate see Eucatropine.
2,2,6,6-TETRAMETHYLPIPERID-4-ONE TOSILATE (tetramethyl-4-oxopiperidine *p*-toluenesulfonate; 'tempidon').
2,2,6,6-TETRAMETHYLQUINUCLIDINE METHIODIDE (imequin; temechine; temequine).
O,O,O',O'-Tetramethyl O,O'-(thiodi-4,1-phenylene)phosphorothioate see Temefos.
Tetramethylthioperoxycarbonic diamide see Thiram.
Tetramethylthiuram disulfide see Thiram.
2,2,5,5-Tetramethyl-α-(o-toloxymethyl)-1-pyrrolidineethanol see Lotucaine.
Tetramethyltrimethylenehexamethylenebis(ammonium bromide)polymer see Hexadimethrine.
Tetramin (tr) see Tetramethylene-1,4-bis-(1-methylpiperidinium iodide).
TETRAMISOLE*** ((±)-2,3,5,6-tetrahydro-6-phenylimidazo(2,1-b)thiazole; tetramisole hydrochloride; tetramizole; McN-JR-8299-11; R-8299; 'anthelvet', 'citarin', 'concurat', 'drofenite', 'nilverm', 'ripercol', 'vadephen').
See also Dexamisole; Levamisole.
Tetramizole see Tetramisole.
Tetramon see Tetrylammonium.
'Tetran' see Oxytetracycline.
'Tetranase' see Tetracycline with bromelains.
Tetranicotinoylfructofuranose see Nicofuranose.
'Tetranitrin' see Erythrityl tetranitrate.
1,2,3,4-TETRANITROCARBAZOLE (Hö-2374; 'holfidal').
'Tetranitrol' see Erythrityl tetranitrate.
Tetranium see Tetrylammonium.
'Tetraolean' see Tetracycline with oleandomycin.
4,7,10,13-Tetraoxahexadecane-1,16-dioylbis(3-carboxy-2,4,6-triiodoanilide) see Iodoxamic acid.
Tetrapon* see Opium alkaloids.
α,α,6,6-Tetrapyrid-2-ylmethano-1,4-cyclopentadienemethanol see Pyrinoline.
TETRASODIUM EDETATE (ethylenediaminetetraacetic acid tetrasodium salt; edetate sodium; tetrasodium EDTA; 'aquamollin', 'calsol', 'distol-8', 'endrate', 'irgalon', 'kalex', 'nervanaid B', 'nullapon', 'syntes-12A', 'tetrine', 'tyclarosol').
Tetrastigmine* see Tetraethylpyrophosphate.

TETRASUL* (2,4,4',5-tetrachlorodiphenyl sulfide; 1,2,4-trichloro-5-[(*p*-chlorophenyl)-thio]benzene; 'animert').
Tetrathion (tr) see Thiram.
Tetraynoic acid see Eicosa-5,8,11,14-tetraynoic acid.
1-TETRAZENE (NH:N.NH.NH$_2$).
2-TETRAZENE(NH$_2$.N:N.NH$_2$).
TETRAZEPAM** (7-chloro-5-cyclohexen-1-yl-1,3-dihydro-1-methyl-2H-1,4-benzodiazepin-2-one; CB-4261; 'myolastan').
TETRAZOLIUM BLUE (3,3'-(3,3'-dimethoxy-4,4'-biphenylene)bis(2,5-diphenyl(2H)-tetrazolium chloride); 3,3'-dianisolebis-[4,4'-(3,5-diphenyltetrazolium chloride)]; ditetrazolium chloride; blue tetrazolium; BT).
Tetrazolium red see 2,3,5-Triphenyltetrazolium chloride.
Tetrazolo(1,5)perhydroazepine see Pentetrazole.
7-[2-(1H-Tetrazol-1-yl)acetamido]-3-[(1,3,4-thiadiazol-2-ylthio)methyl]-2-cephem-2-carboxylic acid see Ceftezole.
m-(1H-Tetrazol-5-yloxy)phenol see Melizame.
3-Tetrazol-5-ylthioxanthen-9-one 10,10-dioxide see Doxantrazole.
'Tetrex' see Hexacycline.
TETRIDAMINE*** (4,5,6,7-tetrahydro-2-methyl-3-methylamino-2H-indazole).
Tetridin (tr) see Pyrithyldione.
'Tetrim' see Rolitetracycline nitrate.
'Tetrine' see Tetrasodium edetate.
TETRIPROFEN*** (*p*-(1-cyclohexen-1-yl)-hydratropic acid; 1-[*p*-(1-carboxyethyl)-phenyl]cyclohexene; 2-[*p*-(cyclohexen-1-yl)phenyl]propionic acid).
'Tetriv' see Rolitetracycline nitrate.
TETROLIC ACID (2-butynoic acid; methylpropiolic acid).
'Tetron' see Tetraethyl pyrophosphate.
'Tetronal' see Dimethylsulfonal.
TETROQUINONE*** (tetrahydroxy-*p*-benzoquinone; tetrahydroxyquinone; HPEK; THQ; 'kelox').
Tetrothalein see Iodophthalein.
TETROXOPRIM*** (2,4-diamino-5-[3,5-dimethoxy-4-(2-methoxyethoxy)benzyl]-pyrimidine).
TETRYLAMMONIUM BROMIDE*** (tetraethylammonium bromide; tetamon; tetramon; tetranium; TEA; TMD-10).
TETRYZOLINE*** (2-(1,2,3,4-tetrahydro-1-naphthyl)-2-imidazoline; tetrahydrozoline; 'tyzanol', 'tyzine', 'visine').
'Tetucur' see Ferropolimaler.
Teturam (tr) see Disulfiram.
'Tevacycline' see Hexacycline.
'Texofors' see under Cetomacrogols.
TGCH see Thioglycolcholine.
TGR see Thioguanosine.
Th-152 see Orciprenaline.
Th-1064 see Dimorpholamine.
Th-1165a see Fenoterol.
Th-1314 see Ethionamide.
Th-1325 see Hydracarbazine.

Th-1395 *see* Glybuthiazole.
Th-1405 *see* Ethionamide sulfoxide.
Th-2131 *see* Pempidine.
Th-2132 *see* Sulfasomizole.
Th-2516 *see* Hydracarbazine with pempidine.
Th-3624 *see* Isonicotinthioamide.
Th-4082 *see* Hydratropic acid.
Th-4114 *see* Phenobutiodil.
Th-4128 *see* 2-Phenylbutyramide.
THA *see* Tacrine.
'Thalamonal' *see* Droperidol with fentanyl.
THALIDOMIDE*** (*N*-(2,6-dioxopiperid-
3-yl)phthalimide; 3-(*N*-phthalimido)-
glutarimide; α-(*N*-phthalimido)glutari-
mide).
THALLIUM SULFATE ('doramu', 'quick-
kill', 'zelio').
THAM *see* Trometamol.
'Thapsin' *see* Calycopterin.
'Thawpit' *see* Carbon tetrachloride.
'Thean' *see* Proxyphylline.
'Thebacetyl' *see* Thebacon.
THEBACON ** (6-acetoxy-4,5-epoxy-
3-methoxy-*N*-methylmorphin-6-ene;
acetyldesmethyldihydrothebaine; acetyl-
dihydrocodeinone; dihydrocodeinone enol
acetate; hydrocodone enol acetate; theba-
codon; 'acedicon', 'acetylcocone', 'cofadi-
con', 'novocodon', 'thebacetyl').
THEBAINE (codeinone (enol) methyl ether;
dimethylmorphine; paramorphine).
'Thebes' *see* Protheobromine.
Thecodine (tr) *see* Oxycodone.
Theelin *see* Estrone.
Theelol *see* Estriol.
'Thefanil' *see* Thenyldiamin.
Thein *see* Caffeine.
'Thekodin' *see* Codeine methyl bromide.
'Thelmesan' *see* Dimantine.
'Thelmin' *see* Piperazine.
'Themalon' *see* Thiambutene.
'Themisone' *see* Atrolactamide.
Thenaldehyde *see* Thiophenecarboxalde-
hyde.
THENALIDINE*** (1-methyl-4-[*N*-
(2-thenyl)anilino]piperidine; 1-methyl-
4-[phenyl-(2-thenyl)amino]piperidine;
thenophenopiperidine; thenopiperidine).
THENALIDINE TARTRATE (AS-716;
'sandosten').
'Thenfadil' *see* Thenyldiamine.
THENIUM CLOSILATE*** (dimethyl-
(2-phenoxyethyl)-2-thenylammonium
p-chlorobenzenesulfonate; thenium closy-
late; BW-611C65; 'ancaris', 'bancaris',
'canopar').
Thenoic acid *see* Thiophenecarboxylic acid.
Thenophenopiperidine *see* Thenalidine.
Thenopiperidine *see* Thenalidine.
p-2-Thenoylhydratropic acid *see* Suprofen.
2-(*p*-2-Thenoylphenyl)propionic acid *see*
Suprofen.
THENYLDIAMINE* (*N*,*N*-dimethyl-*N*'-
(2-pyridyl)-*N*'-(3-thenyl)ethylenediamine;
dethylandiamine; WIN-2848; 'tenfidil',
'thefanil', 'thenfadil').
Thenylpyramine *see* Methapyrilene.

THEOBROMINE (3,7-dimethylxanthine;
santheose).
Theobromineacetic acid *see* Theobrominyl
acetic acid.
**THEOBROMINE CALCIUM SALICYL-
ATE** (calcium theobromsal; theosalicin).
THEOBROMINE SODIUM SALICYLATE
(salnabrom; theobromsal).
THEOBROMIN-1-YLACETIC ACID
(1-(carboxymethyl)theobromine; theobromineacetic acid).
See also (2-Bromoethyl)trimethylammo-
nium theobromin-1-ylacetate; Dextropropoxyphene theobromin-1-ylacetate.
Theobromsal *see* Theobromine sodium
salicylate.
Theoclate(s)* *see* Teoclate(s).
'Theocor' *see* Protheobromine.
THEODRENALINE*** (7-[2-[2-(3,4-di-
hydroxyphenyl)-2-hydroxyethylamino]-
ethyl]theophylline; L-theodrenaline
hydrochloride; 7-[2-(β,3,4-trihydroxy-
phenethylamino)ethyl]theophylline;
noradrenalinetheophylline).
See also Cafedrine with theodrenaline.
'Theo-heptylon' *see* Heptaminol theophyl-
lineacetate.
Theomedrine *see* Chlormerodrin theo-
phylline.
'Theon' *see* Proxyphylline.
Theophyllamine* *see* Aminophylline.
THEOPHYLLINE (1,3-dimethylxanthine).
See also below and Carbocisteine with theo-
phylline; Proscillaridin with theophylline.
Theophyllineacetic acid *see* Theophyllinyl-
acetic acid.
Theophylline-aminoisobutanol *see*
Bufylline.
Theophylline cholinate *see* Choline
theophyllinate.
Theophylline-diethylenediamine *see*
Theophylline-piperazine.
THEOPHYLLINE EPHEDRINE*** (com-
pound of theophylline with (−)-ephe-
drine).
See also Etophylline with theophylline
ephedrine.
Theophylline-ethylenediamine *see*
Aminophylline.
Theophylline-isobutanolamine *see*
Bufylline.
Theophylline-merodrin *see* Chlormerodrin-
theophylline.
Theophylline-methylglucamine *see*
Theophylline-meglumine.
THEOPHYLLINE-PIPERAZINE
(theophylline-diethylenediamine).
Theophylline piperazine acetate *see*
Acefylline piperazine.
Theophylline-piperazine ethanoate *see*
Acefylline piperazine.
THEOPHYLLINE SODIUM GLYCINATE
(1 mol. theophylline with 2 mol. Na amino-
acetate).
THEOPHYLLIN-7-YLACETIC ACID
(7-(carboxymethyl)theophylline; theo-
phyllineacetic acid).

See also Heptaminol theophyllinylacetate; Sodium theophyllinylacetate.

'Theoxylline' *see* Choline theophyllinate.

'Thephorin' *see* Phenindamine.

'Therabloat' *see* Poloxalene.

'Theralene' *see* Alimemazine.

'Theraleptique' *see* Dimorpholamine.

'Therapas' *see* Calcium benzamidosalicylate.

'Theraplix' *see* Glybuzole.

'Theraptique' *see* Dimorpholamine.

'Theratuss' *see* Pipazetate.

'Therminol' *see* Polychlorinated biphenyl mixture.

'Thermogene' *see* Capsaicin.

'Theruhistin' *see* Isothipendyl.

THETIN (2,2-dihydro-1,2-oxathietan-4-one).

'Theuralon' *see* Diethylthiambutene.

Thiabendazole* *see* Tiabendazole.

Thiabenzonium *see* Tibezonium iodide.

Thiabutizide *see* Butizide.

THIACETARSAMIDE SODIUM***
(disodium salt of *S,S*-diester of *p*-carbamoyldithiobenzenearsonous acid with mercaptoacetic acid; disodium salt of *p*-[bis-(carboxymethylmercapto)arsino]benzamide; 'arsenamide').

THIACETAZONE* (4'-formylacetanilide thiosemicarbazone; *p*-acetamidobenzaldehyde thiosemicarbazone; amithiozone; ambathizon; thioacetazone; tibon; RP-4207; Sdt-1-41; SHCH-87; TbI/698).

Thiachroman *see* Thiochroman.

Thiachromane *see* Meticrane.

'Thiactin' *see* Thiostrepton.

Thiacyclobutane *see* Thietane.

Thiadenol *see* Tiadenol.

9-Thia-1,10-diazanthracene *see* Pyrido-(3,2-b)(1,4)benzothiazine.

'Thiadipon' *see* Bentazepam.

THIALBARBITAL* (5-allyl-5-(2-cyclohexen-1-yl)-2-thiobarbituric acid; thialbarbitone; thiohexallymal; 'intranarcon', 'kemithal').

Thialbarbitone *see* Thialbarbital.

Thialbutone* *see* Buthalital.

Thialisobumal *see* Buthalital.

THIAMAZOLE* (1-methyl-2-imidazolethiol; 2-mercapto-1-methylimidazole; methylmercaptoimidazole; methimazole; mercazolyl; thymidazole; timidazole).

THIAMAZOLE METHIODIDE ('jomezol').

THIAMBUTENE* (3-amino-1,1-bis(2-thienyl)-1-butene; 'themalon').

THIAMBUTOSINE* (1-(*p*-butoxyphenyl)-3-(*p*-dimethylaminophenyl)-2-thiourea; 4-butoxy-4'-dimethylaminothiocarbanilide; C-15095-E).

Thiamethonium *see* Tiametonium.

'Thiameton' *see* Tiametonium.

THIAMINE** (3-(4-amino-2-methyl-5-pyrimidylmethyl)-5-(2-hydroxyethyl)-4-methylthiazolium chloride; aneurine; vitamin B$_1$).

Thiamine acetylthiooctyl disulfide *see* Octotiamine.

Thiamine allyl disulfide *see* Allithiamine.

Thiamine monophosphate *see* Mono-phosphothiamine.

THIAMINE PHOSPHORIC ESTER PHOSPHATE SALT ('umbeon').

Thiamine propyl disulfide *see* Prosultiamine.

Thiamine pyrophosphate *see* Cocarboxylase.

Thiamine tetrahydrofurfuryl disulfide *see* Fursultiamine.

Thiamiprine *see* Tiamiprine.

Thiamizide* *see* Tiamizide.

Thiamorpholine *see* Thiomorpholine.

THIAMPHENICOL* (D(+)-*threo*-2-dichloroacetamido-1-(*p*-methylsulfonylphenyl)-1,3-propanediol; D(+)-*threo*-2,2-dichloro-*N*-[β-hydroxy-α-(hydroxymethyl)-*p*-(methylsulfonyl)phenethyl]acetamide; dextrosulfenidol; thiophenicol; CB-8053; WIN-5063-2; 'glitisol', 'thiocymetin').

Thiamphenicol aminoacetate *see* Thiamphenicol glycinate.

THIAMPHENICOL GLYCINATE (thiamphenicol aminoacetate; 'neomyson G', 'urfamicina', 'urfamycin').

THIAMYLAL* (5-allyl-5-(1-methylbutyl)-2-thiobarbituric acid sodium derivative; 5-allyl-5-isoamyl-2-thiobarbituric acid sodium derivative; thiamylal sodium; 'surital', 'thiethamyl', 'thioseconal').

Thianide (tr) *see* Ethionamide.

'Thiantoin' *see* Thyphenytoin.

Thiasine *see* Thioneine.

Thiasolucin *see* Noprylsulfamide.

'Thiaver' *see* Epitizide.

Thiaxanthene *see* Thioxanthene.

1,4-Thiazan *see* Thiomorpholine.

Thiazenone *see* Tiazesim.

Thiazesium* *see* Tiazesim.

Thiazinamon *see* Thiazinamium.

THIAZINAMIUM* ((1-methyl-2-phenothiazin-10-ylethyl)trimethylammonium chloride (or other salt)); promethazine methochloride; thiazinamon; RP-3554; 'multergan', 'multezin', 'padisal').

THIAZOLIDINE (tetrahydrothiazole).

Thiazolidine-4-carboxylic acid *see* Timonacic.

Thiazolidine-2,4-dicarboxylic acid *see* Tidiacic.

4-THIAZOLINE-2-THIONE (2-mercaptothiazoline; 'thyroidan').

THIAZOLINOBUTAZONE (phenylbutazone compound (salt) with 2-amino-2-thiazoline; LAS-11871; 'fordonal').

2-Thiazol-4-ylbenzimidazole *see* Tiabendazole.

2-Thiazol-4-yl-5-benzimidazolecarbamic acid isopropyl ester *see* Cambendazole.

N-Thiazol-2-yl-*p*-phenosulfonamide *see* Phenosulfazole.

5-[*p*-(2-Thiazolylsulfamoyl)phenylazo]-salicylic acid *see* Salazosulfathiazole.

4'-(Thiazol-2-ylsulfamoyl)succinanilic acid *see* Succinylfathiazole.

N^1-Thiazol-2-ylsulfanilamide *see* Sulfathiazole.

Thiazolsulfone *see* Thiazosulfone.

Thiazon *see* Dazomet.
THIAZOSULFONE*** (*p*-aminophenyl
2-amino-5-thiazolyl sulfone; 2-amino-
5-sulfanilylthiazole; thiazolsulfone; 'promizole').
2-Thiazylamine *see* Aminothiazole.
THIBENZAZOLINE (benzimidazole-1,3-
dimethanol-2-thione; 1,3-bis(hydroxymethyl)benzimidazole-2-thione; 'thyreocordon').
'Thibenzole' *see* Tiabendazole.
'Thibetine' *see* Trolnitrate.
Thidoxol *see* Tioxolone.
7-(2-Thienylacetamido)cephalosporanic
acid *see* Cefalotin.
N-[7-(2-Thienylacetamido)ceph-3-em-
3-ylmethylpyridinium]-4-carboxylate
see Cefaloridine.
Thienylacetic acid *see* Thiopheneacetic
acid.
α-Thien-3-ylcyclohexaneacetic acid
2-hexamethyleniminoethyl ester *see*
Cetiedil.
Thienylglycolic acid *see* Thiopheneglycolic
acid.
6-(Thienylmalonamido)penicillanic acid
see Ticarcillin.
THIETANE (trimethylene sulfide; thiacyclobutane; thiethane).
'Thiethamyl' *see* Thiamylal.
Thiethane *see* Thietane.
THIETHYLPERAZINE*** (2-ethylthio-
10-[3-(4-methylpiperazin-1-yl)propyl]-
phenothiazine; thietylperazine; tiethyl-
perazine).
THIETHYLPERAZINE MALEATE*
(thiethylperazine dimaleate; GS-95;
'torecan').
Thietylperazine *see* Thiethylperazine.
Thifen (tr) *see* Thiphen.
Thifenamil* *see* Tifenamil.
'Thifor' *see* Endosulfan.
THIHEXINOL METHYLBROMIDE***
(*trans*-[(4-hydroxydi-2-thienylmethyl)cyclo-
hexyl]trimethylammonium bromide;
trans-α,α-(dithien-2-yl)-4-dimethylamino-
cyclohexyl methyl carbinol bromide;
5-[(4-dimethylaminocyclohexyl)hydroxy-
methyl]-*trans*-2,2'-bithiophene methyl
bromide).
'Thilatazin' *see* Perphenazine.
'Thilaven' *see* Ammonium sulfobituminate.
'Thilorbin' *see* Fluorescein.
Thimerfonate *see* Sodium timerfonate.
'Thimerosal' *see* Thiomersal.
'Thimet' *see* Phorate.
Thimethaphan *see* Trimetaphan camsilate.
'Thimul' *see* Endosulfan.
Thioacetazone*** *see* Thiacetazone.
THIOAMBUCAINE (4-amino-2-butoxy-
benzoate ester of 2-diethylaminoethane-
thiol; WIN-3800).
Thioamobarbital *see* Thioethamyl.
Thioarsphenamine *see* Sulfarsphenamine.
Thiobaral (tr) *see* Thiobarbital.
THIOBARBITAL (5,5-diethyl-2-thiobar-
bituric acid; thiobaral; 'ibition', 'sedo-

thyron', 'thiothyr', 'thiotyr', 'thyreosedine').
Thiobenzoic acid benzyl thioester *see*
Tibenzate.
'Thiobilin' *see* Tidiacic plus sorbitol.
2,2'-Thiobis(4-chlorophenol) *see* Fenticlor.
2,2'-Thiobis(4,6-dichlorophenoxide) *see*
Bithionol.
THIOBUTABARBITAL (5-ethyl-5-(1-
methylpropyl)-2-thiobarbituric acid;
5-*sec*-butyl-5-ethyl-2-thiobarbituric acid;
'inactin', 'inaktin', 'narkothion', 'veno-
barbital').
Thiobutazine *see* Butizide.
Thiobutone *see* Buthalitone.
THIOCAINE (2-diethylaminoethyl ester of
p-aminothiolbenzoic acid).
Thiocarbamide *see* Thiourea.
*N*¹-Thiocarbamylsulfanilamide *see*
Sulfathiourea.
THIOCARBANILIDE (1,3-diphenyl-2-
thiourea).
THIOCARBOXIM* (2-cyanoethyl
N-[[(methylamino)carbonyl]oxy]ethan-
imidothioate; 2-cyanoethyl *N*-(methyl-
carbamoyloxy)acetimidothioate; 'talcord').
Thiocarlide* *see* Tiocarlide.
THIOCHOLINE ((2-mercaptoethyl)tri-
methylammonium hydroxide or salts).
Thiocholine acetate *see* Acetylthiocholine.
THIOCHROMAN (dihydrobenzothiopyran;
thiachroman).
'Thiochrysine' *see* Sodium aurotiosulfate.
Thiocol *see* Sulfogaiacol.
THIOCOLCHICOSIDE** (4-acetamido-
15-glucopyranosyloxy-13,14-dimethoxy-
8-methylthio-7-oxotricyclo(10.4.0.0⁵,¹¹)-
hexadeca-1(12),5,8,10,13,15-hexaene;
2,10-di(demethoxy)-2-glucosyloxy-10-
methylthiocolchicine; 2,14-bis(desmethoxy)-
2-glucosidoxy-14-methylthiocolchicine;
'coltromyl').
'Thiocolciran' *see* Deacetylthiocolchicine.
'Thiocron' *see* Amidithion.
THIOCTIC ACID (α-lipoic acid; 6,8-di-
thiooctanoic acid; thiooctanoic acid;
5-(1,2-dithiolan-3-yl)valeric acid; acetate-
replacing factor; pyruvate-oxidation factor;
protogen A; 'heparlipon', 'thioctidase').
Thioctic acid trometamol ester *see*
Trometamol thioctate.
'Thioctidase' *see* Thioctic acid.
THIOCYANIC ACID (rhodanic acid; sulfo-
cyanic acid).
'Thiocymetin' *see* Thiamphenicol.
'Thiodan' *see* Endosulfan.
Thiodemeton *see* Disulfoton.
3,3'-Thiodialanine *see* Lanthionine.
Thiodiethylenebis(ethyldimethylam-
monium iodide) *see* Tiametonium iodide.
THIODIGLYCOL*** (2,2'-thiodiethanol;
bis(2-hydroxyethyl) sulfide; 'tedegyl').
'Thiodin' *see* Thiosinamine ethiodide.
Thiodiphenylamine *see* Phenothiazine.
O,*O*'-Thiodi(*p*-phenylene) phosphoro-
thioate *see* Tetrafenphos.
O,*O*'-(Thiodi-*p*-phenylene) *O*,*O*,*O*',*O*'-
tetramethyl bis(phosphorothioate)

see Temefos.

THIODIPIN (tr) (1,4-piperazinediylbis-[bis(1-aziridinyl)phosphine sulfide]; *N,N*'-diethylenebis(*N,N*'-diethylene-phosphorothioic diamide); 1,4-bis[(*N,N*'-bisethylene)diamidothiophosphoryl]-piperazine).

2,2'-Thiodipyridine 1,1'-dioxide *see* Dipyrithione.

THIOETHAMYL (5-ethyl-5-(3-methyl-butyl)-2-thiobarbituric acid; 5-ethyl-5-isoamyl-2-thiobarbituric acid; thioamobarbital; V-7; 'venesetic').

Thioethanolamine *see* Mercaptamine.

THIOFURADENE* (1-(5-nitrofurylidene-amino)imidazoline-2-thione; 'furidin').

Thiofuran *see* Thiophene.

Thiofurfuran *see* Thiophene.

'Thiogenal' *see* Methitural.

Thioglucose S-gold derivative *see* Aurothioglucose.

(1-Thio-β-D-glucopyranosato)(triethyl-phosphine)gold 2,3,4,6-tetraacetate *see* Auranofin.

THIOGLYCOLCHOLINE (choline thioglycolate ester; TGCH).

THIOGLYCOLIC ACID (2-mercaptoacetic acid).

Thioguanine* *see* Tioguanine.

6-Thioguanine *see* Tioguanine.

6-Thioguanine riboside *see* Thioguanosine.

THIOGUANOSINE (2-amino-9-(β-D-ribofuranosyl)purine-6-thiol; thioguanine riboside; tioguanine riboside; TGR; NSC-29422; SK-18615).

Thiohexallymal* *see* Thialbarbital.

THIOHEXAMIDE* (1-cyclohexyl-3-(*p*-methylthiobenzenesulfonyl)urea).

THIOHEXETHAL (5-ethyl-5-hexyl-2-thiobarbituric acid).

Thioinosine *see* Mercaptopurine riboside.

'Thiola' *see* Tiopronin.

Thiole *see* Thiophene.

Thiolhistidine-betaine *see* Thioneine.

Thiolosystox *see* Demeton-S.

THIOMALIC ACID (mercaptosuccinic acid).

Thiomebumal* *see* Thiopental.

'Thiomedon' *see* Acetylmethionine.

'Thiomerin' *see* Mercaptomerin.

THIOMERSAL* (sodium salt of *o*-(ethyl-mercurithio)benzoic acid; sodium ethyl-mercurithiosalicylate; mercurothiolate; thimerosal; thiomersalate).

THIOMERSAL TANNATE ('amertan').

Thiomersalate* *see* Thiomersal.

Thiomesterone* *see* Tiomesterone.

Thiomethibumal* *see* Methitural.

THIOMETON* (*S*-[2-(ethylthio)ethyl] *O,O*-dimethyl phosphorodithioate; dithiomethon; dithiometon; M-81; 'aasystem', 'Duphar dimeaat', 'ekatin', 'intrathion', 'intration', 'luxan', 'sysmeton').

Thiometon ethyl *see* Disulfoton.

THIOMORPHOLINE (tetrahydro-1,4-thiazine; parathiazan; thiamorpholine; 1,4-thiazan).

'Thiomucase' *see* Chondroitinase.

THIONAZIN* (*O,O*-diethyl *O*-pyrazinyl phosphorothioate; *O,O*-diethyl *O*-1,4-diazinyl phosphorothioate; 'cynem', 'nemafos', 'nemaphos', 'zinophos').

THIONEINE (thiohistidine trimethyl-betaine; methyl ester betaine of 2-mercapto-*N,N*-dimethylhistidine; thiolhistidine-betaine; ergothioneine; ergothionone; sympectothion; thiasine; thiozone).

'Thionembutal' *see* Thiopental.

'Thionex' *see* Endosulfan.

THIONINE (7-amino-3-imino(3H)pheno-thiazine; Lauth's violet).

THIONINE CHLORIDE (3,7-diamino-phenothiazonium chloride).

THIONOL (7-hydroxy(3H)phenothiazin-3-one; hydroxyphenothiazone).

N-Thiononicotinoylamphetamine *see* Thiophenatin.

Thionosystox *see* Demeton-O.

Thiooctanoic acid *see* Thioctic acid.

Thiooxazolidinone *see* Oxazolidinethione.

Thiopanic acid *see* Pantolactone.

THIOPENTAL SODIUM* (sodium derivative of 5-ethyl-5-(1-methylbutyl)-2-thiobarbituric acid; penthiobarbital; pentothiobarbital; thiomebumal; thio-pentobarbital; thiopentemal; thiopentone; RP-245; V-5; 'farmotal', 'intraval', 'leopental', 'nesdonal', 'penthotal', 'pharmothal', 'thionembutal', 'thiotal', 'thiothal', 'tio-pentemal', 'tranapal', 'trapanal').

Thiopentemal* *see* Thiopental.

Thiopentone* *see* Thiopental.

Thioperazine *see* Thioproperazine.

THIOPHANATE* (diethyl 4,4'-*o*-phenyl-enebis(3-thioallophanate); 4,4'-*o*-phenyl-enebis(3-thioallophanic acid) diethyl ester; 1,2-bis(3-carbethoxy-2-thioureido)benzene; 1,2-bis(3-ethoxycarbonyl-2-thioureido)-benzene; 1,1'-*o*-phenylenebis[3-(ethoxy-carbonyl)-2-thiourea]; diethyl [1,2-phenylenebis(iminocarbonothioyl)]bis-(carbamate); NF-35; 'cercobin', 'topsin').

THIOPHANATE-METHYL* (dimethyl-4,4'-*o*-phenylenebis(3-thioallophanate); 4,4'-*o*-phenylenebis(3-thioallophanic acid) dimethyl ester; 1,2-bis(3-carbomethoxy-2-thioureido)benzene; 1,2-bis(3-methoxy-carbonyl-2-thioureido)benzene; 1,1'-*o*-phenylenebis[3-(methoxycarbonyl)-2-thiourea]; dimethyl [1,2-phenylenebis-(iminocarbonothioyl)]bis(carbamate); methyl thiophanate; NF-44; 'topsin M').

Thiophan sulfone *see* Sulfolane.

THIOPHENATIN (tr) (*N*-thiononicotinoyl-amphetamine; *N*-(2-phenylisopropyl)-thionicotinamide; tiofenatin).

THIOPHENE (divinylene sulfide; thiofuran; thiofurfuran; thiole; thiotetrole).

2-THIOPHENEACETIC ACID (thienyl-acetic acid).

THIOPHENECARBOXYALDEHYDE(S) (thenaldehyde(s)).

THIOPHENECARBOXYLIC ACID(S) (thenoic acid(s)).

2-THIOPHENECARBOXYLIC ACID
(α-thenoic acid).

2-THIOPHENEGLYCOLIC ACID (thienyl-glycolic acid).

6-(Thiophenemalonamido)penicillanic acid *see* Ticarcillin.

Thiophenicol *see* Thiamphenicol.

THIOPHENOBARBITAL (5-ethyl-5-phenyl-2-thiobarbituric acid; thiophenobarbital sodium).

Thiophenylpyridylamine *see* Pipazetate *and* Pyrido(3,2-b)(1,4)benzothiazine.

Thiophos-3422 *see* Parathion.

Thiophosphamide *see* Thiotepa.

Thiophosphoramide *see* Phosphorothioic triamide.
See also Phosphoramidothioic acid; Phosphoramidodithioic acid.

Thiophosphoric acid *see* Phosphorothioic acid.

Thioproline *see* Timonacic.

THIOPROPAZATE*** (10-[3-[4-(2-acetoxyethyl)piperazin-1-yl]propyl]-2-chlorophenothiazine; thiopropazate dihydrochloride; SC-7105; 'artalan', 'dartal', 'dartalan', 'dartan').

THIOPROPERAZINE*** (*N,N*-dimethyl-10-[3-(4-methylpiperazin-1-yl)propyl]-2-phenothiazinesulfonamide; 2-(dimethyl-sulfamoyl)-10-[3-(4-methylpiperazin-1-yl)-propyl]phenothiazine; thioperazine; RP-7843; 'cephalmin').

THIOPROPERAZINE MESILATE (thioproperazine methanesulfonate; 'cephalmin', 'majeptil', 'vontil').

Thiopurinol *see* Tisopurine.

THIOQUINOX* (1,3-dithiolo(4,5-b)-quinoxaline-2-thione; chinothionat; 'eradex').

THIORIDAZINE*** (10-[2-(1-methyl-piperid-2-yl)ethyl]-2-(methylthio)pheno-thiazine; thioridazine hydrochloride; TP-21; 'mallorol', 'malloryl', 'mellaril', 'melleretten', 'melleril').
See also Dihydroergotoxine with thiorid-azine.

Thioridazine dioxide *see* Sulforidazine.

Thioridazine oxide *see* Mesoridazine.

Thiosalan* *see* Tiosalan.

'Thiosan' *see* Thiram.

'Thioseconal' *see* Thiamylal.

Thiosinamide *see* Thiosinamine.

THIOSINAMINE (1-allyl-2-thiourea; rhodallin; thiosinamide; 'aminosin', 'rodallin').

THIOSINAMINE ETHIODIDE ('iodolysin', 'thiodin', 'tiodin').

THIOSINAMINE SALICYLATE ('cicatri-cine', 'fibrolysine', 'salicylysin', 'thiosinyl').

'Thiosinyl' *see* Thiosinamine salicylate.

'Thiospasmin' *see* Hexasonium.

'Thiosporin' *see* Sulfomyxin.

THIOSTREPTON (bryamycin; thiactin).

Thiosulfates *see* Calcium thiosulfate; Sodium thiosulfate.

Thiosulfites *see* Diethyl thiosulfite.

'Thiosystox' *see* Disulfoton.

'Thiotal' *see* Thiopental.

THIOTEPA*** (tris(1-aziridinyl)phosphine sulfide; *N,N',N''*-triethylenephosphoro-thioic triamide; triethylenethiophosphor-amide; tris(ethylenimino)thiophosphate; thio-TEPA; TSPA; tio-TEF; STEPA; TESPA; NSC-6396; 'girostan', 'ledertepa', 'oncotiotepa', 'tespamin', 'tifosyl', 'tiofosyl').

THIOTETRABARBITAL*** (5-ethyl-5-(1-ethylbutyl)-2-thiobarbituric acid).

Thiotetrole *see* Thiophene.

'Thiothal' *see* Thiopental.

'Thio-theo' *see* Carbocisteine with theo-phylline.

6-THIOTHEOPHYLLINE (1,3-dimethyl-6-thioxanthine; 1,3-dimethylpurin-2-one-6-thione).

Thiothixene* *see* Tiotixene.

'Thiothyr' *see* Thiobarbital.

'Thiotyr' *see* Thiobarbital.

THIOURACIL (2-thiouracil; 'antagothyroil', 'deracil').

THIOUREA (2-thiourea; thiocarbamide).

4-(Thiovanilloyl)morpholine *see* Vantiolide.

THIOXANTHENE (thiaxanthene).

N-(2-Thioxanthen-9-ylethyl)amphetamine *see* Tixadil.

'Thioxidrene' *see* Citiolone.

Thioxolone* *see* Tioxolone.

2-Thioxo-4-thiazolidinone *see* Rhodanine.

Thiozine *see* Thioneine.

Thipendyl *see* Isothipendyl.

Thiphencillin *see* Tifencillin.

THIRAM** (bis(dimethylthiocarbamoyl) disulfide; tetramethylthiuram disulfide; tetramethylthioperoxycarbonic diamide; tetrathion; TMTD; TMTDS; SQ-1489; 'arasan', 'fernasan', 'methyl-tuad', 'nobecutane', 'nomersan', 'pomarsol', 'pomasol', 'puralin', 'rezifilm', 'tersan', 'thiurad', 'thiuramyl', 'thiosan', 'thylate', 'tiuramyl', 'tuad', 'tulisan').
See also Benomyl plus thiram.

'Thitrol' *see* 4-(4-Chloro-2-methylphenoxy)-butyric acid.

'Thiurad' *see* Thiram.

'Thiuramyl' *see* Thiram.

'Thiuranide' *see* Disulfiram.

'Thiuretic' *see* Hydrochlorothiazide.

'Thixokon' *see* Sodium acetrizoate.

'Thonzide' *see* Tonzonium.

Thonzonium* *see* Tonzonium.

THONZYLAMINE*** (*N-(p*-methoxy-benzyl)-*N',N'*-dimethyl-*N*-pyrimidin-2-yl-ethylenediamine; histazylamine; thonzyl-amine hydrochloride; thonzylamine chloride).

Thonzylamine hexadecyl bromide *see* Tonzonium.

'Thoragol' *see* Bibenzonium.

'Thorazine' *see* Chlorpromazine.

THORIUM DIOXIDE SOL ('thorotrast').

'Thorotrast' *see* Thorium dioxide sol.

Thozalinone* *see* Tozalinone.

THPP *see* Diponium bromide.

THQ *see* Tetroquinone.

THREITOL (*threo*-1,2,3,4-butanetetrol).

D-**Threityl dimesilate** *see* Dihydroxybusulfan.
L-**Threityl dimesilate** *see* Treosulfan.
THREONINE (2-amino-3-hydroxybutyric acid).
'**Thrombocid**' *see* Sodium polyanhydromannuronic acid sulfate.
Thrombocytin *see* Serotonin.
'**Thrombodym**' *see* Neodymium sulfoisonicotinate.
'**Thromboliquin**' *see* Heparin.
'**Thrombolysin**' *see* Fibrinolysin.
'**Thrombophob**' *see* Heparin.
'**Thrombossoine-heparin**' *see* Diarbarone.
Thrombotonin *see* Serotonin.
'**Thrombovar**' *see* Sodium tetradecyl sulfate.
'**Thrombo-vetren**' *see* Heparin.
THS-839 *see* Denatonium.
3-Thujanone *see* Absinthol.
α-**THUJAPLICIN** (3-isopropyl-2,4,6-cycloheptatriene-2-ol-1-one; 3-isopropyltropolone).
β-**THUJAPLICIN** (4-isopropyl-2,4,6-cycloheptatrien-2-ol-1-one; 4-isopropyltropolone; hinokitiol).
γ-**THUJAPLICIN** (5-isopropyltropolone).
Thujone *see* Absinthol.
THURFYL NICOTINATE* (tetrahydrofuryl ester of nicotinic acid; nicotafuryl; 'trafuril').
THURFYL SALICYLATE (tetrahydrofuryl ester of salicylic acid).
Thuyon *see* Absinthol.
'**Thybon**' *see* Liothyronine sodium.
'**Thylate**' *see* Thiram.
'**Thylin**' *see* Nifenazone.
'**Thymergix**' *see* Pyrovalerone.
Thymic acid *see* Thymol.
Thymidazole (tr) *see* Thiamazole.
THYMIDINE (thymine 2-desoxyriboside).
THYMIDYLIC ACID (thymidine phosphate).
THYMINE (5-methyluracil; 2,4-dihydroxy-5-methylpyrimidine).
Thymine desoxyriboside *see* Thymidine.
THYMOHYDROQUINONE (*p*-cymene-2,5-diol; 2-isopropyl-5-methylhydroquinone).
THYMOL (2-isopropyl-5-methylphenol; 1-hydroxy-2-isopropyl-5-methylbenzene; 3-*p*-cymenol; *m*-thymol; thymic acid).
m-**Thymol** *see* Thymol.
Thymolated silver sulfone *see* Diathymosulfone.
THYMOQUINONE (*p*-cymene-2,5-dione; *p*-mentha-3,6-diene-2,5-dione; 2-isopropyl-5-methylbenzoquinone).
Thymosulfone *see* Diathymosulfone.
o-**THYMOTIC ACID** (3-isopropyl-6-methylsalicylic acid; 3-hydroxy-2-*p*-cymenecarboxylic acid; *o*-thymotinic acid).
See also Cetylpyridinium *o*-thymotate.
Thymotinic acid *see* Thymotic acid.
Thymoxamine* *see* Moxisylyte.
Thymyloxymethylimidazoline *see* Tymazoline.
'**Thyodan**' *see* Endosulfan.
'**Thyonex**' *see* Endosulfan.

Thypendyl *see* Isothipendyl.
THYPHENYTOIN (5-phenyl-5-(2-thienyl)-hydantoin; phetenylate; phethenylate; thyphenytoin sodium; 'thiantoin').
'**Thyreocordon**' *see* Thibenzazoline.
'**Thyreosedine**' *see* Thiobarbital.
'**Thyreostat II**' *see* Propylthiouracil.
THYROACETIC ACID (α-[4-(4-hydroxyphenoxy)phenyl]acetic acid).
Thyrocalcitonin *see* Calcitonin.
'**Thyrochlorate**' *see* Potassium perchlorate.
'**Thyroidan**' *see* 4-Thiazoline-2-thione.
'**Thyrolar**' *see* Liotrix.
Thyromedan* *see* Tyromedan.
THYRONAMINE (β-(4-hydroxyphenoxy)-phenethylamine).
THYRONINE (2-amino-4-[(4-hydroxyphenoxy)phenyl]propionic acid; 3-[4-(4-hydroxyphenoxy)phenyl]alanine).
THYROPROPIC ACID*** (4-(4-hydroxy-3-iodophenoxy)-3,5-diiodohydrocinnamic acid; 3-[4-(4-hydroxy-3-iodophenoxy)-3,5-diiodophenyl]propionic acid; triiodothyropropionic acid; triprop; 'triopron').
'**Thyrosan**' *see* Aminothiazole.
Thyrotrophic hormone *see* Thyrotrophin.
THYROTROPHIN** (thyrotrophic hormone; thyrotropin; TSH; TTH).
Thyrotrophin releasing hormone synthetic *see* Protirelin.
Thyroxin *see* Thyroxine.
THYROXINE (3,5,3',5'-tetraiodothyronine; 3-[(4-hydroxy-3,5-diiodophenoxy)-3,5-diiodophenyl]alanine; thyroxin).
See also Dextrothyroxine sodium; Levothyroxine sodium.
TIABENDAZOLE*** (2-thiazol-4-ylbenzimidazole; thiabendazole; G-491; MK-360; 'mertect', 'mintezol', 'minzol', 'polival', 'tecto', 'thibenzole').
TIADENOL*** (2,2'-(decamethylenedithio)-diethanol; 1,10-bis(2-hydroxyethylthio)-decane; 1,16-dihydroxy-3,14-dithiahexadecane; thiadenol; LL-1558; 'fonlipol').
Tiadenol bis(clofibrate) *see* Tiafibrate.
TIAFIBRATE*** (clofibric acid diester with 2,2'-(decamethylenedithio)diethanol; tiadenol bis(clofibrate)).
TIAMENIDINE*** (2-(2-chloro-4-methyl-thien-3-ylamino)-2-imidazoline; 2-chloro-3-(2-imidazolin-2-ylamino)-4-methyl-thiophene; HOE-440).
Tiameton* *see* Tiametonium.
TIAMETONIUM IODIDE*** (thiodiethylenebis(ethyldimethylammonium iodide); thiamethonium iodide; tiameton; 'thiameton').
TIAMIPRINE*** (2-amino-6-(1-methyl-4-nitroimidazol-5-ylthio)purine; 6-(1-methyl-4-nitroimidazol-5-ylthio)guanine; imidazolylthioguanine; ITG; BW-57-323; NSC-38887; 'guaneran').
TIAMIZIDE** (4-chloro-*N*-methyl-3-methyl-sulfamoylbenzamide; diapamide; thiamizide; CI-456; D-1593; 'vectren').
TIAMULIN** ([[2-(diethylamino)ethyl]thio]-acetic acid 8-ester with octahydro-5,8-

dihydroxy-4,6,9,10-tetramethyl-6-vinyl-3a,9-propano-3aH-cyclopentacycloocten-2(4H)-one).

TIANAFAC** (5-chloro-3-methylbenzo(b)-thiophene-2-acetic acid; 5-chloro-3-methylbenzo(b)thien-2-ylacetic acid; L-8109).

TIAPIRINOL*** (tetrahydro-2-[3-hydroxy-5-(hydroxymethyl)-2-methylpyrid-4-yl]-2H-1,3-thiazine-4-carboxylic acid; 4-(4-carboxytetrahydro-2H-1,3-thiazin-2-yl)-2-hydroxy-5-hydroxymethyl-2-methyl-pyridine).

TIAPRIDE*** (N-(2-diethylaminoethyl)-5-(methylsulfonyl)-o-anisamide; N-(2-diethylaminoethyl)-2-methoxy-5-(methyl-sulfonyl)benzamide); tiapride hydrochloride; FLO-1347).

TIAPROFENIC ACID** (5-benzoyl-α-methyl-2-thiopheneacetic acid; 2-(5-benzoylthien-2-yl)propionic acid; 5-benzoyl-2-(1-carboxyethyl)thiophene; 'surgam').

TIARAMIDE*** (4-[(5-chloro-2-oxobenzo-thiazolin-3-yl)acetyl]-1-piperazineethanol; 5-chloro-3-[[[4-(2-hydroxyethyl)piperazin-1-yl]carbonyl]methyl]benzothiazolin-2-one; 1-[[(5-chloro-2-oxobenzothiazolin-3-yl)-methyl]carbonyl]-4-(2-hydroxyethyl)-piperazine).

TIAZESIM*** (5-(2-dimethylaminoethyl)-2,3-dihydro-2-phenyl-1,5-benzothiazepin-4(5H)-one; thiazesim; thiazesim hydro-chloride; thiazenone; SQ-10496).

Tiazon (tr) *see* Dazomet.

TIAZURIL** (2-[4-[(p-chlorophenyl)thio]-3,5-xylyl]-as-triazine-3,5(2H,4H)-dione; CP-25673).

Tibamide *see* Tybamate.

TIBENZATE** (S-benzyl thiobenzoate).

'Tiberal' *see* Ornidazole.

TIBEZONIUM IODIDE*** (diethyl-methyl[2-[[4-[p-(phenylthio)phenyl]-3H-1,5-benzodiazepin-2-yl]thio]ethyl]-ammonium iodide; thiabenzonium iodide; thiabenzonium; Rec 15/0691).

TIBOLONE*** (17α-ethynyl-17-hydroxy-7α-methyl-5(10)-estren-3-one; 17-hydroxy-7α-methyl-19-nor-17α-pregn-5(10)en-20-yn-3-one; 7α-methylnoretynodrel; Org OD-14).

Tibon (tr) *see* Thiacetazone.

TIBRIC ACID** (2-chloro-5-[(cis-3,5-dimethylpiperidino)sulfonyl]benzoic acid; 1-[(3-carboxy-4-chlorophenyl)sulfonyl]-3,5-dimethylpiperidine; CP-18524).

TIBROFAN*** (4,4',5-tribromo-2-thiophene-carboxanilide).

'Tibutol' *see* Ethambutol.

TICARBODINE** (α,α,α-trifluoro-2,6-dimethyl-1-piperidinethiocarboxy-m-toluidide; EL-974).

TICARCILLIN** (N-(2-carboxy-3,3-dimethyl-7-oxo-4-thia-1-azabicyclo(3.2.0)-hept-6-yl)-3-thiophenemalonamic acid; 6-(thiophenemalonamido)penicillanic acid; (α-carboxy-3-thenyl)penicillin; (α-carboxy-

3-thienylmethyl)penicillin; 6-(thienyl-malonamido)penicillanic acid; BRL-2288; 'triacilline').

TICLATONE*** (6-chloro-1,2-benzisothi-azolin-3-one; 'landromil').

TICLOMAROL** (3-[5-chloro-α-(p-chloro-β-hydroxyphenethyl)-2-thenyl]-4-hydroxy-coumarin).

TICLOPIDINE** (5-(o-chlorobenzyl)-4,5,6,7-tetrahydrothieno(3,2-c)pyridine).

'Tidemol' *see* Buformin.

TIDIACIC*** (2,4-thiazolidinedicarboxylic acid).

TIDIACIC PLUS SORBITOL ('thiobilin').

TIEMONIUM IODIDE*** (4-(3-hydroxy-3-phenyl-3-thien-2-ylpropyl)-4-methyl-morpholinium iodide; 'visceralgine').

TIENILIC ACID*** (2-[2,3-dichloro-4-(2-thenoyl)phenoxy]acetic acid.

Tietylperazine* *see* Thiethylperazine.

TIFEMOXONE*** (tetrahydro-6-(phenoxy-methyl)-2H-1,3-oxazine-2-thione).

Tifen (tr) *see* Tifenamil.

TIFENAMIL*** (S-2-diethylaminoethyl diphenylthioacetate; thiphenamil; tifen; tiphen; tifenamil hydrochloride; B-23; 'trocinate').

TIFENCILLIN*** (6-(phenylthioacetamido)-penicillanic acid or its potassium salt; phenylthiomethylpenicillin; potassium thiphencillin; thiphencillin; L-26383).

'Tiferron' *see* Sodium pyrocatecholdisul-fonate.

TIFLOREX** ((±)-N-ethyl-α-methyl-m-[(trifluoromethyl)thio]phenethylamine; (±)-N-ethyl-m-[(trifluoromethyl)thio]-amphetamine).

TIFORMIN*** (4-guanidinobutyramide; tyformin; tyformin hydrochloride; HL-523; 'augmentin').

'Tifosyl' *see* Thiotepa.

'Tigan' *see* Trimethobenzamide.

TIGESTOL*** (17α-ethynyl-5(10)-estren-17-ol; 19-nor-17α-pregn-5(10)-en-20-yn-17-ol).

TIGLIC ACID (trans-α,β-dimethylacrylic acid; 2-methyl-2-butenoic acid; 2-methyl-crotonic acid; crotonic acid).

TIGLOIDINE*** (pseudotropine 2,3-dimethylacrylate; tiglylpseudotropine; 'tiglyssin').

Tiglyltropine *see* Tropigline.

'Tiglyssin' *see* Tigloidine.

'Tiguvon' *see* Fenthion.

'Tiicarex' *see* Quintozene.

TILETAMINE*** (2-ethylamino-2-thien-2-ylcyclohexanone; 2-(1-ethylamino-2-oxo-cyclohexyl)thiophene; tiletamine hydro-chloride; CI-634).

Tilidate* *see* Tilidine.

TILIDINE** (ethyl DL-trans-2-dimethylamino-1-phenyl-3-cyclohexene-1-carboxylate; tilidate; tilidine hydrochloride; Gö-1261; W-5759A; 'valoron').

See also Dextilidine.

'Tillam' *see* Pebulate.

TILORONE*** (2,7-bis(2-diethylamino-

ethoxy)fluoren-9-one; bis(DEAE)-
fluorenone; NSC-143969).

TIMEPIDIUM BROMIDE*** (3-(dithien-
2-ylmethylene)-5-methoxy-1,1-dimethyl-
piperidinium bromide; 5-methoxy-1,1-
dimethyl-3-(dithien-2-ylmethylene)-
piperidinium bromide; methoxytipepidine
methobromide; SA-504).

Timerfon* *see* Sodium timerfonate.

Timet (tr) *see* Phorate.

Timidazol (tr) *see* Thiamazole.

'Timodyne' *see* Mefexamide.

TIMOLOL*** ((−)-1-*tert*-butylamino-3-
(4-morpholino-1,2,5-thiadiazol-3-yloxy)-2-
propanol; (−)-3-(3-*tert*-butylamino-2-
hydroxypropoxy)-4-morpholino-1,2,5-
thiadiazole).

TIMOLOL MALEATE (timolol hydrogen
maleate; MK-950; 'blocadren').

TIMONACIC*** (thiazolidine-4-carboxylic
acid; thioproline; 'hepaldine', 'heparegene').

TIMOPRAZOLE** (2-[(pyrid-2-ylmethyl)-
sulfinyl]benzimidazole).

'Timosulfon' *see* Diathymosulfone.

'Timovan' *see* Prothipendyl.

'Tinactin' *see* Tolnaftate.

'Tinaderm' *see* Tolnaftate.

'Tin anti-slime' *see* Bis(tributyltin) oxide.

'Tindal' *see* Acetophenazine.

TINIDAZOLE*** (1-(2-ethylsulfonylethyl)-
2-methyl-5-nitroimidazole; ethyl
2-(2-methyl-5-nitroimidazol-1-yl)ethyl
sulfone; CP-12574; 'fasigyn', 'simplotan').

TINOFEDRINE*** (α-[1-[(3,3-dithien-3-yl-
allyl)amino]ethyl]benzyl alcohol).

TINORIDINE*** (2-amino-6-benzyl-3-
ethoxycarbonyl-4,5,6,7-tetrahydrothieno-
(2,3-c)pyridine; ethyl 2-amino-6-benzyl-
4,5,6,7-tetrahydrothieno(2,3-c)pyridine-3-
carboxylate; Y-3642; 'nonframin').

'Tinox' *see* Demephion-S.

TIN OXIDE (colloidal tin oxide with tin;
'oxistan', 'oxstan', 'salostan', 'stannoxyl',
'stannacné', 'vi-stannyl').

'Tintorane' *see* Warfarin.

'Tiobicina' *see* Thiacetazone.

TIOCARLIDE*** (4,4′-bis(isopentyloxy)-
thiocarbanilide; 4,4′-diisoamyloxythio-
carbanilide; N,N′-bis(4-isopentyloxy-
phenyl)thiourea; thiocarlide; DATC;
'isoxyl', 'soxidyl').

Tiodan (tr) *see* Endosulfan.

'Tiofenatin' *see* Thiophenatin.

'Tiofos' *see* Parathion.

Tiofosfamide *see* Thiotepa.

'Tiofosyl' *see* Thiotepa.

TIOGUANINE*** (2-aminopurine-6-thiol;
2-amino-6-mercaptopurine; 6-thioguanine;
BW-50-71; NSC-752; 'lanvis').

Tioguanine riboside *see* Thioguanosine.

TIOMESTERONE*** (1α,7α-diacetylthio-
17β-hydroxy-17-methylandrost-4-en-3-one;
1α,7α-bis(acetylthio)-17α-methylandrost-
4-en-17β-ol-3-one; thiomesterone; 'embadol', 'emdabol').

'Tionidel' *see* Ethylmorphine.

'Tio-pentemal' *see* Thiopental.

TIOPRONIN** (N-(2-mercaptopropionyl)-
glycine; α-mercaptopropionylglycine;
'thiola').

TIOSALAN*** (3,4′,5-tribromo-2-mercapto-
benzanilide; thiosalan).

Tio-TEF (tr) *see* Thiotepa.

TIOTIXENE*** (N,N-dimethyl-9-[3-(4-
methylpiperazin-1-yl)propylidene]thio-
xanthene-2-sulfonamide; thiothixene;
P-4657 B; 'navane', 'orbinamon').

'Tiotrifar' *see* Anethole trithione.

TIOXACIN** (6-ethyl-2,3,6,9-tetrahydro-
3-methyl-2,9-dioxothiazolo(5,4-f)quinoline-
8-carboxylic acid).

**Tioxacin 2-(4-methylpiperid-1-yl)ethyl
ester** *see* Metioxate.

TIOXOLONE*** (6-hydroxy-1,3(2H)-benz-
oxathiol-2-one; thioxolone; thidoxol;
HBT; OL-1; OL-110; 'camyna', 'stepin').

**TIOXOLONE WITH HYDROCORT-
ISONE** ('psoil').

TIPEPIDINE*** (3-(di-2-thienylmethylene)-
1-methylpiperidine; 'antupex', 'asverin',
'delta-asverin', 'di-neumobron').

TIPEPIDINE CITRATE ('asverin C').

TIPEPIDINE HIBENZATE (tipepidine
compound with 4′-hydroxybenzophenone-
2-carboxylic acid; 'asverin H').

Tiphen (tr) *see* Tifenamil.

TIPINDOLE** (2-dimethylaminoethyl
1,3,4,5-tetrahydrothiopyrano(4,3-b)-
indole-8-carboxylate).

TIPINDOLE METHIODIDE (K-206).

TIPRENOLOL*** (1-isopropylamino-3-[o-
(methylthio)phenoxy]-2-propanol; DU-
21445).

TIQUINAMIDE** (5,6,7,8-tetrahydro-3-
methylquinoline-8-thiocarboxamide;
Wy-24081).

'Tirian' *see* Proguanil.

'Tiron' *see* Sodium pyrocatecholdisulfonate.

TIROPRAMIDE*** (DL-α-benzamido-p-[2-
(diethylamino)ethoxy]-N,N-dipropyl-
hydrocinnamamide).

'Tisercin' *see* Levomepromazine.

'Tisercinetta' *see* Levomepromazine
maleate.

TISOCROMIDE*** (N-(3-dimethylamino-
1,3-dimethylbutyl)-6,7-dimethoxy-2,1-
benzoxathian-3-carboxamide 1,1-dioxide;
6,7-dimethoxy-N-(3-dimethylamino-1,3-
dimethylbutyl)-2,1-benzoxathian-3-
carboxamide 1,1-dioxide).

'Tisomycin' *see* Cycloserine.

TISOPURINE** (1H-pyrazolo(3,4-d)-
pyrimidine-4-thiol; 4-mercaptopyrazolo-
(3,4-d)pyrimidine; thiopurinol).

TISOQUONE*** (4-ethyl-3,4-dihydro-4-
phenylthioisocarbostyril; 4-ethyl-3,4-
dihydro-4-phenyl-1(2H)-isoquinoline-
thione).

'Titriplex' *see* Disodium edetate.

Tiuram *see* Disulfiram.

'Tiuramyl' *see* Thiram.

TIXADIL*** (N-(α-methylphenethyl)thio-
xanthene-9-ethylamine; α-methyl-N-

(2-thioxanthen-9-ylethyl)phenethylamine;
N-(2-thioxanthen-9-ylethyl)amphetamine).
'Tixantone' *see* Lucanthone.
TIZOLEMIDE** (2-chloro-5-[4-hydroxy-
3-methyl-2-(methylimino)thiazolidin-4-yl]-
benzenesulfonamide; 4-(4-chloro-3-
sulfamoylphenyl)-4-hydroxy-3-methyl-2-
(methylimino)thiazolidine).
TIZOPROLIC ACID** (2-propyl-5-
thiazolecarboxylic acid).
TM-10 *see* Xylocholine.
β-**TM-10** *see* *β*-Methylxylocholine.
TM-4049 *see* Malathion.
TMB-4 *see* Trimedoxime bromide.
TMBAC *see* Sodium capobenate.
TMD-10 *see* Tetrylammonium.
TMT *see* (+)-Atromepine.
TMTDS *see* Thiram.
'Tobradistin' *see* Tobramycin.
TOBRAMYCIN*** (antibiotic from *Str.
tenebrarius*; *O*-3-amino-3-deoxy-*α*-D-
glucopyranosyl-(1→4)-*O*-[2,6-diamino-
2,3,6-trideoxy-*α*-D-*ribo*-hexopyranosyl-
(1→6)]-2-deoxystreptamine; nebramycin
factor 6; L-47663; 'gernebcin', 'nebcin',
'obracine', 'tobradistin').
TOCAMPHYL*** (diethanolamine salt of
mono-D-camphoric ester of *p*,*α*-dimethyl-
benzyl alcohol).
'Toce' *see* Diethadione.
'Toclase' *see* Pentoxyverine.
TOCOFERSOLAN*** (mono(2,5,7,8-tetra-
methyl)-2-(4,8,12-trimethyltridecyl)-
6-chromanyl succinate polyoxyethylene
ether; tocopherol succinate polyoxyethylene
ether; D-*α*-tocopherol polyethyleneglycol
1000 succinate; tocophersolan; TPGS).
TOCOFIBRATE*** (tocopheryl clofibrate).
α-**TOCOPHEROL** (2,5,7,8-tetramethyl-2-
(4,8,12-trimethyldecyl)-6-chromanol;
5,7,8-trimethyltocol; *α*-tocopherol acetate,
phosphate or succinate; antisterility
vitamin; vitamin E).
α-**TOCOPHEROL NICOTINATE**
('renacin').
**Tocopherol succinate polyoxyethylene
ether** *see* Tocofersolan.
TOCOPHERONIC ACID (lactone of
2-(5-carboxy-3-hydroxy-3-methylpentyl)-
3,5,6-trimethylbenzoquinone).
Tocophersolan* *see* Tocofersolan.
Tocopheryl clofibrate *see* Tocofibrate.
α-**TOCOPHERYLQUINONE** ('eutrophyl').
'Tocosamine' *see* Sparteine.
'Tocosine' *see* Tyramine.
TOCOTRIENOL (2-methyl-2-(4,8,12-tri-
methyltrideca-3,7,11-trienyl)-6-chromanol).
TOCP *see* Tricresyl phosphate.
'Tod'l' *see* Hexachlorophene.
TODRALAZINE** (ethyl 2-phthalazin-1-
ylcarbazate; 1-carbethoxy-2-phthalazino-
hydrazine; 1-ethoxycarbonyl-2-phthalazin-
1-ylhydrazine; ethyl 2-phthalazin-1-
ylhydrazinecarboxylate; todrazoline;
CEPH; 'binazin').
Todrazoline *see* Todralazine.
'Tofacin' *see* Tofenacin.

'Tofazine 5OW' *see* Simazine.
TOFENACIN*** (*N*-methyl-2-(*o*-methyl-
α-phenyl benzyloxy)ethylamine; *N*-methyl-
2-(*o*-methylbenzhydryloxy)ethylamine;
tofenacin hydrochloride; *N*-demethyl-
orphenadrine; 'elamol', 'tofacin').
TOFESILATE(S)** (1,2,3,6-tetrahydro-1,3-
dimethyl-2,6-dioxopurine-7-ethane-
sulfonate(s)).
TOFETRIDINE** ((−)-1,2,3,4,4a,5,6,10b-
octahydro-9-methoxy-10b-methylphen-
anthridine).
TOFISOLINE*** (1-(3,4-dimethoxyphenyl)-
4-ethyl-6,7-dimethoxy-3-methyliso-
quinoline 2-imide).
TOFISOPAM*** (1-(3,4-dimethoxyphenyl)-
5-ethyl-7,8-dimethoxy-4-methyl-5H-2,3-
benzodiazepine).
'Tofranil' *see* Imipramine.
'Togamycin' *see* Spectinomycin.
Togholamine *see* Triacanthine.
'Toilax' *see* Bisacodyl.
'TOK E25' *see* Nitrofen.
'Toladryl' *see* *p*-Methyldiphenhydramine.
Tolamidol *see* Tolamolol.
TOLAMOLOL*** (*p*-[2-[[2-hydroxy-3-(*o*-
toloxy)propyl]amino]ethoxy]benzamide;
1-[2-(4-carbamoylphenoxy)ethylamino]-3-
(2-methylphenoxy)-2-propanol; tolamidol;
UK-6558-01).
'Tolanate' *see* Inositol hexanitrate.
TOLAZAMIDE*** (1-(hexahydro-1H-
azepin-1-yl)-3-(*p*-toluenesulfonyl)urea;
1,1-hexamethylene-4-(*p*-toluenesulfonyl)-
semicarbazide; U-17835; 'norglycin',
'tolinase').
TOLAZOLINE*** (2-benzyl-2-imidazoline;
phenylmethylimidazoline; benzazoline;
benzolin; tolazoline hydrochloride).
'Tolazul' *see* Tolonium.
'Tolbet' *see* Tolbutamide.
TOLBOXANE*** (5-methyl-5-propyl-2-*p*-
tolyl-1,3,2-dioxaborinane; 2-methyl-
2-propyl-1,3-propanediol *p*-tolylborate;
p-tolylborate of 2-hydroxymethyl-2-
methyl-1-pentanol; 'clamil', 'clarmil').
TOLBUTAMIDE*** (1-butyl-3-(*p*-toluene-
sulfonyl)urea; 1-butyl-3-tosylurea;
butamid; tolbutylurea; D-860; HLS-831;
U-2043; 'arcosal', 'artosin', 'diabetol',
'diabuton', 'dolipol', 'glicotron', 'glycotron', 'hypoglycone', 'ipoglicone', 'mobenol', 'orabet', 'oralin', 'orinase',
'pramidex', 'rastinon', 'tolbet', 'toluina').
See also Metformin with tolbutamide.
'Tolbutaphen' *see* Phenformin plus tolbutamide.
Tolbutylurea *see* Tolbutamide.
TOLCICLATE*** (*O*-(1,2,3,4-tetrahydro-
1,4-methanonaphth-6-yl) *m*,*N*-dimethyl-
thiocarbanilate).
Tolclotide* *see* Disulfamide.
TOLDIMFOS*** (4-dimethylamino-*o*-tolyl-
phosphinic acid).
'Tolectin' *see* Tolmetin.
TOLFENAMIC ACID*** (*N*-(3-chloro-*o*-
tolyl)anthranilic acid; 'clotam').

Tolhexamide *see* Glycyclamide.
o-**TOLIDINE** (4,4′-diamino-3,3′-dimethyl-
biphenyl; 3,3′-dimethylbenzidine).
'Tolinase' *see* Tolazamide.
TOLINDATE*** (*O*-indan-5-yl *m,N*-
dimethylthiocarbanilate; 'dalnate').
TOLIPROLOL*** (1-isopropylamino-3-
(*m*-toloxy)-2-propanol; 1-isopropylamino-
3-(3-methylphenoxy)-2-propanol; MHIP;
ICI-45763; Kö-592; 'doberol').
TOLMETIN*** (1-methyl-5-*p*-toluoyl-
pyrrole-2-acetic acid; 'tolectin').
'Tolnaftal' *see* Tolnaftate.
TOLNAFTATE*** (2-naphthyl *N*-methyl-
N-(3-tolyl)thionocarbamate; *O*-2-naphthyl
m,N-dimethylthiocarbanilate; 'dermoxin',
'focusan', 'naphthiomate-T', 'tinactin',
'tinaderm', 'tolnaftal', 'tonoftal').
'Tolnate' *see* Prothipendyl.
Tolocinium* *see* Toloconium metilsulfate.
TOLOCONIUM CHLORIDE (trimethyl-
(1-*p*-tolyldodecyl)ammonium chloride;
'desogen').
TOLOCONIUM METILSULFATE***
(trimethyl(1-*p*-tolyldodecyl)ammonium
methylsulfate; tolocinium; tolytrimonium).
TOLONIDINE*** (2-(2-chloro-*p*-toluidino)-
2-imidazoline; 2-chloro-*N*-(2-imidazolin-
2-yl)-*p*-toluidine).
TOLONIUM CHLORIDE*** (3-amino-
7-dimethylamino-2-methylphenazathio-
nium chloride; dimethyltoluthionine
chloride; toluidine blue; CI-925; Schultz-
1041; 'blutene chloride', 'klot', 'tolazul').
TOLOXATONE** (5-hydroxymethyl-3-
m-tolyloxazolidin-2-one).
TOLOXYCHLORINOL*** (1,1′-(3-*o*-toloxy-
propylenedioxy)bis(2,2,2-trichloroethanol);
1,3-bis(2,2,2-trichloro-1-hydroxyethoxy)-
3-*o*-toloxypropane; compound 1318;
'myavan').
3-(*o*-Toloxy)-1,2-propanediol *see*
Mephenesin.
**1,1′-(3-*o*-Toloxypropylenedioxy)bis-
(2,2,2-trichloroethanol)** *see* Toloxychlorinol.
TOLPENTAMIDE*** (1-cyclopentyl-3-
(*p*-toluenesulfonyl)urea; BH-135).
TOLPERISONE*** (2,4′-dimethyl-3-
piperid-1-ylpropiophenone; 2-methyl-3-
piperid-1-yl-1-(*p*-tolyl)-1-propanone;
β-methyl-γ-(*p*-tolyl)-1-piperidinepropa-
none; PMP; 'mydeton', 'mydocalm').
TOLPIPRAZOLE*** (5-methyl-3-[2-(4-*m*-
tolylpiperazin-1-yl)ethyl]pyrazole; 1-[2-
(5-methylpyrazol-3-yl)ethyl]-4-*m*-tolyl-
piperazine; H-4170).
TOLPOVIDONE (ω-(*p*-iodobenzyl)-2-
(2-oxopyrrolidin-1-yl) ethamer).
TOLPOVIDONE(131I)*** (tolpovidone
labeled with radioiodine; radiotolpovidone;
'raovin').
TOLPRONINE*** (3,6-dihydro-α-(*o*-toloxy-
methyl)-1(2H)pyridineëthanol; 1-(1,2,3,
6-tetrahydropyrid-1-yl)-3-(*o*-(toloxy)-
2-propanol; 1-(△³-piperidino)-3-*o*-toloxy-
2-propanol; tolpronine hydrochloride;

'proponesin').
TOLPROPAMINE*** (*N,N*-dimethyl-3-
phenyl-3-(*p*-tolyl)-1-propylamine; 'prag-
man', 'tylagel').
TOLPYRINE (methylphenazone; methylantipyrine; tolylantipyrine).
TOLPYRINE SALICYLATE ('tolysal').
TOLPYRRAMIDE*** (*N*-(*p*-toluene-
sulfonyl)-1-pyrrolidinecarboxamide;
N-tosylpyrrolidinecarboxamide; 1-tetra-
methylene-3-(*p*-toluenesulfonyl)urea).
TOLQUINZOLE*** (2-ethyl-1,3,4,6,7,11b-
hexahydro-10-methyl-2H-benzo(a)quin-
olizin-2-ol).
'Tolseron' *see* Guaifenesin.
TOLUAMIDE(S) (toluic acid amide(s);
ar-methylbenzamide(s)).
TOLUENE (methylbenzene).
p-**Toluenesulfonic acid,** esters and salts
see Tosilate(s).
N-(*p*-**Toluenesulfonyl)-1-pyrrolidine-
carboxamide** *see* Tolpyrramide.
α-**Toluic acid** *see* Phenylacetic acid.
m-**TOLUIC ACID** (*m*-methylbenzoic acid).
p-**TOLUIC ACID** (*p*-methylbenzoic acid).
TOLUIDINE(S) (*ar*-methylaniline(s);
aminotoluene(s)).
Toluidine blue *see* Tolonium.
TOLUIDINE RED (1-(2-nitro-*p*-tolylazo)-
2-naphthol).
'Toluina' *see* Tolbutamide.
Toluquinone *see* Methylbenzoquinone.
Toluylene *see* Stilbene.
TOLUYLENE DIISOCYANATE (2,4-
diisocyanatotoluene; TDI; 'desmodur T').
'Tolvin' *see* Mianserin.
'Tolvon' *see* Mianserin.
TOLYCAINE*** (methyl 2-(2-diethylamino-
acetamido)-*m*-toluate; 6-carbomethoxy-*N*-
(2-diethylaminoacetyl)-*o*-toluidine; tolycaine hydrochloride; 'baycaine').
m-**Tolyl acetate** *see* *m*-Cresyl acetate.
Tolylantipyrine *see* Tolpyrine.
o-**Tolylazo-*o*-toluidine diacetate** *see*
Diacetazotol.
1-(4-*o*-Tolylazo-*o*-tolylazo)-2-naphthol *see*
Scarlet red.
p-**Tolylboric acid ester with 2-hydroxy-
methyl-2-methyl-1-pentanol** *see* Tolboxane.
m-**Tolylcarbamic acid 3-[(methoxycarbonyl)amino]phenyl ester** *see*
Phenmediphan.
(1-*p*-**Tolyldodecyl)trimethylammonium
methyl sulfate** *see* Toloconium methylsulfate.
m-**TOLYL METHYLCARBAMATE**
('tsumacide').
p-**Tolyl methyl carbinol** *see* *p,*α-Dimethyl-
benzyl alcohol.
Tolylphenazone *see* Tolpyrine.
Tolyl phosphate *see* Tricresyl phosphate.
**2-[3-[4-(*o*-Tolyl)piperazin-1-yl]propoxy]-
pyridine** *see* Toprilidine.
1-*p*-Tolyl-2-propylamine *see* *p*-Methyl-
amphetamine.
(−)-*N*-[(*p*-**Tolylsulfonyl)carbamoyl]-**

amphetamine *see* Tosifen.
'Tolysal' *see* Tolpyrine salicylate.
Tolytrimonium *see* Toloconium metilsulfate.
'Tomanol' *see* 4-Isopropylaminophenazone
with phenylbutazone.
Tomarin *see* Coumafuryl.
'Tomatotone' *see* p-Chlorophenoxyacetic acid.
'Tomil' *see* Promazine.
'Tomorin' *see* Coumachlor.
'Tonarsin' *see* Disodium methanearsonate.
'Toness' *see* Proxazole.
'Tonhormon' *see* Epinephrine ascorbate.
'Tonibral' *see* Deanol hemisuccinate.
Tonka bean camphor *see* Coumarin.
'Tonofosfan' *see* Sodium 4-dimethylamino-
o-toluenephosphonite.
'Tonoftal' *see* Tolnaftate.
'Tonolyt' *see* Carisoprodol.
'Tonophosphan' *see* Sodium 4-dimethyl-
amino-o-toluenephosphonite.
'Tonuron' *see* Chlorothiazide.
TONZONIUM BROMIDE*** (hexadecyl-
[2-[(p-methoxybenzyl)-2-pyrimidinyl-
amino]ethyl]dimethylammonium bromide;
thonzonium bromide; thonzylamine
hexadecyl bromide; thonzylamine cetyl
bromide; NC-1264; 'thonzide').
'Topicorte' *see* Desoximetasone.
'Topisolone' *see* Desoximetasone.
'Topocaine' *see* Cyclomethycaine.
TOPRILIDINE*** (1-(3-pyrid-2-yloxy-
propyl)-4-(o-tolyl)piperazine; 2-[3-[4-(o-
tolyl)piperazin-1-yl]propoxy]pyridine;
HOE-757).
'Topsin' *see* Thiophanate.
'Topsin M' *see* Thiophanate-methyl.
'Topsym' *see* Fluocinonide.
'Topsyne' *see* Fluocinonide.
'Toquilone' *see* Methaqualone.
TOQUIZINE** (9-(3,5-dimethylpyrazole-1-
carboxamido)-4-ethyl-4,6,6a,7,8,9,10,10a-
octahydro-7-methyl-indolo(4,3-fg)quino-
line; N-(4-ethyl-4,6,6a,7,8,9,10,10a-octa-
hydro-7-methylindolo(4,3-fg)quinolin-9-yl)-
3,5-dimethylpyrazole-1-carboxamide;
L-44106).
'Torak' *see* Dialifos.
'Torantil' *see* Diamine oxidase.
'Torantyl' *see* Diamine oxidase.
TORASEMIDE** (1-isopropyl-3-[(4-m-
toluidinopyrid-3-yl)sulfonyl]urea; 3-[[(iso-
propylcarbamoyl)amino]sulfonyl]-4-
(m-toluidino)pyridine).
'Tordon' *see* Picloram.
'Torecan' *see* Thiethylperazine maleate.
'Torelle' *see* Fospirate.
'Torental' *see* Pentoxifylline.
'Toriseptin' *see* Sulfamethylthiazole.
'Torque' *see* Neostanox.
Torutilen *see* Vitamin T.
'Toryn' *see* Caramiphen edisilate.
TOSACTIDE*** (α$^{1-28}$-corticotrophin
(human); ACTH human synthetic;
octacosactrin; 'homactid', 'humacthid').
TOSIFEN** ((−)-1-(α-methylphenethyl)-3-
(p-tolylsulfonyl)urea; (−)-α-methyl-N-
[(p-tolylsulfonyl)carbamoyl]phenethyl-

amine; (−)-N-[(p-tolylsulfonyl)carbamoyl]-
amphetamine).
TOSILATE(S)** (p-toluenesulfonate(s);
tosylate(s)).
See also Bretylium tosilate; Pempidine
tosilate; Trethinium tosilate; Troxonium
tosilate; Troxypyrrolium tosilate; Xylam-
idine tosilate.
'Tosmilen' *see* Demecarium bromide.
TOSYL-L-ARGININE METHYL ESTER
(methyl ester of p-toluenesulfonyl-L-
arginine; TAM; TAME).
Tosylate(s) *see* Tosilate(s).
TOSYLCHLORAMIDE SODIUM***
(sodium derivative of N-chloro-p-toluene-
sulfonamide trihydrate; chloramine-T;
sodium sulfaminochloride).
N-**Tosylpyrrolidinecarboxamide** *see*
Tolpyrramide.
'Totacef' *see* Cefazolin.
'Totacillin' *see* Ampicillin.
'Totapen' *see* Ampicillin.
TOTAQUINE (quinium; mixture of
cinchona alkaloids).
See also Quinetum.
'Totocillin' *see* Ampicillin with dicloxacillin.
'Totokaine' *see* Butamin.
'Totril' *see* Ioxynil octanoate.
Tox-47 *see* Parathion.
'Toxakil' *see* Camphechlor.
'Toxaphene' *see* Camphechlor.
'Toxichlor' *see* Chlordane.
Toxicodendron quercifolium *see* Poisonoak
extract.
Toxilic acid *see* Maleic acid.
'Toxivers' *see* Piperazine adipate.
'Toxogenin' *see* Obidoxime chloride.
'Toxogonin' *see* Obidoxime chloride.
TOXOPYRIMIDINE (6-amino-5-hydroxy-
methyl-2-methylpyrimidine; 4-amino-
2-methyl-5-pyrimidinemethanol).
'Toxynil' *see* Ioxynil.
'Toyomycin' *see* Chromomycin.
TOZALINONE*** (2-dimethylamino-5-
phenyl-2-oxazolin-4-one; thozalinone;
CL-39808; 'stimsen').
TP *see* Testosterone propionate.
2,4,5-TP *see* Fenoprop.
Tp-21 *see* Thioridazine.
TPB *see* Bithionol.
TPD *see* Prosultiamine.
TPGS *see* Tocofersolan.
TPN *see* Nadide phosphate *and* Chlorothalonil.
TPN-12 *see* Sulforidazine.
TPP *see* Testosterone phenylpropionate.
TPS-23 *see* Mesoridazine.
TPTC *see* Fentin chloride.
TPTH *see* Fentin hydroxide.
TPTZ *see* 2,3,5-Triphenyltetrazolium
chloride.
TR-495 *see* Methaqualone.
'Tracebyl' *see* Iobenzamic acid.
'Tradone' *see* Pemoline.
'Trafuril' *see* Thurfyl nicotinate.
'Tral' *see* Hexocyclium metilsulfate.
'Tralgon' *see* Paracetamol.
TRALONIDE*** (9,11-dichloro-6,21-

difluoro-16,17-dihydroxypregna-1,4-diene-3,20-dione 16,17-acetonide; 9,11-dichloro-6,21-difluoropregna-1,4-diene-16,17-diol-3,20-dione 16,17-acetonide).

TRAMADOL** ((±)-*trans*-2-dimethyl-aminomethyl-1-(*m*-methoxyphenyl)-cyclohexanol; (±)-*trans*-1-(*m*-anisyl)-2-dimethylaminomethylcyclohexanol; (±)-*trans*-3-(2-dimethylaminomethyl-1-hydroxy-cyclohexyl)anisole; tramadol hydro-chloride; CG-315; K-315).

TRAMAZOLINE*** (2-(5,6,7,8-tetrahydro-1-naphthylamino)-2-imidazoline; tram-azoline hydrochloride; KB-77; KB-227; 'biciron', 'rhinogutt', 'rhinospray').

TRAMAZOLINE WITH OXYTETRA-CYCLINE (K80-KBOT; 'oxy-biciron').

'**Tranapal**' *see* Thiopental.

'**Trancalgyl**' *see* Ethenzamide.

'**Trancin**' *see* Fluphenazine.

'**Tranco-gesic**' *see* Chlormezanone with acetylsalicylic acid.

'**Trancopal**' *see* Chlormezanone.

TRANEXAMIC ACID*** (*trans*-4-(amino-methyl)cyclohexanecarboxylic acid; AMCHA; CL-65336; 'amchafibrin', 'amikapron', 'anvitoff', 'cyclocapron', 'cyclokapron', 'exacyl', 'frenolyse', 'ugurol').

'**Tranid**' *see* 5-Chloro-6-oxonorbornane-carbonitrile *O*-(methylcarbamoyl)oxime.

'**Tranpoise**' *see* Mephenoxalone.

'**Tran-Q**' *see* Hydroxyzine.

'**Tranquilin**' *see* Benactyzine.

'**Tranquisan**' *see* Perphenazine.

'**Tranquo-alupent**' *see* Orciprenaline with oxazepam.

Transamine (tr) *see* Tranylcypromine.

'**Transannon**' *see* Conjugated estrogens.

'**Transbilix**' *see* Adipiodone meglumine.

'**Transbronchin**' *see* Carbocisteine.

Transclomifene *see* Zuclomifene.

Transclomiphene* *see* Zuclomifene.

'**Transcycline**' *see* Rolitetracycline.

TRANSFERRIN (β-metal-binding globulin; siderophilin).

'**Transithal**' *see* Buthalital.

'**Transoddi**' *see* Cinametic acid.

'**Transren**' *see* Sodium anhydromethylene-citrate.

TRANTELINIUM BROMIDE*** (8-methyl-tropinium bromide xanthene-9-carboxylate; N-640; 'gastrixone').

'**Tranvet**' *see* Propiomazine.

'**Tranxene**' *see* Dipotassium clorazepate.

'**Tranxilene**' *see* Dipotassium clorazepate.

'**Tranxilium**' *see* Dipotassium clorazepate.

TRANYLCYPROMINE*** (DL-*trans*-2-phenylcyclopropylamine; tranylcypro-mine sulfate; transamine; SK&F-385; 'parnate', 'tylciprine').

TRANYLCYPROMINE WITH TRIFLUOPERAZINE ('parstelazine', 'parstelin').

'**Trapanal**' *see* Thiopental.

TRAPIDIL*** (7-diethylamino-5-methyl-*s*-triazolo(1,5-a)pyrimidine; trapymin;

'rocornal').

Trapymin *see* Trapidil.

'**Trascolan**' *see* Aprotinin.

'**Trasentin**' *see* Adiphenine.

'**Trasentin-6H**' *see* Drofenine.

'**Trasentine-A**' *see* Drofenine.

'**Traserit**' *see* Apicycline.

'**Trasicor**' *see* Oxprenolol.

'**Trasylol**' *see* Aprotinin.

Traubenzucker *see* Glucose.

'**Traumanase**' *see* Bromelains.

'**Traumanase-cyclin**' *see* Tetracycline with bromelaine.

'**Trausabun**' *see* Melitracen.

'**Travase**' *see* Sutilains.

TRAZITILINE*** (1-(9,10-dihydro-9,10-ethano-9-anthryl)-4-methylpiperazine; 9,10-dihydro-9-(4-methylpiperazin-1-yl)-9,10-ethanoanthracene).

TRAZODONE*** (2-[3-[4-(*m*-chlorophen-yl)piperazin-1-yl]propyl]-*s*-triazolo(4,3-a)-pyridin-3(2H)-one; AF-1161; 'trittico').

TREBENZOMINE** ((±)-*N,N*,2-trimethyl-3-chromanamine; (±)-3-(dimethylamino)-2,3-dihydro-2-methylbenzopyran; trebenzomine hydrochloride; CI-686).

'**Treburon**' *see* Mepesulfate.

'**Trecator**' *see* Ethionamide.

'**Tredum**' *see* Fenpentadiol.

'**Treflan**' *see* Trifluralin.

TRELOXINATE*** (methyl 2,10-dichloro-12H-dibenzo(d,g)(1,3)dioxocin-6-carboxyl-ate).

'**Tremaril**' *see* Metixene.

'**Tremblex**' *see* Dexetimide.

'**Tremerad**' *see* Clioxanide.

'**Tremin**' *see* Trihexyphenidyl.

'**Tremonil**' *see* Metixene.

TREMORINE (1,4-dipyrrolidin-1-yl-2-butyne).

TRENBOLONE*** (17β-hydroxyestra-4,9,11-trien-3-one; 4,9,11-estratrien-17β-ol-3-one; 17β-hydroxy-19-norandrosta-4,9,11-trien-3-one; 19-norandrosta-4,9,11-trien-17β-ol-3-one; trienbolone; trienolone).

TRENBOLONE CYCLOHEXYL-METHYLCARBONATE ('hexabolan').

TRENGESTONE*** (6-chloro-9β,10α-pregna-1,4,6-triene-3,20-dione; 6-chloro-1,6-didehydroretroprogesterone; Ro 4-8347; 'retroid').

'**Trenimon**' *see* Triaziquone.

'**Trentadil**' *see* Bamifylline.

'**Trental**' *see* Pentoxifylline.

TREOSULFAN*** (L-threitol 1,4-dimethane-sulfonate; L-threityl dimesilate; L-*threo*-1,2,3,4-butanetetrol 1,4-bis(methanesul-fonate) ester; L-dihydroxybusulfan; NSC-39069).

'**Trepidone**' *see* Mephenoxalone.

TREPIRIUM IODIDE*** (2-carboxy-1,1-dimethylpyrrolidinium iodide ester with choline iodide; *N*-methylproline choline ester iodide methiodide; choline iodide 1,1-dimethylpyrrolidinium iodide 2-carboxylate).

'**Trescatyl**' *see* Ethionamide.

445

'**Trescillin**' *see* Propicillin.
'**Tresochin**' *see* Chloroquine diphosphate.
'**Trest**' *see* Metixene.
TRESTOLONE** (17β-hydroxy-7α-methyl-estr-4-en-3-one; 7α-methylestr-4-en-17β-ol-3-one; 7α-methylnandrolone; 7α-methyl-19-nortestosterone).
TRETAMINE** (2,4,6-tris(1-aziridinyl)-*s*-triazine; 2,4,6-tris(ethylenimino)-*s*-triazine; triethanomelamine; triethylenemelamine; triethylenimino-*s*-triazine; TEM; TET; Hö-1/193; M-9500; NSC-9706; R-246; SK-1133; 'persistol', 'triamelin').
TRETHINIUM TOSILATE** (2-ethyl-1,2,3,4-tetrahydro-2-methylisoquinolinium *p*-toluenesulfonate; trethinium tosylate).
TRETHOCANIC ACID** (3-hydroxy-3,7,11-trimethyldodecanoic acid; 3-hydroxy-3,7,11-trimethyllauric acid).
TRETINOIN** (*all-trans*-retinoic acid; 3,7-dimethyl-9-(2,6,6-trimethyl-1-cyclo-hexen-1-yl)nona-2,4,6,8-tetraen-1-oic acid; vitamin A acid; retinoic acid; 'aberel', 'airol', 'dermairol', 'eudyna', 'retin-A').
TRETOQUINOL** ((−)-1,2,3,4-tetrahydro-1-(3,4,5-trimethoxybenzyl)-6,7-iso-quinolinediol; trimetoquinol; trimetho-quinol; tretoquinol hydrochloride; AQ-110; AQL-208; 'inolin').
'**Trevintix**' *see* Protionamide.
'**TRH-Roche**' *see* Protirelin.
TRH synthetic *see* Protirelin.
Tri *see* Trichloroethylene.
'**Tri-6**' *see* Lindane.
'**Tri-abrodil**' *see* Sodium acetrizoate.
TRIAC (3,3',5-triiodothyroacetic acid; α-[4-(4-hydroxy-3-iodophenoxy)-3,5-diiodophenyl]acetic acid; 'triacana').
'**Triacana**' *see* Triac.
TRIACANTHINE (togholamine).
TRIACETIC ACID (3,5-diketohexanoic acid).
TRIACETIN** (glyceryl triacetate; 'enzactin', 'glyped', 'vanay').
1,8,9-Triacetoxyanthracene *see* Dithranol triacetate.
2',3',5'-Tri-*O*-acetyl-6-azauridine *see* Azaribine.
Triacetyloleandomycin *see* Troleandomycin.
'**Triacilline**' *see* Ticarcillin.
'**Triadenyl**' *see* Adenosine triphosphate.
TRIALLATE* (*S*-(2,3,3-trichloroallyl) diisopropylcarbamothioate; *S*-(2,3,3-trichloro-2-propenyl) bis(1-methylethyl)-carbamothioate; 'avadex BW').
'**Triamar**' *see* Diiodohydroxyquin glycolylar-sanilate.
TRIAMCINOLONE** (9α-fluoro-11β,16α,17,21-tetrahydroxypregna-1,4-diene-3,20-dione; 9α-fluoro-1,4-pregnadiene-11β,16α,17α,21-tetrol-3,20-dione; 9α-fluoro-16α-hydroxyprednisolone; fluoxypredni-solone; CL-19823; 'adcortyl', 'aristodan', 'delphicort', 'kenacort', 'ledercort', 'orion', 'polcortolon').
See also below and Demeclocycline with triamcinolone; Fenticlor with triam-

cinolone; Prednisone with triamcinolone.
TRIAMCINOLONE ACETONIDE*
(triamcinolone cyclic 16,17-acetal with acetone; 9α-fluoro-11β,21-dihydroxy-16α,17α-isopropylidenedioxypregna-1,4-diene-3,20-dione; 'albicort', 'aristoderm', 'kenacorta', 'kenalog', 'volon A').
Triamcinolone acetonide dimethyl-butyrate *see* Triamcinolone hexacetonide.
TRIAMCINOLONE ACETONIDE WITH NEOMYCIN ('cidermex').
TRIAMCINOLONE ACETONIDE SODIUM PHOSPHATE* (triamcinolone acetonide 21-disodium phosphate; CL-61965; CL-53381; CL-106359; 'aristosol').
Triamcinolone cyclic 16,17-acetal with acetone *see* Triamcinolone acetonide.
Triamcinolone cyclic 16,17-acetal with acetophenone *see* Amcinafide.
Triamcinolone cyclic 16,17-acetal with acrolein *see* Acrocinonide.
Triamcinolone cyclic 16,17-acetal with cyclopentanone, 21-acetate *see* Amcinonide.
Triamcinolone cyclic 16,17-acetal with 3-pentanone *see* Amcinafal.
TRIAMCINOLONE DIACETATE* (triamcinolone 16,21-diacetate; RP-8357; 'aristocort', 'solutedarol', 'tedarol').
TRIAMCINOLONE WITH HALQUINOLS ('remiderm').
TRIAMCINOLONE HEXACETONIDE** (triamcinolone acetonide 21-(2,3-dimethyl-butyrate); CL-34433; TATBA; 'aristospan', 'hexatrione', 'lederspan').
'**Triamelin**' *see* Tretamine.
2,4,7-Triamino-6-(2-furyl)pteridine *see* Furterene.
2,4,7-Triamino-6-phenylpteridine *see* Triamterene.
1,4,7-Triamino-5-phenylpyrimido(4,5-d)-pyrimidine *see* Ampyrimine.
Triamino-*s*-triazine *see* Melamine.
TRIAMIPHOS* (*P*-(5-amino-3-phenyl-1H-1,2,4-triazol-1-yl)-*N,N,N',N'*-tetramethyl-phosphonic diamide; 5-amino-1-(bis-dimethylaminophosphoryl)-3-phenyl-1,2,4-triazole; 'wepsyn').
TRIAMPYZINE** (2-dimethylamino-3,5,-6-trimethylpyrazine; triampyzine sulfate; W-3976B).
TRIAMTERENE** (2,4,7-triamino-6-phenylpteridine; 'dyren', 'dyrenium', 'dytac', 'iatropur', 'jatropur', 'teriam', 'triamteril', 'triamteryl').
See also Benzthiazide with triamterene; Hydrochlorothiazide with triamterene.
'**Triamteril**' *see* Triamterene.
'**Triamteryl**' *see* Triamterene.
Triantoin *see* Mephenytoin.
'**Triap**' *see* Tricyanoallylamine.
TRIARIMOL* (α-(2,4-dichlorophenyl)-α-phenyl-5-pyrimidinemethanol; EL-273).
'**Triavil**' *see* Amitriptyline with perphenazine.
2,5,8-Triazaeicosane-1-carboxylic acid *see* Dodicin.
TRIAZENE (HN:N·NH₂).

s-**TRIAZINE** (1,3,5-triazine).
Triazinearsinic acid *see* Melarsen.
as-**Triazine-3,5-dione** *see* Azauracil.
s-**Triazine-2,4-dione-6-carboxylic acid** *see*
Azaorotic acid.
s-**Triazinetriol** *see* Cyanuric acid.
TRIAZIQUONE*** (2,3,5-tris(1-aziridinyl)-
p-benzoquinone; 2,3,5-triethylenimino-
1,4-benzoquinone; A-163; Bayer-3231;
NSC-29215; Riker-601; 'trenimon').
TRIAZOLAM** (8-chloro-6-(*o*-chloro-
phenyl)-1-methyl-4H-s-triazolo(4,3-a)(1,4)-
benzodiazepine; U-33030).
1H-1,2,4-Triazol-3-amine *see* Amitrole.
1,2,4-Triazole-3-carboxamide riboside
see Ribavirin.
v-**Triazolo(3,4-d)pyrimidine** *see* 8-Aza-
purine.
Triazotion (tr) *see* Azinphos-ethyl.
'**Triazure**' *see* Azaribine.
'**Triazurol**' *see* Chlorazanil.
'**Trib**' *see* Co-trimoxazole.
TRIBENOSIDE*** (ethyl 3,5,6-tri-*O*-
benzyl-D-glucofuranoside; benzylglucofuranoside; glucofuranoside; Ba-21401;
'glyvenol', 'procto-glyvenol').
Tribromoethanol *see* Bromethol.
3,3',5-Tribromo-6-hydroxybenzanilide
see Tribromsalan.
3,4',5-Tribromo-2-mercaptobenzanilide
see Tiosalan.
3,4',5-Tribromosalicylanilide *see* Tribromsalan.
4,4',5-Tribromo-2-thiophenecarboxanilide
see Tibrofan.
TRIBROMSALAN*** (3,4',5-tribromo-
salicylanilide; 3,5-dibromo-6-hydroxy-
benz-*p*-bromanilide; 3,4',5-tribromo-6-
hydroxybenzanilide; 'diaphene', 'temasept
IV', 'tuasal 100').
See also Dibromsalan with tribromsalan.
'**Tribunil**' *see* Methabenzthiazuron.
'**Triburon**' *see* Triclobisonium.
TRIBUTYL PHOSPHOROTRITHIOATE
(DEF).
TRIBUTYL PHOSPHOROTRITHIOITE
('folex', 'merphos').
TRIBUZONE** (4-(4,4-dimethyl-3-oxo-
pentyl)-1,2-diphenyl-3,5-pyrazolidinedione;
4-[2-(2,2-dimethylpropionyl)ethyl]-3,5-
pyrazolidinedione; 1,2-diphenyl-4-(2-
pivaloylethyl)-3,5-pyrazolidinedione;
1,2-diphenyl-4-(4,4,4-trimethyl-3-oxo-
butyl)-3,5-pyrazolidinedione; trimetazone;
trimethazone; 'benetazone').
Tricaine *see* Cinchocaine.
TRICAMBA* (2,3,5-trichloro-6-methoxy-
benzoic acid; metriben; 'banvel T').
TRICARBALLYLIC ACID (1,2,3-propane-
tricarboxylic acid; carboxyglutaric acid).
Tricarbocyanine-II *see* Indocyanine green.
Tricetamide* *see* Trimeglamide.
'**Trichex**' *see* Metronidazole.
'**Trichlofos**' *see* Triclofos.
TRICHLORAMIC ACID (2-amino-2-
3,3,3-trichlorohydroxypropionic acid;
trichloroisoserine).

See also Ethyl trichloramate.
Trichlorfon *see* Metrifonate.
TRICHLORMETHIAZIDE*** (6-chloro-
3-(dichloromethyl)-3,4-dihydro-1,2,4-benzo-
thiadiazine-7-sulfonamide 1,1-dioxide;
trichloromethylhydrochlorothiazide; trichloromethiazide; 'esmarin', 'eurinol',
'fluitran', 'flutra', 'metahydrin', 'naqua').
TRICHLORMETHINE*** (tris(2-chloro-
ethyl)amine; 2,2',2''-trichlorotriethyl-
amine; trimustine; tris-*N*-lost; HN3;
NSC-30211; R-47; SK-100; TS-160;
'lekamin', 'sinalost', 'trillekamin',
'trimitan').
TRICHLORMETHINE *N*-**OXIDE** (TEAO).
Trichlormethylfos *see* Chlorpyrifos-methyl.
Trichloroacetaldehyde monohydrate
see Chloral hydrate.
Trichloroacetonitrile *see* Chlorocyano-
hydrin.
S-(**2,3,3-Trichloroallyl**) **diisopropylcarbamothioate** *see* Triallate.
TRICHLOROBENZOIC ACID (2,3,6-
trichlorobenzoic acid; 2,3,6-TBA;
'trysben').
See also Dimethylamine trichlorobenzoate.
**1,1,1-Trichloro-2,2-bis(*p*-chlorophenyl)-
ethane** *see* DDT.
**1,1,1-Trichloro-2,2-bis(*p*-chlorophenyl)-
ethanol** *see* Dicofol.
**1,1,1-TRICHLORO-2,2-BIS(*p*-FLUORO-
PHENYL)ETHANE** (DFDT; 'gix').
**1,1,1-Trichloro-2,2-bis(*p*-methoxy-
phenyl)ethane** *see* Methoxychlor.
Trichlorobutanediol *see* Butylchloral
hydrate.
Trichlorobutylidene glycol *see* Butylchloral
hydrate.
3,4,4'-Trichlorocarbanilide *see* Triclocarban.
**1,1,1-Trichloro-2-(*o*-chlorophenyl)-2-(*p*-
chlorophenyl)ethane** *see* *o*,*p*'-DDT.
**1,2,4-Trichloro-5-(*p*-chlorophenyl-
sulfonyl)benzene** *see* Tetradifon.
**1,2,4-Trichloro-5-[(*p*-chlorophenyl)thio]-
benzene** *see* Tetrasul.
**3,5,6-Trichloro-2-[(diethoxyphosphino-
thioyl)oxy]pyridine** *see* Chlorpyrifos.
1,1,1-TRICHLOROETHANE (methylchloroform; 'chlorothene', 'drano liquid').
1,1,2-TRICHLOROETHANE (vinyl trichloride).
Trichloroethene *see* Trichloroethylene.
Trichloroethyl carbamate *see* Trichlorourethan.
Trichloroethyl dihydrogen phosphate
see Triclofos.
TRICHLOROETHYLENE*** (1,1,2-tri-
chloroethylene; ethinyl trichloride; trichloroethene; tri).
**1,1'-(2,2,2-Trichloroethylene)bis(4-
methoxybenzene)** *see* Methoxychlor.
**1,2-*O*-(2,2,2-Trichloroethylidene)-α-D-
glucofuranose** *see* Chloralose.
Trichloroethyl phosphate *see* Triclofos.
**9,11β,21-Trichloro-6α-fluoro-16α,17-
dihydroxypregna-1,4-diene-3,20-dione**

447

cyclic acetal with acetone *see* Triclonide.

9,11β,21-Trichloro-6α-fluoropregna-1,4-diene-16α,17-diol-3,20-dione cyclic acetal with acetone *see* Triclonide.

N-(2,2,2-Trichloro-1-formamidoethyl)-aniline *see* Chloraniformethan.

2,2,2-Trichloro-4′-hydroxyacetanilide *see* Triclacetamol.

β,β,β-Trichloro-α-hydroxy-p-acetophenetidide *see* Cloracetadol.

2,4,4′-Trichloro-2′-hydroxydiphenyl ether *see* Triclosan.

p-(2,2,2-Trichloro-1-hydroxyethoxy)-acetanilide *see* Cloracetadol.

17β-(2,2,2-Trichloro-1-hydroxyethoxy)-androst-4-en-3-one *see* Cloxotestosterone.

17β-(2,2,2-Trichloro-1-hydroxyethoxy)-estra-1,3,5(10)-trien-3-ol *see* Cloxestradiol.

7-[2-(2,2,2-Trichloro-1-hydroxyethoxy)-ethyl]theophylline *see* Triclofylline.

N-(2,2,2-Trichloro-1-hydroxyethyl)-carbamic acid ethyl ester *see* Carbocloral.

3-(2,2,2-Trichloro-1-hydroxyethyl)-5,5-diphenyl-4-imidazolidinone *see* Triclodazol.

(2,2,2-Trichloro-1-hydroxyethyl) estradiol ether *see* Cloxestradiol.

6-O-(2,2,2-Trichloro-1-hydroxyethyl)-α,D-glucopyranose 1→4 polymer with α-D-glucopyranose *see* Amicloral.

(2,2,2-Trichloro-1-hydroxyethyl)-phosphonic acid dimethyl ester *see* Metrifonate.

(2,2,2-Trichloro-1-hydroxyethyl) testosterone ether *see* Cloxotestosterone.

2,4,4′-Trichloro-α-imidazol-1-yl-α,α′-ditolyl ether *see* Econazole.

2,4,5-Trichloro-1-(3-iodo-2-propyn-1-yl-oxy)benzene *see* Haloprogin.

Trichloroisocyanuric acid *see* Symclosene.

Trichloromethiazide *see* Trichlormethiazide.

2,3,5-Trichloro-6-methoxybenzoic acid *see* Tricamba.

Trichloromethyl chloroformate *see* Diphosgene.

2-Trichloromethyl-1,3-dioxane-5,5-dimethanol *see* Penthrichloral.

Trichloromethylhydrochlorothiazide *see* Trichlormethiazide.

N-(Trichloromethylthio)-4-cyclohexene-1,2-dicarboximide *see* Captan.

2-(Trichloromethylthio)-1H-isoindole-1,3-(2H)-dione *see* Folpet.

N-(Trichloromethylthio)phthalimide *see* Folpet.

N-(Trichloromethylthio)tetrahydro-phthalimide *see* Captan.

4,5,7-Trichloro-2-[3-(methylthio)-1,2,4-thiadiazol-2-ylthio]benzimidazole *see* Subendazole.

TRICHLORONAT* (O-ethyl O-(2,4,5-trichlorophenyl) ethylphosphonothioate; fenophosphon; trichloronate; 'agrisil', 'apritox', 'phytosol').

Trichloronitromethane *see* Chloropicrin.

TRICHLOROPHEN (tr) (2,6-bis(5-chloro-2-hydroxybenzyl)-4-chlorophenol; trichlosal; G-610).

2,4,5-TRICHLOROPHENOL ('dowicide 2').

2,4,6-TRICHLOROPHENOL ('dowicide 2S', 'omal').

2,4,5-Trichlorophenolate(s) *see* Triclofenate(s).

2,4,5-Trichlorophenol piperazine compound *see* Triclofenol piperazine.

2,4,5-TRICHLOROPHENOXYACETIC ACID (2,4,5-T).
See also Chlorinated phenoxyacetic acid mixture.

2-(2,4,5-Trichlorophenoxy)ethyl 2,2-dichloropropionate *see* Erbon.

2-(2,4,5-Trichlorophenoxy)propionic acid *see* Fenoprop.

2,4,5-Trichlorophenyl γ-iodopropargyl ether *see* Haloprogin.

2,4,5-Trichlorophenyl 3-iodo-2-propynyl ether *see* Haloprogin.

Trichlorophone *see* Metrifonate.

Trichlorophos *see* Triclofos.

S-(2,3,3-Trichloro-2-propenyl) bis(1-methylethyl)carbamothioate *see* Triallate.

1,1,2-TRICHLORO-1,2,2-TRIFLUORO-ETHANE ('arcton-63', 'frigen-113', 'genetron-113').

Trichlorotriethylamine *see* Trichlormethine.

TRICHLOROURETHAN (trichloroethyl carbamate; 'voluntal').

Trichlorphon* *see* Metrifonate.

'Trichloryl' *see* Triclofos.

Trichlosal *see* Trichlorophen.

'Trichocid' *see* Aminitrozole.

'Trichofuron' *see* Furazolidone.

'Trichojel' *see* Aminoacridine.

'Trichomol' *see* Metronidazole.

'Trichomon' *see* DDT.

'Trichomonacid' *see* Metronidazole.

TRICHOMONACIDE (tr) (4-(4-diethyl-amino-1-methylbutylamino)-6-methoxy-2-(4-nitrostyryl)quinoline).

'Trichomycin' *see* Hachimycin.

'Trichonat' *see* Hachimycin.

Trichopol (tr) *see* Metronidazole.

'Trichorad' *see* Aminitrozole.

'Trichoral' *see* Aminitrozole.

'Trichosept' *see* Hachimycin.

TRICIN (4′,5,7-trihydroxy-3′,5′-dimethoxy-flavone).

TRICLACETAMOL*** (2,2,2-trichloro-4′-hydroxyacetanilide).

TRICLAZATE*** (1-methyl-3-pyrrolidinyl-methyl benzilate; benzilate of 1-methyl-3-pyrrolidinemethanol).

'Tricleryl' *see* Triclofos.

TRICLOBISONIUM CHLORIDE*** (hexamethylenebis[dimethyl-[1-methyl-3-(2,2,6-trimethylcyclohexyl)propyl]-ammonium chloride]hemihydrate; Ro-5-0810/1; 'treburon').

TRICLOCARBAN*** (3,4,4′-trichlorocar-banilide; TCC; 'aseptanide', 'centracid', 'cutisan', 'nobacter', 'septivon', 'solu-

448

bacter').

TRICLODAZOL*** (5,5-diphenyl-3-(2,2,2-trichloro-1-hydroxyethyl)-4-imidazolidinone).

TRICLOFENATE(S)** (2,4,5-trichlorophenolate(s)).
See also Alazanine triclofenate.

TRICLOFENOL PIPERAZINE*** (piperazine di(2,4,5-trichlorophenoxide); CI-416; piperazine compound with 2,4,5-trichlorophenol; IN-29-5931; 'ranestol').

TRICLOFOS* (2,2,2-trichloroethyl dihydrogen phosphate; trichloroethanol phosphate; trichloroethyl phosphate).

TRICLOFOS SODIUM (trichloroethyl sodium phosphate; sodium triclofos; trichlorophos; trichlofos sodium; 'trichloryl', 'tricloryl', 'triclos').

TRICLOFYLLINE*** (7-[2-(2,2,2-trichloro-1-hydroxyethoxy)ethyl]theophylline; 7-[2-(1-hydroxy-2,2,2-trichloroethoxy)-ethyl]theophylline).

TRICLONIDE** (9,11β,21-trichloro-6α-fluoropregna-1,4-diene-16α,17-diol-3,20-dione cyclic acetal with acetone; 9,11β,21-trichloro-6α-fluoro-16α,17-dihydroxy-pregna-1,4-diene-3,20-dione cyclic acetal with acetone; RS-4464).

Triclorfon *see* Metrifonate.

'Tricloryl' *see* Triclofos.

'Triclos' *see* Triclofos sodium.

TRICLOSAN** (5-chloro-2-(2,4-dichlorophenoxy)phenol; 2,4,4'-trichloro-2'-hydroxydiphenyl ether; cloxifenol; CH-3565; GP-41353; 'cidal', 'irgasan DP 300', 'sterlifix').

'Tricofuron' *see* Furazolidone.

'Tricoloid' *see* Tricyclamol.

'Tricoperidol' *see* Trifluperidol.

'Tricornox' *see* Benazolin.

'Tricoryl' *see* Trolnitrate.

'Tricranolin' *see* Chlorocarvacrol.

TRICRESOL (mixture of *o*-, *m*- and *p*-cresols).

TRICRESYL PHOSPHATE (mixture of tris(*o*-, *m*- and *p*-cresyl) esters of phosphoric acid; tolyl phosphate; tritolyl phosphate; TCP; PX-917; 'celluflex', 'kronitex', 'lindol').

TRI-*o*-CRESYL PHOSPHATE (TOCP).

Tricyanic acid *see* Cyanuric acid.

1,1,3-TRICYANOALLYLAMINE (tricyano-2-propenylamine; tricyanoaminopropene; 'triap').

Tricyanoaminopropene *see* Tricyanoallylamine.

TRICYCLAMOL CHLORIDE*** ((±)-1-(3-cyclohexyl-3-hydroxy-3-phenylpropyl)-1-methylpyrrolidinium chloride; procyclidine methochloride; L-14045; 'elorine', 'lergine', 'tricoloid', 'vagosin').

Tricyclo(3.3.1.1³,⁷)decane *see* Adamantane.

1-Tricyclo(3.3.1.1³,⁷)dec-1-yl-2-azetidine-carboxylic acid *see* Carmantadine.

Tricyclohexylhydroxystannane *see* Cyhexatin.

Tricyclohexylhydroxytin *see* Cyhexatin.

3,5,7,8-Tridecatetraene-10,12-diynoic acid *see* Mycomycin.

TRIDEMORPH* (2,6-dimethyl-4-tridecyl-morpholine; 'calixin').

'Tridesilon' *see* Desonide.

'Tridesonit' *see* Desonide.

'Tridigal' *see* Lanatoside(s).

Tridihexethide *see* Tridihexethyl chloride.

TRIDIHEXETHYL CHLORIDE ((3-cyclo-hexyl-3-hydroxy-3-phenylpropyl)triethyl-ammonium chloride; tridihexethide; 'claviton').

TRIDIHEXETHYL IODIDE*** ((3-cyclo-hexyl-3-hydroxy-3-phenylpropyl)triethyl-ammonium iodide; 1-cyclohexyl-3-diethyl-amino-1-phenyl-1-propanol ethiodide propethon; tridihexide; 'pathilon').

Tridihexide *see* Tridihexethyl iodide.

'Tridione' *see* Trimethadione.

'Trieffortil' *see* Etilefrine.

Trienbolone *see* Trenbolone.

TRIETAZINE* (2-chloro-4-diethylamino-6-ethylamino-*s*-triazine; 6-chloro-*N*,*N*',*N*'-triethyl-1,3,5-triazine-2,4-diamine).

Trienolone *see* Trenbolone.

'Tri-ervonum' *see* Megestrol acetate with ethinylestradiol.

TRIETHANOLAMINE (2,2',2''-nitrilotriethanol; 2,2',2''-trihydroxytriethylamine trolamine).

Triethanolamine trinitrate *see* Trolnitrate.

Triethanomelamine *see* Tretamine.

Triethylaminoethanol chloride *see* Triethyl(2-hydroxyethyl)ammonium chloride.

Triethylcholine *see* Triethyl(2-hydroxyethyl)-ammonium chloride.

TRIETHYLENE GLYCOL (3,6-dioxa-octane-1,8-diol; triglycol).

Triethylene glycol diglycidyl ether *see* Etoglucid.

Triethylenemelamine *see* Tretamine.

Triethylenephosphoramide *see* Tepa.

Triethylenethiophosphoramide *see* Thiotepa.

Triethylenimine thiophosphoramide *see* Thiotepa.

Triethyleniminobenzoquinone *see* Triaziquone.

Triethylenimino-*s*-triazine *see* Tretamine.

Triethyl(3-hydroxy-2,3-dimethylpropyl)-ammonium iodide *p*-butoxybenzoate *see* Quateron.

TRIETHYL(2-HYDROXYETHYL)AM-MONIUM CHLORIDE ((2-hydroxy-ethyl)triethylammonium chloride; choline triethyl analog; triethylaminoethanol chloride; triethylcholine; TEC).

Triethyl(2-hydroxyethyl)ammonium *p*-toluenesulfonate 3,4,5-trimethoxy-benzoate *see* Troxonium tosilate.

N,N',N'-Triethyl-N-(2-hydroxyethyl)-ethylenediamine *p*-aminobenzoate *see* Amoxecaine.

TRIETHYL ORTHOFORMATE (triethoxy-methane; ethyl orthoformate; aethylis

449

formias; 'aethon', 'aethussan', 'ethone').

Triethyl[2-(p-styrylphenoxy)ethyl]ammonium iodide see Stilonium iodide.

Triethyl[2-(trimethoxybenzoyloxy)ethyl]ammonium *p*-toluenesulfonate see Troxonium tosilate.

TRIFENMORPH[*] (*N*-(triphenylmethyl)-morpholine; tritylmorpholine; triphenmorph; WL-8008; 'frescon').

TRIFEZOLAC[**] (1,3,5-triphenylpyrazole-4-acetic acid).

TRIFLOCIN[**] (4-(3-trifluoromethylanilino)-nicotinic acid; 4-(α,α,α-trifluoro-*m*-toluidino)nicotinic acid; 4-(3-trifluoromethylanilino)pyridine-3-carboxylic acid; *N*-(3-carboxypyridin-4-yl)-α,α,α-trifluoro-*m*-toluidine; CL-65562; JDL-38).

TRIFLUBAZAM[***] (1-methyl-5-phenyl-7-trifluoromethyl-1H-1,5-benzodiazepine-2,4(3H,5H)-dione; ORF-8063; WE352).

TRIFLUMIDATE[***] (ethyl *m*-benzoyl-*N*-(trifluoromethylsulfonyl)carbanilate; 3-[*N*-carboxy-*N*-(trifluoromethylsulfonyl)-amino]benzophenone ethyl ester; BA-4223; MBR-4223).

TRIFLUOMEPRAZINE[***] (10-[3-(dimethylamino)-2-methylpropyl]-2-(trifluoromethyl)phenothiazine; triflutrimeprazine; SK&F-5354-A).

TRIFLUOPERAZINE[***] (10-[3-(4-methylpiperazin-1-yl)propyl]-2-trifluoromethylphenothiazine; trifluoromethylperazine; trifluperazine; trifluoperazine dihydrochloride; trifluoperazine hydrochloride; triftazine; SK&F-5019; 'eskazinyl', 'jatroneural', 'stelazine', 'terfluzine'). *See also* Tranylcypromine with trifluoperazine.

α,α,α-**Trifluoro-2,6-dimethyl-1-piperidinethiocarboxy-*m*-toluidide** see Ticarbodine.

α,α,α-**Trifluoro-2,6-dinitro-*N*,*N*-dipropyl-*p*-toluidine** see Trifluralin.

Trifluoroethyl vinyl ether see Fluroxene.

Trifluoromethane see Fluoroform.

α,α,α-**Trifluoro-*p*-[3-(methylamino)-1-phenylpropoxy]toluene** see Fluoxetine.

2-(3-Trifluoromethylanilino)nicotinic acid see Niflumic acid.

4-(3-Trifluoromethylanilino)nicotinic acid see Triflocin.

1-[2-(4'-Trifluoromethylbiphenyl-4-yloxy)ethyl]pyrrolidine see Boxidine.

2,2,2-Trifluoro-1-methylethyl 2-cyanoacrylate see Flucrilate.

Trifluoromethylhydrothiazide see Hydroflumethiazide.

α,α,α-**Trifluoro-2-methyl-4'-nitro-*m*-propionotoluamide** see Flutamide.

Trifluoromethylperazine see Trifluoperazine.

8-Trifluoromethylphenothiazine-1-carboxylic acid see Flutiazin.

4-[3-(2-Trifluoromethylphenothiazin-2-yl)propyl]-1-piperazineethanol see Fluphenazine.

2-[[1-[3-[2-(Trifluoromethyl)pheno-

thiazin-10-yl]propyl]piperid-4-yl]oxy]ethanol** see Flupimazine.

6,6,9-Trifluoro-16α-methylprednisolone see Cormetasone.

6,6,9-Trifluoro-16α-methylpregna-1,4-diene-11β,17,21-triol-3,20-dione see Cormetasone.

6α-Trifluoromethylpregn-4-ene-17-ol-3,20-dione see Flumedroxone.

Trifluoromethylpromazine see Triflupromazine.

N-(8-Trifluoromethylquinolin-4-yl)-anthranilic acid 2,3-dihydroxypropyl ester** see Floctafenine.

N-[7-(Trifluoromethyl)-4-quinolyl]anthranilic acid 2-[4-(α,α,α-trifluoro-*m*-tolyl)piperazin-1-yl]ethyl ester** see Antrafenine.

Trifluoromethylthiazide see Flumethiazide.

4-[3-(6-Trifluoromethyl-4H-thieno(2,3-b)-(1,4)benzothiazin-4-yl)propyl]-1-piperazineethanol see Flutizenol.

α,α,α-**Trifluoro-3-nitro-4-(*p*-nitrophenoxy)toluene** see Fluorodifen.

α,α,α-**Trifluoro-*m*-salicylotoluidide** see Salfluverine.

α,α,α-**Trifluoro-*N*-salicyloyl-*m*-toluidine** see Salfluverine.

TRIFLUOROTHYMIDINE (2'-deoxy-5-trifluoromethyluridine; F_3TDR).

2-(α,α,α-Trifluoro-*m*-toluidino)nicotinic acid see Niflumic acid.

4-(α,α,α-Trifluoro-*m*-toluidino)nicotinic acid see Triflocin.

N-[[4-(α,α,α-Trifluoro-*m*-toluidino)-pyrid-3-yl]sulfonyl]propionamide** see Galosemide.

N-(α,α,α-Trifluoro-*m*-tolyl)anthranilic acid** see Flufenamic acid.

N-(α,α,α-Trifluoro-*m*-tolyl)anthranilic acid esters** see Colfenamate; Etofenamate.

2-(α,α,α-Trifluoro-*p*-tolyl)-1,3-indandione see Fluindarol.

6-(α,α,α-Trifluoro-*p*-tolyl)-3-morpholinone see Flumetramide.

2-[4-(α,α,α-Trifluoro-*m*-tolyl)piperazin-1-yl]ethyl *N*-[7-(trifluoromethyl)-4-quinolyl]anthranilate see Antrafenine.

4-(α,α,α-Trifluoro-*p*-tolyl-3-pyrrolidin-1-yl)propiophenone see Boxidine.

6,6,9-Trifluoro-11β,17,21-trihydroxy-16α-methylpregna-1,4-diene-3,20-dione see Cormetasone.

2-($\alpha^3,\alpha^3,\alpha^3$-Trifluoro-2,3-xylidino)nicotinic acid see Flunixin.

Trifluperazine see Trifluoperazine.

TRIFLUPERIDOL[***] (1-[3-(*p*-fluoro-benzoyl)propyl]-4-(*m*-trifluoromethyl-phenyl)-4-piperidinol; 4'-fluoro-4-[4-hydroxy-4-(*m*-trifluoromethylphenyl)-piperidino]butyrophenone; 4'-fluoro-4-[4-hydroxy-4-(α,α,α-trifluoro-*m*-tolyl)-piperid-1-yl]butyrophenone; triperidol; flumoperon; McN-JR-2498; R-2498; 'psichoperidol', 'tricoperidol', 'triperidol', 'trisedyl').

TRIFLUPROMAZINE[***] (10-(3-dimethyl-

450

aminopropyl)-2-trifluoromethylphenothi-
azine; trifluoromethylpromazine; fluopromazine; triflupromazine hydrochloride;
MC-4703; SK&F-4648-A; 'adazine',
'fluorofen', 'flurofen', 'nivoman', 'psyquil',
'siquil', 'vespral', 'vesprin', 'vetame').

TRIFLURALIN* (α,α,α-trifluoro-2,6-dinitro-
N,N-dipropyl-p-toluidine; 2,6-dinitro-N,N-
dipropyl-4-trifluoromethylaniline; 'treflan').

Triflutrimeprazine *see* Trifluomeprazine.

TRIFOLIN (kaempferol 3-galactoside.)

'Triformol' *see* Paraformaldehyde.

Triftazine (tr) *see* Trifluoperazine.

'Trigemine' *see* Butylchloralamidopyrine.

'Trigeminin' *see* Butylchloralamidopyrine.

'Trigenolline' *see* Trigonelline.

TRIGENTISIC ACID ('rehibin').

Triglycol *see* Triethylene glycol.

TRIGLYCOLLAMIC ACID (nitrilotriacetic
acid).
See also Bismuth sodium triglycollamate;
Sodium triglycollamate.

TRIGONELLINE (nicotinic acid N-methyl-
betaine; 'caffearin', 'coffearine', 'gynesin',
'trigenolline').

TRIHEXYPHENIDYL*** (α-cyclohexyl-α-
phenyl-1-piperidinepropanol; 1-cyclo-
hexyl-1-phenyl-3-piperid-1-yl-1-propanol;
benzhexol; hexyphenidyl; trihexyphenidyl
hydrochloride).

2′,3′,4′-Trihydroxyacetophenone *see*
Gallacetophenone.

1,8,9-Trihydroxyanthracene *see* Dithranol.

1,2,3-Trihydroxybenzene *see* Pyrogallol.

1,3,5-Trihydroxybenzene *see* Phloroglucinol.

3,4,5-Trihydroxybenzoic acid *see* Gallic
acid.

**1-(2,3,4-Trihydroxybenzyl)-2-seryl-
hydrazine** *see* Serine trihydroxybenzyl-
hydrazide.

**3β,12,14-Trihydroxy-5β-card-20(22)-
enolide 3-(acetylglucosyltridigitoxo-
side)** *see* Lanatoside C.

**3β,12,14-Trihydroxy-5β-card-20(22)-
enolide 3-(4′′′-acetyltridigitoxoside)**
see Acetyldigoxin.

**3β,12β,14β-Trihydroxy-5β-card-20(22)-
enolide 3-(4′′′-O-methyltridigitoxoside)**
see Medigoxin.

**3β,12,14-Trihydroxy-5β-card-20(22)-
enolide 3-tridigitoxoside** *see* Digoxin.

3,6,7-Trihydroxycholanic acid *see*
Hyocholic acid.

3,7,12-Trihydroxycholanic acid *see* Cholic
acid.

Trihydroxycyanidine *see* Cyanuric acid.

**3,4,5-Trihydroxycyclohexene-1-carboxylic
acid** *see* Shikimic acid.

**3,4,5-Trihydroxy-2,2-dimethyl-6-chrom-
anacrylic acid δ-lactone 4-acetate
3-(2-methylbutyrate)** *see* Visnadine.

**11β,17,21-Trihydroxy-6,16α-dimethyl-
2′-phenyl-2′H-pregna-2,4,6-trieno-
(3,2-c)pyrazol-20-one 21-acetate** *see*
Cortivazol.

**11β,17,21-Trihydroxy-6,16α-dimethyl-2′-
phenyl-2′H-pregna-2,4,6-trieno(3,2-c)-**

pyrazol-20-one 21-(m-sulfobenzoate)
see Cortisuzol.

Trihydroxyethylrutin *see* Troxerutin.

4′,5,7-Trihydroxyflavanone *see* Naringenin.

**11β,17,21-Trihydroxy-B-homo-A-
norpregn-1-ene-3,6,20-dione** *see*
Oxisopred.

**2′,4′,6′-Trihydroxy-3-(p-hydroxyphenyl)-
propiophenone** *see* Phloretin.

**4′,5,7-Trihydroxy-3′-methoxyflavanon-
3-ol** *see* 3-Methyltaxifolin.

**2,3,3′-Trihydroxy-4′-methoxystilbene
2-glucoside** *see* Rhapontizin.

1,3,8-Trihydroxy-6-methylanthraquinone
see Frangula-emodin.

**β,4,4′-Trihydroxy-α-methyldiphenethyl-
amine** *see* Ritodrine.

**11β,17,21-Trihydroxy-16-methylene-
pregna-1,4-diene-3,20-dione** *see*
Prednylidene.

**11β,17α,21-Trihydroxy-16-methylene-
pregna-4,6-diene-3,20-dione** *see*
Isoprednidene.

3,5,6-Trihydroxy-1-methylindole *see*
Adrenolutin.

**11β,17α,21-Trihydroxy-6α-methylpregna-
1,4-diene-3,20-dione** *see* Methylpredni-
solone.

**3α,11α,16β-Trihydroxy-29-nor-8α,9β,13α,
14β-dammara-17(20),24-dien-21-oic
acid 16-acetate** *see* Fusidic acid.

**3β,5,14-Trihydroxy-19-oxo-5β-card-
20(22)-enolide 3-D-cymaro-D-glucoside**
see Strophanthin.

2,4,5-Trihydroxyphenethylamine *see*
6-Hydroxydopamine.

**7-[2-(3,4,β-Trihydroxyphenethylamino)-
ethyl]theophylline** *see* Theodrenaline.

**7-[3-[(β,3,5-Trihydroxyphenethyl)amino]-
propyl]theophylline** *see* Reproterol.

2,4,5-Trihydroxyphenylalanine *see*
6-Hydroxydopa.

**11β,17α,21-Trihydroxypregna-1,4-diene-
3,20-dione** *see* Prednisolone.

**11β,17α,21-Trihydroxypregn-4-ene-3,20-
dione** *see* Hydrocortisone.

2′,4′,6′-Trihydroxypropiophenone *see*
Flopropione.

**9α,11α,15-Trihydroxy-5-cis-13-$trans$-
prostadienoic acid** *see* Dinoprost.

**β,3,5-Trihydroxy-N-(3-theophyllin-7-
ylpropyl)phenethylamine** *see* Reproterol.

2,4,6-Trihydroxy-s-triazine *see* Cyanuric
acid.

**cis-3α,11α,16β-Trihydroxy-4α,8,14-tri-
methyl-18-nor-5α,8α,9β,13α,14β-
cholesta-17(20),24-dien-21-oic acid
16-acetate** *see* Fusidic acid.

Triiodoethanoic acid *see* Iophenoxic acid.

Triiodomethane *see* Iodoform.

**2,4,6-Triiodo-3-[2-[2-[2-[2-(2-methoxy)-
ethoxy]ethoxy]ethoxy]acetamido]-
benzoic acid** *see* Iotrizoic acid.

**4-[2,4,6-Triiodo-3-(morpholinocarbonyl)-
phenoxy]butyric acid** *see* Iobutoic acid.

**2-[2,4,6-Triiodo-3-(2-oxopyrrolidin-1-yl)-
benzyl]butyric acid** *see* Iolidonic acid.

2-(2,4,6-Triiodophenoxy)butyric acid *see* Phenobutiodil.

3,3′,5-Triiodothyroacetic acid *see* Triac.

L-3,5,3′-Triiodothyronine *see* Liothyronine.

Triiodothyropropionic acid *see* Thyropropic acid.

'Triiodyl' *see* Sodium acetrizoate.

Triiotrast (tr) *see* Sodium acetrizoate.

3,7,12-Triketocholanic acid *see* Dehydrocholic acid.

'Trikranolin' *see* Chlorocarvacrol.

'Trilafan' *see* Perphenazine.

'Trifalon' *see* Perphenazine.

TRILINOLEIN (glyceryl trilinoleate; linoleic acid triglyceride).

'Trillekamin' *see* Trichlormethine.

'Trilombrine' *see* Iophenoxic acid.

'Trilon' *see* Trisodium edetate.

'Trilon A' *see* Sodium triglycollamate.

TRILOSTANE** (4α,5-epoxy-17β-hydroxy-3-oxo-5α-androstane-2α-carbonitrile).

'Trimaton' *see* Metam-sodium.

TRIMAZOSIN** (2-hydroxy-2-methylpropyl 4-(4-amino-6,7,8-trimethoxyquinazolin-2-yl)piperazine-1-carboxylate).

TRIMEBUTINE*** (β-dimethylamino-β-ethyl phenethyl alcohol 3,4,5-trimethoxybenzoate; 2-dimethylamino-2-phenylbutyl 3,4,5-trimethoxybenzoate; 'polibutin').

TRIMEBUTINE MALEATE ('debridat').

TRIMECAINE** (N-(α-diethylaminoacetyl)-2,4,6-trimethylaniline; 2-diethylamino-2′,4′,6′-trimethylacetanilide; 2-diethylaminoacetomesidide; N-(α-diethylaminoacetyl)mesidine; mesocaine; mesdicaine).

'Trimedone' *see* Trimethadione.

TRIMEDOXIME BROMIDE*** (1,1′-trimethylenebis(4-formylpyridinium bromide)dioxime; 1,3-bis(4-hydroxyiminomethylpyridinium)propane dibromide; dipyroxime; TMB-4).

TRIMEGLAMIDE** (N′,N′-diethyl-N-(4,4,5-trimethoxybenzoyl)glycinamide; N-(diethylcarbamoylmethyl)-3,4,5-trimethoxybenzamide; trimethoxybenzoylglycine diethylamide; tricetamide; R-548).

'Trimelarsan' *see* Melarsonyl potassium.

TRIMEPERIDINE*** (1,2,5-trimethyl-4-phenyl-4-propionoxypiperidine; promedol; dimethylmeperidine).

TRIMEPRANOL (tr) (1-(4-acetoxy-2,3,5-trimethylphenoxy)-3-isopropylamino-2-propanol; 4-(2-hydroxy-3-isopropylaminopropoxy)-2,3,6-trimethylphenyl acetate; VUFB-6453).

Trimeprazine* *see* Alimemazine.

Trimeprimine* *see* Trimipramine.

Trimepropimine *see* Trimipramine.

TRIMETAMIDE*** (N-(2-amino-6-methylpyrid-3-ylmethyl)-3,4,5-trimethoxybenzamide).

TRIMETAPHAN CAMSILATE*** (1,3-dibenzyldecahydro-2-oxoimidazo(4,5-c)-thieno(1,2-a)thiolium 10-camphorsulfonate; D-3,4-(1,3-dibenzyl-2-ketoimidazolido)-1,2-trimethylenethiophanium D-camphorsulfonate; 4,6-dibenzyl-5-oxo-1-thia-4,6-diazatricyclo(6,3,0,0³,⁷)undecanium D-camphorsulfonate; méthioplégium; trimethaphan; thimethaphan; trimetaphan camphorsulfonate; trimetaphan camsylate; Nu-2222; Ro-2-2222; 'arfonad').

TRIMETAZIDINE*** (1-(2,3,4-trimethoxybenzyl)piperazine; S-4004; 'vastarel').

Trimetazone *see* Tribuzone.

TRIMETHADIONE*** (3,5,5-trimethyl-2,4-oxazolidinedione; troxidone; trimethin; trimetin).

Trimethaphan *see* Trimetaphan.

Trimethazone *see* Tribuzone.

TRIMETHIDINIUM METHOSULFATE*** ((+)-3-(3-dimethylaminopropyl)-1,3,8,8-tetramethyl-3-azabicyclo-(3.2.1)octane methyl sulfate methosulfate; N-methyl-N-(3-trimethylaminopropyl)-camphidinium dimethylsulfate; camphidonium; Ha-106; Wy-1395; 'ostensin').

Trimethin (tr) *see* Trimethadione.

Trimethoate *see* Prothoate.

TRIMETHOBENZAMIDE*** (N-[p-(2-dimethylaminoethoxy)benzyl]-3,4,5-trimethoxybenzamide; 4-(2-dimethylaminoethoxy)-N-(3,4,5-trimethoxybenzoyl)-benzylamine; trimethobenzamide hydrochloride; Ro-2-9578; 'tigan').

TRIMETHOPRIM*** (2,4-diamino-5-(3,4,5-trimethoxybenzyl)pyrimidine; BW-56-72; Ro 5-6846; WR-5949; 'syraprim'). *See also* Co-trimoxazole; Sulfadimidine with trimethoprim; Sulfaperin with trimethoprim.

Trimethoquinol *see* Tretoquinol.

6-(3,4,5-Trimethoxybenzamido)caproic acid *see* Capobenic acid.

6-(3,4,5-Trimethoxybenzamido)hexanoic acid *see* Capobenic acid.

1,3,5-TRIMETHOXYBENZENE (trimethylphloroglucinol). *See also* Phloroglucinol with 1,3,5-trimethoxybenzene.

3,4,5-TRIMETHOXYBENZOIC ACID (trimethylgallic acid).

3,4,5-Trimethoxybenzoic acid, esters and salts *see* (*also*) Megallate(s).

2,4,6-Trimethoxybenzoic acid 2-morpholinoethyl ester *see* Mofloverine.

Trimethoxybenzoyl-6-aminocaproic acid *see* Capobenic acid.

Trimethoxybenzoylglycine diethylamide *see* Trimeglamide.

Trimethoxybenzoylmorpholine *see* Trimetozine.

1-[3-(2,4,6-Trimethoxybenzoyl)propyl]-pyrrolidine *see* Buflomedil.

Trimethoxybenzylimidazoline *see* Phedrazine.

Trimethoxybenzylpiperazine *see* Trimetazidine.

2′,4,4′-Trimethoxychalcone *see* Metochalcone.

3,4,5-Trimethoxycinnamamide *see* Cintramide.

4-(3,4,5-Trimethoxycinnamoyl)-1-piper-azineacetic acid *see* Cinepazic acid.

4-(3,4,5-Trimethoxycinnamoyl)-1-piper-azineacetic acid ethyl ester *see* Cinepazet.

3,4,5-Trimethoxyphenethylamine *see* Mescaline.

3,4,5-Trimethoxy-N-(1-phenoxymethyl-2-pyrrolidin-1-ylethyl)benzamide *see* Fepromide.

4-[[2-(3,4,5-Trimethoxyphenyl)-2-methyl-1,3-dioxolan-4-yl]methyl]morpholine *see* Trioxolane.

2′,4′,6′-Trimethoxy-4-pyrrolidin-1-ylbutyrophenone *see* Buflomedil.

3′,4′,5′-Trimethoxy-3-(3-pyrrolin-1-yl)-acrylophenone *see* Roletamide.

Trimethylacetic acid *see* Pivalic acid.

2-(2,2,2-Trimethylacetyl)-1,3-indandione *see* Pindone.

2,4,5-Trimethylaniline *see* Pseudocumidine.

2,4,6-Trimethylaniline *see* Mesidine.

6,6,9-Trimethyl-9-azabicyclo(3.3.1)non-3β-yl dithien-2-ylglycolate *see* Mazaticol.

1,3,5-Trimethylbenzene *see* Mesitylene.

2-(1,7,7-Trimethylbicyclo(2.2.1)hept-2-yl)-3,4-xylenol *see* Xibornol.

N,N,2-Trimethyl-3-chromanamine *see* Trebenzomine.

3,3,5-Trimethylcyclohexyl lactate *see* Ciclactate.

Trimethylcyclohexyl mandelate *see* Cyclandelate.

***trans*-3,3,5-Trimethylcyclohexyl nicotinate** *see* Ciclonicate.

3,3,5-Trimethylcyclohexyl salicylate *see* Homosalate.

N,N-2-Trimethyl-3,4-diphenyl-3-propionoxy-1-butylamine *see* Dextro-propoxyphene; Levopropoxyphene.

N,N,1-Trimethyl-3,3-dithien-2-ylallyl-amine *see* Dimethylthiambutene.

3,7,11-Trimethyldodeca-2,4-dienoic acid 2-propynyl ester *see* Kinoprene.

3,7,11-Trimethyl-2,6,10-dodecatrien-1-ol *see* Farnesol.

Trimethylene *see* Cyclopropane.

Trimethylenebis(clofibrate) *see* Simfi-brate.

1,1′-Trimethylenebis(4-formyl-pyridinium bromide) dioxime *see* Trimedoxime bromide.

4,4′-(Trimethylenedioxy)bis(3-bromo-benzamidine) *see* Dibrompropamidine.

***p,p′*-(Trimethylenedioxy)dibenzamidine** *see* Propamidine.

Trimethylene oxide *see* Oxetane.

Trimethylene sulfide *see* Thietane.

Trimethylgallic acid *see* 3,4,5-Trimethoxy-benzoic acid.

6,6,9-Trimethylgranatoline dithienyl-glycolate *see* Mazaticol.

N-1,5-Trimethyl-4-hexenylamine *see* Isometheptene.

7,8,10-Trimethylisoalloxazine *see* Lumiflavine.

2,2,3-Trimethyl-3-(methylamino)-norbornane *see* Mecamylamine.

Trimethylmyristylammonium bromide *see* Tetradonium bromide.

Trimethyloctadecylammonium penta-chlorophenate *see* Octriphenate.

Trimethylolaminomethane *see* Trometamol.

Trimethylolmelamine *see* Hexamethylol-melamine.

3,5,5-Trimethyloxazolidine-2,4-dione *see* Trimethadione.

6,6,9-Trimethyl-3-pentylbenzo(c)-chromen-1-ol *see* Cannabinol.

6,6,9-Trimethyl-3-pentyl-6H-dibenzo-(b,d)pyran-1-ol *see* Cannabinol.

α,α,β-Trimethylphenethylamine *see* Pentorex.

N,α,α-Trimethylphenethylamine *see* Mephentermine.

3,4,α-Trimethylphenethylamine *see* Xylopropamine.

3,4,5-TRIMETHYLPHENYL METHYL-CARBAMATE (3,4,5-hemimellitinol methylcarbamate ester; OMS-597).

3,4,5-TRIMETHYLPHENYL METHYL-CARBAMATE PLUS 2,3,5-ISOMER (methylcarbamates of 3,4,5-hemimellitinol and isopseudocumenol; SD-8530; 'landrin').

N,3,3-Trimethyl-1-phenyl-1-phthalan-propylamine *see* Talopram.

1,2,5-Trimethyl-4-phenyl-4-piperidinol propionate *see* Trimeperidine.

1,2,5-Trimethyl-4-phenyl-4-propionoxy-piperidine *see* Trimeperidine.

Trimethylphloroglucinol *see* 1,3,5-Trimethoxybenzene.

1,2′,6-Trimethylpipecolanilide *see* Mepivacaine.

2,6,6-Trimethyl-4-piperidinol benzoate *see* Eucaine B.

4,5,8-Trimethylpsoralen *see* Trioxysalen.

17β-(Trimethylsiloxy)androst-4-en-3-one *see* Silandrone.

2-(TRIMETHYLSILYL)ETHYL ACETATE (acetylsilicocholine).

5,9,13-Trimethyltetradeca-4,8,12-tri-enoic acid 3,7-dimethylocta-2,6-dienyl ester *see* Gefarnate.

Trimethyltetradecylammonium bromide *see* Tetradonium bromide.

Trimethyl(1-p-tolyldodecyl)ammonium methyl sulfate *see* Toloconium metil-sulfate.

Trimethylvinylammonium hydroxide *see* Neurine.

Trimetin (tr) *see* Trimethadione.

'Trimeton' *see* Pheniramine.

Trimetoquinol *see* Tretoquinol.

TRIMETOZINE** (4-(3,4,5-trimethoxy-benzoyl)morpholine; A-22370; PS-2383; 'opalene', 'trioxasin', 'trioxazine').

TRIMETURON* (methyl N′-(p-chloro-phenyl)-N,N-dimethylcarbamimidate; O-methyl derivative of 1-(p-chlorophenyl)-3,3-dimethylpseudourea).

TRIMIPRAMINE** (5-(3-dimethylamino-

2-methylpropyl)-10,11-dihydro-5H-dibenz(b,f)azepine; trimeprimine; trimeprimine; IL-6001; RP-7162; 'stangyl').
TRIMIPRAMINE MALEATE ('surmontil').
'Trimitan' see Trichlormethine.
'Trimlen' see Sulfaperin with trimethoprim.
'Trimol' see Piroheptine.
'Trimon' see Stibophen.
TRIMOPAM* ((+)-2,3,4,5-tetrahydro-7,8-dimethoxy-3-methyl-1-phenyl-1H-3-benzazepine).
TRIMOPAM MALEATE (trimopam hydrogen maleate; Sch-12679).
TRIMOXAMINE*** (α-allyl-3,4,5-trimethoxy-N-methylphenethylamine; trimoxamine hydrochloride; NAT-327; NDR-5523A).
Trimustine* see Trichlormethine.
Trinitroglycerin see Glyceryl trinitrate.
Trinitrophenol see Picric acid.
Trinitroresorcinol see Styphnic acid.
'Trinophenon' see Picric acid.
'Triodan' see Iopanoic acid.
'Triognost' see Sodium acetrizoate.
TRIOLEIN OZONIDE ('oilzo').
'Triomet' see Liothyronine.
'Triomiro' see Iodamide.
'Trional' see Methylsulfonal.
'Trionine' see Liothyronine.
'Triopac' see Sodium acetrizoate.
'Triopron' see Thyropropic acid.
Triorthocresyl phosphate see Tricresyl phosphate.
'Triosil' see Sodium metrizoate.
'Triosol' see Sodium metrizoate.
'Triostam' see Sodium antimonyl gluconate.
'Triostib' see Sodium antimonyl gluconate.
'Triothyrone' see Liothyronine sodium.
'Trioxasin' see Trimetozine.
3,6,9-TRIOXAUNDECANE (bis(2-ethoxyethyl)ether).
'Trioxazine' see Trimetozine.
3,7,12-Trioxocholanic acid see Dehydrocholic acid.
TRIOXOLANE* (4-[[2-methyl-2-(3,4,5-trimethoxyphenyl)-1,3-dioxolan-4-yl]-methyl]morpholine; 2-methyl-4-morpholinomethyl-2-(3,4,5-trimethoxyphenyl)-1,3-dioxolane).
Trioxsalen* see Trioxysalen.
Trioxymethylene see Paraformaldehyde.
TRIOXYSALEN*** (6-hydroxy-β,2,7-trimethyl-5-benzofuranacrylic acid δ-lactone; 4,5,8-trimethylpsoralen; trioxsalen; 'neosoralen', 'trisoralen').
TRIPARANOL*** (2-(p-chlorophenyl)-1-[p-(2-diethylaminoethoxy)phenyl]-1-(p-tolyl)ethanol; α-(p-chlorobenzyl)-p-(2-diethylaminoethoxy)-p'-methylbenzhydrol; MER-29).
'Tripavlon' see Clofibrate.
TRIPELENNAMINE*** (N-benzyl-N',N'-dimethyl-N-(2-pyridyl)ethylenediamine; diaminobenzpyrylum).
'Triperidol' see Trifluperidol.
Triphenmorph see Trifenmorph.
Triphenyl carbinol see Tritanol.

1,1,2-TRIPHENYLETHYLENE (α-phenylstilbene).
Triphenylhydroxytin see Fentin hydroxide.
Triphenylmethanol see Tritanol.
Triphenylmethylamine see Tritylamine.
N-(Triphenylmethyl)morpholine see Trifenmorph.
3-(Triphenylmethylthio)-L-alanine see Tritylthioalanine.
1,3,5-Triphenylpyrazole-4-acetic acid see Trifezolac.
2,3,5-TRIPHENYLTETRAZOLIUM CHLORIDE (red tetrazolium; tetrazolium red; RT; TPTZ; TTC; 'uroscreen').
Triphenyltin see Fentin.
Triphosadenine see Adenosine triphosphate.
Triphosphopyridine nucleotide see Nadide phosphate.
Triple tetracycline see Tetracycline with chlortetracycline and demeclocycline.
'Tripoton' see Pheniramine.
TRIPRENE* ((E,E)-S-ethyl 11-methoxy-3,9,11-trimethyldodeca-2,4-dienethioate; 'altorick').
TRIPROLIDINE*** (trans-2-(3-pyrrolidin-1-yl-1-p-tolylpropenyl)pyridine; trans-1-pyrid-2-yl-3-pyrrolidin-1-yl-1-p-tolyl-1-propene; BW-295C51; 'actidil', 'pro-actidil').
See also Pseudoephedrine with triprolidine.
Triprop see Thyropropic acid.
'Triptide' see Glutathione.
'Triptil' see Protriptyline.
TRIPYRAPHENE (4,4',4''-tris(1,2-diphenyl-3,5-pyrazolidinedione); 4,4-bis(3,5-dioxo-1,2-diphenylpyrazolidin-4-yl)-1,2-diphenyl-3,5-pyrazolidinedione; tripyrazolidinyl; DA-369).
Tripyrazolidinyl see Tripyraphene.
'Triraupin' see Rescinnamine.
Tris see Trometamol.
'Trisaminol' see Trometamol.
Tris(p-aminophenyl)methanol see Pararosaniline.
2,3,5-Tris(1-aziridinyl)-p-benzoquinone see Triaziquone.
Tris(1-aziridinyl)phosphine oxide see Tepa.
Tris(1-aziridinyl)phosphine sulfide see Thiotepa.
Tris(1-aziridinyl)-s-triazine see Tretamine.
Tris(2-chloroethyl)amine see Trichlormethine.
3,3,3-TRIS(p-CHLOROPHENYL)-PROPIONIC ACID 4-METHYL-PIPERAZIDE (LZ-544; 'hetolin').
Tris[di(hydroxymethyl)amino]triazine see Hexamethylolmelamine.
N,N',N''-Tris[[4-(dimethylamino)-1,4,4a,5,5a,6,11,12a-octahydro-3,5,6,10,12,12a-hexahydroxy-6-methyl-1,11-dioxo-2-naphthacenecarboxamido]methyl]-polymyxin E see Colimecycline.
p,p',p''-Tris(dimethylamino)triphenylmethane chloride see Crystal violet.
Tris(2,2-dimethylaziridin-1-yl)phosphine oxide see Hexamethyltepa.

S,S',S''-Tris(dimethylcarbamodithioato)-iron see Ferbam.

4,4',4''-Tris(1,2-diphenyl-3,5-pyrazolidine-dione) see Tripyraphene.

'Trisedyl' see Trifluperidol.

Trisethyleniminobenzoquinone see Triaziquone.

Trisethylenimino phosphate see Tepa.

Trisethylenimino thiophosphate see Thiotepa.

3',4',7-Tris(2-hydroxyethyl)rutin see Troxerutin.

Tris(hydroxyethyl)rutoside* see Troxerutin.

Tris(hydroxymethyl)aminomethane gluconate aluminate see Aloglutamol.

1,1,1-Tris(hydroxymethyl)methylamine see Trometamol.

1,1,1-Tris(hydroxymethyl)propane trinitrate see Propatylnitrate.

'Trisillac' see Magnesium trisilicate.

'Trisix' see Lindane.

2,3,3-Tris(p-methoxyphenyl)-N,N-dimethylallylamine see Aminoxytriphene.

N,N',N''-Tris(2-methyl-1-aziridinyl)-phosphine oxide see Metepa.

1,1,1-Tris(nitratomethyl)propane see Propatylnitrate.

Tris-N-lost see Trichlormethine.

Trisodium 4'-anilino-8-hydroxy-1,1'-azonaphthalene-3,5',6-trisulfonate see Anazolene sodium.

TRISODIUM EDETATE (trisodium salt of ethylenediaminetetraacetic acid; edetate trisodium; 'chelaton', 'complexon', 'komplexon', 'limclair', 'plexochrom', 'sequestrene', 'trilon', 'versene').

'Trisomin' see Magnesium trisilicate.

'Trisophene' see Hexachlorophene.

'Trisoralen' see Trioxysalen.

Tris(polyethyleneglycol 300) sorbitan ethers see Polyoxyethylene 20 sorbitan.

'Trisweet' see Aspartame.

TRITANOL (triphenylmethanol; triphenyl carbinol).

'Tritheon' see Aminitrozole.

'Trithio' see Anethole trithione.

Trithio-(p-methoxyphenyl)propene see Anethole trithione.

'Trithion' see Carbofenotion.

'Tritisan' see Quintozene.

Tritolyl phosphate see Tricresyl phosphate.

'Triton(s)' see Tyloxapol.

TRITOQUALINE* (7-amino-4,5,6-triethoxy-3-(5,6,7,8-tetrahydro-4-methoxy-6-methyl-1,3-dioxolo(4,5-g)isoquinolin-5-yl)phthalide; 1-(3-amino-4,5,6-triethoxy-phthalid-3-yl)-1,2,3,4-tetrahydro-8-methoxy-2-methyl-6,7-methylenedioxy-isoquinoline; L-554; 'hypostamine', 'inhibistamin').

'Tritox' see Fluoroacetic acid and DDT with lindane and methoxychlor.

'Trittico' see Trazodone.

TRITYLAMINE ((triphenylmethyl)amine).

Tritylmorpholine see Trifenmorph.

TRITYLTHIOALANINE (3-(triphenyl-methylthio)-L-alanine; 3-(tritylthio)-L-alanine; NSC-83265).

'Triumbren' see Acetrizoic acid.

'Triurol' see Sodium acetrizoate.

'Trivastal' see Piribedil.

'Trivetrin' see Sulfadoxine with trimethoprim.

'Trix' see Lindane with DDT.

'Trizma' see Trometamol.

TRIZOXIME* (5-benzyl-4,5-dihydro-4-oxo-1H-1,2,5-benzotriazepine-3-carboxamidoxime).

'Trobicin' see Spectinomycin.

TROCIMINE* (octahydro-1-(3,4,5-tri-methoxybenzoyl)azocine).

'Trocinate' see Tifenamil.

TROCLOSENE* (dichloro-s-triazine-2,4,6-(1H,3H,5H)-trione; dichloroisocyanuric acid).

TROCLOSENE POTASSIUM* (troclosene potassium derivative; potassium dichloroisocyanurate; potassium troclosene; ACL-59).

TROCLOSENE SODIUM (troclosene sodium derivative; sodium dichloroiso-cyanurate; sodium troclosene; ACL-60).

'Trodax' see Nitroxinil meglumine.

'Trofodermin' see Clostebol acetate with neomycin.

'Troformone' see Methandriol.

TROFOSFAMIDE* (3-(2-chloroethyl)-2-[bis(2-chloroethyl)amino]tetrahydro-2H-1,3,2-oxazaphosphorine 2-oxide; Asta-4828).

'Trofozim' see Cobamamide.

Trolamine* see Triethanolamine.

TROLEANDOMYCIN* (oleandomycin triacetate ester; triacetyloleandomycin; Wy-651; 'aovine', 'cyclamycin', 'evramicina', 'evramycin', 'oleanbel', 'spectro-bact', 'tao').

'Trolen' see Fenclofos.

'Trolene' see Fenclofos.

TROLNITRATE* (2,2',2''-nitrilotriethanol trinitrate; aminotrate phosphate; triethanol-amine trinitrate; triethanolamine trinitrate biphosphate; nitranol; 'angitrit', 'bentonyl', 'metamine', 'nitralettae', 'nitretamine', 'nitroduran', 'nitro-tabletten', 'ortin', 'praenitrona', 'thibetine', 'tricoryl').

'Trolone' see Sultiame.

'Trolovol' see Penicillamine.

'Tromal' see Butacetin.

TROMANTADINE* ((N-adamant-1-yl)-2-(2-dimethylaminoethoxy)acetamide; tromantadine hydrochloride; D-41; 'viru-Merz').

'Tromasedan' see Bendazol.

'Trombo-vetren' see Heparin.

'Tromcardin' see Magnesium aspartate with potassium aspartate.

TROMETAMOL* (2-amino-2-hydroxy-methyl-1,3-propanediol; 1,1,1-tris(hydroxy-methyl)methylamine; trimethylolamino-methane; tromethamine; THAM; tris; 'pehanorm', 'talatrol', 'trisaminol', 'trizma').

See also Dinoprost trometamol.

Trometamol gluconate aluminate *see* Aloglutamol.

TROMETAMOL THIOCTATE ('lipotam').

Tromethamine* *see* Trometamol.

'Tromexan' *see* Ethyl biscoumacetate.

'Tronothane' *see* Pramocaine.

TROPACIN (tr) (tropine diphenylacetate; tropazine).

Tropacocaine *see* Pseudotropine benzoate.

TROPANE (8-methyl-8-azabicyclo(3.2.1)-octane; 2,3-dihydro-8-methylnortropidine; 8-methylnortropane).

3α-Tropanol *see* Tropine.

3β-Tropanol *see* Pseudotropine.

DL-Tropanyl 2-hydroxy-1-phenyl-propionate *see* Atropine.

(−)-3α-Tropanyl 2-methyl-2-phenyl-hydracrylate *see* Atromepine.

TROPATEPINE** (3-dibenzo(b,e)thiepin-11(6H)-ylidene-1αH,5αH-tropane; SD-12417; 'lepticur').

Tropazine (tr) *see* Tropacin.

TROPENTANE (tr) (tropine phenylcyclo-pentanecarboxylate).

TROPENZILINE BROMIDE** (7-methoxy-8-methyltropinium bromide benzilate; tropenzilium; MTS-263; 'palerol').

Tropenzilium *see* Tropenziline.

Tropethydryline *see* Etybenzatropine.

'Trophenium' *see* Phenactropinium.

'Trophicard' *see* Potassium magnesium aspartate.

'Trophozym' *see* Cobamamide.

TROPIC ACID (2-phenylhydracrylic acid; 3-hydroxy-2-phenylpropionic acid).

(±)-Tropic acid 9-isopropylgranatoline ester *see* Ipragratine.

TROPICAMIDE** (N-ethyl-2-phenyl-N-pyrid-4-ylmethylhydracrylamide; N-ethyl-N-pyrid-4-ylmethyltropamide; tropic acid N-ethyl-N-(γ-picolyl)amide; bistropamide; 'mydriacyl', 'mydrin').

TROPIGLINE** (tropyl 2,3-dimethylacrylate; tiglyltropine; 2-methyl-2-butenoyltropine; tropine tiglate).

'Tropin' *see* Atropine methobromide.

TROPINE (2,3-dihydro-3α-hydroxy-8-methylnortropidine; 3-hydroxy-8-methyl-nortropane; 3-hydroxy-8-methyl-8-azabi-cyclo(3.2.1)octane; 3-hydroxytropane; 3α-tropanol).

Tropine atrolactate *see* Pseudoatropine.

Tropine benzhydryl ether *see* Benzatropine.

2-Tropinecarboxylic acid *see* Ecgonine.

Tropine chlorobenzhydryl ether *see* Clobenztropine.

Tropine dimethylacrylate *see* Tropigline.

Tropine diphenylacetate *see* Tropacin.

Tropine 3-(p-hydroxyphenyl)-2-phenyl-propionate acetate *see* Tropodifene.

Tropine isatropate *see* Belladonnin.

Tropine β-isomer *see* Pseudotropine.

Tropine mandelate *see* Homatropine.

Tropine α-methylmandelate *see* Pseudo-atropine.

Tropine 2-methyl-2-phenylhydracrylate *see* Atromepine.

Tropine methyltropate *see* Atromepine.

Tropine phenylcyclopentanecarboxylate *see* Tropentane.

Tropine tiglate *see* Tropigline.

Tropine DL-tropate *see* Atropine.

Tropine L-tropate *see* Hyoscyamine.

'Tropino' *see* Atropine oxide.

TROPIRINE** (3α-[(5H-benzo(4,5)cyclo-hepta(1,2-b)pyridyl)-5-oxy]tropane; 5-(3α-tropyloxy)-5H-benzo(4,5)cyclohepta-(1,2-b)pyridine).

'Tropital' *see* Piperonal bis[2-(2-butoxy-ethoxy)ethyl]acetal.

TROPODIFENE** (tropine 3-(p-hydroxy-phenyl)-2-phenylpropionate(ester)acetate (ester)).

TROPOLONE (2,4,6-cycloheptatrien-1-one-2-ol).

'Tropotox' *see* Sodium 4-(4-chloro-2-methylphenoxy)butyrate.

5-(3α-Tropyloxy)-5H-benzo(4,5)cyclo-hepta(1,2-b)pyridine *see* Tropirine.

TROSPIUM CHLORIDE** (3α-hydroxy-spiro(1αH,5αH-nortropane-8,1'-pyrrolidi-nium) chloride benzilate; 8α-benziloyloxy-6,10-ethano-5-azoniaspiro(4.5)decane chloride; 8α-hydroxy-6,10-ethano-5-azoniaspiro(4.5)decane chloride benzilate; azoniaspiro(3α-benziloyloxynortropane-8,1'-pyrrolidine) chloride; AS-XVII; MG-42799; 'spasmex').

TROXERUTIN** (3',4',7-tris(2-hydroxy-ethyl)rutin; tris(hydroxyethyl)rutoside; trihydroxyethylrutin; vitamin P_4; Z-12001; 'paroven', 'varemoid', 'venoruton'). *See also* Carbazochrome with troxerutin.

Troxidone* *see* Trimethadione.

Troxone* *see* Troxonium tosilate.

TROXONIUM TOSILATE** (triethyl-[2-(3,4,5-trimethoxybenzoyloxy)ethyl]-ammonium p-toluenesulfonate; triethyl-(2-hydroxyethyl)ammonium p-toluenesul-fonate 3,4,5-trimethoxybenzoate; troxone).

Troxypyrrole* *see* Troxypyrrolium tosilate.

TROXYPYRROLIUM TOSILATE*** (1-ethyl-1-[2-(3,4,5-trimethoxybenzoyloxy)-ethyl]pyrrolidinium p-toluenesulfonate; 1-ethyl-1-(2-hydroxyethyl)pyrrolidinium p-toluenesulfonate 3,4,5-trimethoxybenzo-ate; troxypyrrole).

'Truxal' *see* Chlorprothixene.

TRUXICURIUM IODIDE** (diethyl-(3-hydroxypropyl)methylammonium iodide α-2,4-diphenyl-1,3-cyclobutanedicarboxyl-ate; truxillic acid diester with diethyl(3-hydroxypropyl)methylammonium iodide).

TRUXILLIC ACID (2,4-diphenyl-1,3-cyclobutanedicarboxylic acid).

Truxillic acid diester with diethyl(3-hydroxypropyl)methylammonium iodide *see* Truxicurium iodide.

Truxillic acid diester with 1-ethyl-1-(3-hydroxypropyl)piperidinium iodide *see* Truxipicurium iodide.

TRUXIPICURIUM IODIDE** (1-ethyl-1-(3-hydroxypropyl)piperidinium iodide α-2,4-diphenyl-1,3-cyclobutanedicarboxyl-ate; truxillic acid diester with 1-ethyl-1-(3-hydroxypropyl)piperidinium iodide).

'**Trypadine**' *see* Dimidium bromide.

TRYPAN BLUE (tetrasodium salt of 4,4'-bis-(8-amino-1-hydroxy-3,6-disulfonaphth-2-ylazo)-3,3'-dimethylbiphenyl; tetra-Na salt of 4,4'-bis-(8-amino-1-hydroxy-3,6-disulfonaphth-2-ylazo)-3,3'-bitolyl; sodium ditolyldiazobis(8-amino-1-naphthol-3,6-disulfonate); benzamine blue; Congo blue; naphthylamine blue; 'benzo blue', 'diamine blue', 'dianil blue', 'niagara blue').

TRYPARSAMIDE* (monosodium salt of *N*-(carbamoylmethyl)arsanilic acid; sodium salt of *N*-phenylglycinamide-*p*-arsonic acid; glyphenarsine; tryparsone; glycarsamide; 'tryponarsyl', 'trypothane').

Tryparsone *see* Tryparsamide.

'**Trypchymase**' *see* Chymotrypsin.

'**Tryponarsyl**' *see* Tryparsamide.

'**Trypothane**' *see* Tryparsamide.

TRYPSIN ('parenzyme', 'parenzymol', 'tryptar', 'trypure').
See also Chymotrypsin with trypsin.

TRYPTAMINE (3-(2-aminoethyl)indole; 3-indoleëthylamine).

'**Tryptanol**' *see* Amitriptyline.

'**Tryptar**' *see* Trypsin.

'**Tryptizol**' *see* Amitriptyline.

TRYPTOPHAN (2-amino-3-indolepropionic acid; 'pacitron').

ʟ-**TRYPTOPHAN WITH PYRIDOXINE** ('optimax').

TRYPTOPHOL (indole-3-ethanol; 3-(2-hydroxyethyl)indole).

'**Trypure**' *see* Trypsin.

'**Trysben**' *see* Trichlorobenzoic acid.

'**Trysben 200**' *see* Dimethylamine trichlorobenzoate.

TS-160 *see* Trichlormethine.

TSAG *see* Sodium antimonyl gluconate.

TSH *see* Thyrotrophin.

Tsiklomitsin (tr) *see* Tetracycline.

TSP *see* Serrapeptase.

TSPA *see* Thiotepa.

'**Tsumacide**' *see* *m*-Tolyl methylcarbamate.

TTC *see* 2,3,5-Triphenyltetrazolium chloride.

TTD *see* Disulfiram.

TTH *see* Thyrotrophin.

'**Tuad**' *see* Thiram.

'**Tuamine**' *see* Tuaminoheptane.

TUAMINOHEPTANE* (2-aminoheptane; 2-heptylamine; 1-methylhexylamine; tuaminoheptane sulfate; 'heptadrine', 'heptamine', 'tuamine').

'**Tuasal 100**' *see* Tribromsalan.

'**Tuazole**' *see* Methaqualone.

'**Tuazolone**' *see* Methaqualone.

Tubatoxin *see* Rotenone.

Tubazid (tr) *see* Isoniazid.

Tuberactinomycin B *see* Viomycin.

Tuberactinomycin N *see* Enviomycin.

'**Tubercazon**' *see* Thiacetazone.

'**Tubercidin**' *see* 7-Deazaadenosine.

TUBERCULOSTEARIC ACID (10-methyl-stearic acid).

'**Tuberlite**' *see* Propham.

TUBOCURARINE CHLORIDE* ((+)-tubocurarine chloride; *Chondrodendrum tomentosum* extract).

Tubocurarine dimethyl ether *see* Dimethyltubocurarine.

'**Tuclase**' *see* Pentoxyverine.

'**Tugon**' *see* Metrifonate.

'**Tulisan**' *see* Thiram.

'**Tumovan**' *see* Prothipendyl.

'**Tunic**' *see* Chlormethazole.

'**Tupen**' *see* Ampicillin with cloxacillin.

'**Tuperson**' *see* Siduron.

'**Turinabol**' *see* Clostebol acetate.

'**Turinal**' *see* Allylestrenol tartrate.

'**Turisynchron**' *see* Metallibure.

'**Turloc**' *see* Meturedepa.

TURPENTINE OIL* (rectified turpentine oil; terebinth oil; camphine).

TURPENTINE OIL OXIDATION PRODUCT ('ozothine').

'**Tuscalman**' *see* Noscapine with guaifenesin.

'**Tuscapine**' *see* Noscapine.

'**Tussal**' *see* Methadone.

'**Tussefane**' *see* Fedrilate.

'**Tussicain**' *see* 3-Amino-2-hydroxypropyl *p*-butylaminobenzoate.

'**Tussilan**' *see* Dextromethorphan.

'**Tussilax**' *see* Diphepanol.

'**Tussilex**' *see* Dropropizine.

'**Tussils**' *see* Noscapine.

'**Tussinol**' *see* Oxeladin.

'**Tussol**' *see* Phenazone mandelate.

'**Tussucal**' *see* Diphepanol.

'**Tussukal**' *see* Diphepanol.

'**Tutocaine**' *see* Butamin.

TV-274B *see* Proscillaridin.

TV-274C *see* Proscillaridin with isosorbide dinitrate.

'**Tween(s)**' *see* Polysorbate(s).

'**Twiston**' *see* Rotoxamine tartrate.

TwSb *see* Sodium stibocaptate.

TYBAMATE* (2-methyl-2-propyltrimethylene butylcarbamate carbamate; 2-hydroxymethyl-2-methylpentyl butylcarbamate carbamate; tibamide; W-713; 'benvil', 'solacen', 'tybatran').

'**Tybatran**' *see* Tybamate.

'**Tyclarosol**' *see* Tetrasodium edetate.

'**Tydantil**' *see* Nifuratel.

'**Tyformin**' *see* Tiformin.

'**Tylagel**' *see* Tolpropamine.

'**Tylcalsin**' *see* Calcium acetylsalicylate.

'**Tylciprine**' *see* Tranylcypromine.

'**Tylenol**' *see* Paracetamol.

'**Tylinal**' *see* Amfepramone.

TYLOSIN* (antibiotic from *Str. fradiae*).

TYLOXAPOL* (polymer of *p*-(1,1,3,3-tetramethylbutyl) phenol with ethylene glycol and formaldehyde; octylphenoxy polyethoxyethanol; ethoxylated *tert*-octylphenol formaldehyde polymer; 'alevaire', 'nonidet P-40', 'pazidett', 'superinone', 'tacholiquin', 'triton A-20', 'triton WR-1339').

TYMAZOLINE* (2-thymyloxymethyl-2-imidazoline; 2-(2-isopropyl-5-methyl-phenoxymethyl)-2-imidazoline; tymazol-

ine hydrochloride; 'pernazene').
Tyraminase *see* Monoamine oxidase.
TYRAMINE (*p*-(2-aminoethyl)phenol;
4-hydroxyphenethylamine; 2-(*p*-hydroxy-
phenyl)ethylamine; *p*-tyramine; tyrosamine; 'mydrial', 'systogene', 'tocosine',
'uteramine').
o-**TYRAMINE** (2-hydroxyphenethylamine).
m-**TYRAMINE** (3-hydroxyphenethylamine).
p-**Tyramine** *see* Tyramine.
'**Tyranton**' *see* Diacetone alcohol.
'**Tyrimide**' *see* Isopropamide.
Tyrocidin with gramicidin *see* Tyrothricin.
'**Tyrogel**' *see* Diiodotyrosine.
TYROMEDAN*** (2-diethylaminoethyl
2-[3,5-diiodo-4-(3-iodo-4-methoxyphen-
oxy)phenyl]acetate; thyromedan hydro-

chloride; SK&F-13364-A).
Tyropanoate *see* Sodium tyropanoate.
Tyrosamine *see* Tyramine.
TYROSINE (3-(*p*-hydroxyphenyl)alanine;
2-amino-3-(*p*-hydroxyphenyl)propionic
acid; α-amino-*p*-hydroxyhydrocinnamic
acid; α-tyrosine).
α-**Tyrosine** *see* Tyrosine.
β-**TYROSINE** (3-(*p*-hydroxyphenyl)-β-ala-
nine; 3-amino-3-(*p*-hydroxyphenyl)-
propionic acid; β-amino-*p*-hydroxyhydro-
cinnamic acid).
TYROTHRICIN*** (antibiotic from
Bacillus brevis; mixture of gramicidin and
tyrocidin).
'**Tyzanol**' *see* Tetryzoline.
'**Tyzine**' *see* Tetryzoline.

U

U-0229 *see* Fenpipramide.
U-0382 *see* Scopolamine methyl bromide.
U-0433 *see* Methoxyphenamine.
U-935 *see* Amiquinsin.
U-1063 *see* Proquinolate.
U-1085 *see* Leniquinsin.
U-1093 *see* Buquinolate.
U-1258 *see* Pregnentrione.
U-1363 *see* Diphenadione.
U-2043 *see* Tolbutamide.
U-4527 *see* Cycloheximide.
U-5641 *see* Parathiazine dioxide.
U-5897 *see* Chlorohydrin.
U-6812 *see* Sodium polyethylene sulfonate.
U-6987 *see* Carbutamide.
U-7720 *see* Diallylmelamine.
U-7800 *see* Fluprednisolone.
U-8344 *see* Uramustine.
U-8471 *see* Medrysone.
T-9361 *see* Hydroxycycloheximide.
U-10149A *see* Lincomycin.
U-10387 *see* Isocarboxazid.
U-10858 *see* Minoxidil.
U-10974 *see* Flumetasone.
U-10997 *see* Mibolerone.
U-11100A *see* Nafoxidine.
U-12062 *see* Dinoprostone.
U-12504 *see* Glypinamide.
U-13933 *see* Asperlin.
U-14583 *see* Dinoprost.
U-14583E *see* Dinoprost trometamol.
U-14743 *see* Porfiromycin.
U-15167 *see* Nogalamycin.
U-17312E *see* Etryptamine.
U-17323 *see* Fluorometholone acetate.
U-17835 *see* Tolazamide.
U-18409E *see* Spectinomycin.
U-19183 *see* Sparsomycin.
U-19646 *see* Chlorphenesin carbamate.

U-19718 *see* Kalafungin.
U-19763 *see* Bolasterone.
U-19920A *see* Cytarabine.
U-21251 *see* Clindamycin.
U-22020 *see* Indoxole.
U-22559A *see* Dexoxadol.
U-24729A *see* Mirincamycin.
U-24973A *see* Melitracen.
U-25179E *see* Clindamycin palmitate.
U-26452 *see* Glibenclamide.
U-26597A *see* Colestipol.
U-28288D *see* Guanadrel.
U-28508 *see* Clindamycin phosphate.
U-28774 *see* Ketazolam.
U-31889 *see* Alprazolam.
U-33030 *see* Triazolam.
U-34865 *see* Diflorasone diacetate.
U-181573 *see* Ibuprofen.
UBIQUINONES (coenzymes Q; mito-
quinones).
'**Ubretid**' *see* Distigmine.
UCB-1402 *see* Decloxizine.
UCB-1414 *see* Etodroxizine.
UCB-1414M *see* Methaqualone with
etodroxizine maleate.
UCB-1474 *see* Chlorbenoxamine.
UCB-1545 *see* Phenetamine.
UCB-1549 *see* Minepentate.
UCB-1967 *see* Dropropizine.
UCB-2073 *see* Etoxeridine.
UCB-2543 *see* Pentoxyverine.
UCB-3412 *see* Dixyrazine.
UCB-3983 *see* Mesna.
UCB-4445 *see* Buclizine.
UCB-4492 *see* Hydroxyzine.
UCB-5033 *see* Brallobarbital.
UCB-5062 *see* Meclozine.
UCB-5067 *see* Oxydipentonium chloride.
UCB-6215 *see* Piracetam.

UCB-79171 *see* Ibuprofen.
'Ucenol LS' *see* Sodium dodecyl sulfate.
'Udieci' *see* Papaveroline meglumine.
UDMH *see* 1,1-Dimethylhydrazine.
'Udolac' *see* Dapsone.
UDP *see* Uridine diphosphate.
Ug-767 *see* Penoctonium bromide.
'Ugurol' *see* Tranexamic acid.
'Ujoviridin' *see* Indocyanine green.
UK-738 *see* Etybenzatropine.
UK-2054 *see* Famotine.
UK-2371 *see* Memotine.
UK-3540 *see* Amedalin.
UK-3557 *see* Daledalin.
UK-4271 *see* Oxamniquine.
UK-6558-01 *see* Tolamolol.
'Ukidan' *see* Urokinase.
'Ulbretid' *see* Distigmine.
'Ulbreval' *see* Buthalital.
'Ulcesium' *see* Fentonium bromide.
'Ulcoban' *see* Benzilonium bromide.
'Ulcostidine' *see* Histidine.
ULDAZEPAM** (2-(allyloxyamino)-7-chloro-5-(*o*-chlorophenyl)-3H-1,4-benzo-diazepine).
Ulexine *see* Cytisine.
'Ulo' *see* Clofedanol.
'Ulpepsan' *see* Aluminium glycinate.
'Ultandren' *see* Fluoxymesterone.
'Ultrabil' *see* Adipiodone.
'Ultrabiotic' *see* Penimepicycline.
'Ultracain' *see* Carticaine.
'Ultracid(e)' *see* Methidathion.
'Ultracillin' *see* Ciclacillin.
'Ultracortenol' *see* Prednisolone pivalate.
'Ultracur' *see* Fluocortolone octanoate.
'Ultralan' *see* Fluocortolone.
'Ultrapen' *see* Propicillin.
'Ultraphen' *see* Clorofene.
'Ultraquinine' *see* Cupreine.
'Ultraren' *see* Iodoxyl.
'Ultraseptyl' *see* Sulfamethylthiazole.
'Ultrax' *see* Sulfametoxydiazine.
'Ultrazeozon' *see* Esculetin.
UM-272 *see* Pranolium iodide.
UMBELLIFERONE (7-hydroxycoumarin).
UML-491 *see* Methysergide.
UMP *see* Uridylic acid.
UMS *see* Uracil methyl sulfone.
UNDECANOIC ACID (hendecanoic acid, undecylic acid).
'Undecap' *see* Undecenoic acid.
10-UNDECENOIC ACID (hendec-10-enoic acid; undecylenic acid).
UNDECENOIC ACID WITH METAL SALTS (undecenoic acid in admixture with its copper and/or zinc salts; zincundecate; 'cunate', 'decilderm', 'declid', 'decylon', 'desenex', 'mycodecyl', 'mycosin', 'mycota', 'pedzyl', 'renselin', 'sevinon', 'undecap', 'undenate', 'undesilin', 'undesal').
Undecylenic acid *see* Undecenoic acid.
Undecylic acid *see* Undecanoic acid.
'Unden' *see* Estrone *and* Propoxur.
'Undenate' *see* Undecenoic acid.
'Undesal' *see under* Undecenoic acid.
'Undesilin' *see under* Undecenoic acid.

'Unephral' *see* Mercuderamide.
'Unidigin' *see* Digitoxin.
'Unidone' *see* Anisindione.
'Unilobine' *see* Lobeline.
'Unipen' *see* Nafcillin.
'Uniprin' *see* Calcium acetylsalicylate.
'Unistat' *see* Sulfanitran.
'Unitensen' *see* Cryptenamine.
UNITHIOL (tr) (2,3-propanedithiol-1-sulfonic acid sodium salt; dimercapto-propane sodium sulfonate; sodium dimer-captopropanesulfonate).
'Unitocin' *see* Sparteine.
'Unitop' *see* Cuprimyxin.
'Unospaston' *see* Diponium bromide.
'Unosulf' *see* Sulfamethoxypyridazine.
'Unstetic' *see* Nalidixic acid.
UR-112 *see* Magnesium clofibrate.
UR-661 *see* Glipentide.
'Urab' *see* Fenuron trichloroacetate.
URACIL (2,4(1H,3H)-pyrimidinedione; 2,4-dihydroxypyrimidine).
6-Uracilcarboxylic acid *see* Orotic acid.
Uracil-chlorethamine *see* Uramustine.
6-URACIL METHYL SULFONE (UMS).
Uracil mustard *see* Uramustine.
Uracil riboside *see* Uridine.
Uracylic acid *see* Uridylic acid.
'Uradal' *see* Carbromal.
'Ural' *see* Carbocloral.
'Uraline' *see* Carbocloral.
'Uralium' *see* Carbocloral.
'Uralysol' *see* Methenamine.
'Uramid' *see* Sulfacarbamide.
URAMIL (5-aminobarbituric acid).
Uramine *see* Guanidine.
URAMUSTINE*** (5-[bis(2-chloroethyl)-amino]uracil; nordopan; uracil mustard; uracil nitrogen mustard; uracil-chlor-ethamine; desmethyldopan; NSC-34462; U-8344).
Uranin *see* Fluorescein disodium.
URAPIDIL*** (6-[[3-[4-(*o*-methoxyphenyl)-piperazin-1-yl]propyl]amino]-1,3-dimethyl-uracil; 1-[3-[(1,3-dimethyl-2,4-dioxo-pyrimidin-6-yl)amino]propyl]-4-(*o*-methoxyphenyl)piperazine).
'Uraseptine' *see* Methenamine.
'Urazine' *see* Methenamine salicylate.
'Urbanyl' *see* Clobazam.
'Urbason' *see* Methylprednisolone.
'Urbazid' *see* Methylarsine bis(dimethyl-thiocarbamate).
UREA (carbamide; carbonyl diamide).
Urea-polypeptide complex *see* Polygelin.
UREA QUINATE (diurea tetrahydroxy-cyclohexanecarboxylate; 'urol').
UREA STIBAMINE (ammonium salt of *p*-ureidobenzenestibonic acid; carbostiba-mide; 'stiburea').
'Urecholine' *see* Bethanechol.
UREDEPA*** (ethyl [bis(1-aziridinyl)-phosphinyl]carbamate; AB-100; 'avinar').
'Uregit' *see* Etacrynic acid.
'Uregyt' *see* Etacrynic acid.
Ureidosuccinic acid *see* *N*-Carbamoyl-aspartic acid.

Ureidobenzene *see* Carbanilamide.
p-Ureidobenzenestibonic acid ammonium salt *see* Urea stibamine.
Ureidoformamide *see* Biuret.
5-Ureidonorvaline *see* Citrulline.
'Urelim' *see* Etebenecid.
'Urese' *see* Benzthiazide.
URETHAN (ethyl carbamate; urethane; NSC-746).
Urethane*** *see* Urethan.
'Urethylane' *see* Methyl carbamate.
'Urex' *see* Methenamine hippurate.
6,6'-Ureylenebis(1-methylquinolinium sulfate) *see* Quinuronium.
8,8'-[Ureylenebis[m-phenylenecarbonyl-imino-(4-methyl-m-phenylene)carbonylimino]]di(1,3,5-naphthalenetrisulfonic acid) *see* Suramin.
'Urfamicina' *see* Thiamphenicol glycinate.
'Urfamycin' *see* Thiamphenicol glycinate.
'Urgilan' *see* Proscillaridin.
'Urgo' *see* Benzalkonium chloride.
URIC ACID (2,6,8(1H,3H,9H)-purinetrione; lithic acid).
URIC ACID OXIDASE (CB-8129; 'uricosydase').
'Uricida' *see* Piperazine.
'Uricosid' *see* Probenecid.
'Uricosydase' *see* Uric acid oxidase.
'Uricovac' *see* Benzbromarone.
URIDINE (uracil riboside).
URIDINE DIPHOSPHATE (UDP).
Uridine monophosphate *see* Uridylic acid.
URIDINE TRIPHOSPHATE (uridine-triphosphoric acid; UPT; 'uteplex').
'Uridione' *see* 5-Bromo-2-phenyl-1,3-indandione.
'Uridognost' *see* Iodoxyl.
URIDYLIC ACID (uridine monophosphoric acid; uridine monophosphate; uracylic acid; UMP).
'Urisol' *see* Methenamine.
'Urispas' *see* Flavoxate.
'Uritone' *see* Methenamine.
Uroboramine *see* Methenamine borate.
UROCANIC ACID (4-imidazoleacrylic acid; urocaninic acid).
Urocanoylcholine *see* Murexine.
'Urocedulamin' *see* Methamine mandelate.
'Urofort' *see* Amanozine.
'Urogenine' *see* Methenamine.
'Urografin' *see* Meglumine diatrizoate.
'Urografin 76' *see* Meglumine diatrizoate with sodium diatrizoate.
UROKINASE*** (plasminogen activator from human urine; 'ukidan', 'win-kinase').
'Urokolin' *see* Acetrizoic acid.
'Urokon' *see* Sodium acetrizoate.
'Urol' *see* Urea quinate.
'Urolocide' *see* Benzyl(hydroxymethyl)-dimethylammonium chloride dodecyl-carbamate.
'Urolucosil' *see* Sulfamethizole.
'Uromandelin' *see* Methenamine mandelate.

'Urombrine' *see* Iodamide.
'Uromiro' *see* Iodamide.
'Uronamin' *see* Methenamine mandelate.
'Uro-nebacetin' *see* Neomycin with sulfamethizole.
'Uropac' *see* Iodoxyl.
'Uropax' *see* Oxolinic acid.
'Uropolin' *see* Meglumine diatrizoate with sodium diatrizoate.
'Uropurgol' *see* Methenamine anhydro-methylenecitrate.
'Uropuryl' *see* Methenamine anhydromethyl-enecitrate.
'Uroscreen' *see* 2,3,5-Triphenyltetrazolium chloride.
'Uroselectan' *see* Iodopyridone.
'Uroselectan-B' *see* Iodoxyl.
'Urosept' *see* Nitrofurantoin.
'Urosin' *see* Allopurinol.
Urosulfan (tr) *see* Sulfacarbamide.
Urosympathin *see* Noradrenaline.
UROTERPENOL ((+)-p-Menthen-8,9-diol).
Urotheobromine *see* Paraxanthine.
'Urotrast' *see* Dimethiodal.
'Urotrate' *see* Oxolinic acid.
'Urotropin' *see* Methenamine.
'Urovison' *see* Meglumine diatrizoate with sodium diatrizoate.
'Urovist' *see* Meglumine diatrizoate.
'Urox' *see* Monuron trichloroacetate.
Uroxin *see* Alloxantin.
Ursin *see* Hydroquinone glucopyranoside.
Ursocholanic acid *see* Cholanic acid.
'Ursocyclin' *see* Oxytetracycline.
'Ursol' *see* Phenylenediamine.
URSOLIC ACID (3β-hydroxy-urs-12-en-28-oic acid; urson).
Urson *see* Ursolic acid.
'Urumbrin' *see* Iodoxyl.
Usnein *see* Usnic acid.
USNIC ACID (2,6-diacetyl-7,9-dihydroxy-8,9a-dimethyldibenzofuran-1,3-dione; usninic acid; usnein).
USNIC ACID SODIUM SALT (bin-7; binan).
'Uspulun' *see* Chlorohydroxymercuriphenol.
'Ustimon' *see* Hexobendine.
'Ustinex PA' *see* Amitrole.
'Uteplex' *see* Uridine triphosphate.
'Uticillin' *see* Carfecillin.
'Uticillin VK' *see* Penicillin V potassium.
UTP *see* Uridine triphosphate.
'Utropine' *see* Methenamine.
UV-284 *see* Sulisobenzone.
UV-531 *see* Octabenzone.
'Uval' *see* Sulisobenzone.
'Uvasol' *see* Hydroquinone glucopyranoside.
'Uviban' *see* Sodium actinoquinol.
'Uvilon' *see* Piperazine.
'Uvinul M-40' *see* Oxybenzone.
'Uvinul MS-40' *see* Sulisobenzone.
'Uvistat 2211' *see* Mexenone.

V

V-5 *see* Thiopental.
V-7 *see* Thioethamyl.
V-12 *see* Methallatal.
Va-1470 *see* Xylazine.
'Vaben' *see* Oxazepam.
VACCENIC ACID (*trans*-11-octadecenoic acid).
'Vadephen' *see* Tetramisole.
'Vadilex' *see* Ifenprodil.
'Vaditon' *see* Aminophenazone ascorbate.
'Vaelo' *see* Diazepam.
'Vagophemanil' *see* Diphemanil metilsulfate.
'Vagoprol' *see* Ibrotamide.
'Vagosin' *see* Tricyclamol.
'Vagospasmyl' *see* Adiphenine.
'Valadol' *see* Paracetamol.
'Valamin' *see* Ethinamate.
VALEPOTRIATE (mixture of acevaltrate, didrovaltrate and valtrate; 'valmane').
VALERIC ACID (1-butanecarboxylic acid; pentanoic acid; valerianic acid; propyl-acetic acid).
VALERIDIN (*N*-isovaleryl-*p*-phenetidine; 'sedatin').
VALEROPHENONE (butyl phenyl ketone).
VALETHAMATE BROMIDE* (2-diethyl-aminoethyl ester methobromide of 3-methyl-2-phenylvaleric acid; S-78; 'epidosin', 'murel', 'resitan').
'Valexon' *see* Phoxim.
'Valibran' *see* Medibazine.
'Validol' *see* Menthyl valerate.
VALINE (*x*-aminoisovaleric acid; 2-amino-3-methylbutyric acid).
'Valisone' *see* Betamethasone valerate.
'Valium' *see* Diazepam.
'Valladan' *see* Benactyzine.
'Valledrine' *see* Alimemazine.
'Vallergan' *see* Alimemazine.
'Vallestril' *see* Methallenestril.
'Valmane' *see* Valepotriate.
Valmethamide *see* Valnoctamide.
'Valmid' *see* Ethinamate.
'Valmidate' *see* Ethinamate.
'Valmorin' *see* Chlorthenoxazine.
VALNOCTAMIDE*** (2-ethyl-3-methyl-valeramide; valmethamide; McN-X-181; 'axiquel', 'nirvanil').
'Valoron' *see* Tilidine.
'Valpin' *see* Octatropine methyl bromide.
Valproate sodium* *see* Sodium valproate.
VALPROIC ACID*** (2-propylpentanoic acid; 2-propylvaleric acid; 2,2-dipropyl-acetic acid; 'labazene').
See also Bismuth valproate; Oxazepam valproate; Sodium valproate.
'Valtomicina' *see* Pipacycline.
'Valtorin' *see* Chlorthenoxazine.
VALTRATE** (1,7a-dihydro-1,6-dihydroxy-spiro(cyclopenta(c)pyran-7(6H),2'-oxirane)-4-methanol 4-acetate 1,6-diisovalerate;

3a,4-dihydro-3,4-dihydroxyspiro(benzo-furan-2(3H),2'-oxirane)-6-methanol 6-acetate 3,4-diisovalerate).
See also Valepotriate.
'Valyl' *see* Diethylvaleramide.
'Valzin' *see* Phenetylurea.
'VAM' *see* Vinycombinum.
VAMIDOTHION* (*O,O*-dimethyl *S*-[[2-[1-methylcarbamoyl)ethyl]thio]ethyl] phosphorothioate; *O,O*-dimethyl *S*-[2-[[1-methyl-2-(methylamino)-2-oxoethyl]thio]-ethyl] phosphorothioate; *O,O*-dimethyl *S*-[[2-[1-(methylaminocarboxy)ethyl]thio]-ethyl] phosphorothioate; 'kilval').
'Vanabol' *see* Metandienone.
'Vanay' *see* Triacetin.
'Vancide-89' *see* Captan.
'Vancide-BN' *see* Sodium bitionolate.
'Vancide Z' *see* Ziram plus 2-benzothiazole-thiol zinc salt.
'Vancocin' *see* Vancomycin.
VANCOMYCIN*** (antibiotic from *Str. orientalis*; 'vancocin').
'Vandid' *see* Etamivan.
'Van Dyke 264' *see* *N*-(2-Ethylhexyl)bicyclo-(2.2.1)hept-5-ene-2,3-dicarboximide.
'Vanectyl' *see* Alimemazine.
'Vanidene' *see* Cyclovalone.
'Vanillal' *see* Homovanillin.
Vanillaldehyde *see* Vanillin.
VANILLAMIDE (4-hydroxy-3-methoxy-benzamide; vanillic acid amide).
VANILLIC ACID (4-hydroxy-3-methoxy-benzoic acid).
Vanillic acid diethylamide *see* Etamivan.
Vanillic aldehyde *see* Vanillin.
Vanillideneisoniazid *see* Ftivazide.
VANILLIN (4-hydroxy-3-methoxybenzalde-hyde; protocatechualdehyde 3-methyl-ether; vanillaldehyde; vanillic aldehyde).
Vanillin isonicotinoylhydrazone *see* Ftivazide.
Vanillylacetone *see* Zingerone.
Vanillylidenebissulfanilamide *see* Vanyldisulfamide.
VANILLYLNONAMIDE (nonanoic acid vanillylamide; HH-50).
VANILMANDELIC ACID (4-hydroxy-3-methoxymandelic acid; 4-hydroxy-3-methoxyphenylglycolic acid; MOMA; VMA).
'Vanilone' *see* Cyclovalone.
VANITOLIDE*** (4-(thiovanilloyl)morpho-line).
'Vanizide' *see* Ftivazide.
'Vanquin' *see* Pyrvinium.
'Vantoc' *see* Cetrimonium.
VANYLDISULFAMIDE*** (4-hydroxy-3-methoxy-1-benzylidenebis(aminophenyl-sulfonamide); $N^4,N^{4'}$-vanillylidenebis-(sulfanilamide)).

461

'Vanzide' *see* Ftivazide.
'Vanzoate' *see* Benzyl benzoate.
'Vapam' *see* Metam-sodium.
'Vapona' *see* Dichlorvos.
'Vaporole' *see* Amyl nitrite.
'Vaporpac' *see* Octodrine.
'Vapotone' *see* Tetraethyl pyrophosphate.
'Varemoid' *see* Troxerutin.
'Variagil' *see* Alimemazine.
'Varicocid' *see* Sodium morrhuate.
'Varidase' *see* Streptodornase with strepto-
   kinase.
'Variotin' *see* Pecilocin.
'Varophen' *see* Promazine.
'Vasalgin' *see* Proxibarbal.
'Vasangor' *see* Propatyl nitrate.
'Vascardin' *see* Isosorbide dinitrate.
'Vascoray' *see* Meglumine iotalamate with
   sodium iotalamate.
'Vascoril' *see* Cinepazet.
'Vasculat' *see* Bamethan.
'Vasculit' *see* Bamethan.
'Vascunicol' *see* Bamethan with inositol
   nicotinate.
'Vasobrix 32' *see* Ethanolamine ioxitalamate
   with meglumine ioxitalamate.
'Vasocordrin' *see* Oxedrine.
'Vasodilian' *see* Isoxsuprine.
'Vasodistal' *see* Cinepazide maleate.
'Vasogen' *see* Dimeticone.
'Vasolan' *see* Verapamil.
'Vasomotal' *see* Betahistine.
'Vasombrix' *see* Ioxitalamic acid.
'Vasopentol' *see* Burodiline.
'Vasophemanil' *see* Diphemanil metilsulfate.
VASOPRESSIN* (antidiuretic hormone;
   β-hypophamine).
   See also Argipressin; Felypressin; Lypressin.
'Vasorbate' *see* Isosorbide dinitrate.
'Vasosuprine' *see* Isoxsuprine.
Vasotocin *see* Argiprestocin.
Vasoton (tr) *see* Oxedrine.
'Vasotran' *see* Isoxsuprine.
'Vasoverin' *see* Pyridinedimethanol bis-
   (methylcarbamate).
'Vasoxine' *see* Methoxamine.
'Vasoxyl' *see* Methoxamine.
'Vastarel' *see* Trimetazidine.
'Vasurix' *see* Meglumine acetrizoate.
'Vasylox' *see* Methoxamine.
'Vatensol' *see* Guanochlor.
'Vatsol OT' *see* Sodium dioctyl sulfosuccinate.
V-C 9-104 *see* Ethoprop.
V-C-13 *see* Dichlofenthion.
'Vectren' *see* Tiamizide.
'Veegum' *see* Aluminium magnesium silicate.
'Vegaben' *see* Chloramben.
Vegetable pepsin *see* Papain.
'Veinartan' *see* Metescufylline.
'Velacycline' *see* Rolitetracycline.
'Velardon' *see* Papain.
'Velban' *see* Vinblastine.
'Velbe' *see* Vinblastine.
'Veldopa' *see* Levodopa.
'Velmol' *see* Sodium dioctyl sulfosuccinate.
'Velosef' *see* Cefradine.
'Velsicol 1068' *see* Chlordane.

'Venacil' *see* Ancrod.
'Venalot' *see* Melilotus extract.
'Vendal neu' *see* Nicomorphine with nalor-
   phine dinicotinate.
'Vendex' *see* Neostanox.
'Vendarcin' *see* Oxytetracycline.
'Venene' *see* Snake venoms.
'Venesetic' *see* Thioethamyl.
'Venin' *see* Snake venoms.
'Venobarbital' *see* Thiobutabarbital.
'Venomin' *see* Viper venom.
Venoms *see* Hemocoagulase *and under names of*
   animals.
'Venopan' *see* Enibomal.
'Venoruton' *see* Monoxerutin.
'Venostasin' *see* Aesculus hippocastanum.
'Venotex' *see* Sodium morrhuate.
'Ventaire' *see* Quinetalate.
'Ventolin' *see* Salbutamol.
'Ventox' *see* Acrylonitrile.
'Venzar' *see* Lenacil.
'Venzonate' *see* Benzyl benzoate.
'Veracillin' *see* Dicloxacillin.
'Veractil' *see* Etymemazine *and* Levome-
   promazine.
'Veradyne' *see* Carsalam.
'Verafem' *see* Medroxyprogesterone acetate
   with ethinylestradiol.
'Veralba' *see* Protoveratrine.
'Veramon' *see* Barbipyrine.
VERAPAMIL*** (5-[(3,4-dimethoxyphen-
   ethyl)methylamino]-2-(3,4-dimethoxy-
   phenyl)-2-isopropylvaleronitrile; 2-(3,4-di-
   methoxyphenyl)-2-isopropyl-2-[3-(*N*-
   methylhomoveratrylamino)propyl]aceto-
   nitrile; iproveratril; D-365; 'cordilox', 'iso-
   ptin', 'vasolan').
VERATRALDEHYDE (3,4-dimethoxybenz-
   aldehyde).
VERATRUM ALBUM (white hellebore).
   See also Protoveratrine.
VERATRUM VIRIDE (green hellebore).
   See also Alkavervir; Cryptenamine.
VERATRYL ALCOHOL (3,4-dimethoxy-
   benzyl alcohol).
VERATRYLAMINE (3,4-dimethoxybenzyl-
   amine).
Veratrylideneisoniazid *see* Verazide.
VERAZIDE*** (1-isonicotinoyl-2-veratryl-
   idenehydrazine; veratraldehyde isonico-
   tinoylhydrazone; isonicotinic acid veratryl-
   idenehydrazide; *N'*-veratrylideneisoniazid).
   See also Opiniazide.
'Vercidon' *see* Dithiazanine iodide.
'Vercyte' *see* Pipobroman.
'Vergonil' *see* Hydroflumethiazide.
'Vericyline' *see* Ampicillin.
'Veriloid' *see* Alkavervir.
'Verina' *see* Buphenine.
'Veripaque' *see* Oxyphenisatine.
'Veritan' *see* Clofenciclan.
'Vermexane' *see* Lindane.
'Vermicompren' *see* Piperazine.
'Vermi-drageletten' *see* Ascaridole.
'Vermisol' *see* Piperazine.
'Vermitin' *see* Niclosamide.
'Vermizene' *see* Piperazine gluconate.

'**Vermizym**' *see* Papain.
'**Vermox**' *see* Mebendazole.
'**Vernam**' *see* Vernolate.
'**Vernine**' *see* Guanosine.
'**Vernitest**' *see* Quinaldine blue.
VERNOLATE (*S*-propyl dipropylcarbamo-
    thioate; 'vernam').
'**Verodigen**' *see* Gitalin.
Verodon (tr) *see* Barbipyrine.
'**Verografin**' *see* Meglumine diatrizoate with
    sodium diatrizoate.
'**Veronal**' *see* Barbital.
'**Veronigen**' *see* Barbital.
'**Verophen**' *see* Promazine.
'**Veropyrin**' *see* Barbipyrine.
'**Veroxil**' *see* Piperazine tartrate.
'**Versaclox**' *see* Cloxacillin with hetacillin.
'**Versamine**' *see* Mecamylamine.
'**Versapen**' *see* Hetacillin.
'**Versene**' *see* Trisodium edetate.
'**Versenic acid**' *see* Edetic acid.
'**Versidyne**' *see* Metofoline.
'**Versulin**' *see* Apigenin.
'**Versus**' *see* Bendazac sodium.
'**Vertigon**' *see* Prochlorperazine.
'**Veryl**' *see* Amobarbital with scopolamine
    methyl nitrate.
'**Vesadol**' *see* Buzepide metiodide with
    haloperidol.
'**Vesalvine**' *see* Methenamine.
'**Vesamin**' *see* Sodium acetrizoate.
'**Vesidryl**' *see* Metochalcone.
'**Vesipaque**' *see* Phenobutiodil.
'**Vesipin**' *see* Acetylsalol.
'**Vesipyrin**' *see* Acetylsalol.
'**Vespazin**' *see* Fluphenazine.
'**Vesperone**' *see* Brallobarbital.
'**Vespral**' *see* Triflupromazine.
'**Vesprin**' *see* Triflupromazine.
'**Vesulong**' *see* Sulfapyrazole.
'**Vetame**' *see* Triflupromazine.
'**Vetomazin**' *see* Methopromazine.
'**Vetranquil**' *see* Acepromazine.
Vetrazin (tr) *see* (3,4-Dimethoxybenzyl)-
    hydrazine.
'**Vetren**' *see* Heparin.
'**Viacil**' *see* Lactobacillus acidophilus.
'**Viadril**' *see* Hydroxydione.
'**Viaductor**' *see* Lorajmine.
'**Vialin**' *see* Mephentermine.
'**Vianol**' *see* Butylated hydroxytoluene.
'**Viarespan**' *see* Fenspiride.
'**Vibatex S**' *see* Polyvinyl alcohol.
'**Vibazine**' *see* Buclizine.
'**Vibeline**' *see* Visnadine.
VIBESATE* (modified polyvinyl plastic
    spray; 'aeroplast').
'**Vibramycin**' *see* Doxycycline.
'**Vibravenös**' *see* Doxycycline.
'**Viccillin**' *see* Ampicillin.
'**Vicryl**' *see* Polyglactin.
Victoria green *see* Malachite green.
VIDARABINE*** (9β-D-arabinofuranosyl-
    adenine; adenine arabinoside; ara-A; CI-
    673).
'**Vidipon**' *see* Cloforex.
VIFILCON A* (methacrylic acid polymer

with ethylene dimethacrylate, 2-hydroxy-
    ethyl methacrylate and 1-vinylpyrrolidin-2-
    one; poly(2-hydroxyethyl methacrylate-*co*-
    ethylene dimethacrylate-*co*-methacrylic
    acid-*co*-1-vinylpyrrolidin-2-one); 2-hydroxy-
    ethyl methacrylate polymer with ethylene
    dimethacrylate, methacrylic acid and 1-
    vinylpyrrolidin-2-one polymer; 'softcon').
'**Vigilor**' *see* Fipexide.
'**Vikane**' *see* Sulfuryl fluoride.
Vikasol (tr) *see* Menadione sodium bisulfite.
'**Vilan**' *see* Nicomorphine.
'**Vilexin**' *see* Fenyramidol.
VILOXAZINE** ([2-(*o*-ethoxyphenoxy)-
    methyl]morpholine; 2-(2-ethoxyphenoxy-
    methyl)tetrahydro-1,4-oxazine; viloxazine
    hydrochloride; ICI-58834; 'vivalan').
VIMINOL*** (1-(*o*-chlorobenzyl)-2-[2-[bis(1-
    methylpropyl)amino]-1-hydroxyethyl]-
    pyrrole; 1-(*o*-chlorobenzyl)-α-[(di-*sec*-butyl-
    amino)methyl]pyrrole-2-methanol; 1-[α-(*N*-
    o-chlorobenzyl)pyrryl]-2-di-*sec*-butylamine
    ethanol; diviminol; Z-424).
VIMINOL *p*-HYDROXYBENZOATE
    ('dividol').
'**Vinactane**' *see* Viomycin.
'**Vinactine**' *see* Viomycin.
'**Vinamar**' *see* Ethyl vinyl ether.
'**Vinarol**' *see* Polyvinyl alcohol.
VINBARBITAL*** (5-ethyl-5-(1-methyl-1-
    butenyl)barbituric acid sodium derivative;
    butenemal; vinbarbitone; 'delvinal',
    'diminal').
Vinbarbitone* *see* Vinbarbital.
VINBLASTINE*** (alkaloid from *Vinca rosea*;
    vincaleucoblastine; vincaleukoblastine;
    vincoblastine; vinblastine sulfate; VLB;
    LE-29060; NSC-49842; 'velban', 'velbe').
    See also Vinglycinate.
'**Vinca 10**' *see* Vincamine.
'**Vincadar**' *see* Vincamine.
Vincaleucoblastine *see* Vinblastine.
Vincaleukoblastine *see* Vinblastine.
VINCAMINE*** (alkaloid from *Vinca minor*;
    'devincan', 'pervincamine', 'vinca 10',
    'vincadar').
Vincoblastine *see* Vinblastine.
VINCOFOS*** (2,2-dichlorovinyl methyl
    octyl phosphate; SD-15803).
VINCRISTINE*** (alkaloid from *Vinca rosea*;
    vincristine sulfate; leurocristine; L-37231;
    NSC-67574; 'oncovin').
VINDESINE** (3-carbamoyl-4-deacetyl-3-
    de(methoxycarbonyl)vincaleukoblastine).
'**Vinesthene**' *see* Vinyl ether.
'**Vinesthesin**' *see* Vinyl ether.
'**Vinethene**' *see* Vinyl ether.
VINGLYCINATE*** (deacetylvinblastine-4-
    (*N*,*N*-dimethylglycinate); vinglycinate
    sesquisulfate; vinglycinate sulfate).
'**Vinicristine**' *see* Vinleurosine.
Vinilin (tr) *see* Polyvinox.
'**Vinisil**' *see* Povidone.
VINLEUROSINE*** (alkaloid from *Vinca
    rosea*; vinleurosine sulfate; L-32645;
    leurosine; 'vinicristine').
'**Vinol**' *see* Polyvinyl alcohol.

463

VINPOLINE** (2-hydroxypropyl 14-deoxy-vincaminate).

VINROSIDINE*** (alkaloid from *Vinca rosea*; vinrosidine sulfate; L-36781).

VINTIAMOL*** (*N*-(4-amino-2-methyl-pyrimid-5-ylmethyl)-N-[2-(2-benzoylvinyl-thio)-4-hydroxy-1-methyl-1-butenyl]-formamide).

VINYCOMBINUM* (75% ethyl ether with 25% vinyl ether; 'ethydan', 'VAM').

'Vinydan' *see* Vinyl ether.

17β-Vinylandrostane *see* Pregn-20-ene.

VINYLBITAL*** (5-(1-methylbutyl)-5-vinyl-barbituric acid; vinylbitone; butyvinal; vinymal; 'bykonox', 'optanox', 'speda').

Vinylbitone' *see* Vinylbital.

Vinyl cyanide *see* Acrylonitrile.

Vinylene (tr) *see* Polyvinox.

17α-Vinyl-4-estren-17β-ol-3-one *see* Norvinisterone.

17α-Vinyl-5(10)estren-17β-ol-3-one *see* Norgesterone.

VINYL ETHER (divinyl ether; 'vinesthene', 'vinesthesin', 'vinethene', 'vinydan').
See also Vinycombinum.

Vinylformic acid *see* Acrylic acid.

Vinylidene chloride *see* 1,1-Dichloroethyl-ene.

17α-Vinylnortestosterone *see* Norvinister-one.

'Vinylofos' *see* Dichlorvos.

5-Vinyl-2-oxazolidinethione *see* Goitrin.

1-Vinylpyrrolidin-2-one polymers *see* Povidone; Vifilcon.

Vinyl trichloride *see* 1,1,2-Trichloroethane.

Vinymal* *see* Vinylbital.

'Vinyzene' *see* Bromchlorenone.

'Viocin' *see* Viomycin.

'Vioform' *see* Clioquinol.

'Viokase' *see* Pancrelipase.

Violaquercitrin *see* Rutoside.

VIOLARIN (tr) (antibiotic from *Actinomyces violaceus*).

'Violen' *see* Fenclofos.

VIOMYCIN** (antibiotic from *Str. puniceus* or *Str. floridae*; viomycin sulfate; florimycin; phlorimycin; 'celiomycin', 'koluphthisin', 'vinactane', 'vinactine', 'viocin', 'vionac-tan').

VIOMYCIN PANTOTHENATE ('viothe-nat').

VIOMYCIN WITH DEXPANTHENOL ('panto-viocin').

'Vionactan' *see* Viomycin.

Viosterol *see* Ergocalciferol.

'Viothenat' *see* Viomycin pantothenate.

'Viozene' *see* Fenclofos.

'Vipericin' *see* Viper venom.

VIPER VENOM ('venomin', 'vipericin').
See also Russell's viper venom.

Viprynium* *see* Pyrvinium.

VIQUIDIL*** (1-(6-methoxyquinolin-4-yl)-3-(3-vinylpiperid-4-yl)-1-propanone; 'desclidium').

'Viramid' *see* Ribavirin.

'Virazene' *see* Phenolsulfazole.

'Virazole' *see* Ribavirin.

'Viregyt' *see* Amantadine.

'Virex' *see* Testosterone.

'Virgimycin' *see* Virginiamycin.

VIRGINIAMYCIN*** (antibiotic from *Str. virginiae*; virginiamycin M_1 plus virginia-mycin S; virgimycin; SK&F-7988; 'stafac', 'staphylomycin', 'staxidin').

VIRGINIAMYCIN M_1 (8,9,14,15,24,25-hexahydro-14-hydroxy-4,12-dimethyl-3-(1-methylethyl)-3H-21,18-nitrilo-1H,22H-pyrrolo(2,1-c)(1,8,4,19)dioxadiazacyclo-tetracosine-1,7,16,22(4H,17H)-tetrone; 8,9,14,15,24,25-hexahydro-14-hydroxy-3-isopropyl-4,12-dimethyl-3H-21,28-nitrilo-1H,22H-pyrrolo(2,1-c)(1,8,4,19)dioxadiaza-cyclotetracosine-1,7,16,22(4H,17H)-tetrone).

VIRGINIAMYCIN S (*N*-[(3-hydroxypyridin-2-yl)carbonyl]-L-threonyl-D-α-amino-butyryl-L-prolyl-*N*-methyl-L-phenylalanyl-4-oxo-L-pipecolyl-L-2-phenylglycine β-lactone; *N*-(3-hydroxypicolinyl)-L-threonyl-D-α-aminobutyryl-L-prolyl-*N*-methyl-L-phenylalanyl-4-oxo-L-pipecolyl-L-2-phenyl-glycine β-lactone).

Viride malachitum *see* Malachite green.

Viride nitens *see* Brilliant green.

VIRIDOFULVIN*** (antibiotic from *Str. viridogriseus*; viridogrisein; 'etamycin').

Viridogrisein *see* Viridofulvin.

'Virobis' *see* Moroxydine.

'Virofral' *see* Amantadine.

'Virugon' *see* Moroxydine.

'Viru-Merz' *see* Tromantadine.

'Virunguent' *see* Idoxuridine.

'Viruseen' *see* Poly(1-methylenepiperazine).

'Virustat' *see* Moroxydine.

Visammin *see* Khellin.

'Visatril' *see* Hydroxyzine.

'Visceralgine' *see* Tiemonium.

'Visergil' *see* Dihydroergotoxine with thioridazine.

'Vi-siblin' *see* Ispagula.

'Visine' *see* Tetryzoline.

'Visken' *see* Pindolol.

VISNADINE*** (3,4,5-trihydroxy-2,2-di-methyl-6-chromanacrylic acid δ-lactone 4-acetate 3-(2-methylbutyrate); 10-acetoxy-9,10-dihydro-8,8-dimethyl-9-(α-methylbutyryloxy)(2H,8H)benzo(1,2-b:3,4-b')dipyran-2-one; 4'-acetoxy-3',4'-di-hydro-3'-(2-methylbutyryloxy)seselin; 'cardine', 'carduben' 'vibeline').

VISNAFYLLINE*** ([2-(9-methoxy-7-methyl-5-oxo-5H-furo(3,2-g)(1)benzopyran-4-yloxy)ethyl]trimethylammonium theo-phylline derivative; kellofylline).

Visnagan *see* Provismin.

Visnagidin *see* Visnagin.

VISNAGIN (4-methoxy-7-methyl(5H)furo-(3,2-g)(1)benzopyran-5-one; 5-methoxy-2-methyl-6,7-furanochromone; desmethoxy-khellin; visnagidin).

'Visotrast' *see* Meglumine diatrizoate with sodium diatrizoate.

'Vi-stannyl' *see* Tin oxide.

'Vistaril' *see* Hydroxyzine.

VISTATOLON*** (antiviral antibiotic from

Penicillium stoloniferum).
Visual purple *see* Rhodopsin.
'Vitacarpine' *see* Pilocarpine.
Vitamin A *see* Retinol.
Vitamin A₁ *see* Retinol.
Vitamin A₂ *see* 3-Dehydroretinol.
Vitamin A acid *see* Tretinoin.
Vitamin A alcohol *see* Retinol.
Vitamin A aldehyde *see* Retinal.
Vitamin Bc *see* Folic acid.
Vitamin Bt *see* Carnitine.
Vitamin Bw *see* Biotin.
Vitamin Bx *see* Aminobenzoic acid.
Vitamin B₁ *see* Thiamine.
Vitamin B₂ *see* Riboflavin.
Vitamin B₃ *see* Nicotinamide.
Vitamin B₄ *see* Adenine.
Vitamin B₅ *see* Pantothenic acid.
Vitamin B₆ *see* Pyridoxine.
Vitamin B₁₂ *see* Cyanocobalamin.
Vitamin B₁₂ₐ *see* Hydroxocobalamin.
Vitamin B₁₂ᵦ *see* Aquocobalamin.
Vitamin B₁₂c *see* Nitritocobalamin.
Vitamin B₁₅ *see* Pangamic acid.
Vitamin C *see* Ascorbic acid.
Vitamin C₂ *see references under* Vitamin(s) P.
Vitamin D₂ *see* Ergocalciferol.
Vitamin D₃ *see* Colecalciferol.
Vitamin D₄ *see* 25-Hydroxycolecalciferol.
Vitamin E *see* Tocopherol.
Vitamin G *see* Riboflavin.
Vitamin H *see* Biotin.
Vitamin H₁ *see* *p*-Aminobenzoic acid.
Vitamin K₁ *see* Phytomenadione.
Vitamin K₁ hydroquinone *see* Phytonadiol.
Vitamin K₂ *see* Farnoquinone.
Vitamin K₃ *see* Menadione.
Vitamin K₄ *see* Acetomenaphthone.
VITAMIN K₅ (4-amino-2-methyl-1-naphthol
  hydrochloride; methylaminonaphthol).
VITAMIN K₆ (2-methyl-1,4-naphthalene-
  diamine dihydrochloride).
VITAMIN K₇ (4-amino-3-methyl-1-naph-
  thol).
Vitamin M *see* Folic acid.
Vitamin(s) P *see* Eriodictyol; Hesperidin;
  Rutoside.
Vitamin P₄ *see* Troxerutin.
Vitamin PP *see* Nicotinamide; Nicotinic acid.
VITAMIN T-COMPLEX (Goetsch's
  vitamin; termitin; torutilin; 'tegotin',
  'temina').
VITAMIN U (methionine methylsulfonium
  chloride or methylsulfate; (3-amino-3-
  carboxypropyl)dimethylsulfonium methyl-
  sulfate; antiulcer vitamin; cabbagin).
'Vita-stain' *see* 2,3,5-Triphenyltetrazolium

chloride.
'Vitatax' *see* Carboxin.
'Vitax F-15' *see* Fluoroacetic acid.
'Vivacalcium' *see* Calcium glutamate.
'Vivactil' *see* Protroptyline.
'Vivactyl' *see* Protroptyline.
'Vivalan' *see* Viloxazine.
'Vivicil' *see* Fluvomycin.
'Vivol' *see* Diazepam.
VK-53 *see* Sulfamethizole.
VK-55 *see* Sulfaethidole.
VK-57 *see* Glyprothiazole.
VLB *see* Vinblastine.
VM-26 *see* Teniposide.
VMA *see* Vanilmandelic acid.
'Vnuran' *see* Demeton-O plus demeton-S.
'Vogalene' *see* Metopimazene.
VOLAZOCINE*** (3-cyclopropylmethyl-*cis*-
  6,11-dimethyl-6,7-benzomorphan; 3-cyclo-
  propylmethyl-1,2,3,4,5,6-hexahydro-*cis*-6,11-
  dimethyl-2,6-methano-3-benzazocine;
  WIN-23200).
'Volenyl' *see* Chlormadinone acetate with
  mestranol.
'Volidan' *see* Megestrol acetate with
  ethinylestradiol.
'Volital' *see* Pemoline.
'Volon A' *see* Triamcinolone acetonide.
'Volpar' *see* Phenylmercuric acetate.
'Volplan' *see* Megestrol acetate with
  ethinylestradiol.
'Voltaren' *see* Diclofenac sodium.
'Voltarol' *see* Diclofenac sodium.
'Voluntal' *see* Trichlorourethan.
'Vonedrine' *see* Phenpromethamine.
'Vontac' *see* Methiomeprazine.
'Vontil' *see* Thiproperazine mesilate.
'Vontrol' *see* Difenidol.
'Voren' *see* Dexamethasone isonicotinate.
'Voronit' *see* Fuberidazole.
'Vortel' *see* Ethomoxane.
'Voveran' *see* Cafedrine with theodrenaline.
'Voxifral' *see* Dequalinium chloride.
'Voxsan' *see* Sodium hypochlorite.
VP-16-213 *see* Etoposide.
VPM *see* Metam-sodium.
VTS *see* Vanillin thiosemicarbazone.
'Vucine' *see* Ethacridine.
VUFB-6453 *see* Trimepranol.
VUFB-6683 *see* Acetergamine tartrate.
VUFB-9977 *see* Oxyprothepine decanoate.
'Vulcacycline' *see* Tetracycline dihydro-
  novobiocin sodium phytate.
'Vulcamycin' *see* Novobiocin.
'Vulkamycin' *see* Novobiocin.
'Vulklor' *see* Chloranil.
'Vydate' *see* Oxamyl.

W

W-32 *see* Phenformin.
W-33 *see* Methapyrilene.
W-37 *see* Buformin.
W-50 *see* Methaphenilene.
W-108/HF-1854 *see* Clozapine.
W-108/HF-2159 *see* Clotiapine.
W-583 *see* Mebutamate.
W-713 *see* Tybamate.
W-1015 *see* Nisobamate.
W-1191-2 *see* Amanozine.
W-1224 *see* Pecazine.
W-1372 *see* Beloxamide.
W-1544 *see* Phenelzine.
W-1548-1 *see* Sulocarbilate.
W-1655 *see* Phenazopyridine.
W-1760A *see* Namoxyrate.
W-1803 *see* Benzolamide.
W-1929 *see* Colistin mesilate.
W-2197 *see* Pentrinitrol.
W-2291A *see* Mimbane.
W-2354 *see* Seclazone.
W-2900A *see* Etozolin.
W-3207B *see* Modaline.
W-3366A *see* Quindonium.
W-3395 *see* Algestone acetonide.
W-3399 *see* Quingestrone.
W-3566 *see* Quinestrol.
W-3580B *see* Ampyzine.
W-3623 *see* Cyprazepam.
W-3676 *see* Sulazepam.
W-3699 *see* Piprozolin.
W-3746 *see* Cetofenicol.
W-3976B *see* Triampyzine.
W-4020 *see* Prazepam.
W-43026A *see* Ciclafrine.
W-4425 *see* Almadrate sulfate.
W-4454A *see* Estrazinol.
W-4540 *see* Quingestanol acetate.
W-4565 *see* Oxolinic acid.
W-4600 *see* Algeldrate.
W-4701 *see* Hexedine.
W-4744 *see* Mecloqualone.
W-4869 *see* Prednival.
W-5750A *see* Tilidine.
W-6439A *see* Suloxifen oxalate.
W-6693 *see* Atrazine.
W-7618 *see* Chloroquine.
W-19053 *see* Etidocaine.
'Warbex' *see* Famphur.
WARFARIN** (3-(α-acetonylbenzyl)-4-hydroxycoumarin; 4-hydroxy-3-(3-oxo-1-phenylbutyl)-2H-1-benzopyran-2-one; coumafene; warfarin sodium; zookumarin; 'actosin', 'alferin', 'coumadin', 'cumarina', 'dicusat', 'kumatoks', 'kumatox', 'marevan', 'neratox', 'nexarato', 'panwarfin', 'pro-thromadin', 'ratofarin', 'rido-rato', 'soraxa', 'sorexa', 'tintorane', 'warfex').
WARFARIN-DEANOL ([3-(α-acetonyl-benzyl)-4-hydroxycoumarinyl] dimethyl-aminoethanol; MD-6134; WDMA;

'adoisine').
'Warfex' *see* Warfarin.
WDMA *see* Warfarin-deanol.
WE-352 *see* Triflubazam.
'Weedazol' *see* Amitrole.
'Weedex' *see* Chloromethylphenoxyacetic acid.
'Weedol' *see* Paraquat.
'Weedone' *see* Disodium methanearsonate.
'Wellbatrin' *see* Bupropion.
Wellcome *etc. see* BW *etc.*
'Welldorm' *see* Dichloralphenazone.
'Wepsyn' *see* Triamiphos.
WG-253 *see* Rimiterol.
WG-537 *see* Flumedroxone acetate.
Wh-3363 *see* Fencarbamide.
Whey factor *see* Orotic acid.
'Whipicide' *see* Ftalofyne.
'Wilpo' *see* Phentermine.
WIN-244 *see* Chloroquine.
WIN-771 *see* Hydroxypethidine.
WIN-1011 *see* Glycobiarsol.
WIN-1344 *see* Gamfexine.
WIN-1539 *see* Ketobemidone.
WIN-1766 *see* Methadone.
WIN-1783 *see* Isomethadone.
WIN-2747 *see* Benzoquinonium.
WIN-2848 *see* Thenyldiamine.
WIN-3046 *see* Isoetharine.
WIN-3459 *see* Propoxycaine.
WIN-3706 *see* Ambucaine.
WIN-3800 *see* Thioambucaine.
WIN-4369 *see* Penthienate.
WIN-5069 *see* Chlorbetamide.
WIN-5063-2 *see* Thiamphenicol.
WIN-5162 *see* Isoprenaline.
WIN-5494-1 *see* Aminoxytriphene.
WIN-5606 *see* Benactyzine.
WIN-8077 *see* Ambenonium.
WIN-8851-2 *see* Sodium tyropanoate.
WIN-9154 *see* Inositol nicotinate.
WIN-9317 *see* Propatylnitrate.
WIN-10448 *see* Quinocide.
WIN-11318 *see* Bupivacaine.
WIN-11450 *see* Benorilate.
WIN-11464 *see* Fludorex.
WIN-11530 *see* Menoctone.
WIN-12267 *see* Dichlormezanone.
WIN-13146 *see* Teclozan.
WIN-13820 *see* Becantone.
WIN-14833 *see* Stanozolol.
WIN-17757 *see* Danazol.
WIN-18320 *see* Nalidixic acid.
WIN-18320-3 *see* Sodium nalidixate.
WIN-18413-2 *see* Solypertine.
WIN-18501-2 *see* Oxypertine.
WIN-19578 *see* Cyanoketone.
WIN-20228 *see* Pentazocine.
WIN-20740 *see* Cyclazocine.
WIN-21904 *see* Alexidine.
WIN-23200 *see* Volazocine.
WIN-24933 *see* Hycanthone.

WIN-25978 *see* Amfonelic acid.
WIN-27914 *see* Nivacortol.
WIN-AM-13146 *see* Teclozan.
'Win-kinase' *see* Urokinase.
'Winstrol' *see* Stanozolol.
Wintergreen oil *see* Methyl salicylate.
Wintersteiner's compound F *see* Cortisone.
'Wintomylon' *see* Nalidixic acid.
WL-8008 *see* Trifenmorph.
WL-17731 *see* Benzoylprop-ethyl.
WL-19805 *see* Cyanazine.
'Wofacain A' *see* Diethylaminoethyl butyl-
aminosalicylate.
'Wofatox' *see* Parathion methyl.
'Wofazurin' *see* Anazolene sodium.
'Wofaverdin' *see* Indocyanine green.
Wood alcohol *see* Methanol.
Woolley's antiserotonin *see* Benanserin.
'Worm guard' *see* Parbendazole.
'Wormin' *see* 1-Bromo-2-naphthol.
WR-4629 *see* Sulfalene.
WR-4873 *see* Sulfadoxine.
WR-5667 *see* Dypnone guanylhydrazone.
WR-5949 *see* Trimethoprim.
WR-25979 *see* Nitroguanil.
WSM-3978G *see* Perhexilene maleate.
WV-569 *see* Octopamine.
WX-2412 *see* Fungimycin.
WX-2426 *see* Chlorphentermine.
Wy-401 *see* Ethoheptazine.
Wy-651 *see* Troleandomycin.

Wy-757 *see* Proheptazine.
Wy-806 *see* Oxetacaine.
Wy-1094 *see* Promazine.
Wy-1359 *see* Propriomazine.
Wy-1395 *see* Trimethidinium.
Wy-2445 *see* Carfenazine maleate.
Wy-2837 *see* Potassium aspartate.
Wy-2838 *see* Magnesium aspartate.
Wy-3263 *see* Iprindole.
Wy-3277 *see* Nafcillin.
Wy-3467 *see* Diazepam.
Wy-3475 *see* Norbolethone.
Wy-3478 *see* Oxybate sodium.
Wy-3498 *see* Oxazepam.
Wy-3707 *see* Norgestrel.
Wy-4036 *see* Lorazepam.
Wy-4426 *see* Oxazepam succinate.
Wy-4508 *see* Ciclacillin.
Wy-5103 *see* Ampicillin.
Wy-8138 *see* Bisoxatin diacetate.
Wy-8678 *see* Guanabenz acetate.
Wy-20788 *see* Penamecillin.
Wy-21743 *see* Oxaprozin.
Wy-21901 *see* Indoramin.
Wy-23409 *see* Ciclazindol.
Wy-24081 *see* Tiquinamide.
'Wyamin' *see* Mephentermine.
'Wydane' *see* Chlordane.
'Wylaxin' *see* Bisoxatin.
'Wyovin' *see* Dicycloverine.
'Wypicil' *see* Ciclacillin.

X

X-40 *see* Exiproben.
X-60 *see* Denaverine.
X-1497 *see* Meticillin.
XA-2 *see* Chlormethine *N*-oxide.
'Xalyl' *see* Diethylvaleramide.
XANOXIC ACID*** (7-isopropoxy-9-oxo-
xanthene-2-carboxylic acid).
Xanthacridine *see* Acriflavine.
XANTHENE (*o,o'*-methylenediphenyl ether;
diphenylmethane oxide).
Xanthene-9-carboxylic acid ester with
8-methyltropinium bromide *see* Trante-
linium bromide.
9-Xanthenecarboxylic acid esters *see*
Methantheline; Trantelinium; Propan-
theline.
9-XANTHENONE (diphenylene ketone
oxide; dibenzo-*γ*-pyrone; xanthone).
XANTHINE (2,6(1H,3H)-purinedione).
Xanthine riboside *see* Xanthosine.
Xanthinol niacinate* *see* Xantinol nicotinate.
Xanthinol nicotinate* *see* Xantinol nicotinate.
XANTHIOL*** (4-[3-(2-chlorothioxanthen-

9-yl)propyl]-1-piperazinepropanol;
'daxid').
Xanthocillin' *see* Xantocillin.
Xanthogen *see* Dixanthogen.
Xanthone *see* Xanthenone.
XANTHOPTERIN (2-amino-4,6-dihydroxy-
pteridine).
Xanthopuccine *see* Tetrahydroberberine.
XANTHOSINE (xanthine riboside).
Xanthotoxin *see* Methoxsalen.
XANTHURENIC ACID (4,8-dihydroxy-
quinaldic acid).
XANTIFIBRATE** (7-[2-hydroxy-3-[(2-
hydroxyethyl)methylamino]propyl]theo-
phylline compound with 2-(*p*-chloro-
phenoxy)-2-methylpropionic acid (1:1);
xantinol clofibrate).
Xantinol clofibrate *see* Xantifibrate.
XANTINOL NICOTINATE*** (7-[2-hydro-
xy-3-[(2-hydroxyethyl)methylamino]-
propyl]theophylline compound with nicotinic acid; xanthinol niacinate; xanthinol
nicotinate; SK-331A; 'complamex', 'complamin', 'landrina', 'metabolan', 'sadamine',
'silpromin', 'xavin').

See also Pentosan polysulfate with xantinol nicotinate.

XANTINOL NICOTINATE WITH B-GROUP VITAMINS ('metabolan').

'Xantociclina' *see* Guamecycline.

XANTOCICLIN*** (antibiotic from *Penicillium notatum*; 1,4-bis(*p*-hydroxyphenyl)-2,3-diisocyanatobuta-1,3-diene; 1,4-bis(*p*-hydroxyphenyl)-2,3-diisonitrilobuta-1,3-diene; xanthocillin).

XANTOFYL PALMITATE*** (β-carotene-4,4'-diol dipalmitate; 'adaptinol').

'Xavin' *see* Xantinol nicotinate.

Xenalamine* *see* Xenazoic acid.

Xenalazone *see* Xenygloxal.

Xenaldial *see* Xenygloxal.

'Xenalvis' *see* Xenylgloxal.

XENAZOIC ACID*** (*p*-(α-ethoxy-*p*-phenylphenacylamino)benzoic acid; xenalamine; CV-58903; LG-278; 'xenovis').

XENBUCIN** (α-ethyl-4-biphenylacetic acid; 2-(*p*-biphenylyl)butyric acid; α-(*p*-xenyl)-butyric acid; 4-diphenylylethylacetic acid; 4-biphenylylethylacetic acid; xenbuficin; Mg-1559; 'liosol').

Xenbucin deanol salt *see* Namoxyrate.

Xenbucin *trans*-**4-phenylcyclohexylamine salt** *see* Butixirate.

Xenbuficin *see* Xenbucin.

XENON (¹³³Xe)*** (radioactive xenon).

'Xenovis' *see* Xenazoic acid.

XENTHIORATE*** (*S*-2-diethylaminoethyl ester of 2-(4-biphenylyl)thiolobutyric acid).

XENYGLOXAL*** (*p,p*'-biphenylenebis-glyoxal hydrate; 4,4'-biphenyldiglyoxyl-aldehyde; xenalazone; xenaldial; 'xenalvis').

XENYHEXENIC ACID*** (2-(4-biphenylyl)-hex-4-enoic acid; diphenhexenic acid; 'desenovis').

Xenylacetic acid *see* Biphenylylacetic acid.

α-(*p*-**Xenyl**)**butyric acid** *see* Xenbucin.

Xenylthiolobutyric acid diethylamino-ethyl ester *see* Xenthiorate.

XENYSALATE*** (2-diethylaminoethyl 3-phenylsalicylate; 2-diethylaminoethyl 2-hydroxybiphenyl-3-carboxylate; biphenamine; xenysalate hydrochloride; 'alvinine', 'diaphine', 'mesalphine', 'sebaclen').

XENYTROPIUM BROMIDE*** (8-(*p*-phenylbenzyl)atropinium bromide; 8-(*p*-biphenylylmethyl)atropinium bromide; atropine *p*-biphenylmethyl bromide; xenytropon; FX-501; N-399; 'gastripon', 'gastropin').

'Xenytropon' *see* Xenytropium bromide.

'Xerene' *see* Mephenoxalone.

'Xeroform' *see* Bismuth tribromphenate.

XIBORNOL*** (6-isobornyl-3,4-xylenol; 6-born-2-yl-3,4-xylenol; 4,5-dimethyl-2-(1,7,7-trimethylbicyclo(2.2.1)hept-2-yl)-phenol; 'nanbacin').

Xilamide *see* Proglumide.

'Xilina' *see* Lidocaine.

XIPAMIDE*** (4-chloro-5-sulfamoyl-2',6'-salicyloxylidide; 4-chloro-2',6'-dimethyl-5-sulfamoylsalicylanilide; Bei-1293; 'aquaphor').

See also Reserpine with xipamide.

XIPRANOLOL*** (1-[di(2,6-xylyl)methoxy]-3-isopropylamino-2-propanol; 3-isopropyl-amino-1-[di(2,6-xylyl)methoxy]-2-propanol; 3-isopropylamino-1-(2,6,2',6'-tetramethyl-benzhydryloxy)-2-propanol; 2-hydroxy-3-isopropylaminopropyl 2,6,2',6'-tetramethyl-benzhydryl ether).

XL-7 *see* Bithionol.

XL-90 *see* Guaifenesin.

XLG *see* Polyglactin.

'Xobaline' *see* Cobamamide.

'Xtro' *see* Atropine oxide.

XXI/07 *see* Chloraniformethan.

Xycaine (tr) *see* Lidocaine.

'Xyde' *see* Proglumide.

XYLAMIDE (*ar,ar*-dimethylbenzamide).

'Xylamide' *see* Proglumide.

XYLAMIDINE* (*N*-[2-(*m*-methoxyphenoxy)-propyl]-2-(*m*-tolyl)acetamidine).

XYLAMIDINE TOSILATE*** (xylamidine *p*-toluenesulfonate hemihydrate; xylamidine tosylate; BW-545C64).

Xylamidine tosylate* *see* Xylamidine tosilate.

XYLAZINE** (2-(2,6-dimethylanilino)-5,6-dihydro-4H-1,3-thiazine; 5,6-dihydro-2-(2,6-xylidino)-1,3-thiazine; Bay-1470; Bayer 1470; Va-1470; 'rompun').

XYLENE (dimethylbenzene).

3,5-XYLENOL (3,5-dimethylphenol; *m*-xylenol).

XYLIDINE (*ar,ar*-dimethylaniline).

2-(2,6-Xylidino)-5,6-dihydro-1,3-thiazine *see* Xylazine.

2-(2,3-Xylidino)nicotinic acid *see* Nixylic acid.

2-(2,6-Xylidino)nicotinic acid *see* Metanixin.

Xyloascorbic acid *see* Ascorbic acid.

'Xylocaine' *see* Lidocaine.

XYLOCHOLINE (choline 2,6-xylyl ether bromide; [2-(2,6-dimethylphenoxy)ethyl]-trimethylammonium bromide; TM-10).

XYLOCOUMAROL*** (4-hydroxy-3-(3,5-xylyl)coumarin; 3-(3,5-dimethylphenyl)-4-hydroxycoumarin).

2,5-XYLOHYDROQUINONE (2,5-di-methylhydroquinone).

XYLOMETAZOLINE*** (2-(4-*tert*-butyl-2,6-dimethylbenzyl)-2-imidazoline; Ba-11391; 'otrivin').

'Xylonest' *see* Prilocaine.

XYLOPININE (tetramethoxyberbine; 5,6,13,13a-tetrahydro-2,3,10,10-tetramethoxy-8H-dibenzo(a,g)quinolizine; (−)-norcoral-ydine).

XYLOPROPAMINE (3,4-dimethylamphet-amine; α,3,4-trimethylphenethylamine).

XYLOXEMINE** (2-[2-(di-2,6-xylyl-methoxy)ethoxy]-*N,N*-dimethylethylamine; 2-[2-[bis(2,6-dimethylphenyl)methoxy]-ethoxy]-*N,N*-dimethylethylamine; BS-6748).

N-**Xylylanthranilic acid** *see* Mefenamic acid.

1-(2,4-Xylylazo)-2-naphthol-3,6-disulfonic acid disodium salt *see* Ponceau MX.

1-*o*-Xylylcyclopentanecarboxylic acid

diethylaminoethyl ester *see* Metcaraphen.

3,4-XYLYL METHYLCARBAMATE (3,4-dimethylphenyl methylcarbamate; 'meobal').

3,5-XYLYL METHYLCARBAMATE (3,5-dimethylphenyl *N*-methylcarbamate; 'cosban').

2,4-Xylylmethyl 2,2-dimethyl-3-(2-methylpropenyl)cyclopropanecarboxylate *see* Dimethrin.

1-(3,5-Xylyloxymethyl)oxazolidin-2-one *see* Metaxolone.

N-**(2,6-Xylyl)phthalamic acid** *see* Ftaxilide.

Y

Y-3042 *see* Tinoridine.
Y-4153 *see* Clocapramine.
Y-6047 *see* Clotiazepam.
Y-6124 *see* Bufetolol.
'Yadalan' *see* Chlorothiazide.
Yageine *see* Harmine.
'Yatren' *see* Chiniofon.
'Yermonil' *see* Ethinylestradiol with lynestrenol.
'Yobin' *see* Yohimbane.
'Yobinol' *see* Yohimbine.
'Yodanodia' *see* Prolonium iodide.
'Yonit' *see* Bitoscanate.
YOHIMBANE (dodecahydrobenz(g)indolo-(2,3a)quinolizine; 'yobin').

YOHIMBIC ACID*** (17α-hydroxyyohimban-16α-carboxylic acid; yohimban-17α-ol-16α-carboxylic acid; yohimboaic acid; yohimboic acid).
Yohimbic acid methyl ester *see* Yohimbine.
YOHIMBINE (16α-carbomethoxyyohimban-17α-ol; Me ester of yohimbic acid; aphrodine; quebrachin; 'yobinol').
α-**Yohimbine** *see* Rauwolscine.
δ-**Yohimbine** *see* Raubasine.
Yohimboaic acid *see* Yohimbic acid.
Yohimboic acid *see* Yohimbic acid.
'Yomesan' *see* Niclosamide.
Yperite *see* Mustard gas.
'Yugocillin' *see* Penicillin G.

Z

Z-10-TR *see* Oxazepam.
Z-100 *see* Propoxur.
Z-203 *see* Strychnine *N*-oxide.
Z-326 *see* Fentonium bromide.
Z-424 *see* Viminol.
Z-867 *see* Dextropropoxyphene theobromin-1-ylacetate.
Z-905 *see* Pinazepam.
Z-1141C *see* Dexamethasone pivalate with phenylmercuric borate.
Z-3011 *see* Monoxerutin.
Z-4942 *see* Ifosfamide.
Z-12001 *see* Troxerutin.
Z-12007 *see* Monoxerutin.
Z-28200 *see* Gliflumide.
'Zactane' *see* Ethoheptazine.
'Zanchol' *see* Florantyrone.
'Zanil' *see* Oxyclozanide.
'Zarontin' *see* Ethosuximide.
'Zaroxolyn' *see* Metolazone.
α-**ZEACAROTENE** (7',8'-dihydro-δ-carotene).
β-**ZEACAROTENE** (7',8'-dihydro-γ-carot-

ene).
Zearalanol *see* Zeranol.
ZEARALENONE (6-(10-hydroxy-6-oxo-*trans*-1-undecenyl)-β-resorcylic acid lactone; F-2).
'Zectran' *see* Mexacarbate.
ZEDALAN (*trans*-3-glyoxylamidoacrylamide oxime; NSC-85680).
See also Streptozocin with zedalan.
'Zelio' *see* Thallium sulfate.
'Zenalosyn' *see* Oxymetholone.
'Zeozon' *see* Esculetin.
ZEPASTINE*** (6,11-dihydro-6-methyl-11-(1αH,5αH-tropan-3α-yloxy)dibenzo(c,f)-(1,2)thiazepine 5,5-dioxide).
'Zepelin' *see* Feprazone.
'Zeph' *see* Phenylephrine.
'Zephiran' *see* Benzalkonium.
'Zephirol' *see* Benzalkonium.
ZERANOL*** ((3S,7R)-3,4,5,6,7,8,9,10,11,12-decahydro-7,14,16-trihydroxy-3-methyl-1H-2-benzoxacyclotetradecin-1-one; 6-(6,10-dihydroxyundecyl)-β-resorcylic acid lactone;

zearalanol; P-1496; 'frideron').

'Zerlate' *see* Ziram.

'Zettyn' *see* Cetalkonium.

ZILANTEL*** (phosphonodithioimidocarbonic acid ethylene dibenzyl P,P,P',P'-
tetraethyl ester; 1,2-ethanediyl bis(phenylmethyl) bis[(diethoxyphosphinyl)carbon-
imidodithioate]; CI-64976).

'Zimate' *see* Ziram.

'Zinamide' *see* Pyrazinamide.

'Zinate' *see* Zineb.

ZINC ACETATE (zincasate; 'zinnax').

Zincasate* *see* Zinc acetate.

Zinc bis(pyridine-2-thiol 1-oxide) *see*
Pyrithione zinc.

Zinc dimethylcarbamodithioate *see* Ziram.

Zinc dimethyldithiocarbamate *see* Ziram.

Zinc ethylenebis(carbamodithioate) *see*
Zineb.

Zinc ethylenebis(dithiocarbamate) *see*
Zineb.

'Zincfrin' *see* Phenylephrine with zinc sulfate.

Zinc octanoate with sodium octanoate *see*
Caprylic compound.

**Zinc octanoate with zinc propionate and
calcium and sodium octanoates and
propionates** *see* Propionate caprylate
mixture.

'Zincogen' *see* Zinc peroxide.

'Zinc omadine' *see* Pyrithione zinc.

ZINC PEROXIDE ('zincogen').

**Zinc propionate with zinc octanoate and
calcium and sodium octanoates and
propionates** *see* Propionate caprylate
mixture.

Zinc pyridinethione *see* Pyrithione zinc.

Zinc pyrithione *see* Pyrithione zinc.

ZINC RICINOLEATE ('grillocin').

ZINC SULFANILATE ('nizin').

ZINC SULFATE ('solvezink').

Zinc sulfate with phenylephrine *see*
Phenylephrine with zinc sulfate.

Zinc tetracosactide *see* Tetracosactide zinc
phosphate complex.

Zincundan (tr) *see under* Undecenoic acid.

Zincundecate *see under* Undecenoic acid.

**ZINC UNDECENATE WITH SALICYL-
ANILIDE** (zincundesal).
See also under Undecenoic acid.

Zincundesal *see* Zinc undecenate with
salicylanilide.

ZINEB* ([[1,2-ethanediylbis(carbamodithioato)](2-)]zinc; zinc N,N'-ethylenebis-
(dithiocarbamate); zinc N,N'-ethylenebis-
(carbamodithioate); 'cynkotox', 'dithane
Z78', 'lonacol', 'parzate zineb', 'zinate').

Zineb with maneb *see* Mancozeb.

Zineb methyl derivative, polymer *see*
Propineb.

ZINGERONE (2-(4-hydroxy-3-methoxy-
phenyl)ethyl methyl ketone; 4-(4-hydroxy-
3-methoxyphenyl)-2-butanone; vanillylacetone; zingiberone).

Zingiberone *see* Zingerone.

'Zinnax' *see* Zinc acetate.

'Zinol' *see* Benzalkonium.

'Zinophos' *see* Thionazin.

ZIPEPROL*** (α-(α-methoxybenzyl)-4-(β-
methoxyphenethyl)-1-piperazineethanol;
1-(2-hydroxy-3-methoxy-3-phenylpropyl)-
4-(2-methoxy-2-phenylethyl)piperazine).

ZIRAM* (S,S'-bis(dimethylcarbamodithioato)zinc; zinc dimethyldithiocarbamate;
zinc dimethylcarbamodithioate; 'corozate',
'fuclasin', 'fuklasin', 'karbam white',
'metasan', 'milbam', 'rhodiacid', 'zerlate',
'zimate', 'zirberk').

**ZIRAM PLUS 2-BENZOTHIAZOLETH-
IOL ZINC SALT** ('vancide Z').

'Zirberk' *see* Ziram.

'Zitofenton' *see* Mannomustine heparinate.

'Zitostop' *see* Mannosulfan.

ZN-6 *see* Fusidic acid.

Zoalene* *see* Dinitolmide.

'Zoamix' *see* Dinitolmide.

ZOLAMINE*** (N-(p-methoxybenzyl)-N',N'-
dimethyl-N-thiazol-2-ylethylenediamine;
2-[(2-dimethylaminoethyl)(p-methoxybenzyl)amino]thiazole).

ZOLAZEPAM** (4-(o-fluorophenyl)-6,8-
dihydro-1,3,8-trimethylpyrazolo(3,4-e)-
(1,4)diazepin-7(1H)-one).

ZOLERTINE*** (1-phenyl-4-(2-tetrazol-5-yl-
ethyl)piperazine; phenpiperazole; MA-
1277).

'Zolicef' *see* Cefazolin.

ZOLIMIDINE** (2-[p-(methylsulfonyl)-
phenyl]imidazo(1,2-a)pyridine;
'gastronilo').
See also Indometacin with zolimidine.

'Zolone' *see* Phosalone.

'Zonol' *see* Benzyl benzoate.

'Zonulysin' *see* Chymotrypsin.

Zookumarin (tr) *see* Warfarin.

'Zoralin' *see* Lindane with DDT.

'Zothelone' *see* Quinuronium.

ZOXAZOLAMINE*** (2-amino-5-chloro-
benzoxazole; McN-485; 'flexin', 'zoxine').

'Zoxine' *see* Zoxazolamine.

ZUCLOMIFENE** (2-[p-(2-chloro-cis-1,2-
diphenylvinyl)phenoxy]triethylamine;
(Z)-2-[p-(2-chloro-1,2-diphenylvinyl)-
phenoxy]triethylamine; (*formerly named*
transclomifene; transclomiphene)).
See also Clomifene; Enclomifene.

'Zwitsalax' *see* Dantron.

'Zyklolat' *see* Cyclopentolate.

ZYLOFURAMINE*** (D-threo-α-benzyl-
N-ethyltetrahydrofurfurylamine).

'Zyloprim' *see* Allopurinol.

'Zyloric' *see* Allopurinol.

'Zymarocan' *see* Hexacamphamine.

'Zymofren' *see* Aprotinin.

'Zytostatika' *see* Inproquone.

'Zytostop' *see* Mannosulfan.